The Team Physician's Handbook

2nd edition

Edited by

Morris B. Mellion, M.D.
Medical Director, Sports Medicine Center, Clinical Associate Professor, Departments of Family Practice and Orthopaedic Surgery (Sports Medicine), University of Nebraska Medical Center; Adjunct Associate Professor, School of Health, Physical Education, and Recreation (HPER) and Team Physician, Men's and Women's Sports, University of Nebraska, Omaha, Nebraska

W. Michael Walsh, M.D.
Orthopaedic Surgeon, Sports Medicine Center; Clinical Associate Professor, Department of Orthopaedic Surgery, University of Nebraska Medical Center; Adjunct Graduate Associate Professor, School of HPER and Team Orthopaedic Surgeon, University of Nebraska, Omaha, Nebraska

Guy L. Shelton, M.A., PT, ATC
Sports Physical Therapist and Administrator, HealthSouth Sports Medicine and Rehabilitation Center of Omaha; Clinical Instructor, Division of Physical Therapy Education, School of Allied Health, University of Nebraska Medical Center, Omaha, Nebraska

HANLEY & BELFUS, INC./Philadelphia
MOSBY/St. Louis • Baltimore • Boston • Carlsbad • Chicago• London • Madrid • Naples • New York • Philadelphia • Sydney • Tokyo • Toronto

Publisher: HANLEY & BELFUS, INC.
Medical Publishers
210 South 13th Street
Philadelphia, PA 19107
(215) 546-7293, 800-962-1892
FAX (215) 790-9330

North American and worldwide sales and distribution:

MOSBY
11830 Westline Industrial Drive
St. Louis, MO 63146

In Canada: Times Mirror Professional Publishing, Ltd.
130 Flaska Drive
Markham, Ontario L6G 1B8
Canada

Library of Congress Cataloging-in-Publication Data

The team physician's handbook / [edited by] Morris B. Mellion,
W. Michael Walsh, Guy L. Shelton. — 2nd ed.
p. cm.
Includes bibliographical references and index.
ISBN 1-56053-174-6 (alk. paper)
1. Sports medicine—Handbooks, manuals, etc. I. Mellion, Morris B. II. Walsh, W. Michael. III. Shelton, Guy L.
[DNLM: 1. Athletic Injuries—handbooks. 2. Sports Medicine—handbooks. QT 29 T253 1997]
RC1211.T43 1997
617.1'027—dc21
DNLM/DLC
for Library of Congress 96-45304
CIP

The Team Physician's Handbook, 2nd ed. ISBN 1-56053-174-6

Last digit is the print number: 9 8 7 6 5 4 3 2 1

Dedication

Being a team physician is often a family affair, which involves both joy and sacrifice. For the many afternoons, evenings, and weekends we spent on home and away sidelines, rather than with them; for the years they spent sitting on hard, cold bleachers supporting us in our labor . . . we lovingly dedicate The Team Physician's Handbook to our families:

Irene, Rosie, and Frank Mellion
Claire, Pat, Ryan, Megan, and Tim Walsh
Beverly, Austin, Franklin, and Wade Shelton

Contents

Part IV: Environment

Part V: Behavioral and Psychological Problems

Part VI: General Medical Problems

Part VII: Injury Prevention, Diagnosis, and Treatment

Part VIII: Specific Sports

Contributors

Mark L. Amundson, M.S., PT, ATC
Physical Therapist, PGA Tour 1994 and 1995; Consultant for Grahammarsh Golf Design, Brookings, South Dakota

Thomas R. Baechle, Ed.D.
Professor and Chairman, Department of Exercise Science, Creighton University, Omaha, Nebraska

Karl Lee Barkley II, M.D.
University Family Physicians, Charlotte, North Carolina; Team Physician, Davidson College

Rodney S. W. Basler, M.D.
Assistant Professor, Internal Medicine/ Dermatology, University of Nebraska Medical Center, Omaha, Nebraska; Team affiliation: University of Nebraska Cornhuskers

James B. Bennett, M.D., FACS
Clinical Associate Professor and Chief, Hand and Upper Extremity Surgery Division, Department of Orthopedic Surgery, Baylor College of Medicine, Houston, Texas; Team Consultant, Houston Oilers Professional Football and Houston Astros Professional Baseball

Kris E. Berg, Ed.D.
Professor and Director of Exercise Physiology Laboratory, School of Health, Physical Education, and Recreation, University of Nebraska, Omaha, Nebraska

Turner A. Blackburn, Jr., M.Ed., PT, ATC
Adjunct Assistant Professor, Department of Physical Therapy, University of Miami, Miami, Florida; Co-Founder and Co-Director, Berkshire Institute of Orthopedic and Sports Physical Therapy, Wyomissing, Pennsylvania; Team affiliations: Albright College, Reading, PA and Wilson High School, Spring Township, PA

Daniel Blanke, Ph.D.
Associate Professor, School of Health, Physical Education, and Recreation, University of Nebraska, Omaha, Nebraska

Warren D. Bowman, M.D., FACP
Clinical Associate Professor of Medicine (WAMI), School of Medicine, University of Washington, Seattle, Washington (retired); Member Emeritus, Department of Hematology and Oncology, Deaconess/Billings Clinic Health System, Inc., Billings, Montana; National Medical Advisor, National Ski Patrol; Immediate Past President, Wilderness Medical Society

David E. Brown, M.D.
Clinical Assistant Professor of Orthopaedic Surgery, Department of Orthopaedic Surgery and Rehabilitation, University of Nebraska Medical Center, Omaha, Nebraska; Team Physician, Wayne State College

Peter J. Bruno, M.D., FACSM
Senior Consultant to the Insall/Scott/Kelly Institute for Orthopaedics and Sports Medicine, New York, New York; Attending Physician, Beth Israel Medical Center–North Division, New York, New York; Board of Trustees, American College of Sports Medicine; Internist, New York Knickerbockers

Melinda Burst, B.S.
Medical Student, University of Nebraska Medical Center, Omaha, Nebraska

Dennis A. Cardone, D.O.
Clinical Assistant Professor, Sports Medicine, Department of Family Medicine, University of Medicine and Dentistry–Robert Wood Johnson Medical School, New Brunswick, New Jersey

Cindy J. Chang, M.D.
Head Team Physician, University of California, Berkeley; Assistant Clinical Professor, Department of Family Medicine, University of California, Davis; Assistant Clinical Professor, Department of Family and Community Medicine, University of California, San Francisco; Team affiliation: University of California at Berkeley

Gerald R. Christensen, M.D.
Associate Clinical Professor, Department of Ophthalmology, University of Nebraska Medical Center, Omaha, Nebraska; U.S. Naval Hospital, Yokosuka, Japan

Brian P. Conroy, M.D.
Department of Orthopaedic Surgery, University of Missouri, Columbia, Missouri

Loren A. Crown, M.D.
Director of Emergency Medicine, Baptist Memorial Hospital–Tipton; Associate Professor, Department of Family Medicine, University of Tennessee, Memphis; Associate Site Director, UT Family Practice Center, Tipton, Tennessee

Leon F. Davis, M.D., DDS
Professor of Surgery, Chief–Section of Oral and Maxillofacial Surgery, University of Nebraska Medical Center, Omaha, Nebraska

Paul W. Esposito, M.D.
Associate Professor of Orthopaedics, Department of Orthopaedic Surgery, University of Nebraska Medical Center, Omaha, Nebraska;

Denise M. Fandel, M.S., ATC
Head Athletic Trainer and Instructor, Department of Intercollegiate Athletics, School of Health, Physical Education, and Recreation, University of Nebraska, Omaha, Nebraska; Courtesy Instructor, Division of Physical Therapy Education, University of Nebraska Medical Center

Thomas P. Ferlic, M.D.
Clinical Assistant Professor, Director of Hand Surgery, Department of Orthopaedic Surgery and Rehabilitation, University of Nebraska Medical Center, Omaha, Nebraska

Karl B. Fields, M.D., CAQ Sports Medicine
Associate Professor, Family Medicine, University of North Carolina, Chapel Hill, North Carolina; Residency and Sports Medicine Fellowship Director, Moses H. Cone Memorial Hospital, Greensboro, North Carolina; Team Physician, Grimsley High School and Consulting Physician, Guilford College, Greensboro, North Carolina

Richard B. Flynn, Ed.D.
Dean and Professor, College of Education, University of Nebraska, Omaha, Nebraska

Thomas Frette, M.A., ATC
Associate Head, Athletic Trainer, and Instructor, School of Health, Physical Education, and Recreation, University of Nebraska, Omaha, Nebraska

James B. Gallaspy, Jr., M.Ed., ATC, LAT
Associate Professor, Curriculum Director of Athletic Training, University of Southern Mississippi, Hattiesburg, Mississippi

James G. Garrick, M.D.
Director, Center for Sports Medicine, and Orthopedic Surgeon, Saint Francis Memorial Hospital, San Francisco, California

Ann C. Grandjean, Ed.D.
Director, The Center for Human Nutrition and Assistant Professor, Sports Medicine Program, Department of Orthopedic Surgery and Rehabilitation, University of Nebraska Medical Center, Omaha, Nebraska

Gary Alan Green, M.D.
Clinical Associate Professor, Division of Family Medicine, University of California and UCLA Medical Center; Team affiliations: UCLA and Pepperdine University

William D. Haffey, M.S.
Supervisor of Football Officials, Nebraska–Iowa Athletic Conference, Omaha Metro Conference, River City Conference, Omaha, Nebraska

Ronnie D. Hald, PT, ATC
Physical Therapist and Athletic Trainer, Phelps Memorial Health Center, Holdrege, Nebraska

Brian C. Halpern, M.D.
Medical Director, Hospital for Special Surgery; Assistant Attending Physician, Sports Medicine, New York Hospital, Cornell Medical Center, and Hospital for Special Surgery, New York, New York; Clinical Assistant Professor and Fellowship Director, Sports Medicine, University of Medicine and Dentistry of New Jersey–Robert Wood Johnson Medical School, New Brunswick, New Jersey; Medical Director, Medical Center of Ocean County Sports Medicine Program; Assistant Team Physician, New York Mets

Richard W. Hammer, M.D.
Primus Clinic, Papillion, Nebraska; Assistant Clinical Professor of Pediatrics, Creighton Medical Center, Omaha, Nebraska; Semi-retired

John M. Henderson, D.O.
Director of Primary Care Sports Medicine, Hughston Sports Medicine Center and Medical Director, Rehabilitation Unit, Hughston Sports Medicine Hospital, Columbus, Georgia; Assistant Professor, Department of Family Medicine, Mercer University School of Medicine, Macon, Georgia; Team affiliations: Columbus Redstixx Baseball, Columbus Cottonmouths Hockey, Columbus State University, Pacelli Catholic High School

Todd Paul Hendrickson, M.D.
Assistant Professor and Director of Medical Student Education, Creighton–Nebraska Department of Psychiatry, University of Nebraska College of Medicine and Creighton University School of Medicine, Omaha, Nebraska

Jerry W. Hizon, M.D., FAAFP
Assistant Clinical Professor, Department of Family and Preventive Medicine, University of California, San Diego, California; Medical Director, San Diego PGA Open at Torrey Pines; Team affiliations: Temecula High School, Palomar College

David O. Hough, M.D.
Director of Sports Medicine and Professor of Family Practice, Michigan State University, East Lansing, Michigan. Dr. Hough died of a heart attack September 26, 1996. We are grateful that we are able to share his expertise with our readers.

Gordon Huie, PA
Supervising Physician Assistant, Insall/Scott/Kelly Institute for Orthopaedics and Sports Medicine, New York, New York; Physician Assistant, New York Knickerbockers

Stephen C. Hunter, M.D.
Clinical Instructor and Clinical Assistant Professor, Department of Orthopaedic Surgery, Tulane University School of Medicine, New Orleans, Louisiana; Staff Physician, Hughston Sports Medicine Clinic, Columbus, Georgia

Kirk S. Hutton, M.D.
Clinical Assistant Professor, Orthopaedic Surgery, University of Nebraska Medical Center, Omaha, Nebraska; Team affiliations: University of Nebraska at Omaha, Dana College, Peru State

Robert John Johnson, M.D.
Director, Primary Care Sports Medicine, Department of Family Practice, Hennepin County Medical Center, Minneapolis, Minnesota

Barry D. Jordan, M.D.
Assistant Professor of Clinical Neurology, Cornell University Medical College, New York, New York; former Medical Director, New York State Athletic Commission

Elizabeth Joy, M.D., FACSM
Clinical Faculty, Department of Family Practice, University of Utah, Salt Lake City, Utah

Michele J. Julin, M.S., PAC
Physician Assistant, Sports Medicine Center, Omaha, Nebraska

Timothy F. Kelly, M.A., ATC
Head Athletic Trainer, Office of the Director of Intercollegiate Athletics, United States Military Academy, West Point, New York

J. B. Ketner, M.D.
Family Practice, Lincoln Family Practice Program, Lincoln, Nebraska

Roger H. Kobayashi, M.D.
Clinical Professor of Pediatrics, Division of Immunology and Allergy, University of California, Los Angeles, California; appointments at UCLA Hospital and Children's Hospital of Omaha

Ai Lan Kobayashi, M.D.
Assistant Clinical Professor of Pediatrics, University of Nebraska Medical Center, Omaha, Nebraska; appointment at Children's Hospital of Omaha

Mark A. Kwikkel, M.A., ATC
Instructor and Head Athletic Trainer, Physical Education, Dana College, Blair, Nebraska; Athletic Training Services Network, Sport Medicine Center, Omaha, Nebraska

Richard W. Latin, Ph.D.
Professor, School of Health, Physical Education, and Recreation, University of Nebraska, Omaha, Nebraska

Benjamin D. Levine, M.D.
Assistant Professor of Medicine and Director, Institute for Exercise and Environmental Medicine, University of Texas Southwestern Medical Center, Dallas, Texas; appointment at Presbyterian Hospital

Wade Lillegard, M.D.
Assistant Clinical Professor, University of Minnesota Center for Sports Medicine, Duluth Clinic, Duluth, Minnesota

Cheryl Lindly, M.A., ATC, PAC
Physician Assistant, Immanuel Hospital, Omaha, Nebraska

James M. Lynch, M.D.
Private Practice, St. Louis, Missouri; formerly Affiliate Professor, Exercise and Sport Science, Pennsylvania State University, University Park, Pennsylvania

James G. Macintyre, M.D., FACSM
Director, Primary Care Sports Medicine Fellowship, The Orthopedic Specialty Hospital, Salt Lake City, Utah

J. Douglas May, M.A., ATC
Athletic Trainer, Department of Athletics, The McCallie School, Chattanooga, Tennessee

David P. McCormick, M.D.
Professor, Department of Pediatrics, University of Texas Medical Branch (UTMB), Galveston, Texas; appointment at UTMB Children's Hospital, Galveston

Chris McGrew, M.D.
Associate Professor, Department of Orthopedics/Sports Medicine Division and Department of Family and Community Medicine, University of New Mexico Health Sciences Center, Albuquerque, New Mexico

Thomas L. Mehlhoff, M.D.
Clinical Assistant Professor, Department of Orthopedic Surgery, Baylor College of Medicine, Houston, Texas; Team Physician, Houston Astros

Joseph Lee Moore, M.D.
Specialty Advisor, Sports Medicine, to Navy Surgeon General, Washington, D.C.; Clinical Assistant Professor, Department of Family Medicine, Uniformed University of the Health Sciences, Bethesda, Maryland; Clinical Instructor, Department of Family and Preventive Medicine, University of California School of Medicine, San Diego; Head, Sports Medicine Department, Naval Hospital, Camp Pendleton, California; Sports Medicine Advisor, U.S. Navy SEALS, Coronado, CA and Marine Corps Combat Development Command, Quantico, Virginia

Thomas A. Nique, M.D., DDS
Private Practice, Lawrence, Kansas

Terry L. Nicola, M.D.
Assistant Professor, Director of Sports Medicine Rehabilitation, Department of Rehabilitation Medicine and Restorative Sciences, University of Illinois College of Medicine, Chicago, Illinois; Associate Team Physician, University of Illinois Flames

Laura E. Peter, M.D.
Undersea/Diving Medical Officer, U.S. Navy, Bremerton, Washington

Lawrence D. Powell, M.D.
Staff Physician, Hughston Sports Medicine Clinic, Columbus, Georgia

James C. Puffer, M.D.
Professor and Chief, Division of Family Medicine, University of California, Los Angeles, California; appointment UCLA Medical Center; Team affiliations: UCLA, Pepperdine University

Margot Putukian, M.D., FACSM
Assistant Professor, Department of Orthopaedics and Rehabilitation, Milton S. Hershey Medical Center, Pennsylvania State University, Hershey; Team Physician, Varsity Sports, Pennsylvania State University, Hershey, Pennsylvania

Amanda Duffy Randall, MSW, LCSW
Private Practice, Omaha, Nebraska

Kristin J. Reimers, M.S., RD
Associate Director, The Center for Human Nutrition, University of Nebraska Medical Center, Omaha, Nebraska

E. Lee Rice, D.O.
Clinical Professor of Family Practice and Sports Medicine, Western University of Health Sciences, Pomona, California; Clinical Professor, Department of Community and Family Medicine, University of California School of Medicine, San Diego, California; Team Physician, USA Volleyball Beach Team, San Diego Gulls Ice Hockey, San Diego Sockers

Stephen G. Rice, M.D., Ph.D., MPH, FACSM, FAAP
Lecturer, Division of Sports Medicine, Departments of Pediatrics and Orthopaedics, University of Washington, Seattle; Director, Sports Medicine Clinic, Harborview Medical Center, Seattle; Attending Physician, Children's Hospital and Medical Center, Seattle, Washington

William O. Roberts, M.D., FACSM
Clinical Associate Professor, Family Practice and Community Health, University of Minnesota, Minneapolis, Minnesota; Private Practice, MinnHealth Family Physicians, White Bear Lake, Minnesota

Wm. MacMillan Rodney, M.D.
Professor and Chairman, Department of Family Medicine, University of Tennessee, Memphis, Tennessee

Sharon J. Rowe, M.A., CTRS
Wellness Coordinator, University of Nebraska Medical Center, Omaha, Nebraska; Certified Aerobics Fitness Instructor

Thomas R. Sachtleben, M.D.
Sports Medicine Fellow, Family Medicine, Moses Cone Hospital, Greensboro, North Carolina; Team Physician, Elon College and Ben L. Smith High School, Greensboro

W. Norman Scott, M.D.
Director, Insall/Scott/Kelly Institute for Orthopaedics and Sports Medicine, New York, New York; Chief, Department of Orthopaedics, Beth Israel Medical Center–North Division, New York, New York; Head Team Physician, New York Knickerbockers

Wayne J. Sebastianelli, M.D.
Associate Professor and Director of Athletic Medicine, Department of Orthopaedics and Rehabilitation, Milton S. Hershey Medical Center, Pennsylvania State University, Hershey; Team Orthopaedic Surgeon, Varsity Sports, Pennsylvania State University, Hershey, Pennsylvania

Craig K. Seto, M.D.
Staff Physician, Martin Army Community Hospital, Fort Benning, Georgia

Guy L. Shelton, M.A., PT, ATC
Sports Physical Therapist and Administrator, HealthSouth Sports Medicine and Rehabilitation Center of Omaha; Clinical Instructor (volunteer), Division of Physical Therapy Education, School of Allied Health Professions, University of Nebraska Medical Center, Omaha, Nebraska

David M. Smith, M.D.
Clinical Assistant Professor, Department of Family Medicine, University of Kansas Medical Center, Kansas City, Kansas; Co-Medical Director, SportsCare at Shawnee Mission Medical Center

Keith L. Stanley, M.D.
Assistant Clinical Professor; Co-Coordinator, Primary Care Sports Medicine Fellowship, University of Oklahoma College of Medicine, Tulsa, Oklahoma

Neal Alan Stansbury, M.D.
Professor, Department of Orthopaedics, Orthopaedic Surgery, Milton S. Hershey Medical Center, Pennsylvania State University, Hershey, Pennsylvania

J. Richard Steadman, M.D.
Clinical Professor, University of Texas Southwestern Medical School, Dallas, Texas; Chairman, U.S. Ski Team Medical Group; Orthopaedic Surgeon, Steadman Hawkins Clinic, Vail, Colorado

William Irwin Sterett, M.D.
Steadman Hawkins Clinic, Vail; Vail Valley Medical Center, Vail, Colorado

James Stray-Gundersen, M.D.
Assistant Professor of Orthopedic Surgery and Physiology, Southwestern Medical School, University of Texas, Dallas, Texas

Jeffrey J. Tiedeman, M.D.
Clinical Assistant Professor, Department of Orthopaedics, University of Nebraska Medical Center, Omaha, Nebraska

David C. Thorson, M.D.

Joseph L. Torres, M.D.
Chairman, Family Practice Department, Columbia Medical Center, Osceola, Florida; Private Practice, Kissimmee, Florida

Harold K. Tu, M.D., DMD
Associate Professor, Oral and Maxillofacial Surgery, University of Nebraska Medical Center, Omaha, Nebraska; appointments at Methodist Hospital, Omaha Veterans Hospital, University of Nebraska Hospital

W. Michael Walsh, M.D.
Orthopaedic Surgeon, Sports Medicine Center; Clinical Associate Professor, Department of Orthopaedic Surgery, University of Nebraska Medical Center; Adjunct Graduate Associate Professor, School of Health, Physical Education, and Recreation, University of Nebraska; Team Orthopaedic Surgeon, University of Nebraska, Omaha, Nebraska

Jerry Weber, M.S., PT, ATC
Head Athletic Trainer and Physical Therapist, University of Nebraska, Lincoln, Nebraska

John M. Wilhite, M.D., Major, USAF, MC
Primary Care/Sports Medicine, Peterson Air Force Base, Colorado Springs, Colorado

Leonard A. Wilkerson, D.O., FAAFP
Director, Center for Family Practice and Sports Medicine, Kissimmee, Florida

Paul D. Zawatsky, M.D.
Suncoast Medical Family Practice, Sarasota, Florida

Preface to First Edition

The Team Physician's Handbook is written for the many thousands of physicians who are fortunate enough to provide care in a wide variety of team, school, league, and club settings. Being a team physician is both an honor and a challenge. It may be an awesome responsibility for the uninitiated. For the family physician, pediatrician, or internist, there may be unique musculoskeletal problems not seen in daily practice. For the orthopedic surgeon, there will be medical and psychological problems that are alien to the operating room and the cast room. And for physicians from other narrowly defined specialties, the broad knowledge base necessary for care of athletes may pose an even greater challenge.

This book is designed to be both a ready reference and a detailed resource for team physicians, athletic trainers, and other health professionals caring for athletes. It is written in outline format with liberal use of bold type to indicate topic headings and critical points. This approach is designed to provide immediate access to a large volume of well-organized, practical information. The book is divided into four major parts. The first part contains general chapters relating to sports, exercise physiology, and a variety of other general concerns. Part II provides in-depth treatment of important general medical problems. Part III describes specific injury prevention, diagnosis, and treatment. It is organized primarily by body part, but there are also chapters on musculoskeletal injuries in general and on athletic taping. Finally, Part IV deals with the sports medicine issues of most of the popular team sports in the United States. In Part IV a chapter on dance has been included, because caring for a group of dancers is a responsibility very similar to that of being a team physician.

The sport-oriented chapters contain a great deal of overlap with the anatomically-oriented injury chapters, as well as with some of the more general chapters in the first two parts of the book. It was decided to permit this overlap in order to provide the reader with sport-specific insights into many of the common injuries.

Preface to Second Edition

The widespread acceptance of The Team Physician's Handbook as the basic resource for team physicians, athletic trainers, physical therapists, and other health professionals caring for athletes has led to its broad expansion in 1997. Since the 1st edition, the published sports medicine literature has almost doubled. Consequently, we have added 14 new chapters, and virtually all of the original ones have been rewritten or thoroughly revised. Additionally, there are many new authors.

The chapter "General Medical Problems in Athletes" has been divided into four separate chapters to give better focus on specific medical problems. Similarly, the chapter "Head and Neck Injuries" has been divided into two distinct entities. New chapters have been added: "The High School Athlete: Setting Up a High School Sports Medicine Program," "High Altitude Training and Competition," "Overtraining," "Exercise Addiction," "Stress Fractures," "Administration and Medical Management of Mass Participation Endurance Events," and "Medical Coverage for Special Olympic Games." New sports chapters include "Ice Hockey" and "Martial Arts"; the skiing chapter has been divided into "Alpine Skiing" and "Cross Country Skiing."

We trust that the 2nd edition's extensive additions and revisions will maintain the role of The Team Physician's Handbook as both a ready reference and detailed resource.

Morris B. Mellion, M.D.
W. Michael Walsh, M.D.
Guy L. Shelton, M.A., PT, ATC

Foreword

The Hanley & Belfus Handbooks are designed to be both ready references and detailed resources for primary care physicians. They use the outline style to concentrate a large quantity of information into a manageable space. The format is "user friendly" with many key issues highlighted in bold print.

Because The Team Physician's Handbook was so well received, it became the model for the Hanley & Belfus Handbook series. The second volume in the series, The Handbook of Pregnancy and Perinatal Care in Family Practice, transcends the traditional boundaries of obstetrics textbooks by combining the care of the mother with the care of the newborn in a single volume. The Women's Healthcare Handbook abandons the limited perspective of the usual gynecology text to provide a "seamless" Handbook for the care of the whole woman, with sections on all of the developmental, preventive, medical, sexual, and emotional issues which challenge women and the physicians who care for them. The Low Back Pain Handbook is a clear, concise, and thorough manual for care of the low back pain patient. It replaces the traditional emphasis on rest with a focus on therapeutic exercise and early return to full activity.

I hope you will avail yourself of the up-to-date information contained in all of the Hanley & Belfus Handbooks.

Morris B. Mellion, M.D.
Handbook Series Editor

Acknowledgments

We would like to express our personal thanks to the many people who have helped us make this book possible. First, thanks go to the student-athletes at the University of Nebraska at Omaha. It has been a pleasure to care for you and to be challenged by your needs, desires, and goals. Mr. Donald Leahy, B.S., M.S., Miss Connie J. Claussen, M.A., and Mr. Robert Danenhauer, B.S., M.S., athletic directors; Ms. Denise M. Fandel, M.S., ATC, and Mr. Thomas A. Frette, M.A., ATC, athletic trainers; and the coaching, training room, and equipment manager staffs have fostered an ideal setting for us to provide team physician services in a variety of extremely competitive men's and women's sports.

A special word of thanks goes to the publishers, Jack Hanley and Linda Belfus, of Hanley & Belfus, Inc., who have provided the highest level of professional support and encouragement for both editions of this book.

We wish to offer special thanks to Michelle L. Sanderson and Keri R. Younker for their endless patience and tireless efforts in working and reworking the manuscripts and organizing and pursuing the logistics of this book.

Finally, we have the deepest appreciation for the opportunity to work with an extremely bright, articulate group of sports medicine and exercise science colleagues, the authors and coauthors of this book. Many support us directly at the University. Others are friends made through the American Medical Society for Sports Medicine and the American Orthopaedic Society for Sports Medicine. The contributing authors share a common devotion to the health and welfare of athletes.

Thank you all very much.

Morris B. Mellion, M.D.
W. Michael Walsh, M.D.
Guy L. Shelton, M.A., PT, ATC

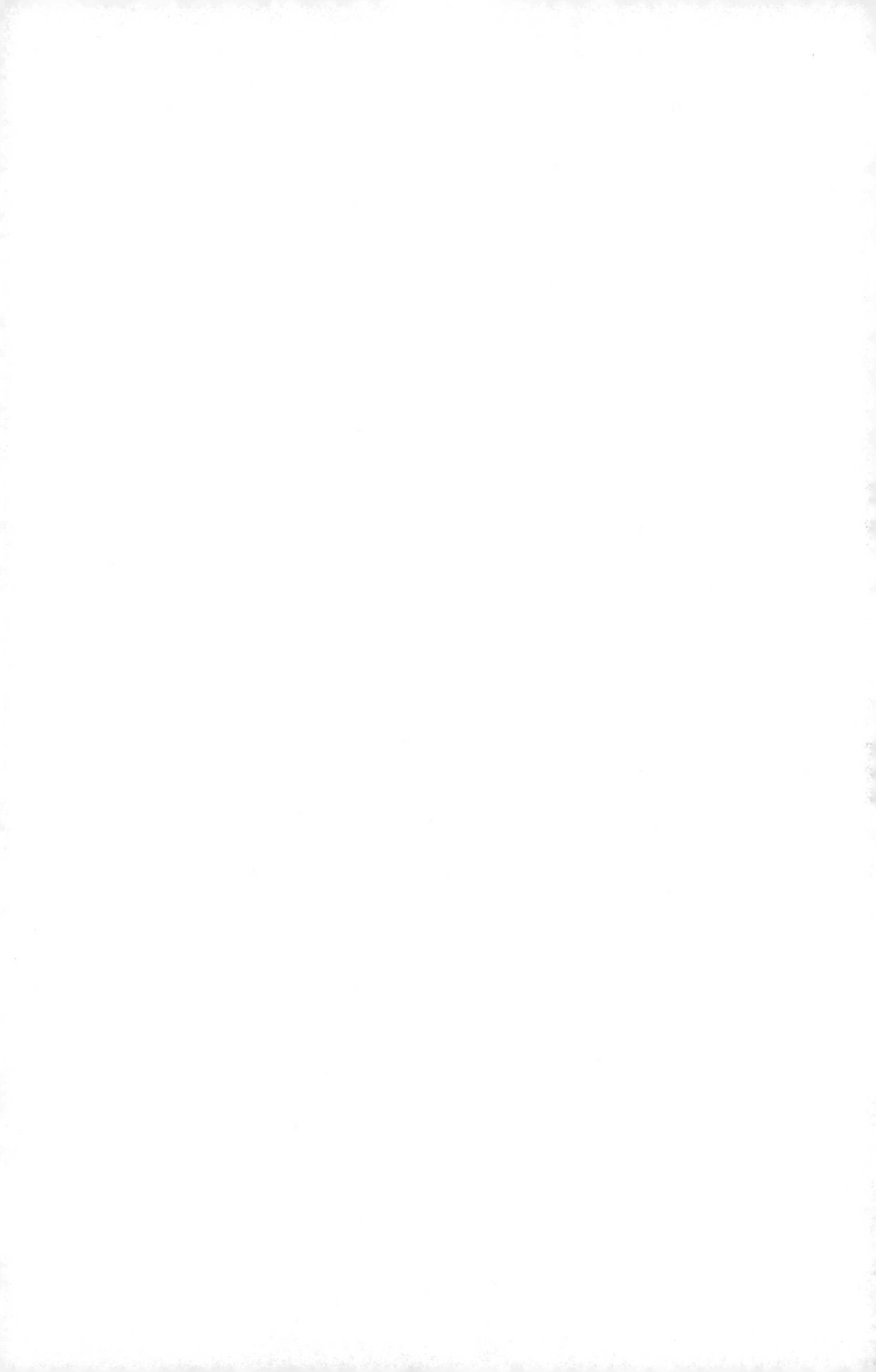

PART I
MEDICAL SUPERVISION OF THE ATHLETE

1: The Team Physician

Morris B. Mellion, M.D., and W. Michael Walsh, M.D.

I. Being a Team Physician: A Special Privilege, an Awesome Challenge

A. **Special role—team physicians have a unique responsibility for important decisions.** They are expected by school, community league, or professional team administrators to make major decisions about athletes' health, qualifications to join the team, and ability to participate safely. These decisions are often made in a setting of intense time pressure. They may affect the competitive success of the team as well as the athlete. They often influence the athlete's mental and economic, as well as physical, well-being. Level of performance, scholarships, and professional opportunities may depend on timely, high-quality medical care.

B. **The team physician addresses the physical, emotional, and spiritual needs of the athlete in the context of the sport and the needs of the team.** Consequently, family physicians, pediatricians, general internists, and other generalists are best suited by training to function as team physicians. When orthopedists, emergency physicians, general surgeons, gynecologists, and other specialists function as team physicians, their success depends on their individual ability and training to meet the athletes' broad range of medical and psychosocial needs.
   1. **To perform effectively, the team physician must maintain a broad, up-to-date knowledge base that addresses athletics as well as medicine.**
      a. **Medicine:**
         i. Musculoskeletal system
         ii. Growth and development
         iii. Cardiorespiratory function
         iv. Gynecology
         v. Dermatology
         vi. Neurology
      b. **Psychology and behavior**
      c. **Pharmacology:**
         i. Therapeutics
         ii. Performance aids
         iii. Recreational drugs
      d. **Exercise science:**
         i. Exercise physiology
         ii. Biomechanics
         iii. Specific sports

C. **The team physician has a range of ethical responsibilities that reflect the many relationships involved in the care of the team. Responsibilities to the athlete, the team, and the institution and its representatives must be balanced.**

1. **Responsibilities to athletes**
   a. **To allow to participate:** The team physician should not arbitrarily disqualify athletes from participation for reasons that are insignificant or out of line with current thinking. Especially in school-based programs, athletes have a right to participate if there is no valid medical contraindication.
   b. **To protect**: Athletes must be protected from injury, reinjury, permanent disability, and themselves. When there is valid medical contraindication to participation or resumption of participation, athletes must be counseled and thoroughly informed. It may be especially difficult to reason with an athlete who has a "participate at any cost" attitude.
   c. **To provide optimal health care**
   d. **To ensure confidentiality**: Confidentiality is often compromised by the relationship to the school or professional club. Seldom may information be held in strict physician-patient confidentiality. However, the team physician must be sensitive to how widely information is disseminated. For example, if an athlete wishes to resign from the team without having the physician tell others the medical reasons for this decision, that wish should be honored.
   e. **It is a cardinal rule that the team physician may not sacrifice the welfare of the athlete to the welfare of the team or the institution.**
2. **Responsibility to the team:** to **facilitate success of the group**, whose members have all dedicated time and effort to the sport
3. **Responsibilities to the coach**
   a. **To facilitate success:** The coach should not view the team physician as an impediment to success, but rather as a part of the team striving for success.
   b. **To educate:** Continuing education about improvements in medical and preventive care is important to eliminate archaic and possibly harmful techniques.
   c. **To protect from possible future liability**
4. **Responsibilities to the institution**
   a. **To facilitate success** in light of financial commitment:
      i. To provide optimal health care for the athletes
      ii. To prescreen scholarship and professional athletes. In this regard, the team physician does not have a doctor-patient relationship and may disqualify athletes who fail to meet physical standards.
   b. **To protect from liability**

D. ***Availability* is a cornerstone for success as a team physician.** Personal availability and a well-organized coverage system are essential.
   1. **On the sidelines:** the front lines of sports medicine, especially for contact sports. A physician who covers a team solely from the stands or the office does not truly deserve the title "team physician."
   2. **In the training room:** It is important to demonstrate interest in the team by seeing athletes in their own environment, rather than only in the physician's environment.
   3. **In the office:** Team physicians may wish to make special accommodations in their office schedules for athletes with urgent problems.
   4. **Nights and weekends:** Most athletic activity goes on outside the normal work day. Team physicians should always be available to coaches or trainers.
   5. **Unstructured time with the athletic trainer and/or coach**

E. **Who serves as team physician?**
   1. **A broad spectrum of generalists and specialists serve as team physicians. The majority are primary care physicians.** The most comprehensive available data, from *The Physician and Sportsmedicine* 1995 survey of 30,597 team physicians, is presented in Table 1.

TABLE 1. *The Physician and Sportsmedicine* Team Physician List, June 1995

	Number	Percentage
Family practice	7788	25.5
Orthopedic surgery	4972	16.2
Osteopathic medicine	3347	10.9
Internal medicine	3078	10.1
General practice	1925	6.3
Pediatrics	1643	5.4
Emergency medicine	1499	4.9
General surgery	1382	4.5
Obstetrics/gynecology	847	2.8
Cardiology	608	2.0
All other specialties	3508	11.5
Total	30,597	100.0

Source: The Physician and Sportsmedicine circulation department.

2. **Some physicians share responsibility by pairing a generalist and a specialist**—for example, team physician and team orthopedist. This situation may be ideal, since the majority of injury problems are musculoskeletal. A generalist (family physician, pediatrician, internist) and an orthopedist should be able to deal effectively with most problems that arise. They can then call upon other specialists as necessary.

F. **Team physicians derive a variety of rewards from service in this capacity.**
   1. **Satisfaction:** immense personal satisfaction
      a. Providing a service to the community
      b. Working with young, motivated patients
   2. **Credibility:** Undoubtedly, affiliation with teams from high school to professional enhances a physician's prestige in the community and may contribute to practice building.
   3. **Remuneration:** Serving as a team physician should be a labor of love. At anything less than a professional team level, most of the time spent is as a volunteer. Above the high school level, some compensation may be a part of the agreement. However, remuneration is extremely variable, ranging from none to a considerable retainer with a professional club. Some colleges and universities provide team physician services through Student Health or an affiliated medical school, but most of these arrangements include large amounts of volunteer time as well. Surgeons may receive surgical fees for procedures performed, but often these services are provided on a discount basis.

G. **Relationship of team physician to institution**
   1. It is important for both physician and institution to establish **an explicit formal relationship between the physician and the school, league, or team.** It should include job description, any fiscal arrangements, and a statement of expectations. Whenever possible, especially if monetary arrangements are involved, it should be in writing. If a formal contract is not appropriate, it is even more critical to discuss these items before the season begins.
   2. **Who hires** or obtains the services of the team physician
      a. Athletic director
      b. Athletic trainer
      c. Business manager or other officer of professional team
   3. **Job description** of team physician
      a. Person to whom team physician reports
      b. Services provided by team physician:
         i. At home
         ii. Away (reimbursement for travel expenses, if any)

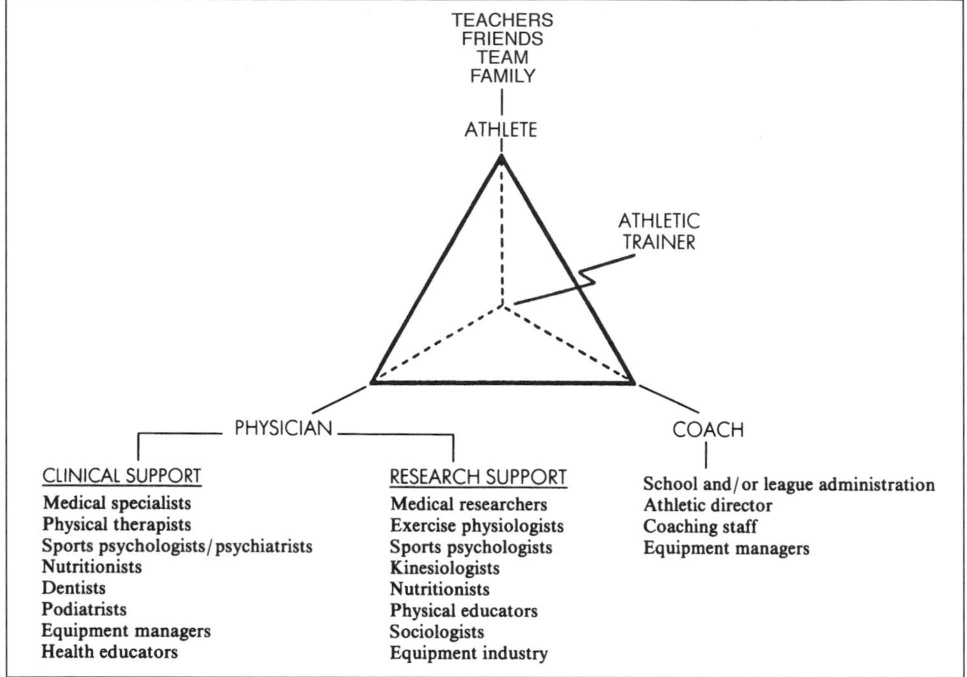

FIGURE 1. The sports medicine team. (Modified from Mellion MB: Office Sports Medicine. Philadelphia, Hanley & Belfus, Inc., 1996.)

c. Remuneration and benefits
d. Any other expectations of the institution or the physician

4. **Principles and guidelines for care. The team physician must:**
   a. **Have professional autonomy over all medical decisions**
   b. Be protected against coercive pressures

II. The Sports Medicine Team

The team physician cares for an athletic team and also serves as a key player on the sports medicine team, which consists of the athlete, the team physician, the coach, and the athletic trainer, when one is available. Each of these individuals has a support system to draw upon. The care of the athlete is a team effort in which the members of the sports medicine team support each other for the benefit of the athlete and the athletic team. Like the athletic team itself, sports medicine services are best provided following a team concept of this kind. (See Figure 1.)

A. **The athlete's support system**
   1. Teammates
   2. Family and significant others
   3. Friends
   4. Teachers
   5. Athletic trainers

B. **The team physician's support systems**
   1. Clinical support
      a. Medical specialists
      b. Physical therapists
      c. Sports psychologists/psychiatrists
      d. Nutritionists
      e. Dentists
      f. Podiatrists
      g. Equipment managers
      h. Health educators

2. Research support
   a. Medical researchers
   b. Exercise physiologists
   c. Sports psychologists
   d. Kinesiologists
   e. Nutritionists
   f. Physical educators
   g. Sociologists
   h. Equipment industry
3. Athletic trainer

C. **The coach's support system**
1. School or league administration, athletic director
2. Coaching staff
3. Athletic trainer
4. Equipment manager

D. **The athletic trainer** occupies a unique position at the center of the athletic health care triangle.
1. Therapist and counselor for the athlete
2. Advisor and friend to the coach
3. Eyes and ears for the team physician
   a. Triage or screening
   b. Supervision of conditioning, care, and rehabilitation
   c. Continuous functional evaluation of the athlete
4. Every high school and college athletic program should have a certified athletic trainer.

III. Roles and Functions of the Team Physician

A. **Medical supervision of athletes:** Herein lies the traditional function of a team physician, which has now been greatly expanded.
1. **Prevention**
   a. The team physician is responsible for the **preparticipation evaluation:**
      i. Qualification of athletes:
         (a) General
         (b) Sport-specific
      ii. Counseling on appropriate sports
      iii. Treatment and rehabilitation of deficits
   b. The team physician is often asked for advice on **proper conditioning techniques** to prevent or rehabilitate injuries:
      i. Preseason and in-season
      ii. General and sport-specific
   c. The team physician may be asked for advice on **protective equipment:**
      i. Selection
      ii. Fit
      iii. Injury and reinjury prevention
2. **Supervision**
   a. On-site coverage—field, gym, arena, pool:
      i. A physician should be present for high-risk situations and high-risk sports.
      ii. When a physician is not available for coverage, an athletic trainer or other personnel trained in prevention, recognition, and initial evaluation and care of injured athletes should be present.
   b. Tournaments
3. **Evaluation**
   a. Preparticipation evaluation
   b. Illness and injury:
      i. On the field
      ii. In the training room
      iii. In the team physician's office

iv. In the student health clinic
v. In the emergency department

4. **Management**
   a. Treatment
   b. Consultation and referral when appropriate

B. **Administration.** The team physician may be expected to perform a variety of administrative functions.
1. **Develop a general system of care for the team.**
2. **Establish guidelines for consultation** with the team physician or referral to a consultant.
3. **Plan and organize the preparticipation evaluation.**
   a. Determine content and standards of the evaluation.
   b. Establish guidelines for participation.
   c. Arrange location.
   d. Secure and coordinate personnel.
4. **Prearrange a system of emergency care.**

C. The team physician should **ensure the availability of:**
1. General medical equipment and supplies
2. Emergency equipment
3. Emergency transport (ambulance present at high-risk events)
4. Referral to hospital staffed to care for anticipated injuries
5. Communication
   a. Telephone on sidelines
   b. Radio

D. **Coordination and medical supervision**
1. Medical personnel
2. Athletic trainers
3. Paramedical personnel

E. **Legal and medicolegal**
1. Contract with school, league, or team
2. Permission to treat minors
3. Liability
   a. Institutional liability
   b. Professional liability
4. Athlete's right to participate
5. Treatment of athletes on out-of-state trips
   a. Legality:
      i. For *major* athletic events, the host state or country generally passes legislation granting visiting team physicians temporary licenses.
      ii. For routine competitions and tournaments, it is recommended that the traveling team physician work through the host team or tournament physician or local physician in the host town.
   b. "Good Samaritan" laws:
      i. No suit has yet been brought against a team physician traveling with a team to another state over the issue of practicing without a license.
      ii. "Good Samaritan" laws focused on the care of athletes have been passed in many states. These laws vary from one jurisdiction to another. They generally do not protect team physicians receiving compensation for their services.
   c. Professional liability insurance coverage

F. **Medical insurance**
1. School, league, or team insurance
2. Dealing with coverage problems

a. Capitated medical care systems—**HMOs, PPOs**
b. Military dependents
c. Coverage for preventive services
d. Coverage for cognitive vs. procedural services

G. **Communication/liaison:** The ideal team physician is a skilled communicator who can often resolve conflicts or enhance cooperation among members of the athletic and sports medicine teams.

1. Certain relationships often require special attention.
   a. Athlete–coach
   b. Athlete–parents
   c. Team physician–parents
   d. Team physician–athlete's family doctor
   e. Athlete–medical colleagues and consultants
   f. Athletic trainer–coach
   g. Injured athlete–press
2. In many settings, it may be beneficial to send a preseason letter to the athletes and/or their parents describing the role of the team physician and what services are provided. Below the college level, such letters should emphasize the importance of the student athlete's own family physician or pediatrician in the student's care.

H. **Education:** The team physician can serve as an educator at many levels and to many audiences in sports medicine.

1. Audiences
   a. Athletes
   b. Coaches
   c. Athletic trainers
   d. Administration, especially athletic directors
   e. Medical personnel:
      i. Medical students
      ii. House officers
      iii. Colleagues and consultants
   f. Paramedical personnel
   g. Parents
   h. General public
2. Methods
   a. One-on-one instruction and preception
   b. In-service training
   c. Lectures, workshops, seminars
   d. Formal instructional courses
   e. Newsletters
   f. Audio and video instructional tapes
   g. Written books and articles in sports and professional journals
   h. Computerized training modules

I. **Research:** Sports medicine is a relatively young discipline with a growing scientific literature. The team physician can improve the health care and safety of athletes by promoting and performing sports medicine research.

J. **Student**

1. Responsibility for remaining current with a body of knowledge that changes rapidly
2. Opportunity to learn about life, sport, and medicine from highly motivated athletes, coaches, and other members of sports medicine team

K. **Healer:** Even in this highly technical era of medicine, the intangible effect of the "laying on of hands" and the supportive care of the team physician are often the keys to recovery and participation for the athlete.

Recommended Reading

1. Albright JP, Noyes FR: Role of the team physician in sports injury studies. Am J Sports Med 16(suppl): S1–S4, 1988.
2. American Academy of Pediatrics: A Self-Appraisal Checklist for Health Supervision in Scholastic Athletic Programs. Elk Grove Village, IL, Amer Acad Ped, 1993.
3. Committee on Sports Medicine and Fitness, American Academy of Pediatrics, Dyment PG (ed): Sports Medicine: Health Care for Young Athletes, 2nd ed. Elk Grove Village, IL, Amer Acad Ped, 1991.
4. Gallup EM: Law and the Team Physician. Champaign, IL, Human Kinetics, 1995.
5. Howe WB: Primary care sports medicine: A part-timer's perspective. Phys Sportsmed 16(1):103–114, 1988.
6. Howe WB: The team physician. Primary Care: Clin Office Pract 18:763–775, 1991.
7. Lombardo JA: Sports medicine: A team effort. Phys Sportsmed 13(4):72–81, 1985.
8. McKeag DB, Hough DO: Primary Care Sports Medicine. Dubuque, IA, Brown & Benchmark, 1993.
9. Samples P: The team physician: No official job description. Phys Sportsmed 16(1):169–175, 1988.
10. Shaffer TE: So you've been asked to be the team physician. Phys Sportsmed 4(12):57–63, 1976.
11. Walsh WM, Mellion MB: The team physician. In DeLee JC, Drez D Jr (eds): Orthopaedic Sports Medicine: Principles and Practice. Philadelphia, WB Saunders, 1994, pp 346–355.

2

The Athletic Trainer and the Training Room

Cheryl Lindly, M.A., ATC, PAC, and Denise Fandel, M.S., ATC

I. Roles of the Certified Athletic Trainer

A. **Responsible** for prevention, emergency care, first aid, evaluation, and rehabilitation of injuries to athletes under his or her care

B. **Liaison** between the team physician, the athlete, the athlete's parents, and coaching staff

C. **Consultant** to the coaching staff on conditioning, nutrition, and protective equipment

II. Education of Certified Athletic Trainer

A. **Methods of achieving certification by the National Athletic Trainers' Association Board of Certification (NATABOC)**

1. **Internship pathway**
    - a. 1500 hours of supervised athletic training experience:
        - i. 25% in high-risk sports
        - ii. Supervised by a NATABOC certified athletic trainer
    - b. Coursework
        - i. Human anatomy
        - ii. Human physiology
        - iii. Exercise physiology
        - iv. Kinesiology
        - v. Nutrition
        - vi. Basic athletic training
        - vii. Advanced athletic training
    - c. Bachelor's degree, usually in a related field
    - d. Passing score on certification exam
2. **Curriculum pathway**
    - a. 800 hours of supervised athletic training experience
    - b. Graduation from approved curriculum

B. **State certification, licensure, and registration**

1. Many, but not all, states certify, license, or register athletic trainers practicing in their states.
2. State certification may or may not reflect the same competencies measured in the NATABOC Certification Exam.

III. Roles and Responsibilities of the Certified Athletic Trainer

A. **Prevention of injuries**

1. Education of athletes and student athletic trainers
2. Conditioning—development of conditioning programs
3. Preseason screening
    - a. Identify factors that put athlete at risk.

b. Correct deficiencies:
   i. "Prehabilitation"—begin work on deficits before injuries occur
   ii. Referral for further workup
4. Taping and bracing—prescribe when needed

B. **Emergency care and first aid**
1. Necessary equipment available
2. Communication procedures for emergency situations—scenarios and procedures rehearsed by entire staff
3. Prompt, accurate triage

C. **Injury evaluation**
1. Acute injuries
2. Chronic injuries
3. Referral to team physician or specialist when appropriate

D. **Treatment**
1. PRICES (see Chapter 37, "Musculoskeletal Injuries in Sports")
2. Qualified use of modalities
   a. Cold or heat
   b. Ultrasound
   c. Electrical stimulation

E. **Rehabilitation** (therapeutic exercise)
1. Development of individual exercise prescriptions
2. Supervision of programs
3. Evaluation and modification in program as progress deems necessary
4. Return to competition—functional testing

IV. How the Athletic Trainer and Physician Function as a Team

A. **Standard operating procedures should be written whenever possible.**
1. Emergency care
2. Transportation
3. Modalities
4. Other treatments and procedures

B. **Coordination of referrals**
1. To physician
2. From physician
3. Between physicians
4. With other health care providers

C. **Game coverage procedures**
1. Establish roles in emergency situations
   a. On-field assessment
   b. Off-field assessment
2. Provide emergency equipment (see Chapter 7, "Injuries and Emergencies on the Field")

D. **Return to play decisions**—define parameters
1. Range of motion
2. Strength
3. Functional ability
4. Functional taping/bracing

E. **Open lines of communication**
1. On treatment and rehabilitation
2. On return to competition
3. On emergency care

V. Training Room Management

A. **Record keeping**
1. Injury reports
2. Home care instructions
3. Referrals
4. Treatment records
5. Rehabilitation progress notes
6. Insurance

B. **Budgeting**—consult with team physician regarding specific needs

C. **Equipment and supplies**
   1. Basic training room supplies and equipment
      a. Taping
      b. Wound care
      c. Rehabilitation devices:
         i. Sandbag weights
         ii. Surgical tubing
         iii. Exercise equipment
         iv. Proprioception boards
      d. Modalities:
         i. Whirlpool
         ii. Ultrasound
         iii. Ice machine or freezer
         iv. Hydrocollator
         v. Electrical stimulator
   2. Emergency equipment and supplies
      a. Spine boards and stretchers
      b. Cervical immobilizer
      c. Splints:
         i. Air
         ii. Rapid evacuation form immobilizer
         iii. Knee immobilizer
      d. Slings:
         i. Shoulder immobilizer
         ii. Clavicle fracture yoke
      e. Crutches

D. **Equipment available for team physician use only**
   1. Prescription medications
   2. Suture kit
   3. Cardiorespiratory emergency medications
   4. Oxygen

E. **Student athletic trainers**
   1. Education
      a. Hands-on experience
      b. Didactic methodology
      c. Preparation for certification examination
   2. Supervision
   3. Establishment of competencies before taping, evaluations, or application of modalities

VI. Professional Relationships With Support Personnel

A. Coaches
B. Administrators
   1. Strength and conditioning coaches
   2. Nutritionists
   3. School nurses
   4. Physical therapists

VII. Summary

The athletic trainer is a vital member of the team of allied medical professionals who care for interscholastic and intercollegiate athletes. It is important for the team physician to understand the potential for a working relationship with the athletic trainer.

With adequate time, space, staffing, and budget, the athletic trainer, with guidance from the team physician, can make a vast improvement in the level of care provided for the athletes through timely evaluation and treatment, patient education, rehabilitation, and emergency care. For the team physician, the athletic trainer acts as a daily liaison with student athletes. As more schools hire certified athletic trainers, the effectiveness of the team physician becomes proportionally greater. We hope that in the years to come educational institutions will see fit both to hire a certified athletic trainer and to expand the role of the team physician, thereby allowing the formation of a health care team whose primary concern is the welfare of the student athlete.

3

Team Hygiene and Personal Equipment

Mark A. Kwikkel, M.A., ATC

I. Importance of Hygiene

The lack of personal hygiene can lead to bacterial, fungal, and even viral infections. Personal hygiene is important not only for athletes, but also for the team physician and other health professionals.

A. **Dealing with large numbers of athletes:** In dealing with athletic teams, numbers can range from seven or eight on the golf or tennis team to well over 130 on the football team. The larger the squad, the higher incidence of hygiene problems.
   1. Lack of personal hygiene can lead not only to infection problems, but also to complaints from other team members of the offensive odors generated by an individual.
   2. Showering with copious amounts of water and deodorant soap should be stressed. Showers before examination by the physician or athletic trainer are a common practice in nonemergency situations.

B. **The locker room environment:** Damp, dark areas are a prime breeding ground for mold, mildew, and bacteria. The shower area, drying area, and sweat-soaked clothing need proper cleaning.

C. **Cleaning and disinfecting the locker room:** The locker room should be disinfected daily with industrial cleaners. A well-trained custodial staff should know the proper techniques for cleaning and disinfecting a locker room.
   1. Daily damp mopping
   2. Carpeted areas vacuumed daily (antifungal carpets recommended)
   3. Biweekly high-pressure steam cleaning
   4. Weekly disinfection of lockers. Custodial personnel should use Occupational Safety and Health Administration (OSHA)–approved products for cleaning and disinfecting the lockers.

II. Personal Equipment

All sports have one thing in common—workout and competition clothing. These items need to be properly laundered. Sports such as hockey, football, wrestling, and lacrosse have special protective equipment that needs special attention.

A. **Proper clothing** for each sport is highly recommended. Clothing should be of a nonbinding nature.

B. **Laundry facilities:** Clothing should be laundered daily. Athletic facilities should be equipped with commercial washers and dryers designed to handle their laundry.
   1. **Washing:** Clothing should be washed in warm water (100–105°F) using heavy-duty detergents, all-fabric bleach, and fabric softener.
   2. **Drying:** Clothing should be **dried completely**. It is highly recommended that a cooling period be used to avoid shrinkage. Clothing should be folded promptly.

3. **Home facilities:** Institutions that cannot provide laundry service should provide **written instructions on the care that should be given the athletic clothing.**
4. **Laundry facilities on road trips:** Many teams need laundry facilities while participating away from home.
    a. Take clothing items to a coin-operated laundry.
    b. Make arrangements with the host team to have items laundered.
    c. Bring extra items of clothing on road trips.
5. **Handling of contaminated laundry:** Quite often, game and practice uniforms become contaminated with bodily fluids, which may contain blood-borne pathogens.
    a. Laundry soiled with blood or other potentially infectious material should be handled with caution.
    b. Handle soiled laundry with gloves and as little as possible.
    c. Laundry should be double bagged and labeled as BIOHAZARD.
    d. Launder soiled articles as recommended by the clothing manufacturer.
6. **Blood on the uniform during competition:** During competition, blood may contaminate the uniform. General rules for most sports both at high school and collegiate levels dictate that either removal of the uniform or cleansing of the stain must be performed before return to competition.
    a. If the uniform is saturated with blood, it must be removed.
    b. If the uniform is not saturated, the stain must be removed using a commercial product. A solution of 50/50 3% hydrogen peroxide and vinegar is most effective.

C. **Cleaning specialized equipment:** Specialized equipment needs to be cleaned periodically with a spray disinfectant/deodorant.
1. Football equipment
    a. Helmets
    b. Shoulder pads
    c. Thigh pads, hip pads, tail pad
    d. Knee pads
2. Wrestling equipment
    a. It is extremely important that the wrestling mat be disinfected before and after each practice and competition.
    b. A chlorine bleach solution (1 part chlorine bleach, 2 parts water) should be kept in a spray bottle near the mat to clean any blood (Thor Germicidal Detergent, Huntington Laboratories, Huntington, IN).
3. The protective equipment of every sport should be disinfected periodically.

III. Athletic Training Room and Examination Areas

The athletic training room and examination areas should be cleaned daily.

A. **Keeping facilities clean:** Usually the facility's custodial staff does general cleaning and disinfecting, yet certain items need to be cleaned daily by the athletic training staff.
1. Disinfection of treatment and taping tables
2. Disinfection of whirlpools
3. Removal of trash
4. Vacuuming or sweeping of floor

B. **Hand washing:** Hands should be washed with soap and water before and after examining athletes, especially following an event or practice when examining a large number of athletes.

IV. HIV/AIDS Concerns in Athletics

With the growing problem of human immunodeficiency virus (HIV) and the acquired immunodeficiency syndrome (AIDS) epidemic, it is important that certain precautions be taken when dealing with blood and open wounds.

A. HIV/AIDS precautions
   1. Use latex gloves when examining and managing open wounds.
   2. Wash hands thoroughly before and after treating an athlete with an open wound.
   3. Use proper eye protection when treating open wounds.
   4. Use chlorine bleach (1 part chlorine bleach, 2 parts water) in spray bottles to clean tables and other surfaces that become contaminated with blood. Paper towels should be discarded in a plastic bag and incinerated as soon as possible.

B. Prevention of HIV transmissions—it is recommended that the **Centers for Disease Control Recommendations for Prevention of HIV Transmission in Health-Care Settings** be read and followed in the physician's office and in the athletic training room.[1,2]

Recommended Reading

1. Centers for Disease Control: Recommendations for prevention of HIV transmission in health-care settings. MMWR 36(suppl 25), 1987.
2. Centers for Disease Control Update: Universal precautions for prevention of transmission of human immunodeficiency virus, hepatitis B virus, and other bloodborne pathogens in health-care settings. MMWR 37:377–388, 1988.
3. NCAA Sports Medicine Handbook, 7th ed. Overland Park, KS, National Collegiate Athletic Association, 1995, pp 24–28.
4. Pfeiffer RP, Mangus BC: Concepts of Athletic Training. Boston, Jones & Bartlett Publishers, 1995, p 259.

4

Coaching and Its Role in Injury Prevention

James B. Gallaspy, Jr., M.Ed., ATC, LAT, and J. Douglas May, M.A., ATC

I. Introduction

A. The coach is a key member of the sports medicine team. His or her responsibilities include the general care and well-being of athletes through good coaching and leadership, preparticipation screening, and a proper playing environment.

B. In schools, conferences, and leagues in which athletic trainers are not available, the coach's role in prevention and care of injuries in athletes is magnified.

II. Optimal Sports Environment

Good coaching and positive leadership are essential.

A. **Leadership**
   1. **Based on positive reinforcement**—tell the athlete what he or she is doing right
   2. **Leadership by example**
   3. **Open, honest communication**
      a. With players
      b. Among coaches
      c. With officials
   4. **Understand and meet the emotional needs** of athletes and fellow coaches. The most emotionally vulnerable athletes generally respond more positively to good coaching and more negatively to poor coaching than their more stable teammates.

B. **Administration**
   1. **Recruit only qualified coaches and assistants.**
   2. **Encourage effectiveness training for coaches.**
      a. Hold coaching clinics for assistants.
      b. Use courses and clinics in the community or region. Common sponsoring organizations include:
         i. Local colleges and universities
         ii. American Coaching Effectiveness Program (P.O. Box 5076, Champaign, IL 61825)
         iii. Little League Baseball, Inc. (P.O. Box 3485, Williamsport, PA 17701)
         iv. National Youth Sports Coaches Association (2611 Okeechobee Road, West Palm Beach, FL 33409)
   3. Insist on teaching only safe athletic techniques.
   4. Obtain services of a team physician and/or a certified athletic trainer whenever possible.

C. **Proper and safe fundamentals**
   1. Coach should **know the individual sport thoroughly** in order to:

a. Teach proper athletic skill techniques.
b. Correct poor mechanics, which might otherwise lead to overuse injuries.
c. Teach other coaches and athletes injury prevention by means of:
i. On-field coaching
ii. Clinics
iii. Written material
d. Stress the proper fundamentals that lead to success.

2. **Good coaching guidelines prevent injury and reduce liability risk.**
a. Advise the athlete (or parents) of inherent dangers of the sport.
b. Supervise constantly and attentively.
c. Properly prepare and condition the athlete.
d. Properly instruct the athlete in the skills of the sport.
e. Insist on safe techniques.
f. Ensure that safe equipment and facilities are used by the athlete at all times.
g. Ensure that proper precautions are taken in extremes of heat and cold. The coach may occasionally even need to cancel practice or competition.
h. **Recognize physical and emotional injury early, and arrange consultation before the problem becomes more severe.**

D. **Officiating and sportsmanship**
1. The coach should appreciate the role of the rules and the officials in prevention of injuries (see Chapter 5, "The Role of Rules and Officials").
2. **The coach should insist that athletes observe the rules and demonstrate proper sportsmanship.**

E. **Conditioning:** The coach is generally responsible for the total conditioning effort, for which the following guidelines are helpful (see also Chapters 14–16).
1. Teach the athletes the importance of all aspects of conditioning for both maximum performance and injury prevention.
2. The conditioning program should contain preseason, in-season, and postseason phases.
3. The conditioning program should contain multiple components, with the emphasis on each determined by the specific sport.
a. Aerobic power
b. Strength—requires special coach training
i. Specific age or maturity group
ii. Flexibility
iii. Proprioception, agility, and coordination

F. **Nutrition** (see Chapter 8, "Sports Nutrition")
1. The coach should understand and teach current valid concepts of nutrition.
2. The coach should attempt to "debunk" popular nutritional myths that may be harmful to the athlete.
3. **The coach is obliged to prohibit the use of banned or harmful substances.**

G. **Weight and body composition**
1. The coach should use and teach **a scientific approach to the issue of weight reduction in athletics. Avoid archaic and/or harmful methods** of body weight manipulation.
a. Bizarre diets
b. Fasting
c. Induced vomiting
d. Purging
e. Diuretics
f. Rubber suits
g. Hot boxes
2. The coach should understand and employ valid methods of assessing weight and body composition.

III. Preparticipation Evaluation

The coach is responsible for ensuring that preparticipation evaluation is performed in compliance with appropriate school, league, or conference regulations.

A. Much of that responsibility may be shared with or assigned to the team physician or athletic trainer; however:
   1. **The coach must ensure that no player practices or competes without proper preseason clearance.**
   2. The coach must ensure **proper follow-up on deficiencies before athletes are permitted to participate.**
      a. Treatment
      b. Rehabilitation
      c. Medical clearance
   3. Similarly, the coach is responsible for the same medical evaluation, treatment, rehabilitation, and clearance pattern for the injured athlete during the season.

B. **Coaches are often major participants in performing the preparticipation evaluation.**
   1. **Conditioning evaluations**
      a. Aerobic power
      b. Strength
      c. Speed
      d. Agility and coordination
   2. **Musculoskeletal evaluations**
      a. Flexibility
      b. Strength
         i. Manual muscle testing
         ii. Muscle girth measurements
      c. Range of motion
   3. **Body composition measurements**
   4. **Nutrition evaluations**

IV. Playing Environment

A. **Temperature** (see Chapters 17 and 18)
   1. The coach should understand the effects of heat and cold on the safety and performance of the athlete.
   2. **The coach is responsible for measuring temperature and humidity and rescheduling or canceling practices or competitions when conditions are not safe.**
   3. The coach is responsible for **preventive measures**, including but not limited to:
      a. Educating the athlete about safety precautions in hot or cold weather
      b. Ensuring proper clothing for the weather
      c. In hot conditions:
         i. Providing adequate fluid replacement
         ii. Providing adequate rest breaks
         iii. Monitoring fluid loss—supervising "weigh-in" and "weigh-out" procedures

B. **Athletic facilities and equipment**
   1. The coach should **set standards for periodic inspection** of athletic facilities and playing surface, particularly before practices and competition.
   2. The coach should ensure that safety devices, such as mats and pads, are properly placed and maintained and that dangerous obstacles are eliminated from the playing area.
   3. The coach should ensure that the playing field or facility is properly lighted for the sport.

4. The coach has responsibilities involving **individual equipment**, which include ensuring that protective equipment is:
    a. Properly selected and high quality
    b. Issued by a well-trained individual who can ensure proper fit
    c. Properly maintained and inspected
    d. Properly used by the athlete

C. **Emergency planning**
1. The coach is responsible for **developing a plan to evaluate, treat, and transport medical emergencies that occur during practice and competition.**
    a. Plan should be in writing
    b. Responsibility may be shared with or assigned to the team physician and/or athletic trainer
    c. Plan should include prior arrangements for transportation of injured athletes and spectators to medical facilities and prior coordination with the referral facility
2. **Coaches should have current American Red Cross advanced first aid and cardiopulmonary resuscitation training, or the equivalent, as minimal preparation for handling athletic emergencies.**

Recommended Reading

1. Anderson MK, Hall SJ: Sports Injury Management. Baltimore, Willians & Wilkins, 1995.
2. Arnheim DD: Essentials of Athletic Training. St. Louis, Times-Mirror, 1987.
3. Arnheim DD, Prentice WE: Principles of Athletic Training, 8th ed. St. Louis, Mosby-Year Book, 1993.
4. Booher JM, Thibodeau GA: Athletic Injury Assessment, 3rd ed. St. Louis, Mosby, 1994.
5. Ellison AE (ed): Athletic Training and Sports Medicine. Chicago, American Academy of Orthopedic Sports Medicine, 1984.
6. Fahey TD: Athletic Training—Principles and Practices. Palo Alto, CA, Mayfield Publishing, 1986.
7. Hirata I: The Doctor and the Athlete, 2nd ed. Philadelphia, JB Lippincott, 1974.
8. Kuland DN: The Injured Athlete. Philadelphia, JB Lippincott, 1982.
9. Pfeiffer RP, Mangus BC: Concepts of Athletic Training. Boston, Jones & Bartlett Publishers, 1995.
10. Zachazewski JE, Magee DJ, Quillen WS: Athletic Injuries and Rehabilitation. Philadelphia, WB Saunders, 1996.

5

The Role of Rules and Officials

William D. Haffey, M.S.

I. The Role of Rules

Rules were developed for the distinct purpose of permitting a congruent transition throughout the length of the contest. **They maintain a consistency in the operation of the mechanics of the contest and a concern for the safety of the participants.** They also provide information by which coaches may instruct players and fans may become more enlightened about the sport. Rules are basic or established criteria by which the officials judge a contest. Rules are divided into several specific areas, each designed to aid in the smooth and normal progress of a contest:

A. **The field of play, court, the pool:** The rules committees involved with establishing the specifications have set up standards that must be adhered to. The specifications for areas of participation allow for consistency between schools and states.

B. **Game equipment:** All equipment, such as goals, bases, mats, ladders, screens, balls, clocks, and yardage chains, used for sport activities must adhere to the standard established by the rules committees.

C. **Player equipment:** The rule books list mandatory equipment that all participants must wear. These items include helmet, mouth pieces, pads, shoes, jerseys, pants, and uniforms. These items are professionally manufactured; alterations may decrease protection for the athlete. The mandatory equipment required for all sports is listed in all rule books.
   a. Game or contest administrators, coaches, and equipment managers must review annually the mandatory equipment that must be worn by participants.
   b. The rule books are reviewed and updated annually.

D. **Illegal equipment:** No player wearing illegal equipment should be permitted to participate. Questions about the legality of a player's equipment are discussed under "The Role of the Official." The list of illegal equipment is for the express purpose of protecting participants in a contest.
   a. Game or contest administrators, coaches, equipment managers, and officials must be knowledgeable about illegal equipment.
   b. The use of illegal equipment should be definitely restricted during practice sessions.

E. **Terminology:** All participants, coaches, fans, and officials should be familiar with terms or phrases expressing certain actions involved in an individual sport.

F. **Control: Rules were developed to control the actions of the participants involved with the contest.** One of the basic fundamentals of the game is that coaches should familiarize each player with the rules involved in the sport. They need not know the technicalities involved with the administration of all the rules, but they should have at least a working knowledge of them.

G. **Violations:** It is a recognized fact that participation in sports activities may result in injury. Some sports are more vigorous than others, and physical contact has to be accepted as a consequence. The safety of participants should receive considerable attention. Those responsible for teaching participants of a sport should see that proper techniques are the only methods taught. It is the responsibility of those involved in administrating an athletic program to see that coaches teach techniques that are within the rules.

H. **Fouls and penalties:** It is recognized in sports that the basic principle behind the enforcement philosophy is that you are entitled to the advantage gained only without the assistance of a foul. The administration of penalties is the responsibility of the official in charge of the contest. Also, coaches should have a basic working knowledge of the fouls and penalties.

II. The Role of the Official

The official is the essential third dimension of an athletic contest. The players and coaches make up the other two dimensions of the triangle. **The official's primary job is to see that a contest progresses according to the stipulated rules and regulations.** He/she must know the rules and mechanics of the sport, have the courage to administer the rules, possess tact and poise to insure confidence, be in physical condition to work the sport, and possess the judgment and common sense to execute instinctive reactions to situations that arise during a contest. **Official's duties** can be divided into two areas:

A. **Pregame duties:** The general pregame duties for officials follow a similar pattern for most contests.
   1. The official, regardless of the contest, should have **a precontest meeting to discuss all facets of the contest.** The precontest meeting should follow a well-planned outline. Another objective of this meeting is to get all officials involved mentally to work the contest. The precontest meeting boils down to a "nuts-and-bolts" meeting.
   2. **Inspect entire area where the activity will take place.** Observe any unusual markings or serious irregularities, and advise the rest of the personnel working the contest. They will take measures to correct or remove any hazardous obstructions within or near the boundary areas of the activity.
   3. **Inspect and approve all equipment**, and see that all equipment necessary for the proper conduct of a contest is in the proper place and condition.
   4. **Check mandatory player equipment.** During the pregame, the officials can spot check player equipment, bandages, and tapes. They can have necessary corrections made before the contest.
      a. **Football:** Before the start of the game, the head coach or a designated representative is responsible for verifying to the referee or umpire (depending on whether it is college or high school) that all the players are in compliance with the rules on mandatory equipment required of all participants. The legality of a player's equipment is determined by the umpire.
         i. National Collegiate Athletic Association (NCAA) Coaches Certification, in football, implies that all players have been informed what equipment is mandatory by rule and what constitutes illegal equipment, have been provided the equipment mandated by rule, have been instructed to wear and how to wear mandatory equipment during the game, and have been instructed to notify the coaching staff when equipment becomes illegal through play during the game.
         ii. In high school, when any required player equipment is missing or when illegal equipment is found, correction must be made before participation.
      b. **Wrestling**
         i. Before a dual meet begins, the referee visits each team's dressing room to inspect contestants for presence of oils, improper clothing, jewelry, long fingernails, and improper grooming. Clarify the rules with the coaches and contestants on request, and review the scores and timekeeper signals and procedures to be used.
         ii. The legality of all equipment, including mats, markings, uniforms, supplementary devices, pads, and taping, is decided by the referee.

c. **Basketball**
   i. The referee does not permit any player to wear equipment that, in his or her judgment, is dangerous to other players.
   ii. Any equipment that is unnatural and designed to increase a player's height or reach, or to gain advantage, should not be used.

d. **Baseball**
   i. Before the start of the game, the umpire-in-chief ascertains legality of all equipment, especially bats and helmets.
   ii. The coach's acceptance of responsibility for players being properly equipped is part of the pregame duties of officials.

e. **Soccer**
   i. The head referee inspects and approves the game balls, field of play, and nets; inquires about local ground rules; and determines if a fair game may be started.
   ii. Illegal equipment should not be worn by any player. This applies to any equipment that, in the opinion of the referee, is dangerous or confusing.

f. **Volleyball**
   i. The referee checks players for proper and legal uniforms and equipment.
   ii. The legality of game equipment is determined by the referee.

B. **Game duties:** General duties involve knowing the rules and mechanics to officiate the sport within the general established guidelines. One of the official's primary concerns, regardless of the sport, is the safety of the participants.

1. **Whenever game and player equipment, or a participant's physical condition, can adversely affect the safety of a player or players, the officials must take precautions to correct the situation.**
2. **During the contest, whenever damaged or illegal equipment is detected, the officials must take steps to correct the problem, in accordance with the stipulated rules.**
3. **Injuries:** There are no known steps to prevent all of the injuries that can and do occur during athletic contest. Specific procedures exist for use when a participant is injured. The following are examples:

a. **Football**
   i. An injured or apparently injured player who is discovered by an official while the ball is dead and the clock is stopped, and for whom the ready-for-play signal is delayed or for whom the clock is stopped, is replaced for at least one down unless the halftime or overtime intermission occurs.
   ii. In college, the player may remain in the game if the team is charged a time-out in the interval between downs. If the team's charged time-outs have been exhausted, the injured player must leave for one down, whether in college or high school. An exception is the blood rule, and the player remains out of the game until the problem has been corrected. Any official may stop the clock for an injured player.

b. **Wrestling**
   i. Wrestlers are entitled to injury time-outs and injury recovery time.
   ii. If a competitor is rendered unconscious, he shall not be permitted to continue after regaining consciousness without the approval of a physician. If a physician recommends that an injured wrestler not continue, even though consciousness is not involved, the physician cannot be overruled.

c. **Track**
   i. A competitor who has been rendered unconscious during a meet is not permitted to resume participation in that meet without written authorization from a physician.

   ii. A competitor who scratches from an event because of illness or injury must have a signed permission from a physician to participate later in the meet. This statement is required by some state athletic associations.

d. **Volleyball**
   i. In case of injury, the referee may interrupt play and, after sufficient time for replacement of the injured player, direct a replay.
   ii. In case of injury to a starting player during warmups, substitution is made without penalty, and no entry is charged to the injured player.

e. **Basketball**
   i. When a player is injured, the official may suspend play after the ball is dead or in control of the injured player's team, or when the opponents complete play.
   ii. When necessary to protect an injured player or players, the official may immediately suspend play.

III. Liability Insurance

A. **Sports officials should consider carrying a liability policy.** It has often been said, with much truth, that in the United States, anyone can sue anyone else for about everything.

B. **Officials working nonprofessional sports should definitely consider carrying liability insurance**.

C. Examples of legal cases involving sports officials:

1. *Daily v. McNesse* (Alabama) This case involved a claim by a high school player who was injured during the course of the game when an opponent intentionally struck him in the groin, resulting in his testicles being removed. The local officials association was sued, based on its failure to supervise the game.
2. *Rapfogel v. Morris County Industrial Recreation Assn.* (New Jersey) This case involved a claim by a fan who was injured by a foul ball and claimed the umpire and the recreational softball league failed to warn her of the danger.
3. *Thomas v. Board of Education of Hamilton* (Ontario, Canada) This case involved a claim against a local football officials association by a high school football player who was injured when he was tackled during a game. The claim was that the local association failed to insure that there was proper medical supervision in attendance at the game to handle such injuries.
4. *Wilhelm v. San Diego Unified School District* (California) This case involved a defamation claim by a high school basketball official who was allegedly defamed by a coach following a game.
5. *Cole v. Atlantic Coast Hockey League* (New York) This case involved a claim by an ice hockey referee who was thrown to the ice by players during a game.
6. *Heimbaugh v. City and County of San Francisco* (California) This case involved a claim by a recreation baseball player that an umpire was negligent for allowing the game to proceed with improper bases. The player slid into the base and was injured.
7. *Wilson v. Anaheim Union High School District* (California) This case involved a claim by a soccer player against the local soccer officials' association for failure to make calls during the game and prior games that would have prevented the reckless actions by a player who injured another player during the course of the game.
8. *Lynch v. Connellsville Area School District* (Pennsylvania) This was a worker's compensation claim by a high school football referee who was injured during the course of the game, which resulted in his leg being amputated. He brought a claim against the Pennsylvania Interscholastic Athletic Association as well as the area school district.
9. *Smith v. Sinsun* (California) This was a claim by a recreational baseball umpire who was attacked with a bat by a player during the game and suffered serious injuries to his eye and face.

10. *Smith v. Cumberland County High School* (Tennessee) This case involved an assault by a fan on a basketball referee at a high school game.
11. *Uhrig v. Township of Cranford, et al.* (New Jersey) This was a claim by a recreational wrestler who was injured when an opponent picked him up and slammed him to the mat. The referee is being sued for his failure to supervise properly.
12. *Frazier v. Rutherford Board of Education* (New Jersey) This was a claim by a high school track participant who was injured when he slipped off the take-off board in the long jump competition. There is a claim against the sports official for failure to make sure that the take-off board was in a safe, clean, and dry condition.
13. *Elvert v. City of Long Beach v. Russ Rendly Sports Officials Association* (California) This case involved a claim by a recreational softball player against the sports officials association for failure to properly train and supervise its umpires. The injury allegedly occurred when he slid into second base and second base was not tied down properly, resulting in a spike going through his leg.
14. *Poole v. Morgan* (Georgia) This case involved an assault on a midget league football umpire by a fan.
15. *Pichardo v. North Patchogue Medford Youth Athletic Association* (New York) This case involved a baseball player being struck and killed by lightning. The parent claimed the North Patchogue Medford Youth Athletic Association Inc. and the Eastern Suffolk Baseball Umpires Association were negligent in allowing the baseball game to continue when the weather in the area became threatening.
16. *Kennel v. Carson City School District* (Nevada) This case involved assault and battery by an opposing high school basketball player. It was alleged that the school district and the referees were negligent.
17. *Harvey v. Ouachita Perish School Board* (Alabama) This case involved an injured football player who blamed officials for an unnecessary roughness injury.

Recommended Reading

1. Bunn JW: The Art of Officiating Sports. Englewood Cliffs, NJ, Prentice-Hall, Inc., 1957.
2. Clegg R, Thompson WA: Modern Sports Officiating. Dubuque, William C. Brown Company, 1979.
3. Goldberger AS: Sports Officiating—A Legal Guide. New York, Leisure Press, 1984.
4. Baseball Rulebook. Shawnee Mission, Kansas, National Collegiate Association, 1995.
5. Basketball Rules. Kansas City, National Federation of State High School Association, 1995/96.
6. Basketball Rules and Interpretations Book. Shawnee Mission, Kansas, National Collegiate Association, 1995/96.
7. Boys Gymnastics Rules. Kansas City, National Federation of State High School Association, 1994/95.
8. Football Case Book. Kansas City, National Federation of State High School Association, 1995/96.
9. Football Officials Manual. Kansas City, National Federation of State High School Association, 1995/96.
10. Football Rules. Kansas City, National Federation of State High School Association, 1995/96.
11. Football Rules and Interpretations Book. Shawnee Mission, Kansas, National Collegiate Association, 1994/95.
12. Girls Gymnastics Rules. Kansas City, National Federation of State High School Association, 1994/95.
13. Ross C, Thomas JD: Sports and the courts. Physical Education and Sports Law Newsletter 11(5), 1990.
14. Ross C, Thomas JD: Sports and the courts. Physical Education and Sports Law Newsletter 13(4), 1992.
15. Ross C, Thomas JD: Sports and the courts. Physical Education and Sports Law Newsletter 13(1), 1992.
16. Soccer Rules. Kansas City, National Federation of State High School Association, 1994/95.
17. Swimming, Diving, and Water Polo Rules. Kansas City, National Federation of State High School Association, 1994/95.
18. Volleyball Rules. Kansas City, National Federation of State High School Association, 1995/96.
19. Track and Field and Cross Country Rules. Kansas City, National Federation of State High School Association, 1996.
20. Wrestling Rules. Kansas City, National Federation of State High School Association, 1995/96.

6

The Preparticipation Physical Evaluation

David M. Smith, M.D.

I. Overview

A. **Responsibility of sports medicine team**
   1. Assist athletes in maintaining health and ensure safe participation in training and competition.
   2. Prevent and treat injuries, illnesses, and underlying conditions as they relate to athletic participation.

B. **Preparticipation physical evaluation (PPE)**
   1. PPE is considered an important first step in fulfilling the above responsibility.
   2. Despite general agreement that PPE is necessary, there is wide variability in recommendations and requirements.
   3. Guidelines for PPE, endorsed by American Academy of Family Physicians, American Academy of Pediatrics, American Medical Society for Sports Medicine, American Orthopaedic Society for Sports Medicine, and American Osteopathic Academy of Sports Medicine, serve as a foundation for the sports medicine team to critically appraise the effectiveness of the PPE.

II. Objectives of the PPE

A. **Primary (essential)**
   1. Detect conditions that may limit participation.
   2. Detect conditions that may predispose to injury.
   3. Meet legal and insurance requirements.

B. **Secondary (ideal)**
   1. Assess general health and identify health-risk behaviors.
   2. Assess physical maturity.
   3. Determine fitness and performance level.

III. Timing and Frequency of the PPE

A. **Variability in recommendations**
   1. Dependent on individual athlete (i.e., age; gender; sport—single or multiple; health—underlying medical conditions, injury history)
   2. Dependent on availability of record from past PPEs (i.e., continuity of care)
   3. Dependent on requirements of state, city, or athletic governing body

B. **General guidelines**
   1. The PPE should be performed at least 6 weeks before the beginning of the sport to allow adequate time to further evaluate identified problems and to treat or rehabilitate any conditions or injuries.
   2. Annual evaluation is recommended.

a. Comprehensive baseline PPE before initiating a new sport or attaining a new level (e.g., entry into high school, college, or professional level)
b. Subsequent annual PPEs may be limited to interim injuries or illnesses but should also include review of cardiopulmonary system and repeat examination of same
c. If in multiple sports during the year, consider more frequent evaluations

IV. Format of the PPE

A. **Office-based**

1. Potential advantages include physician–patient familiarity, privacy, and continuity of care.
2. Disadvantages may include greater cost, limited appointment time, and lack of communication of pertinent information back to school athletic staff.

B. **Group screening-station** (Table 1)

1. Potential advantages include specialized personnel, time and cost efficiency, and good communication with school athletic staff.
2. Disadvantages may include rushed examinations, lack of privacy, and inadequate follow-up of identified problems.

V. Personnel

A. **Physicians**

1. Primary care physicians perform the majority of PPEs because of their ability to evaluate all organ systems (i.e., cardiopulmonary, musculoskeletal, neurologic, ophthalmologic, gastrointestinal, genitourinary, dermatologic).
2. Specialists such as orthopedic surgeons, cardiologists, and ophthalmologists or optometrists are key consultants and may be on-site during the screening-station format examination.

B. **Ancillary**

1. Medical staff, including athletic trainers, physical therapists, nurses, exercise scientists, dietitians, and sports psychologists may be involved, especially in the screening-station format PPE.
2. Nonmedical staff, including coaches, school administrators, and community volunteers, are especially helpful in the screening-station format PPE.

TABLE 1. Required and Optional Stations and Personnel for Group Screening-Station Preparticipation Physical Evaluation

Required Stations	Personnel
Sign-in, height and weight, vital signs, vision	Ancillary personnel (coach, nurse, community volunteer)
History review, physical examination (medical and orthopedic), clearance	Physician
Optional Stations	**Personnel**
Orthopedic examination (specific)	Physician
Flexibility	Trainer or therapist
Body composition	Physiologist
Strength	Trainer, coach, therapist, physiologist
Speed, agility, power, balance, endurance	Trainer, coach, physiologist

From Preparticipation Physical Evaluation (monograph). Kansas City, MO, American Academy of Family Physicians, American Academy of Pediatrics, American Medical Society for Sports Medicine, American Orthopaedic Society for Sports Medicine, American Osteopathic Academy of Sports Medicine, 1992, with permission.

VI. Medical History (see Fig. 1A)

A. The **medical history** is the cornerstone of the PPE and may identify up to 75% of problems affecting athletes.

B. The **cardiovascular** questions under #4 are key questions designed to identify conditions (e.g., hypertrophic cardiomyopathy, Marfan's syndrome, premature atherosclerotic heart disease) that may limit athletic participation (see Table 2 for **cardiovascular causes of sudden death in athletes**).

   1. *"Have you ever passed out during or after exercise?"* Exertional syncope is considered a "red flag" for the potential cardiovascular conditions that may cause sudden death.
   2. *"Has anyone in your family died of heart problems or a sudden death before age 50?"* Familial premature death from cardiovascular disease or sudden death should raise suspicion for hypertrophic cardiomyopathy, Marfan's syndrome, prolonged Q-T syndrome, and familial hyperlipidemia.

C. Specific questions regarding **health-risk behaviors**, such as alcohol, tobacco, and illicit drug use; sexually transmitted diseases and unwanted pregnancies; pathogenic weight control behaviors; and use of ergogenic aids for performance enhancement, are not included on the medical history form to avoid incriminatory feelings and thus inaccurate responses.

   1. A general question such as *"Are there any concerns you would like to discuss (nutrition, weight problems, training techniques, steroids or other performance-enhancing agents, tobacco, alcohol, other drugs, birth control, sexually transmitted diseases, family problems, school problems, or problems with friends or peers, stress, or anything else)?"* may open the door for identifying health-risk behaviors.
   2. Specific questions such as *"Do you use seat belts on a regular basis?"* and *"Has any physician discussed the importance of preventive care (Pap smears, breast self-exams, testicular self-exams, cholesterol screening)?"* may identify poor health habits or lack of understanding of the importance of preventive health maintenance.

D. The rest of the questions on the medical history form are self-explanatory but may be supplemented if necessary.

   1. Consider supplemental questions to question #15 for female athletes at risk for **female athlete triad syndrome (interrelatedness of disordered eating, amenorrhea, and osteoporosis)**.
      a. *"What do you consider your ideal weight?"*
      b. *"What do you do to control your weight?"*
      c. *"Do you worry about your weight?"*
   2. Review each question with the athlete to ensure full understanding and accurate responses.
   3. Have parent or guardian review and sign form to increase accuracy of responses by the athlete.

TABLE 2. Cardiovascular Causes of Sudden Death in Athletes

Common	Uncommon
Hypertrophic cardiomyopathy*	Aortic stenosis*
Anomalous coronary artery	Mitral valve prolapse*
Atherosclerotic heart disease	Myocarditis
Marfan's syndrome (aortic rupture)*	Right ventricular dysplasia
Idiopathic concentric left ventricular hypertrophy	Conduction system abnormalities
	Amyloidosis
	Sarcoidosis
	Cardiac tumors

* Screenable by history and physical examination.

FIGURE 1A. Preparticipation Physical Evaluation Form.

History Date ____________

Name ______________________ Sex______ Age________ Date of birth __________

Grade ________ Sport ______________ ______________ ______________

Personal physician ______________ ______________ ______________

Address Physician's phone

Explain "Yes" answers below:

	Yes	No
1. Have you ever been hospitalized?	☐	☐
Have you ever had surgery?	☐	☐
2. Are you presently taking any medications or pills?	☐	☐
3. Do you have any allergies (medicine, bees or other stinging insects)?	☐	☐
4. Have you ever passed out during or after exercise?	☐	☐
Have you ever been dizzy during or after exercise?	☐	☐
Have you ever had chest pain during or after exercise?	☐	☐
Do you tire more quickly than your friends during exercise?	☐	☐
Have you ever had high blood pressure?	☐	☐
Have you ever been told that you have a heart murmur?	☐	☐
Have you ever had racing of your heart or skipped heartbeats?	☐	☐
Has anyone in your family died of heart problems or a sudden death before age 50?	☐	☐
5. Do you have any skin problems (itching, rashes, acne)?	☐	☐
6. Have you ever had a head injury?	☐	☐
Have you ever been knocked out or unconscious?	☐	☐
Have you ever had a seizure?	☐	☐
Have you ever had a stinger, burner or pinched nerve?	☐	☐
7. Have you ever had heat or muscle cramps?	☐	☐
Have you ever been dizzy or passed out in the heat?	☐	☐
8. Do you have trouble breathing or do you cough during or after activity?	☐	☐
9. Do you use any special equipment (pads, braces, neck rolls, mouth guard, eye guards, etc.)?	☐	☐
10. Have you had any problems with your eyes or vision?	☐	☐
Do you wear glasses or contacts or protective eye wear?	☐	☐
11. Have you ever sprained/strained, dislocated, fractured, broken or had repeated swelling or other injuries of any bones or joints?	☐	☐
☐ Head ☐ Shoulder ☐ Thigh ☐ Neck ☐ Elbow ☐ Knee ☐ Chest		
☐ Forearm ☐ Shin/calf ☐ Back ☐ Wrist ☐ Ankle ☐ Hip ☐ Hand ☐ Foot		
12. Have you had any other medical problems (infectious mononucleosis, diabetes, etc.)?	☐	☐
13. Have you had a medical problem or injury since your last evaluation?	☐	☐

14. When was your last tetanus shot? ______________

When was your last measles immunization? ______________

15. When was your first menstrual period? ______________

When was your last menstrual period? ______________

What was the longest time between your periods last year? ______________

Explain "Yes" answers:

____

____

____

____

____

____

I hereby state that, to the best of my knowledge, my answers to the above questions are correct.

Date ______________

Signature of athlete ______________

Signature of parent/guardian ______________

FIGURE 1B. Preparticipation Physical Evaluation Form *(continued)*.

Physical Examination

Date ______

Name ______ Age ______ Date of birth ______

COMPLETE / LIMITED

Height ______ Weight ______ BP ____ / ____ Pulse ______

Vision R 20/____ L 20/____ Corrected: Y N Pupils ______

	Normal	Abnormal findings				Initials
Cardiopulmonary						
Pulses						
Heart						
Lungs						
Tanner stage	1	2	3	4	5	
Skin						
Abdominal						
Genitalia						
Musculoskeletal						
Neck						
Shoulder						
Elbow						
Wrist						
Hand						
Back						
Knee						
Ankle						
Foot						
Other						

Clearance:

A. Cleared

B. Cleared after completing evaluation/rehabilitation for: ______

C. Not cleared for: ☐ Collision
☐ Contact
☐ Noncontact ____ Strenuous ____ Moderately strenuous ____ Nonstrenuous

Due to: ______

Recommendation: ______

Name of physician ______ Date ______

Address ______ Phone ______

Signature of physician ______

From Preparticipation Physical Evaluation (monograph). Kansas City, MO, American Academy of Family Physicians, American Academy of Pediatrics, American Medical Society for Sports Medicine, American Orthopaedic Society for Sports Medicine, American Osteopathic Academy of Sports Medicine, 1992, with permission.

VII. Physical Examination (see Fig. 1B)

A. The **physical examination** should be comprehensive yet focused on pertinent findings from the medical history.

B. **Physical examination form** is general in scope but should not limit the clinician if additional exam is deemed pertinent.

1. Head/eyes/ears/nose/throat (HEENT) section omitted from form but should not imply that this is not important.
   a. Pupils (for anisocoria), conjunctiva (for anemia), and visual acuity required in all athletes.
   b. Swimmers (otitis externa), scuba divers (otic barotrauma), and wrestlers (auricular hematoma) need ear exams.
   c. Allergy sufferers and athletes with history of nose trauma need nasopharynx exams.
   d. Smokeless tobacco users need oropharynx exams.
   e. Clinical judgment based on history determines necessity of HEENT in all other athletes.
2. Cardiovascular assessment is essential for both initial PPE and subsequent annual reevaluations.
   a. Blood pressure measurement (with appropriate cuff size)—if elevated (rule of thumb: > 125/75 in those < 10 years and > 135/85 in those ≥ 10 years), follow-up blood pressure later in examination or at follow-up appointment
   b. Palpation of upper and lower extremity pulses—brachial-femoral delay screens for coarctation of aorta
   c. Heart auscultation in two positions (supine and standing/sitting) and with provocative maneuvers (Valsalva, deep inspiration, squat-to-stand, stand-to-squat) helps differentiate functional (e.g., pulmonic flow murmurs) from pathologic (e.g., aortic stenosis, hypertrophic cardiomyopathy) murmurs.
   d. Ectopic beats that disappear with exercise are generally benign but need electrocardiogram to confirm.
3. Musculoskeletal examination is important to identify musculotendinous, bone, or joint problems that may limit athletic participation or predispose an athlete to acute injury or long-term complications (e.g., shoulder instability, anterior cruciate deficient knee, unrehabilitated ankle sprain, juvenile rheumatoid arthritis).
   a. In the absence of historical findings, a general musculoskeletal screening examination may be performed (Table 3).
   b. Any positive responses to the musculoskeletal history mandates a complete examination of that particular joint or region.
   c. Consider sports-specific musculoskeletal examination (e.g., shoulder exam for throwers, tennis players, swimmers; knee exam for basketball, football, and soccer players).
   d. Consider screening for flexibility (e.g., back, hamstrings, Achilles) because clinical anecdotal evidence suggests that increasing flexibility reduces risk of overuse problems (e.g., mechanical back pain, patellofemoral pain, medial tibial stress syndrome), but studies do not support decreased risk of acute injury (i.e., sprains, strains, dislocations).
4. Negative history and musculoskeletal examination obviates need for complete neurologic screening examination. If positive history for neurologic problems (e.g., concussions, brachial plexopathy, seizures), more detailed examination is warranted.

C. **Fitness and performance evaluation**

1. Considered a secondary (ideal) objective of the PPE
2. More frequently performed in a group screening-station format

TABLE 3. Musculoskeletal Screening Examination

Position and Functional Motion	Observation
Patient facing examiner	Symmetry of upper and lower extremities and trunk
Neck flexion, extension, right and left lateral flexion and rotation	Cervical spine range of motion
Resisted shoulder shrug	Trapezius strength
Resisted shoulder abduction	Deltoid strength
Shoulder internal and external rotation with arms 90° abducted	Glenohumeral range of motion
Elbow flexion and extension	Elbow range of motion
Elbow and wrist pronation and supination with arms adducted at side and elbows 90° flexed	Elbow and wrist range of motion
Make a fist then spread fingers	Hand and finger range of motion
Patient facing away from examiner	Symmetry of upper and lower extremities and trunk
Back flexion with knees straight	Thoracic and lumbosacral vertebral spine motion and curvature and hamstring flexibility
Lower extremity examination with patient facing examiner, then contraction of quadriceps simultaneously	Alignment of lower extremities and symmetry of muscle tone
Squat and "duck walk" 4 steps	Hip, knee, and ankle motion and general lower extremity strength and balance
Patient standing on toes (facing away from examiner) and then heels (facing examiner)	Calf muscle symmetry, leg strength, and balance

Adapted from Preparticipation Physical Evaluation (monograph). Kansas City, MO, American Academy of Family Physicians, American Academy of Pediatrics, American Medical Society for Sports Medicine, American Orthopaedic Society for Sports Medicine, American Osteopathic Academy of Sports Medicine, 1992, with permission.

3. Measures any or all of the following parameters:
   a. Body composition—skinfold, underwater weighing, circumferences
   b. Flexibility—sit-and-reach, goniometry
   c. Strength—manual muscle testing; hand or leg dynamometer; bench press or leg press; pushups, pullups, or situps
   d. Endurance—12–minute run, 1.5–mile run
   e. Power—vertical jump, standing broad jump
   f. Speed—40–yard dash
   g. Agility—agility run
   h. Balance—stork stand, balance beam walking
4. Vision performance testing has been added in some settings.
   a. Dynamic visual acuity
   b. Visual tracking or pursuit
   c. Depth perception
   d. Eye–hand and eye–body coordination

VIII. Routine Screening Tests

A. Must differentiate between what constitutes routine **screening** versus **diagnostic** testing (e.g., a complete blood count in an asymptomatic female athlete is a *screening test*, whereas a complete blood count in a female athlete with poor eating habits, heavy menstrual periods, fatigue, and pale conjunctiva becomes a *diagnostic test*).
   1. Does the burden of suffering resulting from the condition warrant screening?
   2. If "yes" to above question, ask the following:
      a. What is the sensitivity of the proposed screening test?
      b. Are the potential risks and cost of the proposed screening test acceptable?
      c. If the screening test identifies the condition, are proven and acceptable methods of treatment available, and is there a clear advantage to initiating this treatment during the asymptomatic phase of the condition?

B. Many **screening tests** have been proposed and have been used in various settings including:

TABLE 4. Classification of Sports by Contact

Contact/Collision	Limited Contact	Noncontact
Basketball	Baseball	Archery
Boxing*	Bicycling	Badminton
Diving	Cheerleading	Body building
Field hockey	Canoeing/kayaking (white water)	Bowling
Football	Fencing	Canoeing/kayaking (flat water)
Flag	Field	Crew/rowing
Tackle	High jump	Curling
Ice hockey	Pole vault	Dancing
Lacrosse	Floor hockey	Field
Martial arts	Gymnastics	Discus
Rodeo	Handball	Javelin
Rugby	Horseback riding	Shot put
Ski jumping	Racquetball	Golf
Soccer	Skating	Orienteering
Team handball	Ice	Power lifting
Water polo	Inline	Race walking
Wrestling	Roller	Riflery
	Skiing	Rope jumping
	Cross-country	Running
	Downhill	Sailing
	Water	Scuba diving
	Softball	Strength training
	Squash	Swimming
	Ultimate frisbee	Table tennis
	Volleyball	Tennis
	Windsurfing/surfing	Track
		Weight lifting

* Participation not recommended.
From Committee on Sports Medicine and Fitness: Medical conditions affecting sports participation. Pediatrics 94:757–760, 1994, with permission.

1. Laboratory—urinalysis, complete blood count, chemistry profile, lipid profile, ferritin, sickle cell trait, human immunodeficiency virus
2. Cardiopulmonary—electrocardiogram, echocardiogram, exercise stress test, spirometry, exercise spirometry
3. Radiographic—chest film, cervical spine, joint x-rays

C. **Conclusion** is that with the available research on athletes **the use of routine screening tests is not recommended and remains unproven**. One exception to this is that individuals with Down's syndrome are still required to have initial screening cervical spine radiographs to exclude atlantoaxial instability before participation in sports. This requirement, however, is being challenged by a study showing no greater risk of morbidity in Down's syndrome athletes with atlantoaxial instability than in those without.

IX. Clearance for Participation

A. To make a **clearance determination** with the information gathered from the medical history, physical examination, and any diagnostic tests, the clinician must be familiar with the demands of the sport.
   1. Classification of sports by degree of contact (Table 4)
   2. Classification of sports by degree of strenuousness (Table 5)

B. Consider the following **four questions** before determining a clearance status:
   1. Will this problem increase the athlete's risk of morbidity or mortality?
   2. Will other participants be at increased risk of morbidity if this athlete is allowed to participate?

TABLE 5. Classification of Sports by Strenuousness

High to Moderate Intensity		
High to Moderate Dynamic and Static Demands	**High to Moderate Dynamic and Low Static Demands**	**High to Moderate Static and Low Dynamic Demands**
Boxing*	Badminton	Archery
Crew/rowing	Baseball	Auto racing
Cross-country skiing	Basketball	Diving
Cycling	Field hockey	Equestrian
Downhill skiing	Lacrosse	Field events (jumping)
Fencing	Orienteering	Field events (throwing)
Football	Ping-pong	Gymnastics
Ice hockey	Race walking	Karate or judo
Rugby	Racquetball	Motorcycling
Running (sprint)	Soccer	Rodeoing
Speed skating	Squash	Sailing
Water polo	Swimming	Ski jumping
Wrestling	Tennis	Water skiing
	Volleyball	Weight lifting
Low Intensity (Low Dynamic and Low Static Demands)		
	Bowling	Golf
	Cricket	Riflery
	Curling	

* Participation not recommended.
From Committee on Sports Medicine and Fitness: Medical conditions affecting sports participation. Pediatrics 94:757–760, 1994, with permission.

3. Will further evaluation, treatment, or rehabilitation allow full participation, and, while these are initiated, can the athlete participate in limited activities?
4. If the problem precludes full, unrestricted participation, can the athlete be cleared for participation in limited activities?

C. Do *not* "cookbook" clearance for sports participation determinations but rather use sound medical judgment in all cases.
   1. Guidelines for medical conditions affecting sports participation (Table 6)
   2. Guidelines for cardiovascular abnormalities and athletic participation[9]

D. **Categorizing clearance determinations**
   1. **Unrestricted clearance**—no restrictions on participation in any activity
   2. **Clearance after completion of specific evaluation or rehabilitation**—problem identified that needs further evaluation or treatment, and until this has been completed, the athlete does not have full clearance
   3. **No clearance**—due to a problem that contraindicates participation in specific sports based on degree of contact or strenuousness

E. **Medicolegal considerations**
   1. Under enactments such as the Americans With Disabilities Act and the Federal Rehabilitation Act, the athlete may have the legal right to participate against medical advice.
   2. In cases in which athletes choose to participate against medical advice, it is highly recommended that an *exculpatory waiver* or *prospective release* be used. Despite questions of validity, these forms of written contracts are intended to demonstrate that the athlete was fully informed of his or her condition and the potential risk of participation, thus releasing the physician of liability in the event of morbidity or mortality caused by participation against medical advice.

TABLE 6. Medical Conditions and Sports Participation

Condition	May Participate?
Atlantoaxial instability (instability of the joint between cervical vertebrae 1 and 2) *Explanation:* Athlete needs evaluation to assess risk of spinal cord injury during sports participation	Qualified Yes
Bleeding disorder *Explanation:* Athlete needs evaluation	Qualified Yes
Cardiovascular diseases	
Carditis (inflammation of the heart) *Explanation:* Carditis may result in sudden death with exertion	No
Hypertension (high blood pressure) *Explanation:* Those with significant essential (unexplained) hypertension should avoid weight and power lifting, body building, and strength training. Those with secondary hypertension (hypertension caused by a previously identified disease), or severe essential hypertension, need evaluation	Qualified Yes
Congenital heart disease (structural heart defects present at birth) *Explanation:* Those with mild forms may participate fully; those with moderate or severe forms, or who have undergone surgery, need evaluation	Qualified Yes
Dysrhythmia (irregular heart rhythm) *Explanation:* Athlete needs evaluation because some types require therapy or make certain sports dangerous, or both	Qualified Yes
Mitral valve prolapse (abnormal heart valve) *Explanation:* Those with symptoms (chest pain, symptoms of possible dysrhythmia) or evidence of mitral regurgitation (leaking) on physical examination need evaluation. All others may participate fully	Qualified Yes
Heart murmur *Explanation:* If the murmur is innocent (does not indicate heart disease), full participation is permitted. Otherwise the athlete needs evaluation (see congenital heart disease and mitral valve prolapse above)	Qualified Yes
Cerebral palsy *Explanation:* Athlete needs evaluation	Qualified Yes
Diabetes mellitus *Explanation:* All sports can be played with proper attention to diet, hydration, and insulin therapy. Particular attention is needed for activities that last 30 minutes or more	Yes
Diarrhea Explanation: Unless disease is mild, no participation is permitted, because diarrhea may increase the risk of dehydration and heat illness. See fever below	Qualified No
Eating disorders Anorexia nervosa Bulimia nervosa *Explanation:* These patients need both medical and psychiatric assessment before participation	Qualified Yes
Eyes Functionally one-eyed athlete Loss of an eye Detached retina Previous eye surgery or serious eye injury *Explanation:* A functionally one-eyed athlete has a best corrected visual acuity of < 20/40 in the worse eye. These athletes would suffer significant disability if the better eye was seriously injured as would those with loss of an eye. Some athletes who have previously undergone eye surgery or had a serious eye injury may have an increased risk of injury because of weakened eye tissue. Availability of eye guards approved by the American Society for Testing Materials (ASTM) and other protective equipment may allow participation in most sports, but this must be judged on an individual basis	Qualified Yes
Fever *Explanation:* Fever can increase cardiopulmonary effort, reduce maximum exercise capacity, make heat illness more likely, and increase orthostatic hypotension during exercise. Fever may rarely accompany myocarditis or other infections that may make exercise dangerous	No

Table continued on following page.

TABLE 6. Medical Conditions and Sports Participation *(Cont.)*

Condition	May Participate?
Heat illness, history of	Qualified Yes
Explanation: Because of the increased likelihood of recurrence, the athlete needs individual assessment to determine the presence of predisposing conditions and to arrange a prevention strategy	
HIV infection	Yes
Explanation: Because of the apparent minimal risk to others, all sports may be played that the state of health allows. In all athletes, skin lesions should be properly covered, and athletic personnel should use universal precautions when handling blood or body fluids with visible blood	
Kidney: absence of one	Qualified Yes
Explanation: Athlete needs individual assessment for contact/collision and limited contact sports	
Liver: enlarged	Qualified Yes
Explanation: If the liver is acutely enlarged, participation should be avoided because of risk of rupture. If the liver is chronically enlarged, individual assessment is needed before collision/contact or limited contact sports are played	
Malignancy	Qualified Yes
Explanation: Athlete needs individual assessment	
Musculoskeletal disorders	Qualified Yes
Explanation: Athlete needs individual assessment	
Neurologic	
History of serious head or spine trauma, severe or repeated concussions, or craniotomy	Qualified Yes
Explanation: Athlete needs individual assessment for collision/contact or limited contact sports, and also for noncontact sports if there are deficits in judgment or cognition. Recent research supports a conservative approach to management of concussion	
Convulsive disorder, well controlled	Yes
Explanation: Risk of convulsion during participation is minimal	
Convulsive disorder, poorly controlled	Qualified Yes
Explanation: Athlete needs individual assessment for collision/contact or limited contact sports. Avoid the following noncontact sports: archery, riflery, swimming, weight or power lifting, strength training, or sports involving heights. In these sports, occurrence of a convulsion may be a risk to self or others	
Obesity	Qualified Yes
Explanation: Because of the risk of heat illness, obese persons need careful acclimatization and hydration	
Organ transplant recipient	Qualified Yes
Explanation: Athlete needs individual assessment	
Ovary: absence of one	Yes
Explanation: Risk of severe injury to the remaining ovary is minimal	
Respiratory	
Pulmonary compromise including cystic fibrosis	Qualified Yes
Explanation: Athlete needs individual assessment, but generally all sports may be played if oxygenation remains satisfactory during a graded exercise test. Patients with cystic fibrosis need acclimatization and good hydration to reduce the risk of heat illness	
Asthma	Yes
Explanation: With proper medication and education, only athletes with the most severe asthma have to modify their participation	
Acute upper respiratory infection	Qualified Yes
Explanation: Upper respiratory obstruction may affect pulmonary function. Athlete needs individual assessment for all but mild disease. See fever above	
Sickle cell disease	Qualified Yes
Explanation: Athlete needs individual assessment. In general, if status of the illness permits, all but high exertion, collision/contact sports may be played. Overheating, dehydration, and chilling must be avoided	

Table continued on following page.

TABLE 6. Medical Conditions and Sports Participation *(Cont.)*

Condition	May Participate?
Sickle cell trait	Yes
Explanation: It is unlikely that individuals with sickle cell trait (AS) have an increased risk of sudden death or other medical problems during athletic participation except under the most extreme conditions of heat, humidity, and possibly increased altitude. These individuals, like all athletes, should be carefully conditioned, acclimatized, and hydrated to reduce any possible risk	
Skin: boils, herpes simplex, impetigo, scabies, molluscum contagiosum	Qualified Yes
Explanation: While the patient is contagious, participation in gymnastics with mats, martial arts, wrestling, or other collision/contact or limited contact sports is not allowed. Herpes simplex virus probably is not transmitted via mats	
Spleen, enlarged	Qualified Yes
Explanation: Patients with acutely enlarged spleens should avoid all sports because of risk of rupture. Those with chronically enlarged spleens need individual assessment before playing collision/contact or limited contact sports	
Testicle: absent or undescended	Yes
Explanation: Certain sports may require a protective cup	

From Committee on Sports Medicine and Fitness: Medical conditions affecting sports participation. Pediatrics 94:757–760, 1994, with permission.

Recommended Reading

1. Ades PA: Preventing sudden death: Cardiovascular screening of young athletes. Phys Sportsmed 20:75–89, 1992.
2. American Academy of Pediatrics, Committee on Sports Medicine and Fitness: Medical conditions affecting sports participation. Pediatrics 94:757–760, 1994.
3. Epstein SE, Maron BJ: Sudden death and the competitive athlete: Perspectives on preparticipation screening studies. J Am Coll Cardiol 7:220–230, 1986.
4. Herbert DL: Prospective releases: Will their use protect sports medicine physicians from suit? Sports Med Stand Malpract Report 6:33–36, 1994.
5. Johnson MD: Tailoring the preparticipation exam to female athletes. Phys Sportsmed 20:61–72, 1992.
6. Kibler WB: The Sport Preparticipation Fitness Examination. Champaign, IL, Human Kinetics Publishers, 1990.
7. Lombardo JA, Robinson JB, Smith DM: Preparticipation Physical Evaluation. Kansas City, MO; American Academy of Family Physicians, American Academy of Pediatrics, American Medical Society of Sports Medicine, American Orthopaedic Society of Sports Medicine, American Osteopathic Academy of Sports Medicine, 1992.
8. Magnes SA, Henderson JM, Hunter SC: What conditions limit sports participation? Phys Sportsmed 20:143–160, 1992.
9. Mitchell JH, Maron BJ, Raven PB (eds): American College of Sports Medicine and American College of Cardiology 26th Bethesda Conference: Recommendations for determining eligibility for competition in athletes with cardiovascular abnormalities. Med Sci Sports Exerc 26:S223–283, 1994.
10. Smith DM: Preparticipation physical examination. Sports Med Arthr Rev 3:84–94, 1995.
11. Tanji JL: The preparticipation exam: Special concerns for the Special Olympics. Phys Sportsmed 19:61–68, 1991.

7

Injuries and Emergencies on the Field

Brian C. Halpern, M.D., and Dennis A. Cardone, D.O.

I. Basic Principles of Emergency Treatment

In any traumatic incident, especially one that occurs on the playing field, rapid evaluation and management are imperative for a good prognosis. Often the initial evaluation and treatment determine the ultimate outcome. **Good medical care is possible in the emergency setting if trained personnel, who are familiar with athletic injuries, are on the field.**

A. **Adequate preparation**

1. A **team leader** should be designated as the person responsible for supervising on-the-field management of an injury. This position is usually filled by the team physician or trainer. He or she designates responsibilities, prearranges a network of referrals and emergency care, and directs the treatment of injury.
2. **Appropriate health care personnel** should be on or readily accessible to the field to assist the team leader. Their training and expertise should include, at least, basic cardiopulmonary resuscitation (CPR) and life support as well as how to transport an injured athlete. The medical care provider should not perform procedures or provide treatment that is beyond his or her training.
3. All necessary **emergency equipment** should be at the site of the potential injury (Table 1). It must be in good operating condition, and all personnel must be trained to use it properly in advance.
4. **Ambulance transportation** to a hospital or neurosurgical center must be immediately available for high-risk sports and "on call" for other sports.
5. **Telephone link-up** to the emergency department, ambulance, and trauma center is necessary for communication between the medical facility and the team leader. Information on the athlete's condition and the estimated time of arrival are vital so that adequate preparation can be made.
6. Various **injury scenarios** should be worked through before their actual occurrence. Once instituted, these strategies promote faster, safer, and more effective care for the injured athlete.

B. **Step-by-step assessment (ABCDE)**

1. A careful but swift initial assessment can save the patient's life and prevent further injury. Maintain close, continued observation by looking, listening, and feeling. Take all the time necessary for the evaluation and use the letters "ABCDE" as a mnemonic for a step-by-step assessment of the patient. Begin with the query "Are you okay?" Touch an arm or leg to see if the patient responds.
2. **The American Heart Association (AHA) has defined the following sequence of events to maximize the chance of survival:**
   a. Recognition of early warning signs
   b. Activation of the emergency medical system
   c. Basic CPR
   d. Defibrillation

TABLE 1. Equipment List

Mandatory for Head, Neck, and Other Neurologic and Orthopedic Trauma		
Spine board	Rescue knife/screwdriver	Sand bags
Stretcher	Rigid cervical collar	Knee immobilizer
Mandatory for Basic CPR and Advanced Cardiac Life Support (usually supplied by the ambulance)		
Oral and nasal airway	Stethoscope	Intravenous tubing
Oxygen with mask	Blood pressure cuff	Retrieval forceps (for foreign body removal)
Suction	18- and 14-gauge catheter	Automated external defibrillator (optional)
Intravenous D5W and Ringer's lactate	Crash cart with cardiac and anaphylactic medications	
Military Anti-Shock Trousers (MAST)	Endotracheal kit	
Cardiac monitor and defibrillator	Communication device (2-way radio or cellular phone)	
For General Care		
Injectable epinephrine	Penlight	Hemostats
Sharps disposal container	Blankets	Suture kit
Steri-Strips	Ace bandages	Alcohol and povidone-iodine (Betadine) swabs
Topical antibiotic	Splints	Eye kit with eye chart
Beta-agonist inhaler	Crutches	Irrigation kit
Scissors	Slings	Scalpel
Foil	Ice	Syringes and needles
Tape	Tongue depressors	Thermometer
Bandages	Gauze	Sterile gloves
Otoscope and ophthalmoscope	Band-Aids	Tampon

e. Intubation

f. Intravenous administration of medications

3. **A = Airway and cervical spine**

a. **Airway:**

i. Look and listen for spontaneous breathing. If the athlete is in the face-down position and the airway cannot be accessed, he must be brought into the face-up position by **the log roll**. The leader of the team controls the head and gives commands while three members roll (one at the shoulders, one at the hips, and one at the knees). The body must be maintained in line with the head and spine during the roll (Fig. 1).

ii. **Establish airway access.**

(a) **Remove the face mask** using sharp knife or screwdriver or snap-offs to gain airway access.

(b) **Institute head-tilt, chin-lift, or jaw-thrust maneuvers** with someone always maintaining in-line traction. The jaw-thrust technique without head tilt is the safest initial approach to opening the airway of the victim with suspected neck injury because it usually can be accomplished without extending the neck.

(c) **Clear the airway** of any material with the finger sweep or with suction. Consider that the tongue has fallen back or that there is a foreign body, such as the player's mouth piece, obstructing the airway.

(d) Insert an **oral or nasal airway** to maintain air exchange if procedures to open the airway, e.g., jaw thrust, fail to provide a clear, unobstructed airway. **Use the oral airway only in an unconscious person.** It can stimulate vomiting in the responsive patient.

(e) Use **supplemental oxygen** with or without the airway in place.

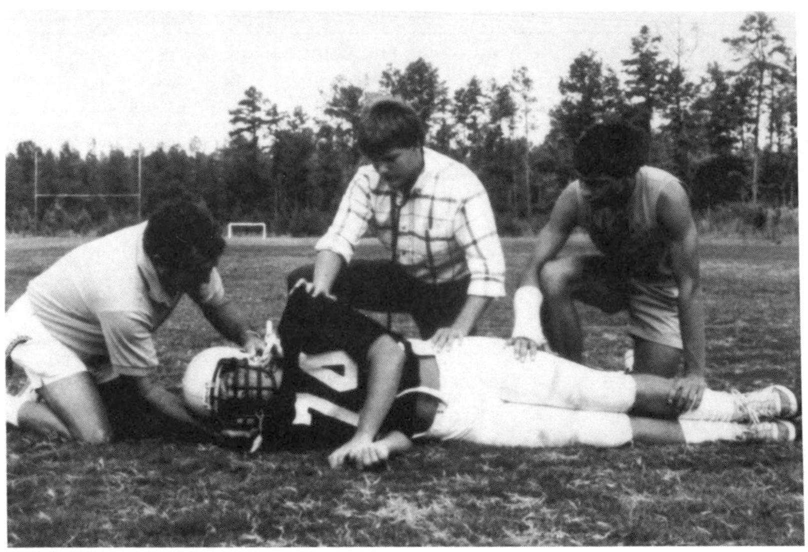

FIGURE 1. The log roll.

b. **Cervical spine:**
   i. **When a player sustains an injury above the clavicle or a head injury that results in an unconscious state, an associated cervical spine injury should be suspected**.
   ii. **The head and neck must be maintained in the neutral position with in-line traction** (Fig. 2).
   iii. **Do not remove the helmet when cervical spine injury is suspected**.
   iv. **In the unconscious athlete in whom cervical spine injury is suspected, do not use ammonia capsules**. The athlete should not be made to awaken and suddenly move.

4. **B = Breathing**
   a. If there is no respiration after the airway is established, proceed with:

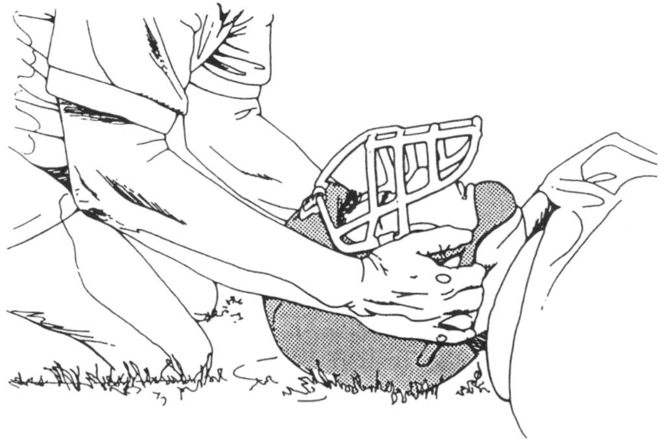

FIGURE 2. In-line traction to maintain head and neck in the neutral position.

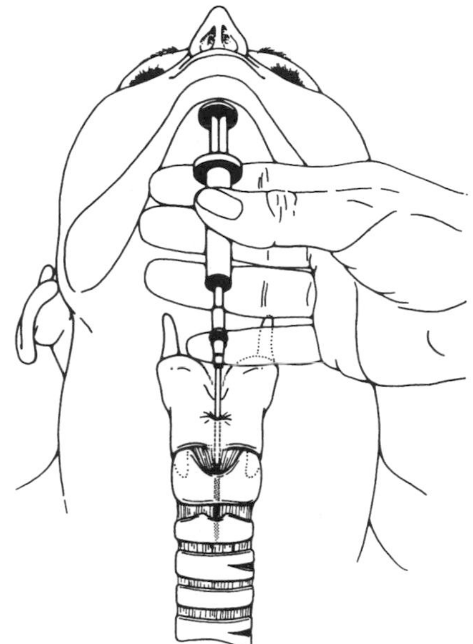

FIGURE 3. Needle cricothyroidotomy.

i. **Artificial ventilation:** During artificial ventilation, the athlete may spontaneously vomit. Suction the airway or do the finger sweep simultaneously with the log roll. Remember, do not extend the neck. Methods of artificial ventilation:
   (a) Mouth-to-mouth
   (b) Mouth-to-mask } Safer than mouth-to-mouth with regard
   (c) Bag-valve-mask } to infectious diseases

ii. **Endotracheal intubation** is another option, but is difficult to perform on the field. Nasotracheal intubation is the preferred method in patients with suspected cervical spine injuries.

b. Continue with artificial ventilation and supplemental oxygen.

c. If stridor, hoarseness, anterior neck pain, bony crepitus, or subcutaneous emphysema occurs, suspect **laryngeal fracture or marked laryngeal edema**. If there is laryngeal edema or massive facial trauma or if ventilation cannot be established with mouth-to-mouth or endotracheal tube, consider **needle cricothyroidotomy**.
   i. Palpate the cricothyroid membrane.
   ii. Puncture the skin with a 14-gauge catheter over the needle, directing it at a 45° angle caudad (Fig. 3).
   iii. Aspiration of air signifies entry into tracheal lumen.
   iv. Ventilate through the catheter.

d. Once spontaneous ventilation occurs, or once artificial ventilation has been adequately established:
   i. Look and listen for asymmetry of the chest wall during respiration (must remove the chest equipment, including jersey and pads).
   ii. **If asymmetry, tachypnea, or labored respiration occurs, consider:**
      (a) **Tension pneumothorax**
         • **Diagnosis**
         Tracheal deviation
         Hypotension
         Unilateral absence of breath sounds
         Distended neck veins
         Cyanosis

- **Treatment**
  Ventilate. Place a large-bore needle into the second intercostal space along the midclavicular line on the involved side. Ultimately a chest tube is indicated, but this is done in the hospital setting.

(b) **Open pneumothorax (sucking chest wound)**
- **Diagnosis**
  Decreased breath sounds
  Open chest wound
- **Treatment**
  Ventilate. Place a piece of foil, cloth, or other item over the wound. Secure it on three sides, leaving the fourth side open (if all sides are taped down, it can cause a tension pneumothorax). Use a chest tube.

(c) **Flail chest**
- **Diagnosis**
  Asymmetry of chest wall movement (usually secondary to multiple rib fractures)
- **Treatment**
  Ventilate. Place patient on the involved side, or place sandbags on the involved side. Intubation and a respirator can be used in a hospital setting.

(d) **Massive hemothorax**
- **Diagnosis**
  Decreased breath sounds
  Shock
  Dullness to percussion
- **Treatment**
  Ventilate
  Chest tube

(e) **Cardiac tamponade**
- **Diagnosis**
  Shock
  Distended neck veins
  Decreased heart sounds
- **Treatment**
  Ventilate
  Massive volume infusion intravenously
  Perform pericardiocentesis in hospital setting

5. **C = Circulation**
   a. Check the **carotid pulse** for quality, rate, and regularity. In the emergency setting, do not bother with the blood pressure cuff. Use the pulse as an estimate of the blood pressure.
      i. When a carotid pulse is palpable, systolic blood pressure is approximately 60 or higher.
      ii. When radial pulse is palpable, systolic blood pressure is approximately 80 or higher.
   b. If the pulse is absent, begin CPR. For adult patients (≥ 8 years old), the compression-to-ventilation ratio is 15:2. The compression rate is 80–100 per minute.
   c. **Defibrillation** has had the single greatest impact on survival statistics. More than 80% of sudden nontraumatic adult cardiac arrests are ventricular fibrillation. **Early defibrillation by nonparamedics is possible with automatic and semiautomatic external defibrillators**. Automatic external defibrillators have reduced response times and improved survival rates.

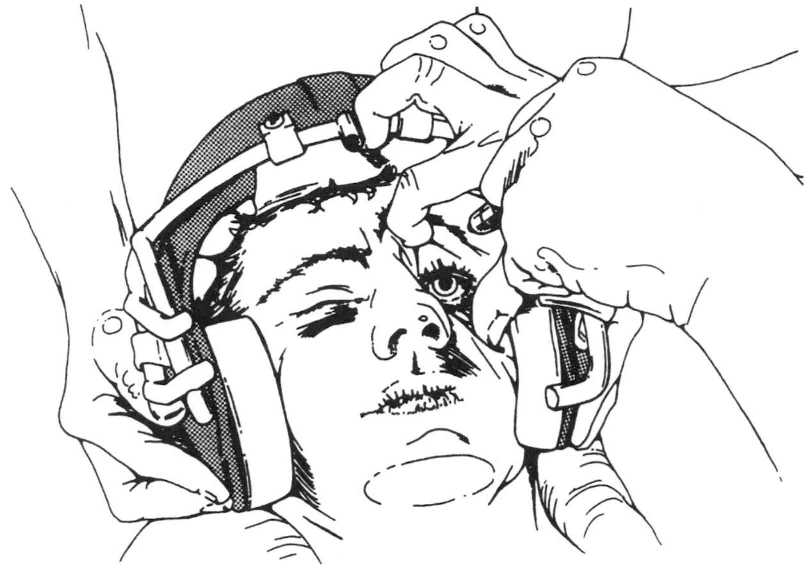

FIGURE 4. Assessing pupillary size and reaction.

   d. If the pulse is present, but weak, do **the capillary blanch test** (if the capillary bed stays white for longer than 2 seconds after release, there is some type of shock):
      i. Check for areas of hemorrhage and apply pressure with gloved hand.
      ii. Rapidly infuse Ringer's lactate.
      iii. Place electrocardiogram leads on the chest and monitor cardiac rate and rhythm.
      iv. Oxygen
      v. MAST (contraindicated in acute pulmonary edema)

6. **D = Disability.** Perform a **limited neurological exam**, assessing the level of consciousness, pupillary size and reaction, extraocular movements, and motor response (Fig. 4). You must record the initial assessment and compare it with subsequent examinations.
   a. **Minimum grading system:**
      A = Alert
      V = Vocal stimuli response
      P = Painful stimuli response
      U = Unresponsive
   b. **Moderate grading system** (Glasgow Coma Scale, Table 2). This system is based on eye opening, verbal, and motor responses. Responsiveness of the patient is expressed by summation of the figures. Lowest score is 3, highest is 15. Score of 7 or less indicates coma.
7. **E = Exposure**
   a. Inspect extremities and other body parts for **bleeding, fractures, and contusions**.
   b. Take blood pressure with blood pressure cuff.

II. Specific Life and Limb Emergencies

A. **Cardiovascular emergencies** (hypovolemia, myocardial infarction, dysrhythmias) Cardiovascular instability is commonly secondary to hypovolemia, but may also be cardiogenic in nature. The initial evaluation and treatment for cardiovascular instability should follow the same method described previously for circulation. The immediate

TABLE 2. Glasgow Coma Scale[15]

Eyes		
Open	Spontaneously	4
	To verbal command	3
	To pain	2
No response		1
Best motor response		
To verbal command	Obeys	6
To painful stimulus	Localizes pain	5
	Flexion-withdraws	4
	Flexion-abnormal (decorticate rigidity)	3
	Extension (decerebrate rigidity)	2
	No response	1
Best verbal response		
Arouse patient with painful stimulus if necessary	Oriented and converses	5
	Disoriented and converses	4
	Inappropriate words	3
	Incomprehensible sounds	2
	No response	1
Total		3–15

goals are to maintain vascular expansion, optimum cardiac filling, and adequate oxygenation. Packed red blood cells should be given early in the course of shock to provide optimum oxygen-carrying capacity. The initial hemoglobin and hematocrit may not be low with blood loss because the diminished red cell mass has not had time to equilibrate with the interstitial fluid that has moved into the vascular tree. Adequate vascular lines are the priority and, if necessary, early surgical intervention should be considered. **The cause of shock must be identified and reversed**.

1. **Hypovolemia** develops as a result of decreased intravascular volume, secondary to external or concealed blood loss. Blood loss leads to decreased preload, which causes decreased cardiac output. The body's response is vasoconstriction to maintain blood pressure. When ¼ to ⅓ of the intravascular volume is lost, the result is hypotension.
   a. **Manifestations:**
      i. Pallor
      ii. Cool extremities
      iii. Tachycardia
      iv. Hypotension
      v. Diaphoresis
      vi. Oliguria
      vii. Decreased sensorium
      viii. Decreased capillary refill
      ix. Metabolic acidosis
      x. Hyperpnea
   b. **Treatment:**
      i. Oxygen should be used at all times.
      ii. Use intravenous fluids to restore intravascular volume:
         (a) Rapidly infuse 1 or 2 L of lactated Ringer's solution or isotonic sodium chloride (0.9%) solution. In severe cases, a colloid plasma substitute should be given.
         (b) Maintain hemoglobin at 12 g/dL through blood replacement. **Estimates of localized blood loss from adult fractures:**

Humerus	**1.0–2.0 L**	**Femur**	**1.0–2.0 L**
Elbow	0.5–1.5 L	Knee	1.0–1.5 L
Forearm	0.5–1.0 L	Tibia	0.5–1.5 L
Pelvis	**1.5–4.5 L**	Ankle	0.5–1.5 L
Hip	**1.5–2.5 L**		

iii. Control external and internal hemorrhage.
iv. Monitor blood pressure, central venous pressure, urine output, electrocardiogram, hemoglobin/hematocrit, arterial blood gases, coagulation profile, and electrolytes.

2. **Cardiogenic emergencies develop as a result of myocardial infarction, dysrhythmia, tamponade, or contusion**.
   a. **Manifestations**—same as hypovolemia
   b. **Treatment:**
      i. Oxygenation
      ii. Decrease myocardial oxygen demand with a cardioselective beta-blocker.
      iii. Improve myocardial contractility with epinephrine, dopamine, or dobutamine intravenously.
      iv. Improve coronary blood flow and decrease left ventricular afterload with intravenous or sublingual nitroglycerin.
      v. Control pain with morphine sulfate 2–4 mg intravenously.
      vi. Manage life-threatening dysrhythmia appropriately:
         (a) Ventricular fibrillation and pulseless ventricular tachycardia—defibrillate/epinephrine intravenously
         (b) Ventricular tachycardia—lidocaine intravenously/cardioversion
         (c) Asystole—epinephrine and atropine intravenously
         (d) Pulseless electrical activity—epinephrine and atropine intravenously
         (e) Bradyarrhythmia with symptoms—atropine intravenously/pacemaker
      vii. Monitor blood pressure, central venous pressure, pulmonary capillary wedge pressure, vascular resistance (systemic and pulmonary), urine output, electrocardiogram, hemoglobin/hematocrit, arterial blood gases, coagulation profile, electrolytes, oxygen consumption, left ventricular stroke work index, and isoenzymes.
3. **Syncope** is a complete loss of consciousness and postural tone with prompt recovery.
   a. The most common type of syncope in athletes is **neurocardiogenic syncope**. The diagnosis is made with tilt table testing. Beta-blockers and disopyramide have proven to be effective treatments.
   b. There are many other causes of syncope in the athlete, such as:
      i. Structural heart disease
      ii. Arrhythmias

B. **Anaphylaxis** is the immediate shocklike, frequently fatal hypersensitivity reaction that occurs within minutes of administration of foreign sera or drugs. It may occur after an **insect sting**.

1. **Manifestations**
   a. Apprehension
   b. Paresthesia
   c. Generalized urticaria or edema
   d. Choking
   e. Cyanosis
   f. Wheezing
   g. Cough
   h. Incontinence
   i. Shock
   j. Fever
   k. Pupillary dilation
   l. Loss of consciousness
   m. Seizures
2. **Treatment:** Follow the algorithm in Figure 5.
3. **Prevention**
   a. Deaths from anaphylaxis can be avoided if correct treatment is provided quickly.
   b. After an episode of anaphylaxis, the cause should be identified and thereafter avoided.
   c. When the cause cannot be identified or avoided, the patient should carry some form of **medical identification tag** and be equipped with a **self-administered epinephrine device**.

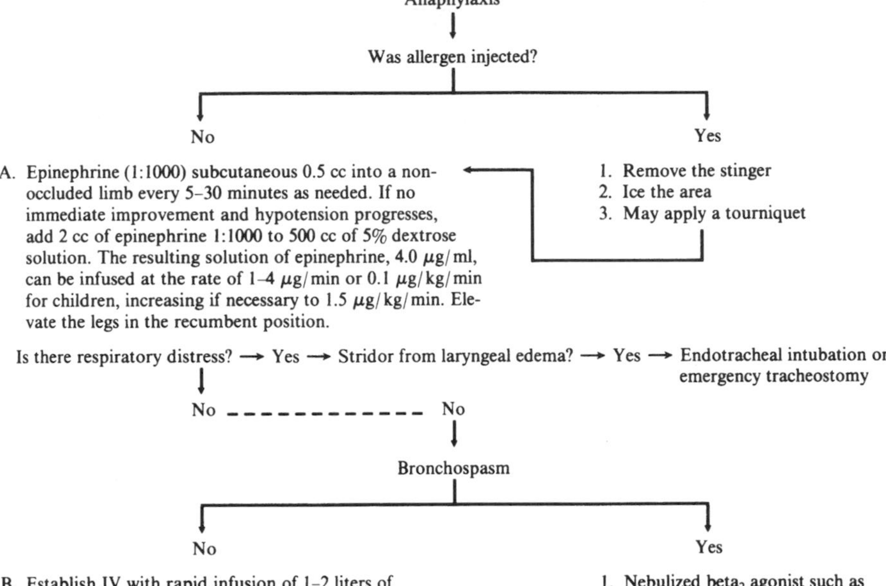

FIGURE 5. Treatment of anaphylaxis.

C. **Central nervous system injuries**
   1. **Head injury:** A major cause of death on the football field is the head injury. This injury can be characterized as either a diffuse brain injury (concussive syndrome) or more focal brain syndromes (epidural, subdural, or intracerebral hematoma). You need to be able to evaluate and treat this quickly.
      a. **Diagnosis and treatment:**
         i. The key elements to assess are loss of consciousness, an abnormal neurologic examination, and retrograde and antegrade amnesia. Memory loss is a more sensitive marker than the level of consciousness. Begin treatment with the ABCDE method that was outlined in the step-by-step assessment, and continue appropriate treatment when a specific diagnosis has been made. For easy reference, use flow diagram in Table 3.
         ii. Rapid alternating movement test
            (a) Physical marker to help delineate the degree of concussion and aid in determining return to sport after a head injury. Performed repeatedly after injury, this returns to normal as concussion signs and symptoms clear.
            (b) Patient is seated with palms of hands on lap. Patient performs as many rapid alternating movement cycles as possible in 15 seconds. One complete cycle is both hands simultaneously moving from palmar surface to dorsal surface and then back to palmer surface. Count the number of cycles that the patient is ale to perform from 5 seconds to 15 seconds (a 10-second period). The first 5 seconds are used for the learning process of performing the test. (This test should be performed at the preparticipation evaluation to set normals for the athlete.)

TABLE 3. Assessment of a Head Injury

	Grade I (mild)		Grade II (moderate)	Grade III (severe)
Diagnosis	*A*	*B*		
Loss of consciousness	–	–	< 5 min	> 5 min
Amnesia (retrograde or antegrade)	–	+	+ > 30 min	+ > 24 hr
Confusion	+	+	+	+
ABCDE	+	+	+	+
Immobilize cervical spine and transport to hospital for radiographic and further evaluation	–/+ if also have neck pain or abnormal neurologic or cervical exam		–/+	+
Observation out of hospital	+	+	+/–	–
Transportation to hospital for neurologic consultation, computed tomography scan, magnetic resonance imaging, and close observation	–	–	–/+	+
Hyperventilation to P_{CO_2} 22–23 mm Hg, Dexamethasone 1 mg/kg, and maintain serum osm to less than 320 osm/L	–	–	–	–/+ if signs of increasing cerebral edema
Return to play the same day if appropriate evaluation on sidelines is negative: no headache, irritability, inability to concentrate or obvious changes in functions (as in normal dexterity, strength, and speed), no photophobia, is first concussion	+	–	–	–

Return to Play

	1st Concussion	2nd Concussion	3rd Concussion
Grade IA	May return same day after 20 min if symptoms clear	May return 1 week after symptoms clear	Terminate season. Noncontact OK next season
Grade IB	May return within 1 week but not that day	May return 1 week after symptoms clear	Terminate season. Noncontact OK next season
Grade II	May return 1 week after symptoms clear	Terminate season	Terminate sport
Grade III	Consider return 1 month after symptoms clear	Terminate season	Terminate sport

2. **Neck injury** usually results in greater morbidity than mortality. A small fraction of sports-incurred neck injuries result in permanent neurologic injury. If handled improperly, an unstable lesion without a neurologic deficit can be converted to one with a neurologic deficit and permanent disability. For assessment, see Figure 6.
3. **Back injury:** For assessment, see Figure 7.

D. **Abdominal and pelvic (gastrointestinal and genitourinary) injuries:** With trauma to the abdomen and pelvis, anticipate possible injury to the spleen, pancreas, liver, bowel, kidney, bladder, urethra, testicles, aorta, or vena cava. The key to successful management is rapid detection of a vascular or visceral injury and control of hemorrhage and abdominal contamination.

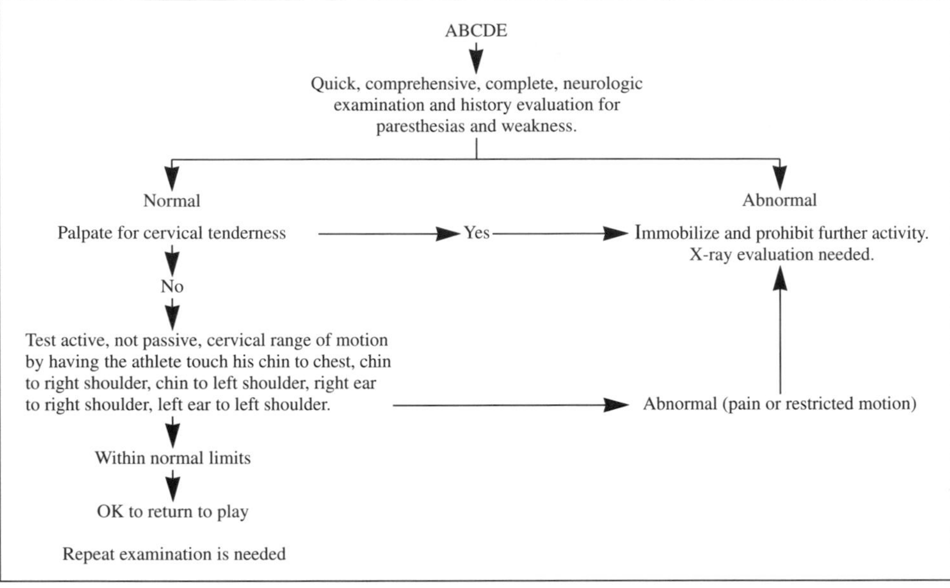

FIGURE 6. Assessment of a neck injury.

1. **Diagnosis** (signs of significant injury)
   a. Decreased bowel sounds
   b. Tender abdomen
   c. Hard or rigid abdomen
   d. Distended abdomen
   e. Flank pain or guarding
   f. Hematuria
   g. Inability to void
   h. Signs and symptoms of shock: hypotension and tachycardia
   i. Abdominal or flank ecchymosis
   j. Referred shoulder pain
2. **Evaluation and treatment**
   a. NPO (nothing by mouth)
   b. Minimal pain medication
   c. Serial hematocrit and white blood cell count determinations
   d. Urinary catheterization
   e. Serial amylase and hematocrit measurements
   f. Serial physical examinations
   g. Plain radiography including upright view
   h. Computed tomography (CT) with contrast
   i. Diagnostic peritoneal lavage
   j. Surgical consultation
3. **Specific examples**
   a. **Spleen**
      i. **Signs and symptoms:**
         (a) Abdominal pain in left upper quadrant
         (b) Left shoulder or neck pain
         (c) Frequently associated with left lower rib fractures
      ii. **Diagnostic workup:**
         (a) Ultrasound
         (b) Spleen scan to detect hemorrhage or intrasplenic hematoma
         (c) CT or arteriography to detect occult hemorrhage or intrasplenic hematoma
   b. **Liver**
      i. **Signs and symptoms:**
         (a) Abdominal pain in right upper quadrant

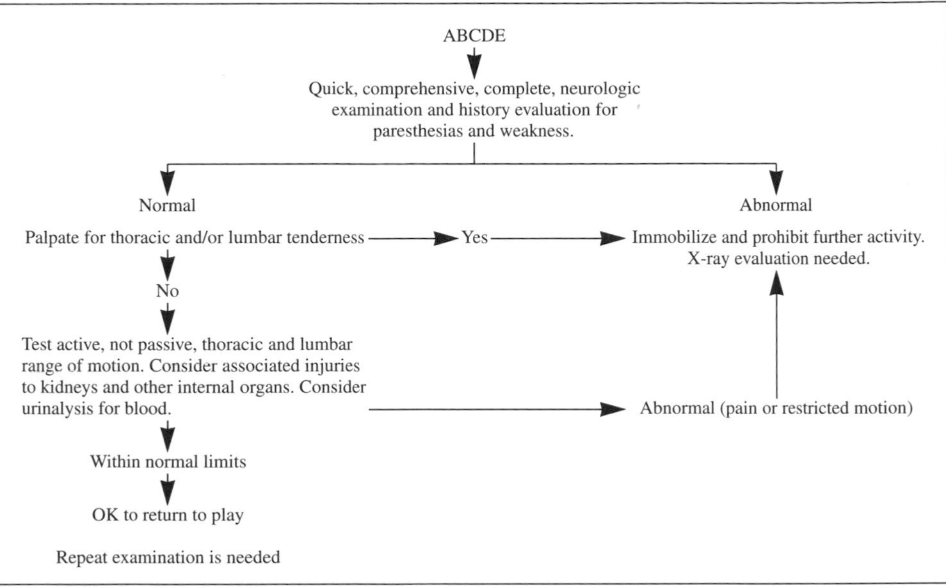

FIGURE 7. Assessment of a back injury.

(b) Right shoulder or neck pain
(c) Possible right lower rib fractures

ii. **Diagnostic workup:**
(a) Ultrasound
(b) Liver scan
(c) CT or arteriography to detect occult hemorrhage or intrahepatic hematoma

c. **Kidney, bladder, urethra**

i. **Signs and symptoms:**
(a) Hematuria
(b) Bloody meatal discharge or inability to void
(c) Flank pain
(d) Associated pelvic fracture

ii. **Diagnostic workup:**
(a) CT with contrast
(b) Intravenous pyelogram—should be done before cystogram because extravasation from cystogram may obscure a lower urethral injury
(c) Urethrogram or cystogram

d. **Testicles** (Fig. 8)

i. **Signs and symptoms:**
(a) Inability to void
(b) Swelling so excessive that the epididymis is indistinguishable from the testes.
(c) If the testicle cannot be transilluminated, there may be a testicular rupture.

ii. **Diagnostic workup:**
(a) Ultrasound of scrotum
(b) Doppler study of testicles
(c) Testicular scan

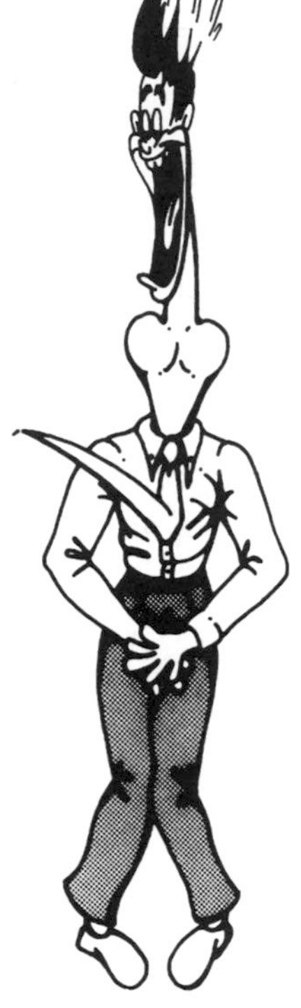

FIGURE 8. Testicular trauma.

iii. **Treatment:**
 (a) For a simple contusion, use ice, scrotal support, analgesics.
 (b) Ambulate when pain and swelling stabilize.

e. **Rectus abdominis muscle contusion or strain**
 i. **Signs and symptoms:**
 (a) Positive bowel sounds
 (b) Differentiate between abdominal wall contusion and visceral injury. Palpate abdomen while the patient tenses rectus muscles by lifting legs and/or head off exam table:
 - Increased pain with superficial palpation is more indicative of an abdominal wall injury.
 - Decreased pain with superficial palpation may be a sign of a visceral injury (the rectus muscles guard the viscus).
 (c) No distention
 (d) No rigidity
 (e) No signs or symptoms of shock
 ii. **Treatment:**
 (a) Ice
 (b) Rest
 (c) Abdominal support

f. **Rectus abdominis muscle hematoma**
 i. **Signs and symptoms:**
 (a) Muscle guarding and tenderness
 (b) Increased abdominal pain with straight leg raising and hyperextension of the back

(c) Nausea and vomiting
(d) Palpable mass in the abdominal wall

ii. **Diagnostic workup** is a CT scan.

iii. **Treatment:**

(a) Ice
(b) Rest
(c) Abdominal support
(d) Surgery only if bleeding continues into the muscle and the hematoma expands

E. **Eye, ear, nose, or throat injuries**

1. **Eye:** Care for ocular trauma or sudden loss of vision begins with a differentiation between potentially blinding problems and a less serious situation.
   a. **Signs and symptoms of serious injury:**
      i. Blurred vision or abnormal visual acuity that does not clear with blinking
      ii. Loss of all or part of the visual field of the eye
      iii. Sharp stabbing or deep throbbing pain
      iv. Double vision after injury
      v. Black or red eye
      vi. Object in the cornea
      vii. An eye that does not move as completely as the opposite eye
      viii. One eye protruding when compared with the opposite eye
      ix. Abnormal pupil size or shape compared with the opposite eye
      x. Layer of blood between the cornea and iris
      xi. Laceration or penetration of eyelid or eyeball
      xii. A dark subconjunctival mass that may indicate scleral rupture
   b. **Treatment for abnormal eye exam:**
      i. Ask patient to shut eye lightly as if sleeping, tape a sterile eye pad in place, and tape a hard shield over the eye pad.
      ii. Transport to eye facility and make sure that the patient does not squeeze eye tightly shut.
2. **Ear**
   a. Signs and symptoms of **cauliflower ear**:
      i. Throbbing, painful, swollen ear
      ii. Organized hematoma
   b. Treatment:
      i. Aspirate the hematoma under sterile technique.
      ii. Compress to area of the hematoma using a collodion pack, plaster of Paris cast, or a silicone mold.
3. **Nose**
   a. Sign and symptom of epistaxis—bleeding from the nose
   b. Treatment:
      i. Nasal area should be covered with cold cloths or ice and compression.
      ii. If bleeding is profuse and not easily stopped, careful packing of the anterior nares may reach the area of bleeding and control it. A regular-size tampon works well for this purpose.
4. **Throat or mouth (tooth avulsion)**
   a. Rinse tooth in milk or saline and replace it intraorally within 30 minutes.
   b. If tooth cannot be replanted, place it in either milk, saline, or saliva.
   c. Patient should be sent immediately to a dentist for further evaluation and treatment.

F. **Extremity injuries**

1. **The following systems must be evaluated in the affected extremity:**
   a. Vascular
   b. Neural
   c. Osseous
   d. Ligamentous
   e. Muscular
   f. Tendinous
   g. Skin and subcutaneous tissue
2. **Management**
   a. **Initial evaluation to detect the following:**
      i. Absent or decreased pulse
      ii. Pallor
      iii. Generalized extremity edema
      iv. Deformity
      v. Local swelling
      vi. Ecchymosis
      vii. Joint laxity
      viii. Obvious soft tissue lacerations or defects
      ix. Decreased motion to command or to painful stimulation
      x. Hypesthesia or anesthesia
   b. **Initial treatment:**
      i. Splint
      ii. Cover wound with moist dressing
      iii. Early reduction of dislocation after neurovascular check
      iv. Early transport, especially after neurovascular injury
      v. Rest, ice, compression, elevation
   c. **Specific injuries**
      i. **Open fractures:**
         (a) Wounds should be covered with sterile dressing that has been soaked in saline or Betadine.
         (b) **The fracture should be splinted without pulling the exposed bone back into the soft tissue. Do not probe the wound. Do not push extruded soft tissue or bone back into the wound**.
         (c) Transport the patient to the hospital to begin antibiotics, tetanus, and repair.
      ii. **Traumatic amputation:**
         (a) **The proximal stump should first be irrigated with lactated Ringer's injection and a pressure dressing applied with sterile gauze.**
         (b) **The amputated part should be irrigated in lactated Ringer's injection, wrapped in sterile gauze, and then placed in a plastic bag or aluminum foil. It should then be cooled, not frozen, by placing it into a container of ice**.
      iii. **Dislocations:**
         (a) **Neurovascular assessment**
         (b) Reduction on the field before marked muscle spasm occurs
         (c) Splint and neurovascular recheck
      iv. **Vascular injury:**
         (a) **Peripheral arterial injury should be suspected in any patient sustaining knee or elbow dislocation, any long-bone fracture (particularly if there is a supracondylar humeral or femoral fracture), or crush injury**.
         (b) Check for external hemorrhage; pulse deficit; ischemic changes, including pallor or cyanosis, coolness, hypesthesia, and partial or complete paralysis; bruit or thrill; and hematoma:
            - Control bleeding by applying direct pressure.
            - Immediate revascularization of ischemic extremity.

v. **Peripheral nerve injury:**
   (a) Primary nerve repair is performed only if the laceration is clean, especially with digital nerves of the hand.
   (b) Traction nerve injury usually has continuity of the nerve, and function gradually returns.

Recommended Reading

1. Araujo D, Rubin A: Instituting the updated CPR protocol. Phys Sportsmed 22(7):51–56, 1994.
2. Bruno LA, Gennarelli TA, Torg JS: Head and neck injuries. Clin Sports Med 6:17–29, 1987.
3. Cantu RC: Guidelines for return to contact sports after a cerebral concussion. Phys Sportsmed 14(10):75–83, 1986.
4. Cloward RB: Acute cervical spine injuries. CIBA Clin Symp 32:1–32, 1980.
5. Colucciello S, Plotka M: Abdominal trauma. Phys Sportsmed 21(6):33–43, 1993.
6. Cowley RA, Dunham CM: Shock Trauma/Critical Care Manual: Initial Assessment and Management. Baltimore, University Park Press, 1982.
7. Deshazo WF: Hematoma of the rectus abdominis in football. Phys Sportsmed 12(9):73–75, 1984.
8. Emergency Cardiac Care Committee and Subcommittees, American Heart Association: Guidelines for cardiopulmonary resuscitation and emergency cardiac care. JAMA 268:2171–2302, 1992.
9. Friedman WA: Head injuries. CIBA Clin Symp 35:1–32, 1983.
10. Graver K: A review of the new guidelines for advanced cardiac life support. Fam Pract Recert 10:55–68, 1988.
11. Haycock CE: How I manage abdominal injuries. Phys Sportsmed 14(6):86–99, 1986.
12. Hoover DL: How I manage testicular injury. Phys Sportsmed 14(4):127–129, 1986.
13. Hugenholtz H, Richard MT: The on-site management of athletes with head injuries. Phys Sportsmed 11(6): 71–80, 1983.
14. Iverson LD, Clawson DK: Manual of Acute Orthopaedic Therapeutics, 2nd ed. Boston, Little, Brown, 1982.
15. Jennett B, Teasdale G: Predicting outcome in individuals after severe head injury. Lancet 1:1031–1034, 1976.
16. Kumamoto DP, Jacob M, Nickelsen D: Oral trauma. Phys Sportsmed 23(5):53–62, 1995.
17. Lehman LB: Nervous system sports-related injuries. Am J Sports Med 15:494–499, 1987.
18. McIntyre KM, Lewis AJ: Textbook of Advanced Cardiac Life Support. Dallas, American Heart Association, 1981.
19. Nelson WE, Gieck JH, Jane JA, Hawthorne P: Athletic head injuries. Athletic Training 19:95–100, 1984.
20. Ormerod AD: Emergency management of anaphylaxis: Treatment and clues to diagnosis. Emergency Decisions March:31–40, 1988.
21. Simons SM: Preventing sudden death. Phys Sportsmed 21(10):53–59, 1993.
22. Swenson TM, Lauerman WC, Donaldson III WF, et al: Cervical spine alignment in the immobilized football player—radiographic analysis before and after helmet removal. Am Orthop Soc Sports Med July 1995.
23. Rubin A: Emergency equipment. Phys Sportsmed 21(9):47–54, 1993.
24. Wagshal A, Huang SS: Syncope in athletes: Sorting through the many causes. J Musculoskel Med 10(4): 21–34, 1993.

8

Sports Nutrition

Ann C. Grandjean, Ed.D., and Kristin J. Reimers, M.S., RD

The dietary objectives for athletes are straightforward: meeting caloric and nutrient needs and maintaining fluid balance. However, situations and conditions specific to sport and sport participation—making weight, travel, long and intensive workouts, demanding schedules—often make meeting these objectives difficult.

To provide sound nutritional information to athletes in the context of pragmatic recommendations, physicians have to consider not only the science behind the nutritional requirements, but also the athlete's lifestyle, training program, preferences, and factors specific to the sport.

Most of the research that serves as the basis of sports nutrition has been conducted on subjects participating in aerobic activity of long duration (endurance). Paradoxically, athletic events requiring sudden bursts of effort separated by periods of relative rest constitute the majority of sports. Thus, the widely published and often repeated guidelines may not be the best recommendation you can offer your athletic patient.

I. Energy Requirements

A. **Ranges**

1. **Energy requirements depend on body size, demands of the sport and period of training, training conditions, age, and nontraining activity level, with body size being the primary determinant.**
2. Whether comparing athletes participating in the same sport or comparing athletes among different sport groups, a wide range of energy intakes is observed. Among the highest energy intake groups are male swimmers, cyclists, triathletes, and basketball players, with intakes as high as 6000 kcal/day reported. Lower energy intake groups include female figure skaters, gymnasts, and dancers, who may consume as few as 1200 kcal/day. Reported on a per kilogram of body weight basis, adolescent swimmers report the highest intakes (65 kcal/kg body weight) and wrestlers during competitive season report the lowest (28 kcal/kg body weight).

B. **Estimating calorie needs:** Without a metabolic chamber, it is difficult if not impossible to determine calorie requirements of an individual accurately due to significant day-to-day, season-to-season, and athlete-to-athlete variation. However, estimates of calorie requirements can be derived using actual calorie intake as the guide, or by using equations.

1. **Energy balance techniques**
   a. Verify energy balance by monitoring body weight. If body weight is stable, the athlete's energy intake = energy output.
   b. Ask the athlete to record accurately (by measuring with household utensils) everything consumed for 3 consecutive days. Results of this recording should estimate energy requirement in the presence of stable body weight.
2. **Factors for estimating daily energy needs:** A simple rule of thumb to estimate energy needs is to multiply the athlete's weight (lb) by one of the following numbers:

Activity level	*Male*	*Female*
Light	17	16
Moderate	19	17
Heavy	23	20

II. Nutrient Requirements

A. Carbohydrate (CHO)

1. **Basis for current recommendations**
   a. It is erroneous to suggest that exact CHO requirements for all situations are known because of wide interindividual and intersport variation.
   b. Most research conducted on CHO requirements has examined runners and cyclists in laboratory settings. Data from these studies have been extrapolated to athletes in other sports because no better data currently exist. As more applicable data become available, current recommendations may change.
2. **Range of requirements**
   a. Research indicates athletes training or competing at high intensities (> 70% $\dot{V}O_2$ max) for prolonged periods of time have a high CHO requirement. Examples include distance runners and triathletes.
   b. Athletes whose training and competitions consist of brief periods of high-energy output, alternated with short periods of rest, such as sprinters, weightlifters, and football players, have lower CHO requirements.
   c. Along this continuum of CHO requirements, actual intakes vary significantly. It is not uncommon to observe a sprinter consuming twice as much CHO as a distance runner. Unless a problem with performance is observed, a drastic change in CHO intake is not indicated.
3. **Meeting CHO needs for various situations**
   a. 200 g/day replaces liver glycogen.
   b. 8–10 g CHO/kg body weight per day maintains muscle glycogen levels in the endurance athlete training aerobically > 90 minutes on most days.
   c. 5 g CHO/kg body weight per day is adequate to support training of athletes involved in intermittent, power, or sprint activities.

B. Protein

1. **Increased requirements:** Although CHO is emphasized and protein deemphasized in the popular press, adequate protein intake is not to be assumed in all athletes. **Research shows that athletes have increased protein requirements compared to their sedentary counterparts.**
2. **Factors that increase an athlete's protein requirements**
   a. **Low-calorie diet:** An important factor affecting protein requirements is the interrelationship of protein and energy (calories). Increasing energy intake improves nitrogen balance. Thus, protein requirements increase as energy intake decreases.
   b. **Vegetarianism:**
      i. Digestibility and amino acid composition of vegetable protein are not equal to animal protein, leading to increased requirements.
      ii. Recommended protein intakes assume a mixed diet containing 65–69% of the protein from meat, poultry, fish, milk, milk products, or eggs.
      iii. As the percentage of protein derived from plant protein increases above 35% of total protein intake, the amount of total protein needed as g/kg body weight also increases.
   c. **Endurance training:**
      i. Utilization of protein as an energy substrate increases during endurance events.
      ii. The amount used is variable based on glycogen stores or CHO consumption.

d. **Resistance training:**
   i. Resistance training and the resulting muscular hypertrophy increase protein requirements.
   ii. The increased need appears to vary with degree of effort and phase of training.
e. **High muscle-to-fat ratio**
f. **Growth**

3. **Estimated protein requirements** (assuming adequate calorie intake and a representative American diet containing both animal and plant proteins):
   a. **Endurance athletes** 0.9–1.4 g/kg body weight per day
   b. **Strength athletes** up to 1.8 g/kg body weight per day
   c. **In general, most athletes meet protein requirements by consuming 1.5– 2.0 g/kg body weight per day.**

C. **Fat** is a concentrated source of energy. It functions as a carrier of fat-soluble vitamins, adds palatability to the diet, and has a protein-sparing effect.
   1. **Fat is a major source of energy during exercise.** A **chief advantage** is the role of fatty acid oxidation in sparing glycogen stores.
   2. Trained subjects oxidize more fat and less CHO than untrained subjects.
   3. Exercise performed under aerobic conditions promotes fat oxidation.

D. **Vitamins**
   1. **Intakes above requirements have not been shown to improve performance in the absence of deficiency.**
   2. **Athletes' requirements are met by the Recommended Dietary Allowance (RDA) except for B vitamins.**
   3. Because of the role of B vitamins in energy-producing metabolic processes, **athletes with high energy expenditure may have increased requirements for B vitamins.**
   4. A reasonable guideline for B vitamin requirements is provided by the Military Recommended Dietary Allowance (MRDA). See Table 1.

E. **Minerals:** A comprehensive review of minerals is not warranted. Iron and calcium, however, are frequently consumed in amounts less than required and therefore deserve further discussion.

F. **Iron**
   1. **Functions:** As a component of hemoglobin, myoglobin, and cytochromes, iron impacts oxygen transport and energy metabolism.
   2. **Incidence of deficiency:** Although frank anemia appears to be no more common in athletes than in nonathletic counterparts, low iron stores are a frequent finding among elite endurance athletes.
   3. **Effects of iron on performance**
      a. **Iron deficiency anemia affects performance** by decreasing the capacity of skeletal muscle to consume oxygen and produce ATP.

TABLE 1. Military Recommended Dietary Allowances for B Vitamins

		MRDAs		RDAs			
Nutrient	Unit	*Men (17–50 yr)*	*Women (17–50 yr)*	*Men (19–24 yr)*	*Men (25–50 yr)*	*Women (19–24 yr)*	Women (25–50 yr)
Thiamin (B_1)	mg	1.6	1.2	1.5	1.5	1.1	1.1
Riboflavin (B_2)	mg	1.9	1.4	1.7	1.7	1.3	1.3
Niacin	mg NE	21.0	16.0	19.0	19.0	15.0	15.0
Vitamin B_6	mg	2.2	2.0	2.0	2.0	1.6	1.6

NE = niacin equivalent.
Adapted from Table 2-1, MRDA for selected nutrients, AR 25–40, 1985, p 2-4, and National Research Council Recommended Dietary Allowances, 1989b, p 284 and Tables 3–4, 3–5, 11–1, pp 29, 33, 253.

b. **Although controversy exists, the majority of data suggest that iron depletion without anemia does not diminish performance.**

4. **Factors contributing to negative iron status**
   a. **Inadequate absorption:**
      i. Iron deficient diet
      ii. Diet high in cereal content and low in animal protein
      iii. Pica or geography
   b. **Blood loss:**
      i. Menstruation
      ii. Pregnancy
      iii. Hemorrhage—wounds, nose, hemorrhoids, gastrointestinal tract
   c. **Rapid growth:**
      i. Childhood
      ii. Adolescence
      iii. Pregnancy
   d. *Note:* With aerobic training, there is an increase in plasma volume that dilutes the red blood cells and lowers hemoglobin levels. This phenomenon is called **dilutional pseudoanemia**:
      i. A beneficial, adaptive change
      ii. Does not require medical supervision
5. **Measuring iron status**
   a. Several blood parameters have been used to measure iron status, including serum ferritin, transferrin saturation, free erythrocyte protoporphyrin, hemoglobin, hematocrit, total iron-binding capacity, and serum iron.
   b. Iron deficiency develops gradually, progressing through several stages before anemia is evident (Fig. 1).
6. **Recommendations for screening**
   a. Draw hemoglobin and hematocrit levels one or two times per year. *Note:* Hemoglobin concentration varies greatly in normal subjects, and lesser degrees of iron store depletion can go undetected if hemoglobin is the only test used.
   b. Combining hemoglobin, hematocrit, and ferritin provides a more sensitive measure of status.
   c. For a complete assessment of iron status, a battery of tests is indicated, including serum ferritin, transferrin saturation, hemoglobin, hematocrit, total iron-binding capacity, and serum iron.

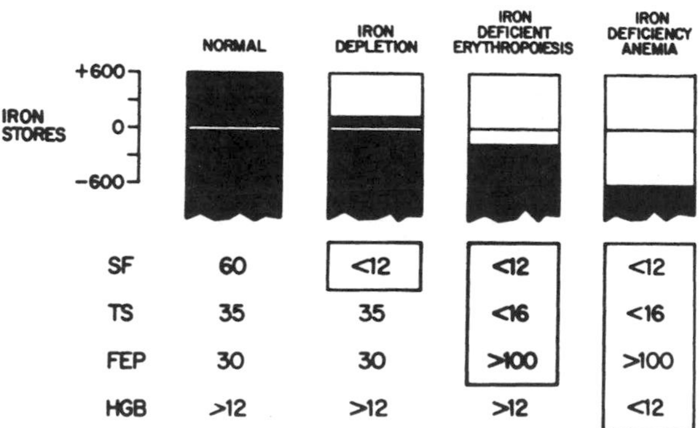

FIGURE 1. Parameters of iron status in relationship to body iron stores (mg). Negative iron stores indicate the amount of iron that must be replaced in circulating red cells before iron reserves can reaccumulate. (From Cook JD, Finch CA: Assessing iron status of a population. Am J Clin Nutr 32:2115–2119, 1979, with permission.)

7. **Dietary treatment:** The athlete should be informed about the types and sources of dietary iron to prevent or augment treatment of iron depletion or deficiency.
   a. Iron is absorbed in two forms by the body—heme and nonheme.
   b. **Heme iron:**
      i. **Absorbed at a higher rate than nonheme:** In an iron-replete individual, approximately 23% of ingested heme iron is absorbed; more if the individual has low iron stores. Dietary factors do not influence heme iron absorption.
      ii. **Sources:** Heme iron is found exclusively in animal tissues, especially organ tissue and red meat (Table 2).
   c. **Nonheme iron**
      i. **Absorbed poorly compared to heme;** approximately 3–8% is absorbed depending on dietary inhibitors, enhancers, and the individual's iron status.
      ii. **Dietary factors that increase absorption:**
         (a) **Animal tissue** (e.g., beef, poultry or fish)
         (b) **Ascorbic acid**
      iii. **Dietary factors that decrease absorption:**
         (a) Polyphenols in tea
         (b) Calcium phosphate
         (c) Phytates
         (d) Bran
         (e) Antacids
      iv. **Sources** (Table 2):
         (a) Cereals
         (b) Bread
         (c) Grains
         (d) Fruit
         (e) Vegetables
8. **Supplementation**
   a. **Treatment of confirmed iron deficiency:**
      i. 300 mg of ferrous sulfate, 1 time/day, gradually increasing to 3 times/day
      ii. If ferrous sulfate is not well tolerated, ferrous fumarate or ferrous gluconate should be prescribed.
      iii. Treatment may also include 250 mg of ascorbic acid 3 times/day.
   b. **Caution:** Overuse and abuse of dietary supplements is not uncommon among athletes. Self-treatment should be discouraged.
   c. If the athlete does not respond to therapy after 3–6 months, further workup is recommended.
9. **Iron overload**
   a. Hereditary hemochromatosis is one of the most common autosomal recessive diseases in populations of Northern European descent.
      i. Definitive diagnosis—liver biopsy
      ii. Indicative—increased serum iron and transferrin saturation; total iron-binding capacity may be depressed
   b. Factors that can increase risk or exacerbate the condition in genetically prone athletes:
      i. Iron-rich diet
      ii. Iron supplement use
      iii. High altitude
      iv. Erythropoietin

G. **Calcium** deserves mention because of the incidence of amenorrhea in female athletes, the role of calcium in bone density, and inadequate consumption by many athletes.
   1. **Role in bone health:** Calcium is important to bone health, in combination with gonadal hormones and physical activity, but does not compensate for either. For example, in amenorrheic women with decreased estrogen levels, who are not on hormone replacement therapy, calcium supplementation does *not* prevent bone loss.

TABLE 2. Dietary Sources of Iron

Heme Sources of Iron

Food (3 oz, cooked, lean only)	*Total Iron (mg)*	*Available Iron (mg)*
Beef		
Liver, pan fried	5.34	0.60
Chuck, arm pot roast, braised	3.22	0.48
Tenderloin, roasted	3.05	0.46
Sirloin, broiled	2.85	0.42
Roundtip, roasted	2.50	0.38
Top round, broiled	2.45	0.37
Top loin, broiled	2.10	0.31
Ground, lean, broiled	1.79	0.27
Eye round, roasted	1.65	0.25
Pork		
Shoulder, blade, Boston, roasted	1.36	0.15
Tenderloin, roasted	1.31	0.15
Ham, boneless, 5–11% fat	1.19	0.14
Loin chop broiled	0.78	0.09
Lamb		
Loin, roasted	2.07	0.31
Leg, shank half, roasted	1.75	0.26
Veal		
Loin, roasted	0.93	0.14
Cutlet, pan fried	0.74	0.11
Chicken		
Liver, simmered	7.20	0.81
Leg, roasted	1.11	0.17
Breast, roasted	0.88	0.13
Turkey		
Leg, roasted	2.26	0.34
Breast, roasted	0.99	0.14
Fish		
Tuna, light meat, canned	2.72	0.31
white meat, canned	0.51	0.06
Halibut, dry heat	0.91	0.10
Salmon, sockeye, dry heat	0.47	0.06
Flounder/sole, dry heat	0.23	0.03
Shellfish		
Oysters, 6 medium, raw	5.63	0.63
Shrimp, moist heat	2.63	0.30
Crab, Alaskan king, moist heat	0.65	0.07

Nonheme Sources of Iron

Food	*Total Iron (mg)*	*Available Iron (mg)*
Cereals		
Raisin bran (enrich), dry, ½ cup	4.50	0.23
Corn flakes (enrich), dry, 1 oz.	1.80	0.09
Shredded wheat, dry, 1 oz.	1.20	0.06
Oatmeal, cooked, ½ cup	0.80	0.04
Whole wheat hot cereal, ½ cup	0.75	0.04
Grains		
Bagel, 1	1.80	0.09
Bran muffin, home recipe, 1	1.40	0.07
Whole wheat bread, 1 slice	1.00	0.05
White rice (enrich), cooked, ½ cup	0.90	0.05
White bread (enrich), 1 slice	0.70	0.04
Brown rice, cooked, ½ cup	0.50	0.03
Fruits		
Apricots, dried, 7 halves	1.16	0.06
Prunes, dried, 3 medium	0.84	0.04
Raisins, 2 Tbsp.	0.38	0.02
Banana, 1 medium	0.35	0.02
Apple, 1 medium	0.25	0.01
Orange, 1 medium	0.13	0.01
Vegetables		
Potato, baked w/skin, 1 medium	2.75	0.14
Peas, cooked, ½ cup	1.26	0.06
Spinach, raw, ½ cup	0.76	0.04
Broccoli, raw, ½ cup	0.39	0.02
Carrots, 1 medium	0.36	0.02
Lettuce, iceberg, ⅛ head	0.34	0.02
Corn, cooked, ½ cup	0.25	0.01
Beans/legumes		
Kidney beans, boiled, ½ cup	2.58	0.13
canned, ½ cup	1.57	0.08
Chickpeas, boiled, 1/2 cup	2.37	0.12
canned, ½ cup	1.62	0.08
Baked beans, canned, plain, ½ cup	0.37	0.02
Meat substitutes		
Tofu, 2½ × 2¾ × 1 in.	2.30	0.12
Egg, whole	1.00	0.05
yolk	0.95	0.05
white	tr	—
Peanut butter, 2 Tbsp.	0.60	0.03
Dairy		
Milk, low fat, 1 cup	0.12	0.01
Yogurt, plain low fat, 1 cup	0.18	0.01
Cheese, cheddar, 1 oz.	0.19	0.01
Molasses		
Cane, blackstrap, 1 Tbsp.	5.05	0.25

From Iron in Human Nutrition. Chicago, National Livestock and Meat Board, 1990, with permission.

TABLE 3. Food Sources of Calcium

Foods*	Serving Size (g)	Calcium Content (mg)	Estimated Absorbable Ca/Serving (mg)
Milk	240	300	96.3
Almonds, dry roasted	28	80	17.0
Beans, pinto	86	44.7	7.6
Beans, red	172	40.5	6.9
Beans, white	110	113	19.2
Broccoli	71	35	18.4
Brussel sprouts	78	19	12.1
Cabbage, Chinese	85	79	42.5
Cabbage, green	75	25	16.2
Cauliflower	62	17	11.7
Citrus punch with CCM	240	300	150
Fruit punch with CCM	240	300	156
Kale	65	47	27.6
Kohlrabi	82	20	13.4
Mustard greens	72	64	37.0
Radish	50	14	10.4
Rutabaga	85	36	22.1
Sesame seeds, no hulls	28	37	7.7
Soy milk	120	5	1.6
Spinach	90	122	6.2
Tofu, calcium set	126	258	80.0
Turnip greens	72	99	51.1
Watercress	17	20	13.4

* Based on ½-cup serving size except for milk, citrus punch, and fruit punch (1 cup) and almonds and sesame seeds (1 oz).
CCM = calcium citrate malate
Adapted from Weaver CM, Plawecki KL: Dietary calcium: Adequacy of a vegetarian diet. Am J Clin. Nutr 59(suppl.):1238S, 1994, with permission.

2. **Intake**
   a. Calcium intake is lower than optimal in many female athletes who restrict calories, strive for low fat intake, or avoid milk and milk products.
   b. **Several factors decrease the bioavailability of calcium**, including fiber, phytates, and oxalates. Table 3 lists total calcium content of foods and the estimated amount of absorbable calcium.
   c. **Current recommendations** developed by a National Institutes of Health (NIH) expert panel for calcium intake to maximize bone mineral density and inhibit bone loss are higher than the RDA, as depicted in Table 4.
3. **Calcium supplementation**
   a. **Indications:**
      i. Athletes unwilling or unable to meet dietary calcium requirements
      ii. Athlete who does not consume milk or milk products probably ingests only about 300 mg calcium/day.
      iii. Supplementation should provide the difference between intake and requirement.
      iv. Most efficient when taken in doses ≤ 500 mg between meals
   b. **Types:**
      i. Calcium carbonate most widely used
      ii. Avoid calcium from fossilized oyster shells or bone meal because of the potential for heavy metal contamination.

TABLE 4. Comparison of NIH Expert Panel Recommendation to the Recommended Dietary Allowance of Calcium

Ages	NIH Expert Panel (mg)	RDA (1989) (mg)
11–24 yr	1200–1500	1200
Women:		
25–49 yr	1000	800
50–65 yr		
Taking estrogen	1000	800
Not taking estrogen	1500	800
65+ yr	1500	800
Men:		
25–64 yr	1000	800
65+ yr	1500	800

c. **Inhibits iron absorption:**
   i. Calcium supplements with meals or with iron supplements decrease iron absorption significantly.
   ii. If iron supplements are also used, calcium supplements should be taken apart from iron.

III. Fluid Balance

A. **Dehydration and thermoregulation**

1. **A lowered blood volume in the dehydrated state results in decreased blood flow to the skin and hinders heat loss.** A fluid loss as little as 1% of total body weight can be associated with an elevation in core temperature during exercise. When dehydration becomes extreme, the body stops sweating in an attempt to conserve remaining blood volume. In this state, core temperatures can rise to lethal levels (Table 5).
2. During intense, prolonged exercise, some athletes can lose up to 6–8 lb (2.7–3.6 kg) of sweat per hour.

B. **Involuntary dehydration**

1. Humans do not maintain fluid balance during periods of physiologic or thermal stress when fluid is consumed as desired. **Thirst is *not* an adequate indicator of water needs during exercise** because an individual is already 1% dehydrated when thirst is sensed.

TABLE 5. Adverse Effects of Dehydration

Percent of Body Weight Loss	
0	
1	Thirst threshold and threshold for impaired exercise thermoregulation leading to decrement in physical work capacity
2	Stronger thirst, vague discomfort and sense of oppression, loss of appetite
3	Dry mouth, increasing hemoconcentration, reduction in urinary output
4	Decrement of 20–30% in physical work capacity
5	Difficulty in concentrating, headache, impatience, sleeplessness
6	Severe impairment in exercise temperature regulation, increased respiratory rate leading to tingling and numbness of extremities
7	Likely collapse if combined with heat and exercise

Adapted from Greenleaf JE, Harrison MH: Water and electrolytes. In Layman DK (ed): Nutrition and Aerobic Exercise. Washington, DC, American Chemical Society, 1986, pp 107–124.

2. Dehydration can be acute or chronic in nature.
   a. **Chronic dehydration** is less visible and potentially more dangerous than acute dehydration. It usually results from several days of cumulative dehydration and commonly occurs during early fall football or soccer practice. Recording athletes' weights on charts before and after training for sports such as basketball, soccer, distance running, or football to monitor hydration is desirable.
   b. **Acute dehydration** can occur in a matter of 2–3 hours. Most commonly, it is seen in endurance athletes such as marathon runners and triathletes.

C. **Deliberate dehydration**
   1. Primarily used by athletes to reduce weight rapidly to reach a desired weight class
   2. Despite potential thermoregulatory dangers posed by dehydration, high-power performance lasting ≤ 30 seconds may not be affected if weight loss through dehydration is ≤ 5% body weight.
   3. Acute dehydration to achieve weight loss followed by rehydration poses less danger than attempts to remain dehydrated for long periods of time. Some athletes, not understanding the importance of fluid balance, try to keep their weight down continually by limiting fluids, sweating, and spitting.

D. **Maintaining and monitoring hydration status**
   1. Most accurate method for determining fluid replacement needs:
      a. Athlete weighs nude and dry before and after activity.
      b. For every pound lost, athlete should consume 1 pint (16 oz, 480 ml) of fluid.
      c. Lost fluid should be replaced and weight normalized before the next episode of exercise.
      d. When the athlete has determined usual sweat loss patterns and is able to match fluid consumption with variable environmental and training conditions, weighing can usually be discontinued, but should not be discouraged, because it gives the athlete a continued objective measure of fluid balance.
   2. **The preferred strategy for maintaining fluid balance at all times during training is to consume fluid before, during, and after training.** The biggest stumbling block for fluid consumption among most athletes is consumption of fluid *during* training and competition. Emphasis on the importance and appropriateness of drinking water during exercise and dispelling myths about risks for cramping or getting "waterlogged" are important educational points when counseling an athlete.
   3. If weighing is not possible or is discontinued, athletes can monitor adequate hydration status indirectly. Fluid balance is indicated by:
      a. Urinating full bladder 4 times/day (average adult's urine volume is 1.2 quart/24 hours)
      b. Light yellow urine, unless taking vitamin or mineral supplement, which may cause urine to be dark yellow
      c. Not experiencing thirst during training

E. **Fluid type**
   1. **Water** can be used by all athletes to meet fluid needs.
   2. **Carbohydrate (CHO)-electrolyte replacement beverages** (sport drinks)
      a. Definition—Sport drinks are commercial preparations, isotonic in nature, that are promoted as a source of CHO and electrolytes and as having antifatigue properties.
      b. CHO—Consumption of CHO along with water can delay fatigue during long-term aerobic activity. CHO solutions containing ≤ 11% CHO from a mix of glucose, fructose, glucose polymers (malodextrins), or sucrose are absorbed quickly and used to maintain blood glucose and hydration status. Normal dilution (as purchased or as directed for powder form) of commercial sport drinks is usually well tolerated.

c. Electrolytes—Addition of electrolytes to sport drinks may aid intestinal absorption but is not physiologically necessary for electrolyte replacement in most cases. Most athletes' diets provide adequate electrolytes. Oral electrolyte replacement is indicated in rare cases, for example, during endurance events of > 3 hours in duration when no food or other source of electrolytes is consumed. Improvement in flavor is perhaps the major benefit of added electrolytes for most athletes.

d. Provision of flavored beverages, in addition to water, may enhance fluid consumption during and after training in all athletes and, as such, may be beneficial from a hydration standpoint. Use of sport drinks by an athlete should be tested during training and not consumed for the first time during competition.

IV. Carbohydrate for Endurance Events and Training

Sources of energy during exercise include a mixture of blood glucose, muscle glycogen, amino acids (primarily branched-chain) and fatty acids. Fatty acids and amino acids are plentiful in the body, regardless of diet. Stores of CHO in the body are limited, however, and the supply depends on dietary intake. Inadequate CHO intake is associated with low muscle glycogen levels, which, in turn, are associated with exhaustion and fatigue during intense, long-term efforts. Research in the area of CHO requirements for endurance athletes has focused not only on daily requirements, but also CHO intake during specific periods of time relative to training and competition:

A. **Precompetition—"CHO loading"**
   1. Goal is to increase muscle glycogen stores via dietary and activity manipulation.
   2. **Current recommendation:** maintain a CHO intake of 8–10 g CHO/kg body weight per day (or more) while tapering training the week before competition, with complete rest the day before.
   3. **Preexercise:** sucrose, glucose, or malodextrin at the level of 1.0–4.5 g/kg 1–4 hours before the activity (correspondingly less CHO closer to the activity) has been documented as performance enhancing and without ill side effects. This method is sometimes used to "top off" energy stores in addition to or in place of CHO loading.
   4. CHO loading offers potential benefits for distance runners, road cyclists, cross-country skiers, some distance swimmers and others who risk depleting glycogen stores. It is *not* recommended for athletes in nonendurance sports.
   5. **Potential side effects**
      a. Increased water retention and weight gain
      b. Stiffness

B. **During competition**
   1. **CHO ingestion during endurance exercise can delay time to fatigue.**
   2. 30–60 g CHO/hour of activity is recommended in the form of sugar or starch.
   3. The CHO may be consumed from a variety of sources, including sport drink, soft drinks, diluted juice, cookies, candy bars, sport bars, fruit, or other foods depending on preferences.

C. **After competition**
   1. **Consumption of CHO as soon as possible (no longer than 2 hours) after a glycogen-depleting training bout or competition speeds the rate of glycogen synthesis.** Rapid resynthesis of muscle glycogen is indicated for athletes who deplete glycogen stores during successive days of prolonged aerobic training or are participating in competitions such as a stage race.
   2. Consuming 1.5 g CHO/kg body weight immediately after exercise and again 2 hours later was shown in one study to maximize glycogen resynthesis. Because the athlete may not be hungry this soon after intense training, some prefer ingesting the CHO in the form of a beverage, for example, conventional soft drinks, fruit juice, or specially formulated high-CHO drinks.

3. **Caution: If the athlete is dehydrated after training, consuming concentrated beverages or food may cause nausea, vomiting, or diarrhea. In this case, the athlete should rehydrate with water or sport drinks before ingesting large amounts of CHO.**

V. Carbohydrate for High-energy Output Alternated with Relative Rest

A. The majority of competitive athletes participate in sports requiring brief periods of high-intensity activity mixed with periods of rest, such as football, basketball, tennis, or wrestling.

B. The CHO requirements of athletes participating in such sports have not been extensively studied.

C. Many successful athletes consume < 5 g CHO/kg body weight per day, suggesting that a high-CHO diet is neither necessary nor beneficial for athletes.

D. Empiric wisdom indicates that the athlete participating in a sport characterized as anaerobic but who also trains aerobically (e.g., a boxer who does road work) may benefit from a CHO intake between 5 and 8 g CHO/kg body weight per day.

VI. Issues of Weight and Body Composition

Although the predominant weight concern with the general public is weight loss, the sports medicine physician is likely to receive as many concerns about weight gain as weight loss.

A. **Weight loss**

1. Athletes who present with the desire to lose weight fall into three categories:
   a. **Relatively lean** but desire to lose body fat for performance or appearance
   b. **Overly fat** who desire to lose body fat for performance and health reasons
   c. **Little or no excess body fat**, but desire to lose weight to compete in lower weight class
2. Considerations when working with each type
   a. **Lean group**—those who are lean by conventional standards, but who desire to reduce body fat for aesthetic or performance reasons:
      i. If the patient is female and amenorrheic, she may already be restricting calories to a point beyond which is physiologically appropriate. If the amenorrhea is related to intense conditioning and not an eating disorder, the decision to restrict calories is based on whether her current eating pattern is already minimal.
      ii. If the patient has passed through adolescence and is trying to achieve prepubescent body fat level, expect difficulty in achieving weight loss.
      iii. If menses ceases, if energy level or performance diminishes, or if weight or fat loss ceases despite continued calorie restriction, reassess adequacy of the diet.
      iv. **The ability to achieve and maintain minimal body fat levels is largely genetic. Some athletes are able to do so while maintaining health and performance. Others experience health and performance problems** (e.g., recurrent illness or injury, amenorrhea, diminished strength and endurance). The clinician must be aware that those athletes who cannot easily achieve low body fat levels may try more extreme methods. Sometimes acceptance by the athlete that he or she has "matured out of" a sport requires counseling and support from the clinician.
      v. See the section on "Gradual weight loss protocol to reduce body fat," later, for general guidelines on fat reduction.
   b. **Overly fat group**—those who need to lose body fat for health and performance:
      i. These athletes require treatment similar to the nonathletic overweight patient.
      ii. If training is already maximal or further aerobic exercise would compromise strength or anaerobic training, calorie reduction is the only viable treatment modality.

c. **Rapid weight loss group**—those who are already very lean but wish to lose weight to compete in desired weight class:

i. **Definition:** The process of rapid weight loss is usually called **"cutting"** and is typically accomplished by restricting food and fluids and increasing sweating for 3 to 10 days before competition. Precompetition dieting and dehydration are followed by refeeding and rehydrating after weigh-in. The practice is repeated with each competition of the season.

ii. **Consequences:** Many athletes practice cutting weight with no adverse consequences. Athletes who experience problems (e.g., get sick, suffer heat illness, can't make the weight) are usually those who attempt to lose too much weight and those who attempt to stay at the lower weight instead of refeeding and rehydrating. Speculation about increased incidence of eating disorders, growth failure, and renal compromise has been asserted. No data exist, however, to support or discount these claims. Earlier claims about reduction in resting metabolic rates in wrestlers who weight-cycle have been refuted; no long-term change in metabolic rate has been observed.

iii. **Guidelines:** Although it is conventional and often indicated for health professionals to advise against this practice, most athletes will cut weight with or without professional guidance. Based on your personal philosophy and the situation at hand, you may or may not find it suitable to offer guidance to the athlete cutting weight. If you believe that providing information will minimize complications in an athlete determined to cut weight, refer to the section on "Rapid weight loss protocol," later, for basic guidelines.

B. **Weight gain**

1. **The key for weight gain is progressive resistance training** (i.e., systematic weightlifting program) and adequate diet. However, genetic predisposition, somatotype, maturity level, and compliance determine progress.
2. **Strength athletes are more vulnerable to steroid experimentation.** Watch for signs and symptoms of use, such as rapid gains in strength and size, increased aggression, acne, hypertension, muscle-tendon tears, abnormal liver function tests, low high-density lipoprotein cholesterol, or premature closure of epiphyses on x-ray.
3. Refer to the section on "Weight gain protocol," later, for a general description of guidelines for your patient.

VII. Precompetition Meal

A. Although there is no magic to the specific foods that comprise a precompetition meal, for many athletes precompetition eating remains mythical. It is important to appreciate an athlete's concerns and beliefs about precompetition eating, while understanding the physiologic aspects.

B. Numerous recommendations on timing, amount, and types of food for precompetition meals appear in sports nutrition publications; however, many of the recommendations are not supported by scientific data and may not be appropriate for all athletes.

C. When advising an athlete about precompetition eating, consider the following points.

1. **Purpose**
   a. **The primary purpose of the precompetition meal is to provide fluid and energy for the athlete during the performance.**
   b. Foods and beverages consumed should not interfere with the physiologic stresses associated with athletic performance.
2. **Timing**
   a. Most athletes report eating 2–3 hours before competition. There are also reports of athletes who:

i. Get uncomfortably hungry if the meal is eaten more than an hour or two before the competition
ii. Have gorged just minutes before breaking world records or winning gold medals
iii. Fast for the 6–12 hours before competition

b. **The timing of precompetition eating varies greatly from athlete to athlete.**

3. **Physiologic considerations**
   a. A relatively empty stomach at the time of competition may be desirous for athletes in a contact sport, in which there is an increased chance of injury.
   b. Fat is one of the primary factors that slows gastric emptying; therefore, the amount of fat can be modulated to achieve the desired results.
   c. CHO loading:
      i. CHO loading before competition may be associated with enhanced endurance for marathon runners, triathletes, or road cyclists.
      ii. It should not be practiced for the first time before a major competition because each athlete reacts differently.
      iii. Refer to the previous section on "Carbohydrate for endurance events and training" for more information on CHO loading.
4. **Practical considerations**
   a. Liquid meals can replace conventional foods, and while suitable in any situation, may be of particular value in situations of limited availability of food and with athletes who have cut weight.
   b. Eating foods that the athlete does not like at a time when nervous tension is high does not enhance performance. Personal preference and tolerance must be considered.
   c. It is important that the athlete consumes food and beverages that:
      i. Are liked
      ii. Are well tolerated
      iii. Are usually eaten
      iv. Are thought to result in a winning performance
   d. Diaries can be useful in helping athletes determine their best precompetition regimen.
   e. **The "winning" precompetition meal regimen is an individual matter.** It is essential for each individual athlete to determine the precompetition regimen that works best for him or her.

D. **The precompetition meal should be individualized!!!**

VIII. Dietary Supplements

Using dietary supplements as ergogenic aids is a practice that has long existed and will likely continue to exist as long as athletes are driven by their competitive nature.

The pervasive practice of dietary supplementation to improve performance has created a marketplace abundant with supplements. As such, it is futile to attempt to review supplements in a product-specific manner. Instead, general comments about the safety of categories of supplements are offered.

A. **Vitamin or mineral supplements:** not innocuous in large amounts as perceived by many athletes. See previous sections on "Vitamins" and "Iron."
B. **Herbs:** Allergic reaction, toxicity resulting from long-term use, and positive drug testing due to ephedrinelike compounds are the major risks.
C. **Amino acids:** Amino acid consumption from pills is usually small relative to dietary intake and as such poses no significant health risk. However, the physician should remain cognizant of the fact that a perceived function associated with amino acids is "natural steroid replacement," so those athletes questioning about or using amino acids may also be contemplating steroid use.

IX. Gradual Weight Loss Protocol to Reduce Body Fat

The clinician should review the following with the patient who needs or desires to lose body fat.

A. **Basic premise:** Create calorie deficit.
B. **Timing:** Best to achieve fat loss during off-season or early preseason.
C. **Rate**
   1. For lean athlete—½ lb per week
   2. For overly fat athlete—up to 2 lb or 1% body weight per week
D. **Realistic schedule:** Based on above rates, significant fat loss takes weeks to months.
E. **To achieve negative calorie balance**
   1. **Diet:** based on usual intake, consider reducing fat, reducing meals eaten out, establishing eating schedules, substituting lower-calorie snacks, and decreasing use of caloric beverages.
   2. **Exercise:** based on current training, determine whether aerobic activity can be increased. Is athlete already at a maximum level of daily training? Will increased aerobic activity impair strength or sprint training? If not, recommend increased aerobic activity.

X. Rapid Weight Loss Protocol

The clinician should review the following with the athlete desiring to cut weight.

A. **Risks of rapid weight loss**
   1. Acute side effects of mild dehydration and low calorie intake
      a. Fatigue
      b. Weakness
      c. Dizziness
      d. Decreased concentration
      e. Mood swings, irritability
      f. Muscle cramps
      g. Muscle tissue loss
      h. Glycogen loss
   2. Potential for diarrhea, cramping, and vomiting during refeeding phase. The greater the weight loss, the greater the possibility for refeeding problems.
   3. Cannot accomplish complete fluid and electrolyte balance and glycogen repletion between weigh-in and competition. The longer the time between weigh-in and competition, the greater the restoration in body fluid and glycogen stores.
B. **The goal is for the clinician and the athlete to work together to establish a routine that works for the athlete in terms of health and performance.** Schedule of competitions, tolerance to dehydration and refeeding, dedication, and competitive status impact the weight-cutting routine. The following serves as a guide when developing an athlete's weight-cutting routine.
   1. If competitions are spaced a week apart, do *not* restrict food and fluid during the first 2–3 days of the week. This only prolongs state of dehydration.
   2. Reduce bulk-forming foods (high-fiber cereal, raw fruits and vegetables, milk and cheese) from the diet a few days before weigh-in.
   3. Twenty-four to 48 hours before weigh-in, decrease food and fluid and increase exercise. The safest routine allows the athlete to weigh the desired weight for the absolute shortest period of time possible.
   4. Immediately after weigh-in, rehydrate with a CHO-electrolyte replacement beverage (Powerade, All Sport, Gatorade, 10-K) or water. Consume more concentrated food or fluid as tolerated. The athlete who has cut >5% body weight may benefit from consumption of canned liquid meals (e.g., Ensure, Sportshake, Exceed, Sustacal) in place of food.
   5. If the athlete feels chronically weak, light-headed, and tired, the weight class may be too low.

6. Recording weight-loss methods, refeeding techniques (what is drunk and eaten and how much), and performance outcome help the athlete develop a routine that is suitable and help determine the viability of practice.

XI. Weight Gain Protocol

A. **Strength training program:** The appropriate progressive, resistance-training program (i.e., lifting weights), with adequate rest between sessions, is the basic impetus to create lean tissue rather than fat tissue. Without training, the dietary component is useless.

B. **Increase calorie intake by approximately 400 calories/day.**

1. **Meal and snack frequency** usually must increase to five to nine eating occasions per day. Skipping breakfast impedes progress. Continuous availability of food allows the athlete to eat whenever and wherever hunger occurs or on the predetermined schedule.
2. **Diet composition:** If total caloric intake is already high, it may be difficult simply to add more food to the diet. If food volume is maximum, the next option is to concentrate calories without adding bulk. Strategies might include adding butter, margarine, peanut butter, sauces, salad dressing, syrup, jam, jelly, sugar, cheese, or powdered milk to foods already eaten. When possible, extra calories should be balanced between CHO, protein, and fat. Supplementing only one nutrient is not advised because of nutrient imbalance and monotony.
3. **High-calorie supplements:** If the athlete is unable to increase calories from traditional food to a level needed for weight gain, supplements are an option. High-calorie shakes, canned beverages, or bars are useful to increase frequency of eating as well as calories. Costs vary greatly. Because the goal is simply "more calories," the exact supplement chosen should be determined by the athlete's preference, product availability, and financial resources.

C. **Increase protein intake?**

1. Athletes who are gaining muscle have increased protein requirements. Many athletes' typical intake meets this increased requirement; however, for some, intake does not meet requirements. Requirements are estimated up to 1.8 g protein/kg body weight and may be higher if the athlete is a vegetarian because of the lower biologic value of plant protein.
2. Protein intake is often deemphasized by health professionals, but protein intake is a priority (real or perceived) for most weight-training athletes. Use of protein powders and amino acid supplements remains prevalent. While usually not a significant or necessary source of protein, the psychological benefit of supplements can be significant. Questions asked of the practitioner regarding supplements or other weight-gain aids deserve adequate attention because they can indicate a curiosity about steroids.

PART II
SPECIAL POPULATIONS
9: Youth Sports Issues

Kris Berg, Ed.D.

I. Fitness and Health Status of American Youth

A. **National Children and Youth Fitness Study**
   1. A random sample of 8800 boys and girls, grades 5–12, in 19 states
   2. Students participating in physical education classes outperformed those who were not on a battery of physical fitness tests.
   3. Students participating in community physical activity/sports programs were more fit than those who did not.

B. **Other national fitness tests**
   1. Lower fitness levels of American youth in the 1980s than previous decades
   2. Increased body fatness in boys and girls is one of the most consistent findings.

C. **Physical activity levels of American youth:** A study using Holter monitoring indicated that American youth in a typical day do not exercise vigorously enough to meet criteria for achieving aerobic fitness.

D. **Cardiovascular disease**
   1. A number of studies indicate that elementary school age children are at risk for coronary heart disease. American youth have significantly higher levels of total cholesterol and body fatness than youth in Third World nations and Japan.
   2. Fatty streaks are evident in prepubescents.

E. **Role of youth sports programs**
   1. Critical role in youth fitness
   2. Physical education programs have been eliminated in some areas and often are poorly funded.

II. Traits of Sound Youth Sports Leagues

A. **Sound Coaching**
   1. **American Coaching Effectiveness Program (ACEP)**
      a. Training program for youth coaches
      b. Offered by many colleges, universities, YMCAs, etc.
      c. Content
         i. First aid
         ii. Safety
         iii. Philosophy of developing all children and deemphasizing winning
         iv. Conditioning
         v. Strategy and skill development
   2. **Handbook for Youth Sports Coaches**
      a. Available from American Alliance Publications, P.O. Box 704, Waldorf, MD 20601
      b. Topics
         i. Goalsetting
         ii. Injury prevention
         iii. Teaching sportsmanship
         iv. Organizing practice

TABLE 1. The Bill of Rights for Young Athletes

Right to participate in sports	Right to participate in safe and healthy environments
Right to participate at a level commensurate with each child's maturity and ability	Right to proper preparation for participation in sports
Right to have qualified adult leadership	Right to an equal opportunity to strive for success
Right to play as a child and not as an adult	Right to be treated with dignity
Right to share in the leadership and decision-making of their sport	Right to have fun in sports

Reprinted with permission of the American Alliance for Health, Physical Education, Recreation and Dance, 1900 Association Drive, Reston, Virginia 22091.

3. **"The Winning Trap: Sports and Our Kids"**—a videotape available from National Association for Sport and Physical Education, 1900 Association Drive, Reston VA 22091

B. **Sound philosophy**
  1. **The Bill of Rights for Young Athletes**
     a. Formulated by the American Alliance for Health, Physical Education, Recreation and Dance (Table 1)
     b. Sound criteria for developing, modifying, and assessing youth sports leagues

C. **Modification of rules to suit developmental level of participants**
  1. Use smaller balls, fields, and courts.
  2. Shorten the duration of games and practices.
  3. Reduce the number of participants playing at one time (e.g., three instead of five basketball players, six instead of 11 soccer players).
  4. Stop play when a rules violation is made and allow the player who normally would be penalized to continue to play without penalty after a brief explanation or demonstration (e.g., a player double-dribbling in basketball is stopped, gven a brief explanation, and given the ball again to continue play).
  5. Do not keep score or win-loss records.
  6. Rotate players to different positions each game.
  7. In baseball and softball, use a batting tee or have a coach pitch to his or her own players.

D. **Constructive role of parents**
  1. Parents play a critical role in encouraging children to participate in sports. Constructive parental support should lead to a happy and voluntary involvement of the child in sports. If, however, a child is driven beyond his or her own wishes by a parent playing the role of a "vicarious athlete," then the effects can be destructive.
  2. Parents who coach must be especially aware not to favor or disfavor their own children. This requires considerable sensitivity.
  3. Classic poor examples of a parent coach are illustrated by a son or daughter who pitches or plays quarterback while other equally skilled children are given secondary roles, and a parent who screams at his or her players or at referees.
  4. ACEP training can greatly assist the parent coach, but the individual's own value system is still likely to be openly expressed in a moment of duress on the playing field. Most coaches need to continually remind themselves of the important duties they have assumed in being a volunteer coach.

E. **Assessing the effect on youth**

  The following questions provide a simple but effective means of assessing a program.
  1. Do children look like the they are having fun during games or while at practice?
  2. Do they like the coaches?

3. Do they speak of playing the sport again? Do they actually play again?
4. Are their skills noticeably better at the end of the season?
5. Are they bothered by losing?
6. Does everyone play at least half the game?
7. Do skilled performers dominate key positions?
   a. Pitcher
   b. First base
   c. Point guard
8. Do skilled performers dominate play?
   a. Score most of the goals or baskets
   b. Dribbling the ball
   c. Passing the ball

III. Trainability of Youth

A. Aerobic power

1. A number of studies have indicated no change in maximum oxygen uptake due to training in children, nor a reduction in trainability due to training.
2. Some suggest that a critical maturational threshold may exist or that children possess an initially high aerobic power not readily improved with training.
3. In most studies not indicating significant gain scores, the exercise was below the intensity, duration, and frequency guidelines used for adults.
4. In most studies demonstrating significant change, adult guidelines were followed.
5. It appears that unless exercise is relatively prolonged and intense, and based on standards recommended for adults, improvement is not likely to occur.

B. Strength and muscular development

1. A maturational threshold has been proposed as a requisite for strength and muscle development.
   a. However, several studies indicate that prepubescents and pubescents (i.e., stages 1 and 2 of Tanner's or Greulich's scale[23]) can significantly increase strength.
   b. Because gains in body weight did not occur in these studies, it is suggested that strength gains in children are induced neurologically as typifies the response by women and the elderly.
2. For decades many physical educators and physicians have warned that weight training was not only ineffective in prepubescents and early adolescents, but that it would damage the epiphyseal plate and soft tissues. The validity of the injury issue was addressed in a recent investigation. Only one training injury occurred in 14 weeks to 32 boys and scintigraphy revealed no bone, epiphysis, or muscle damage.
3. It appears that prepubescents are not only strength trainable but when closely supervised, injury is infrequent.
4. The importance of close supervision is supported by the observation that roughly half of some 35,000 weight training injuries requiring visits to an emergency room occurred in 10–19 year olds, most of whom were training at home.

C. Recommendations

1. If wishing to elicit gains in aerobic fitness, adult standards should be used, i.e., 15–20 minutes duration three or more times weekly at or above 50% of $\dot{V}O_2$max.
2. Recommendations for safe development of strength in youth have been made by the American Orthopedic Society for Sports Medicine (Table 2).
   a. Elimination of overhead lifts while standing should be added to their recommendations because of the undue pressure placed on the lumbar spine.
   b. Sitting presses, for example, develop the same upper body muscles as the standing press, but are much safer because of reduced spinal hyperextension.

TABLE 2. Strength-training Recommendations for Prepubescent Boys and Girls

Equipment

1. Strength-training equipment should be of appropriate design to accommodate the size and degree of maturity of the prepubescent.
2. It should be cost effective.
3. It should be safe, free of defects, and inspected frequently.
4. It should be located in an uncrowded area free of obstructions with adequate lighting and ventilation.

Prescribed Program

1. Training is recommended two to three times a week for 20- to 30-minute periods.
2. No resistance should be applied until proper form is demonstrated. Six to fifteen repetitions equal one set; one to three sets per exercise should be done.
3. Weight or resistance is increased in 1- to 3-lb increments after the prepubescent does 15 repetitions in good form.

Program Considerations

1. A preparticipation physical exam is mandatory.
2. The child must have the emotional maturity to accept coaching and instructions.
3. There must be adequate supervision by coaches who are knowledgeable about strength training and the special problems of prepubescents.
4. Strength training should be a part of an overall comprehensive program designed to increase motor skills and level of fitness.
5. Strength training should be preceded by a warm-up period and followed by a cool-down.
6. Emphasis should be on dynamic concentric contractions.
7. All exercises should be carried through a full range of motion.
8. Competition is prohibited.
9. No maximum lift should ever be attempted.

American Orthopaedic Society for Sports Medicine: Strength-training Workshop. Indianapolis, IN, August, 1985.

IV. Sex Differences

A. Body composition

1. Throughout childhood, girls have slightly more body fat than boys.
2. At puberty, boys rapidly gain muscle mass and lose about 3–5% of body fat between ages 12 and 17, whereas girls gain some lean body mass as well as fat.
3. Typical body fatness for older teenage girls is about 20–25%, whereas athletic girls will often have less than 16–18%.
4. Body fatness greatly affects athletic performance. Consequently, exercise is valuable, because by facilitating weight control, other factors are also positively affected.
   a. Aerobic power
   b. Heat tolerance
   c. Ability to handle body parts
      i. Agility
      ii. Power
      iii. Speed
5. Body fatness probably influences a person's overall like or dislike for physical activity.

B. Physique and performance

1. Boys and girls are similar in height and weight until puberty.
2. By maturation, men are considerably heavier and taller, and possess more muscle mass than women.
3. The onset of these changes is so rapid that boys and girls are usually separated in competition well before even the early maturers reach puberty. Third grade is a commonly cited time for this separation.
4. Adolescent growth differs in early and late maturers.
   a. Growth rate (e.g., peak height velocity) is greater the earlier the spurt occurs, but growth also ceases earlier, leading to a reduction in adult height.
   b. Early maturing boys are typically more muscular with shorter legs, whereas early maturing girls have shorter legs and narrower shoulders.
5. The adolescent growth spurt provides the average man with major athletic advantages in comparison to women.
   a. Strength
   b. Speed

c. Power
d. Aerobic power
e. Recent world records in track and swimming place the woman's performance at about 6–14% below that of the man's.

C. **Aerobic power**
1. After puberty, endurance performance of girls typically decreases, whereas it increases in boys.
2. In boys, increased androgen secretion leads to increased protein synthesis.
a. Greater hypertrophy of skeletal and cardiac muscle
b. Greater red blood cell and hemoglobin production
c. Adolescent and adult males consequently have greater heart size and weight than females, even when expressed relative to body size.
d. Net result is an aerobic power and endurance typically about 20–25% greater in males than females.
e. Group data usually exaggerate the difference, whereas comparison of elite females, who are lean, highly trained, and genetically endowed, with elite males results in much smaller differences.

D. **Cultural expectations**
1. Most physical activity surveys of children and adolescents show boys to be more active in organized sports as well as in recreational physical activity than girls.
2. American culture seems to promote sports and exercise as basic to the male's general development.
3. Only in the last decade or so have females been widely encouraged to participate in sport.
4. Societal norms regarding females and exercise seem to have changed dramatically.
5. The increased participation of girls coupled with appropriate coaching and facilities will likely continue to increase the need for sound sports programs for girls.

V. Differences Between Youth and Adults

A. **Children should not be treated as miniature adults.**
1. They are remarkably different physically, emotionally, socially, and psychologically.
2. Although the physical differences are obvious, the others may be less so.
a. For example, it is a common error of many youth coaches to presume that all the participants on a team have winning as their primary goal. However, surveys indicate that most children would rather play a lot on a losing team than play minimally on a winning team.
b. Similarly, children do not typically wish to strive for optimal physical conditioning. Spending excessive time on intense and elaborately designed conditioning does not suit the needs and interests of most children below age 13.

B. **Heat tolerance is less in children.**
1. Reduced sweating capacity
2. Greater body surface area to weight ratio—detrimental when ambient temperature exceeds body temperature

C. **Walking and running efficiency is considerably lower.** From age 8 to 18, efficiency of locomotion increases about 1% per year.

D. **Effect of maturation rate on sports performance**
1. Most female athletes tend to initiate menarche later than nonathletes.
2. Prepubertal sex characteristics such as leanness seem to be advantageous in many sports.
3. Early maturing boys seem to prevail in team sports in which height, weight, and strength are requisites for success. Several classic studies show that boys competing

in the Little League World Series were above average in skeletal growth, and the more mature boys tended to play the critical positions, including pitcher.

4. Grouping of youngsters to promote equality of competition
   a. Age and grade level are the predominant modus operandi.
   b. Maturation should be taken into consideration.

E. **Recommendations**

1. Emphasize fun and skill development. Lacking this, further participation in sports is hampered, as may be the physical activity pattern in adulthood.
2. Begin specific conditioning work only when youth are old enough to understand its purpose and are willing to subject themselves to vigorous, demanding exercise.
   a. Err on the side of too little rather than too much to reduce the incidence of injury and encourage enjoyment.
   b. Consider conditioning below age 13 to be primarily for the sake of exposure to conditioning.

Recommended Reading

1. American Academy of Pediatrics: Fitness in the preschool child. Pediatrics 58:88–89, 1976.
2. American College of Sports Medicine: Position statement on the recommended quantity and quality of exercise for developing and maintaining fitness in healthy adults. Med Sci Sports Exerc 10(3):vii–x, 1978.
3. Bar-Or O: Pediatric Sports Medicine for the Practitioner: From Physiological Principles to Clinical Applications. New York, Springer-Verlag, 1983.
4. Berg K, LaVoie J, Latin R: Physiological training effects of playing youth soccer. Med Sci Sports Exerc 17:656–660, 1985
5. Berg K, Sady S, Beal D, et al: Developing an elementary school CHD prevention program. Phys Sportsmed 11:99–105, 1983.
6. Brooks G, Fahey T: Fundamentals of Human Performance. New York, Macmillan, 1987.
7. Consumer Product Safety Commission National Electronic Injury Surveillance System: Report for January 1 through December 31, 1979.
8. Duda M: Prepubescent strength training gains support. Phys Sportsmed 14:157–161, 1986.
9. Gilliam TB, Freedson PS, Geenen DL, and Shahraray B: Physical activity patterns determined by heart rate monitoring in 6–7 year old children. Med Sci Sports Exerc 13:65–67, 1981.
10. Gilliam TB, Katch VL, Thorland W: Prevalence of coronary heart disease risk factors in active children, 7 to 12 years of age. Med Sci Sports Exerc 9 (Spring):21–25, 1977.
11. Greene L, Osness WL: Health education: Sunflower style. Health Education 10 (November–December): 34–35, 1979.
12. Hale C: Physiological maturity of little league baseball players. Res Q 27:276–282, 1956.
13. Hamilton P, Andrew GM: Influence of growth and athletic training on heart and lung functions. Eur J Appl Physiol 36:27–38, 1976.
14. Kobayashi K, Kiamura K, Miura M, et al: Aerobic power as related to body growth and training in Japanese boys: Longitudinal study. J Appl Physiol 44:666–672, 1978.
15. Kraemer W, Fleck S: Strength Training for Young Athletes. Champaign, IL, Human Kinetics, 1993.
16. Krogman W: Maturation age of 55 boys in the little league world series. Res Q 30:54–49, 1959.
17. Martens R: The uniqueness of the young athlete: Psychological considerations. Am J Sports Med 8:382–385, 1980.
18. Martens R, Christina RW, Harvey JS, Sharkey BJ: Coaching Young Athletes. Champaign, IL, Human Kinetics, 1981.
19. Moritani T, DeVries H: Neural factors versus hypertrophy in the time course of muscle strength gain. Am J Physical Med 58:115–124, 1979.
20. Pate RR, Blair SN: Exercise and the prevention of atherosclerosis: Pediatric implications. In Strong WB (ed): Atherosclerosis: Its Pediatric Aspect. New York, Grune & Stratton, 1978.
21. Ross J, Gilbert G: The National Children and Youth Fitness Study: A summary of findings. Journal of Physical Education, Recreation and Dance. 56 (January):3–8, 1985.
22. Rowland T: Exercise and Children's Health. Champaign, IL, Human Kinetics, 1990.
23. Sailors M, Berg K: Comparison of responses to weight training in pubescent boys and men. J Sports Med Physical Fit 27:30–37, 1987.
24. Washington R, VanGundy J, Cohen C, et al: Normal aerobic and anaerobic exercise data for North American school-age children. J Pediatr 112:223–233, 1988.
25. Weltman A, Janney C, Clark R, et al: The effects of hydraulic resistance training in pre-pubertal males. Med Sci Sports Exerc 18:629–638, 1986.

10

The High School Athlete: Setting Up a High School Sports Medicine Program

Stephen G. Rice, M.D., Ph.D., MPH, FACSM, FAAP

I. Overview

A. **Reasons athletic health care is well established at college and professional levels**
   1. Awareness of needs and the obligation to meet responsibilities
   2. Commitment to solve "problem" by meeting responsibilities
      a. Risk management and loss control are central concerns to organization
      b. Well-being and health of the athlete optimize on-field performance
   3. Attention to detail routinely practiced
   4. Control in all situations is usual operating procedure of the organization
   5. Adequate financial resources available
   6. Professional personnel secured in adequate quantity
      a. Certified athletic trainers
      b. Qualified team physicians:
         i. Primary care physicians with certificate of added qualification (CAQ) or fellowship training (ideal)
         ii. Orthopedists (ideally with sports orthopedic fellowship)
         iii. Other specialists with vast experience in sports medicine
      c. Other allied health professionals:
         i. Certified strength and conditioning coaches
         ii. Nutritionists
         iii. Psychologists
         iv. Optometrists
         v. Dentists
         vi. Exercise physiologists
         vii. Physical therapists
   7. Policies delineated and enforced routinely

B. **Reasons athletic health care in secondary schools is clearly inferior**
   1. Lack awareness of scope of "problem"
   2. Assume obligations are met by minimal standards and effort by external agencies
      a. Preparticipation physical examinations required
      b. Team physician or ambulance present at home varsity football games
   3. Resist change—do not like to establish new policies
   4. Lack adequate financial resources; thus seek assistance at little or no expense
   5. Unwilling to exert effort routinely, as in daily preparedness and record keeping
   6. Seek "quick fix," "big splash," easy solutions
   7. Turnover of personnel (school board, superintendent, principal, athletic director, coaches); lack of continuity leads to lack of policy
   8. Avoid real, long-range, long-term, permanent change—too hard to commit
   9. Not a priority—too many other issues

C. **Common pitfalls for high schools**
   1. Lack of knowledge among coaches and athletic directors about sports medicine
   2. Lack of standards—unclear exactly what is expected; seek low standards
   3. Poor communication with medical community
   4. No overall single system of care—each coach does own thing
   5. Lack of leadership—maintain status quo

D. **Solution—goals and requirements**
   1. Goals
      a. Proper health care for athletes
      b. Minimize liability through a risk management (loss control) policy
   2. Requirements
      a. Knowledge
      b. Organization
      c. Attention to detail (commitment)

E. **Approaches to improving current high school athletic health care**
   1. **Three key elements** to the solution (three legs to a stool)
      a. School
      b. Medical community
      c. Certified athletic trainer (ATC)
   2. **Commitment of a school is critical**
      a. School as a unit—operates a single athletic program
      b. Solution must be internal as well as external
         i. Obligations and knowledge of athletic directors and coaches
         ii. Use of student trainers in preparedness and athletic first aid
         iii. Institution of policies, guidelines, and procedures for daily use
         iv. Record-keeping system
      c. Team physicians and outside clinics *alone* cannot provide the constant daily health care needed for all athletes in all sports at all athletic venues.
   3. **Athletic trainer—the key person**
      a. **Not automatically the entire solution**
      b. Cannot be present at all athletic venues simultaneously
      c. Needs support and a system to work under
         i. Educated coaches
         ii. Educated corps of student trainers (who can cover all venues)
         iii. Knowledgeable and supportive administration
         iv. Policies and procedures
         v. Record-keeping, accountability, and quality assurance system
      d. Should insist on medical supervision and support by team physician
      e. Should have adequate budget
      f. Reasonable schedule demands because turnover may be likely after a few years (burn-out, or starting a family)
   4. **School should assume responsibility for operating safe program**
      a. Know obligations and commit to meeting them.
      b. Develop a system with clear written policies, procedures, and mandates.
      c. Hire a National Athletic Trainers Association (NATA)–certified athletic trainer as best person to coordinate and operate the program.
      d. Seek assistance of medical community:
         i. Know what is desired from physicians, physical therapists, and clinics.
         ii. Ask *entire* medical community to get involved.
         iii. Seek broad assistance and coverage for all sports:
            (a) Physical exams as well as preseason fitness screening
            (b) Weekly school visits

(c) Event coverage
(d) Therapy treatments

e. Appreciate who is in charge (who is the consumer).

5. **Role of team physician and medical community**
   a. Written contract—yes or no:
      i. Delineates responsibilities and expectations
      ii. Helps ensure that school has given careful thought to its obligations
      iii. Good communication leads to good working relationships.
   b. Monetary compensation—yes or no:
      i. If compensated, may nullify Good Samaritan immunity
      ii. Amount of compensation offered frequently meager
      iii. Compensation recognizes value of assistance provided.
   c. Responsibilities
   d. Jurisdiction—are your decisions final?
   e. Primary duty—to athlete or to school?
   f. Insurance and liability coverage:
      i. Personal coverage under personal or clinic policy
      ii. Personal coverage by school or organization
      iii. Good Samaritan Law immunity may cover team physician in some states:
         (a) Team physician not really a Good Samaritan under strict definition—"someone without obligation who steps forward to render emergency care"
         (b) Has clearly defined responsibility to athletes and school
         (c) Event coverage is evidence of that responsibility
         (d) May be covered by "good intent, no compensation" concern
         (e) Good Samaritan immunity extends only to "emergency care" rendered during event coverage; protection does not extend to preparticipation physical examinations, weekly injury clinics at the school, and return-to-play clearance exams.
      iv. Potential responsibility and liability for athletic trainer's actions:
         (a) Need to clarify issue with school district
         (b) NATA-certified athletic trainers generally function "under direct medical supervision of a physician."
         (c) In those states that have not specifically defined the "scope of practice" for athletic trainers through licensure, certification, or registration, team physician needs to assess implications and responsibilities of "direct medical supervision." An analogous supervisory situation may be the physician-physician's assistant relationship.
   g. Degree of involvement:
      i. Set policy with athletic director and athletic trainer. Form medical advisory board with school district.
      ii. Provide advice to program.
      iii. Provide medical coverage at games.
      iv. Develop an emergency contact plan.
      v. Conduct preseason physical examinations.
      vi. Visit school/athletes regularly.
      vii. Educate coaches and athletic trainers.
      viii. Support for athletic trainer's authority:
         (a) Medical-legal supervisor of certified athletic trainer
         (b) Role in writing job description
         (c) Role in interviewing and hiring
         (d) Role in job evaluation
         (e) Role in quality assurance—chart review and case studies

6. **Athletic trainers:** getting a job isn't easy (but it's getting easier!)
   a. Scenario—submits resume and NATA pamphlets as to why a certified athletic trainer is necessary
   b. Athletic trainer may be perceived as salesman:
      i. Identifying "a problem I didn't know existed"
      ii. Offering a solution to problem
   c. Funding a factor—usually low-paying, entry-level job
   d. If athletic trainer is hired, under what conditions?
      i. Full-time trainer or part-time?
      ii. Teacher and trainer? How many classes?
      iii. How many working hours per week, including games?
      iv. Medical backup and supervision
      v. Whose decision is final regarding return to play?
      vi. Adequate budget for supplies
      vii. Quality of training room
      viii. Written job description
      ix. Job performance evaluation (accountability and quality assurance)
      x. Potential for career advancement
      xi. Library fund and continuing education

II. Athletic Health Care System

A. **Generic model system:** developed by examining what makes college and professional sports programs successful in handling athletic health care and adapting to high school level
   1. Can be installed at **any** school
      a. Large or small; urban, suburban, or rural
      b. Especially helpful in remote, poor, rural areas
      c. Also effective for large urban districts
   2. Can work with or without other health professionals; however, quality of system is greatly improved with addition of trainer and team physician.

B. **Model system developed under strict guidelines of U.S. Department of Education**
   1. Development from 1978–1982; national dissemination from 1983–1995
   2. Rigorously tested and evaluated with new evaluation methodologies
      a. Full evaluation is repeated with each new adopting school
      b. Large data bank for injuries from all high school sports
   3. Validated by U.S. Department of Education review panels in 1982, 1987, and 1995; potentially a gold standard to adopt, or to compare with existing program
   4. Approved for national dissemination via competitive grants in 1983, 1988, 1990, and 1993 by U.S. Department of Education through the National Diffusion Network (NDN), a consortium of "proven programs that work"
      a. Don't have to reinvent the wheel
      b. Schools know and recognize NDN programs in all areas of education:
         i. "Proven educational programs that work"
         ii. Rigorously tested, transportable, cost-effective
         iii. Have a track record with most school districts nationally
   5. Orientation is practical; specific forms, protocols, lists

C. **Six key elements of the Athletic Health Care System:** What would a certified athletic trainer do if newly hired by a high school to start a program? Install these six key elements, in some fashion.
   1. **Assessment**
      a. Thorough evaluation of current program
      b. Standards for care delineated

c. Areas of assessment
  i. Staff training
  ii. Athletic facilities
  iii. Athletic equipment
  iv. Emergency preparedness
  v. Central training room
  vi. Provision of athletic health care services
  vii. Record keeping
d. Self-assessment initially followed by an outside evaluation:
  i. Similar concept and methodology to assessments by:
    (a) Joint Commission on Accreditation of Health Organizations (JCAHO)
    (b) Educational assessments
  ii. Formal written report issued
  iii. Action plan developed based on weaknesses and deficiencies
e. Assessment frequency—every 3–5 years

2. **Education**
  a. **Education of coaches**
    i. More states introducing coach education requirements
    ii. National Coaching Standards promulgated in 1995 by National Association for Sport and Physical Education (NASPE)
    iii. Scope of knowledge
      (a) Cardiopulmonary resuscitation—annual recertification
      (b) Red Cross First Aid—is it relevant?
      (c) Sports medicine and athletic training
        • Content (prevention, injury management); organization
        • Length—hours, days (30–35 hours)
        • Methods: didactic (lectures, slides, videos, CD-ROM), demonstration, laboratories, and supervised practice
        • Course for "soldiers on the front lines every day"
    iv. Sensitivity of coaches:
      (a) Toward injuries and injured athletes:
        • Old school—"no pain, no gain"; no practice, no play
        • New school—recognize injury, treat, and fully rehabilitate; pain-free participation only
      (b) Sports psychology
    v. Receptivity to installing a new system, athletic trainer, or team physician:
      (a) Personal knowledge still required even though more support available:
        • Prevention and preparedness
        • Recognition of injuries and applying sports first aid
        • Insisting on full treatment and rehabilitation
      (b) Share responsibilities—don't dump everything onto athletic trainer.
      (c) Recognize need to defer to knowledge of objective health professionals (certified athletic trainer or team physician) when present.
  b. **Education of student trainers**
    i. Assist coaches and certified athletic trainers in daily tasks
    ii. Courses in summer and/or during school year
    iii. May be funded through vocational education monies
    iv. Provides career opportunities in health care fields
  c. **Education of athletic directors and other key administrative personnel**
    i. Athletic administration courses:
      (a) Athletic Health Care System, National Leadership Institute—1 week course held annually each summer

- Also attended by team physicians, athletic trainers, coaches, physical therapists, school nurses, and risk managers
- Contact: Stephen G. Rice, MD, Athletic Health Care System, Sports Medicine, Box 354060, University of Washington, Seattle, WA 98195-4060; 206-543-6734; FAX 206-543-6573.

(b) National Certification for Athletic Administrators through National Federation of State High School Associations

ii. Organizational management of operating safe athletic program
iii. Safety, health care, and liability issues stressed
iv. Course for "general," who must supervise the entire athletic program
v. Broader scope than perspective of athletic trainer alone

3. **Central training room**
   a. Treatment facility:
      i. May also be rehabilitation room
      ii. Not weight room or conditioning center
   b. Physical parameters of room:
      i. Size—square footage
      ii. Location within building—proximity to gymnasium and lockers
      iii. Access for boy and girl athletes
      iv. Lighting
      v. Heating and ventilation
      vi. Plumbing and drainage
      vii. Electricity
   c. Equipment and supplies
   d. Layout of room for smooth traffic flow
   e. Stocking, storage, inventory, and budgeting
   f. Security
   g. Daily operations
   h. Educational resource center—posters and books
4. **Standard procedures**
   a. **Preseason screening and preparticipation physical examination; coordinate with medical community, athletic trainer, and coaches:**
      i. Establish fitness expectations or requirements:
         (a) Flexibility
         (b) Muscle strength in legs and shoulders
         (c) Muscle endurance
         (d) Aerobic capacity
         (e) Body composition
      ii. Know athletes:
         (a) Chronic illnesses (asthma, diabetes, seizures)
         (b) Differences from other athletes based on screening exam
         (c) Response to pain:
            - High pain threshold—hide injuries; rarely report
            - Low pain threshold—constant injury reporting
         (d) Plays within capabilities and rules versus takes excessive risks
         (e) Mental "toughness"—psychological and emotional make-up
      iii. Athlete education
         (a) Weight gain—anabolic steroids and supplements
         (b) Weight loss—fat, not water or muscle mass; eating disorders
         (c) Nutrition
         (d) Wellness and general health
         (e) Substance abuse

(f) High-risk behaviors
iv. Guidelines for athletes—in season, off-season, summer fitness
b. **Communication:**
i. Location of telephones, wireless (cellular) telephone, pagers
ii. Lists of key people and telephone numbers widely disseminated
iii. Whom to notify in case of emergencies
iv. Emergency information cards for every athlete
v. Lists of hospitals, clinics, physicians—addresses and phone numbers
c. **Preparedness:**
i. Emergency information cards for every athlete
ii. Checklists to ensure proper materials available daily:
(a) First aid kit supply list
(b) Sideline equipment list
(c) Communication supplies—sideline notebook
d. **Area safety:**
i. Safety inspections at start of year and season
ii. Daily inspections of playing surface and surroundings
e. **Evaluation procedure for injuries**
f. **Written action plan for emergencies:**
i. Written policy statement—what to do in case of an emergency
ii. Define specific medical emergencies
iii. Emergency map—prepared in advance
(a) How to get emergency response vehicle to site
(b) How to drive to appropriate medical facility
iv. Paramedical units—Medic One versus Aid Unit:
(a) Medic One—800–1000 hours of training
(b) Aid Unit—100 hours of training
(c) Be sure to ask for most appropriate assistance.
v. Written note should always accompany injured athlete.
vi. Call ahead to hospital when appropriate—talk directly to emergency room physician.
vii. Notify parents, guardians and personal physicians.
g. Protocols and guidelines
h. Steps to recovery and full rehabilitation—as policy
i. Criteria for return to play—as policy

5. **Record keeping**
a. Purposes:
i. Injury surveillance
ii. Document care and treatments given
iii. Communicate among persons involved in athlete's health care
iv. Protection regarding medical-legal liability
v. Inventory supplies and cost justification
vi. Quality assurance and accountability
b. Forms:
i. Athlete emergency information card
ii. Attendance and injuries (daily report as part of injury surveillance system):
(a) Note all athletes absent, ill, or injured
(b) Healthy athletes who are present—leave box blank
(c) Completed daily; submitted monthly
iii. Training room treatment log:
(a) All treated athletes sign in daily
(b) Trainers record (check off) treatments received

iv. Athlete injury report—two part, four-copy NCR (no-carbon-required) form:
  (a) From coach, athletic trainer, or team physician to parents, athlete's personal physician, or hospital emergency department
    • One part gives information to health care provider
    • Other part receives findings or advice from provider
  (b) Copies to coach, athletic trainer or athletic director, team physician, provider
v. Sports injury report or individual charts for athletes:
  (a) Can be "charting" for athletic trainer or team physician
  (b) Uses date of evaluation as the filing point
  (c) With three-copy NCR form, copies for coach, athletic trainer or athletic director, and team physician
vi. Master daily injury list—all sports:
  (a) List of all athletes not at full participation
  (b) All those on limited participation and no participation recorded
  (c) Includes diagnosis, limitations, treatments, and rehabilitation

6. **Evaluation and feedback, technical assistance**
  a. **Needs assessment**
  b. **Education**—knowledge gain in courses for coaches and student trainers:
    i. Pretest/posttest comparison—document significant knowledge gains
    ii. Compare to established norms among similar trainees
  c. **Prevention**—emergency preparedness and sideline safety:
    i. Observation technique
    ii. Checklist for first aid kit contents
    iii. Checks for stretching, area safety, emergency equipment, presence of water, emergency information and written action plan, availability of athletic trainers and coaches to care for athletes
    iv. Printed report to return to school
    v. Compare results to established norms among similar schools
  d. **Injury data—injury surveillance:**
    i. Tabulate data, determine injury rates (Table 1):
      (a) Numerator—number of injuries, body part or injury type
      (b) Denominator (measure of risk)—number of participants or athletic exposures
    ii. Follow year-to-year trends within school and sports
    iii. Compare self to others in data bank—this year and against prior years
    iv. Actual findings may challenge "conventional wisdom"; nearly 60,000 athletes followed over 13 years in 2.5 million athletic exposures:
      (a) Girls cross country has the highest injury rate of all sports.
      (b) Fall sports have more injuries than spring sports.
      (c) Girls sports have more injuries than identical boys sports.
      (d) Cross country and soccer (boys and girls) are in the highest tier of injuries along with football, wrestling, and gymnastics.
    v. Provide basis for epidemiologic studies
  e. **Case studies:**
    i. Technique for monitoring quality of care rendered from moment of injury through return to play
    ii. Questionnaire to gather data from coach, athlete, and athletic trainer
    iii. Narrative prepared
    iv. Specific evaluation criteria developed and shared with evaluators
    v. Blind review by expert evaluators in sports medicine
    vi. Areas of evaluation:

TABLE 1. Injury Data Analysis: All Years, Fall 1979 through Spring 1992

Rank*	Sport	Season	Total Athletes	Injury Rate/100 Athletes/ Season	Injury Rate/1000 Athletes/ Season	Significant Injury Rate/ 1000 Athletic Exposures (1 wk)	Major Injury Rate/ 1000 Athletic Exposures (3 wk)	Percent of Different Athletes Injured
1	Girls' cross country	Fall	1299	61.4	17.3	3.3	0.9	33.1
2	Football	Fall	8560	58.8	12.7	3.1	0.9	36.7
3	Wrestling	Winter	3624	49.7	11.8	2.6	1.0	32.1
4	Girls' soccer	Fall	3186	43.7	11.6	2.9	0.7	31.6
5	Boys' cross country	Fall	2481	38.7	10.5	2.3	0.5	24.6
6	Girls' gymnastics	Winter	1082	38.9	10.0	2.3	0.7	26.2
7	Boys' soccer	Spring	3848	36.4	9.5	2.1	0.4	25.2
8	Girls' basketball	Winter	3634	34.5	7.1	1.7	0.5	24.2
9	Girls' track	Spring	3543	24.8	6.2	1.6	0.3	18.0
10	Boys' basketball	Winter	3874	29.2	5.5	1.3	0.3	22.9
11	Volleyball	Fall	3444	19.9	5.4	1.1	0.3	16.1
12	Softball	Spring	2957	18.3	4.8	1.2	0.3	14.8
13	Boys' track	Spring	4425	17.3	4.4	1.1	0.3	13.6
14	Baseball	Spring	3397	17.1	4.2	1.0	0.3	14.4
15	Fastpitch	Spring	134	11.9	2.4	1.2	0.6	11.9
16	Coed swimming	Winter	4004	8.3	2.2	0.5	0.2	6.4
17	Coed tennis	Fall/ Spring	4096	7.0	1.9	0.4	0.1	5.8
18	Coed golf	Fall/ Spring	2170	1.4	0.8	0.0	0.0	1.3
Total			59,758	30.6	7.6	1.8	0.5	21.1

* Ranking based on injury rate/1000 athletic exposures. Data contributed by 21 different high schools. Copyright, Stephen G. Rice, MD, 1993.

(a) Time frames:
- Moment of injury
- Later that day—before going home or to hospital
- Next day until rehabilitation over
- Day of return to play

(b) Categories of activities
- Injury recognition
- Transport
- Examination and assessment
- First aid and treatments
- Communication and advice
- Documentation—record keeping

vii. Identify strengths and weaknesses in care

viii. Overall quality assurance evaluation—process of health care provided

D. **Adoption process**

1. **Goal of permanent change and long-term results**
   a. Fidelity to install all six key elements
   b. Local control—identify local resources to maintain implementation and establish "ownership"
   c. Self-sufficiency from continued fidelity

2. **Adoption begins with awareness**
   a. Parents and boosters
   b. School boards
   c. Superintendents
   d. Curriculum directors
   e. Principals
   f. Risk managers/business managers
   g. Athletic directors
   h. Coaches
   i. Physicians
   j. Athletic trainers
   k. Sports medicine clinics
   l. Regional and state organizations
   m. Media
3. Networking
   a. Helps to generate a standard for quality of care for athletes
   b. Identifies other health professionals interested in bringing program to their area
   c. Spreads via the ripple effect through "disciples" with fidelity to concept
4. Adoption specifics
   a. Athletic Health Care System staff travels nationally to install system in individual schools or states.
   b. Individuals may come to summer National Leadership Institute for a week to learn in detail how to implement system in their locale with or without direct help of Athletic Health Care System staff.

Recommended Reading

1. Bloom M: Girls' cross country taking a heavy toll, study shows. New York Times, December 4, 1993, p 1.
2. Dougherty K, Rice SG: Cross country: A high risk sport? Cross Country Journal 11(6):1–8, 1994.
3. France R: Today's athletic training: Built on tomorrow's needs. The First Aider 61(1):6, 1991.
4. National Association for Sports and Physical Education (NASPE): National Standards for Athletic Coaches. Dubuque, Kendall/Hunt Publishing Company, 1995.
5. Ray R: Management Strategies in Athletic Training. Champaign, IL, Human Kinetics Publishers, 1994.
6. Rice SG (ed): Training Course Syllabus for the Athletic Health Care System. Seattle, HMS Publishing Services, 1988.
7. Rice SG: Epidemiology and mechanisms of sports injuries. In Teitz CT (ed): Scientific Foundations of Sports Medicine. Philadelphia, B.C. Decker, 1989, pp 3–23.
8. Rice SG: Organization of a sports medicine program. In Athletic Training and Sports Medicine, 2nd ed. Park Ridge, IL, American Academy of Orthopaedic Surgeons, 1989, pp 25–35.
9. Rice SG: An injury surveillance system. Sports Medicine Digest 13(8):1–2, 1991.
10. Rice SG: Dr. Rice responds to his study. Cross Country Journal 12(3):1–8, 1994.
11. Rice SG (ed): Administrative Manual for the National Leadership Institute. Seattle, Athletic Health Care System, University of Washington, 1995.
12. Rice SG, Foley WE: Assessment Manual—Athletic Health Care System, 3rd ed. Seattle, Athletic Health Care System, University of Washington, 1992.
13. Rice SG, Schlotfeldt JD, Foley WE: The athletic health care and training program: A comprehensive approach to the prevention and management of athletic injuries in high schools. West J Med 142:352–357, 1985.
14. Swenson EJ Jr: Setting up a high school sports medicine program. J Musculoskel Med 8(9):14–30, 1991.

11

Women in Sports

Elizabeth A. Joy, M.D., FACSM, and James G. Macintyre, M.D., FACSM

Fitness is not just for athletes; fitness is for everyone. We tell this to our patients every day, trying to encourage them to a lifestyle including regular exercise. An active lifestyle is important in women's health. Exercise begun in childhood and adolescence is more likely to be continued into adulthood. A woman's exercise goals and needs change throughout her life. Adolescent and young adult women are at risk for the female athlete triad. Exercise during pregnancy becomes an issue for women in their childbearing years. The interaction of exercise and menopause is important in the older woman. Female athletes are at risk for injuries as a result of their sporting activities. Injuries may be activity and/or age dependent. Early recognition and treatment of illness or injury as well as encouragement and appropriate patient education allow for safe participation in sports and exercise.

I. Female Athlete Triad

A. This is a term used to describe the relationship between **disordered eating**, **altered menstrual function**, and **abnormalities in bone mineralization**. The pressure placed on young female athletes to excel in sports has prompted some to adopt unhealthy eating habits to achieve unrealistic body composition. This puts them at risk for the development of the other two associated disorders, amenorrhea and osteoporosis. Athletes whose sports emphasize thinness or leanness tend to be at greater risk for the development of the triad. The prevalence of the complete triad among female athlete groups is largely unknown. Some small studies have demonstrated prevalence rates for disordered eating as high as 62% in certain athlete groups. The incidence of amenorrhea in the general population of premenopausal women is thought to be 2–5%. Studies of runners and dancers cite prevalence rates of 10–15%. The incidence of osteoporosis among female athletes is unknown. A large body of evidence now suggests, however, that bone not formed, or bone that is lost, may not be completely regained. Researchers have identified women in their 20s with bone densities comparable to women in their 60s, 70s, and 80s! Given these figures, it is important that health practitioners recognize the athlete at risk for the triad, pursue the appropriate evaluation, and prescribe adequate treatment.

B. **Disordered eating:** the spectrum of abnormal eating habits practiced by many individuals to lose or maintain their weight

1. Disordered eating behavior is **largely fueled by misconception** of athletes, nonathletes, coaches, parents, and peers who believe that thinner is better: "If I'm thinner, I'll run faster, jump higher, be more popular, be happier." The consequences of this behavior are significant.
   a. Some studies indicate that 20% of untreated anorectics die as a result of their disease.
   b. The medical and social costs of untreated eating disorders is significant in terms of prolonged inpatient or outpatient treatment and treatment of associated medical problems.

2. **Medical evaluation and treatment**
   a. **Medical history**
      i. **Eating behavior and medication use**
         (a) Restricting:
            - Average daily intake
            - Meals/day
            - Calories/day
            - Eliminated foods—fats, dairy, protein
         (b) Bingeing:
            - Frequency of binges
            - Foods binged on
            - Binge trigger foods
         (c) Purging activities:
            - Self-induced vomiting
            - Laxatives, diuretics, ipecac
            - Excessive exercise and exercise history—type, frequency, duration
         (d) Other medications:
            - Diet pills
            - Oral contraceptives
            - Nonsteroidal anti-inflammatory drugs (NSAIDs)—use may indicate ongoing injury, which may be indicative of disordered eating or poor nutrition
            - Anabolic steroids
            - Tobacco, alcohol, illicit drugs
      ii. **Weight**—current, ideal, most and least in the past year
      iii. **Menstrual history:**
         (a) Menarche
         (b) Last menstrual period
         (c) Skipped menstrual periods
         (d) Number menstrual periods in the past year
      iv. **Family history:**
         (a) Disordered eating
         (b) Obesity
         (c) Depression or anxiety
         (d) Substance abuse
      v. **Psychological history:**
         (a) Life stresses
         (b) Self-esteem and control issues
         (c) Ability to complete activities of daily living
         (d) Symptoms of depression (fatigue, sleep problems, suicidal ideation)
      vi. **Review of systems**
         (a) Anorexia nervosa—symptoms due to starvation and dehydration:
            - Lightheadedness, syncopal episodes
            - Weakness
            - Palpitations
            - Overuse injuries
            - Decreased school, work, sport performance
         (b) Bulimia nervosa—symptoms due to purging activity:
            - Frequent sore throats, dental or periodontal disease
            - Bloating
            - Abdominal pain
            - Diarrhea, constipation

- Gastrointestinal bleeding (upper—Mallory-Weiss tears due to self-induced vomiting; lower—rectal bleeding from finger manipulation of the rectum and/or frequent use of laxatives)
- Overuse injuries
- Decreased school, work, sport performance

b. **Physical examination** (pelvic examination indicated in women with alteration in menstrual function)

i. **Physical signs—anorexia nervosa** (secondary to starvation and dehydration):

(a) Hypotension
(b) Bradycardia
(c) Lanugo hair
(d) Dry skin, hair, nails
(e) Lower extremity edema

ii. **Physical signs—bulimia nervosa** (secondary to purging activities):

(a) Parotid gland hypertrophy
(b) Dental caries, peridontal disease
(c) Pharyngeal erythema
(d) Conjunctival petechiae
(e) Scars on the dorsum of hands
(f) Rectal fissures

iii. **Laboratory studies and tests**

(a) **Standard:**

- Complete blood count (anemia)
- Electrolytes (abnormalities associated with use of diuretics, laxatives, self-induced vomiting, undernourishment)
- Blood urea nitrogen, creatinine (dehydration)
- Calcium, magnesium, phosphorus, cholesterol, albumin, total protein (nutritional laboratory tests)
- Urinalysis

(b) **Optional:**

- Urine pregnancy test (if patient amenorrheic)
- Hormonal studies—follicle-stimulating hormone (FSH), estradiol (if patient amenorrheic)
- Thyroid function tests (if patient amenorrheic)
- Electrocardiogram—bradycardia (heart rate < 50 bpm), history of syncope or near syncope, arrhythmia, significant electrolyte abnormalities, weight < 25% of ideal body weight
- Bone density evaluation (history of stress fractures; may also be used as an educational/motivational tool in patients who may be reluctant to take hormone therapy in light of low estrogen state, amenorrhea, and stress fractures)
- Calorimetry (may be useful in the patient with "unexplained" weight loss)

c. **Treatment:** need to determine level of treatment (inpatient versus outpatient)

i. **Indications for inpatient treatment:**

(a) Significant hypotension
(b) Significant arrhythmia
(c) Repeated syncopal episodes
(d) Severe electrolyte disturbances (potassium < 2.5 mg/dl)
(e) Weight < 25% below ideal body weight
(f) Suicidal intent
(g) Purging > 5 times/day

(h) Severe body image disturbance
(i) Failure to respond to outpatient treatment after 3 months
(j) Concurrent alcohol/drug abuse
(k) Poor patient support system, inadequate outpatient treatment facilities

ii. **Outpatient treatment:**
(a) **Set a weight goal**—below height of 5 feet, 100 lbs; add 5 lbs for each inch over 5 feet
(b) **Behavior contract:**
- No skipping meals
- Decreased or no purging
- Decreased or no exercise
- Avoidance of "lite" or low-fat products

(c) **Medications:**
- Multivitamin, calcium 1000 mg/day, iron 325 mg 2–3 times/day
- Hormone replacement therapy (amenorrhea)
- Laxatives, fiber (history of laxative abuse)
- Antidepresssants (selective serotonin reuptake inhibitors)
- Antiemetics (may be useful in bulimics)

(d) **Referrals:**
- Nutritionist—daily eating record for 7 days completed by patient before initial visit
- Psychologist—indicated for those patients with body image disturbance and those with comorbid mental illness
- Dentist—dental caries, peridontal disease

(e) **Activity restriction:**
- < 10% ideal body weight—restrict competition
- < 25% ideal body weight—restrict practice and competition

(f) **Physician follow-up:**
- Every 1–2 weeks
- Vital signs, weight
- Laboratory tests—hemoglobin, electrolytes if indicated

C. **Exercise-induced menstrual disorders**

1. **Spectrum of menstrual dysfunction related to exercise**
a. Delayed menarche
b. Shortening of luteal phase
c. Anovulation
d. Oligomenorrhea
e. Amenorrhea

2. **Definitions**
a. **Delayed menarche**
i. Average age menarche in United States is 12.8 years (normal range 10 to 16 years)
ii. American Academy of Pediatrics defined delayed menarche as > 16 years or 1 year beyond average of mother and sisters
iii. Age of menarche in athletic females is later than in nonathletic females. Numerous studies have established that menarche occurs later in athletes than in nonathletes:
(a) Some have concluded from these observations that participation in sports delays sexual maturation; however, the majority of studies supporting this theory have been retrospective and inherently biased.
(b) Others have believed that the later age of menarche in athletes is due to social rather than physiologic influences.

(c) Athletic competition often favors the later maturer, who is leaner and has less body mass.
(d) Early maturing girls may be socialized away from sports.

b. **Luteal phase suppression**
   i. Shortening of the luteal phase (normal range 12–17 days) results in decreased serum progesterone levels.
   ii. Menstrual cycle length is essentially normal.
   iii. Incidence in sedentary population is 16%; athletic population 33%.
   iv. Intermediate or end point of menstrual dysfunction?
   v. Side effects of luteal phase suppression are unknown.
   vi. Inadequate luteal phase accounts for 3–4% of infertility.
   vii. In runners, more miles per week paralleled greater shortening of the luteal phase.

c. **Anovulation**
   i. Tends to affect younger women with immature hypothalamic–pituitary–ovarian (HPO) axis
   ii. May have regular menses; most often oligomenorrheic, sometimes amenorrheic
   iii. Not recognized in regularly menstruating woman until she tries to get pregnant
   iv. Appears to be reversible with altered lifestyle

d. **Oligomenorrhea**
   i. Defined as irregular, infrequent menstruation:
      (a) 6–9 menstrual periods per year
      (b) Cycle length > 35 days, < 90 days
   ii. Intermediate form of amenorrhea:
      (a) Anovulatory
      (b) Low circulation estrogens
      (c) Similar adverse effects as amenorrhea

e. **Amenorrhea**
   i. Defined by the American College of Sports Medicine as absence of 3–12 consecutive menstrual periods
   ii. Most extreme form of menstrual dysfunction associated with exercise
   iii. **Diagnosis of exclusion**
   iv. Always consider pregnancy as cause

3. **Oligomenorrhea and amenorrhea**
   a. **Described in all sports**
   b. **Incidence**
      i. 2–5% sedentary
      ii. 10–50% runners (mileage and intensity)
      iii. 15–40% dancers (level of performance, competitiveness)
   c. **Risk factors**
      i. Age—younger females (with immature HPO axis)
      ii. Activity—runners (26%); cyclists (12%); swimmers (12%)
      iii. Intensity—more strenuous exercise
      iv. Mileage—more miles per week
      v. History of menstrual irregularity
      vi. Prepubertal training
      vii. Delayed menarche
      viii. Low body weight/weight loss; low body fat/fat loss—seems to play a role, but does not in itself cause altered menstrual function
      ix. Nulliparity
      x. Never used oral contraceptive pills—twice as likely to suffer a stress fracture than those who have used oral contraceptives

 xi. Diet—deficient in protein and total calories. **Poor nutrition may be the most important factor in individuals with exercise amenorrhea.**
 xii. Eating disorders
 xiii. Psychological stress—studies contradictory
 xiv. Genetic/hereditary factors—may play a role in age of menarche
 xv. Total number of risk factors—the more risk factors an athlete has, the more likely she has exercise-related menstrual dysfunction.

d. **Etiology of exercise-induced menstrual dysfunction**
 i. Decreased pulsatile release of gonadotropin-releasing hormone (GnRH) from the hypothalamus
 ii. Leads to decreased luteinizing hormone (LF) and FSH pulses from the anterior pituitary

e. **Causes of GnRH pulse inhibition**
 i. Beta-endorphins—difficult to correlate serum and cerebrospinal fluid levels, role uncertain
 ii. Cortisol—increased in both exercise and anorexia, may play a role
 iii. Catecholestrogens—formed by the hydroxylation of estrogen and functions as a circulating catecholamine
 iv. Melatonin—levels are significantly increased in women with hypothalamic amenorrhea, role uncertain
 v. Androgens—levels increase immediately following training, but mean and 24-hour levels no different than in controls, role uncertain
 vi. Prolactin—no evidence for hyperprolactinemia in athletic amenorrhea

f. **Consequences of oligomenorrhea and amenorrhea**
 i. Osteoporosis
 ii. Stress fractures
 iii. Endometrial hyperplasia—may be seen in the euestrogenic, oligomenorrheic, anovulatory athlete
 iv. Other injuries—increased incidence of soft tissue injuries

g. **Osteoporosis:** Drinkwater and colleagues looked at lumbar bone density in amenorrheic and cyclic athletes.
 i. Previously amenorrheic athletes who became cyclic increased their bone mass but not to the level of the athletes who had never been amenorrheic.
 ii. Athletes who remained amenorrheic continued to lose bone density over the study period.

h. **Stress fractures**
 i. Consequences of impact exercise and decreased bone mineral density
 ii. A study of college female distance runners showed 48% amenorrheic athletes suffered stress fractures, compared with only 29% of regularly menstruating runners.

4. **Evaluation of menstrual dysfunction**
 a. Menstrual history
 i. Menarche
 ii. Menstrual periods per year
 iii. Flow length
 iv. Last menstrual period
 b. Training schedule
 i. Sessions per week
 ii. Miles per week
 iii. Intensity
 iv. Competitive activities
 c. Diet

i. Calories/day
ii. Protein intake
iii. Calcium intake

d. Eating disordered behavior

e. Drugs
i. Oral contraceptive pills
ii. Steroids
iii. Diuretics
iv. Laxatives
v. Diet pills
vi. Thyroid medications
vii. Vitamins
viii. Illicit drugs
ix. Alcohol
x. NSAIDs

f. Injuries
i. Stress fractures
ii. Overuse injuries

g. Psychological stress

5. **Physical examination**

a. Height, weight (body fat), hirsutism, parotid gland enlargement, dentition, hands and fingers, pelvic examination

b. **Adolescent female:** Physical examination of the adolescent female with amenorrhea may indicate the underlying pathology.
i. No breasts, no uterus—should prompt chromosomal evaluation (rare)
ii. No breasts, normal uterus—suggests gonadal dysgenesis, hypogonadotropic hypogonadism, resistant ovarian syndrome
iii. Normal breasts, no uterus—suggests testicular feminization
iv. Normal breasts, normal uterus—suggests secondary amenorrhea

c. **Laboratory examination**
i. Urine pregnancy test, thyroid-stimulating hormone (TSH), prolactin (routine)
ii. Progestin challenge test:
(a) Administer medroxyprogesterone (Provera) 10 mg orally for 5 days.
(b) Two to 5 days later patient should have a withdrawal menstrual bleed. This indicates a positive test and implies adequate levels of circulating estrogen.
iii. FSH/LH:
(a) FSH/LH high—ovarian failure; FSH/LH low—athletic amenorrhea
(b) Not necessary to order on a routine basis. Need to order if progestin challenge test negative.
iv. In the patient who has a history of regular menstrual periods yet becomes amenorrheic during a period of increased training:
(a) If urine pregnancy test is negative, can assume amenorrhea is due to training.
(b) If amenorrhea persists longer than 3–6 months or patient develops stress fracture, need to consider hormone replacement therapy.
(c) Observe patient after training decreases—if spontaneous menstruation returns, no further workup or treatment needs to be pursued.

6. **Treatment**

a. **Alter lifestyle**
i. **Decrease training, increase body weight.**
ii. Most athletes are reluctant to do this. Those with clinically significant weight loss, however, should be required to meet recommended weights before return to practice or competition.

b. **Hormonal treatment**
   i. Euestrogenic, anovulatory—Medroxyprogesterone 10 mg, days 15–25. Every 3 months is probably adequate withdrawal.
   ii. Hypoestrogenic, amenorrheic—oral contraceptives, cyclic conjugated estrogens (Premarin) and medroxyprogesterone. This will probably provide adequate amounts of estrogen to prevent, and perhaps restore, bone mineral losses.

c. **Diet**
   i. Increase total calories—consider nutrition consultation
   ii. Increase protein intake (1–2 g/kg/day)
   iii. Adequate calcium intake (1500 mg/day)

D. **Osteoporosis**

1. **Pathophysiology**
   a. **Metabolic causes** (hypoestrogenism)
      i. Athletic amenorrhea
      ii. Menopause
      iii. Hyperprolactinemia
   b. **Medical illnesses**
      i. Hypothyroidism or hyperthyroidism
      ii. Malnutrition
      iii. Chronic illnesses
      iv. Renal insufficiency
      v. Hyperparathyroidism
      vi. Connective tissue disorders
      vii. Malignancy
   c. **Medications**
      i. Corticosteroids
      ii. Excessive thyroid replacement
      iii. Thiazide diuretics
   d. **Diet and habits**
      i. Excessive caffeine intake
      ii. Inadequate calcium intake
      iii. Alcohol abuse
      iv. Tobacco use
      v. Prolonged bed rest, inadequate weight-bearing exercise
      vi. Low body mass (decreased daily bone stress)
2. **Bone density determination:** Dual energy x-ray absorptiometry (DEXA) is gold standard—more precise and uses a smaller radiation dose than either dual-photon absorptiometry or computed tomography.
3. **Exercise**—mechanism of action
   a. Increases bone density by increasing mechanical stress on bone.
   b. Stronger muscles exert greater forces; therefore, resistance training has been shown to improve bone density.
   c. Non–weight-bearing aerobic exercise (e.g., swimming) does not seem to positively impact on bone density.
   d. Weight-bearing exercise without adequate nutrition or adequate levels of estrogen has less of a positive effect.
   e. The optimal amount of exercise to improve or maintain bone health has yet to be determined.
4. **Amenorrhea**
   a. Delayed menarche (> 16 years of age)—low estrogen state during a time of peak bone mass accumulation leads to inadequate primary bone acquisition.

b. Secondary amenorrhea—premature loss of estrogen leads to premature bone loss.
c. Menopause—most bone loss occurs in the first 4–6 years following menopause.

5. **Treatment**
   a. Hormone replacement therapy
      i. Oral contraceptives
      ii. Cyclic estrogen and progesterone therapy
   b. Calcium—1000 to 1500 mg/day
   c. Weight-bearing exercise, resistance training
   d. Vitamin D
   e. Calcitonin, alendronate for significant osteoporosis

II. Exercise During Pregnancy

A. Pregnancy is a normal condition for women, and **exercise should be part of normal pregnancy**. The goals of exercise during pregnancy should be to maintain maternal fitness levels, while minimizing risk to the developing fetus. Previously sedentary women may start an exercise program during their pregnancy, and regular exercisers may continue with most prepregnant exercise programs. Exercise guidelines are tailored to each individual woman. As a woman's pregnancy changes, so must her exercise regimen. **The primary concern with exercise during pregnancy is safety.** The original American College of Obstetricians and Gynecologists (ACOG) guidelines for exercise during pregnancy were published in 1986. In February 1994 (ACOG Technical Bulletin 189), the guidelines were revised and liberalized after numerous studies demonstrated maternal benefits and no fetal or neonatal risks with exercise during pregnancy (Table 1).

B. **Contraindications to exercise during pregnancy**

1. **Absolute obstetric contraindications**
   a. Pregnancy-induced hypertension
   b. Premature rupture of membranes
   c. Preterm labor during the prior or current pregnancy or both
   d. Incompetent cervix or cerclage
   e. Persistent 2nd or 3rd trimester bleeding
   f. Intrauterine growth retardation
2. **Absolute medical contraindications**
   a. Hemodynamically significant heart disease
   b. Uncontrolled hypertension
   c. Uncontrolled renal disease
   d. Hemodynamically significant anemia
   e. Uncontrolled diabetes mellitus
3. **Relative obstetric contraindications**
   a. Multiple gestations
   b. Previous history of miscarriage (more than 1)
   c. Breech position in the 3rd trimester
   d. History of precipitous labor
4. **Relative medical contraindications**
   a. Malnutrition
   b. Cardiac arrhythmia
   c. Anemia
   d. History of extremely sedentary lifestyle
   e. Active thyroid disease

C. **Benefits of exercise during pregnancy**

1. **Physical**
   a. Maintenance or improvement of maternal fitness
   b. Control of excess weight gain
   c. Improved appearance and posture
   d. Increased energy
   e. Improved sleep
   f. Less backache
   g. Fewer problems with varicose veins
   h. Less water retention
   i. Possible decreased labor complications and shortened labor
   j. More rapid postpartum recovery

TABLE 1. American College of Obstetricians and Gynecologists Guidelines for Exercise During Pregnancy and the Postpartum Period

1986	1994
Regular activity (3 times/week) is preferable to intermittent activity. Competitive activity is discouraged	Regular activity (3 times/week) is preferable to intermittent activity
Vigorous exercise should not be performed in hot, humid weather or during times of febrile illness. Maternal core temperature should not exceed 38°C. Liquids should be taken liberally before, during, and after exercise to prevent dehydration	Pregnant women who exercise in the first trimester should augment heat dissipation by ensuring adequate hydration, appropriate clothing, and optimal environmental surroundings
Ballistic movements (jerky, bouncy motions) should be avoided. Exercise on a wooden or carpeted surface Deep flexion or extension of joints should be avoided because of connective tissue laxity. Activities that require jumping, jarring motions or rapid changes in direction should be avoided because of joint instability	Morphologic changes in pregnancy should serve as a relative contraindication to types of exercise in which balance could be detrimental to maternal or fetal well-being, especially in the third trimester. Further, any type of exercise involving the potential for even mild abdominal trauma should be avoided
Vigorous exercise should be preceded by a 5-minute period of muscle warm-up	
Vigorous exercise should be followed by a period of gradually declining activity. Stretches should not be taken to the point of maximal resistance	
Maternal heart rate should not exceed 140 beats per minute Strenuous activities should not exceed 15 minutes' duration	Women should be aware of the decreased oxygen available for aerobic exercise during pregnancy. They should be encouraged to modify the intensity of exercise according to maternal symptoms. Pregnant women should stop exercising when fatigued and not exercise to exhaustion. Weight-bearing exercises may under some circumstances be continued at intensities similar to those before pregnancy throughout pregnancy. Non–weight-bearing exercises such as cycling or swimming minimize the risk of injury and facilitate the continuation of exercise during pregnancy
No exercises should be performed in the supine position after the fourth month of gestation	Women should avoid exercise in the supine position after the first trimester. Such a position is associated with decreased cardiac output in most pregnant women. Prolonged periods of motionless standing should also be avoided
Exercises that employ the Valsalva maneuver should be avoided	
Caloric intake should be adequate to meet the needs of both pregnancy and exercise	Pregnancy requires an additional 300 kcal/day to maintain metabolic homeostasis. Thus, women who exercise during pregnancy should be particularly careful to ensure adequate diet
Women who have sedentary lifestyles should begin activity at very low intensity and advance activity very gradually	Many of the physiologic and morphologic changes of pregnancy persist 4–6 weeks postpartum. Thus, prepregnancy exercise routines should be resumed gradually

2. **Psychological**
    a. Improved mental outlook and self-image
    b. Improved sense of control
    c. Relief of tension

D. **Exercise prescription—safety, individualization, flexibility**

1. **Sedentary women**
    a. Mode—walking, bicycling, stair climbing, aerobic dance, water aerobics, swimming

   b. Intensity—65–75% maximum heart rate; perceived exertion = moderately hard
   c. Duration—30 minutes
   d. Frequency—minimum of three times per week
2. **Recreational athletes and regular fitness exercisers**
   a. Mode—same; running or jogging, cross country skiing, downhill skiing, water skiing, horseback riding, dance, aerobic dance instruction, ice or roller skating, tennis
   b. Intensity—65–85% maximum heart rate; perceived exertion = moderately hard to hard
   c. Duration—30–60 minutes
   d. Frequency—three to five times per week
3. **Elite athletes**
   a. Mode—same; some competitive activities
   b. Intensity—75–85% of maximum heart rate; perceived exertion = hard
   c. Duration—60–90 minutes
   d. Frequency—four to six times per week

III. Exercise and Menopause

A. **Menopause—cessation of menstrual function**

B. **Climacteric—broader term, describing the gradual change from reproductive to nonreproductive stages of life**
   1. 35–45 years climacteric begins
   2. 46–55 years perimenopause, ovarian failure begins
   3. > 56 years postmenopause

C. **Menopausal symptoms**
   1. **Reproductive system**
      a. Cessation of menstruation
      b. Vaginal dryness
      c. Stress incontinence
      d. Decreased breast tissue mass and tissue elasticity
   2. **Cardiovascular:** increased cholesterol, low-density lipoproteins, and triglycerides; decreased high-density lipoproteins
   3. **Skeletal system**—osteoporosis
      a. 33–50% of all postmenopausal women develop osteoporosis.
      b. 1.3 million fractures per year occur as a result of osteoporosis at a cost of $10 billion.
   4. **Integumentary system**
      a. Wrinkling of skin
      b. Thinning, graying of hair
   5. **Psychological**
      a. Depression and anxiety
      b. Insomnia
   6. **Other:** vasomotor instability—85% of women experience hot flashes.

D. **Regular exercise**
   1. **Starting an exercise program:** Before engaging in vigorous physical activity, women > 50 years of age who have two or more coronary risk factors or symptoms suggestive of cardiovascular disease should undergo a complete physical examination and a graded exercise stress test.
   2. **Cardiovascular exercise to improve health and fitness**
      a. Types—continuous aerobic exercise using large muscle groups, e.g., walking, jogging, aerobic dancing, swimming
      b. Frequency—regular exercise preferable to intermittent exercise; minimum of three sessions per week

c. Duration—20 minutes of continuous aerobic activity
d. Intensity—65–85% of maximal heart rate
e. Benefits
   i. Improved lipid profiles
   ii. Increased bone mass (seen with weight-bearing exercise and resistance training)
   iii. Decreased anxiety and depression, improved sleep
   iv. Decreased vasomotor instability
   v. Maintenance of weight
f. Stress incontinence risk—to maintain/improve continence, perform Kegel exercises: 25 repetitions/set
   8 counts/repetition
   2–3 sets/day

3. **Strength training**
   a. Falls due to loss of balance are a leading cause of morbidity and mortality in the elderly. Falls are the primary cause of death in people > 64 years of age. There is a 20–40% decrease in isometric muscle strength by the age of 60.
   b. Studies have demonstrated strength gains up to 195% in women following a 24-week strength training program.
   c. Types—heavy resistance training; major muscle groups (3 days/week)
   d. Benefits—improved strength, balance, and bone density
4. **Flexibility exercise:** benefits—improved balance, biomechanics

E. **Nutrition and medications**
   1. Calcium: 1000–1500 mg/day
   2. Hormone replacement therapy—cyclic estrogen and progesterone
   3. Adequate dietary intake—age, size, and activity level dependent

IV. Musculoskeletal Injuries in Athletic Women

Musculoskeletal injuries account for up to 40% of the conditions seen in the average general practitioner's office. There are two broad categories: overuse injuries and overstress injuries. Overstress injuries are the acute injuries associated with single episodes of macrotrauma to the bones or soft tissues. These include ligamentous sprains and muscular strains as well as bony fractures. It is important to remember that a fracture is merely a soft tissue injury associated with a broken bone. The general principles of soft tissue treatment and rehabilitation still apply.

A. **Overstress (acute injuries)**
   1. **Dealing with acute injuries involves the PRICE principle.**
      a. **Protection from further injury:** accomplished with the use of casting, splints, and braces. General sports medicine principles attempt to minimize the use of immobilization for treatment of injuries to effect more rapid rehabilitation and return to activities. Notwithstanding, casts and splints are occasionally necessary for treating fractures, but rigid immobilization is rarely indicated for the treatment of soft tissue injuries alone. There are numerous braces that allow for protected motion yet still allow joint mobility to avoid the effects of immobilization on the joint cartilage and on muscle and tendon strength and function.
      b. **Rest:** Acutely injured structures should be rested, although absolute rest should generally be avoided. Continued athletic performance is unwise on the acutely injured limb because this may provoke increased swelling, further injury, and prolonged disability. Although the injury should be rested, this does not mean that the rest of the body cannot be exercised. It is good from both a psychological and a physiologic point of view to continue on with exercise that does not stress the injured area, including cycling, swimming, or deep water running. These activities can maintain cardiovascular fitness as well as allow for protected range of motion.

c. **Ice:** Ice is an excellent treatment for acute soft tissue injuries. Ice relieves pain, controls edema, and reduces inflammation. Heat should never be applied to acute injuries because it tends to provoke an increase in local swelling and should be reserved for use after 5–7 days. When persistent swelling is present, heat can be a useful adjunct but should always be followed by ice, commonly referred to as "contrast therapy."

d. **Compression:** Acute injuries should generally receive compression to minimize edema. This may come in the form of an Ace Bandage with a compression pad over an acute muscle injury or taping to provide support and compression for injuries such as ankle sprains. Remember the importance of distal circulation and avoid distal edema when dealing with compression of proximal injuries. This is especially important in the older athlete, in whom the possibility of venous stasis and deep venous thrombosis is increased. If compression of the proximal portion of the leg is used, it is advisable to use a Jobst stocking or compression device to provide some compression to the lower, more dependent part of the leg.

e. **Elevation:** Acutely injured limbs should be elevated above the heart whenever practical to prevent edema and assist in pain relief.

2. **Ankle sprains**
   a. **Definition:** injury to the ligamentous supports of the ankle
   b. **Causes:** Ankle sprains are the most common musculoskeletal injury, with thousands occurring every day. Women are particularly vulnerable to ankle sprains because they generally have tight heel cords, which maintain the foot in a plantarflexed position, in which there is reduced stability of the talus within the ankle mortice. High-heeled shoes present a similar risk.
   c. **Signs and symptoms** See Chapter 50, "Ankle and Leg Injuries."
   d. **Treatment** See Chapter 50, "Ankle and Leg Injuries."
3. **Anterior cruciate ligament injury**
   a. **Definition:** The anterior cruciate ligament is an intra-articular structure joining the tibia to the femur. It is the primary restraint for anterior translation of the tibia on the femur as well as for rotational movements. It is a secondary restraint for varus and valgus stress and can be injured alone or in combination with other ligamentous structures, depending on the knee position and the magnitude and direction of the injuring force. Because of its location within the joint, it does not heal on its own and may require surgical reconstruction in some women.
   b. **Causes**
      i. Knee injuries are common in a wide variety of contact and noncontact sports. Particularly troublesome for women is the noncontact injury to the anterior cruciate ligament, which occurs with attempts to decelerate, cut, or pivot on a planted foot.
      ii. **The exact reasons why female athletes are at particularly high risk for anterior cruciate injuries are not clear, but a number of theories have been proposed:** Smaller ligament size, a narrowed intercondylar notch, inadequate strength, ligamentous hyperlaxity, defects of neuromuscular coordination, and hormonally induced laxity during certain phases of the menstrual cycle. All of these should be considered conjecture at present because anterior cruciate ligament injuries are likely multifactorial in nature.
   c. **Signs and symptoms** See Chapter 49, "Knee Injuries."
   d. **Physical findings and radiographic findings** See Chapter 49, "Knee Injuries."
   e. **Treatment** See Chapter 49, "Knee Injuries."

B. **Overuse injuries**

1. In contrast to traumatic injuries, overuse injuries result from repetitive microtrauma to bony, ligamentous, or musculotendinous structures. They generally arise from the inability of the body to absorb the forces generated by the repeated cyclic loading of the musculoskeletal structures. Although it might seem that these injuries occur in a random fashion, it is possible to identify numerous factors involved in their causation. Several factors are related to the athletes themselves, including strength and flexibility, biomechanics and alignment, individual variations in bony and ligamentous structures and previous injuries that have been incompletely rehabilitated and have led to imbalances or functional asymmetries. Factors that are considered extrinsic to the athlete include training methods, shoes and equipment, and training surfaces.
2. **Etiologic factors**
   a. **Inadequate strength and flexibility:** The muscles are the shock absorbers for the joints. They are required to absorb the forces involved with repeated impacts or movements. If there is inadequate strength or endurance of the muscular structures, fatigue results and overload can occur to the muscles, ligaments, tendons, or bones. Inadequate flexibility can cause relative tissue tightness, leading to the improper mechanics or imbalances of the forces acting on the joints. This is specifically true for injuries to the knee and shoulder. Imbalances in muscle strength between major groups can lead to a tendency to acute muscle tears and injuries. Individuals who have too much joint laxity can be predisposed to injury unless muscular support and balance are optimized. This is especially common in throwers and swimmers.

   b. **Functional biomechanics and alignment:** To fully understand the problem of overuse injuries, it is important to remember that the injured joint or structure is only one part of the kinetic chain of muscles and joints that are involved in performing the motion or action. This is particularly true for the knee in running and for the shoulder in throwing. It is important to consider the other structures both above and below the injured area when dealing with these types of injuries. Incomplete rehabilitation of previous injury may cause abnormal or restricted motion, predisposing the injury in another part of the chain. In running sports, the alignment and biomechanics of the lower limb can lead to problems, especially when associated with excess pronation or supination.

   c. **Hormonal and nutritional status:** As previously discussed, highly trained women can be at risk for the development of the female athlete triad of disordered eating, amenorrhea, and osteoporosis. Lower circulating estrogen levels can lead to increased osteoclast activity with bone resorption and increased risk of stress fractures. Nutritional deficiencies can lead to loss of muscle mass and early muscle fatigue, predisposing to overuse injuries.

   d. **Training methods:** The most common cause of injuries is inappropriate training methods, which usually take the form of doing too much activity too soon. Training errors include excessive duration or intensity of training, failure to allow adaptation to new training levels, failure to recognize the specificity of training when changing activities, and failure to allow for individual differences in adaptation and performances.

   e. **Training shoes and equipment:** Many individuals suffer running-related injuries because of the use of inappropriate footwear. Footwear design is generally a compromise between motion-control features and shock absorption. Increases in one often lead to decreases in the other. Problems arise when women buy footwear that is not appropriate for their type of individual biomechanics, foot type, or activity. Problems can also arise in other sports when bicycles are not properly adjusted to an individual's size or alignment or when racquets are not properly sized and selected.

f. **Training surface** is important for running sports. Excessively hard surfaces, such as concrete, result in more impact than relatively soft-packed trails, leading to overuse injuries. Similarly, aerobic dance classes performed on hard surfaces can lead to injury. Running on banked surfaces or cambered roadsides can also lead to injury.

3. **Treatment** for overuse injuries depends on three steps. Unfortunately, many athletes are treated only until their symptoms resolve and are sent back to activities without being completely rehabilitated. All the steps are important, and failure to deal with any one of the factors can lead to repeated injuries.
   a. **Relief of symptoms**
      i. Ice massage, anti-inflammatory medications, and physical therapy
      ii. Modified rest
   b. **Correct underlying factors**
      i. Any factor that has been identified as the cause of the injury should be corrected.
      ii. Specific strengthening or flexibility exercises
      iii. Appropriate footwear or equipment or possibly a supportive orthotic, gait retraining, or the proper alignment and adjustment of equipment to the individual's biomechanics
      iv. Treat joint mobility and strength deficiencies proximal and distal to the joint in question to ensure the proper function of all segments required in the activity.
      v. Braces may be important to allow an earlier return to activities or help alleviate the symptoms in ongoing activities.
   c. **Reintroduction of activities** Activities must be restarted gradually, with training reintroduced at a lower level with a progressive buildup of frequency, intensity, and duration. Reinjuries often occur if training is reintroduced too quickly. Proprioceptive training is important, especially in the treatment of ankle and foot injuries and knee injuries.

4. **Shoulder impingement syndrome**
   a. **Definition:** Impingement is a group of syndromes with a common end point of tendinitis of the rotator cuff or inflammation of the subacromial bursa.
   b. **Causes:** It was once thought that impingement was solely anatomic in basis, resulting from the pinching of the cuff and bursa underneath the bony and ligamentous subacromial arch. It is now recognized that impingement can result from other factors, such as primary tendonopathies, glenohumeral instability, muscle weakness and imbalances, capsular laxity, poor scapulothoracic stability, acromioclavicular arthritis, and abnormal movement patterns of the shoulder because of tightness of the posterior capsule. Women are particularly susceptible to calcific tendinitis and to impingement caused by postural defects.
      i. **Impingement may be due to acute calcific tendinitis.** This is a disorder of unknown cause that often affects women in their 30s and 40s:
         (a) Awake spontaneously at night with excruciating shoulder pain
         (b) Loss of active abduction
         (c) Exquisite tenderness over the involved tendon
         (d) Radiographic findings of calcification
         (e) Trauma not thought to play a role in this disorder
      ii. **Acute trauma can lead to rotator-cuff tendinitis and subacromial bursitis.** This is common with a fall on an outstretched hand or elbow. This axial load on the humerus forcibly impinges the cuff and bursa onto the acromial arch and leads to injury and subsequent symptoms.
      iii. **Rotator cuff tears can mimic the symptoms of impingement, producing both pain and weakness.** In older women, attritional tears can occur with

relatively minor trauma following years of impingement. In younger women, they can occur following acute trauma. A high index of suspicion is necessary for diagnosis.

c. **Signs and symptoms** See Chapter 43, "Shoulder Injuries."

d. **Physical findings and radiographic findings** See Chapter 43, "Shoulder Injuries."

e. **Treatment** See Chapter 43, "Shoulder Injuries."

5. **Lateral epicondylitis**

a. **Definition:** Lateral epicondylitis is inflammation, degeneration, and microtears at the muscle-bone interface at the origin of the common extensor bundle from the lateral epicondyle.

b. **Causes**

i. Although classically known as tennis elbow, most cases do not arise as a result of tennis, but rather from other repeated activities involving the elbow and forearm. In tennis, extensor overload often results from poor hitting technique, especially on the back hand; improper racquet sizing with a grip too small or too large; and poor flexibility around the elbow with extensor contracture.

ii. Poor posture can be a major contributing factor, especially in women who spend prolonged periods of time working at a keyboard. Women who were tall for their age in school or who are large-breasted often adopt a "poke neck" posture with protracted scapulae, hunched shoulders, increased thoracic kyphosis, and cervical lordosis.

(a) **Underlying factors should be addressed:**

- Treatment of neck dysfunction and postural problems
- In individuals with repetitive stress injuries from the use of keyboards, proper seating posture and the ergonomics of the work station should be addressed. This includes support for the forearms to allow the wrist to adopt a relaxed position on the keys without excessive flexion or extension. Computer monitors should generally be moved up to eye level to avoid the hunched, "poke-neck" posture.

(b) Women should be encouraged to "sit tall" through elevating and protracting their sternum, which causes them to retract their scapulae and shoulders. Thoracic stretching exercises to improve extension and reduce kyphosis are important. Figure-of-eight straps are occasionally helpful in reinforcing the proper posture by maintaining the scapulae and shoulders in a retracted position. On the job, repetitive tasks should be interrupted frequently to allow for stretching and relaxation of the muscles.

c. **Signs and symptoms** See Chapter 44, "Elbow Injuries."

d. **Physical findings** See Chapter 44, "Elbow Injuries."

e. **Treatment** See Chapter 44, "Elbow Injuries."

6. **Stress fractures**

a. **Definition:** Stress fractures represent the end point of a continuum of bony stress reactions to repetitive loading. When a mechanical load is applied to a bone, remodeling accelerates to maintain skeletal integrity. Early in this process, osteoblastic activity to lay down new bone generally lags behind osteoclastic resorption, resulting in a net loss of bone and the development of microfractures. In most instances, the bone is able to adapt to the new level of stress; however, when loading is increased too rapidly, the imbalance can be of sufficient magnitude to lead to a clinically significant weakening of the bone.

b. **Causes—the etiology of stress fractures is multifactorial.** The primary factors are similar to those of all overuse injuries as previously described. Women seem to have a greater predisposition to stress fractures than men. Numerous reasons have been postulated, including differences in bone mass, lower muscle-to-body mass ratio, lower levels of musculoskeletal strength and cardiovascular fitness, and hormonal and endocrine factors. Although none of these theories has been properly validated in a prospective study, there is consensus that there is a **significant relationship between stress fractures, reproductive hormone levels, and bone mass**. There is significant concern that women suffering from the female athlete triad are at a greater risk for stress fractures during their athletic career and that they have significant risk for premature osteoporotic fractures later in life.

i. Stress fractures comprise up to 10% of all sports injuries and represent a higher proportion of running injuries. They can occur in some areas of the spine as well as in almost every bone of the appendicular skeleton. The most common site is the tibia, followed by the tarsals, metatarsals, and femur.

ii. Stress fractures that are considered to be at high risk for complications include the shaft and neck of the femur, the proximal tibia, the base of the fifth metatarsal , and the tarsal navicular. Women seem to be at particular risk for femoral stress fractures, which can go on to completion and displace if they are not diagnosed and treated with appropriate rest and rehabilitation.

c. **Signs and symptoms**

i. Stress fractures usually present with **pain**, initially following activity, then during and after activity, and finally with the activities of daily living. Night pain is a common feature that should alert the clinician to the possibility of a stress fracture. The pain is often poorly localized and may be easy to dismiss due to the lack of physical findings.

ii. Femoral stress fractures may produce dull aching in the anterior or lateral hip with pain radiating down the leg. There is usually no point tenderness, although this can occasionally be found in shaft fractures in thin women. Gentle hopping on the affected leg reproduces the hip pain, although this must be performed with caution in individuals who are acutely symptomatic:

(a) Femoral neck fractures can occasionally present with decreased hip flexion and internal rotation.

(b) Unfortunately, some femoral stress fractures present acutely with displacement because the athlete or her physician has ignored the warning signs of persistent and increasing pain.

d. **Radiographic findings** often lag several weeks behind the clinical picture and are frequently negative in the early symptomatic stages. It is therefore essential to understand that a negative x-ray study does not rule out a stress fracture.

i. Technetium radionuclide bone scans are quite sensitive to stress fractures and can be positive as little as 3 days after the onset of the injury. They represent the most cost-effective means to diagnose stress fractures.

ii. Magnetic resonance imaging is also sensitive but is much more expensive.

e. **Treatment:** Stress fractures are treated with modified rest.

i. Ambulation is permitted for the activities of daily living, but all other weight-bearing activities and skeletal loading are ceased until symptoms have abated.

ii. Alternate forms of nonimpact activity are substituted.

iii. During the period of relative rest, underlying factors are corrected, and strength training is undertaken.

iv. Once the athlete has been pain free in normal daily activities for 14 days, she is allowed to reintroduce weight-bearing activities gradually. Some authors recommend crutches and non–weight-bearing and even surgical fixation of femoral neck stress fractures, but there are large series showing successful treatment with the aforementioned regimen if the athlete is compliant.

7. **Low back pain**
   a. **Definition:** Low back pain affects virtually every women at some stage in her life. Management is often frustrating and depends on an accurate diagnosis and then treatment specific to the diagnosis. Fortunately, almost all back pain is self-limiting, and even in the absence of an accurate diagnosis, excellent treatment results are frequently obtained with conservative management.
   b. **Causes:** The cause of low back pain is multifactorial in nature. The pain can arise from any of the structures in the back, including the muscles, ligaments, facet joints, intervertebral disc, or sacroiliac joints.
      i. **Acute back pain** can involve any of these structures and usually is instigated by one acute episode of lifting or twisting. Falls can also cause acute pain.
      ii. **Chronic overuse syndromes** can also occur with the back. These are predisposed by poor posture, including increased lumbar lordosis, tightness of the hamstrings and iliopsoas, and poor strength of the abdominal and paraspinal musculature. Women may be predisposed to lumbosacral problems because of increased lumbar lordosis, which may be exaggerated by the wearing of high heels and exacerbated by pregnancy.
      iii. **There are two significant sources of low back pathology that are more common in women:**
         (a) **Pelvic instability is a mechanical disorder arising from sacroiliac joint dysfunction.** It is a common source of back pain during pregnancy and can also occur in running and a variety of other sports.
         (b) **Spondylolysis** is a bony stress reaction or stress fracture to the pars interarticularis of the lumbar spine that is common in gymnasts, divers, and dancers.
8. **Pelvic instability—sacroiliac joint dysfunction**
   a. **Causes:** Sacroiliac joint dysfunction is a common and frequently overlooked condition. The pelvic ring is composed of the innominate bones, which meet at the symphysis anteriorly and articulate with the sacrum posteriorly at the sacroiliac joints.
      i. Conventional medical wisdom frequently maintains that the sacroiliac joint is immobile, despite numerous studies which have demonstrated that **movement does indeed occur**.
      ii. **Movement is increased during pregnancy** because of hormonal effects on ligamentous laxity.
      iii. **Excessive mobility can lead to instability and lumbopelvic pain.** The pain can be variously attributed to mechanical stresses on ligamentous structures, facet joints, discs, and muscles.
      iv. The **most common dysfunctions occur with anterior subluxation and rotation of the innominate**, leading to an asymmetry in the pelvic ring structure. Some patients show an upslip pattern in which the innominate is subluxated superiorly. Less common are posterior rotations. Once the subluxation has been corrected, these patients may demonstrate an underlying hypermobile sacroiliac joint that allows the subluxation and then locking into a position at the extremes of motion.
   b. **Signs and symptoms:** Sacroiliac dysfunction and pelvic instability can present with pain in either an acute or chronic fashion with the clinical presentation determined by the actual site and type of dysfunction.
      i. In pregnancy, the **back pain may have a gradual onset** with activities of daily living or acutely with a twisting motion. Some women suffer significant pain and disability, which, if untreated, can leave them bedridden for the duration of their pregnancy.

ii. In athletic women, there may be a **history of trauma**, often a fall onto the buttocks, or an axial load onto one leg, such as can occur with stepping unexpectedly off a curb or into a hole in the ground. Overstriding during downhill running or performing kicks or vigorous hip flexion or extension movements in dance may also lead to sacroiliac joint dysfunction. It is not uncommon to see dysfunction following motor vehicle accidents in which the patient has braced the legs against the brake pedal or floor in anticipation of impact.

iii. The **pain is often localized to the sacroiliac joint itself but may be found in the buttocks, pubic symphysis, lower abdomen, or lateral thigh**. Occasionally, there is pain referred to the posterior thigh and lower leg and foot. This can mimic pain of a protruded intervertebral disc, which creates a common source of confusion because many individuals interpret leg pain as originating only from discs. Sacroiliac joint pain differs in that there are no associated neurologic findings. Additionally, sacroiliac joint pain is often discontinuous within the leg, with discrete areas of pain that do not radiate in a continuous bandlike fashion. Pressure over the sacroiliac joint can also reproduce leg symptoms in some individuals. Movement is painful, with extension often more painful than flexion. Prolonged sitting can cause pain in the low back and buttocks.

iv. Patients occasionally complain of **increased pain with cough or sneeze**. This is often thought to indicate disc pathology; however, pelvic instability because of sacroiliac joint dysfunction can also cause pain with this maneuver. A good way of distinguishing them is to have the patient cough while the pelvis is being stabilized by a compressive force across the iliac crests to support the sacroiliac joint. If this abolishes the cough-induced pain, it suggests that the pain may be due to a sacroiliac dysfunction.

v. Patients with sacroiliac dysfunction often present with a **secondary injury arising from gait alterations** but admit to underlying activity-related back pain. Patients may also complain that they feel as if they are out of alignment and that their gait is abnormal, but many do not admit to this sensation unless specifically questioned.

vi. Dysfunction of the sacroiliac joint leads to **compensatory changes at other sites in the axial skeleton**, including sacral torsion, rotation of the lumbar vertebrae, and frequently secondary rotations of thoracic and even cervical vertebrae. These can manifest themselves as pain at sites distant from the sacroiliac joint as well as in the characteristic findings of flexible dual scoliosis and rotations of the upper thorax and shoulder girdle. If the sacroiliac joint remains unstable and malaligned, it does little good to try to correct more proximal problems in the upper back or neck until the sacroiliac is treated.

c. **Physical examination**

i. The most common finding is that of **tenderness** over the sacroiliac joint, which can be assessed by applying direct pressure while the patient is lying prone.

ii. There is often local tenderness over the region of the posterior-superior iliac spine.

iii. **Asymmetric positioning** of the levels of the anterior and posterior superior iliac spines in the frontal plane.

iv. Additional clues are **leg lengths** that are asymmetric and change when the patient goes from a supine position to a long sitting position in which the patient sits upright on the table with the hips flexed to 90° and the knees extended.

   v. An asymmetric **range of hip motion** is also suggestive of a sacroiliac dysfunction. Usually one hip has a predominant range of external rotation and the other predominant range of internal rotation.
   vi. **Hamstring flexibility** is affected by a sacroiliac joint dysfunction, with the hamstring on the side of the anterior rotation having a reduced flexibility relative to the other.

d. **Radiographic findings**
   i. Imaging for low back pain is controversial. The diagnosis of sacroiliac joint dysfunction must be made on a clinical basis, using history and detailed physical examination, with imaging studies of little use in its management. In the patient with acute, nontraumatic low back pain without neurologic signs or symptoms suggestive of systemic problems such as infection or neoplasm, it is generally recommended that plain x-rays be performed only after the failure to respond to 6 weeks of conservative treatment. With current cost consciousness, this would appear to be a good policy, although it may be difficult to convince patients to take this approach.
   ii. There is a high prevalence of radiographic abnormalities in the asymptomatic population, with magnetic resonance imaging demonstrating disc disease in up to 30% of 30-year-olds. As a general rule of thumb, imaging should be reserved for cases in which it will change management of the patient.

e. **Treatment**
   i. The treatment of almost all lumbosacral problems is directed toward relief of symptoms, followed by restoration of strength and flexibility.
   ii. Patients who maintain mobility within the limits of their pain tolerance have the most rapid recovery time.
   iii. Acetaminophen and NSAIDs are used for symptomatic relief.
   iv. Ice massage over the lumbosacral region is often effective.
   v. Physical therapy is occasionally helpful, although the use of modalities alone for symptomatic relief for any longer than a few days should be discouraged.
   vi. Mobilization has been shown to be effective in some cases.
   vii. Strengthening and pelvic stabilization drills are essential. Muscle tone must be improved in the abdominals and paraspinals.
   viii. Specific treatment of sacroiliac joint dysfunction and pelvic instability consists of correcting the underlying dynamics and positional defects of the pelvis.
   ix. Sacroiliac support belts place a compressive force around the pelvis and stabilize the sacroiliac joint. They are useful in treating pelvic instability, especially during pregnancy.

9. **Spondylolysis**
   a. **Causes:** Spondylolysis is a defect of the pars interarticularis and is thought to arise from repetitive extension and flexion of the spine. **Both the pathology and clinical presentation of spondylolysis are variable.** There are many asymptomatic cases, with 6% of the population having radiographic evidence of a pars defect, although there are higher rates in adolescent athletes, especially gymnasts, dancers, and divers. The specific pathology is on a continuum and may range from an asymptomatic fibrous defect discovered on an x-ray to a stress fracture with disabling pain. It is thus **important to correlate the clinical findings with any imaging studies**.
   b. **Signs and symptoms:** Spondylolysis usually presents with **activity-related low back pain**, usually exacerbated by extension or twisting, which loads the posterior elements of the spine. It is often unilateral and relieved by rest, although night pain may occur in acute cases.

i. Adolescents with spondylolysis usually demonstrate defective posture with lumbar hyperlordosis, poor abdominal tone, tight hip flexors, and weak hamstrings.
ii. Unilateral extension of the back frequently reproduces pain.
iii. There is occasional unilateral tenderness over the posterior elements on the involved side.

c. **Radiographic findings**
i. Radiographs frequently show the characteristic "Scotty dog" lesion on the oblique view, but they must be interpreted with caution because of the high prevalence of asymptomatic lesions.
ii. The technetium radionuclide bone scan is the diagnostic test of choice, and improved diagnostic accuracy can be gained through the use of single-photon emission computed tomography (SPECT), which can accurately localize the lesion to the pars.
iii. **A positive x-ray with a negative bone scan should prompt the clinician to search for another cause of the patient's back pain, including sacroiliac joint dysfunction, which is common in this group of athletes.**

d. **Treatment**
i. The treatment of spondylolysis is controversial and depends on the stage of the pathology.
ii. There is general agreement that the offending activities should be stopped. Some authors recommend cessation of all activities, but it seems more reasonable and equally effective to maintain activities that can be performed on a pain-free basis.
iii. Hamstring stretching is important during the rehabilitation period.
iv. Bracing of the lower back is often used. Some advocate prolonged (> 3 months) bracing to allow injured areas to heal, whereas others recommend short-term (4–6 weeks) bracing during the period when the patient is symptomatic.

10. **Patellofemoral knee pain**

a. **Definition:** Patellofemoral pain represents a spectrum of disorders of the patellofemoral joint. The exact source of the pain is unknown, although it is variously postulated to come from the subchondral bone, the patellar retinaculum, and the synovium about the knee joint. Other structures that can produce anterior knee pain are the patellar tendon origin, peripatellar plicas, and occasionally arthrosis of the patellofemoral joint.

b. **Causes**
i. **Bony problems:**
(a) Dysplastic femoral condyles
(b) Patellar abnormalities of size, shape and height
(c) Underlying cause is thought to be poor patellar tracking, leading to abnormal distribution of the patellofemoral joint reactive forces

ii. **Soft tissue causes:**
(a) Generalized ligamentous laxity with poor patellar tracking leading to lateral patellar compression syndrome
(b) Tightness of the hamstrings, which leads to an increase in patellofemoral joint reactive forces
(c) Deficiency of the vastus medialis obliquus, leading to lateralization of patellofemoral tracking
(d) **Biomechanical factors**
- Genu valgum and increased Q angle leading to lateral pull of the patella. Some authors report that women are particularly predisposed to patellofemoral pain because of their wider pelvis and higher Q angles.

This has not been borne out by research that controlled for both normal and injured subjects.

- Excess pronation leading to obligatory internal torsion of the tibia on the femur and lateral tracking of the patella.
- Restrictions of hip or foot mobility that may lead to patellar tracking abnormalities, reinforcing the notion that it is important to examine the entire kinetic chain in patients with overuse injuries.

c. **Signs and symptoms** See Chapter 49, "Knee Injuries."

d. **Physical findings and radiographic findings** See Chapter 49, "Knee Injuries."

e. **Treatment** See Chapter 49, "Knee Injuries."

Recommended Reading

1. American College of Obstetricians and Gynecologists Technical Bulletin: Exercise during pregnancy and the postpartum period. No. 189. Washington, DC, American College of Obstetricians and Gynecologists, 1994.
2. American College of Sports Medicine: The female athlete triad: Disordered eating, amenorrhea, bone mineral disorders. Preliminary summary. Washington, DC, American College of Sports Medicine, 1992.
3. Barrow GW, Subratta S: Menstrual irregularity and stress fractures in collegiate female distance runners. Am J Sports Med 16:209–216, 1988.
4. Bonen A, Keizer HA: Athletic menstrual cycle irregularity: Endocrine response to exercise and training. Phys Sportsmed 12:78–93, 1984.
5. Brukner P, Khan K: Clinical Sports Medicine. Sydney, McGraw-Hill, 1993.
6. Clapp JF: Exercise in pregnancy: A brief clinical review. Fetal Med Rev 2:89–101, 1990.
7. DeLee JC, Drez D (eds): Orthopedic Sports Medicine: Principles and Practice. Philadelphia, WB Saunders, 1994.
8. Drinkwater BL, et al: Bone mineral density after resumption of menses in amenorrheic athletes. JAMA 256:380–382, 1986.
9. Giannini AJ, et al: Anorexia and bulimia. Am Fam Phys Apr:1169–1176, 1990.
10. Joy EA: Exercise during pregnancy. MN Fam Phys 48:12–13, 1983.
11. Joy EA, et al: Outpatient management of disordered eating (parts I and II). Your Patient and Fitness 9(Feb/Mar), 1995.
12. Kibler WB, Chandler TJ, Stracener ES: Musculoskeletal adaptations and injuries due to overtraining. Excer Sport Sci Rev 20:99–126, 1992.
13. Lee D: The Pelvic Girdle: An Approach to the Examination and Treatment of the Lumbo-Pelvic-Hip Region. New York, Churchill-Livingstone, 1989.
14. Loucks AB: Effects of exercise training on the menstrual cycle: Existence and mechanisms. Med Sci Sports Exerc 22:275–279, 1990.
15. Macintyre JG, Lloyd-Smith DR: Overuse running injuries. In Renstrom P (ed): I.O.C. Encyclopedia of Sports Medicine, Volume 4: Sports Injuries—Basic Principles of Prevention and Care. Oxford, Blackwell Scientific Publications, 1993, pp 139–160.
16. Magee DJ: Orthopedic Physical Assessment. Philadelphia, WB Saunders, 1981.
17. Marshall P, Hamilton W: Cuboid subluxation in ballet dancers. Am J Sports Med 20(2):169–175, 1992.
18. Myburgh KH, et al: Are risk factors for menstrual dysfunction cumulative? Phys Sportsmed 20:114–125, 1992.
19. Olson BR: Exercise-induced amenorrhea. Am Fam Phys 39(2):213–221, 1989.
20. Otis CL: Pathogenic weight control in athletes. Sports Med Dig 11(2):7, 1989.
21. Otis CL: Recognizing the athlete with an eating disorder. Sports Med Dig 11(4):4, 1989.
22. Reid DC: Sports Injury, Assessment and Rehabilitation. New York, Churchill Livingstone, 1992.
23. Reider B (ed): Sports Medicine: The School-Age Athlete. Philadelphia, WB Saunders, 1991.
24. Woerman AJ: Evaluation and treatment of the lumbar-pelvic-hip complex. In Donatelli R, Wooden MJ (eds): Orthopedic Physical Therapy. New York, Churchill Livingstone, 1989.

12

The Mature Athlete*

Wade Lillegard, M.D., David O. Hough, M.D., and Chris McGrew, M.D.

In 1960, there were approximately 16 million Americans aged 65 years and older. This increased to more than 31 million by 1990 and is predicted by the U.S. Census Bureau to rise to 75 million by 2040. As the U.S. population ages, health care providers will be increasingly challenged to meet the special needs of the elderly, especially in helping them to remain more functional. Aging is associated with decreased muscular strength and endurance, leading to declining functional capacity and quality of life. **A large component of this decline is likely not the result of aging per se, but of the sedentary lifestyle associated with aging.** Regular physical activity may increase life expectancy by 1–2 years. More importantly, it can improve function and quality of life as an individual ages. Unfortunately, only approximately 10% of the adult population engages in light to moderate exercise for at least 30 minutes per day, and only 29% of the population over 65 years old report doing any regular exercise, including walking. Fifty-eight percent of the population is considered sedentary.

Mature athletes can and do participate in a wide variety of sports, competing in community, regional, and national levels of competition, including the Senior Olympics, at the highest level. Physicians may inappropriately tell their older patients with exercise-related problems to stop their activity altogether. This chapter looks at the importance and benefits of exercise in older people and evaluates the types of injuries seen in this population. The growing importance of the aged and their role in society makes it imperative that the health professional understands their needs and problems.

I. Principles of Exercise Prescription for the Mature Athlete

A. **Before instituting an exercise program in the elderly, consider the following:**
   1. The exercise **goals** of the patient
   2. The **availability** of equipment and facilities
   3. **Cost** of the program
   4. Performing a thorough **assessment of the patient's health**
      a. Appropriate history and physical examination
      b. Assessment of nutritional status, present activity level, smoking habits, alcohol use, and weight problems
      c. Diseases that lead to decreased exercise tolerance
      d. Orthopedic problems and disabilities that produce physical limitations
      e. Any history of prior injury and rehabilitation
      f. Present status of the patient's physical condition and training status
      g. Medications that may interfere with or alter the exercise response
   5. **Laboratory testing**—urinalysis, electrocardiogram

* Editor's note: This chapter is written from a slightly different perspective than the rest of the book. As group or "team" activities and competitions have become popular for older adults, many of the physicians who care for younger athletes are asked by older patients for advice about safe exercise. "The Mature Athlete" provides insights and guidelines for exercise prescription and participation in a more senior population.

6. **Assessing risk** of exercise using graded exercise testing
   a. Major risks for cardiovascular disease (CVD):
      i. Cholesterol level > 240 mg
      ii. Blood pressure > 160/90 mmHg
      iii. Cigarette smoker
      iv. Diabetes
      v. Family history of CVD in parents or siblings younger than 55 years old
   b. Major symptoms or signs of cardiopulmonary disease:
      i. Ischemic chest pain or discomfort
      ii. Shortness of breath out of proportion to exertion
      iii. Lightheadedness or syncope
      iv. Orthopnea and paroxysmal nocturnal dyspnea
      v. Ankle edema
      vi. Palpitations or tachycardia
      vii. Claudication
   c. Recommendations for graded exercise testing for patients wanting to start a moderate exercise program (40–60% functional capacity, also called $\dot{V}O_2max$, or METs):
      i. Patients with known CVD
      ii. Patients with 2 or more major risk factors or signs for CVD, with symptoms
   d. Recommendations for graded exercise testing for patients wanting to start a vigorous exercise program (> 60% $\dot{V}O_2max$):
      i. Men over 40, women over 50
      ii. Patients with 2 or more risk factors or signs for CVD
      iii. Patients with known CVD
   e. The risk of graded exercise testing in the elderly may be higher than that in the young population because of the increased incidence of coronary artery disease. After age 65, 30% of patients develop myocardial ischemia during exercise, and the use of a modified graded exercise testing protocol is warranted.

B. **Physical changes of aging** (Table 1)
   1. **Cardiac**
      a. Increased left ventricular wall thickness and cardiac mass—minimal to no change in left ventricular cavity dimension
      b. Decreased left ventricular diastolic functional reserve:
         i. Decreased passive filling
         ii. Increased dependence on atrial kick

TABLE 1. Age-Related Decreases in Functional Status

Cardiovascular system	↓ Maximum heart rate	10 beats/minute/decade
	↓ Maximum cardiac output	20–30% by 65 years old
	↓ Vessel compliance	↑ Blood pressure 10–40 mmHg
Respiratory system	↑ Residual volume	30–50% by 70 years old
	↓ Vital capacity	40–50% by 70 years old
Nervous system	↓ Number of motor units (type II)	1–3%/year after 60 years old
	↓ Nerve conduction	1–15% by 60 years old
	↓ Proprioception and balance	35–40% ↑ in falls by 60 years old
Metabolism	↓ Maximum O_2 uptake	9%/decade
Musculoskeletal system	↑ Bone loss	
	> 35 years old	1%/year
	> 55 years old	3–5%/year
	↓ Muscle strength	10–15%/decade after > 60 years old
	↓ Flexibility	Degenerative disease or inactivity
	↓ Muscle mass	24–36% by 65–90 years old

c. Unchanged **resting** cardiac output and heart rate
d. Smaller increase in ejection fraction with exercise—decreased $\dot{V}O_2max$
e. Decreased vascular compliance—prevalence of hypertension (> 150/95) is 50% of patients over 80.

2. **Metabolic**
   a. Decreased $\dot{V}O_2max$:
      i. Decreased stroke volume
      ii. Decreased maximal heart rate
      iii. Decreased peripheral O_2 extraction
   b. Increased potential for developing heat stress
3. **Ventilation**
   a. Decreased arterial CO_2 elimination
   b. Decreased pulmonary venous blood oxygenation
   c. Increased work of breathing:
      i. Increased rib cage rigidity
      ii. Decreased lung tissue elasticity
   d. Decreased vital capacity and increased residual volume
4. **Neuromuscular**
   a. Decreased muscle mass—decreased number of type II motor units and type II muscle fiber area
   b. Decreased maximal isometric strength

C. **Benefits of regular exercise in the mature athlete**
   1. Improved muscle tone, range of motion, posture, coordination, and physical work capacity
   2. Increased $\dot{V}O_2max$ and decreased blood pressure
   3. Improved weight control and body image and decreased incidence of depression
   4. Reduction in the incidence of low back pain
   5. Improvement in the prevention of accidents
   6. Improved social contacts and sleep patterns
   7. Improved functional ability and more independence

D. **Purpose of exercise evaluation**
   1. Determine the appropriate exercise (type, frequency, intensity, and duration) for the patient. The importance of graded exercise testing for patients in this age group should be noted.
   2. Evaluate any chronic health problem that may compromise the patient's physical capacity.
   3. Acknowledge medical conditions that preclude vigorous physical activity, and understand absolute contraindications for exercise participation.
   4. Instruct the patient to start all exercise programs gradually and increase activity levels based on the exercise evaluation.

E. **Guidelines for patient education**
   1. Specificity about the exercise prescribed—importance of including aerobic and strength training
   2. Exercise three to four times a week with a proper warm-up and cool-down period; avoid hot or humid weather
   3. A gradual increase in activity from week to week
   4. Significance of muscle and joint pain and the importance of fatigue

F. **Goals of the exercise program**
   1. Increased cardiovascular fitness, endurance, flexibility, balance, and strength through walking, jogging, swimming, biking, and strength training
   2. Minimize deconditioning and disuse changes previously attributable to aging
   3. Increase self-esteem

G. **Special concern—to avoid unnecessary injury**

1. Avoid running, jumping rope, and weight lifting in selected patients.
2. Avoid isometric exercise if the patient has congestive heart failure.
3. Exercise within the aerobic limits established by the graded exercise testing.
4. Establish a target heart rate of 60–75% of maximum heart rate.
5. Inform patients with decreased visual or hearing acuity about the dangers of exercising without special precautions (e.g., traffic).
6. Keep resistance below 80% of 1 RM (repetition maximum).

II. Common Musculoskeletal Problems of the Mature Athlete

A. **Common injuries**

1. The following problems account for the largest number of visits to physicians: low back injuries, acute cervical strains, bursitis and tendinitis of the shoulder, patellofemoral dysfunction, and chronic ankle injuries. Treatment is discussed elsewhere.
2. **Possible contributing factors and disease processes contributing to musculoskeletal complaints**
   a. **Decreasing flexibility with aging—primary cause is disuse.** Regular stretching and exercises involving full range of joint motion may retard process.
   b. **Decreased nerve conduction and reaction time**—15% decrease between age 30 and 70. Patients should progress slowly to allow for neuromuscular adaptation.
   c. **Decreased hearing or vision associated with unsteady gait**—use of a stationary bicycle may be helpful for those with balance problems.
   d. **Degenerative joint disease**—increased incidence with aging, almost ubiquitous over age 65. Studies show that jogging is not a causal factor of degenerative joint disease. If symptomatic, may need to use non–weight-bearing form of exercise, such as cycling or water exercises.
   e. **Rheumatoid arthritis**—increased incidence with aging; more prevalent in women than in men. Similar recommendations for non–weight-bearing exercises as for degenerative joint disease.
   f. **Gout**—increased incidence over age 60; more prevalent in men than in women; should curtail activity during acute attack, using adequate rest periods, appropriate splinting, and medications.
   g. **Decreased muscle mass**—results in decreased strength and shock absorption. Regular exercise helps maintain lean muscle mass.
   h. **Osteoporosis**—more significant for women; may predispose older individuals to increased fractures, especially in the hip, vertebral column, and forearm. Regular weight-bearing exercise may play an important role in prevention.

B. **Principles of injury treatment**

1. Proper analysis of contributing factors with **appropriate modification or correction** is required in the following:
   a. **Specific movements or activities:** A tennis player with tennis elbow requires instruction in proper back-hand technique.
   b. **Training patterns:** A runner with an overuse injury such as posterior tibialis stress syndrome (shin splints) should reduce mileage and increase strength work and stretching.
   c. **Biomechanical factors:** A runner with excessive subtalar joint pronation may benefit from a properly designed orthotic.
   d. **Equipment:** A bicyclist with knee pain may need an adjustment in seat height and use of lower resistance gears.
2. **Appropriate use of rest (either relative or absolute)**
   a. For a prescribed period of time or related to symptom relief (nonaggravating activities are allowed)

b. May be expressed in terms of percent of decrease in activity—often reduced by increments of 15–25% of usual activities until symptoms disappear
c. Followed by a gradual return to activity (increase activity by increments of 15–25% over the course of 3 to 6 weeks)
d. With increased age of patient, probably need to increase recovery time

3. **Provision of an appropriate and aggressive rehabilitation program**
    a. Use of simple, inexpensive equipment (such as free weights or elastic tubing) that can be used at home along with printed material showing rehabilitation methods may increase compliance and recovery.
    b. Rehabilitation should also include range-of-motion and flexibility exercises.

III. Exercise Prescription for the Sedentary Adult

The goal of an exercise program should be firmly established before recommending an activity. Exercise can be used to improve overall health, improve cardiorespiratory fitness, increase strength and flexibility, provide socialization, or enhance athletic performance. The level of activity required to promote general health is significantly less than that required for improving cardiorespiratory fitness. **All-cause and cardiovascular mortality rates have been shown to decrease with modest increases in the amount of habitual physical activity.** This relationship is essentially linear, which means that any increase in activity is beneficial, and more is better. Improvements in cardiovascular fitness require a volume overload to the heart resulting from repetitive use of large muscle groups at a moderate to high intensity over time (aerobic exercise). Most activities of daily living are enhanced by strength training. **The best exercise program is one that a patient enjoys doing and will do on a regular basis.**

Reduction of other risk factors for heart disease also should be employed. Lowering dietary cholesterol, avoiding cigarettes, and treating hypertension when present should be routine advice for the patient prone to develop heart disease. A comprehensive approach that includes these behavioral modifications, treatment techniques, and a regular exercise program can significantly change the long-term health of the active individual.

A. **Prescription for improved general health**

Every U.S. adult should accumulate 30 minutes or more of moderate-intensity (3 to 6 METs) physical activity on most, and preferably all, days of the week.

1. Most adults do not need to be cleared by their physician before starting a moderate intensity (40-60% $\dot{V}O_2max$) program.
2. Thirty minutes can be accomplished by adding relatively short bouts of exercise throughout the day (e.g., home repair, mowing, climbing stairs)
3. Sedentary individuals should incorporate a few minutes per day and gradually increase to 30 minutes.

B. **Contraindications for exercise training and testing**

1. Exercise testing is useful in patients when the physician must decide whether closer monitoring of the exercise program is indicated. Patients in this category should undergo a medically supervised test for functional capacity.
2. Patients with the following conditions require supervised stress testing:
    a. Recent myocardial infarction or post–coronary artery bypass surgery
    b. Presence of a pacemaker—fixed rate or demand
    c. Use of chronotropic or inotropic cardiac medications
    d. Presence of morbid obesity combined with multiple coronary risk factors
    e. Occurrence of ST segment depression at rest
    f. Severe hypertension
    g. Intermittent claudication
3. Conditions, both medical and environmental, that require moderation of activity or caution in prescribing exercise are listed in Tables 2 and 3.

TABLE 2. Conditions Requiring Caution in Exercise Prescription

Viral infection or cold
Chest pain
Irregular heart beat
Exercise-induced asthma
Prolonged, unaccustomed physical activity
Conduction disturbances (left bundle branch block, complete atrioventricular block, or bifascicular block with or without first-degree block)

4. In general, many patients in the mature athlete age group require some form of exercise testing before instituting an exercise program.

C. **Intensity of exercise**
   1. The **most important variable** in any exercise prescription is intensity, but it also is the most difficult factor to determine.
   2. Intensity is expressed as a percentage of maximum heart rate (MHR), heart rate (HR) reserve (MHR minus resting HR), or functional capacity ($\dot{V}O_2$max or METs).
   3. **The intensity rate for proper training depends on the initial fitness level of the adult.**
      a. Unconditioned individuals have a low threshold for improving functional capacity, whereas conditioned patients require a greater intensity level to increase aerobic fitness.
      b. Determining intensity by heart rate:
         i. MHR is determined through a linear relationship between the HR and $\dot{V}O_2$max. Intensity is expressed as a percentage of MHR (HR_{max}), where HR_{max} = (220 – age ± 15 beats):
         ii. Intensity levels of 60–90% of MHR can induce training. These values correspond to approximately 50–85% of functional capacity.
         iii. The **Karvonen method** is the preferred method of determining intensity and is based on the MHR formula of 220–age ± 15 beats:
            (a) Calculate the training heart rate (THR) as follows: THR = $[(0.60 \text{ to } 0.90) \times (HR_{max} - HR_{rest})] + HR_{rest}$, where (0.60 to 0.90) represents a potential range of training intensities from 60% to 90% of MHR.
            (b) The mature athlete should begin exercise at low intensity levels and gradually increase as fitness improves.
            (c) The Karvonen method is advantageous over simple measures of MHR because variability in the athlete's resting heart rate is accounted for in the formula. Table 4 shows average maximum heart rates and THR for various age groups.

D. **Exercise prescription using METs:** generally reserved for mature patients with some from of disability, for whom calculation by percent of MHR is not adequate for defining an exercise level.
   1. MET is a unit used to describe exercise intensity.

TABLE 3. Conditions Requiring Moderation of Activity

Extreme heat and high relative humidity
Extreme cold, especially when strong winds are present
Following heavy meals
Exposure to high altitudes (greater than 1700 meters)
Significant musculoskeletal injuries

TABLE 4. Average Maximum Heart Rates by Age and Recommended Target Heart Rates for Normal Asymptomatic Participants During Exercise

Age (yrs)	20–29	30–39	40–49	50–59	60–69
HRmax	190	185	180	170	160
Peak THR 0.9 (HR_{max} – 75) + 75	179	174	170	161	152
Lowest THR 0.6 (HR_{max} – 75) + 75	144	141	138	132	126
Average THR 0.7 (HR_{max} – 75) + 75	155	152	149	141	135

Modified from the American College of Sports Medicine: Guidelines for Graded Exercise Testing and Exercise Prescription, 4th ed. Philadelphia, Lea & Febiger, 1991. Reprinted from Fox E: The Physiological Basis of Physical Education and Athletics, 3rd ed. Philadelphia, Saunders College Publishing, 1981, p 412, with permission.

a. One MET is equivalent to O_2 consumption at rest in a sitting position.
b. One MET = 3.5 ml/kg/min

2. Maximum MET (MMET) = $\frac{\dot{V}O_2max\ (ml/kg/min)}{3.5\ ml/kg/min}$
3. Training intensity (TMET) should be between 0.5 and 0.85 MMET.
   a. Low intensity = 0.5 MMET
   b. High intensity = 0.85 MMET
4. Metabolic cost (in METs) of various activities is readily available (Table 5). This is useful when prescribing exercise prognosis in this patient group.
5. Energy expenditure can be calculated per session as follows (because 1 MET = 1 kcal/kg/hr): energy expenditure (kcal) = METs × time in activity (in hours) × body weight (in kg). Use this formula to determine how many kcal are burned in each exercise session.

E. **Cycle ergometry**

1. Cycle ergometry is used as an alternative to treadmill testing to determine O_2 uptake at given uploads.
   a. Calculations are based on the liner relationship of heart rate and O_2 uptake ($\dot{V}O_2$) at varying workloads.
   b. The ergometer is used when the patient has problems with walking or jogging on the treadmill. It is a good alternative when proper protocols are followed.
2. Maximum oxygen concentration ($\dot{V}O_2max$) is calculated based on a projected workload at the predicted or known MHR of the mature athlete.
   a. You must have at least two submaximal $\dot{V}O_2$ determinations.
   b. The heart rate at submaximal workloads should be 125–170 beats/minute for the best prediction of $\dot{V}O_2$.
3. **Bicycle ergometry protocol principles**
   a. Multistage tests are more valid than single-stage tests.
   b. Adjust the workload for the mature athlete's age, sex, and level of conditioning.
   c. Complete at least two stages with the HR 125–170, depending on predicted MHR.
   d. Each stage should last 3 minutes (or longer if the heart rate is not stable [within 5 beats/min]).
   e. Calculations of $\dot{V}O_2$ are made from simple graphs.

F. **Duration of exercise**

1. Ideal duration of exercise for most mature athletes is 20–60 minutes of continuous aerobic activity at a moderate intensity.

TABLE 5. Average Work Intensities for Activities Suitable for Exercise Prescription

	Average Work Intensity	
Activity	***METs***	***Kcal/hr (75 kg)***
Walking, 0% grade		
2.5 mph	3.0	225
3.0 mph	3.3	240
3.5 mph	3.5	262
4.0 mph	4.6	345
Jogging		
4.5 mph	5.7*	375–490
5.0 mph	8.4	630
6.0 mph	10.0	750
7.0 mph	11.4	855
8.0 mph	12.8	960
Cycling (ergometer)		
300 kpm	3.7	278
450 kpm	5.0	375
600 kpm	6.0	450
750 kpm	7.0	525
900 kpm	8.5	630
1050 kpm	10.0	750
1200 kpm	11.0	825
1500 kpm	11.3	1010
Swimming, crawl†		
20 yd/min	6.0	420
30 yd/min	9.0	675
40 yd/min	12.0	900
Games (average intensity)		
Basketball	7–15	525–1125
Volleyball	5–12	375–900
Soccer	7–15	525–1125
Handball	8–12	600–900
Tennis	6–10	450–750

* Metabolic cost of jogging at 4–5 mph is variable owing to the transition between fast walk and jog.
† Metabolic cost of swimming is highly variable owing to efficiency, buoyancy, and technique; values may vary by 25%.
From Hanson PG, Giese MD, Corliss RJ: Clinical guidelines for exercise training. Postgrad Med 67:120, 1980, with permission.

2. Exercise sessions should be gradually extended from an initial 15–20 minutes as cardiovascular endurance improves. In this age group, instruct the patient to start with walking before jogging and gradually work the patient into a "walk-jog" program.
3. Once initial fitness programs are underway, you should instruct the patient to extend the exercise session up to 60 minutes.
4. Fat utilization increases significantly after approximately 20 minutes of light-to-moderate exercise, enhancing body fat reduction during longer periods of aerobic exercise.
5. The mature athlete should avoid high-intensity exercise of short duration because this may lead to increased musculoskeletal injury and the possibility of adverse cardiovascular events.

G. **Frequency of exercise**
1. A minimum of three exercise sessions per week is necessary to achieve an aerobic effect (allows sufficient rest to prevent musculoskeletal overuse syndromes).
2. In the obese and in adults with low functional capability (< 3 METs), prescribe repeated exercise sessions of 5 minutes each, several times per day. As functional capacity improves, one or two longer daily sessions should be undertaken.

3. As functional capacity improves, increase to three or more sessions per week.
4. Easier days must then be included during which the duration and intensity of exercise are reduced.
5. Exercise sessions should not exceed 5 days per week.
    a. Progression from 3 to 5 days per week should occur gradually over a 4-week period.
    b. No more than two intense sessions should occur per week.
6. Exercising 7 days per week does not further improve aerobic power and may serve to initiate overuse problems. **One exception is the obese adult** who needs daily low-intensity exercise to reduce body fat.

H. **Exercise mode**
1. Exercise activities that use large muscle groups in a rhythmic and continuous manner are the preferred type of aerobic exercise.
    a. Jogging and running, swimming, bicycling, or cross-country skiing programs
    b. Less intense activities such as golf, bowling, and archery offer little training stimulus because heart rates rarely exceed 100 beats/minute.
    c. Rope skipping may produce excessively high heart rates and should be avoided in patients with restricted to moderate exercise intensity levels.
    d. Tennis and squash are adequate training stimuli if the skill level is sufficiently high. Squash, however, involves rapid starting and stopping, increases systolic blood pressure and myocardial oxygen demands, and should be prescribed only in healthy, risk-free patients.
2. Strength-training programs should be of sufficient intensity to elicit a strength-training effect while minimizing musculoskeletal injury and an elevated blood pressure response.
    a. At least one set of 8–12 repetitions of 8 to 10 exercises that condition the major muscle groups at least 2 days per week.
    b. Avoid sustained isometric activities against heavy resistance because they are strongly discouraged in unconditioned, hypertensive, and coronary-prone patients.

I. **Monitoring exercise:** The mature athlete should be instructed to stop after 3–5 minutes of exercise. Measure the radial pulse for 6 seconds; then add a zero to yield the HR.
1. Wrist palpation avoids the possibility of reflex hypotension that may occur with overly vigorous carotid massage.
2. The pulse should be counted immediately after stopping because HR decreases rapidly after exercise has stopped.

J. **Progression of the exercise program**
1. As cardiovascular and musculoskeletal fitness improves, increase the intensity, frequency, and duration of exercise. Increase only one variable in any one session.
2. The rate of progression depends on the athlete's age (in general, the older the patient, the slower the progression), functional capacity, overall health status, and exercise goals.
3. Typically, an exercise program is divided into three stages.
    a. **Initial conditioning phase:** duration 2–10 weeks; average approximately 6 weeks
        i. **Purpose**—transition from sedentary to active lifestyle; if patient is already fairly active, duration of this phase may be short.
        ii. **Emphasis**—avoiding undue discomfort, which is discouraging to new athletes.
        iii. **Content:**
            (a) Stretching and light calisthenics for warm-up and cool-down, with low-level aerobic activities sandwiched in between.

(b) The aerobic phase should initially be 5–10 minutes in duration. The total workout in this phase should progress by 2–3 minutes every 1–2 weeks up to 20 minutes.
(c) Training intensity is usually low, approximately 50–60% of functional capacity

iv. **Basis for progression:**
(a) **Objective:** decrease in steady-state HR at a given intensity (3 to 8 bpm); voluntary adaptation of a slightly faster pace by the patient and improvement in functional capacity
(b) **Subjective:** decrease in fatigue and perceived exertion; improved movement patterns, more relaxed facial expression

b. **Improvement phase:** up to 6 months or more after initial conditioning phase
i. **Purpose**—major physical adaptation
ii. **Emphasis**—gradual increase in intensity and duration of exercise
iii. **Content:**
(a) Intensity and duration alternately increased
(b) Intensity gradually increased from 50–60% to 70–85% of $\dot{V}O_2max$ for a given duration
(c) When tolerance of the new intensity is achieved, duration can increase, usually in increments of 2–5 minutes per workout. The duration is increased gradually to 30–45 minutes, depending on the intensity level.
iv. Instruct the patient that further improvements in fitness occur more slowly than during initial conditioning phase.

c. **Maintenance phase:** next 6 months
i. **Purpose**—sustaining the gains made through prior conditioning program
ii. **Emphasis**—long-term adherence to the exercise program and avoiding injury
iii. **Content:**
(a) Review of exercise goals—weight control, cardiovascular fitness, competition
(b) Introduction of a variety of other aerobic activities to maintain interest and avoid overuse injuries
(c) The patient exercises at 70–85% of functional capacity ($\dot{V}O_2max$) for 30–45 minutes three to five sessions per week
(d) Monitor progress with a training diary and follow-up exercise testing if appropriate.
iv. Emphasize the fact that musculoskeletal **overuse injuries are common with rapid progression of exercise programs.**
v. Adequate rest periods between exercise periods are important to avoid overuse problems.

Recommended Reading

1. Paffenbarger RS, Hyde RT, Wing AL: Physical activity and physical fitness as determinants of health and longevity. In Bouchard C, Shephard RJ, Stephens TS, et al (eds): Exercise, Fitness, and Health. Champaign, IL, Human Kinetics Books, 1990, pp 33–48.
2. Astrand P-O: Why exercise? Med Sci Sports Exerc 24(2):153–162, 1992.
3. American College of Sports Medicine: Guidelines for Exercise Testing and Prescription, 4th ed. Philadelphia, Lea & Febiger, 1991.
4. Barry HC: Exercise prescriptions for the elderly. Am Fam Phys 34(3):155–162, 1986.
5. Elkowitz EB, Elkowitz A: Prescribing exercise for the elderly. J Fam Pract Recert 8:117–130, 1986.
6. Laslett LJ, Amsterdam EA, Mason DT: Exercise testing in the geriatric patient. Ann Intern Med 112:56, 1980.
7. Mean WF, Hartwig R: Fitness evaluation and exercise prescription. J Fam Pract 13:1039–1050, 1981.

8. Lakatta EG: Changes in cardiovascular function with aging. Eur Heart J 11(suppl C):22–29, 1990.
9. Williams RS: How beneficial is regular exercise? J Cardiovasc Med 119:1112–1120, 1982.
10. Smith EL, Gilligan C: Physical activity prescription for the older adult. Phys Sportsmed 11(8):91, 1983.
11. Hanson PG, Giese MD, Corliss RJ: Clinical guidelines for exercise training. Postgrad Med 67:120–138, 1980.
12. Panush RS, Holtz HA: Is exercise good or bad for arthritis in the elderly? South Med J 87(5):S74–S78, 1994.
13. Lee IM, Hsieh C-C, Paffenbarger RS: Exercise intensity and longevity in men: The Harvard Alumni Health Study. JAMA 273:1179–1184, 1995.
14. Simons-Morton BG, Pate RR, Simons-Morton DS: Prescribing physical activity to prevent disease. Postgrad Med 83(1):165, 1988.
15. Pate RR, Pratt M, Blair SN, et al: Physical activity and public health: A recommendation from the Centers for Disease Control and Prevention and the American College of Sports Medicine. JAMA 273:402–407, 1995.
16. Smith LK: Medical clearance for vigorous exercise. Postgrad Med 83(1):146, 1988.
17. American College of Sports Medicine: Position stand on the recommended quantity and quality of exercise for developing and maintaining cardiorespiratory and muscular fitness in healthy adults. Med Sci Sports Exerc 22:265–274, 1990.

13

Medical Coverage for Special Olympics Games

David P. McCormick, M.D.

I. Background

A. **History:** Special Olympics was originated by Eunice Kennedy Shriver, who developed sports for mentally retarded athletes at her home in the early 1960s. Over the next 8 years, the program was further developed, and with the help of the Joseph P. Kennedy Foundation, the games were expanded throughout the United States and many foreign countries.

B. **Mission:** to provide sports training and competition for persons with mental retardation age 8 years through adult. Children between the ages of 5 and 8 years may participate in the training, but may not participate in competition.

C. **Goals**
   1. Physical fitness
   2. Social development
   3. Acceptance into larger society

D. To be eligible, the person must:
   1. Have been identified by an agency or professional as having mental retardation.
   2. Have a cognitive delay as determined by standardized measures.
   3. Have significant learning or vocational problems due to cognitive delays that require or have required specially designed instruction.

E. **Range of functioning:** 55% of athletes participating in Special Olympics are in a high-functioning range, with IQs > than 50.

F. **Special Olympics movement:** Programs exist in all 50 states, the District of Columbia, and Puerto Rico. A total of 131 Special Olympics programs are accredited throughout the world, and worldwide Special Olympics serves more than 1 million people with mental retardation. About 550,000 athletes compete in chapters in the United States. Games are held at local, regional, state, national, and international levels. Special Olympics International Winter and Summer Games are held every 4 years. Local games attract 300–600 athletes, and International Games are attended by 1500–6000 athletes.

G. **Relationship to the International Olympic Committee (IOC):** The IOC recognizes Special Olympics International (SOI) as a representative of the interests of athletes with mental retardation. Under an act of the U.S. Congress known as the Amateur Sports Act, the U.S. Olympic Committee (USOC) is authorized to grant membership status to other organizations that conduct amateur athletic training and competition for individuals with disabilities. Under this authority, the USOC has granted recognition to SOI. SOI may use the term "Olympics."

II. Organization of Games

A. **Levels of participation:** During competition, Special Olympics athletes are divided by sex, age, and ability. "Developmental" sports are available for athletes with severe limitation in adaptive skills.

B. **Coaches** consist of special education teachers, athletic instructors, parents, and other volunteers. Coaches typically have an extensive knowledge of the physical and mental characteristics of each athlete. The ratio of athlete to coach in Special Olympics programs is usually quite low (roughly 4:1); at the First World Winter Games in Salzburg, Austria, Team USA numbered 148 athletes and 38 coaches.

C. **Volunteers** play an important role by providing support services during Special Olympics Games. Volunteers serve as guides, escorts, water and supply carriers, and communications assistants.

D. **Administration:** At all levels of competition, safety and health issues are coordinated by medical committees that consist of health volunteers such as physicians, nurses, physical therapists, trainers, and occupational therapists. The medical committee typically works closely with the Special Olympics executive director, the games committee, and the competition manager to provide health supervision and emergency care at competitions.

III. Preparticipation Physical Examination

A. **Requirements**

1. **Preparticipation questionnaire:** The parent, guardian, or adult athlete must complete a preparticipation questionnaire that provides important personal health information. The licensed examiner signs the form after completing the physical examination.
2. **All athletes:** questionnaire and physical examination required on entry into the program
3. **For athletes with special medical problems**, physical examination required every 3 years
   a. Heart disease, heart defect, or high blood pressure
   b. Chest pain or fainting spells
   c. Seizures/epilepsy
   d. Diabetes
   e. Down syndrome
4. **Athlete develops a new medical problem:** Physical examination is required the first time a new problem is encountered that could pose a risk for the athlete during sports participation.
   a. Parent or sibling under 40 died of heart disease
   b. Absence of vision or blind in one eye
   c. Absence of one kidney or testicle
   d. Concussion or serious head injury
   e. Heat stroke or exhaustion
   f. Impaired motor ability
   g. Other problem that would interfere with participation

B. **Pertinent medical and developmental issues**

1. **Preparticipation questionnaire** documents the following:
   a. Use of a wheelchair
   b. Allergy to medication, food, or insect sting or bite
   c. Special diet (7% of athletes)
   d. Exercise-induced wheezing
   e. Tendency to bleed easily
   f. Emotional, psychiatric, or behavioral problem
   g. Serious bone or joint disorder
   h. Sickle cell trait or disease
   i. Hearing aid or hearing loss
   j. Contact lenses or eyeglasses

k. Dentures or false teeth
l. Immunizations up-to-date
m. Date of last tetanus shot
n. Medications—name, amount, date prescribed, and number of times a day medication needs to be taken (30% of athletes are using medication)

2. **Communication:** Many Special Olympics athletes have expressive and receptive language deficiencies. Five percent of athletes are nonverbal. As a result, the athlete may be unable to describe symptoms clearly. Caregivers should take additional time to establish communication; review the health record; speak with the athlete's coach; and use gestures, signing, or other means to accomplish communication.

C. **Use of preparticipation questionnaire**

1. **At competitions:** Coaches must ensure that questionnaires are updated and brought to all competitions.
2. **Review of questionnaires:** Forms are reviewed by medical team before competition and when athlete reports for injury or illness care.

D. **Down syndrome**

1. **Definition:** Down syndrome is the single most common diagnosis among mentally retarded individuals, occurring at a rate of 1.4 per 1000 live births. Approximately 15–30% of Special Olympics athletes have Down syndrome. The syndrome is caused by an abnormality in cell division that results in reduplication of chromosome number 21 in cells of the body. Down syndrome is associated with a constellation of abnormalities, including mental retardation, gastrointestinal defects, heart defects, joint and ligament laxity, epicanthal folds, simian crease, premature senility, and susceptibility to infectious diseases. The life expectancy is usually abbreviated, but some individuals with Down syndrome survive many decades.
2. **Atlantoaxial instability:** There is evidence from medical research that up to 15% of individuals with Down syndrome have a laxity of the transverse ligament of C-1 (atlas), which stabilizes the articulation of the odontoid process of C-2 (axis) with C-1. If this ligament is excessively lax, C-1 may spontaneously sublux forward on C-2 resulting in compression of the cervical spinal cord. Individuals with Down syndrome have experienced spontaneous subluxation and catastrophic spinal cord injury during surgical procedures that require general anesthesia and endotracheal intubation. Spinal cord injuries have also occurred after a fall or blow to the head.
3. **Diagnosis:** Atlantoaxial subluxation is diagnosed with a lateral x-ray film of the cervical spine in flexion, neutral, and extension. The distance between the anterior ramus of C-1 and the dens of C-2 should not exceed 4.0 mm.
4. **Restrictions:** All Down syndrome athletes must receive a diagnostic x-ray of the cervical spine before entering sports participation. Individuals with atlantoaxial instability should be referred for neurosurgical consultation and may not participate in sports training and competition activities that result in hyperextension, radical flexion, or direct pressure on the neck or upper spine. Such sports include butterfly stroke and diving in swimming, pentathlon, high jump, equestrian sports, gymnastics, soccer, squat lift, alpine skiing, and any warm-up exercise placing undue stress on the head and neck.

IV. Special Olympics Official Sports

A. **Official summer and winter sports** (Table 1)

B. **Demonstration sports:** Before a sport becomes a Special Olympics official sport, it must first be classified as a demonstration sport, and at least 12 national programs must have included the sport in their national games or tournaments. As of 1992, the demonstration sports were those listed in Table 1.

TABLE 1. Official Special Olympics Sports

Summer	Winter
Aquatics (swimming and diving)	Alpine skiing
Athletics (track and field)	Cross country skiing
Basketball	Figure skating
Bowling	Floor hockey
Cycling	Speed skating
Equestrian sports	
Football (soccer)	**Demonstration**
Gymnastics	Badminton
Roller skating	Golf
Softball	Powerlifting
Tennis	Table tennis
Volleyball	Team handball

V. Epidemiology of Injury and Illness

A. Factors that may predispose to injury or illness

1. **Screening for factors:** 44% of abnormalities can be identified by preparticipation questionnaire, 26% by both questionnaire and physical examination, and 29% by physical examination only. About 50% of athletes have no medical problem detected on preparticipation history and physical examination.
2. **Eyes:** 12–17% of Special Olympics athletes have eye problems, such as monocular vision, cataracts, myopia, amblyopia, and blindness.
3. **Hearing:** 6% of athletes have hearing loss or a hearing problem.
4. **Seizures:** 12–16% of athletes have a seizure disorder.
5. **Musculoskeletal:** 6% have problems such as prior scoliosis surgery (Harrington rods), recurrent dislocations, congenital amputee, atlantoaxial instability, excessive ligament laxity, history of fracture or sprain, and spasticity.
6. **Medical:** 6% have medical problems such as those listed under section III, B. Other problems are varied. Some examples include thyroid disease, cardiac arrhythmias, mitral valve prolapse, ventricular septal defect, celiac disease, and phenylketonuria.
7. **Emotional and behavioral:** Concomitant with mental retardation, athletes have a higher prevalence of mental disorders, such as attention deficit disorder and conduct problems.

B. Summer sports

1. **Surveillance data:** Table 2 lists injury and illness events recorded at the International Summer Special Olympics Games, Baton Rouge, Louisiana, 1983.
2. **Claims reported in summer sports:** Insurance claim data were reported by Perlman and were collected from 12 states, July 1992–October 1993, representing a pool of 389,000 athletes. On the average, each Special Olympic athlete participated in 1.6 sports. During the time period, 340 claims were filed. Four of 13 sports (basketball, track/field, softball, and soccer) accounted for 81% of the injury claims. Sixty-three percent of the athletes participated in these sports.
3. **Triage experience at Summer International Games:** 87% of athletes seen at the first aid stations at the Baton Rouge games were treated and released, 10% were referred to the infirmary, 2% were referred to the training room for further observation, and 1% were referred to the hospital.
4. **Injury rate for summer sports:** vary depending on many factors. Rates for summer sports are approximately 0.4 reported injury per 1000 participant hours.

C. Winter sports

1. **Surveillance data:** Table 3 lists injury and illness events recorded by the Team USA physicians at the First International Special Olympics Winter Games in Salzburg and Schladming, Austria, 1993.

TABLE 2. Injury and Illness Events at International Summer Special Olympics Games, 1983, Baton Rouge, Louisiana*

Diagnosis	Number (%)
Heat-related illness	302 (22%)
Abrasion, laceration, contusion	287 (21%)
Sprain, strain	280 (20%)
Other illness	146 (10.6%)
Gastrointestinal illness	115 (8.0%)
Respiratory illness	70 (5.0%)
Other injury	57 (4.0%)
Other routine services such as allergy shot, x-ray, or physical examination	33 (2.4%)
Behavioral/psychiatric	26 (1.9%)
Seizure disorder	22 (1.6%)
Dental injury or illness	15 (1.0%)
Closed head or neck injury	12 (0.9%)
Fracture or dislocation	8 (0.6%)

* A total of 2150 athletes competed in 7000 events.

2. **Relative safety of winter sports:** calculated for Team USA at the Austrian winter games. Injury rates per participant were calculated by dividing the number of injuries reported by the number of athletes participating in each sport.
   a. Alpine skiing: 20/28 = .71
   c. Floor hockey: 11/35 = .31
   b. Speed skating: 7/28 = .25
   d. Figure skating: 3/29 = .10
   e. Cross country skiing: 1/28 = .04
3. **Are athletes with Down syndrome at greater risk?** Athletes with Down syndrome who participated in the First International World Winter Games were not more likely to experience an injury or illness occurrence than other athletes.

VI. Medical and Safety Requirements at Competitions

A. **Sport-specific medical and safety requirements:** contained in the Official Special Olympics Sports Rules[9]

B. **Minimum medical coverage at large competitions**
   1. **Emergency medical technician** must be in attendance at the first aid area at all times.
   2. **Physician** must be on-site or on immediate call at all times.
   3. **Other allied health personnel:** At regional, national, and international competitions, athletes compete at higher levels of intensity, which places them at greater risk for athletic injury. Athletes at such games should be attended by personnel skilled in the assessment and treatment of musculoskeletal injury, such as general and sports medicine physicians, orthopedic surgeons, trainers, and physical therapists.
   4. **Equipment and transportation:** An ambulance, resuscitator, source of oxygen, and other appropriate medical equipment must be available at all times.

C. **Minimum safety precautions at competitions**
   1. **Heat and sun:** Precautions must be exercised to avoid heat-related illnesses and sunburn.
   2. **Environment and weather:** Precautions must be taken when competitions are held at high altitudes, including providing training recommendations for athletes before the competition and properly equipping the competition venues. Teams should have adequate time to adjust to altitude, temperature, and humidity.

TABLE 3. Injury and Illness Diagnoses and Health Station Visits Recorded by Team USA Physicians at the First International Special Olympics Winter Games, Salzburg and Schladming, Austria, 1993

Sport	Number/Diagnosis	Total Each Sport (% Total Visits)
	Injury Visits	
Speed skating	5 abrasion	7 (9%)
	1 patellofemoral syndrome	
	1 contusion	
	1 ankle sprain	
Figure skating	3 contusion	3 (4%)
Floor hockey	5 abrasion	11 (14%)
	4 abrasion	
	1 sprain	
	1 patellar subluxation	
Alpine skiing	5 contusion	20 (25%)
	4 abrasion	
	3 blister	
	3 sprain	
	2 muscle strain	
	1 lateral meniscus	
	1 wind burn	
	1 shoulder injury	
Cross country skiing	1 ankle sprain	1 (1%)
Subtotal injury visits		42 (53%)
	Illness Visits	
	10 respiratory illness	
	8 dehydration	
	5 behavioral/psychiatric	
	5 gastrointestinal illness	
	4 dermatologic problem	
	3 canker sores, gingivitis	
	1 eye	
	1 menstrual problem	
Subtotal illness visits		37 (47%)
Total visits		79 (100%)

3. **Fluids:** The Special Olympics athlete often lacks the normal perception of thirst. Ample water or other liquids must be available and encouraged by coaches, volunteers, and health care teams. Caffeinated drinks are not recommended for rehydration. Adequate toilet facilities should be readily available at all events.
4. **Medications:** Athletes must receive the medications prescribed. Coaches should have access to medical consultation in case medications are lost or if adjustments are needed because of time zone crossings while en route to games.

D. **Communication**
1. **On site:** a two-way wireless radio system connecting site venues with first-aid station
2. **Between competition site and support facilities:** radio or telephone communication to the nearest hospital emergency room

E. **Transportation**
1. **On the field:** golf carts or other appropriate transportation to transport injured or ill athletes to a centralized first-aid station if sports venues are at some distance
2. **Ambulance:** to transport athlete safely to the hospital if necessary

3. **Helicopter:** Life-flight has been used at International Winter Games where emergency facilities are distant from the downhill and crosscountry ski venues.

F. **Medical liaison** at large competitions, such as national and international games, includes:
1. Individual team primary care physicians or nurses
2. Access to medical subspecialists such as orthopedic surgeon, emergency medicine physician, ophthalmologist, pediatrician, family medicine physician, internal medicine physician, cardiologist, dermatologist, and neurologist
3. Availability of translators to communicate with foreign language–speaking athletes

G. **Equipment and supplies** See Chapter 7, "Injuries and Emergencies on the Field," Table 1.

H. **Insurance:** Many athletes are covered by their family's insurance; however, SOI has an umbrella insurance plan that covers medical costs of emergency care required at games, if necessary.

VII. Injury and Illness Prevention

A. **Training:** Adequate training, including muscle and cardiovascular conditioning, as suggested in other chapters, promotes the safe participation of the Special Olympics athlete in sports.

B. **Other specific preventive measures**
1. **Protective gear:** The Special Olympics athlete should be provided with adequate protective padding and gear appropriate to each sport and to the athlete's condition.
   a. Protective polycarbonate **eyewear** is recommended for athletes playing projectile or ball sports.
   b. Athletes who wear glasses while playing contact or collision sports should wear safety eyewear.
   c. Individualize recommendations for protection and participation of the one-eyed athlete in contact or collision sports or projectile or ball sports.
2. **Seizure precautions:** required around swimming pools, water hazards, equestrian events, certain gymnastics events, and alpine skiing. Especially while swimming, a qualified lifeguard should be alongside at all times. In competition, the swimmer should be in outside lanes. A seizure while in or around the water is the greatest hazard in all of Special Olympics.
3. **Vaccines:** Flu vaccine and measles vaccine status should be reviewed, especially for athletes participating in regional, national, and international games.
4. **Injury surveillance:** Careful and complete injury and illness reporting and review by medical committees should be carried out during and after large competitions to document specific needs for health intervention and injury prevention.

Recommended Reading

1. Birrer RB: The special Olympics: An injury overview. Phys Sportsmed 12(4):95–97, 1984.
2. Burke SW, Roberts JM, Johnston CE, et al: Chronic atlanto-axial instability in Down syndrome. J Bone J Surg 67A(9):1356–1360, 1985.
3. Emes C, Page S: Training Special Olympics athletes: A pilot study. Percept Mot Skills 75(2):41, 1992.
4. Goldberg MJ: Spine instability and the Special Olympics. Clin Sports Med 12(3):507–515, 1993.
5. Harley EH, Collins MD: Neurologic sequelae secondary to atlantoaxial instability in Down syndrome: Implications in otolaryngologic surgery. Arch Otolaryngol Head Neck Surg 120(2):159–165, 1994.
6. Klein T, Gilman E, Zigler E: Special Olympics: An evaluation by professionals and parents. Ment Retard 31(l):15–23, 1993.
7. McCormick DP, Ivey FM Jr, Gold DM, et al: The preparticipation sports examination in Special Olympics Athletes. Texas Med 84(4):39–43, 1988.
8. McCormick DP, Niebuhr VN, Risser WL: Injury and illness surveillance at local Special Olympics games. Br J Sports Med 24 (4):221–224, 1990.

9. Official Special Olympics Summer [Winter] Sports Rules: 1992–1995, rev. ed. Washington, DC, Special Olympics International, 1992.
10. Perlman SP: Special Olympics athletes and the incidence of sports-related injuries. J Mass Dent Soc 43(4):44, 1994.
11. Pitetti KH, Campbell KD: Mentally retarded individuals—a population at risk? Med Sci Sports Exerc 23(5):586–592, 1990.
12. Pueschel SM: Atlanto-axial instability: Sport and Down syndrome. Lancet 1:980, 1983.
13. Pueschel SM, Scola FH: Epidemiological radiographic and clinical studies of atlantoaxial instability in individuals with Down syndrome. Pediatrics 80:555–560, 1987.
14. Robson HE: The Special Olympic games for the mentally handicapped—United Kingdom 1989. Br J Sports Med 24(4): 225–230, 1990.
15. Wekesa M, Onsongo J: Kenyan team care at the Special Olympics. Br J Sports Med 26(3):128–133, 1992.

PART III
CONDITIONING

14: Preseason Conditioning: Aerobic Power

Richard W. Latin, Ph.D.

Cardiovascular fitness is an important aspect of physical fitness for endurance athletes. Aerobic power is the maximum capability to transport and use oxygen and is an index of cardiovascular efficiency. Training programs for aerobic power improvement need to stress the physiologic components of the oxygen transport system.

I. Physiologic Components of Oxygen Uptake ($\dot{V}O_2$)

$\dot{V}O_2$ may be mathematically and physiologically defined as:

$$\dot{V}O_2 = HR \times SV \times a - \overline{v}O_2 \text{ difference}$$

The system has a central and peripheral component.

A. **Central component**
   1. Heart rate (HR)
   2. Stroke volume (SV)
   3. Cardiac output (CO) = HR × SV
   4. A primary component to high $\dot{V}O_2$ is dictated by the heart's ability to pump a large volume of blood.

B. **Peripheral component**
   1. Arterial–mixed venous oxygen difference ($a - \overline{v}O_2$ difference)
   2. The ability of tissues to extract and use oxygen for ATP resynthesis is another primary component of $\dot{V}O_2$. This is particularly true for muscles that are being recruited during an activity.

C. **Maximum oxygen uptake ($\dot{V}O_2$max)**
   1. The measure of $\dot{V}O_2$max represents the maximum capabilities of the oxygen transport system.
   2. It is generally expressed in milliliters of O_2 consumed per kilogram of body mass per minute (ml/kg/min). It may also be expressed in L/min.

II. Training Principles

A. **Specificity of training**
   1. One of the most important conditioning principles. The athlete should train in a manner similar to how he or she would compete. There are metabolic and neuromuscular components.
   2. Metabolic—stress the metabolic pathways that would be responsible for the bioenergetics (ATP resynthesis) of a particular exercise task.
   3. Neuromuscular—recruit the motor units that would be similarly recruited for a given exercise task.
   4. Training specificity is best accomplished by having an individual practice using movement patterns and speeds similar to a given exercise task, e.g., a marathoner

TABLE 1. Summary of American College of Sports Medicine Guidelines for Quantity and Quality of Exercise Programs for Healthy Adults

Component	Recommendation
Frequency	3–5 days/week
Duration	20–60 min
Intensity	60–90% HRmax 50–85% $\dot{V}O_2$max or 50–85% HRRmax
Mode	Any exercise using large muscle groups that is continuous and rhythmic in nature

would train by performing long endurance runs as opposed to short high-intensity sprints, or a cyclist would train by cycling not running. Both exercises use leg muscles but different recruitment patterns.

B. **Overload:** For adaptive improvement to occur, work stresses must be greater than normally encountered.

C. **Progression:** a gradual, systematic increase in training intensity or volume as improvement occurs

D. **Individuality:** No two individuals respond or adapt similarly to the same training program. Allowances for initial fitness levels, responses to training, etc. need to be considered.

III. Aerobic Training Guidelines

A. **Guidelines:** The American College of Sports Medicine (ACSM) has proposed guidelines that may be used to train successfully athletes or persons interested in health-related aerobic fitness. These guidelines address intensity, frequency, duration, and mode of aerobic exercise (Table 1).

B. **Intensity of exercise training**

1. Selecting an appropriate intensity
   a. No exact method exists to establish a starting exercise intensity.
   b. Perceived exertion ratings may allow for an adjustment in initial exercise intensities.
   c. Refer to Table 2 for suggested guidelines.
2. HR as an indicator of intensity
   a. Using HR provides a reasonably accurate means of assessing exercise intensity. However, one must use a valid means of quantifying HR such as telemetry, exercise cardiotachometer, or a careful palpation technique.
   b. Consideration should be given to conditions or situations that may affect HR, e.g., medications, heat, altitude, emotional state, overtraining, and cardiovascular drift.
3. Heart rate reserve (HRR) method
   a. 50–85% of HRR plus the resting rate (HRrest) may be used to establish appropriate exercise intensities.

TABLE 2. Suggested Initial Training Intensities

Fitness Level	HRmax	HRR and %$\dot{V}O_2$
Beginner (unconditioned)	60–70%	50–65%
Intermediate (recreational athlete)	70–80%	65–75%
Advanced (competitive athlete)	80–90%+	75–85%+

TABLE 3. Calculation of Aerobic Training Heart Rate by Heart Rate Reserve*

Step	Calculation
Compute age predicted HR	220 – 20 = 200
Compute HRR	200 – 60 = 140
Select training intensity	80%
Calculate percent of reserve	140 × 0.80 = 112
Add resting HR	112 + 60 = 172
Target HR	172 beats/min

* Example is for a 20-year-old with a resting HR = 60 beats/min. A corresponding target HR by the HRmax method would be 200 × 0.80 = 160 beats/min.

b. Values may be obtained by using the formula developed by Karvonen:
   i. HRmax = 220 – age (or other appropriate equations or testing methods)
   ii. HRR = HRmax – HRrest
   iii. Select intensity: 50–85% of HRR
   iv. Add result to HRrest for exercise target HR
   v. See Table 3 for sample calculation.

4. HRmax: 60–90% of HRmax may be used to establish appropriate exercise intensities.
5. Percent of $\dot{V}O_2$ as an indicator of intensity: Using $\dot{V}O_2$ provides an accurate means of assessing exercise intensity. It is not subject to excessive variation and quantification as is HR and may be the method of choice when $\dot{V}O_2$max may be accurately determined. However, it is difficult to apply this method to some modes of exercise, e.g., swimming, cross country skiing.
6. Percent $\dot{V}O_2$max method
   a. Workloads that require an oxygen cost of 50–85% of the $\dot{V}O_2$max may be used to establish appropriate exercise intensities.
   b. Determination of $\dot{V}O_2$max is required:
      i. A maximal exercise test using indirect open circuit calorimetry provides the most accurate measure of $\dot{V}O_2$max. This may be time or cost prohibitive.
      ii. A field test may be used to estimate $\dot{V}O_2$max, e.g., Astrand cycle or step test.
   c. Workloads may be established by two methods:
      i. Plot the workload or HR/$\dot{V}O_2$ relationship obtained during a maximal test (Fig. 1).
      ii. Algebraically determine the oxygen cost of exercise from the equations reported by ACSM.[1]
   d. $\dot{V}O_2$ for horizontal running:
      $\dot{V}O_2$ (ml/kg/min) = speed (m/min) × 0.2 + 3.5 ml/kg/min
   e. $\dot{V}O_2$ of cycle ergometry:
      $\dot{V}O_2$ (ml/min) = power load (kg/min) × 2 + (3.5 × kg body mass)
   f. Example calculation:
      i. Athlete B has a $\dot{V}O_2$max = 60 ml/kg/min
      ii. Equation for oxygen cost for running on horizontal surface: $\dot{V}O_2$ = speed (m/min) × 0.2 + 3.5 ml/kg/min
      iii. Selected training intensity 80% of $\dot{V}O_2$max: 60 ml/kg/min × 0.80 = 48 ml/kg/min
      iv. Running for $\dot{V}O_2$ = 48 ml/kg/min:
         (a) 48 ml/kg/min = speed (m/min) × 0.2 + 3.5 ml/kg/min
         (b) 44.5 ml/kg/min = speed (m/min) × 0.2
         (c) 222.5 = speed (m/min) or 8.3 mph or 7:14 per mile pace
      v. Athlete B may run at a 7:14 per mile pace for an appropriate training intensity.

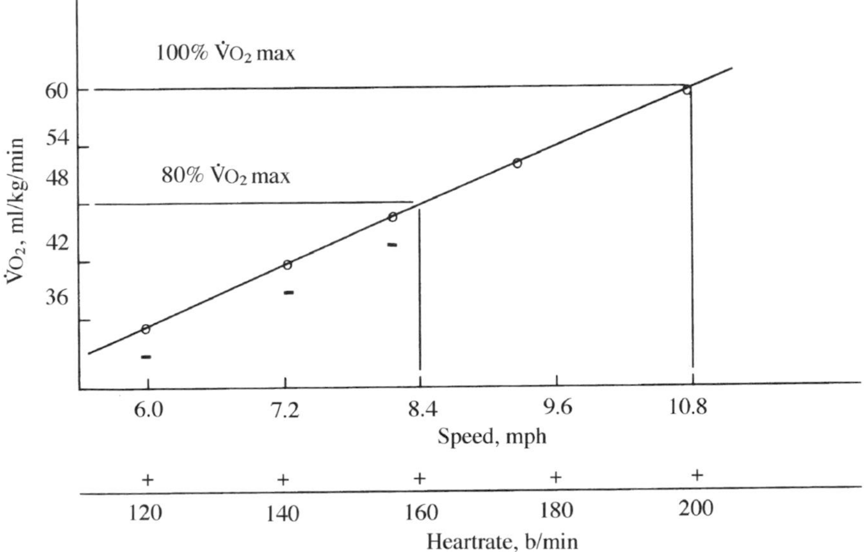

FIGURE 1. Relationship between $\dot{V}O_2$ and heart rate or workload.

C. **Frequency of exercise training**
   1. Suggested training frequencies are 3–5 days per week.
   2. Endurance athletes may train 5–6 days per week. For health-related aerobic fitness or in sports in which aerobic demand is not as great, 3 days per week is recommended.

D. **Duration of exercise training**
   1. The suggested duration of an individual training session is 20–60 minutes.
   2. Twenty minutes is the minimal duration required for maintenance or improvement to occur, and 60 minutes or longer may be required in training sessions for long endurance athletes.

E. **Mode of exercise training**
   1. Exercises that use large muscle groups and that are continuous and rhythmic in nature should be used to improve aerobic power.
   2. Exercises that require heavy muscle contractions such as weight training produce little changes in $\dot{V}O_2$max.

F. **Effects of exercise mode**
   1. **Central adaptations**—relatively nondiscriminatory changes. HR, SV, and CO adaptations may occur regardless of aerobic exercise mode. Therefore, this component to improving $\dot{V}O_2$max is nonspecific.
   2. **Peripheral responses**—highly task-specific changes. Neuromuscular recruitment of specific motor units and appropriate blood flow shunts are essential to peripheral physiologic and biochemical adaptations that allow for greater tissue utilization of oxygen and improvement of $\dot{V}O_2$max.
   3. Although a runner may maintain the central component of the oxygen transport system by cycling, the peripheral component is not adequately stimulated because neuromuscular recruitment and blood flow shunts are not the same. This violates one of the tenets of exercise specificity. However, it may be important to consider that many modes of exercise may be used interchangeably if only the health and fitness of the central component (heart) is of concern.

G. **Overload and progression**
1. Intensity, frequency, and duration may be manipulated to impose progressive overload.
2. Intensity of exercise has the greatest influence on improvements of aerobic power.
3. From the standpoint of progression, frequency should be emphasized first, keeping duration and intensity constant until the desired times per week can be safely (to minimize injury) achieved.
4. Once the frequency is established, increasing the duration of exercise is emphasized, keeping intensity constant, until a desired length of time is achieved.
5. Finally, intensity is manipulated. As fitness levels improve, gradual increases in the intensity of exercise stimulate improvement in aerobic power.
6. Any abrupt increases in exercise frequency, duration, and especially intensity should be avoided. This predisposes the athlete to an underpreparation injury.

H. **Improvement**
1. The amount of improvement in $\dot{V}O_2max$ to expect from training is highly individualized and inversely related to the initial fitness level. An untrained individual may experience a 20–25% increase in $\dot{V}O_2max$ in an 8- to 12-week training period. A trained individual may observe a 5% or less improvement in the same time period. Table 4 contains norms for $\dot{V}O_2max$.
2. A genetically determined peak $\dot{V}O_2max$ may occur in 18–24 months of intense training. Up to 70% of this may be achieved in about 3 months.
3. Improvement in endurance performance when $\dot{V}O_2max$ fails to increase is accomplished by athletes being able to sustain exercise at a higher percent of their $\dot{V}O_2max$ with less fatigue. Higher percent utilization of $\dot{V}O_2max$ is synonymous with a higher lactate threshold (LT) or point at which there is an onset of blood lactate accumulation.
4. Percent utilization of $\dot{V}O_2max$ and LT are excellent predictors of endurance performance among individuals with similar $\dot{V}O_2max$.

IV. Methods of Training

A. **When to begin training** is dictated by the type of sport and when a peak level of conditioning is desired. Athletes in sports such as cross country, track, and swimming may use the season itself as a conditioning period aiming to peak at the season's end for a championship meet. If a season were 10 weeks long, serious training might start 2 or 3 weeks before its beginning. Knowing that it requires 8–12 weeks of training to obtain significant levels of improvement, an athlete's training agenda may be planned accordingly.

B. **How much training is needed** is also dictated by the sport. A football player requires minimal aerobic fitness and may dedicate three times per week for about 15–20 minutes to this type of conditioning, whereas a 10-km running specialist may train six times per week for about 40 to 60 minutes using a variety of high-intensity methods during half of those sessions. Therefore, the amount of aerobic conditioning is influenced by the aerobic metabolic demand of the sport or event.

TABLE 4. Aerobic Fitness Classifications $\dot{V}O_2max$ (ml/kg/min)

	Male Ages		Female Ages	
Category	***13–19***	***20–29***	***13–19***	***20–29***
Poor	Below 39	Below 36	Below 30	Below 27
Good	40–50	37–47	31–40	28–37
Excellent	51–59	48–56	41–50	38–47
Highly trained	60–80	57–80	51–65	48–65

C. **Long slow duration training:** emphasis on duration rather than intensity. Intensities are typically about 65–75% of HRR + HRrest or 60–70% of $\dot{V}O_2$max or HRmax. This approach may be used for general conditioning or as a training mode on days following intense workouts. This type of training should not be used exclusively for the competitive athlete because it lacks the specific neuromuscular and metabolic stress necessary under competitive conditions. An example of this would be a middle distance runner running 8 miles at a 7:30 per mile pace.

D. **Long fast duration training:** typified by higher intensity, moderate duration forms of exercise. Intensities are generally 80–90% of HRR + HRrest or 80–85% of $\dot{V}O_2$max or HRmax. The athlete maintains a pace just at or below a racing speed. Because the intensity is higher than long slow duration training and the metabolic and neuromuscular components are specific to racing conditions, greater improvements can be made using this training mode. The physical and psychological demands of this type of training are great; therefore, alternating slow and fast workouts or other training variations is recommended. An example of this type of training is a middle distance runner running 4 miles at a 5:30 per mile pace.

E. **Interval training:** intervals of intense exercise interspersed with recovery. An athlete may maintain levels of intensity at or above racing conditions for an extended time period. This makes interval training a high-quality conditioning mode that exemplifies the tenets of exercise specificity.
   1. Exercise intervals—aerobic training intervals are typically 3–5 minutes in duration performed at or above race paces.
   2. Recovery intervals—suggested recovery times are from one to one half the exercise interval time. An example is 3 minutes of exercise with 3 minutes of recovery. Recovery time may also be judged sufficient when the athlete's HR has returned to about 120–130 beats/min.
   3. Type of recovery—low level activity (30–50% of $\dot{V}O_2$max) between exercise intervals hastens the removal of lactic acid and thus expedites recovery.
   4. Number of intervals—the suggested number of intervals is dictated by their length, e.g., shorter intervals such as 3 minutes may be repeated 5 to 10 times, and longer intervals such as 5 minutes may be repeated 4 to 8 times.

F. **Combination programs:** Most successful programs incorporate all three of the previously described methods. Typically, intensive training days or weeks are followed by a corresponding number of easier days or weeks. This is necessary from not only physiologic but also psychological standpoints. See Fox and coworkers for an excellent discussion of conditioning programs.

V. Other Training Considerations

A. **Muscle glycogen depletion and restoration:** Some endurance athletes become chronically glycogen depleted, which causes their performance to suffer. This is largely due to overtraining, inadequate rest, and failure to take in an adequate amount of dietary carbohydrates. It takes approximately 48 hours while eating diets high in carbohydrates for complete restoration from a significantly depleted state to occur. No exhaustive training should take place during this time.

B. **Multiple daily training sessions:** Little scientific evidence exists to support that training two or three times per day is better than a single workout. Although more research in this area is necessary, it is generally recommended that the athlete participate in one high-quality training session on scheduled days.

C. **Training quantity versus quality:** The "more is better" attitude is adopted by many endurance athletes. This stance invites overtraining injuries as well as decreased performance. Runners reporting 150 miles per week or so are probably training by the long slow duration method, which is not as productive for improvement. Although no method exists to establish a "perfect" training regimen, the emphasis should be on quality workouts interspersed with adequate low-intensity recovery days. An excellent example of successful high-quality training is demonstrated by a former U.S. Olympic steeplechase runner and medalist. This athlete reported to train only about 35 miles per week for his 3-km event.

Recommended Reading

1. American College of Sports Medicine: Guidelines for Exercise Testing and Prescription. Baltimore, Williams & Wilkins, 1995.
2. American College of Sports Medicine: Position statement on the participation of the female athlete in long distance running. Med Sci Sports 11:9, 1979.
3. American College of Sports Medicine: Position statement on the recommended quantity and quality of exercise for developing cardiorespiratory and muscular fitness in healthy adults. Med Sci Sports Exerc 22:265, 1990.
4. Fox E, Bowers R, Foss M: The Physiological Basis for Exercise and Sport. Madison, WI, WC Brown & Benchmark, 1993.
5. Wilmore J, Costill D: Training for Sport and Activity. Dubuque, IA, William C. Brown, 1988.

15

Preseason Strength Training

Thomas R. Baechle, Ed.D., and Brian P. Conroy, M.D.

This chapter identifies and describes the variables employed in designing safe, effective preseason strength training programs. These design variables should be carefully manipulated with regard to the demands of the sport, the athlete's capacities and limitations, and the goals of the training program. The following information assumes that the length of the preseason period is 8 weeks.

Strength training is only part of total athletic conditioning. It is a means to an end and not an end in itself. Improvement in sports performance, not simply developing superior strength, should be the ultimate goal. Strength training should be integrated into the total conditioning program to provide an optimal environment for improvements in agility, power, speed, speed endurance, speed strength, and flexibility while avoiding overtraining.

I. Strength Training Principles

A. **Overload and progressive overload principles**

1. "Overload" means imposing a greater stimulus than that to which the body is accustomed.
2. **Overload is the stimulus** needed for physiologic adaptation and maximal gains.
3. Introducing overload in a systematic manner is referred to as **progressive overload**. Theoretically, each training session should involve a greater overload than the previous one. In reality, one should recognize the need for variation in training. Well-conceived programs do involve progressively greater overload, but also have time for recovery and adaptation.
   a. The use of variation in training sessions is referred to as **cycling** and is based on the concept of periodization.
   b. **Periodization** is the systematic organization of the entire training process, e.g., method of training, loads, volumes, and variation needed over an extended period of time.

B. **SAID principle (*S*pecific *A*daptation to *I*mposed *D*emands)**

1. **Adaptations occurring in response to training are specific to the type of training undertaken.** For example, long distance training is associated with increases in mitochondria number and size, with little or no change in muscular strength levels. Conversely, sprint training has a minimal effect on mitochondria but produces increased leg strength.
2. The extent of change is dictated largely by the level of imposed demands and the fitness and training levels of the athlete at the onset of training.

C. **Specificity concept**

1. Specificity is an application of the SAID principle. It refers to **training in a specific manner to produce a specific outcome**. Its application involves determining the specific or unique demands of the sport, then designing a strength training program that stimulates the appropriate adaptation and improved performance in the sport.

2. In using the specificity concept, the following demands or characteristics of the sport are considered:
   a. **Strength:** ability to produce maximal force in a one-time, all-out effort
   b. **Speed strength:** ability to produce high forces at fast velocities
   c. **Muscular endurance:** ability to perform muscular work over an extended period of time without undue fatigue
   d. **Speed endurance:** ability to produce high forces at fast velocities repeatedly over an extended period of time
   e. **Cardiovascular endurance:** ability of the heart and vessels to transport, the lungs to oxygenate, and the muscles to use oxygen efficiently over an extended period of time
   f. **Power:** ability to exert force rapidly, defined as **P = work/time**
   g. **Range of movement (flexibility):** ability to move a joint through its entire range of movement
   h. **Metabolic demands:** refers to determining the predominant energy system involved in a particular form or intensity of exercise
3. Manipulation of the program design variables allows emphasizing or deemphasizing improvement in these eight characteristics.

II. Program Design Variables

A. **Choices of exercises for the preseason program**
   1. Definitions
      a. **Core exercises:** involve two or more joints and large muscle groups
      b. **Secondary exercises:** involve smaller muscle groups
      c. **Power or quick lift exercises:** core exercises distinguishable by their ballistic nature and recruitment of *power zone* muscles (thighs to rib cage)
   2. To **select exercises appropriately**, apply the specificity concept as follows:
      a. **Give emphasis to those exercises that work the same muscle groups, in a similar range of motion, as the movements involved in the sport.**
      b. **The choice of power or quick lift exercises is essential in developing speed strength for sports involving explosive movements.**
   3. Attempt to include at least one exercise for thighs, calf, upper and lower back, shoulders, arms, abdomen, chest, and neck for wrestling and football.
   4. Include at least one power exercise (power clean, hang clean, snatch, push press) to improve neuromuscular coordination and power among the power zone muscles.
   5. For preseason training, include 2 or 3 power movement exercises, 3 or 4 additional core exercises, and 4–6 secondary exercises.
   6. Although the off-season program uses a greater number of core exercises, the preseason program includes sport-specific or secondary exercises, e.g., wrist curls (baseball, softball), pullovers (volleyball), neck exercises (football, wrestling).
   7. Core and secondary exercises commonly included in strength training programs are listed in Table 1. Baechle and colleagues[2] is an excellent resource for details on how to perform the exercises listed in Table 1 correctly.

B. **Order of the exercises**
   1. The order in which exercises are performed is important because it may affect the intensity of effort.
      a. An appropriate arrangement provides better recovery, thereby enabling the athlete to work more intensely.
      b. An appropriate arrangement may also help reduce the incidence of injury (e.g., low back exercises before power cleans or squats could predispose the athlete to injury).

TABLE 1. Core and Secondary Exercises Commonly Included in Strength Training Programs*

Core Exercises		
Power movements—quick lifts		
Power snatch	Hang clean	High pull, from floor and hang
Power clean	Push press	
Hang snatch	Push jerk	
Other		
Squat, front and back	Dead lift, with bent and straight legs	Standing overhead press, in front and behind the neck
Quarter squat, front and back	Bench press	
Leg press, hip sled	Incline press	Bent-over row
Secondary Exercises		
Leg extension	Hyperextension	Tricep press-down
Leg curl	"Good morning"	Reverse curl
Lunge forward, lateral, and step through	Pull-over	Dumbbell fly
	Lateral front raise	Neck exercises
Heel raise	Shoulder shrug	
Bent-knee twisting sit-up	Bicep curl	

* Almost all of the exercises listed can be performed with a dumbbell(s).

2. Exercise order should follow these guidelines:
   a. Core exercises first, then secondary exercises
   b. Power exercises first, then strength exercises
   c. Low back and abdominal exercises last
3. Once priorities (e.g., power exercises before strength exercises) have been established, next consider the order of exercises within both core and secondary exercise categories. Common approaches include:
   a. Alternating push and pull exercises
   b. Alternating upper body exercises with lower body exercises
4. Table 2 shows how the same 12 exercises might be arranged or ordered into a 3-day-a-week and 4-day-a-week program.
5. Should athletes strength train before or after practice? During the **preseason** and **off-season**, athletes should **strength train first**, then practice the sport. **In season**, athletes should strength train **after practice**.

C. **Number of repetitions/sets (volume)**
   1. Definitions
      a. **Repetitions:** number of times an exercise is performed before a period of rest
      b. **Set:** the completion of one series of repetitions, followed by a rest period or a different exercise
      c. **Volume** = sets × repetitions
   2. Using the specificity concept, volume guidelines for the core exercises presented in Table 3 may be summarized as follows:
      a. For **power**, assign 3–6 sets of 1–3 repetitions.
      b. For **muscle strength**, assign 3–5 sets of 3–8 repetitions.
      c. For **muscle hypertrophy**, assign 3–6 sets of 8–12 repetitions.
      d. For **muscular endurance**, assign 2 sets of 15–20 repetitions.
   3. Volume guidelines for secondary exercises are 2–3 sets of 8–12 repetitions.
   4. Table 3 shows that volumes are lowest when training for power and strength and highest when training for hypertrophy and muscular endurance.
      a. Muscular endurance requirements of certain sports are best acquired through drills and participation in the sport, rather than through development in the weight room.
      b. For this reason, loads less than 60% are not presented in Table 3.

TABLE 2. Order of Exercise: 3- and 4-Day-a-Week Programs

For purposes of comparison, the same 12 exercises are ordered/arranged in 3- and 4-day-a-week programs.

3-Day-a-Week (Monday, Wednesday, Friday) Program

Type of Exercise*	Exercise	Muscle Area†
C,P	Power clean‡	TB
C,P	Hang clean‡	TB
C	Bench press‡	CH
C	Back squat‡	LG
C	Bent-over row	UB
C	Overhead press	SH
S	Bicep curl	A-A
S	Tricep press-down	A-P
S	Leg extension	L-A
S	Leg curl	L-P
S	Hyperextensions	LB
S	Bent-knee sit-ups	AB

The above would be considered a long workout during the preseason for some teams (representing approximately 1.5 h). Should the amount of workout time need to be reduced, the clean from a hang position and the triceps press-down could be deleted without having a significant negative effect.

4-Day-a-Week Split Program

Type*	Monday–Thursday	Muscle Area†	Type	Tuesday–Friday	Muscle Area
C,P	Power clean	TB, LG, UB, LB	C	Bench press	CH, SH, A-P
C,P	Hang clean	TB, LG, UB, LB	C	Bent-over row	UB, A-A
C	Back squat	TB, LG	C	Overhead press	SH, A-P
S	Leg extension	L-A	S	Bicep curl	A-A
S	Leg curl	L-P	S	Tricep press-down	A-P
S	Hyperextension	LB	S	Bent-knee sit-ups	AB

* Type of exercises: C = core; P = power; S = secondary exercises.
† Muscle area: TB = total body; CH = chest; LG = leg; UB = upper back; SH = shoulder; A-A = arm-anterior; A-P = arm-posterior; L-A = leg-anterior; L-P = leg-posterior; LB = lower back; AB = abdominal.
‡ Exercises to be cycled. For wrestling or football, include neck exercises.

5. As the season draws nearer, the number of sets typically becomes smaller as the loads become heavier. More emphasis and time are given to practicing skills and strategies of the sport.

D. **Resistance or load assignments**

1. Calculating assignments of resistance or loads typically involves use of a percentage of maximum strength, expressed as the athlete's 1 repetition maximum (**1 RM** = the maximum amount of weight lifted for 1 repetition).
   a. If the athlete or coach is not comfortable with the actual performance of a 1 RM, the **predicted 1 RM** may be obtained by having the athlete perform as many repetitions as is possible with a weight that allows 10 or fewer repetitions resulting in muscular failure occurring during the last repetition.

TABLE 3. Specificity Concept Applied to Program Design Variables

Intensity Classification	Outcome of Training	% of 1 RM	Repetition Range	Sets	Rest Between Sets
High	Power	80	1–3	3–6	2–4 min
High	Strength	80–90	3–8	3–6	2–4 min
Moderate	Hypertrophy	70–80	8–12	3–6	30–90 sec
Light	Muscular endurance	60–70*	12–15 +	2–3	30 sec or less

* Although it is common to see percentages of less than 60% recommended for developing muscular endurance, especially in circuit training programs, the authors' opinions are that endurance activities associated with the sport, not strength training, should be predominantly relied on to produce the needed changes in sport-specific muscular endurance.

TABLE 4. Prediction of the 1 Repetition Maximum (1 RM)

Repetitions Completed	Repetition Factor
1	1.00
2	1.07
3	1.10
4	1.13
5	1.16
6	1.20
7	1.23
8	1.27
9	1.32
10	1.36
11	1.40
12	1.43

Adapted from Lombardi VP: Beginning Weight Training: The Safe and Effective Way. Dubuque, IA, William C. Brown, 1989, p 201.

b. Predict the 1 RM by multiplying the weight lifted times the repetition factor (that corresponds to the number of repetitions performed) found in Table 4.
c. For example, consider an athlete that places 100 pounds on the bench press and is able to complete six but not seven strict repetitions (6 RM). The repetition factor to the right of six repetitions in Table 4 is 1.20, which when multiplied by 100 gives 120 pounds as the predicted 1 RM in the bench press.

2. Using the specificity concept, the 1 RM resistance or load guidelines presented in Table 3 may be summarized as follows:
   a. For **power**, assign a load that approximates 80% of the 1 RM.
   b. For **muscle strength**, assign a load that approximates 80–90% of the 1 RM.
   c. For **muscle hypertrophy**, assign a load that approximates 70–80% of the 1 RM.
   d. For **muscle endurance**, assign a load that approximates 60–70% of the 1 RM.
   e. **Note:** These percentages are useful as a general guideline to identify the correct weight to use in the exercises selected. Be aware that in certain exercises, such as the leg press, higher percentages of the 1 RM may be needed for the athlete to reach muscular failure in the repetition range that corresponds to the desired training outcome (e.g., repetition range for strength is three to eight repetitions) as described in Table 3.
3. A second method that can be used for developing resistance or load assignments is simply to decide on a specific number of repetitions to be performed and determine, by trial and error, a load that permits that number of repetitions to be completed.
   a. For example, consider an athlete scheduled to use a weight that permits eight repetitions in each of the three sets (three sets, eight repetitions) to achieve the training outcome of increased strength.
   b. The load for this athlete is correct if he or she is able to complete eight repetitions in the first two sets and between 6 and 10 repetitions in the last set.
   c. If fewer than 6 or greater than 10 repetitions are performed in the last set, the load should be decreased or increased. **Note:** The athlete should complete only the predetermined number of repetitions in the preceding sets, then perform as many repetitions as possible in the last set to maximize strength gains and to determine if the load needs to be adjusted.

E. **Rest periods**

1. Table 3 shows application of the specificity concept in determining lengths of rest periods between sets.

2. Longer rest periods (2–4 minutes) are more appropriate for strength and power development, whereas rest periods for muscle endurance are 30 seconds or less. The rest periods for hypertrophy fall somewhere in between.

F. **Frequency of training:** Once exercises have been selected, decide when they will be performed during the week.
   1. The three common approaches are:
      a. To work out **3 days a week** (Mondays, Wednesdays, Fridays or Tuesdays, Thursdays, Saturdays) and perform all exercises each day
      b. To work out **4 days a week** (Mondays, Tuesdays, Thursdays, Fridays), splitting up exercises into body parts, working some on Mondays and Thursdays and some on Tuesdays and Fridays (split program)
      c. To work out **6 days a week**, dividing exercises into three categories, performing each twice a week, but not 2 days in succession
   2. Only the 3- and 4-day-a-week programs are discussed here. These programs are presented in Tables 2, 5, and 6.

G. **Variation**
   1. Varying training loads and volumes is important. **By varying loads or volumes there is a greater chance of sufficient recovery, optimal adaptation, and maximum gains.** There is less chance that overtraining signs and symptoms will occur.

TABLE 5. 3-Day-a-Week, 8-Week Training Cycle (for Selected Core Exercise)*

Week	Variables	Monday (Heavy)	Wednesday (Light)	Friday (Moderate)
1	% 1 RM	60	50	55
	Sets	3	3	3
	Reps	10	10	10
2	% 1 RM	70	60	65
	Sets	3	3	3
	Reps	8	7	7
3	% 1 RM	75	68	72
	Sets	4	3	3
	Reps	6	8	7
4	% 1 RM	70	60	65
	Sets	3	3	3
	Reps	8	8	7
5	% 1 RM	80	70	76
	Sets	3	3	4
	Reps	5	8	6
6	% 1 RM	85	72	80
	Sets	4	4	4
	Reps	4	7	5
7	% 1 RM	90	75	83
	Sets	4	4	4
	Reps	2	5	4
8	No training on Monday and Friday. Test for 1 RM on Wednesday and recalculate the loads for the next cycle using the new 1 RM			

* All exercises are performed each day. The cycle pertains to loads and volumes for selected core exercises. Two to three sets of 8–12 repetitions are recommended for secondary exercises and other core exercises.

Note: No more than 5 repetitions in a set should be performed in power movement exercises, such as the power snatch or power clean from the floor position, and no more than 6 repetitions in a set in partial movement exercises, such as the snatch or clean from a hang.

TABLE 6. 4-Day-a-Week, 8-Week Split Program Training Cycle (for Selected Core Exercises)*

Week	Variables	Monday (Heavy)	Tuesday (Light)	Wednesday	Thursday (Light)	Friday (Heavy)
1	% 1 RM Sets Reps	60 3 10	55 3 8	Rest	55 3 8	60 3 10
2	% 1 RM Sets Reps	65 3 8	60 3 7	Rest	60 3 7	65 3 8
3	% 1 RM Sets Reps	75 4 6	68 3 8	Rest	68 3 8	75 4 8
4	% 1 RM Sets Reps	70 3 8	60 3 7	Rest	60 3 7	70 3 8
5	% 1 RM Sets Reps	80 3 5	70 3 8	Rest	70 3 8	80 3 5
6	% 1 RM Sets Reps	85 4 4	72 4 7	Rest	72 4 7	85 4 4
7	% 1 RM Sets Reps	90 4 2	75 4 5	Rest	75 4 5	90 4 2
8		No training on Monday, Tuesday, Thursday, and Friday. Test for 1 RM on Wednesday and recalculate the loads for the next cycle using the new 1 RM.				

* Exercises are performed on the following days: Mondays, Thursdays—shoulder, upper back, chest, arms, abdomen; Tuesdays, Fridays—power movements, legs, lower back. The cycle pertains to loads and volumes for selected core exercises. Two to three sets of 8–12 repetitions are recommended for secondary exercises and other core exercises.

Note: No more than 5 repetitions in a set should be performed in power movement exercises, such as the power snatch or power clean from the floor position, and no more than 6 repetitions in a set in partial movement exercises, such as the snatch or clean from a hang.

2. Tables 5 and 6 show variation of load and volume within the week and from week to week, with increasingly greater intensities as the 8-week cycle of training continues.
   a. Percentages of the 1 RM are used to create the variation in training loads presented in Tables 5 and 6.
   b. Variations of load and volume are typically used only with core exercises; however, cycling of certain highly sport-specific secondary exercises may be beneficial as well.
3. Training loads and volumes in a **3-day-a-week program** can be varied in the following manner (Table 5):
   a. Monday—heavy loads
   b. Wednesday—light loads
   c. Friday—moderate loads
4. The **4-day-a-week (split) program** can be used in the following manner (Table 6):
   a. Monday—heavy loads; Thursday—light loads: Performing power cleans, hang cleans, back squat, leg curls, leg extensions, and hyperextensions
   b. Tuesdays—light loads; Friday—heavy loads: Performing overhead presses, bent-over rows, bench presses, bicep curls, tricep press-down, and bent-knee sit-ups
5. The **8-week cycles** presented in Tables 5 and 6 assume that the athletes have been strength training during the off-season.

6. Should the preseason be longer than 8 weeks, another cycle can be developed using the guidelines presented, or the cycles outlined in Tables 5 and 6 may be expanded to cover the entire preseason.
   a. Succeeding cycles should begin with 2 weeks of high volumes and light loads, then progress to heavier loads with a tapering in the volume of exercise.
   b. The 1 RM determined during the 8th week of the cycle should be used in assigning training loads for the next cycle.
7. **Be aware that:**
   a. **Power movements** (e.g., snatches, high pulls from the floor, power snatches) **are very stressful exercises.**
   b. Repetitions for **power exercises** should not exceed five repetitions in a set.
   c. Repetitions for **partial power exercises** (e.g., hang cleans, hang snatches, partial pulls) should not exceed six repetitions in a set.

H. **Progression**
1. As the training cycle continues, the 1 RM should theoretically increase; therefore, training loads based on a percentage of the original 1 RM may underestimate the athlete's current capabilities.
   a. **Retesting the 1 RM** during the 8th week of the periodization model is typically sufficient; however, if an athlete is progressing rapidly, which often occurs among new trainees, prediction of a new 1 RM during the cycle and recalculation of the appropriate training loads may optimize strength gains.
   b. Predicting a new 1 RM during the cycle can be accomplished by having the athlete complete the normal warm-up sets, then perform as many repetitions as is possible with a weight that allows 10 or fewer repetitions resulting in muscular failure occurring during the last repetition.
   c. The 1 RM may then be predicted by multiplying the weight lifted times the repetition factor (which corresponds to the number of repetitions performed) found in Table 4.
2. In secondary exercises in which the training load is based solely on a repetition range rather than using a greater percentage of the 1 RM, progression should occur in the following manner:
   a. When the athlete can complete two or more repetitions above the intended number of repetitions in the last set of two consecutive workouts, it is time to increase the load used in that exercise.
   b. Typically, increasing the weight by 5 pounds is sufficient; however, exercises involving large muscle groups and exercises involving small muscle groups may require greater or lesser than a 5-pound weight increase.
3. The key is to **observe athletes on a daily basis**, being alert to situations requiring modifications in training intensities.

III. Plyometric Training

A. **Role of plyometric exercises in preseason strength training program**
1. When training for explosive sports, supplementing the strength training program with plyometric exercises, which develop speed strength, greatly facilitates the conversion of the strength gained in the weight room to functional sport-specific strength and power.
2. **Plyometrics are exercises designed to:**
   a. Enhance the athlete's ability to reach maximal force over the shortest period of time
   b. Increase the forces that an athlete can generate at high velocities of movement
   c. Improve the recruitment patterns of the strength-trained motor units in a sport-specific manner
3. Preseason plyometric training has been reported to have the additional benefit of reducing in-season muscle soreness while not increasing the preseason injury rate.

B. **Description:** Plyometric exercises are characterized by the athlete rapidly decelerating the body (or an object such as a medicine ball) followed immediately by an explosive effort to move the body or object in the opposite direction.

C. **How plyometrics work:** The mechanism by which plyometric exercises improve sports performance is through enhancement of the functioning of the stretch-shortening cycle.
   1. The active muscle is forcibly lengthened to store elastic energy immediately before the concentric contraction (shortening) of the muscle.
   2. Prestretching the muscle before a concentric contraction activates a neural reflex that increases the power of the concentric contraction, thereby improving the athlete's potential power output and reaction time.

D. **General considerations and prerequisites for plyometric training**
   1. **Because of the explosive nature of plyometric training, a baseline level of strength relative to an athlete's body weight is required for an athlete to perform plyometric exercises safely and effectively.**
      a. Plyometric exercises are appropriate only after an athlete has spent several weeks to months in both sprint training and resistance exercise training and has achieved a high level of strength relative to body weight.
      b. It has been recommended that certain high-intensity plyometric exercises such as depth height (in-depth jumps) for large athletes (> 100 kg) be performed from heights no greater than 0.5 meter.
   2. Footwear and landing surfaces used in plyometric drills must have good shock-absorbing qualities.
   3. Absence of predisposing previous injuries to ankles, knee, or lower back

E. **Plyometric program design variables**
   1. **Exercise selection**
      a. A plyometric training program for athletes should include **sport-specific exercises:**
         i. Analyze the athlete's sport skills and identify the importance of horizontal, lateral, and vertical movements as well as upper versus lower body demands.
         ii. Select a plyometric exercise that mimics the targeted sport skill (e.g., squat jumps for basketball or volleyball and zigzag hops for soccer).
         iii. Allerheiligen[1] provides illustrations and descriptions of how to perform correctly many commonly used plyometric exercises.
      b. Less demanding drills should be mastered before attempting more complex and intense drills.
   2. **Frequency of training**
      a. 1–3 days per week for each body segment trained, keeping the total number of training sessions per week in perspective with the overall training program
      b. Plyometric drills affecting a particular muscle and joint complex should not be performed on consecutive days.
   3. **Exercise arrangement**
      a. **Generally, plyometric exercises are not performed on the same body area on days when heavy resistance exercise or other intense activities are scheduled** (i.e., day 1—strength train the lower body and perform upper body plyometric exercises; day 2—strength train the upper body and perform lower body plyometric exercises).
      b. A thorough set of **warm-up** exercises should be performed before beginning a plyometric training session. The warm-up should progress from generalized aerobic or calisthenics exercises and static stretches to dynamic stretches followed by submaximal activities (e.g., nonexplosive jumps performed with a pause between repetitions) that mimic the plyometric exercise to be performed.
      c. During preseason training, plyometric exercises should be performed before practice sessions, strength training, sprinting training, or other fatiguing activities.

4. **Intensity of exercise:** To gauge the relative intensity of the exercises selected, consider the following guidelines.
   a. **Depth jumps are the highest intensity** form of plyometric exercises, with the intensity of the exercise being relative to:
      i. Body weight of athlete
      ii. Height that center of gravity is raised above ground for jump
   b. Single leg bounding is more intense than double leg bounding
   c. Vertical jumping is more intense than horizontal jumping
   d. High-speed activities are more intense than low-speed activities
5. **Volume of exercise**
   a. Typically expressed as the number of **foot or hand contacts per training session**
   b. The following are examples of the total number of foot contacts of low to moderate intensity plyometric exercises to be completed during one training session for athletes at different levels of training:
      i. Beginner 80–100
      ii. Intermediate 100–120
      iii. Advanced 120–140
   c. In general, the volume of the exercise must decrease relative to the increase in intensity to avoid overtraining (Table 7).
6. **Recovery**
   a. **Complete metabolic recovery** should be obtained between sets and exercises.
   b. Complete recovery should be achieved by resting 2–3 minutes between sets and exercises.
   c. Plyometric drills should not be performed when an athlete is fatigued.
   d. Wait at least 48 hours before repeating plyometric exercises for the same body segment.
7. **Progression:** Progressive overload directed at the stretch shortening cycle involves advancement to more complex exercises, higher-intensity exercises, and a greater volume of exercise.
   a. Progression of exercise **complexity**—single leg bounding to single leg zigzag hops
   b. Progression of exercise **intensity**—double leg bounding to single leg bounding
   c. Progression of exercise **volume**—80 foot contacts per training session to 100 foot contacts per session or increasing from two to three training sessions per week
   d. To keep the preseason injuries to a minimum, make small adjustments in the above-mentioned variables and allow adequate time for adaptations to occur.

IV. Overtraining Considerations

A. Overtraining is a condition characterized by a plateau or drop-off in athletic performance.
B. **Characteristics of overtraining**
   1. Extremes in **muscle soreness and stiffness**
   2. **Inability to complete training sessions** that normally would be completed

TABLE 7. Guidelines for Intensity and Volume of Plyometric Training Programs

Intensity	Sets × Reps	Volume of Drills/Sessions
Low	10 × 12	Very high
Moderate	7 × 10	High
High	5 × 8	Moderate
Very high	3 × 6	Low

Modified from Stone M, O'Bryant H: Weight Training: A Scientific Approach. Minneapolis, Burgess International, 1987, p 98.

3. **Higher** than normal **resting heart rate**
4. Greater **susceptibility** to colds and other illnesses
5. Unexplained **loss in body weight**
6. **Loss of appetite**
7. **Higher** than normal resting **blood pressure**

C. **Ways to avoid overtraining**
1. Consider stress imposed on the body by the total program (plyometric exercises, running, agility drills, practice sessions), not just strength training.
2. Increase training intensity gradually.
3. Provide adequate recovery time.
4. Ensure proper nutrition.
5. Ensure adequate sleep.
6. Incorporate sufficient variety into the training program.

V. Total Program

A. Although it is beyond the scope of this chapter, it is important to mention that well-designed programs consider all requirements (running, jumping, agility, speed, speed endurance, strength speed, power, and flexibility) of the sport.

B. Designing a total program that integrates the training for each of these requirements at the same time, at the correct intensity, and within the context of the sport season requires considerable effort and knowledge.

Recommended Reading

1. Allerheiligen WB: Speed development and plyometric training. In Baechle TR (ed): Essentials of Strength Training and Conditioning. Champaign, IL, Human Kinetics, 1994, pp 314–344.
2. Baechle TR, Earle RW, Allerheiligen WB: Strength training and spotting techniques. In Baechle TR (ed): Essentials of Strength Training and Conditioning. Champaign, IL, Human Kinetics, 1994, pp 345–401.
3. Baechle TR, Groves BR: Weight Training Instruction: Steps to Success. Champaign, IL, Leisure Press, 1992.
4. Fleck S, Kraemer W: Resistance Training. Urbana, IL, Human Kinetics, 1987.
5. Garhammer J: Sports Illustrated Strength Training. New York, Harper & Row, 1986.
6. Lombardi VP: Beginning Weight Training: The Safe and Effective Way. Dubuque, IA, William C. Brown, 1989, p. 201.
7. Stone MH: Literature review: National Strength and Conditioning Association position statement: Explosive exercises and training. NSCA J 15(3):6–15, 1993.
8. Stone M, O'Bryant H: Weight Training: A Scientific Approach. Minneapolis, Burgess International, 1987.
9. Wathen D: Literature review: National Strength and Conditioning Association position statement: Explosive/plyometric exercises. NSCA J 15(3):16–19, 1993.

16

Preseason Conditioning: Flexibility

Daniel Blanke, Ph.D.

Flexibility is the ability to move the joints of the body through the range of motion (ROM) for which they are intended. Although there is little evidence that excessive flexibility improves performance, there is some indication that **lack of flexibility can hamper performance and may lead to injury**. It is therefore important that an athlete maintains adequate flexibility. Because changes in the ROM are best developed over a long time, it is important for an athlete to include flexibility training in a preseason conditioning program.

I. General Principles of Flexibility

A. **Definition of terms**

1. **Stretch**—increasing the length of a tissue
2. **Stretching**—the process of increasing the length of a tissue
3. **Elastic stretch**—a temporary increase in the length of a tissue that returns to its original length when the stress is removed
4. **Plastic stretch**—a more permanent increase in the length of a tissue that remains elongated after the stress is removed
5. **Flexibility training**—a program of stretching exercises designed to increase the ROM of the targeted joints to a desired level. Once that level is attained, flexibility training can be used to maintain the desired ROM.

B. **Characteristics of connective tissue**

1. Connective tissue is one of the most widely varied types of tissue. Although cartilage, bone, blood, and lymph are types of connective tissue, the connective tissue that is found in tendons, ligaments, intramuscular and extramuscular layers of fascia, and joint capsules is the type of connective tissue of concern in flexibility training. This type of connective tissue is **primarily collagenous fibers** arranged in a protein-polysaccharide ground substance. It possesses both **elastic and plastic properties** and is referred to as dense or collagenous connective tissue. References made to connective tissue in this chapter imply this dense or collagenous type of connective tissue.
2. Connective tissue exhibits **high tensile strength** and therefore is **difficult to elongate.**
3. Connective tissue is primarily responsible for limiting joint ROM. It is therefore the **target of flexibility training**. Joint flexibility can be increased through stretching exercises that increase the length of the connective tissue structures.

C. **Plastic versus elastic stretch**

1. When connective tissue is stretched, some of the elongation is elastic and some is plastic. Once the force causing the stretch in the connective tissue is removed, the elastic elements return to their resting length, whereas the plastic components remain elongated.
2. **Flexibility training should be designed to produce plastic rather than elastic deformation.** Plastic deformation results in a more permanent change in length of the tissue.

3. **Low force loads applied for long periods of time result in a greater incidence of plastic deformation.** Flexibility training should therefore reflect these force and time requirements.

D. **Specificity** of flexibility training

1. The amount of flexibility in any joint is **specific to that joint** and is not a general characteristic.
2. Increasing flexibility in any joint does not result in an increase in any other joint. To increase flexibility of any joint, stretching exercises that increase the length of the connective tissue surrounding and crossing that joint are necessary.

E. Effects of **temperature** on flexibility training

1. **Stretching connective tissue under conditions of elevated temperature results in greater plastic deformation.** It is difficult to elevate tissue temperature deep within large muscles with topical application of heat. In a clinical environment, deep heating methods of diathermy or ultrasound may be beneficial, but in the nonclinical environment, the **temperature is best elevated through several minutes of muscle activity.**
2. To gain maximum benefit of plastic deformation of connective tissue after stretching, the connective tissue should be allowed to **cool while the stress is applied.** This implies that the most effective flexibility training can be done after the tissue temperature has been elevated then allowed to cool during the training period. This substantiates the normal practice of training for increased flexibility during the cool-down portion of an exercise bout.

F. Effects of **age** on flexibility: tends to **increase until young adulthood, then decrease with age.**[3] The effects of aging on flexibility can be reduced by consistently participating in a program designed to maintain or enhance flexibility.

G. Effects of **gender** on flexibility: **Females tend to be more flexible than males of the same age.** The difference in flexibility between males and females of the same age is partly due to the differences in muscle mass and quantity of connective tissue, but also is due to the greater tendency for girls and women to participate in activities such as dance, slimnastics, and gymnastics, which typically promote flexibility.

H. Effects of **habitual movement patterns** on flexibility: Moving the joint through a limited ROM decreases the flexibility of the joint over time due to **adaptive shortening** of the muscle and connective tissue. The elastic nature of connective tissue causes it to shorten when no load is applied. To reduce the potential for limited ROM, it is important to exercise the joint through full ROM whenever possible. Habitual movement patterns have the greatest effect on flexibility.

I. **Retention of flexibility:** The greatest loss of flexibility occurs in the first 2 weeks after termination of flexibility training. After 4 weeks, the athlete continues to lose flexibility but still is more flexible than before starting a flexibility training program. It is therefore **important to train for flexibility on a regular basis**. If training is not possible because of illness or injury, flexibility deteriorates, but the increases in joint ROM gained in flexibility training are not completely eroded even after 4 weeks of inactivity.

J. **Stretch reflex**

1. The stretch reflex is a protective reflex caused by the action of the muscle spindles. When a muscle is stretched rapidly, especially at its greatest length, the muscle spindle sends a stimulus to the central nervous system, which, in turn, sends a stimulus back to the muscle. The muscle responds by contracting. The force of contraction is somewhat related to the speed of the muscle as it is being stretched. The purpose of this reflex is to **protect the muscle and associated joints from injury by limiting the ROM of the muscle.**
2. The stretch reflex can hamper flexibility training by actively contracting the muscle that is in the process of being elongated. If the muscle contracts vigorously while

being stretched quickly, an injury can result. **Slow movements that reduce the intensity of the contraction and delay the activity of the stretch reflex until reaching maximum ROM are more desirable than fast movements, which elicit the stretch reflex.** Flexibility training that uses slow movements therefore reduces the incidence of injury.

K. **Preseason versus in-season flexibility training**
   1. **Considerable time is required to develop a significant increase in the flexibility of a joint.** This necessitates that the majority of flexibility training be done **preseason or off-season.**
   2. Essentially, it is **important to maintain flexibility during the entire off-season. Preseason workouts can then be used to increase flexibility for the upcoming season.** This pattern results in a progressive increase in flexibility over an athletic career. An athlete that begins flexibility training with the first practice and stops with the last game begins to demonstrate the improvements in flexibility only late in the season. This pattern results in a progressive decrease in flexibility over an athletic career.

II. Role of Flexibility in Injury Prevention

A. **Optimal flexibility**
   1. Optimal flexibility is extremely difficult to define. It depends more on the expected activity and is therefore a **relative term rather than an absolute value**. Optimal flexibility for a gymnast may be considerably different than optimal flexibility for a marathon runner. Also, optimal flexibility must be identified at a specific joint because flexibility is not a general factor and is joint specific.
   2. Optimal flexibility can be described as **the required amount of flexibility or ROM at the joint that allows for maximum performance of the defined activity while protecting the joint from acute or chronic injury.** This definition allows for differing amounts of flexibility at any joint depending on the activity level of the joint and yet does not encourage excessive flexibility, which can result in acute or chronic joint injury.

B. **Flexibility versus stability**
   1. **Although lack of flexibility can result in a poor performance, there is little evidence that excessive flexibility can result in outstanding performance.** The amount of flexibility necessary at a joint is dictated by the maximum ROM experienced during the performance of the activity. If this ROM is less than the ROM normally exhibited by a nonathlete of this age and sex, the athlete should be encouraged to maintain the flexibility expected to match the nonathlete. If the ROM is greater than that normally exhibited by a nonathlete of this age and sex, the athlete must increase his or her flexibility to meet the demands of the sport or activity in which he or she is participating.
   2. There is a **concern over excessive increases of flexibility.** Just because a little bit is good does not imply a lot is better. There is a **tradeoff between flexibility and stability.** Increasing flexibility can lead to decreased stability. This is especially evident when the flexibility increases are the result of lengthening of the connective tissue structures that stabilize the joint. Athletes should be encouraged to maintain flexibility at the level necessary for maximum performance in their chosen activity but not in excess of that amount because excessive flexibility can be associated with a decrease in stability and therefore a greater tendency for injury.
   3. **Permanently elongating connective tissue results in some mechanical weakening of the tissue.** Flexibility training with **low stress applied over a long period of time results in less mechanical weakening** than training of a short duration with a large amount of force.

C. **Muscle strain versus joint sprain:** When lack of flexibility is noted in an athlete, the athlete is more prone to muscle strain, whereas an athlete with a large amount of flexibility at a joint may be more prone to joint sprain. Increasing flexibility in the athlete with limited ROM helps reduce the incidence of muscle strains. Excessive increase in the flexibility of an athlete increases the likelihood of joint sprains while reducing the tendency for muscle strains.

III. Role of Flexibility in Performance Enhancement

The quality of a performance is affected by many variables, including lack of flexibility. Swimmers lacking flexibility in the ankles or shoulders are not able to orient the foot or arm to the water for maximum push, pull, or lift. Divers lacking low back and hamstring flexibility are not able to achieve the tight pike position necessary to rotate rapidly or secure a high score. The gymnast lacking flexibility, similar to the diver, is not able to achieve certain positions, which definitely can affect the athlete's score. **The coach or athlete must evaluate an activity to determine the maximum ROM necessary for optimum performance, and then increase flexibility during the off-season to this required level.**

IV. Techniques for Improving Flexibility

A. Several techniques to increase flexibility have been shown to work if practiced regularly. In contrast to training to increase strength, **flexibility training should be practiced daily or more than once per day.** Some techniques are more conveniently practiced with a partner, whereas others are easily practiced alone. At least one technique increases the chance of muscle and joint injury and therefore is not advocated. Choice of the technique to use should be made by the athlete or coach in light of what will be practiced regularly, because that is the most crucial factor.

B. **Static stretching** is done by slowly moving the joint to the end of the ROM and holding the position for 5–60 seconds. Taylor and associates recommend four stretches of 15–20 seconds per stretch. It is important when moving to the end of the ROM to stop at the point of moderate discomfort and before pain. As a result of the slow movement, there is a reduced tendency to elicit the stretch reflex. **Static stretch is therefore one of the safest techniques for increasing flexibility.**

C. **Static stretching with contraction of the antagonist** is done by slowly moving the joint to the end of the ROM, then isometrically contracting the antagonist muscle group for 3–30 seconds. This is the muscle group directly opposite the muscle being stretched. It is again important to move the joint to the point of moderate discomfort and no further. **This techniques enjoys all the benefits of static stretching with the added benefit of further reducing the tendency to elicit the stretch reflex by actively contracting the antagonist muscle group.** By the action of reciprocal inhibition, there is a release of an inhibitory transmitter substance at the spinal cord to reduce the activity of the muscle being stretched.

D. **Static stretching with contraction of the agonist (proprioceptive neuromuscular facilitation [PNF])** is performed by slowly moving the joint to the end of the ROM, then isometrically contracting the agonist muscle group (the one being stretched) for 3–30 seconds. It must be an isometric contraction, so that no movement occurs in this group. **It is theorized that the isometric contraction relaxes the muscle, possibly through the action of the Golgi tendon organ, and therefore allows additional ROM at the joint.** Minimally the isometric contraction puts an additional stretch on the connective tissue surrounding the joint and therefore allows greater ROM.

E. **Static stretching with contraction of the agonist followed by contraction of the antagonist (PNF)** is performed by slowly moving the joint to the end of the ROM and isometrically contracting the agonist muscle group for 5–30 seconds. As with the previous PNF method, this is contraction of the muscle group being stretched. This is followed by relaxing the agonist and contracting the antagonist muscle group, the group opposite the group being stretched, for 5–30 seconds while attempting to stretch the muscle group even more.

F. Ballistic stretching is performed by quickly moving the joint to the end of the ROM. It often uses **bouncing, jerking movements or momentum to force the joint beyond its normal ROM**. The movements may be described as pulsing, bobbing, swinging, or kicking movements. Although ballistic stretching has been shown to increase flexibility, it is **not recommended because of the increased potential for injury** due to the additional forces that are present with movement. These forces are in the direction opposite to the direction of the forces incurred in stretching the muscle and therefore can lead to muscle or connective tissue tears or bone avulsion.

V. Identifying Flexibility Requirements of Selected Sports

A. **Evaluation**

1. The flexibility required for any activity can be determined by identifying the ROM required for each movement of the activity. It therefore becomes **important to analyze the activity carefully** to determine the maximum ROM necessary for performing the activity.
2. As an example, jogging requires little ROM at the hip, knee, ankle, foot, shoulder, elbow, or trunk. When the speed of the jog is increased to running, the ROM of each joint increases. Sprinting demands even greater ROM at the joints with the largest differences occurring at the knee and hip. **The flexibility requirement increases as the ROM of the joint increases.**
3. Sports such as diving, dance, and gymnastics require a large amount of flexibility, especially in the wrists, shoulders, back, and hips, because of the ROM necessary for performance of many of the component activities. Because showing flexibility is part of the scoring system for diving and gymnastics and part of the aesthetic value of dance, inadequate flexibility results in lower scores, whereas optimal flexibility allows for higher scores.
4. After identifying the flexibility requirements of a sport, the next task is to **develop the appropriate flexibility training program.** A series of flexibility exercises that increase the flexibility of the joints to the level necessary for optimal performance of the sport must be identified.
5. The **technique of flexibility training** also needs to be identified. The athlete can then begin to increase flexibility with daily training.

B. **Each sport or game, because of the inherent activity, has a certain flexibility requirement.** Sports that require considerable upper body motion have a greater requirement for the upper body, whereas those with considerable lower body activity require more lower body flexibility. Some sports require rotational flexibility, whereas others require only linear flexibility training. Anderson, Alter, and Beaulieu have identified flexibility training programs for a variety of sport activities as well as detailed descriptions of flexibility exercises for every joint.

VI. Flexibility Myths and Misconceptions

A. **Flexibility exercises to avoid:** These exercises are identified as placing excessive pressure on the spinal discs, the arterial system, knee ligaments, or the sciatic nerve. Beaulieu identifies high-risk flexibility exercises; Anderson identifies the correct and incorrect position for stretching specific joints.

1. **Yoga plow**—places excessive strain on the neck and lower back
2. **Hurdler's stretch**—applies excessive pressure to the medial collateral ligament of the knee when performed with one hip joint abducted and inwardly rotated, the knee flexed, and the leg outward rotated

3. **Full head circles**—applies excessive pressure to the cervical vertebrae and discs
4. **Toe touching**—applies excessive pressure to the lumbar discs when performed from a standing position with the knees fully extended
5. **Bridge ups or back bends**—hyperextension of the back applies excessive force to vertebrae and discs

B. **Flexibility myths**

1. **Pulsing is better than bouncing.** It is a myth that rapid pulsing, which is essentially short bounces at the end of the ROM, is a desirable technique to improve flexibility. This technique is occasionally taught in conjunction with dance exercise. It is still **ballistic** in nature and therefore a less desirable technique for improving flexibility.
2. **Flexibility training should be used for warm-up.** To reduce the chance of muscle injury and increase the effect of flexibility training, the muscle temperature should be elevated before stretching. The temperature of the muscle can be most easily elevated by exercise. **Easy, rhythmic exercise should precede easy stretching in the warm-up portion of an exercise bout. Flexibility training is most effective after an exercise bout when the muscle temperature is most elevated.**

VII. Summary

Flexibility training should be a part of the conditioning program for **every athlete**. **Significant increases in the level of flexibility take 6–12 weeks to develop.** Although flexibility training should take place during the season of competition, it **must be started preseason and should be continued throughout the year**. Flexibility training should take place **daily**. Each session should begin with several minutes of warm-up exercises designed to **increase the temperature of the muscle.** The warm-up exercises should be followed by **specific exercises designed to increase the flexibility of the joints that are used in the activity** for which the athlete is training. The technique used for flexibility training is up to the discretion of the athlete or coach. **Ballistic training should be avoided.**

Recommended Reading

1. Alter M: Science of Stretching. Champaign, IL, Human Kinetics, 1988.
2. Anderson B: Stretching. Bolinas, CA, Shelter Publications, 1984.
3. Anderson B, Burke E: Scientific, medical, and practical aspects of stretching. Clin Sports Med 10:63–86, 1991.
4. Beaulieu J: Stretching for All Sports. Pasadena, CA, Athletic Press, 1980.
5. Beaulieu J: Developing a stretching program. Phys Sportsmed 9(11):59–66, 1981.
6. Chandler J, Kibler W, Uhl T, et al: Flexibility comparison of junior elite tennis players to other athletes. Am J Sports Med 18:134–136, 1990.
7. Donovan G, McNamara J, Gianoli P: Exercise Danger. Dubuque, IA, Kendall/Hunt, 1988.
8. Etnyre B, Lee E: Comments on proprioceptive neuromuscular facilitation stretching techniques. Res Q 58:184–188, 1987.
9. Etnyre B, Lee E: Chronic and acute flexibility of men and women using three different stretching techniques. Res Q 59:222–228, 1988.
10. Hamilton W, Hamilton L, Marshall P, Molnar M: A profile of the musculoskeletal characteristics of elite professional ballet dancers. Am J Sports Med 20:267–272, 1992.
11. Knapik J, Bauman C, Jones B, et al: Preseason strength and flexibility imbalances associated with athletic injuries in female collegiate athletes. Am J Sports Med 19:76–80, 1991.
12. Knapik J, Jones B, Bauman C, Harris J: Strength, flexibility and athletic injuries. Sports Med 14:277–278, 1992.
13. Kravitz L, Heyward V: Flexibility training. Fitness Management 11(2):32–38, 1995.
14. Marieb E: Human Anatomy and Physiology, 3rd ed. Redwood City, CA, Benjamin/Cummings, 1995.
15. Nelson K, Cornelius W: The relationship between isometric contraction durations and improvement in shoulder joint range of motion. J Sports Med Phys Fitness 31:385–388, 1991.
16. Rasch P: Kinesiology and Applied Anatomy, 7th ed. Philadelphia, Lea & Febiger, 1989.
17. Sapega A, Quedenfeld T, Moyer R, Butler R: Biophysical factors in range-of-motion exercise. Phys Sportsmed 9(12):57–64, 1981.

18. Smith A, Stroud L, McQueen C: Flexibility and anterior knee pain in adolescent elite figure skaters. J Pediatr Orthop 11:77–82, 1991.
19. Smith C: The warm-up procedure: To stretch or not to stretch. J Orthop Sports Phys Ther 19:12–17, 1994.
20. Taylor D, Dalton J, Seaber A, Garrett W: Viscoelastic properties of muscle-tendon units. Am J Sports Med 18:300–308, 1990.
21. Thomas T, Zebas C: Scientific Exercise Training. Dubuque, IA, Kendall/Hunt, 1984.
22. Wang S, Whitney S, Burdett R, Janosky J: Lower extremity muscular flexibility in long distance runners. J Orthop Sports Phys Ther 17:102–107, 1993.
23. Wilson G, Wood G, Elliott B: The relationship between stiffness of the musculature and static flexibility. Int J Sports Med 12:403–407, 1991.

PART IV
ENVIRONMENT

17: Safe Exercise in the Heat and Heat Injuries

Morris B. Mellion, M.D., and Guy L. Shelton, M.A., PT, ATC

I. Heat Transfer and Heat Dissipation

A. **Increased heat load** of exercise
1. Muscles can generate 20+ times as much energy at maximal activity as at rest, leading to huge increases in heat load.
2. At maximum exercise, the human body's work efficiency is approximately 25%; therefore, roughly 75% of muscle energy consumption is converted to heat rather than work.
3. Well-conditioned endurance athletes can generate and dissipate 1033 Kcal of heat per hour safely into the environment.

B. **Peripheral mechanisms—minor effect**
1. A small amount of heat produced by muscle is transferred passively by **conduction** through tissue to overlying skin.
2. Some heat from muscle is carried by **convection** via the venous blood in superficial veins en route to the heart.

C. **Central mechanisms—major effect**
1. Most of the heat produced in exercise is transported by the blood from the working muscles to the venae cavae and then the heart. The warmed blood from the muscles mixes with the venous return from the rest of the body and enters the heart to form the cardiac output, much of which is pumped to the vessels of the skin for heat dissipation.
   a. Blood has a high **heat capacity**. It can transport a relatively large quantity of heat with only a moderate increase in temperature.
   b. Early in exercise, heat production exceeds heat loss, producing an increase in body core temperature.
   c. The rise in core temperature is sensed by **thermodetectors** in the hypothalamus, the spinal cord, and limb muscles and provides the stimulus to initiate sweating and increase skin blood flow. High ambient temperature or severe radiant heat from the sun may trigger the heat-dissipating mechanisms before exercise is begun.
2. Skin blood flow transfers heat by **convection** to the skin, where it is lost by:
   a. **Evaporation** of sweat
   b. **Radiation**
   c. **Convection**
   d. **Conduction**
3. **Radiation and convection** dissipate most of the heat when the ambient temperature is less than 68°F (20°C), and **evaporation accounts for most of the heat loss when the temperature is above 68°F**.

a. In heavy exercise, evaporation can account for up to 85% of heat loss.
b. The **evaporative heat loss** of 1 L of water at 86°F (30°C) is 580 Kcal.
c. A 70-kg athlete sweats 1 to 2 L/hour during intense exercise in the heat. Larger athletes may sweat considerably more.
d. Above 95°F (35°C), convection and radiation do not contribute to heat loss.
e. At high temperatures, radiation causes heat gain.

4. After the heat-dissipating mechanisms are brought into play, the core temperature reaches a plateau, where it remains until the exercise's demand is past. In elite athletes, the equilibrium between heat production and heat dissipation may be as high as 104°F without diminished performance.
5. If the heat-dissipating mechanisms fail or if there is an overwhelming heat stress, the core temperature may continue to rise, even to dangerous levels.

D. **Conflicting demands for cardiac output and plasma volume during exercise in the heat:**

1. In the first 10–20 minutes of exercise, approximately 15% of the intravascular fluid volume is shunted to the working muscles.
2. Increases of skin blood flow for cooling also shunt blood from the central circulation and effectively lower central plasma volume. Skin blood flow may be 15–25% of cardiac output during intense exercise in a hot environment.
3. Sweating can easily produce losses of 1 to 2 L/hour, thus causing further losses in plasma volume.
4. As plasma volume (or central blood volume) decreases, there is less blood returning to the heart to be pumped. Therefore, stroke volume and cardiac output decrease. If this process were to continue, the system would collapse.
5. The process can be changed favorably by:
   a. Reducing exercise overload (slowing down)
   b. Building plasma volume by drinking water or other specific hypotonic fluids
   c. Shifting blood flow away from skin. If this shift is too great, core temperature may rise dangerously.

E. **Dehydration**

1. Sweat is **hypotonic**; very little salt is lost. Even less salt is lost in the well-conditioned, heat-acclimatized athlete.
2. Loss of sweat increases electrolyte concentration in the remaining plasma, which is **hypertonic**.
3. Taking salt pills or drinking salty (normotonic or hypertonic) solutions may make the plasma more hypertonic.
4. Water reduces the hypertonic state of the plasma back to normal osmolality.
5. For most exercise situations, **cold water** is the best fluid replacement. Generally, obtaining salt only from the normal sodium content of a well-balanced diet is adequate.
6. **For prolonged or repetitive endurance exercise in the heat,** there is growing evidence that a **hypotonic salt solution** may retard dehydration and speed rehydration. The addition of carbohydrate in the form of up to 7% glucose polymer may also be helpful.
7. Thirst is not an adequate guide for fluid consumption in humans. For optimum hydration, the athlete should drink before, during, and after exercise. (See Chapter 8, "Sports Nutrition" for a detailed discussion of fluid, electrolyte, and carbohydrate replacement.)

F. **Metabolic considerations—Hubbard's "energy depletion model"**

1. **Premise:** Thermally driven metabolic events can drain an individual's energy supply, even in a state of euhydration.
2. **Three major contributing mechanisms:**
   a. Elevated skeletal muscle temperature increases the muscle metabolic rate and magnifies the energy cost of force development.

b. Elevated temperature causes increased cell membrane permeability with leakage of sodium and potassium ions. The compensatory transmembrane ion pumping necessary to restore homeostasis causes a large energy drain. Evidence for the increased membrane permeability comes from elevations of serum creatine kinase and lactate dehydrogenase.
c. Intracellular lactic acidosis develops, promoting fatigue and cell swelling.

3. This model demonstrates a **"fundamental problem with energy availability."** The heat load increases the metabolic rate and decreases metabolic efficiency. Muscle weakness and fatigue occur with extreme energy deficiency, and muscles fail to relax and remain contracted. Muscle weakness, tightness, and fatigue are common symptoms of heat illness.

G. **Thermoregulation in women**

1. **Some evidence** exists that women exercising in the heat demonstrate better thermoregulation than men.
   a. Better maintenance of plasma volume and serum electrolytes
   b. Less sweat electrolyte loss
2. Heat dissipation may be reduced in postovulatory (luteal) phase in reproductive-age women because of increased temperature set-point and possibly smaller plasma volume.
3. **Estrogen replacement therapy** in postmenopausal women may lower the resting core temperature and the threshold for onset of sweating and cutaneous vasodilatation during exercise.

H. **Acclimation and training effect**

1. **Acclimation** to exercise in heat
   a. Adults: four–seven sessions of exercise in heat, 1–4 hours per session
   b. Children slightly longer
2. The **training effect** related to increased level of physical conditioning also contributes to improved capacity for exercise in the heat, owing to:
   a. Increased basal plasma volume
   b. Lower salt sodium concentration
3. **Physiologic effects of acclimation to exercise in the heat combined with physical conditioning**
   a. **Heat dissipation** (Table 1):
      i. Earlier initiation of sweating
      ii. Increased rate of sweating
      iii. Increased maximum sweating capacity
      iv. Lower sweat sodium concentration
   b. **Cardiovascular effects:**
      i. Increased basal plasma volume
      ii. Decreased heart rate at given work load and heat stress
   c. **Metabolic effects:**
      i. Increased aldosterone production
      ii. Increased urinary sodium excretion
      iii. Increased skeletal muscle mitochondrial density

TABLE 1. Sweat Rate and Sweat Na^+ Concentration in Humans

	Maximal Sweating Rate	Na^+ Concentration	Maximal Na^+ Loss/Hour
Unacclimatized	1.5 L/hr	100 mEq/L	150 mEq/hr
Acclimatized	2.5 L/hr	75 mEq/L	175 mEq/hr

From Anderson RJ, Reed G, Knochel J: Heatstroke. Adv Intern Med 28:115–141, 1983, with permission.

iv. Increased skeletal muscle myoglobin
v. Increased skeletal muscle glycogen

d. **Thermal effects:**
   i. Increased exercise capacity in the heat
   ii. Lower core and skin temperature at given work load and heat stress
   iii. Reduced perceived intensity of exercise
   iv. Increased thermal comfort

I. **Exercise, fever, and antipyretics**
1. Core temperature elevations caused by **fever** and illness are additive to those caused by exercise.
   a. Therefore, **cardiac output and aerobic capacity are both reduced in the febrile athlete.**
   b. **Exercise with a fever may be dangerous, especially in the heat.**
2. Core temperature elevations caused by exercise cannot be reduced by using aspirin, acetaminophen (Tylenol), or other **antipyretics**.

II. Exertional Heat Illness

A. Six exertional heat syndromes
1. **Heat edema** is a transitory peripheral swelling that occurs when an unacclimated individual is exposed to heat.
2. **Heat syncope** is a transient hypovolemic syncopal episode.
3. **Heat cramps, heat exhaustion, and heatstroke** form a progression of increasingly severe heat illnesses caused by dehydration, electrolyte losses, and failure of the body's thermoregulatory mechanism.
4. **Hyponatremic collapse** is a recently described syndrome attributed to excessive hypotonic fluid consumption in ultraendurance athletes. It is reported in marathoners as well.

B. **Heat edema**
1. In **unacclimated individual**
   a. Exercise in hot environment
   b. Marked peripheral vasodilatation and sweating
   c. Decreased plasma volume
   d. Increased aldosterone production
   e. Sodium and water retention
   f. Transitory dependent edema (hands and feet)
2. Generally resolves over first few days of heat exposure

C. **Heat syncope**
1. Syncope (fainting) or lightheadedness usually seen at the end of a race. The athlete is maximally vasodilated; when activity is stopped, **much of the blood volume "pools" in the lower extremities.** Consequently, the heart has too little venous return to pump an adequate supply to the brain.
2. **Predisposing factors**
   a. Ending exercise without cool-down
   b. Dehydration
   c. Lack of acclimatization
   d. The same phenomenon may occur when going from the cold (such as a cold bath) to hot sauna or whirlpool.
3. **Treatment**
   a. Lie down and elevate legs slightly.
   b. Rest in a cool place.
   c. Drink cold water.
4. **Complications**—rare

D. **Heat cramps**
   1. Muscular tightening and spasm seen during or after intense, prolonged exercise in heat
      a. May be exquisitely painful
      b. Lower extremity muscles most common, but any muscles may be affected, including abdominals and intercostals
   2. **Predisposing factors**
      a. Lack of acclimatization. Also seen in well-conditioned athletes in long or repetitive endurance events.
      b. Ongoing negative sodium balance—the already sodium-depleted athlete loses additional sodium in sweat and replaces the accompanying volume loss with water, producing even further dilutional hyponatremia.
      c. Diuretics, especially first few weeks of therapy
   3. **Treatment**
      a. Rest and cooling down
      b. Massage (knead) affected muscles.
      c. Oral hypotonic salt solution—1 teaspoon table salt/1 quart water
      d. If sodium replenishment fails to resolve heat cramps, evaluate potassium, calcium, and magnesium levels.
   4. **May be warning sign of impending heat exhaustion**

E. **Heat exhaustion**
   1. A serious acute heat injury with hyperthermia caused by dehydration, hyponatremia, or both. It may progress to become a form of exercise-associated collapse. Sweating mechanisms are generally working, but the amount of sweating may be reduced because of dehydration. Core temperature is significantly elevated, but generally < 103°F.
   2. **Two patterns**
      a. **Sodium depletion heat exhaustion:**
         i. Unacclimated athletes
         ii. Sweat losses replaced with water
         iii. **Inadequate dietary sodium intake**
         iv. Process develops over several days, but symptom onset is acute.
         v. **Symptoms:**
            (a) Fatigue
            (b) Profound weakness
            (c) Lightheadedness
            (d) Sweating
            (e) Muscle cramps
            (f) Occasional flu-like symptoms (headache, myalgias, nausea, vomiting, or diarrhea)
         vi. **Signs:**
            (a) Moderate, if any, temperature elevation
            (b) Tachycardia
            (c) Occasional hypotension
         vii. **Mental status**—generally clear or mildly impaired and loss of consciousness is rare
      b. **Water depletion heat exhaustion:**
         i. Due to exercise in the heat with inadequate water intake
         ii. **Symptoms:**
            (a) Thirst
            (b) Headache
            (c) Mild anxiety
            (d) Muscle weakness
            (e) Generalized fatigue
            (f) Neuromuscular incoordination

iii. **Signs:**
   (a) High fever
   (b) Decreased skin turgor
   (c) Tachycardia
   (d) Hypotension (often severe)

iv. **Mental status**—confused, often agitated

v. **Sweating mechanism intact**, but sweating may be reduced because of hypernatremia and increased serum osmolarity.

3. **Pure sodium depletion or water depletion forms of heat exhaustion are rare in athletes. Generally, they have a mix of the two syndromes.**
4. Treatment
   a. Rest
   b. Rapid cooling
   c. Fluid and electrolyte replacement:
      i. Hypotonic oral fluids
      ii. D5W/½ normal saline intravenously:
         (a) Start with 1 L over 30–60 minutes.
         (b) Measure serum sodium. If markedly elevated, hydrate cautiously to avoid inducing cerebral edema.

F. **Heatstroke—a medical emergency**

1. Exercise-associated collapses characterized by extreme hyperthermia with thermoregulatory failure and profound central nervous system dysfunction.
   a. **Core temperature ≥ 105°F**
   b. Often as high as 107–108°F
   c. **Delayed core temperature measurements, however, may be considerably lower—even normal.**
2. **Traditionally described presentation—patient hot, flushed, and dry with failed sweating mechanism**
3. **It is now known that in most cases of heatstroke, the sweating mechanism is still functioning.**
4. **Level of mental status impairment differentiates heatstroke from heat exhaustion.** In heatstroke, there is progressive moderate to severe impairment.
   a. Heat exhaustion: mild confusion or agitation
   b. "Mild" heat stroke: moderate levels of confusion, disorientation, agitation
   c. Severe heatstroke: hysterical behavior, delirium, seizures, coma
5. **Not spontaneously reversible**
   a. **Thermoregulatory failure prevents control of elevated core temperature without external cooling**, even in those heatstroke patients who retain the ability to sweat.
   b. Progresses to cardiovascular and central nervous system collapse in the absence of prompt intervention
6. **Complications** extend to all major organ systems (Table 2).
7. **Multiple electrolyte and metabolic abnormalities**
   a. Hyperkalemia or hypokalemia
   b. Hypernatremia or hyponatremia
   c. Hypocalcemia
   d. Hyperphosphatemia
   e. Hypoglycemia
   f. Lactic acidosis
   g. Uremia
8. **May be part of a continuum with heat exhaustion, but in some individuals the sweating mechanism stops functioning at a relatively low level of heat exposure.** In these patients, exertional heatstroke **may be a variant of malignant hyperthermia.**
9. **Predisposing factors**
   a. Genetic predisposition
   b. Dehydration—acute and chronic

TABLE 2. Severe Complications of Heatstroke

Cardiovascular	Gastrointestinal	Musculoskeletal
Arrhythmias	Diarrhea and vomiting	Rhabdomyolysis
Myocardial infarction	Hepatocellular necrosis	Myoglobinemia
Pulmonary edema	Upper gastrointestinal bleeding	**Pulmonary**
Shock		Hyperventilation
Central Nervous System	**Hematologic**	Respiratory alkalosis
Confusion	Fibrinolysis	Adult respiratory distress syndrome
Coma	Thrombocytopenia	Pulmonary infarction
Seizures	Disseminated intravascular coagulation	**Renal**
Cerebral or spinal infarction		Acute renal failure

From Mellion MB, Shelton GL: Thermoregulation, heat illness, and safe exercise in the heat. In Mellion MB (ed): Office Sports Medicine, 2nd ed. Philadelphia, Hanley & Belfus, 1996, pp 45–57.

c. Lack of acclimatization to heat—often seen on an exceptionally hot spring day
d. Negative sodium balance over time may be a factor.
e. Frequently occurs near a race finish line, where the already dehydrated athlete increases speed, causing increased muscle heat production, increased muscle blood flow, secondarily decreased skin blood flow, and a resultant rise in core temperature.

10. **Treatment**
    a. **Before treating patient with exercise-associated collapse, determine body temperature.**
        i. **In moderate to cool ambient temperatures, collapse may be due to hypothermia.**
        ii. **Only hyperthermic patients should be cooled.**
        iii. **Warm hypothermic patients.**
    b. **Immediate external cooling in the field:**
        i. Wet patient down with a tepid or cool spray (or a single layer of wet cheesecloth or thin sheeting) and use a large fan to speed evaporation.
        ii. Remove patient's clothing and pack him or her in ice (less effective, but may be best option in the field).
        iii. Immerse in ice water bath and vigorously massage extremities.
    c. **Monitor rectal temperature:** External cooling may be discontinued when the core temperature drops to 102°F and stabilizes.
    d. **Place intravenous line early, but avoid massive fluid administration before cooling.**
        i. Cooling techniques:
            (a) Cause vasoconstriction
            (b) Increase venous return
            (c) Increase cardiac output
        ii. If patient remains hypotensive after cooling, give 250- to 500-ml boluses of normal saline by rapid infusion and monitor blood pressure. Occasionally, judicious use of pressor agents may be necessary.
    e. Sophisticated **emergency or intensive care facility** necessary for the following (especially in heatstroke patients):
        i. Airway management
        ii. Oxygenation with or without respirator
        iii. Careful fluid and electrolyte administration
        iv. Circulatory support
        v. Cardiac, hemodynamic, and laboratory monitoring
    f. Dantrolene may be helpful in some subsets of patients:

i. Known malignant hyperthermia
ii. Patients on neuroleptic agents with exertional heatstroke

G. **Hyponatremic exercise-associated collapse**
1. **Hyponatremia common in ultraendurance athletes**
a. Incidence of decreased serum sodium 9–29%
b. **Etiology not yet proven:**
i. **Water intoxication** most likely
ii. Other postulated causes:
(a) Sodium depletion
(b) Heat exhaustion
(c) Atrial natriuretic peptide
(d) Antidiuretic hormone excess
c. **Most hyponatremic competitors tolerate their electrolyte abnormality without collapse.**
2. **Hyponatremic exercise-associated collapse is a proven entity** in ultraendurance events and marathons. **Its incidence is currently undefined.**
3. **Measure serum sodium**, whenever possible, before administering intravenous fluids in ultraendurance and marathon athletes with exercise-associated collapse.
a. Do not withhold intravenous fluids, however, from other hyperthermic heat exhaustion and heatstroke victims.
b. Remember, **cooling** is the primary treatment for hyperthermia.

H. **Populations at increased risk for heat injury** (Table 3)
1. **Healthy individuals**
a. Poorly acclimatized
b. Poorly conditioned
c. Inexperienced competitor (limited judgment about heat risk)
d. **Salt or water depleted**
e. **Large or obese:**
i. Generate more heat for same level of activity
ii. Dissipate heat less efficiently (due to lower body surface-to-mass ratio)
iii. Obese individuals demonstrate higher tissue temperature elevations from the same heat load because adipose tissue has a lower specific heat than lean tissue.
iv. Obese individuals have fewer heat-activated sweat glands in skin overlying adipose tissue.
f. **Children:**
i. Sweat less

TABLE 3. Populations at Increased Risk for Exertional Heatstroke

Healthy individuals	Acute illnesses	Medications
Poorly acclimatized	Febrile illnesses	Anticholinergics
Poorly conditioned	Gastrointestinal illnesses	Antidepressants: tricyclics, monoamine oxidase inhibitors
Inexperienced competitor	**Chronic illnesses**	Antihistamines
Salt or water depletion	Alcoholism and substance abuse	Beta-blockers
Large or obese	Cardiac disease	Diuretics
Age extremes: children, elderly	Cystic fibrosis	Neuroleptics
Previous heat injury	Diabetes, uncontrolled	
Sleep-deprived	Eating disorders	
	Hypertension, uncontrolled	
	Skin problems with impaired sweating	
	Thyrotoxicosis	

From Mellion MB, Shelton GL: Thermoregulation, heat illness, and safe exercise in the heat. In Mellion MB (ed): Office Sports Medicine, 2nd ed. Philadelphia, Hanley & Belfus, 1996, pp 45–57.

ii. Require greater core temperature increases to trigger sweating
iii. Acclimatize more slowly
iv. Lower cardiac output at given metabolic rate; therefore, may lack adequate blood flow for both muscle and cooling needs
v. High surface area-to-body mass ratio:
(a) Works as advantage ordinarily
(b) When sun is hot or ambient temperature is high, however, children absorb relatively more heat from the environment.
vi. Transition to adult thermoregulation begins after puberty.

g. **Elderly:**
i. Age-related limitation on full heat acclimatization—reduced vasodilatory response may begin as early as age 50.
ii. Decreased maximum heart rate with age leads to decreased maximum cardiac output.
iii. Reduced thirst response after water deprivation
iv. Frequently, reduced fitness level

h. **Previous heat injury**
i. **Postovulatory phase of menstrual cycle** in reproductive-age women
j. **Sleep deprivation:**
i. Decreased sweat rate
ii. Decreased skin blood flow response to heat load

2. **Acute illnesses**
a. **Fever:**
i. Reduced cardiac output
ii. Increased metabolic demand for blood flow throughout body
b. **Gastrointestinal illnesses:**
i. Increased blood flow to gastrointestinal tract competes with skin blood flow for cardiac output.
ii. Dehydration and electrolyte disturbances

3. **Chronic illnesses**
a. Cardiac disease
b. Cystic fibrosis
c. Diabetes, uncontrolled
d. **Eating disorders:**
i. Fluid and electrolyte problem
ii. Compulsive overexercising
e. Hypertension, uncontrolled
f. Malignant hyperthermia

4. **Abuse of alcohol and other substances**
a. Alcohol:
i. Acute effect
ii. Residual effect persists on thermoregulation capacity
b. Amphetamines
c. Cocaine—**acute cocaine intoxication may be difficult to differentiate from heatstroke.**
d. Hallucinogens
e. Laxatives
f. Narcotics

5. **Medications**
a. Anticholinergics
b. Antihistamines
c. Beta-blockers
d. Diuretics
e. Neuroleptics, especially tricyclic antidepressants and monoamine oxidase inhibitors

III. Prevention of Heat Illness

A. **Medical history and evaluation:** Identify those individuals at increased risk.
   1. **Further workup or treatment**
      a. Acute illness
      b. Chronic illness
      c. Substance abuse
   2. **Risk factor correction**
      a. Acclimation
      b. Conditioning:
         i. Preseason conditioning (strength, endurance, skills acquisition)
         ii. Increased awareness of heat stress signs and symptoms in workout situations
         iii. Delay full participation until minimum conditioning level met.
      c. Obesity:
         i. Weight loss program is best done in the off-season.
         ii. During season, peak performances are often required; this is difficult if calorie restriction is enforced.
         iii. Calorie restriction might make it more difficult to take in proper electrolyte replacement through diet.
      d. Sleep deprivation:
         i. Delay participation until adequate rest is achieved.
         ii. Allow time for adequate sleep and rest during season.
   3. **Participant education—athlete, coach, parent**
      a. Inexperienced athlete
      b. Obese athlete
      c. Child athlete
      d. Elderly athlete
      e. Athlete with previous heat illness
      f. Athlete on certain medications
      g. All others with risk factors
   4. **Activity restriction**
      a. Used in situations (specified previously) in which other modifications do not allow safe participation
      b. Temporary restrictions may be imposed until certain risk factors are corrected.
      c. Restrictions may be absolute or relative, depending on each individual situation.

B. **Atmospheric conditions**
   1. **High heat and humidity**
      a. Severely limit body's ability to dissipate heat
      b. Exercising athlete cannot go by "how hot or humid it feels" to judge the environmental heat stress.
   2. Increased awareness of atmospheric conditions needed—**objective measures.**
      a. **Weather reports:**
         i. U.S. Weather Service
         ii. Local radio and television stations
         iii. Provide approximate temperature and humidity readings
         iv. Table 4 and Figure 1 show how relative degrees of heat stress can be determined.
         v. Simple and convenient
         vi. These remote temperature and humidity readings do not allow for variances due to local geography or distance between the weather reporting site and the workout area.
      b. **Sling psychrometer** (Fig. 2):
         i. Measures dry-bulb (DB) and wet-bulb (WB) temperature at the activity site
         ii. Relative humidity is then determined from a chart supplied with the instrument

TABLE 4. Heat Stress (Apparent Temperatures in °F)

Relative humidity (%)		Air Temperatures (°F)										
		70	75	80	85	90	95	100	105	110	115	120
	0%	64	69	73	78	83	87	**91**	**95**	**99**	**103**	**107**
	10%	65	70	75	80	85	**90**	**95**	**100**	**105**	**111**	**116**
	20%	66	72	77	82	87	**93**	**99**	**105**	**112**	**120**	**130**
	30%	67	73	78	84	**90**	**96**	**104**	**113**	**123**	**135**	**148**
	40%	68	74	79	86	**93**	**101**	**110**	**123**	**137**	**151**	
	50%	69	75	81	88	**96**	**107**	**120**	**135**	**150**		
	60%	70	76	82	**90**	**100**	**114**	**132**	**149**			
	70%	70	77	85	**93**	**106**	**124**	**144**				
	80%	71	78	86	**97**	**113**	**136**					
	90%	71	79	88	**102**	**122**						
	100%	72	80	**91**	**108**							

Danger zone = > 90°F (boldface temperatures above).
Adapted from National Weather Service: Heat Wave. U.S. Department of Commerce, National Oceanic and Atmospheric Administration, NOAA/PA 85001, 1985.

   iii. Table 4 and Figure 1 show how relative degrees of heat stress can be determined.
   iv. Readily available, reasonably inexpensive, accurate, portable, and easy to use

c. **Heat index thermometer** (Fig. 3):
   i. Measures DB, WB, and black bulb (BB) temperatures
   ii. BB thermometer provides measure of radiant heat gained
   iii. Web Bulb Global Temperature (WBGT) index calculated using the following formula:

$$\text{WBGT} = 0.7\ (\text{WB}) \times 0.1\ (\text{DB}) \times 0.3\ (\text{BB})$$

   iv. The WBGT index is compared to published guidelines that indicate relative levels of heat stress risk and provide suggestions for activity modification.

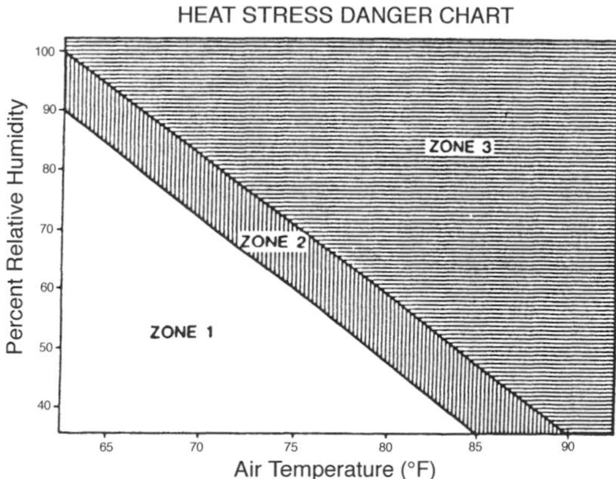

FIGURE 1. Heat stress danger chart. Environmental conditions in **zone 1** are fairly safe for participation. Normal heat stress precautions should be taken. In **zone 2**, moderate heat stress precautions should be taken. Workouts should be less intense, shorter, and with more frequent fluid breaks. More careful observation of individuals at increased risk. In **zone 3**, heat stress danger is at its greatest. Workouts should be rescheduled to a cooler part of the day. Workouts should be relatively easy. Light clothing and a minimum of equipment should be worn. Extra fluids for everyone and close observation for early heat injury symptoms are essential. (Adapted from Fox EL, Mathews DK: The Physiological Basis of Physical Education and Athletics, 3rd ed. Philadelphia, Saunders College Publishing, 1981.)

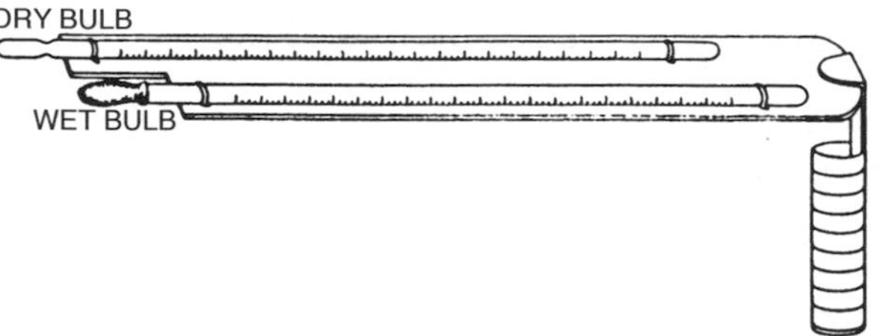

FIGURE 2. Sling psychrometer. Wick on wet bulb is moistened with distilled water and the unit is rotated overhead. Evaporative cooling causes the wet bulb temperature to decrease. The dry bulb and wet bulb readings are used to determine percent relative humidity.

C. **Workout schedule**
   1. Identifying adverse environmental conditions has absolutely no benefit unless appropriate steps are taken to **adjust the practice or competition schedule.**
   2. **Reschedule** workouts, practices, and competitions to cooler time of day or **cancel** altogether.
   3. **Alter** practices and workouts.
      a. Decreased intensity
      b. Shorter duration
      c. More frequent breaks

D. **Clothing**
   1. Restrictive clothing and bulky protective equipment block skin surface area.
      a. **Reduce cooling by:**
         i. Radiation
         ii. Convection
         iii. Evaporation
      b. Examples:
         i. Helmets
         ii. Heavy, long-sleeved uniforms
         iii. Protective pads
         iv. Rubberized workout suits

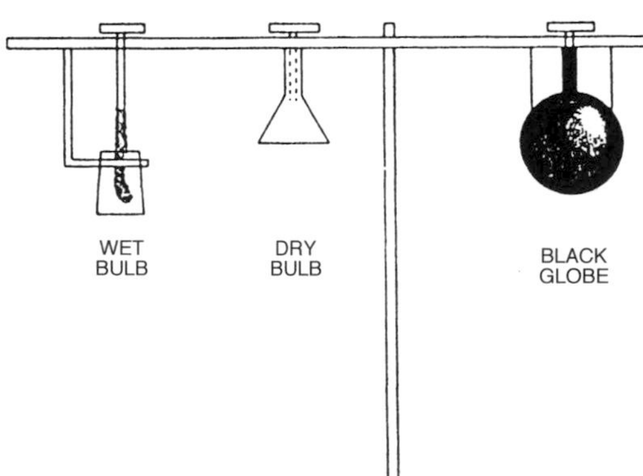

FIGURE 3. Heat index thermometer. Homemade unit consists of three thermometers mounted on a board. The bulb of the wet thermometer is enclosed in a moistened wick. The bulb of the dry thermometer is in an inverted funnel to shield it from direct sunlight. The bulb of the black globe thermometer is enclosed in a black copper globe to absorb radiant energy. An electronic heat index thermometer is also commercially available (Reuter-Strokes, Cambridge, Ontario).

2. **Some oil-based or gel-based sunscreens may block evaporative cooling.**
3. **Useful strategies**
    a. Short-sleeved, loose-fitting, open weave or mesh jerseys allow better evaporation. Short midriff T-shirts, especially under football shoulder pads.
    b. Practice or play in shorts when possible.
    c. Light-colored uniforms reflect sunlight.
    d. Change uniforms so soaked with sweat that they block evaporation from the skin.
    e. Wearing no shirt:
        i. Benefit—better heat loss from evaporation and convection
        ii. Risk—more radiant heat gain

E. **Body weight**
1. **Acute weight loss = dehydration**
    a. > 2% affects performance
    b. > 3% affects thermoregulatory capacity
2. **Nude weight measured and charted before and after practice or competition**
    a. Supervised and checked by athletic trainer or coach
    b. **Caution indicated when:**
        i. Workout weight loss > 3%
        ii. Athlete fails to regain previous day's weight loss by workout time the next day.
3. Athletes with large or persistent acute weight loss should be restricted from activity until rehydrated.

F. **Observe:**
1. Athletes at increased risk for heat illness
2. Overachiever—may be less aware of the early signs of heat illness
3. Unacclimatized athletes
4. Inexperienced athletes
5. Athletes with excessive practice weight loss

G. **Education**
1. All involved with athletics and fitness should have a basic understanding of heat illness and its causes, treatment, and prevention.
2. **Medical personnel**
    a. Should be able to provide sound advice on prevention, recognition, and treatment of various types of heat illness
    b. Good communication among coaches, athletes, and medical staff is essential.
3. **Coaches**
    a. Should set aside myths that can contribute to additional heat stress
    b. Should be trained to recognize early signs of heat illness and apply appropriate first-aid measures
    c. Are responsible to coordinate prevention program in absence of an athletic trainer
3. **Athletes**
    a. Should be able to recognize the symptoms of heat illness in themselves
    b. Should be aware of initial treatment
    c. Should understand heat illness prevention principles
    d. Should understand how to adjust training program to allow for heat
    e. Should understand how to consider personal medical conditions and their effect on ability to adapt to heat stress

H. **Fluid replacement**
1. **Most important factor in preventing heat stress syndromes**
2. Indicators of adequate hydration
    a. Postworkout body weight equal to preworkout body weight
    b. After workout, urine clear and unconcentrated
3. See Chapter 8, "Sports Nutrition" for details on fluid and electrolyte replacement.

Recommended Reading

1. American College of Sports Medicine: Position stand on prevention of thermal injuries during distance running. Med Sci Sports Exerc 19(5):529–533, 1987.
2. Anderson RJ, Reed G, Knochel J: Heatstroke. Adv Intern Med 28:115–141, 1983.
3. Anderson RJ, DeLuca JP, Hubbard RW: Time course of recovery and heat acclimation ability of prior exertional heatstroke patients. Med Sci Sports Exerc 22:36–48, 1990.
4. Barner HB, Masar M, Wettach GE, Wright DW: Field evaluation of a new simplified method for cooling heat casualties in desert. Milit Med 149:95–97, 1984.
5. Bar-Or O: Climate and the exercising child. In Bar-Or O (ed): Pediatric Sports Medicine for the Practitioner. From Physiologic Principles to Clinical Applications. New York, Springer-Verlag, 1983, pp 260–299.
6. Barr SI, Costill DL, Fink WJ: Response to clinical commentary. Med Sci Sports Exerc 24:626, 1992.
7. Cadarette BS, Sawka MN, Toner MM, Pandolf KB: Aerobic fitness and the hypohydration response to exercise-heat stress. Aviat Space Environ Med 55:507–512, 1984.
8. Convertino VA: Blood volume: Its adaptation to endurance training. Med Sci Sports Exerc 23:1338–1348, 1991.
9. Costrini A: Emergency treatment of exertional heatstroke and comparison of whole body cooling techniques. Med Sci Sports Exerc 22:15–18, 1990.
10. Costrini AM, Pitt HA, Gustafson AB, Uddin DE: Cardiovascular and metabolic manifestations of heat stroke and severe heat exhaustion. Am J Med 66:296–302, 1979.
11. Eichner ER: Sacred cows and straw men [editorial]. Phys Sportsmed 19(7):24, 1991.
12. Epstein Y: Heat intolerance: Predisposing factor or residual injury? Med Sci Sports Exerc 22:29–35, 1990.
13. Falk B, Bar-Or O, MacDougall JD: Thermoregulatory responses of pre-, mid-, and late-pubertal boys to exercise in dry heat. Med Sci Sports Exerc 24:688–694, 1992.
14. Fortney SM, Vroman NB: Exercise, performance and temperature control: Temperature regulation during exercise and implications for sports performance and training. Sports Med 2:8–20, 1985.
15. Gisolfi CV, Wenger CB: Temperature regulation during exercise: Old concepts, new ideas. Exerc Sports Sci Rev 12:339–372, 1984.
16. Gonzalez RR, Cena K: Evaluation of vapor permeation through garments during exercise. J Appl Physiology 58:928–935, 1985.
17. Goodpaster BH, Sinning WE, Reommich J, et al: The residual effects of alcohol consumption on thermoregulation in heat acclimated males. Med Sci Sports Exerc 25 (5 suppl):S28, 1993.
18. Hiller WDB: Dehydration and hyponatremia during triathlons. Med Sci Sports Exerc 21(5 suppl):S219–S221, 1989.
19. Hiller WDB, O'Toole ML, Massimino F: Plasma electrolyte and glucose changes during the Hawaiian ironman triathlon. Med Sci Sports Exerc 17:219, 1985.
20. Hirata K, Nagasaka T, Hirai A, et al: Effects of human menstrual cycle on thermoregulatory vasodilation during exercise. Eur J Appl Physiol 54:559–565, 1986.
21. Hubbard RW: Heatstroke pathophysiology: The energy depletion model. Med Sci Sports Exerc 22(1):19–28, 1989.
22. Hubbard RW, Armstrong LE: An introduction: The role of exercise in the etiology of exertional heatstroke. Med Sci Sports Exerc 22:2–5, 1989.
23. Jardon OM: Heat stroke, stress, and malignant hyperthermia. Neb Med J 70:195–199, 1985.
24. Kenney WL: Physiologic correlates of heat intolerance. Sports Med 2:279–286, 1985.
25. Kenney WL, Johnson JM: Control of skin blood flow during exercise. Med Sci Sports Exerc 24:303–312, 1992.
26. Knochel JP: Dog days and siriasis: How to kill a football player. JAMA 233:513–515, 1975.
27. Knochel JP, Dotin LN, Hamburger RJ: Pathophysiology of intense physical conditioning in a hot climate: I. Mechanisms of potassium depletion. J Clin Invest 51:242–255, 1972.
28. Kobayashi Y, Ando Y, Takeuchi S, et al: Effects of heat acclimatization of distance runners in a moderately hot environment. Eur J Appl Physiol 45:189–198, 1980.
29. Meyer F, Bar-Or O, MacDougall JD, et al: Electrolyte loss in sweat and urine during exercise in the heat: Effects of gender and maturation. Med Sci Sports Exerc 23(4 suppl):S68, 1991.
30. Meyers EF, Meyers RW: Thermic stress syndrome. JAMA 247:2098–2099, 1982.
31. Millard M, Sparling PB, Rosskopf LB, et al: Gender differences in fluid requirements during prolonged running in the heat? Med Sci Sports Exerc 24(5 suppl):S63, 1992.
32. Milne CJ: Rhabdomyolysis, myoglobinuria and exercise. Sports Med 6:93–106, 1988.
33. Nadel ER: Recent advances in temperature regulation during exercise in humans. Fed Proc 44:2286–2292, 1985.
34. Noakes TD: Hyponatremia during endurance running: A physiological and clinical interpretation. Med Sci Sports Exerc 24:403–405, 1992.
35. Noakes TD, Berlinski N, Solomon E, Weight L: Collapsed runners: Blood biochemical changes after IV fluid therapy. Phys Sportsmed 19(7):70–82, 1991.

36. Noakes TD, Goodwin N, Rayner BL, et al: Water intoxication: A possible complication during endurance exercise. Med Sci Sports Exerc 17:370–375, 1985.
37. Noakes TD, Myburgh KH, Du Plessis J: Metabolic rate, not percent dehydration, predicts rectal temperature in marathon runners. Med Sci Sports Exerc 23:443–449, 1990.
38. Pivarnik JM, Miriachal CJ, Spillman HT, et al: Menstrual cycle phase affects temperature regulation during endurance exercise. Med Sci Sports Exerc 22(2 suppl):S119, 1990.
39. Roberts WO: Exercise-associated collapse in endurance events: A classification system. Phys Sportsmed 17(5):49–56, 1989.
40. Sawka MN, Gonzalez RR, Pandolf KB: Effects of sleep deprivation on thermoregulation during exercise. Am J Physiol 246(1 pt 2):R72–R77, 1984.
41. Shapiro Y, Magazanik A, Udassin R, et al: Heat intolerance in former heatstroke patients. Ann Intern Med 90:913–916, 1979.
42. Shapiro Y, Seidman DS: Field and clinical observations of exertional heat stroke patients. Med Sci Sports Exerc 22:6–14, 1990.
43. Simon HB: Hyperthermia. N Engl J Med 329:483–487, 1993.
44. Stephenson LA, Kolka MA: Thermoregulation in women. Exerc Sports Sci Rev 21:231–262, 1993.
45. Wailgum TD, Paolone AM: Heat tolerance of college football linemen and backs. Phys Sportsmed 12(5):81–86, 1984.
46. Wheeler KB: Effect of hypohydration on performance—fluid and electrolyte requirements. NSCA J 10(5):46–48, 1988.

18

Safe Exercise in the Cold and Cold Injuries

Warren D. Bowman, M.D., FACP

I. Physiologic Changes During Cold Exposure

A. Humans have evolved to adapt less readily to cold than to heat. Inhabitants of cold regions show evidence of a limited amount of adaptation, such as high metabolic rates (Eskimos), the ability to work with the hands in cold water for long periods due to an unusually strong cold-induced vasodilation response (Eskimos and Gaspé Peninsula fishermen), and the ability to sleep naked on the ground at temperatures close to freezing (Tierra del Fuegan Indians and Australian aborigines). Anecdotal reports, such as John Harlin preparing for the North Face of the Eiger, attest to the value of skiing barehanded and carrying snowballs in the unprotected hands. For optimum performance in cold weather, however, **behavioral changes** are more important than **physiologic changes.**

B. **Heat gain and loss.** Humans, as homeotherms, must control their body temperatures within narrow limits (75–105°F [24–40°C]) for survival and within even more narrow limits for the level of function needed for optimum physical performance.

1. **Body temperature is the net result of opposing mechanisms** that tend to increase or decrease body heat production, body heat loss, and the addition of heat available from the outside.
2. **When exposed to the cold**, the body behaves as though it were made up of **two separate compartments**:
   a. **The core** (heart, lungs, liver, central nervous system)
   b. **The shell** (skin, muscles, and extremities). Shell changes designed to protect the core temperature, such as vasoconstriction, may put the shell at risk from cold injury such as frostbite.
3. **The body produces heat in three major ways.**
   a. **Basal biochemical reactions, amounting to 40–60 Kcal/m^2/hr.**
   b. **Muscular activity** includes **shivering**, an involuntary mechanism that can increase basal heat production up to 6 times; **vigorous exercise**, which can increase it up to 10 times; and **semiconscious activity**, such as foot stamping.
   c. **Nonshivering thermogenesis**, which is a weak form of augmented heat production caused by:
      i. A slow increase in thyroxine secretion causing an increase in the rate of cellular metabolism
      ii. Increased secretion of epinephrine and norepinephrine, which act on brown fat to increase uncoupling of oxidative phosphorylation. In humans, significant brown fat is found solely in infants; adult heat production can be increased only 10–15% through this process.
4. **The body loses heat by four mechanisms.**
   a. **Conduction:** direct transfer of heat by contact between the body and a colder object

b. **Convection:** transfer of heat when air or water of a lower temperature moves across the body surface
c. **Evaporation:** loss of heat when water or other volatile liquid on the body surface is transformed into vapor. As a result of the high heat of vaporization of water (0.580 Kcal/g), considerable heat can be lost through this mechanism.
d. **Radiation:** loss of heat by infrared rays to a cooler object not in contact with the body
e. In addition, a small amount of heat is lost when **inspired air** is warmed to body termperature before being expired.

5. **When the body is exposed to cold,** cold receptors in the skin are stimulated and warm receptors are inhibited, causing regulatory centers in the hypothalamus to increase heat production through shivering and initiation of nonshivering thermogenesis and to limit heat loss by decreasing sweating and reducing shell circulation. The most important and efficient methods of maintaining body temperature in the cold, however, are **behavioral ones**, such as exercising, eating, adding clothing, seeking shelter, and adding heat from outside sources such as a stove or fire.
   a. The **shell cooling** resulting from reduced shell circulation can **interfere with the ability to perform well athletically** because it weakens and slows muscle contractions and delays nerve conduction time.
   b. Cold, stiff muscles require a longer, more careful warm-up period to prevent injury.
6. **Wind chill.** The athlete must consider not only the actual temperature, but also the effect of wind in accelerating heat loss. This refers both to natural wind and to the air movement created by a moving body.
   a. The greatest effect of wind is exerted in the first 20 mph—greater wind speeds have little additional effect (Fig. 1). Heat loss at these low velocities is not linear but is proportional to the **square root** of the wind speed.
   b. The **danger point** is around –10°F (–23°C), a temperature below which the amount of air movement created by such activities as running, bicycling, and skiing can cause rapid frostbite of exposed body parts, such as the cheeks, chin, and ears.

C. **Effect of cooling on the organ systems**

1. As the skin and muscles cool, **shivering** begins and increases in violence. **Below 90°F (32°C), shivering gradually ceases** as the muscles become cooler and stiffer.
2. As the body temperature falls **below 95°F (35°C)**, the rates of essential biochemical reactions slow.
   a. **Regulatory center cooling** slows the heart and breathing rates. The cardiac output and blood pressure fall.
   b. **Central nervous system cooling leads to a decrease in cerebral blood flow,** dilation of the pupils, and obtundation of the sensorium, leading to stupor and eventually coma.
   c. **Oxygen consumption decreases** to 50% of normal at 82°F (28°C) and 22% of normal at 64°F (18°C).
3. **Polyuria (cold diuresis)** occurs as shell vasoconstriction increases core blood volume.
4. **Acidosis develops** because of carbon dioxide retention, increased lactate production, decreased tissue perfusion, and starvation.
5. **Insulin activity decreases.**
6. **The myocardium becomes more irritable. Atrial fibrillation** is a common (benign) arrhythmia; **ventricular fibrillation** is a hazard, especially **below 82°F (28°C)**.
7. **The ECG** in mild hypothermia may show sinus bradycardia; prolongation of the P-R, QRS, and Q-T intervals; nonspecific ST-T changes; and the J waves of Osborne.

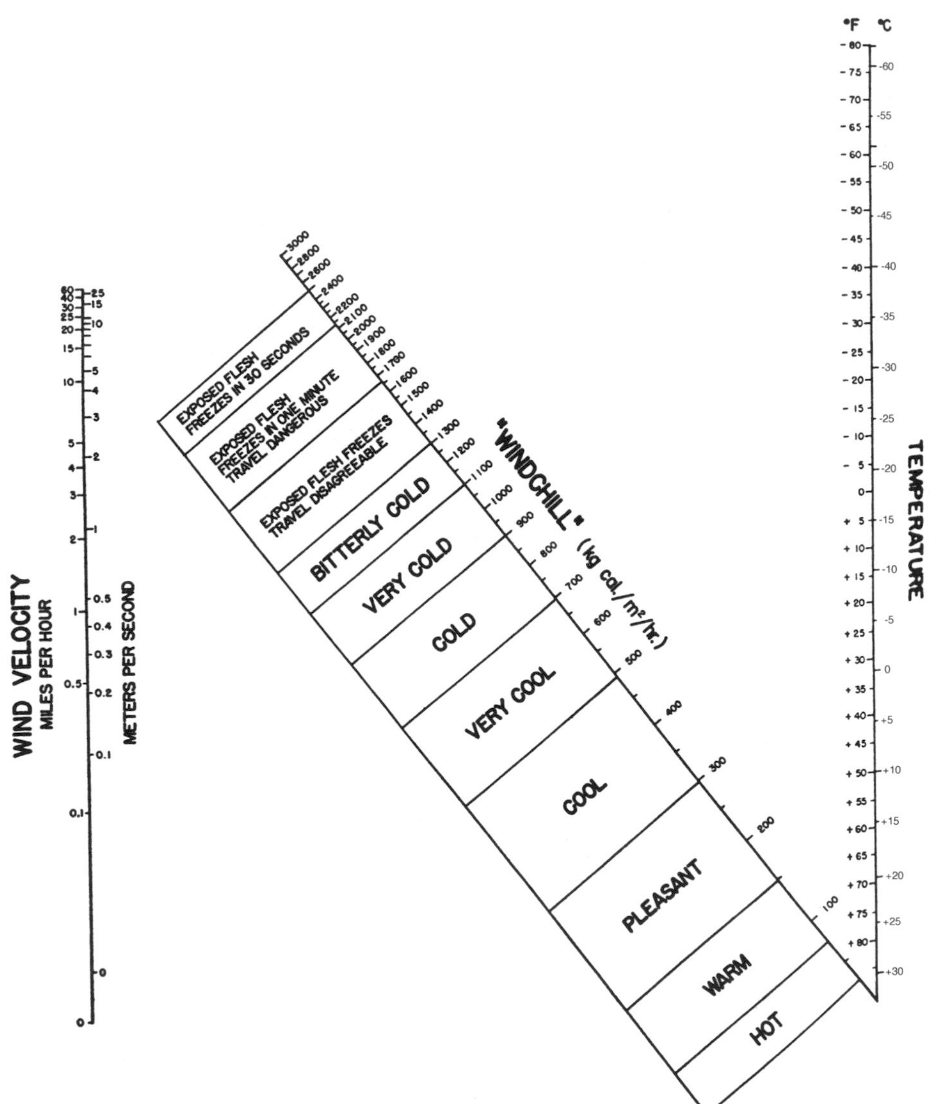

FIGURE 1. Line chart showing windchill and state of comfort under varying conditions of temperature and wind velocity. The numbers along the right-hand margin of the diagonal center block refer to the "windchill factor"—the rate of cooling in kilogram-calories per square meter per hour of an unclad, inactive body exposed to specific temperatures and wind velocities. Windchill factors above 1400—the value at which exposed flesh freezes—are very dangerous. (From Consolazio CF, et al: Metabolic Methods. St. Louis, The C.V. Mosby Company, 1951, with permission.)

D. **Localized cold injury can occur at temperatures both above and below freezing;** the latter is more of a concern in sports medicine. Temperatures below the freezing point for tissue (about 24.8°F [–4°C]) can cause injury both from local freezing and from interference with circulation.

1. **Blood vessel spasm and vessel wall damage** occur first, slowing circulation and causing loss of plasma into interstitial spaces.

2. As the temperature continues to drop, extracellular **ice crystals** appear, causing osmotic changes that produce cell dehydration and shrinkage and increase the concentration of electrolytes.
3. Circulatory stasis progresses because of sludging, spasm, and clots in small blood vessels, eventually leading to ischemic tissue death.

II. Prevention of Cold Injury

This can be accomplished by increasing body heat production and decreasing body heat loss; the latter is the most energy-efficient method. If these fail, heat must be added from the outside.

A. **Increased heat production** can be achieved by **eating** and by **increasing muscular activity.**
   1. **Eating** provides both the "specific dynamic action" of the digestive process and calories from the food. Regular nutritious meals keep glycogen and fat stores replenished. During prolonged exercise, provision should be made for **snacks at regular intervals**.
   2. **Muscular activity** may be involuntary (shivering) or by exercise. Good nutrition and physical conditioning are necessary if prolonged muscular activity or sustained shivering is required to stay warm.

B. **Decreasing heat loss**
   1. **The "layer principle" of clothing** adapts well to outdoor sports. This means wearing several (three or more) thin layers of insulation rather than one or two thick layers. Clothing can then be adjusted to maintain an optimal microclimate of still, warm air next to the body, preventing chilling and overheating with excessive sweating (which diminishes the insulative value of clothing).
   2. The **preferred fabrics** for cold weather sport clothing are those that have **high insulating properties that are not diminished significantly by becoming wet.** These fabrics include wool, wool/synthetic blends, polypropylene, treated polyesters such as Capilene, and hollow polyesters such as Thermastat.
      a. **Cotton should not be worn** because it has poor insulating ability, which is markedly decreased if it becomes wet.
      b. Pile garments and those containing a filler such as down, Dacron, Hollofil, and Thinsulate are less useful during exercise because their thickness produces excessive insulation, leading to overheating; they are more useful when worn during the warm-up or cool-down periods. Tight garments, which may be more aerodynamic, nevertheless interfere with the insulating value of underlying clothing by compressing its loft: the "Lycra look" may be "cool" but is colder than the "Pillsbury Doughboy look."
   3. **Wind protection** is essential and is provided by wearing a windproof outer jacket and pants. Preferred garments are those made from fabrics that are also water-repellent, such as Gore-Tex. The jacket should have a **hood** with a drawstring.
   4. **Protection for special body parts.** Parts at risk are those that are normally exposed, such as the face (nose, cheeks, eyelids, chin), or that have a large surface area-to-volume ratio, such as the ears, extremities, fingers, toes, male genitalia, and nipples.
      a. **Blood supply to the head is not decreased by cold exposure, leading to considerable heat loss from radiation if the head is uncovered.**
      b. **Wear a cap**, preferably the ski type, that can be pulled down over the ears.
      c. The **exposed face, which can be subject to frostbite at low temperatures, can be covered** with a face mask, balaclava, or a "neck gaiter" that can be pulled up over the lower face.
      d. Under extreme cold conditions, **the cornea of the eye can freeze,** possibly requiring a corneal transplant. This can be prevented by **wearing ski goggles**.

e. Athletes who wear glasses may wish to use contact lenses, remembering that at extreme cold temperatures these may actually freeze to the eyeball.
f. Glasses and goggles tend to fog unless well ventilated; this can be prevented to some extent by treating them with antifog preparations.
g. **Hands** should be protected, with polypropylene or wool gloves at moderate temperatures and wool or pile mittens with windproof shells at lower temperatures.
h. Athletic **shoes** should be sized large enough to admit a suitable number of socks. For cold weather running, wear an inner pair of polypropylene socks and at least one outer pair of heavy wool socks, especially when running in snow, in which the feet may become wet.
i. Because trunk cooling leads to vasoconstriction in the skin and extremities, **prevent cold hands and feet by adequate trunk insulation**, thereby insuring a greater supply of warm blood to the extremities. Insulate well high heat loss areas in which there are large blood vessels close to skin, such as the groin and sides of the neck, or in which there is little natural insulation, such as the sides of the chest.
j. Women should wear insulated bras to prevent cold injury to nipples; men should wear shorts with insulated, windproof front panels to prevent cold injury to genitals.

5. **Avoid wetting** by rain, snow, or perspiration because heat loss is increased both by evaporation and by the resulting decrease in the insulating ability of wet clothing. A water-repellent jacket and pants should be worn during activities in rain or wet snow.
6. If conditions are bad enough, it may be better to **cancel the workout and get out of the weather**. The combination of wind and cold rain or wet snow, as in a blizzard around 32°F (0°C), is particularly dangerous; the effects are compounded by fatigue and hunger.
7. **Warming up.** Cold muscles, tendons, and joints are more prone to strains and sprains because they are stiffer and less coordinated. Injury can be prevented by proper warm-ups.
   a. **Because the body should be warm before warm-up exercises begin, they are preferably performed indoors before outdoor activity.**
   b. If performed outdoors, protective clothing should be worn to prevent cooling.
   c. If the body shell is cool before exercises are started, the warm-up activity should start less abruptly and be done slower and for a longer time.
8. **Cold weather water sports** include rafting, kayaking, canoeing, wind-surfing, small-boat sailing, and long distance swimming. Aside from **drowning**, the major hazard is **hypothermia**—most often resulting from an unexpected capsizing. Remember that water is an excellent conductor, causing heat loss at a rate of 25 to 32 times that of cold air at the same temperature. Participants should wear wet or dry suits and suitable personal flotation devices.

III. Types of Cold Injury

A. Hypothermia

1. **Diagnosis:** Hypothermia, or "exposure," exists when the body core temperature falls below 95°F (35°C).
   a. Anticipate hypothermia when suitable climatic conditions exist, and suspect it when an athlete shivers; appears clumsy, apathetic, or confused; has slurred speech; stumbles; and drops things (Table 1).
   b. Hypothermia is more of a danger to athletes exposed to cold for long periods of time, such as long distance runners and Nordic ski racers, especially those who are slowing down late in a race because of fatigue or injury. Any injured or ill athlete who has been exposed to cold weather or cold water, however, is suspected to have hypothermia until proved otherwise.

TABLE 1. Hypothermia

°F	°C	Signs and Symptoms
99–96	37–35.6	Intense shivering. Impaired ability to perform complex tasks.
95–91	35–32.8	Violent shivering, dysarthria, sluggish thinking, amnesia
90–86	32.4–30	Shivering ceases, muscular rigidity supervenes. Movements jerky, sensorium dull
85–81	29.8–27	Coma, areflexia, atrial fibrillation
< 78	< 25.6	Failure of cardiac and respiratory center control. Pulmonary edema, ventricular fibrillation. Death

   c. **Low-reading thermometers should be available in first-aid kits during cold weather athletic events.**

2. **Field first aid and prehospital management**
   a. For purposes of field first aid, **hypothermic patients are divided into those with mild hypothermia (rectal temperature ≥ 90°F [32°C]) and those with moderate to severe hypothermia (rectal temperature < 90°F [32°C]).** In previously healthy athletes, the recovery rate from mild hypothermia should be close to 100%. The recovery rate from moderate to severe hypothermia is lower; the most common cause of death is probably ventricular fibrillation.
   b. In all cases of definite or suspected hypothermia, **get the patient out of the cold and wind and into a tent or other shelter and prevent further heat loss.**
      i. **Replace wet clothing with dry:**
         (a) In severely affected patients, cut off clothing to avoid the type of jostling that may precipitate ventricular fibrillation.
         (b) Insulate the patient with dry clothing, blankets, or a sleeping bag; cover the head; and do **not** let him or her sit, stand, or walk until rewarmed.
      ii. Make arrangements for speedy transport to a hospital in all but the mildest cases.
   c. **Field first aid then depends on the patient's measured or estimated core temperature.** If no thermometer is available, core temperature can be estimated by noting the level of consciousness and whether shivering is present.
      i. A patient **who is still shivering** likely has a core temperature ≥ 90°F (32°C).
      ii. A patient **who is obtunded and not shivering** is likely colder than 90°F (32°C).
3. **Mild hypothermia.** Previously healthy athletes with mild hypothermia can almost always be safely rewarmed on the spot by any means available.
   a. An effective method is to allow them to shiver themselves warm inside a sleeping bag in a warm shelter.
   b. Slow external rewarming devices, such as hot water bottles, heating pads, or canteens full of hot water (all carefully wrapped to avoid causing burns) or a small, charcoal-burning stove developed by the Norwegian army (Heatpak), can be used, or one or two healthy persons can get into a sleeping bag or blanket roll with the patient. Although these external methods have been shown experimentally to slow rewarming because they inhibit shivering—theoretically limiting their value—extensive positive field experience supports their use.
   c. Hot tubs (around 110°F [43°C]) can be used if available.
   d. Special devices have been developed that deliver heated, humidified air or oxygen (e.g., UVIC Heat Treat, Res-Q-Aire). The amount of heat delivered is not great and, theoretically, their main value would be to prevent heat loss through the airway. Again, however, extensive field experience supports their use.

e. Hot (preferably noncaffeinated) drinks are useful (mainly for morale purposes) after the patient has been partly rewarmed and is able to swallow.

4. **Moderate to severe hypothermia.** In this case, **the best field results are obtained by preventing further heat loss** (by one of the methods listed previously, which can be applied during transportation) and **transporting the patient to definitive medical care rather than attempting field rewarming.**
   a. Avoid active rewarming methods, such as a hot tub or electric blanket. These patients remain relatively stable for a number of hours if treated gently and **not allowed to get any colder. Once rewarming starts, serious electrolyte, metabolic, and cardiovascular changes occur that are impossible to diagnose or treat in the field.**
   b. Because these patients are dehydrated, **start an intravenous infusion** of 5% glucose/normal saline if available, warmed at least to body temperature.
   c. **The usual procedures of basic life support should be followed except that cardiopulmonary resuscitation (CPR) should not be given unless ventricular fibrillation is likely.** Advanced life support is given according to American Heart Association criteria.
      i. In severe hypothermics, the presence of a heartbeat may be difficult to document without a cardiac monitor. Spend 30 seconds searching for a pulse or heartbeat before deciding it is absent.
      ii. In severe hypothermia, the chest may be rigid and incompressible.
      iii. Transport of the patient to definitive medical care is important. It is difficult to give continuous CPR in a patient being transported by litter—intermittent CPR during frequent stops is probably preferable.
      iv. Closed chest cardiac massage, if given, is **likely to precipitate ventricular fibrillation if it does not already exist.**
   d. Because blood pressure is normally low in hypothermia and does respond to rewarming, do not use the pneumatic antishock garment (PASG) without a strong indication, such as an unstable fractured pelvis.
   e. Handle the hypothermic gently during transport, avoiding sudden bumps and changes of direction.
5. **In-hospital treatment.** With close attention to hydration, oxygenation, acid–base balance, and cardiac monitoring, mild to moderate hypothermics (rectal temperature 85°F [29°C]) or above can be rewarmed externally with heated, humidified oxygen and an electric blanket, the Bair Hugger warmer, or a plumbed device such as the Blanketrol. Severe hypothermics are best treated with central core rewarming techniques, such as peritoneal dialysis or partial cardiopulmonary bypass.

B. **Frostbite:** actual localized freezing of body tissues to variable depth depending on the temperature, length of exposure, amount of insulation, adequacy of circulation, contact with metal, wetting, and other factors. The most commonly affected parts are those at the body periphery or those that have a large surface area-to-volume ratio or exposed position. Frostbite can be a danger to Alpine and Nordic ski racers; gatekeepers at Alpine races; and cold-weather distance athletes such as speed skaters, bicyclers, and runners. Team sports held outdoors in cold weather, such as football, soccer, field hockey, and bobsledding, can also result in frostbite in poorly dressed participants. Figure skating and ice hockey, which are usually held in indoor rinks, are less of a hazard because the air is warmer and natural wind is absent.

1. **Diagnosis:** Frostbite is generally divided into **superficial** and **deep**.
   a. **Superficial frostbite**, mild cases of which are sometimes called "frostnip," involves the outer layers of the skin.
      i. **Symptoms include a burning feeling followed by numbness.**

   ii. **Inspection** shows a grayish or pale area of skin, usually on the face or extremities. The deeper tissues **can be felt to be soft and pliable**. After thawing, the area becomes red, sensitive, and swollen to varying degrees. In more severe cases, a few small blebs may appear. A few days later, the skin is shed by flaking or peeling.

  b. **Deep frostbite** is a less common but much more serious injury that should be seen rarely, if at all, during well-managed athletic events. It is most common in the ears, nose, fingers, toes, and extremities.
   i. **The affected part typically becomes painfully cold, then stops hurting, becomes numb, and "feels like a block of wood."**
   ii. **Inspection** shows a cold, firm, rigid, pale, or waxy member resembling a piece of chicken removed from the freezer. After thawing, blisters develop within hours to days and may have a startling appearance.

 2. **First aid and prehospital management**
  a. **Superficial frostbite can be thawed on the spot** by direct body heat such as a warm hand on the frozen cheek or a frozen finger held inside a jacket in the patient's axilla.
   i. **Attention should then be paid as to why the frostbite occurred.**
   ii. The patient should put on protective clothing and in many cases be taken to a shelter where general body warming can be performed. As mentioned previously, additional trunk insulation is desirable because an increase in core temperature causes peripheral vasodilation, increasing the amount of warm blood available to the shell.
  b. **Deep frostbite is best rewarmed under controlled conditions in a hospital.**
   i. Experience has shown that the least tissue damage results if rewarming is rapid and is performed in a water bath at a temperature of 102–108°F (39–42°C).
   ii. During transport, keep the patient warm but do not actively rewarm the frozen part.
   iii. Refreezing should be avoided because it inevitably leads to tissue loss.

IV. Miscellaneous Cold-related Illnesses

For a detailed discussion of these conditions, appropriate medical textbooks should be consulted.

A. **Raynaud's syndrome:** not rare in young athletes, especially women. It is characterized by bilateral episodic spasms of digital blood vessels in response to cold exposure or emotion. It can be due to an underlying disease or anatomic abnormality and can be a long-term complication of frostbite, but is usually idiopathic. The fingers are most commonly affected.
 1. **Signs and symptoms**
  a. During the ischemic phase, the affected digits are cold, pale, and numb.
  b. This phase is followed by hyperemia with redness, throbbing pain, and swelling.
 2. **Treatment and prevention**
  a. Attacks can be terminated by warming the affected extremity.
  b. The patient should have a **thorough medical evaluation** to rule out an underlying condition, such as collagen vascular disease, occlusive arterial disease, thoracic outlet compression syndromes and other neurologic conditions, cryoglobulinemia, and cold agglutinin disease.
  c. **Smoking should be avoided.**
  d. During cold exposure, the trunk should be well insulated to prevent reflex extremity vasoconstriction, which can precipitate Raynaud's phenomenon. Boots and socks should be well chosen, and mittens should be worn instead of gloves.
  e. Attacks can be prevented to some extent by prophylactic use of calcium channel blockers, angiotensin-converting enzyme inhibitors, vasodilators such as prazosin and tolazoline, or resperpine.

B. **Cold-induced bronchospasm.** Exposure to cold, dry air during cold-weather sports such as cross country skiing is a common contributor to exercise-induced bronchospasm (see Chapter 33). Attacks can frequently be prevented by the prophylactic use of bronchodilators, such as long-acting theophylline preparations, beta$_2$-agonists, or cromolyn, singly or in combination. Salmeterol, a recently developed, long-acting bronchodilator, administered by two inhalations 30–60 minutes before exercise, appears to protect many patients for up to 12 hours.

C. **Cold-agglutinin disease** may be idiopathic or due to a viral infection or lymphoproliferative disorder, but in an athlete it is most frequently due to a *Mycoplasma* infection.
   1. **Signs and symptoms,** which are due to intravascular agglutination of red blood cells by an antibody that is activated by cold exposure, include cyanosis and pain or numbness of exposed body parts, such as the ears and fingers.
   2. It is differentiated from Raynaud's syndrome by the lack of initial blanching followed by hyperemia. In the mycoplasmal variety, which is self-limited, there is commonly a history of recent upper respiratory infection, particularly bronchitis.
   3. **Treatment** is warming.
   4. **Prevention** is same as for Raynaud's syndrome.

Recommended Reading

1. American Heart Association: 1996 Handbook of Emergency Cardiac Care for Health Providers. AHA, 1996.
2. Bowman WD: Outdoor Emergency Care: Comprehensive First Aid for Nonurban Settings, 2nd ed. Denver, National Ski Patrol, 1993.
3. Crawshaw LI: Thermoregulation. In Auerbach PS (ed): Wilderness Medicine. St. Louis, Mosby-Year Book, 1995, pp 38–50.
4. Danzl DF, Pozos RS: Current concepts: Accidental hypothermia. N Engl J Med 331:1756–1760, 1994.
5. Danzl DF, Pozos RS, Hamlet MP: Accidental hypothermia. In Auerbach PS (ed): Wilderness Medicine. St. Louis, Mosby-Year Book, 1995, pp 51–103.
6. Fuentes RJ, Rosenberg JM (eds): Exercise-induced asthma and the athlete. In Athletic Drug Reference '94. Durham, NC, Clean Data, 1994, pp 161–177.
7. Giesbrecht G, et al: Treatment of mild immersion hypothermia by direct body to body contact. J App Physiol 76(6):2373–2379, 1994.
8. Giesbrecht G: The respiratory system in a cold environment. Aviat Space Environ Med 66:890–902, 1995.
9. Guyton AC: Body temperature, temperature regulation, and fever. In Textbook of Medical Physiology. Philadelphia, WB Saunders, 1991, pp 797–808.
10. Lereim I: Sports at Low Temperatures. Federation Internationale de Ski, Worbstrasse 210, Postfach, CH-3073, Gumligan, Switzerland, 1988.
11. Lloyd EL: Cold stress in sport. In Hypothermia and Cold Stress. Rockville, MD, Aspen, 1986, pp 310–318.
12. McCauley RL, Smith DJ, Robson MC, et al: Frostbite and other cold-induced injuries. In Auerbach PS (ed): Wilderness Medicine. St. Louis, Mosby-Year Book, 1995, pp 129–145.
13. Paton BC: Cold injuries. In Strauss RH (ed): Sports Medicine, 2nd ed. Philadelphia, WB Saunders, 1991, pp 359–388.
14. Stamford B: Smart dressing for cold weather workouts. Phys Sportsmed 23:105–106, 1995.

19

Sports Surfaces

Richard B. Flynn, Ed.D.

It is generally accepted that the type of surface on which an activity or sport is played can affect the quality of performance. Other aspects of the game influenced by the playing surface include speed, costs, player comfort, and player safety. Unfortunately, there is no one surface that satisfactorily meets the needs of participants for all indoor and outdoor activities. Each activity has its own unique characteristics requiring a particular type of surface for optimal performance. Economic considerations often dictate a common surface be used to support a variety of activities, especially at recreational and amateur levels. Planners of formal sports facilities are urged to consult with the various governing organizations regarding rules, regulations, and standards that may affect the type of surface necessary for sanctioned participation in a particular sport. The purpose of this chapter is to outline some of the surfaces used for different sporting activities, relate surface selection to player performance and safety, and identify factors to be considered in the selection of sports surfaces.

I. General Considerations

A. **Range of surfaces:** hundreds available as possible choices for sporting events. Some of these surfaces are natural and are formed from products found in nature, whereas others are more complex, requiring processing or the use of synthetic materials.

1. **Natural surfaces**
   a. Earth—loams, sand, sand-clay, clay-gravel, fuller's earth, stabilized earth
   b. Turf (grass)—bluegrass mixtures, bent, fescue, Bermuda
   c. Aggregates—gravel, graded stone, graded slag, shell, cinders
   d. Masonry—flagstone (sandstone, limestone, granite), brick
   e. Wood flooring—usually polished hard woods
   f. Miscellaneous—tanbark, sawdust, shavings, cotton-seed hulls
2. **Nonnatural surfaces**
   a. Asphalt—penetration-macadam, asphaltic concrete (cool and hot poured), sheet asphalt, natural asphalt, sawdust asphalt, vermiculite asphalt, cork asphalt, other patented asphalt mixes.
   b. Synthetics—rubber, synthetic resins, rubber asphalt, chlorinated butyl-rubber, mineral fiber, plastics, vinyl.
   c. Concrete—monolithic, terrazzo, pre-cast.

B. **Factors influencing choice of surfaces:** In general, safety, the appropriateness of the surface properties for the specified sport, and the material properties related to wear and maintenance all need to be considered when selecting a surface.[3] Additional factors that may influence the choice of surface:

1. Expected multiplicity of use
2. Durability and longevity
3. Dustless and stainless
4. Reasonable initial cost and economy

5. Ease and cost of maintenance
6. Pleasing appearance
7. Nonabrasiveness
8. Resiliency and consistency of resiliency
9. Year-round usage
10. Color and color stability
11. Impact absorption
12. Effects of temperature and sun (for outdoor surfaces)
13. Tensile strength
14. Texture

C. **Ideal surface conditions:** No one surface satisfactorily meets the needs of all activities. Each activity has its own surface requirements that dictate what type of materials can be used. Ideally, most sports or activities need the following conditions to be met:
   1. A surface that provides appropriate traction
   2. A surface that is smooth and even
   3. A surface that provides consistent hardness
   4. A surface that has enough spring to prevent injuries

D. **Base system:** serves as the foundation for the sports surface, and can influence the costs, longevity, and safety of the overall surface. It should be as carefully selected as the visible surface.

E. **Surface selection process**
   1. Specify requirements of the activity, material, and base system.
   2. Select information from multiple manufacturers.
   3. Compare alternatives, and clarify advantages and disadvantages.
   4. Visit sites with the various surfaces.
   5. Tentatively select a surface.
   6. Ascertain the manufacturers' reputability, support after the sale, years in business.
   7. Identify potential installers and similarly investigate their reputation.
   8. Clarify maintenance requirements and costs.
   9. Clarify total costs for initial installation.
   10. Calculate life-cycle costs.
   11. Solicit bids.
   12. Require the manufacturer to oversee the installation process to ensure compliance.

II. Surfaces for Outdoor Sporting Events

A. **Outdoor field events:** Football, soccer, baseball, field hockey, and lacrosse are all played on outdoor fields. The surface material, whether natural or artificial, is critical to the use and success of the field as a site for practice and games.
   1. **Surface requirements**
      a. Smooth and uniform
      b. Resilient enough to prevent injuries, but hard enough to facilitate running
      c. Providing traction
   2. **Surface options**
      a. **Grass**—bluegrass mixtures, bent, fescue, and Bermuda are popular natural fields for athletics.
         i. **Advantages** of grass:
            (a) Attractiveness
            (b) Resiliency
            (c) Nonabrasiveness
            (d) Relatively dust free
            (e) Cool temperature maintained by surface even in hot weather
            (f) Generally regarded as safe

ii. **Disadvantages** of grass
(a) Difficult to maintain when there is intense usage
(b) Expense of watering (can be costly in some parts of the United States)
(c) Field cannot be used, without damage, when wet or frozen.
(d) Field must be given time to recuperate after heavy use.
(e) Requires scheduled aeration, fertilization, deep watering, seeding, and trimming.

b. **Synthetic turf** is a good choice if a field would otherwise be dirt or mud for most of the season. Synthetic turf is a tufted or knit carpet made from nylon or polypropylene. The composition of the subcarpet base varies in thickness and resiliency. Embedded in, or bonded to, the subcarpet base are plastic fibers resembling grass. The density and height of the blades vary with anticipated use. Innovations in synthetic turf include the use of more porous materials that facilitate better drainage, and now with some materials there is no grain, or direction, in the field. "Sand-filled" turf systems are an option designed to reduce the potential for injury.

i. **Advantages** of synthetic turf:
(a) Consistently smooth and uniform surface
(b) Greatly expands the effective use of an area (allows multiuse including recreational activities and instructional classes rather than just formal athletics)
(c) Provides opportunity for use under all but most adverse weather conditions
(d) Generally regarded as safe
(e) Provides economic benefits through reduced acreage requirements
(f) Increased use and decreased maintenance costs
(g) Many top regional, state, national, and international events are conducted on synthetic surfaces, providing for greater uniformity in performance.
(h) Does not cause allergies
(i) No bald spots

ii. **Disadvantages** of synthetic turf:
(a) Initial costs are high, sometimes double or triple depending on grading, subsurface, installation process, and selected material.
(b) Maintenance, although minimal in some cases, is necessary. When required, it is both costly and time-consuming. Maintenance is reduced if measures are taken to reduce or eliminate vehicular and pedestrian traffic and security measures are taken to reduce vandalism and misuse.
(c) Aspects of the weather do affect outdoor synthetic surfaces. Extreme temperatures may alter the resiliency of the surface. The character of the composition may also alter over a short period of time either from temperature extremes or ultraviolet exposure.
(d) Limited research studies have indicated a heat buildup on the surface that may affect the performer.
(e) Surface is abrasive

3. **Relationship between turf type and injuries:** Many studies over the years have compared injury rates on artificial versus natural turf. A review of the research suggests there may be a slightly higher injury rate on artificial turf. However, as developments in artificial turf have taken place over the years, it appears progress is being made toward artificial turf becoming safer. In addition, there are **subfactors that affect injury rates:**

a. May be greater frequency of play on synthetic surfaces
b. Varying surface pad thicknesses

c. Different equipment padding
d. Different types of injuries
e. Varying coaching methods
f. Inaccurate recording of injuries
g. Varying shoe-turf interactions

B. **Outdoor basketball**
1. **Surface requirements**
a. Smooth
b. Hard
2. **Recommended options**
a. Asphaltic concrete:
i. Durable
ii. Can be used year-round
iii. Dust-free
iv. Drains quickly
v. Marks easily and with a high degree of permanence
vi. Neat appearance
vii. Colors easily
viii. Easy to maintain
b. Portland cement concrete:
i. More expensive to install
ii. May crack when used in an extreme cold climate
c. Synthetic surfaces:
i. Same advantages as asphaltic concrete
ii. Aesthetically pleasing
iii. More expensive to install

C. **Outdoor tennis**
1. **Factors to consider in selecting a surface**
a. Player preference
b. Maintenance cost and amount of maintenance required
c. Initial construction cost
d. Surface on which player can slide or not slide
e. Length of time until resurfacing is required
f. Resurfacing cost
g. Softness of surface desired for player comfort
h. Surface adaptability for other uses
i. Fast or slow surface
j. Uniformity of ball bounce
k. Effect of color on glare and heat absorption
l. Drying time after rain
m. Availability of service from court builder
n. Color fastness of surface and its effect on ball discoloration
o. Effect of abrasive surfaces on ball, rackets, shoes, and falling players
p. Quality of lines and markings
q. Hazards, maintenance of lines
2. **Classification of tennis court surfaces**
a. Pervious construction (permits water to filter through the surface):
i. Fast dry (fine crushed aggregate)
ii. Clay
iii. Grass
iv. Others (dirt, grit)
b. Impervious construction (water does not penetrate, but runs off the surface):

- i. Noncushioned
  - (a) Concrete
  - (b) Asphalt:
    - Hot-plant mix
    - Emulsified asphalt mix
    - Combination of hot-plant and emulsified mix
    - Penetration macadam
    - Asphalt job mix
  - (c) Others (wood)
- ii. Cushioned construction
  - (a) Asphalt bound systems:
    - Hot-leveling course and hot-cushion course
    - Cold-leveling course and cold-cushion course
  - (b) Synthetic
    - Elastomer
    - Textile
  - (c) Others

D. **Outdoor track**

1. **Options**
   - a. Natural or aggregate materials
   - b. Asphalt-bound
   - c. Latex or latex-bound
   - d. Polyurethane or polyurethane-bound
   - e. Premanufactured rubber mats
2. **Factors for consideration**
   - a. Cost for the foundation and drainage
   - b. Cost of the surface
   - c. Color options:
     - i. Performance is enhanced on colors other than black.
     - ii. Surface temperature is reduced on nonblack surfaces, in turn lengthening surface life.
     - iii. A color surface change in a nonblack surface indicates need for maintenance.
     - iv. A nonblack surface is "treated" better by athletes and spectators.

III. Surfaces for Indoor Sporting Events

A. **Multipurpose use:** The best choice of flooring depends on expected use. Wood is an excellent all-round surface, although it lacks the flexibility that might be demanded by extensive community use of the facility. Synthetic surfaces are excellent for all normal game-type activities and can better accommodate chairs, tables, and booths. Some activities require specialized flooring, such as dance, weight training, and body conditioning.

1. **Surface options**
   - a. Wood
   - b. Synthetic:
     - i. Prefabricated
     - ii. Poured-in-place
   - c. Carpet
2. **Life-cycle costs:** Variability in initial costs and maintenance costs affects choice of a multipurpose activity surface.
3. **Advantages and disadvantages of various options** (see "Surface options," next page)

B. **Basketball/volleyball**
   1. **Surface requirements**
      a. Hard, but resilient
      b. Smooth and even
   2. **Surface options:** Wood or synthetic flooring of a nonslip nature is best for volleyball and basketball. Maintenance of all gymnasium flooring is an ongoing and costly necessity.
      a. **Wood** (generally hard northern maple)—over an extended time period, the costs per square foot for wood flooring may be less than for most synthetic floors.[2]
         i. **Advantages:**
            (a) Natural resiliency due to organic nature
            (b) Variability in resilience based on choice of subflooring (floating systems with foam or rubber underlayment, sleeper systems and spring systems under plywood)
            (c) Can be sanded to accept a wide variety of finishes
            (d) Traction is superb for basketball, volleyball, and other sports
            (e) Properly maintained wood floor can outlast the building
         ii. **Disadvantages:**
            (a) High initial cost
            (b) Maintenance costs can be high (but with new polyurethane finishes, maintenance costs are decreasing).
            (c) Can warp when exposed to moisture
            (d) Is not as versatile as some synthetics (e.g., too smooth for indoor tennis)
      b. **Synthetics** (plasticized polyvinyl chlorides or polyurethanes)—generally polyurethanes possess most of the desirable characteristics in a synthetic floor surface.[10]
         i. **Advantages:**
            (a) Prefabricated floors are uniform in thickness (poured-in-place floors may not be).
            (b) Prefabricated floors are durable (poured-in-place floors may disintegrate, harden, shrink, and crack as a result of ultraviolet rays and evaporating chemicals).
            (c) Resilient
            (d) Available in a wide variety of colors, textures, and amount of traction
            (e) Initial cost usually lower than wood
            (f) Unaffected by moisture
            (g) Not slippery when wet
            (h) Versatile for multiple uses
         ii. **Disadvantages:**
            (a) Can be difficult to keep clean
            (b) Ultraviolet rays can cause disintegration in some cases.
            (c) Plasticizers in poured-in-place floors may cause unpleasant odors.
            (d) Poured-in-place floors can be difficult to repair in worn areas.
            (e) Poured-in-place floors may not be uniform thickness.

C. **Dance**
   1. **Surface requirements**
      a. Has shock-absorbing qualities
      b. Will "give" under impact to some degree and absorb some of the impact energy in doing so
      c. Will not deform permanently or dent under pressure or impact in normal use
      d. Should not be "dead" or softly yielding as sand is, but should return some bounce to shoe

e. Should not be absolutely rigid or hard and should not give impression of being so
f. Nonslippery but smooth and permitting of gliding
g. Constructed for easy cleaning

2. **Design options for subflooring** (seven major types)
   a. **Anchor sleeper construction:** 2 × 3 inch or 2 × 4 inch sleepers of varying lengths leveled and anchored to the concrete substrate with mechanical fasteners
   b. **Resilient rubber-padded sleeper with floating floor:** 2 × 3 inch sleepers with resilient rubber or vinyl pads attached to the underside of the sleeper
   c. **Spring-coil:** resembles a miniature coil spring used in the automobile industry but is designed specifically for flooring applications
   d. **Spring-leaf:** resembles the leaf spring suspension of an automobile, only it is smaller
   e. **Resilient foam underlayment:** sheets of varying thicknesses and densities deaden sound and absorb shock. Subflooring is laid over foam sheeting.
   f. **Multilayered basket-weave sleeper or joist construction:** stacked layers of 1 × 4 inch or 2 × 3 inch alternating perpendicular to one another
   g. **Mastic set floor:** Different compositions provide cushioning but little return of energy. Mastic can be applied under subfloor components at various thicknesses.
3. **Surface materials** laid over the subfloor systems vary greatly, but all are intended to have proper surface friction, uniformity of surface, and long-term performance.
   a. Wood products:
      i. Northern hard-strip maple
      ii. Strip oak
      iii. Pine
      iv. Fir
      v. Birch
   b. Synthetic products:
      i. Vinyl roll sheet goods
      ii. Linoleum
      iii. Portable synthetic flooring mats
   c. Coatings/wood finishes:
      i. Varnish
      ii. Linseed or tung oil
      iii. Epoxy ester (preferred when dance involves street shoes)
      iv. Polyurethane
      v. Moisture-cure urethane
      vi. Penetrating oil—modified urethane
      vii. Natural uncoated wood

D. **Aerobics**
1. **Surface requirements**
   a. Compliance
   b. Foot stability
   c. Traction
   d. Resiliency
   e. Impact independence (ability to isolate the absorption of impact energy)
2. **Surface options**
   a. **Foam systems with carpet**
      i. **Advantages:**
         (a) Low cost
         (b) Self-installation
         (c) Generally low maintenance cost
         (d) Quieter
         (e) Often can be used for multipurposes
         (f) Carpeting provides a good surface to lie down on and is perceived aesthetically as softer to dance on.
         (g) Good on compliance characteristics

ii. **Disadvantages:**
(a) Limited life expectancy of the foam
(b) Hygiene problems related to the carpet covering
(c) Some carpet coverings inhibit foot glide and pivot.
(d) Less resilience

b. **Hardwood floor systems.** If hardwood flooring is used, it should be such that greater resiliency than the typical gymnasium flooring is offered.

i. **Advantages** of hardwood:
(a) Ideal for lateral movements
(b) Provides considerable shock absorption
(c) Dependent on underlayment of the subflooring
(d) Can be beautiful depending on type of wood and finish
(e) Long life expectancy (30 years possible)
(f) Good for foot stability, surface traction, and resilience

ii. **Disadvantages:**
(a) Cost
(b) Periodic maintenance requirements
(c) Usually require mats or carpeting over the wood
(d) More restrictive use (avoid tables, chairs, and street shoes)
(e) Less compliant

c. Carpeting over hardwood flooring

d. Multipurpose synthetics (polyurethane or microcell foam):
i. Easy to clean
ii. Wears well
iii. Provides good shock absorbency
iv. Provides good traction
v. One-fourth the price of wood flooring
vi. Microcell foam is available in interlocking sections that are movable.

E. **Tennis**

1. **Surface requirements:** Tennis can be played indoors on any firm surface of sufficient size for a tennis court. The composition of a synthetic surface can be altered to offset the bounce of the tennis ball. A surface constructed for playing basketball usually proves to be too fast for tennis competition, but suffices for beginning instruction.

2. **Synthetic options**

a. **Carpet**—textile materials that are installed permanently or rolled out as a temporary surface
i. Coated for wearability
ii. Generally fast playing
iii. Allows a low bounce
iv. Allows a quiet game
v. Required minimal maintenance

b. **Modular surfacing**—interlocking gridwork of various chemical compositions, the most common being a combination of polypropylene and rubber
i. Usually 1 square foot in size
ii. Can form a new surface over an existing court
iii. Requires minimal maintenance
iv. Quiet, cushioned effect
v. Durable
vi. Relatively higher in cost
vii. Not recommended for tournament play because variations in temperature can cause expansion and contraction

c. Synthetic sand-filled turf—made of loosely woven polypropylene fibers with a rubber-like backing, filled with graded sand; appearance like a grass court
   i. Consistency of bounce
   ii. Easy on the legs
   iii. Minimal maintenance
   iv. Can be laid over deteriorated surfaces
   v. Sand may shift during the course of play
   vi. Has a tendency to absorb odors
d. Removable court surfaces—12-foot-wide strips of various synthetic surfaces
e. Asphalt-bound

F. **Racquetball/handball/squash:** Floors should be hardwood, as in standard gymnasium construction.

G. **Indoor tracks:** Alternative surfaces for indoor tracks include polyurethane or polyurethane-bound and latex or latex-bound, both of which can be either premanufactured or poured-in-place.

H. **Weight lifting:** Rubberized floor surfaces and indoor/outdoor carpeting can both be good choices for flooring in a weight lifting/training area.

I. **Wrestling/martial arts:** Flooring is preferably resilient underneath the wrestling mats. Concrete is not recommended.

J. **Archery:** Recommended flooring for archery activity areas is "hardwood, tongue-and-groove floor, with boards running the length of the shooting area."

IV. Standards

There are various standards for surfaces that may be applicable to a given situation. Some standards are voluntary; others are requirements for legitimate play.

A. **Governance body standards.** If the sport being played needs to be in compliance with a specific governing body's regulations to be considered a valid game, there may be surface requirements in addition to the space and lining requirements (e.g., the National Collegiate Athletic Association or the United States Tennis Association). These standards need to be verified in advance of design and construction of an athletic facility.

B. **ACSM standards.** The American College of Sports Medicine (ACSM) has issued standards for health and fitness facilities that are, at this time, voluntary. The primary standards associated with surfaces address the following issues:
   1. Proper surface for each planned activity
   2. Floor surfaces designed and constructed to address specific activities projected for facility
   3. Flooring periodically checked and maintained
   4. Floor surfaces clean and free of oil, wax, liquid, and dust, which can cause slippery conditions
   5. Floor surfaces meet standards established by the Americans with Disabilities Act Guidelines for Buildings and Facilities

C. **DIN standards.** The Deutsches Institut Fur Normung (DIN) standards are voluntary and should be interpreted flexibly, but do provide good guidelines for safe play. There are different standards for different types of flooring. The standards address:
   1. Shock absorption
   2. Deflection
   3. Ball bounce
   4. Surface friction
   5. Rolling load

V. Safety, Shoes, and Accessibility

The public's increased interest in exercise has raised the level of consciousness concerning sports injury prevention and treatment. Often because of poor or inappropriate surfaces or the wrong shoe-to-surface match, a large number of individuals have suffered injuries to feet, ankles, knees, hips, and back while attempting to improve the condition of their heart and lungs. Owing in part to publicity and encouragement provided by sports medicine personnel and facility planners, surface manufacturers have become increasingly aware of the relationship between surfaces and safety. Additionally, the issue of access is now gaining national attention because of the Americans with Disabilities Act. Individuals with and without disabilities want access to safe spaces and facilities for sports and leisure activities.

A. **Safety considerations** should address the following surface conditions:
   1. Smooth
   2. Secure
   3. Clean
   4. Level
   5. Appropriate match of surface to use
   6. Firm
   7. Adequate support for wheelchair accessibility
   8. Dry—abrasive, nonskid, slip-resistant flooring impervious to moisture where water is used (pools, laundry, shower area)

B. **Shoes in relation to playing surfaces.** Shoe technology is rapidly evolving. Different players need different shoes.
   1. College teams have tended to adopt "team" shoes in the past, and high school and younger teams have tried to emulate this pattern.
   2. Sports shoes, however, should be selected and fitted for each individual on the basis of their foot, their sport, and the predominant surface.
   3. It should be noted that some shoes that may be suited well for one surface or activity may not be appropriate for another surface or activity and may lead to not only poorer performance, but also an increased chance for injury.

C. **American with Disabilities Act.** The Americans with Disabilities Act Guidelines specify the necessity for the following conditions:
   1. Firm, stable, and slip resistant surfaces and routes that are accessible for disabled individuals. For example, routes for travel to a playground cannot be made of loose-fill products such as wood chips.
   2. Floors should be a common level throughout a facility or must be accessible via ramps, passenger elevators, or special access lifts.
   3. Carpeting or carpet tiles should be a maximum of ½ inch deep. Carpet edges must be fastened to the floor.

VI. Conclusion

Many variables associated with surfaces and flooring affect the performance and safety of sports and physical activities. The team physician needs to be aware of the best match between surfaces and the various activities to reduce the chance that players are placed in at-risk situations; reduce the opportunity and extent of injuries; and reduce the liabilities on behalf of the team, facility, and physician.

More research and study related to sports surfaces are needed. Expressed concern for safety and injury prevention has prompted an increase in the amount of research on sports surfaces and shoe performance, and some manufacturers have sought market advantage by making significant improvements in their products. All sports participants, from casual to highly competitive, stand to benefit from an increase in both research and product improvement.

Recommended Reading

1. Americans with Disabilities Act (ADA) Accessibility Guidelines for Buildings and Facilities; Final Guidelines, 56 Fed Reg 35,408 (1991) (to be codified at 36 C.F.R. 1911), 1991.
2. Berg R: Floored. Athletic Business 18(4):9, 1994.
3. CDDS Seminar: Research activities into synthetic surfaces. Cologne, Germany, 1988, p 143.
4. Choosing the right aerobics surface. Athletic Business 11(4):78–83, 1987.
5. Court sentences. Athletic Business 10(8):30–36, 1986.
6. Dance Facilities. Washington, D.C., American Alliance for Health, Physical Education and Recreation, 1972.
7. Di Geronimo JW: We've learned the hard way. Athletic Business 9 (8):64–75, 1985.
8. Ellison T: Sport floor dynamics, Athletic Business, 16(4):54–60, 1993.
9. Ferguson M: Great strides in flooring. Athletic Business 13(11):60–62, 1989.
10. Flynn RB (ed): Facility Planning for Physical Education, Recreation, and Athletics. Reston, VA, American Alliance for Health, Physical Education, Recreation and Dance, 1993.
11. Handbook of Sports and Recreational Building Design. London, The Architectural Press, 1981.
12. Hay C: Cushioning, control features mark aerobics shoes' development: Sports Mednotes. Omaha, NE, University of Nebraska Medical Center Sports Medicine Program, 1989, p 2.
13. Kniley S: The turf game, Athletic Business 18(9):56–60, 1994.
14. Miller DA: Sports surface specs. Athletic Business 12(8):72–78, 1988.
15. On solid ground: The importance of proper flooring. IRSA Club Business, 1986, pp 35–37.
16. Penman KA: Planning Physical Education and Athletic Facilities in Schools. New York, John Wiley & Sons, 1977.
17. Schmid S: Grounds for action. Athletic Business 18(7):16–18, 1994.
18. Seals G: A study of dance surfaces. Clin Sports Med 2:557–561, 1983.
19. Sol N, Foster C (eds): ACSM'S Health/Fitness Facility Standards and Guidelines. Champaign, IL, Human Kinetics Books, 1992.
20. Sports surface improvements. Athletic Business 13(7):35, 1989.
21. U.S.T.A. Facilities Committee: Tennis Courts 1984–85. Lynn, MA, H.O. Zinman, Inc. for the United States Tennis Association, 1984.

20

High-Altitude Training and Competition

Benjamin D. Levine, M.D., and James Stray-Gundersen, M.D.

High altitude presents a unique challenge to athletic competition. Athletes must cope with hypoxia, cold, and dehydration, yet still maintain maximal performance. The timing of altitude exposure and the degree of acclimatization are also critical to a successful outcome. This physiologic adaptation to high altitude may, in fact, be beneficial, and altitude training is frequently used by elite athletes in an attempt to improve sea-level performance.

I. High-Altitude Environment

A. Barometric pressure is reduced, with a parallel decrease in the inspired partial pressure of oxygen (P_IO_2); **hypobaric hypoxia is thus the most prominent physiologic manifestation of high altitude.** The range of terrestrial altitudes may be characterized as follows:
   1. 0 to 1000 m—sea level
   2. 1000 to 2000 m—low altitude
   3. 2000 to 3000 m—moderate altitude
   4. 3000 to 5000 m—high altitude
   5. 5000 to 8848 m—extreme altitude

B. Temperature decreases at a rate of approximately 6.5°C/1000 m.

C. Other features include:
   1. Dry air (increasing the risk of dehydration)
   2. Decrease in air density and therefore air resistance
   3. Increase in the amount of ultraviolet light (4% per 300 m) increasing the risk of sunburn

II. Effect of High Altitude On Exercise

A. Physiologically defined by the "oxygen cascade": the **environment** (determined by altitude achieved) to the **alveoli** (a function of ventilation and the hypoxic ventilatory response), across the **pulmonary capillary** (limited by diffusion), to be transported by the **cardiovascular system** (a function of cardiac output and hemoglobin concentration), and diffused into **skeletal muscle** (dependent on muscle capillarity and biochemical state), to be used by muscle **mitochondria** (influenced by oxidative enzyme activity) for aerobic respiration and ATP production.

B. **Altitude-induced hypoxia reduces the amount of oxygen available to do physical work.**
   1. **Maximal aerobic power ($\dot{V}O_2$max) is reduced by approximately 1% for every 100 m above 1500 m in normal individuals.**
   2. **For endurance-trained athletes, this effect is even greater—reductions in $\dot{V}O_2$max and performance can be identified at altitudes as low as 500 m.**

a. Occurs because of diffusion limitation in both lung and skeletal muscle exacerbated by high pulmonary and systemic blood flow (cardiac output) of endurance athletes. Severe hypoxemia results even from base training pace ($SaO_2 < 80\%$ at 6 min/mile pace at 2700 m).
b. Running velocity, $\dot{V}O_2$, heart rate, and lactate are lower during interval training at altitude.
c. Running velocity and $\dot{V}O_2$ are lower during typical base training at altitude, but heart rate is the same as training at sea level, and lactate is slightly higher.

3. **During submaximal exercise at high altitude, ventilation, lactate, and heart rate are greater for the same absolute work rate, increasing the sensation of dyspnea and fatigue.**
4. **Peak** blood lactate concentration is **lower** in individuals acclimatized to high altitude—termed "the lactate paradox."

C. **Altitude affects endurance athletes and sprinters in different ways.**

1. **Endurance events** requiring high levels of aerobic power (> 2 minutes)—performance is impaired at altitude because of a reduction in $\dot{V}O_2$max.
2. **Mixed events** requiring high sustained power outputs (30 seconds to 2 minutes)—performance may or may not be impaired at altitude depending on the interplay of oxidative and glycolytic energy pathways.
3. **Sprint and field events** requiring short bursts of high-intensity activity (≤ 30 seconds)—energy sources are not dependent on oxygen transport. The reduced air resistance at altitude thus actually improves sprint performance.

III. Acclimatization Process

A. Chronic exposure to altitude stimulates acclimatization, which includes adaptations that improve **submaximal** work performance at altitude. At high and extreme altitudes (4000 m and above), $\dot{V}O_2$max never returns to sea-level values despite prolonged acclimatization. At low altitudes (below 2000 m), maximal oxygen uptake may approach sea-level values after 1–2 weeks, at least in nonathletic populations.

1. Increases in alveolar ventilation and reductions in mixed venous oxygen content maximize exercise capacity at altitude—**begins immediately on ascent.**
2. Hyperventilation causes a respiratory alkalosis, which stimulates renal excretion of bicarbonate **over the first week** to normalize acid-base balance.
3. Sympathetic activation acutely **(minutes to hours)** increases heart rate and cardiac output so that tissue oxygen delivery remains close to sea-level values at rest and during submaximal work. By **2–3 weeks**, systemic and regional blood flow have returned toward sea-level values as oxygenation improves.
4. Oxygen carrying capacity of the blood increases due to an increase in hemoglobin and hematocrit—**early** (1–2 days) increases owing to plasma volume reduction; **later** (weeks to months) increases owing to increases in red cell mass. **This critical adaptation offsets the reduction in oxygen availability, thereby restoring oxygen transport toward normal sea-level values.**
5. Peripheral uptake of oxygen by skeletal muscle is facilitated by increased capillary density, mitochondrial number, myoglobin concentration, and 2,3-diphosphoglycerate (2,3-DPG).
6. Buffer capacity of skeletal muscle is increased.
7. Substrate utilization is enhanced by increasing mobilization of free fatty acids and increasing utilization of blood glucose, thus sparing muscle glycogen.

B. **For competitions at altitude**

1. **Acclimatization** is critical and clearly improves performance **at altitude**.
2. If possible, adequate time for acclimatization should be allowed to maximize performance at altitude (1–2 weeks).

3. If adequate time for acclimatization is not possible, anecdotal experience among athletes suggests that competing immediately on arrival at altitude may be best.

C. **For competitions at sea level**
   1. Living at altitude and training at altitude has not been shown to improve performance at sea level.
   2. **Living at altitude and training as close to sea level as possible (living high–training low) does improve sea-level performance.**
   3. Performance is best immediately on return to sea level and remains high at least up to 3 weeks after return.

D. Recreational athletes who hike, climb, or mountain bike but are not interested in athletic competition are also affected by the hypoxia of altitude. For recreational athletes, **sea-level** training is effective at increasing the ability to perform **at altitude**.

IV. Failure of Acclimatization—High-Altitude Illness and Overtraining

A. **Acute mountain sickness:** With moderate or higher altitudes (> 2000 m) and rapid ascent rates (> 300 m sleeping altitude/day above 3000 m), a maladaptive state called acute mountain sickness (AMS) may develop.
   1. Symptoms
      a. Headache
      b. Nausea
      c. Anorexia
      d. Fatigue
      e. Difficulty sleeping
   2. Usually mild and self-limited; rest and analgesics are sufficient treatment.
   3. No evidence that competitive athletes are at any greater risk of developing AMS than nonathletes, although exercise may exacerbate the development of AMS, and physical activity should be reduced appropriately in symptomatic individuals.
   4. For patients who do not improve with rest, the addition of supplemental oxygen or descent to a lower altitude virtually always results in prompt symptom relief.
   5. Other effective treatments include acetazolamide, dexamethasone, and simulated descent using a portable hyperbaric bag.
   6. The problem is best prevented by:
      a. Limiting the rate of ascent
      b. Allowing for rest or acclimatization days
      c. Maintaining adequate hydration
      d. Avoiding alcohol or sedatives during the early acclimatization phase
      e. Limiting training volume and intensity during the first few days at altitude
   7. The use of drugs to prevent AMS is discouraged in endurance athletes who are going to moderate altitude (below 3000 m) unless a clear history of recurrent AMS is obtained.

B. **Severe high-altitude illness:** In some individuals, AMS may progress to a more severe and life-threatening form, including high-altitude pulmonary (HAPE) or cerebral (HACE) edema.
   1. **HAPE** is characterized by:
      a. **Dyspnea at rest**
      b. Cyanosis
      c. Severe hypoxemia
      d. Noncardiogenic pulmonary edema
   2. **HACE** is characterized by:
      a. Vomiting
      b. **Ataxia**
      c. Reduction in the level of consciousness
      d. In some cases, frank coma

3. Both of these syndromes can result quickly in death—**immediate descent is mandatory.** High flow supplemental oxygen or a portable hyperbaric bag if available may be useful adjunctive therapy while descending or if descent is delayed.
4. Both HAPE and HACE are rare at the moderate altitudes to which most athletes are exposed (< 0.1%).

C. **Overtraining:** Another potentially serious problem with training at altitude is the increased risk of overtraining. It is helpful to make the analogy between exercise training and the pharmacologic administration of a medication (see Fig. 1). Any medication has a specific dose-response relationship, accompanied by a toxic/therapeutic range. These parameters define the optimal dose and frequency of administration to maximize benefit but minimize side effects and toxicity. Exercise can be thought of conceptually as a medication, with a training response that is proportional to volume and intensity (ED 50), but a clear toxic effect of too much exercise characterized by musculoskeletal injury and the systemic effects of overtraining (LD 50).

Overtraining may be precipitated by:

1. **Inappropriately hard workouts**
   a. Base pace too fast because of narrowed training zones and/or athlete inexperience
   b. Intervals too hard—run at maximal speed rather than 105% race pace
   c. Recovery exercise too hard, i.e., not recovery pace
2. **Inadequate recovery**
   a. Dehydration
   b. Sleep disturbance
   c. Too short recovery times either between workouts or between intervals within a hard workout

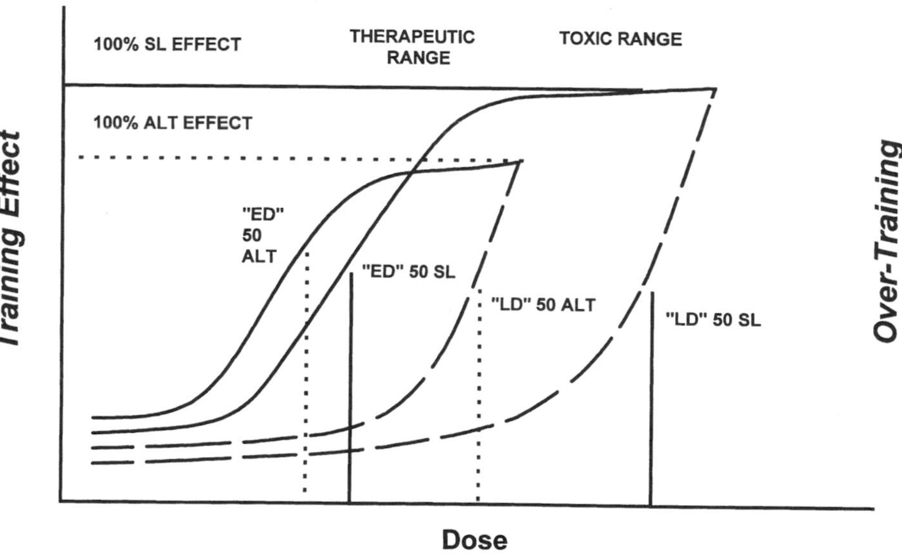

FIGURE 1. Toxic-therapeutic range of exercise training: the effect of high altitude. Although the mechanical stress of exercise is likely to be less at altitude due to the reduction in training speed, the metabolic stress may well be greater, at least with regard to the effect of hypoxia on the central nervous system. Thus, exercise training at altitude narrows the toxic/ therapeutic range of exercise, possibly enhancing the training effect, but also increasing the risk of toxicity.
SL = sea level; ALT = altitude; ED = effective dose at which 50% of the maximal response is achieved; LD = lethal dose at which 50% of the maximal toxicity is achieved.

V. Practical Strategies for Implementing Altitude Training

A. From a practical perspective, the critical questions to answer for athletes and coaches are: what are the **"indications"** for altitude training, and, if indicated, what is the appropriate **"dose"** of altitude and training?

1. **Indications**

a. **Which athletes should use altitude training?** The evidence is best for events in which $\dot{V}O_2$ max is important for performance, i.e., endurance athletes in events lasting longer than 2–3 minutes; sprint athletes may, however, benefit from neuromuscular/kinesthetic training from the faster speeds allowed by the reduced air resistance. Because a supervised training camp by itself is such a powerful stimulus for training, even in elite athletes, athletes who are already well trained with a solid base and regular interval work are likely to obtain the most specific benefit from the altitude per se. **Altitude training is not a substitute for a focused, well-designed training program with appropriate rest and nutrition.**

b. **Which athletes should not use altitude training?**

i. Team sports that depend more on strategy and technique for success are unlikely to derive much benefit from altitude training for sea-level performance (e.g., water polo, baseball, soccer, field hockey, handball).

ii. Sports that depend on normal air resistance for fine motor skill are likely to be impaired by altitude training (e.g., basketball, archery, tennis); such sports may require an adjustment period both at altitude and on return to sea level to compensate for differences in projectile movement through air.

iii. Swimming is most controversial. The extremely low mechanical efficiency of swimming makes the key to successful performance in swimming **biomechanics** rather than **physiology**. Therefore, despite the fact that many swimmers attempt to use altitude training, there is no evidence for its benefit.

iv. Iron-deficient athletes should not engage in altitude training (see "Nutritional factors," next page).

2. **Dose**

a. **How high to live?** 2500–3000 m to maximize acclimatization and minimize complications (muscle wasting and AMS). Some sports scientists have described a technique of sleeping in a nitrogen-enriched environment to simulate high altitude.

b. **How long to reside at altitude?** Erythropoietin levels increase acutely, are clearly still elevated after 2 weeks, and are back to sea level values by 4 weeks. Therefore, 3–4 weeks appears necessary to develop sufficient acclimatization, particularly for competition at sea level. A sample training camp based on a 4-week mesocycle is presented in Table 1. Some athletes use multiple shorter cycles,[8] although there is no evidence that an altitude-specific effect persists for more than a few weeks after an altitude training camp.

c. **How high to train?**

i. **Interval training**—Definitely as low as possible, preferably below 1500 m

ii. **Base training**—Possibly could be performed at altitude to minimize travel requirements in the living high–training low approach. **Base training must be performed at relatively easy pace to prevent overtraining. Careful monitoring of heart rate and/or blood lactate during training may help ensure the correct training pace.**

d. **When to compete on return to sea level?** Immediately on return appears best, particularly if high-intensity training has been done low. Some reacclimatization may be necessary (2–3 weeks) to restore sea-level running speed if interval training has been done at altitude. Although athletes often report "feeling better" after such a reacclimatization period, there is no clear evidence that performance is correspondingly improved.

TABLE 1. Sample Training Camp Based on 4-Week Mesocycle

Week 1 (Acclimation Week 2200–2500 m)	
Mon.	Base training
Tues.	Base training PM base training
Wed.	Base training
Thurs.	Base training
Fri.	Base training
Sat.	Base training (or off)
Sun.	Long run
0/1/8 (# hard/# long/# total workouts)	

Week 2 (Medium Week)	
Mon.	Base training
Tues.	5 × 1000 m 105% 5 K race pace PM recovery run
Wed.	Base training
Thurs.	Base training
Fri.	Easy run
Sat.	5 K road race PM recovery run
Sun.	Base training
2/0/9	

Week 3 (Hard Week)	
Mon.	Long run
Tues.	Base training
Wed.	5 × 1000 m 105% 5 K race pace PM recovery run Diet log
Thurs.	Base training PM base training
Fri.	Base training PM hill drills Pliometrics
Sat.	Base training
Sun.	Long run
2/2/11	

Week 4 (Easy Week)	
Mon.	Easy run
Tues.	5 × 1000 m 105% 5 K race pace PM recovery run
Wed.	Base training
Thurs.	Base training
Fri.	Base training
Sat.	Off
Sun.	Long run
1/1/7	

Mesocycle = a period incorporated into an athlete's training plan for the year (macrocycle) which typically includes increasing volume and intensity, followed by a period of rest and recovery.

B. **Nutritional factors, particularly iron stores, play a critical role in the ability to respond to altitude training.**

1. Many athletes (male and female) have reduced iron stores based on a **low serum ferritin**. Such athletes are unable to increase the volume of red cell mass (blood volume – plasma volume) and do not increase $\dot{V}O_2$; thus, they are unable to obtain the potential benefits of altitude acclimatization.
2. Simple measurement of hemoglobin or serum iron is inadequate because they do not reflect bone marrow iron stores. Because iron is also a critical moiety in myoglobin as well as mitochondrial cytochromes, iron deficiency may not only compromise oxygen carrying capacity, but also may inhibit oxygen extraction (a-v O_2 difference) and reduce O_2 flux, thereby limiting $\dot{V}O_2$max and performance, even in nonanemic athletes. **Iron stores (ferritin) must be normal before undertaking a period of altitude training.**
3. High doses of oral iron (150–400 mg elemental iron/day in divided doses) are usually required to maintain ferritin levels during altitude training. Even athletes with normal iron stores at the start of an altitude training program experience rapid falls in serum ferritin at altitude and must be supplemented and monitored closely.
4. Best tolerated in liquid, pediatric preparation—Feosol, 15 ml dissolved in orange juice and mixed with 500 mg vitamin C, one to three times per day, 1/2 hour before or 1–2 hours after a meal. May use more frequent administration of smaller doses if gastrointestinal upset develops.

Recommended Reading

1. Adams WC, Bernauer EM, Dill DB, Bomar JB: Effects of equivalent sea-level and altitude training on $\dot{V}O_2$max and running performance. J Appl Physiol 39(2):262–265, 1975.

2. Balke B, Nagle FJ, Daniels JT: Altitude and maximum performance in work and sports activity. JAMA 194(6):176–179, 1965.
3. Berglund B: High-altitude training, aspects of haematological adaptation. Sports Med 14:289–303, 1992.
4. Brooks GA, Butterfield GA, Wolfe RR, et al: Increased dependence on blood glucose after acclimatization to 4,300 m. J Appl Physiol 70:919–927, 1991.
5. Buskirk ER: Physiology and performance of track athletes at various altitudes in the United States and Peru. In Goddard RF (ed): The Effects of Altitude on Physical Performance. Chicago, Athletic Institute, 1966, pp 65–72.
6. Buskirk ER, Kollias J, Akers RF, et al: Maximal performance at altitude and return from altitude in conditioned runners. J Appl Physiol 23(2):259–266, 1967.
7. Daniels J, Oldridge N: The effects of alternate exposure to altitude and sea level on world-class middle distance runners. Med Sci Sports Exerc 2:107–112, 1975.
8. Dick FW: Training at altitude in practice. Int J Sports Med 13(suppl 1):S203–206, 1992.
9. Dill DB, Adams WC: Maximal oxygen uptake at sea level and at 3,090-m altitude in high school champion runners. J Appl Physiol 30(6):854–859, 1971.
10. Faulkner JA, Daniels JT, Balke B: Effects of training at moderate altitude on physical performance capacity. J Appl Physiol 23(1):85–89, 1967.
11. Faulkner JA, Kollias J, Favour CB, et al: Maximum aerobic capacity and running performance at altitude. J Appl Physiol 24(5):685–691, 1968.
12. Green HJ, Sutton JR, Cymerman A, et al: Operation Everest II: Adaptations in human skeletal muscle. J Appl Physiol 66:2454–2461, 1989.
13. Hackett PH, Roach RC, Sutton JR: High altitude medicine. In Auerbach PS, Gehr EC (eds): Management of Wilderness and Environmental Emergencies. St. Louis, CV Mosby, 1989, pp 1–34.
14. Hannon JP, Shields JL, Harris CW: Effects of altitude acclimatization on blood composition of women. J Neurophysiol 26:540–547, 1969.
15. Harper KM, Stray-Gundersen J, Schecter MB, Levine BD: Training at moderate altitude causes profound hypoxemia during exercise in competitive runners. Med Sci Sports Exerc 27:S110, 1995.
16. Levine BD, Engfred K, Friedman DB, et al: High altitude endurance training: Effect on aerobic capacity and work performance. Med Sci Sports Exerc 22:S35, 1990.
17. Levine BD, Stray-Gundersen J: A practical approach to altitude training: Where to live and train for optimal performance enhancement. Int J Sports Med 13(suppl 1):S209–S212, 1992.
18. Levine BD, Stray-Gundersen J: Training at moderate altitude increases blood oxygen content, maximal oxygen uptake and running performance. In Sutton JR, Houston CS, Coates G (eds): Hypoxia and the Brain. Burlington, VT, Queen City Printers, 1995.
19. Levine BD, Stray-Gundersen J, Duhaime G, et al: Living high—training low: The effect of altitude acclimatization/normoxic training in trained runners. Med Sci Sports Exerc 23:S25, 1991.
20. Maher JT, Jones LG, Hartley LH: Effects of high altitude exposure on submaximal endurance capacity of men. J Appl Physiol 37:895–898, 1974.
21. Mariburl H, Schobersberger W, Humpeler E, et al: Beneficial effects of exercising at moderate altitude on red cell oxygen transport. Pflugers Arch 406:594–599, 1986.
22. Mizuno M, Juel C, Bro-Rasmussen T, et al: Limb skeletal muscle adaptation in athletes after training at altitude. J Appl Physiol 68(2):496–502, 1990.
23. Peronnet F, Thibault G, Cousineau DL: A theoretical analysis of the effect of altitude on running performance. J Appl Physiol 70:399–404, 1991.
24. Reeves JT, Wolfel EE, Green HJ, et al: Oxygen transport during exercise at altitude and the lactate paradox: Lessons from Operation Everest II and Pikes Peak. Exerc Sports Sci Rev 20:275–296, 1992.
25. Saltin B: Aerobic and anaerobic work capacity at 2300 meters. Med Thorac 2:107–112, 1970.
26. Saltin B, Grover RF, Blomqvist CG, et al: Maximal oxygen uptake and cardiac output after 2 weeks at 4,300 m. J Appl Physiol 25:400–409, 1968.
27. Schultz WW, Stray-Gundersen J, Schecter M, Levine BD: Vigorous oral iron supplementation can maintain iron stores during altitude training. Med Sci Sports Exerc 26:S181, 1994.
28. Squires RW, Buskirk ER: Aerobic capacity during acute exposure to simulated altitude, 914-2286 meters. Med Sci Sports Exerc 14:36–40, 1982.
29. Stine TA, Levine BD, Taylor S, et al: Quantification of altitude training in the field. Med Sci Sports Exerc 24:S103, 1992.
30. Stray-Gundersen J, Alexander C, Hochstein A, et al: Failure of red cell volume to increase to altitude exposure in iron deficient runners. Med Sci Sports Exerc 24:S90, 1992.
31. Stray-Gundersen J, Hochstein A, Levine BD: Effect of 4 weeks altitude exposure and training on red cell mass in trained runners. Med Sci Sports Exerc 25:S171, 1993.
32. Stray-Gundersen J, Levine BD: Altitude acclimatization/normoxic training (high/low) improves sea-level endurance performance immediately on descent from altitude. Med Sci Sports Exer 26:S64, 1994.
33. Stray-Gundersen J, Mordecai N, Levine BD: O2 transport response to altitude training in runners. Med Sci Sports Exercise 27:S202, 1995.

34. Sutton JR, Reeves JT, Wagner PD, et al: Operation Everest II: Oxygen transport during exercise at extreme simulated altitude. J Appl Physiol 64:1309–1321, 1988.
35. Terrados N, Jansson E, Sylven C, Kaijser L: Is hypoxia a stimulus for synthesis of oxidative enzymes and myoglobin? J Appl Physiol 68(6):2369–2372, 1990.
36. Terrados N, Melichna J, Sylven C, et al: Effects of training at simulated altitude on performance and muscle metabolic capacity in competitive road cyclists. Eur J Appl Physiol 57:203–209, 1988.
37. Terrados N, Mizuno M, Andersen H: Reduction in maximal oxygen uptake at low altitudes; role of training status and lung function. Clin Physiol 5(suppl. 3):75–79, 1985.
38. Torre-Bueno JR, Wagner PD, Saltzman HA, et al: Diffusion limitation in normal humans during exercise at sea level and simulated altitude. J Appl Physiol 58:989–995, 1985.
39. Wagner PD: Algebraic analysis of determinants of VO2max. Respir Physiol 93:221–237, 1993.
40. Weil JV, Jamieson G, Brown DW, Grover RF: The red cell mass–arterial oxygen relationship in normal man. J Clin Invest 47:1627–1639, 1968.
41. Young AJ, Evans WJ, Cymerman A, et al: Sparing effect of chronic high-altitude exposure on muscle glycogen utilization. J Appl Physiol 52:857–862, 1982.

PART V
BEHAVIORAL AND PSYCHOLOGICAL PROBLEMS

21: The Role of Sports Psychology/Psychiatry

Todd P. Hendrickson, M.D., and Sharon J. Rowe, M.A., CTRS

I never hit a shot, not even in practice, without having a very sharp in-focus picture of it in my head.

-Jack Nicklaus, Professional Golfer

If you are relaxing and subconsciously thinking about your coming race, you are going to perform at just about 100% efficiency.

-Mark Spitz, Olympic Swimmer

The committed athlete of the future will be able to achieve peak performance ONLY through the use of a comprehensive mental AND physical training program.

-Marilyn King, Olympic Pentathlete

Everyone can vividly remember a special time in their athletic lives when everything they did was perfect, effortless, and focused, with an overwhelming rush of excitement and power that accompanied a task that was extraordinarily well done.

Most athletes, whether competitive or recreational, will acknowledge that mental factors and psychological mastery account for 60 to 90% of any given athletic performance. Understanding the role of sports psychology/psychiatry as a major influence on sport behavior and sport performance must be a priority in any sport training program that is designed to maximize both physical and mental preparation. By understanding the effects of psychological factors on behavior or the psychological factors that participation has on the performer, we can evaluate, assess, and assist the athlete in his/her environment.

Understanding the psychological aspects of sport and sport behavior can help us identify strengths and weaknesses, solve performance problems, improve self-esteem, provide a framework for the appropriate use of intervention techniques, and ultimately enhance the performance of the athlete through the facilitation of personal growth.

I. Historical Background

The study of sport psychology is not new; it has only been within the past 25 to 30 years that it has been scientifically linked to excellence in performance. Much of this progress can be attributed to experts in the U.S. and Soviet Union:

1895—George W. Fritz' investigation of reaction time raises the questions of why physical education needs an understanding of psychology and what psychological benefits can be derived from participating in physical education.

1925—Coleman R. Griffith is hired by the University of Illinois to help coaches improve players' performance. He is intrigued by the psychological effects of Knute Rockne's "pep talks," and the "mental toughness" of football player Red Grange.

1930-1940s—Soviet and American experts study the profound psychological ramifications of the Nazi Holocaust and its survivors; specifically their ability to tap into hidden reserves to find the strength to go on in spite of heinous, abusive treatment.

1950s—Soviet Alexander Romen's basic research using ancient yogic techniques to teach Soviet cosmonauts to control psychophysiological processes while in space leads to programs for teaching optimal sports performance. This field of inquiry comes to be known as "self-regulation training."

American John Lawther's research in motor learning stimulates interest about motivation, team cohesion, interpersonal relationships; and motor control.

1960s—Bruce Ogilvie pioneers clinical work with athletes in their environment(s) focusing on motivation, motives of participation, performance decrements, and the integration of intervention strategies to enhance performance in athletes.

Nov., 1976—*Track and Field News* reports that mental training sessions were being employed by Soviet weight lifters. This report was filed after unprecedented success by Soviet and East German athletes in the 1976 Olympic Games.

1980s—Comprehensive mental training programs begin to flourish and are accepted as legitimate forms of sport training. Performance enhancement programs become more widespread.

II. Evaluation and Assessment of the Athlete

For the most effective care, thorough evaluation of the athlete and assessment of the clinical problem are necessary before formulating a management program and selecting therapeutic techniques.

A. **The clinician's qualifications**
   1. Emphasis should be placed on the qualifications of the clinician providing services (i.e., educational background, specialized training, and clinical experience in the field of sports psychology).
      a. Sport psychologist (now a recognized field)
      b. Clinical psychologist
      c. Psychiatrist
      d. Therapists, counselors

B. **The scope of clinical problems encountered: the client**
   1. Clients seen may exhibit a range of behaviors, thoughts, and feelings that can either complicate or facilitate personal growth through various mental training programs or interventions.
   2. Clinically, the impression via the evaluation of an athlete may range from mental healthiness (most athletes) to mental illness (i.e., depression, substance abuse, personality disorder, anorexia nervosa, etc.)
   3. Ethical principles of complete confidentiality must be maintained.
   4. The client is the consumer.

C. **The role of the clinician**
   1. **Service**—Provision of services for crisis intervention, stress management, psychological skills training (i.e. performance enhancement), group and individual psychotherapy, pharmacotherapy, etc.
   2. **Educational**—Care must be taken to provide information to clients regarding theoretical principles being used (i.e., intervention techniques, therapy, expectations of treatment, etc.) so that the client may be able to function independently and with autonomy (i.e., without you). Didactics and group teaching can be extremely helpful when working with athletes.

3. **Research**—One must be able to validate principles being applied through reproducibility and consistency.

D. **Goals of the evaluation and assessment**
   1. **Diagnosis** is a major goal. Categorization according to the DSM-IV R multiaxial system (if applicable) should be done with each case.
   2. **Treatment planning** is based on the patient's needs and capacity for responding to various types of treatment.
   3. **Psychological understanding of the patient** is critical regardless of diagnosis or treatment. This allows for greater empathetic communication and affords insight into the patient's likely response to treatment.
   4. **A working alliance** or rapport with the patient is fostered by a thorough evaluation by the treating clinician.

E. **Use of the biological-psychological-sociological model**
   1. **Biological:** medical history, medical status, familial history, current physical skill level/development, and overall physiology of the athlete.
   2. **Psychological assessment** should include:
      a. **Mental Status Examination** (a measure of psychological fitness)
         i. General attitude and behavior (i.e., appearance)
         ii. Speaking style and form
         iii. Affect (emotional tone)
         iv. Mood
         v. Thought content (what the patient thinks about)
         vi. Cognitive function (ability to calculate, concentrate, reason, and abstractly think)
         vii. Insight (into self and/or problems)
         viii. Judgment (right versus wrong)
      b. **Problem-solving skills**
      c. **General reaction to stress**
      d. **Athlete's overall perception of SELF**
   3. **Sociological assessment** should include analysis of the patient's athletic and nonathletic environment. This includes social support systems, family dynamics, interpersonal relationships, substance abuse history, educational background, cultural background, childhood development, and sport-performance experiences (successful and unsuccessful).

F. **Evaluation and assessment procedure**
   1. **The clinical interview with a biopsychosocial orientation**
   2. **Direct observation of the athlete** (i.e., field study) is a prerequisite for complete evaluation, as one must see the athlete in action to develop a "feel" for how the athlete responds to various internal and environmental stimuli. This can be facilitated through the use of videography (videotape).
   3. **Data gathering**, with the permission of the athlete, can be helpful to comprehend how others see the athlete (i.e., reports from coaches, parents, friends, other athletes).
   4. **Psychological testing** may be helpful in organizing an overall picture of the athlete, although it may not be indicated in all clinical cases. This testing can be extremely beneficial when diagnostic issues are confusing, or when treatment is meeting with resistance (i.e., refractoriness to treatment).
      a. **Personality** can be assessed through the use of the Minnesota Multiphasic Personality Inventory (MMPI), which helps to establish longstanding behavioral patterns and adaptation to life stressors. There are also numerous new tools being tested that give us information about personality traits and their interaction with sport-specific situations.

b. **Mood assessment** may give valuable feedback regarding an athlete's subjective feeling about himself/herself.
   i. POMS (Profile of Mood States)
   ii. HDRS (Hamilton Depression Rating Scale)

c. **Anxiety**, which can be crippling to the athlete and may deter performance capabilities, can be identified as well. In most cases, behavior is believed to be determined by the reciprocal interaction of personal traits and the characteristics of different situations. This can be especially helpful in understanding the anxiety-performance relationship.
   i. State/Trait Anxiety Inventory
   ii. Sport Competition Anxiety Test (SCAT)
   iii. Competitive State Anxiety Inventory (CSAI)

d. **Stress** may be evaluated through the use of the Holmes Rate Scale, which helps to identify causes of stress.

e. **Motivational assessment** can be accomplished through goal analysis and behavioral assessment.

f. **Thought disorders** (i.e., psychosis, delusional thinking) may be assessed via the:
   i. MMPI
   ii. SCL-90 (Symptom Checklist-90)
   iii. The Rorschach

g. **Conclusion**

Evaluation and assessment of the athlete can be complex yet challenging. If done appropriately and comprehensively, it can serve as the foundation on which to build individualized programs for performance enhancement and personal growth of the athlete. Once again it should be pointed out that there are numerous intervention techniques available today that profess to enhance performance in athletes. However, care should be taken to evaluate and assess *each* athlete appropriately so that any intervention techniques used will reap maximum benefits for the athlete.

III. Psychiatric Disorders Seen in Athletic Populations

A. **Major depression** (principal disorder of affect and mood)

1. **Clinical features:** usually of insidious onset; may see symptoms of subjective depression, loss of pleasure, suicidal thoughts, loss of appetite, sleep disturbance, self-reproach, lack of energy, dysphoric (depressed) mood, and feelings of guilt.
   a. In children, one tends to see more somatic symptoms and psychomotor agitation.
   b. In adolescents, one sees more frequent anorexia, weight loss, hypersomnia, and hopelessness.

2. **Differential diagnosis:** substance abuse (especially cocaine withdrawal, sedative-hypnotic usage, and anabolic steroid use), anxiety disorders, eating disorders. This type of depression is usually *not* related to specific psychosocial stressors as seen in adjustment disorders.

3. **Treatment**
   a. Referral to mental health professionals is often appropriate.
   b. Psychosocial therapy (i.e., individual, group, family)
   c. Pharmacotherapy may be indicated, especially if significant disturbance in ability to function on a daily basis is noted. A combination approach of pharmacotherapy and psychotherapy is usually very effective and may be the quickest resolution to symptoms.

B. **Adjustment disorder** may be considered if the psychiatric symptoms (including symptoms of depression) seem to be related to a recent (within 3 months) psychosocial stressor(s) and will usually remit when the stress is over. This syndrome is commonly seen in sport-related situations.

1. Injury, career termination, death of a loved one, loss of a relationship, change in playing status (i.e., demotion of status), change of a coach, change of academic status (i.e., high school to college), loss of a "big game," situational anxiety (i.e., "preperformance anxiety")
2. Chronic adjustment disorders may be seen in overuse/overstraining syndromes, burnout, and failed physical rehabilitation (i.e., knee injuries).
3. **Treatment**
   a. Psychosocial therapy (individual or group) can be extremely helpful with this "reactive" depression through a supportive and nurturing approach. Allow time for transition as this clinical situation usually abates.
   b. Pharmacotherapy is rarely indicated here. However, symptomatic treatment of insomnia (initial) or severe anxiety can be facilitated with low-dose benzodiazepine therapy (i.e., lorazepam, temazepam). This type of therapy should be considered short-term (2–3 weeks).

C. **Anxiety disorders**

1. **Description.** Anxiety is characterized by subjective feelings of anticipation, dread, or apprehension or a sense of impending disaster associated with varying degrees of autonomic arousal and reactivity. Anxiety can lead to changes in behavior, playing an important role in learning and adaptation.
2. **Generalized anxiety**
   a. Unrealistic or excessive anxiety and worry about various life circumstances
   b. Symptoms of motor tension (trembling, restlessness, easy fatiguability)
   c. Symptoms of autonomic hyperactivity (shortness of breath, dry mouth, sweating)
   d. Symptoms of vigilance and scanning ("on edge")
   e. **Differential diagnosis:** hyperthyroidism, hypertension, caffeinism, unstable angina, substance abuse, stimulants, alcohol withdrawal, major depression, adjustment disorder
   f. **Treatment**
      i. **Pharmacologic:** benzodiazepines are the treatment of choice. Tolerance develops to the sedative effects but not to their anxiolytic properties. These medications do have addictive properties. Combined treatment with antidepressant medication has also been useful.
      ii. **Psychosocial:**
         (a) Behavioral therapy (i.e. systematic desensitization, relaxation training, biofeedback) can be especially helpful
         (b) Individual psychotherapy
            - Psychoanalytical
            - Cognitive (identification of irrational beliefs/thoughts)
3. **Obsessive compulsive disorder (OCD) is characterized by the presence of recurrent obsessions and compulsions with near magical thinking.**
   a. **Obsessions are thoughts or images that are involuntary, intrusive, and anxiety provoking. They often have sexual, violent, or derogatory connotations, provoke severe anxiety, and may be described as ego-alien.**
   b. **Compulsions** are impulses to perform a variety of stereotyped behaviors or rituals that serve to reduce anxiety or get rid of obsessions (usually the patient experiences a sense of relief upon completing the act). The diagnosis of OCD should be made when these symptoms cause marked distress to the individual or interfere with social or occupational functioning. OCD is often chronic, beginning in childhood to young adulthood with marked variability in dysfunction. In athletes, it is common to see obsessive-compulsive personality traits/characteristics, but less common to see the full-blown disorder.

c. **Differential diagnosis:** schizophrenia, major depression, exercise addiction, compulsive gambling, substance abuse (esp. alcohol abuse), obsessive-compulsive personality disorder

d. **Treatment**

i. **Psychosocial:**

(a) Behavioral therapy—exposure, modeling, response prevention, thought stopping

(b) Supportive psychotherapy, psychoanalytic psychotherapy

ii. **Pharmacotherapy:**

(a) Antidepressants (imipramine, clomipramine, fluoxetine, fluvoxamine, sertraline, paroxetine) are a mainstay of the treatment plan.

(b) Monoamine oxidase inhibitors (i.e., Nardil, Parnate)

(c) Anxiolytics may be used as adjuncts if anxiety is excessive.

D. **Panic disorders**

1. **Panic vs. anxiety.** Panic is beyond normal experience, has a sudden onset without a clear precipitant, and is usually associated with physical symptoms (notably activation of the autonomic nervous system). Panic has a catastrophic quality that is not present in anxiety. These individuals have a sense of "impending doom" and may think they are going to die. Disorientation may be seen. Symptoms may last from a few minutes to a few hours.

2. **Panic disorder with agoraphobia**

a. Panic symptoms *with* a fear of being in places or situations from which escape might be difficult (or embarrassing), or in which help might not be available in the event of a panic attack.

b. **Common situations:** outside home alone, being in a crowd, travel in a bus/train/car. May be seen in athletes who are fearful to travel away from home environment.

c. **Differential diagnosis:** cardiac arrhythmias, hypoglycemia (seen in athletes who have used dietary restriction), vertigo, drug alcohol intoxication/withdrawal, hypochondriasis, generalized anxiety disorder, performance anxiety (adjustment disorder), hyperthyroidism

d. **Laboratory tests:**

i. Provocative—lactate infusion induces panic.

ii. Echocardiography—mitral valve prolapse syndrome may be seen in 8-20% of patients with panic disorder.

e. **Pharmacotherapy:** based on severity of attack, frequency, and amount of dysfunction (i.e., progressive) noted. May be especially useful (along with psychotherapy) for those who also have prominent depressive symptoms.

i. Antidepressants (monoamine oxidase inhibitors, imipramine)

ii. Benzodiazepines (especially alprazolam [Xanax]) are most helpful because of their rapid onset and can be useful in early treatment at a time when psychosocial dysfunction is at its greatest.

iii. Beta-blockers (propranolol [Inderal])—contraindicated in athletes with asthma; relative contraindication with heart disease (conduction abnormalities) and diabetes (masks hypoglycemia)

iv. Serotonin-specific reuptake inhibitors (antidepressants) have proven effective, often in combination with a benzodiazepine.

f. **Psychosocial therapy:** This supportive and insight-oriented approach can be helpful in dealing with the psychosocial complications of the panic attacks.

E. **Phobias.** Seen more commonly in athletes than one might think. When panic attacks are present, they generally precede and are more troublesome than phobic symptoms—this combined disorder is now seen as primarily a panic disorder.

1. **Agoraphobia** *without* history of panic disorder
   a. **Pharmacotherapy**—if panic occurs, same as for panic disorder with agoraphobia (see previous page)
   b. **Psychosocial therapy**
      i. Behavioral therapy
         (a) Relaxation response (progressive muscle relaxation, hypnosis, meditation, self-hypnosis, biofeedback, massage)
         (b) Exposure treatment (systematic desensitization, flooding)
      ii. Cognitive therapy
      iii. Psychodynamic psychotherapy
      iv. Support groups, family therapy
2. **Social phobia.** Some individuals may have specific fears (fear of speaking in public), whereas others may have more general fears of being embarrassed, humiliated, scrutinized, or unable to perform while in public or at social functions (fear of being judged in competition). Key to diagnosis is that anxiety increases as the individual approaches the situation, which may be avoided or be endured with extreme anxiety. In sport situations, the anxiety is usually represented as tremulousness, or saying inappropriate things while in the competitive, feared environment.
   a. **Pharmacotherapy** (usually used only if refractory to psychotherapy)
      i. Benzodiazepines, i.e., anxiolytics
      ii. Propranolol (has been on the list of "banned" substances in international competition if used for enhancement of performance)
   b. **Psychosocial therapy**
      i. Desensitization through gradual exposure to the anxiety-provoking situation/stimuli. Use of the anxiety hierachy is essential.
      ii. Propranolol (has been on the list of "banned" substances in international competition(s) if used for enhancement of performance)
3. **Simple phobia.** Usually starts in childhood. A persistent fear of a circumscribed stimulus (object or situation) other than the fear of having a panic attack (as in panic disorder), or of humiliation in social situations (as in social phobia). Exposure to the stimulus produces an immediate anxiety response. Avoidant behavior becomes more and more disruptive to the person's normal routine.
   a. **Pharmacotherapy is usually ineffective** unless panic symptoms are present.
   b. **Psychosocial**—as above, desensitization (progressive exposure) is vital, and insight-oriented approaches may be helpful as adjuncts.
4. **General considerations of anxiety-related phenomena**
   a. Generalized anxiety—anxiety is chronic
   b. Obsessive-compulsive—anxiety when behaviors/thoughts resisted
   c. Panic disorder—anxiety of sudden onset, without clear precipitants
   d. Phobias—anxiety when confronting stimuli
   e. Post-traumatic stress disorder—anxiety when trauma recalled

F. **Post-traumatic stress disorder** is defined by the temporal relationship between a recognizable traumatic event and the development of symptoms that result in impairment of psychological, social, and physical function. Stressors involved are generally outside the range of normal experience (rape, sexual abuse, assault, traffic accidents, natural disasters, extraordinary athletic injury, etc.) and are not frequently seen in athletic populations.
1. **Clinically one would see disturbances in these three areas:**
   a. Traumatic event is re-experienced
   b. Numbing of general responsiveness
   c. Persistent symptoms of increased arousal
2. In the athlete, it is not unusual to see **symptoms of physiologic reactivity (increased arousal)** upon exposure to events that symbolize an aspect of the traumatic

event (i.e., a gymnast is "paralyzed" on the balance beam after having been previously abducted by a motorcyclist). Exaggerated startle responses are common as well as irritable, oppositional behavior and difficulty concentrating.

3. **Normal response to moderate trauma** (not necessarily out of range of human experience)—anxiety, depression, psychosomatic reactions
4. **Common phases of response to severe trauma**
   a. Outcry (ranges from acute alarm to stunned ability to take in the meaning)
   b. Denial (weeks to months)—withdrawal, sleep disturbances, somatic symptoms
   c. Intrusive (fear, anxiety)—startle responses, increased reactivity
   d. Working through (mourning of the loss or injury)—examination of the meaning of the trauma; consideration of plans for coping in the future
   e. Completion—recognize the impact of the trauma, hopeful about the future, resumption of normal activities
   f. This process may take up to 2 years to work through. Delayed forms have a worse prognosis.
5. **Differential diagnosis**—adjustment disorder, substance abuse, brief reactive psychosis, panic disorder, major depression with anxiety (all separate but overlapping)
6. **Prevention/treatment**
   a. Assistance immediately following the trauma; supportive role
   b. Support groups
   c. Psychotherapy with an empathetic approach aimed at helping individual recognize connection between the trauma and other life conflicts is generally successful.
   d. Pharmacotherapy may be needed in severe cases, especially if depression or anxiety is prominent.

G. **Personality disorders**

1. **General considerations.** Everyone has a personality style or certain personality traits that distinguish them from others. This is of course not to say that everyone has a personality disorder. Personality traits are enduring patterns of perceiving, relating to, and thinking about the environment and oneself, and are exhibited in a wide range of important social and personal contexts. Personality disorders become evident when these traits become inflexible and maladaptive, and cause either significant impairment in social or occupational functioning or subjective distress. Usually this maladaptive behavior is evident by adolescence or young adulthood. Most personality disorders can be grouped into these areas:
   a. **Odd, eccentric behavior**—paranoid, schizoid, schizotypal (rare in healthy athletes)
   b. **Dramatic, emotional, or erratic behavior**—histrionic (hysterical), narcissistic, antisocial, borderline (more common)
   c. **Anxiety, fear as manifestations**—avoidant, dependent, compulsive, passive-aggressive (more common)
2. **Clinical considerations in athletes**
   a. Manifestations of a personality disorder often develop under extreme or persistently stressful situations that are perceived as harmful to the athlete's self.
      i. **Injury** (i.e., patient sabotages rehabilitation by overworking or missing appointments)
      ii. **Consistently poor performances with resultant worry** (i.e., acting out behavior at practice, not obeying rules, getting into fights, backstabbing, not listening, being consistently late for practice, etc.)
      iii. **Demotion in playing status** due to objective drop off in actual performance (i.e., may have grandiose ideas of playing abilities/competence, narcissistic, with claims that the coach is off track or that others are out to get him/her, blaming of others)

b. Frequently, one of the first and earliest signs that a personality disorder may be affecting an athlete is the subjective feeling in the *coaches* or *sports physician* of anger, frustration, and lack of being in control in dealing with the athlete's needs. This can be a very important insight to be aware of, and its recognition may be the difference between treatment success and failure.

3. **Specific disorders**
   a. **Borderline:** The clinical picture here is dramatic, with a pervasive pattern of mood instability, stormy interpersonal relationships, and disturbed self-image. Impulsivity, inappropriate anger, identity disturbance, chronic feeling of emptiness, and self-abusive behavior (drug use, suicidal gestures, rehabilitative abuse) may be seen. These are extremely challenging patients that probably need to be referred to a mental health specialist as part of the overall treatment plan. **Helpful hints:**
      i. Be consistent with your treatment plan.
      ii. Keep all scheduled appointments.
      iii. Use a "team" approach.
      iv. Explain all procedures. Try to be an empathetic listener without guaranteeing promises that you cannot keep (i.e., false hope).
   b. **Narcissistic:** tendency to display rage, hypersensitivity to slights, boredom, and exploitive behavior are common. The narcissistic patient is usually aloof and arrogant, accompanied by a sense of entitlement (being special—"I get something for nothing in return"), with brooding preoccupations with issues of self-esteem. **Helpful hints:**
      i. Remember that the patient is in psychological pain.
      ii. A straightforward approach is necessary here, as one wants to avoid excessive joking around with the person in order to insure treatment compliance.
      iii. Be "up-front" with behaviors that seem exploitive.
   c. **Histrionic:** behavioral features of self-dramatization, emotional expressiveness, drawing attention to oneself, craving activity and stimulation, overreacting to minor events, and irrational outbursts—all occurring against a background of dependence and manipulation. **Helpful hints:**
      i. Avoid seductive interactions.
      ii. Encourage the patient to express "real" feelings about his/her treatment.
   d. **Passive-aggressive:** Characteristically, this person procrastinates, resists demands for adequate performance, finds excuses for delays, and finds fault with those he/she depends on, yet refuses to separate him/herself from dependent relationships. Passive, self-detrimental behavior may be an expression of personal conflicts through retroflexed anger. Lack of assertiveness and indirectness of need are common. Frequently, the clinician becomes enmeshed in trying to support the patient's many claims of unjust treatment. **Helpful hints:**
      i. Fulfilling the demands of such patients is often to support their disorder, but refusing their demands is to reject them.
      ii. Try to point out consistently the probable consequences of passive-aggressive behaviors as they occur.
      iii. Try not to get enmeshed in issues outside the treatment plan.
   e. **Other personality disorders seen in athletes**
      i. **Antisocial**
      ii. **Obsessive-compulsive (personality disorder)**—obsessions and compulsions are NOT seen as intrusive by the patient, although these traits may be disruptive to others.
      iii. **Dependent**
      iv. **Avoidant**

4. **Management**
   a. **Psychotherapeutic modalities are the primary intervention.**
      i. **Individual psychotherapy** attempts to overcome resistance to establish a more healthy self.
      ii. **Family therapy** is especially helpful for adolescents and young adults when the family situation is enmeshed.
      iii. **Group therapy** is especially helpful when control is needed for acting-out or impulsive behavior.
   b. **Pharmacotherapy** has some usefulness here if there are symptoms of psychosis, major depression, or agitation (i.e., borderline personality disorder). The serotonin-specific reuptake inhibitors (i.e., Sertraline-Zoloft) have shown to be helpful in treating agitated and impulsive behavior in patients with personality disorders. One should avoid the tricyclic antidepressants due to their toxicity in overdose.

H. **Eating disorders** (see Chapter 23, "Eating Disorders")
1. Anorexia nervosa
2. Bulimia nervosa

I. **Psychoactive substance abuse**
1. **Alcohol**
2. **CNS stimulants**
   a. Cocaine
   b. Amphetamine
3. **CNS depressants**—benzodiazepines, barbiturates, meprobamate (Miltown), ethchlorvynol (Placidyl), glutethemide (Doxiden)
4. **Anabolic steroids** (see Chapter 22, "Drugs and Doping in Athletes")
5. **Opioids**—heroin, morphine, methadone, meperidine (Demerol), propoxyphene (Darvon), hydromorphone (Dilaudid), oxycodine (Percocet, Percodan), pentazocine (Talwin)
6. **Hallucinogens**—LSD, mescaline, psilocybin
7. **Arylcyclohexylamines**—phencyclidine (PCP)
8. **Cannabinoids**—marijuana, hashish

J. **Disorders of childhood and adolescence**

In addition to the disorders of adulthood previously discussed (which also apply to children and adolescents), there are a few clinical syndromes that one may see specifically in the child or adolescent who is also a competitive athlete. **Interestingly, because of the time and energy commitment to sport performance by young athletes, it is often in their sport performance and behavior that we see hints that may suggest underlying psychopathology.**

1. **Symptoms and behaviors that may be indicative of underlying conflict**
   a. **Persistent oppositional behavior**—defiant, devious (breaking rules, talking back)
   b. **Excessive fear**—anxiety and extreme resistance to participate (especially with new skill acquisition)
   c. **Excessive anxiety**—need for constant reassurance, lots of self doubt, somatic concerns—stomach problems, sickness, absence from practice, inability to relax
   d. **Persistent irritability, defensiveness, mood changes**—possibly verbal and physical fights with coaches, teammates, parents. May be indicative of depression, anxiety, substance abuse, etc.
   e. **Lying, cheating, behavior**—may be indicative of low self-esteem, personal problems, family problems
   f. **Frequent, seemingly hard-to-understand injuries**—may be indicative of confusion or dissatisfaction in the athlete owing to conflicts of interest, interpersonal problems, unmanageable stress, or true questions regarding the motives for participation in sport (i.e., "Am I doing this for myself or someone/something else?")

2. **Evaluation of the child/adolescent—special considerations**
   a. **Care must be taken to consider the physiological and psychological development of the athlete** (i.e., developmental ages) in order to gain a true idea of what the problem is and the appropriateness of intervention strategies.
   b. **Family and social context(s)** are extremely important variables in these age groups. An example is **"the vicarious athlete"** where parents and/or coaches influence the young athlete in various ways (through pushing, discipline, manipulation) in an attempt, usually unconscious, to fulfill their own unmet needs.
   c. **Sources of information** must include the client, family, coaches, and school representatives.
   d. **Always include a substance abuse history as well as history of sexual and/or physical abuse** (as deemed appropriate).
3. **Clinical syndromes**
   a. **Attention deficit hyperactivity disorder**
      i. **Clinically manifested as:**
         (a) Attention deficits (high distractibility, can't concentrate)
         (b) Hyperactivity (high motor activity, "on the move constantly")
         (c) Coordination problems (in both fine and gross motor systems)
         (d) Impassivity (sudden change in interest, stealing, substance abuse)
         (e) Perceptual problems (poor school performance in youngster with normal IQ)
         (f) Immature and domineering behavior
      ii. **Evaluation.** Careful listing of symptoms and conditions upon their occurrence, pediatric evaluation, testing of motor skills and attention span, IQ testing, school and parent reports
      iii. **Sports context.** Disorder may be seen in a young athlete who can't seem to sit still or follow instructions, or in an athlete that appears to have a disproportionate problem with learning and developing certain motor skills (i.e., beam routines in gymnastics, baseball swing, shooting baskets, etc.).
      iv. **Treatment:**
         (a) **General**—individual may need special education programs, special activities to enhance coordination and sensory organization, or supportive and directive psychotherapy if child views self as abnormal or worthless.
         (b) **Pharmacotherapy**—methlyphenidate (Ritalin), dextroamphetamine (Cylert)—**after psychiatric consultation**
   b. **Oppositional defiant disorder**
      i. **General**—not uncommonly seen in young athlete populations. Typically, one will see temper outbursts, frequent challenging/arguing of authority (i.e., the coach), easily annoyed by others, angry outbursts, use of obscenity, blaming of others for own mistakes, "bossy stubbornness." Chronic oppositional behavior almost always interferes with interpersonal relationships and school and athletic performance.
      ii. **Differential diagnosis**—rule out major depression and conduct disorder.
      iii. This behavior can be both normal and adaptive at specific developmental stages and in response to situational crises. If related to a significant stressor, this is an adjustment disorder. However, in the disorder the symptoms are usually prolonged and not transient in nature.
      iv. **Treatment:**
         (a) Individual therapy and counseling with parents/coaches—emphasis is to help understand self-destructive nature of behavior and work on self-esteem (which is typically low).
         (b) Family therapy can be helpful for identification of stressors and patterns of behavior.

(c) **Helpful hint:** It is easy to be angry and turned off by this type of problem because this athlete/person threatens your authority. Remember, the youngster is *telling you something*, and a more understanding and empathetic approach is desirable. A one-to-one approach may help the youngster open up to you.

c. **Conduct disorder**
The essential feature is a "persistent pattern of conduct in which the basic rights of others and major age-appropriate societal norms or rules are violated." This is one of the disruptive behavior disorders (along with attention deficit hyperactivity disorder and oppositional defiant disorder).
   i. **Clinically, behavior patterns are repetitive, persistent**, and include stealing (with confrontation of the victim), lying, running away overnight, fire-setting, forced entry, destruction of other's property, cruelty to animals, sexual abuse, substance abuse, use of weapons in fights, frequent physical fights, and lack of regard for other people's sense of autonomy.
   ii. **Treatment approach**—referral to mental health system for evaluation and treatment. This person may need more acute care (i.e., hospitalization).

d. **Specific developmental disorders** (reading, arithmetic, language, etc.)

IV. Intervention Strategies

A. **General concepts.** It is important to note that there are numerous intervention strategies available for athletes to use in their attempts to solve problems, change or examine certain behaviors, relax, and enhance/maximize their overall performance both on and off the field. Care must be taken to individualize each athlete's program to maximize its effectiveness and to allow the athlete to take as active a part in the program as possible. An educational approach in which one carefully teaches the athlete the concepts of the various intervention techniques has been shown to be very helpful, in that it allows the athlete to take a dynamic, active part in his/her own growth and development through the use of these techniques. In order for the techniques to work, the athlete must believe in your ability to give him/her accurate information and he/she must be able to develop a trusting, nurturing, and empathetic relationship with you. Feedback from the sports medicine professional and the athlete is critical; **listen to the athlete**.

B. **Relaxation training**
   1. **Concept.** One must realize that increased anxiety levels may hamper sport-related performance by causing muscular tension, nausea, inappropriate focus attention (i.e., easy distractibility), autonomic hyperarousal, and decreased psychological flexibility (i.e., resistance to change). Relaxation techniques can be helpful skills (they take practice, as do physical skills) in an attempt to decrease anxiety-arousal levels and to minimize the stress-related anxiety that is common to nearly all sport behaviors.
   2. **Types of relaxation training**
      a. **Deep breathing** is the most natural technique to use. When an athlete is tense or nervous, breathing typically will involve the upper chest and the accessory muscles of respiration. When relaxed, the athlete will use more diaphragmatic (i.e., stomach) breathing. The athlete should breathe at his/her own rate, deeply and slowly. As breathing becomes deeper and slower, the athlete will notice that he/she becomes more and more relaxed.
      b. **Progressive muscle relaxation (Jacobsen)** is usually used with deep breathing exercises and is based on understanding high and low muscle tension, the relative differences between the two, and the subsequent control over muscle relaxation that one can obtain with practice. It is helpful to move slowly through each muscle group until the desired relaxation response is obtained (tense toes, relax

toes, tense quadriceps, relax quadriceps, etc.). Initially, this exercise is best done in a comfortable position and quiet location, but with practice the technique can be used even during competition. Background music without lyrics may be a helpful adjunct for the relaxation process (soothing). It is also helpful to practice this technique at least once or twice each day (especially before and after workouts, prior to bedtime, before competition, etc.) when learning the process. One must be patient!

c. **Biofeedback** is a type of training that involves necessary physiological feedback (i.e., blood pressure, skin temperature, etc.) via a visual or auditory signal that indicates the athlete's present state of tension. Biofeedback can promote self-awareness by helping athletes become more aware of what causes tension, anxiety, and pain. This awareness can then help to give the athlete alternative ways of responding to particular stressors through the practice of new responses outside biofeedback sessions.

d. **Autogenic training (Johannes Schultz)**
   i. The word autogenic comes from the Greek words meaning "self-create," implying that one should be able to have control over self with the help of one's own concentration. The starting point for autogenic training is the learned ability to exert control over mind and body through thought.
   ii. Involves the use of self-suggestions or self-statements that are implemented to help with self-development (i.e., change behavior, improve attitude/mood, intensify motivation, etc.). Examples: "My mind is crystal clear"; "I feel secure"; "I feel strong, active, on the offensive." The self-suggestions can come in several forms: verbal (from oneself), verbal in the form of an imagined thought, auditory (i.e., audiotape), and visual (words as symbols). Once again, it is easier to achieve success with this technique while in a relaxed state, as described above.

e. **Other techniques:**
   i. **Yoga**
   ii. **Meditation**
   iii. **Massage**
   iv. **Exercise**

3. **Uses of relaxation training techniques**
   a. **Especially helpful for anxiety and stress-related phenomena** (i.e., anxiety, mood-depression, irritability, distractibility)
   b. Helpful in **pain management** and its relationship to injury and subsequent rehabilitation
   c. Athlete should confer with his/her physician prior to initiation of a regular relaxation training program.
   d. Relaxation is a helpful preliminary exercise to learn if the athlete is planning to use visualization (visual imagery) as a part of a regular training program.
   e. Once again, if there are any questions regarding the implementation of these techniques, athlete should consult with his/her sport psychologist/psychiatrist/therapist.

C. **Visual/mental imagery (visualization)**

1. **Concept.** Many athletes have reported that just prior to performance they try to mentally picture themselves going through the forthcoming activity in their mind. Most athletes have an ability to picture in their mind certain aspects (either mechanical-technical or emotional) of their performance without even trying very hard to do so. Visualization can involve creating mental images of oneself, a particular idea, or a desired/experienced emotional response/feeling. **The "visualization," in other words, can be used to produce mechanical and technical images of one's**

performance (past, present, future), or it can be used in a kinesthetic fashion to produce images of control, comfort, and relaxation (i.e., emotional).

This conceptual technique can be used with or without relaxation techniques, but relaxation often increases its effectiveness and adds to the learning effect of the training.

The use of visual imagery and its effectiveness remains controversial with regard to its direct effect on performance. Controlled studies are difficult to reproduce, and there are few observable data (reliance primarily on self-reports) to interpret when one is talking about the images we create in our minds. However, there is a growing body of athletes at all levels that personally attest to its effectiveness in their own training program(s). This technique will continue to stimulate research and development as a viable intervention tool in helping athletes maximize their performance.

2. **Visual-motor-behavioral rehearsal (Suinn)**
   a. This technique combines deep breathing, muscle relaxation, and visualization in a step-by-step process of gaining control over arousal, stress-related anxiety, negative thoughts/disruptive thoughts, and energy levels (i.e., directing one's energy).
   b. It is designed to allow flexibility of thought processes in a relaxed state within each athlete so that he/she may maximize sport performance by learning how to appropriately direct thoughts and emotional energy with regard to performance.

D. **Hypnosis** is a form of attentive, receptive focal concentration with a sense of parallel awareness and a constriction in peripheral awareness. During this focused attention, the athlete is relatively open to receiving information and exploring the mind-body relationship. This approach can help facilitate the evaluation of an athlete's psychological resources for change and also help to adjust therapeutic strategies to the athlete's personal style and abilities. More specifically, hypnosis has proven effective in the reduction of stress-related anxiety, a phenomenon encountered by nearly all competitive athletes.

E. **Cognitive training/self-regulation**

Most, if not all, athletes have specific vulnerabilities, particular stressors impinging on these vulnerabilities, and habitual patterns of reacting to various situations. Cognitive training can help identify, test the reality of, and correct distorted perceptual conceptualizations of certain beliefs. Cognitive training is based on the underlying theoretical rationale that the way individuals structure their experiences determines how they feel and behave.

The sports therapist plays a vital role in the training, as the proximal goal is to modify the athlete's bias in interpreting personal life experiences and making future predictions. This is attempted through a series of techniques including the **identification of automatic thoughts** (rapid thoughts usually preceding some affect such as anger, anxiety, etc.), **identification of cognitive errors** (arbitrary inferences, over-generalizations, etc.) **reality testing,** and **monitoring anxiety**, all of which are intended to give the athlete a healthier set of self-referring statements and beliefs (i.e., improve self-esteem/self concept).

1. **A model of self-regulation (Kirschenbaum)**
   a. **Problem identification** (verbally noted, expressively written down)
   b. **Commitment to change** (to self and others)
   c. **Implementation/execution**—specific plans are set up and carried out systematically, e.g., change in training routine, use of relaxation training, regular use of positive self-statements
   d. **Self-monitoring of progress**, including progression and setback, e.g., use of feedback for constant reevaluation (videotape, verbal feedback, performance diaries)

e. **Generalization**—improvement and success in certain, specific areas may "generalize" to other areas of performance and/or life skills management

2. **Uses**
   a. Stress management, anxiety reduction
   b. Correcting performance flaws (technical or emotional)
   c. Breaking bad habits or undesired patterns of behavior
   d. Performance enhancement, personal growth (life skills management)
   e. Communication problems
   f. Negative attitudes, thoughts
3. Another cognitive model—covert conditioning/modeling

F. **Desensitization training**

1. Desensitization is the gradual ability to tolerate or become insensitive to negative disturbances/situations that typically create a sense of heightened arousal that is uncomfortable (anxiety, fear, panic, etc.).
2. It is helpful to **analyze performance behavior** and identify which situation(s) stimulate the exaggerated arousal that is uncomfortable. Examples might include:
   a. Balance beam series in front of judges
   b. A technical free-throw in front of a hostile crowd during a basketball game
   c. Teeing off at the first hole of the last round of a match-play golf tournament
   d. Wrestling an opponent one has never been able to beat
3. A hierarchy of situations can then be identified and arranged by the athlete along a continuum of least anxious (bottom of the list) to most anxious (top of the list).
4. With the use of relaxation techniques, the athlete then "desensitizes" him/herself to each situation, starting on the bottom of the list, until the situation can be tolerated with little/no anxiety. Interestingly, this process can be done either via de novo exposure (i.e., actual performance) or through the use of imagery (i.e., imagined situations), or a combination of both.
5. Once the anxiety-provoking situation is tolerated, the athlete moves up the list systematically until the desired performance is obtained.
6. **Uses.** The training is especially helpful for situational anxiety (e.g., free throws in basketball, hitting with two strikes in baseball) and phobias (e.g., fear of being harshly judged, fear of heights). This technique is used in various sport contexts to acclimate athletes to potentially stressful situations. For example:
   a. A professional football team practices with loudspeakers that bring in sound similar to that to be experienced in the upcoming game, which will be in a noisy, domed stadium.
   b. A gymnast practices her backhand spring series on a lower-set balance beam (with padding and with a spotter) before moving up to the competition balance beam (without padding, without a spotter).
   c. A baseball team plays intrasquad games with real-game situations prior to the start of the season.

G. **Motivational goal setting** is the systematic use of short/intermediate/long-term goals that are identifiable and realistic. The goals should be directed toward desired behavior(s) intended to enhance performance, facilitate personal growth, and feel good. It is important to set goals that have emotional or affective significance—"It feels good," "I want to do this badly," "I need to do this to improve my performance"—in order to facilitate compliance with goal-setting programs.

In addition, goal-setting programs will lose their effectiveness if they are not periodically re-evaluated and if there is no feedback mechanism put into place (e.g., contact with coaching staff regarding updates on goal-directed behavior).

It can be helpful to conceptualize goals and/or behavior into four major areas.

1. Before goals are set, one should identify **areas of strength and weakness (i.e., a "needs" assessment).** This can be done on an individual or team basis.
   a. Athletic/physical—athletic, physical skills
   b. Academic/professional/vocational—school, sport, work
   c. Social—self, friends family, coaches, significant others, etc.
   d. Spiritual—faith, religion
2. **Set goals that are performance-related** (e.g., increased strength, increased speed, improved form, a particular score/time) rather than strictly outcome-related (e.g., win-lose, national championship). Although general outcome goals can be important in a motivational setting, they are often difficult to put into objective form and can be difficult to apply to the daily setting of practice (physical and mental).
3. **Set goals that are realistic but allow athletes to be a little bit grandiose about what they think they are capable of doing.** Confer with teammates and/or coaches to make sure that they objectively concur with what the athlete thinks he/she is capable of. This process can be extremely helpful and allow the athlete to take risks that will not automatically result in failure.
4. **Be creative with goal-setting.** Make it challenging but fun and enjoyable. Structure the environment for motivational training:
   a. Provide opportunity for skill development and fitness development.
   b. Create practices/games that are fun/exciting.
   c. Allow for socialization needs (i.e., friendship).
   d. Provide a realistic view of success and personal growth.
   e. Allow for athlete's feedback.
   f. Provide constructive/specific criticism and positive reinforcement.
   g. Put a premium on open communication.
   h. Promote the use of self-evaluation.

H. **Psychological skills training** (PST) consists of techniques and strategies designed to teach and develop mental skills that facilitate high quality performance, a positive approach to sport competition, and personal growth. The premise is that athletes are generally mentally healthy, but they may benefit from learning cognitive skills that help them cope with the demands of sport and its competitive environment.

This process takes practice and patience. It requires receptiveness from the group/individual being worked with (players, coaches, trainers, etc.).

The process typically requires several years for players and teams to reach maximum effectiveness and for its acceptance into a regular practice/competition routine.

PST is based on an educational model that attempts to identify the key psychological skills that are usually needed to facilitate personal growth. Many of these skills may be sport-specific. The program then helps individuals develop these skills through the implementation of training methods (such as visual imagery, goal-setting, and arousal control).

1. **Typical PST program (adapted from Vealey) for a sports team**
   a. Overview, presentation of concepts, format
   b. Psychological skill assessment
      i. **Volition**—why this is important to me
      ii. **Awareness of self**—use of self-monitoring, self-inventories (i.e., strengths, weaknesses) in major life skills areas (academic, athletic, social, spiritual)
      iii. **Self-esteem (Riedler)**—understanding of oneself and adaptability to change
      iv. **Arousal**—anxiety
      v. **Attentional focus**—concentration
      vi. **Stress management**—learning to anticipate stressful events
      vii. **Communication skills/interpersonal skills**
      viii. **Motivation**—concepts of goal-setting

ix. **Leadership**—personal challenge
x. **Lifestyle management**

c. **Methods of development**
   i. **Physical practice** (no substitute)
   ii. **Education**
   iii. **Intervention strategies** (imagery, relaxation, thought control, cognitive-behavioral problem-solving, etc.)

d. **Application to the sport setting** as well as life skills management—**sport-specific** vs. general

e. **Constant use of feedback regarding effectiveness of program** during and after the season
   i. Adjustments for competition, variations in performance, problem areas that need more emphasis, injury, etc.
   ii. Use of videotape, self-report evaluations

f. **Allowance for individual sessions as needed** (coaches, players), especially for crisis intervention

g. **Use of coaching staff to help implement program**

h. **Collection of data for evaluation, research**

V. Future Directions in Sports Psychology/Psychiatry

A. A shift to more community service-based programs
B. Premiums placed on certification and training for sports therapists
C. Integration into sports medicine
D. Acceptance at all competitive levels. Programs will become commonplace for the individual athlete and sports team.
E. Work with athletes at all levels, not just the elite athlete, with special focus on youth development
F. Increased competition for services rendered
G. Practical application of knowledge through research
H. Educational development with coaches, athletes, and parents
I. More research with the "non"-athlete
J. Expansion of tools available to assess and assist athletes (e.g., psychometric testing, computer-assisted programs)

22

Drugs and Doping in Athletes

Gary A. Green, M.D., and James C. Puffer, M.D.

I. Definition

Doping is the administration to, or the use by, a competing athlete of any substance foreign to the body or any physiologic substance taken in abnormal quantity or by an abnormal route of entry into the body, with the sole intention of increasing in an artificial and unfair manner the athlete's performance in competition.[1]

II. Historical Perspective

A. 1960—Danish cyclist Kurt Enemar Jensen dies during Summer Olympics in Rome from amphetamines and Roniacol

B. 1964—International Olympic Committee (IOC) adopts definition of "doping"[2]

C. 1964—Tokyo becomes the first Olympiad to perform a trial of nonpunitive drug testing. Several athletes found to be using foreign substances, and this leads to the establishment of a banned substance list, which has been modified and expanded repeatedly (Table 1).

D. 1968—Formal drug testing adopted for the Summer and Winter Olympics. Drug testing has been present at every Olympiad since, and the results are listed in Table 2.

E. 1972—U.S. swimmer Rick DeMont stripped of gold medal for using ephedrine to treat underlying asthma

F. 1986—Cocaine-related deaths of Maryland basketball player Len Bias and Cleveland Browns football player Don Rogers give impetus to expand drug testing for intercollegiate athletes

G. 1988—Canadian Olympian Ben Johnson stripped of his gold medal following a positive drug test for stanazolol

H. 1991—Former NFL football player Lyle Alzado attributes terminal brain tumor to his massive use of anabolic-androgenic steroids and human growth hormone (hGH).

III. Prevalence of Drugs in Athletics

A. The scope of the problem has been investigated using self-report surveys at various institutions. The purpose is to determine the prevalence of drug use and if athletes' drug use differs from the general population.

1. 1981—National Collegiate Athletic Association (NCAA)–sanctioned study of the Big Ten conference surveyed 1140 male athletes competing in four sports as compared to the general student population. Alcohol and marijuana use was similar (80% and 20% for both groups). However, 2% of the athletes, as compared to none of the nonathletes, admitted to using anabolic steroids.[3]
2. 1983—Clement[4] surveyed 1687 Canadian Olympic athletes
   a. 5% used anabolic steroids.
   b. 21% considered using anabolic steroids.
   c. 10% used psychomotor stimulants.
   d. 57% used alcohol.
   e. 23% used marijuana.
   f. 4% used cocaine.

TABLE 1. Banned Substance List

Doping classes
- Stimulants
  - Psychomotor stimulants
  - Sympathomimetic amines
  - Miscellaneous central nervous system stimulants (including caffeine)
- Narcotics
- Anabolic steroids
- Beta-blockers
- Diuretics
- Growth hormone

Doping methods
- Blood doping
- Pharmacologic, chemical, and physical manipulation of the urine

Classes of drugs subject to certain restrictions
- Alcohol*
- Local anesthetics†
- Corticosteroids‡
- $Beta_2$-agonists§

* Not prohibited but levels (breath or blood) may be requested by an international federation.
† Permitted when medically indicated and documented in writing to IOC Medical Commission.
‡ Banned except when used topically, via inhalation, locally, or intraarticularly and documented in writing to IOC Medical Commission (oral, intravenous, and intramuscular use banned).
§ Permitted in the aerosol or inhalant form for the treatment of asthma.

3. Anderson and colleagues[5] from Michigan State first evaluated 2039 intercollegiate athletes in 1985 and have since repeated the study in 1989 and 1993. Table 3 lists the percentage of athletes reporting the use of each drug in the previous 12 months. Periodic surveys are necessary to assess the patterns of drug use among the recreational and ergogenic substances.

TABLE 2. Olympic Game Doping Results

	Positive	No. Athletes Tested
Grenoble, 1968	0	86
Mexico City, 1968	1	668
Sapporo, 1972	1	211
Munich, 1972	7	2079
Montreal, 1976	11*	2061
Lake Placid, 1980	0	N/A
Moscow, 1980	0	2200
Sarajevo, 1984	1†	408
Los Angeles, 1984	16‡	1520
Calgary, 1988	1	422
Seoul, 1988	10	1601
Albertville, 1992	0	523
Barcelona, 1992	8§	1871
Lillehammer, 1994	0	529

* Eight samples positive for anabolic steroids
† Positive for anabolic steroids
‡ Ten samples positive for anabolic steroids. Five of these samples were positive for the “A” test, but were never confirmed by a second “B” test.
§ Two samples positive for clenbuterol, three positive for increased T:E ratio
Personal communication from Don Catlin, M.D., UCLA Olympic Laboratory

TABLE 3. Drug Use by Intercollegiate Athletes

	Percent of Athletes		
Drug	***1985***	***1989***	***1993***
Alcohol	88	89	88
Amphetamines	8.1	2.8	2.1
Anabolic steroids	4.4	4.9	2.5
NSAID/pain medications	27.7	34.3	30.1
Barbiturates/tranquilizers	2.1	1.9	1.4
Cocaine	17	5	1
Marijuana	36	28	21
Smokeless tobacco	20	28	27

NSAID—Nonsteroidal anti-inflammatory drug.
Data from Anderson WA, Albrecht RR, McKeag DB: Second replication of a national study of the substance use and abuse habits of college student-athletes. Report to NCAA, Mission, KS, 1993.

4. A study comparing college athletes with nonathletic peers revealed that athletes appear to be at higher risk for certain maladaptive lifestyle behaviors, including quantity of alcohol consumed, driving while intoxicated with alcohol or other drugs, and riding with an intoxicated driver.[6]

B. Based on these studies, various types of substances and doping methods as they relate to their use and abuse by athletes are explored in this chapter.

IV. Anabolic Steroids

A. **Definition:** testosterone or testosterone-like synthetic drugs that result in both anabolic and androgenic effects, e.g., increase protein synthesis (anabolism) and enhance the development of male secondary sexual characteristics (androgenic)

B. **History.** Originally developed in the 1930s and used in World War II to help restore positive nitrogen balance to starvation victims.[7] Also, reportedly used by German troops to increase aggressiveness.[8] Introduced to world class athletics in the 1950s.[9]

C. **Prevalence**

1. 1988—Buckley and coworkers[10] surveyed 12th-grade male students from 150 high schools across the United States and received 3403 responses, which corresponded to a 50% response rate.
   a. 6.6% used or had used anabolic steroids.
   b. 21% had obtained the drugs from a health professional.
   c. 35% of the users of anabolic steroids were not involved in a school-sponsored sport.
   d. The data from Buckley's study indicate that anabolic steroid use is prevalent in high schools and has broken out beyond traditional "power sports." Additional data from Buckley's study are provided in Tables 4 and 5.
2. There are probably at least 1 million anabolic steroid users in the United States today involved in a $100 million black market industry.[11]

TABLE 4. Age of Respondents at First Use of Anabolic Steroids

Age	Percent
<15	38
16	33
17	26
>18	3

Data from Buckley WE, et al: Estimated prevalence of anabolic steroid use among high school seniors. JAMA 260:3441–3445, 1988.

TABLE 5. Main Reasons for Using Anabolic Steroids

Reason	Percent
Improve performance	47
Appearance	27
Prevent or treat sports injury	11
Social	7
Other	8

Data from Buckley WE, et al: Estimated prevalence of anabolic steroid use among high school seniors. JAMA 260:3441–3445, 1988.

3. Two surveys of anabolic steroid use among male competitive bodybuilders revealed prevalence rates of 54% and 38%.[12,13]
4. 1992—The International Weightlifting Federation eliminates all previously recognized weightlifting records, believing they were all achieved with the aid of anabolic steroids. The Federation starts over and institutes stringent testing procedures and penalties.[14]

D. **Mechanism of action**
1. Anabolic steroids are bound by cytoplasmic proteins and transported to the nucleus. This activates DNA-dependent RNA polymerase and results in the production of messenger RNA for protein synthesis.[15]
2. Anabolic steroids may also have an anticatabolic effect that occurs by attenuating the effects of cortisol. It is postulated that this results from anabolic steroids displacing cortisol from receptors, allowing the athlete to train at a high level.[16]
3. It has also been proposed that anabolic steroids act by increasing the motivation of athletes through heightened aggressiveness.[16]

E. **In vivo studies of athletes and anabolic steroids**
1. There have been numerous studies of anabolic steroids and male athletes that support both improvement in strength[17–21] and no significant improvement in strength.[22–25] A review of these studies by the American College of Sports Medicine in 1984 led to the following conclusions:[26]
   a. In the presence of an adequate diet, anabolic steroids can contribute to increases in body weight and lean mass.
   b. The gains in muscular strength achieved through high-intensity exercise and proper diet can occur by increased use of anabolic steroids in some individuals.
   c. Anabolic steroids do not increase aerobic power.
2. Meta-analysis of 30 studies of anabolic steroids performed between 1966 and 1990 found that only 16 were randomized, used placebos, and made objective measurements of strength and percent of change in strength and were thus included in the analysis. These studies concluded that while anabolic steroids may slightly enhance muscle strength in previously trained athletes, results for the low steroid dosages studied cannot be generalized to steroid-using athletes using megadose regimens.[27]

F. **Potential therapeutic uses.** It is believed that true medical indications account for fewer than 3 million prescriptions per year.[28] In 1990, anabolic steroids were added to Schedule III of the Controlled Substances Act. **Indications include:**
1. Refractory anemias
2. Hereditary angioedema
3. Palliation therapy in advanced breast carcinoma
4. Replacement therapy in hypogonadal males
5. May also be useful with constitutional delay of growth, as an adjunct to growth hormone therapy and osteoporosis.

TABLE 6. Two-Month History of Anabolic Steroid Use by a Bodybuilder

Drug	Dose	Therapeutic Dose
Methandrostenolone (Dianabol)	75 mg subcutaneously every other day	5 mg daily
Methenolone (Primabolin)	150 mg subcutaneously every other day	
Oxandrolone (Anavar)	20 mg orally daily	2.5–10 mg daily
Oxymetholone (Anadrol)	100 mg orally daily	5–10 mg daily

Data from Tennant F, Black DL, Voy RO: Anabolic steroid dependence with opioid-type features. N Engl J Med 319:578, 1988.

G. **Dosage**
  1. **When used by athletes, doses may be taken in amounts that are 10 to 40 times the therapeutic dose.**
  2. Athletes frequently use combinations of anabolic steroids (**"stacking"**) or cycling in a pyramidal fashion to achieve maximum affect.[29] Table 6 describes the 2-month drug history of a bodybuilder.[30]

H. **Adverse reactions**
  1. **Gastrointestinal**—hepatocellular dysfunction, peliosis hepatis,[26] case reports of hepatocellular carcinoma.[31] Hepatic effects are increased with the 17-α-alkylated compounds that are consumed orally.
  2. **Cardiovascular**—increase in total cholesterol and low-density lipoprotein (LDL) cholesterol; decrease in high-density lipoprotein (HDL) cholesterol; hypertension;[26] reported cases of myocardial infarction[32,33] and cerebrovascular accident[34]
  3. **Psychological effects**—changes in libido, mood swings, aggressive behavior.[26] A dependence pattern with opioid-type features has been reported.[30,35] Pope and Katz[36] interviewed 41 bodybuilders and football players who had used anabolic steroids and found that according to DSM III-R criteria:
     a. Nine subjects (22%) displayed a full affective syndrome
     b. Five subjects (12%) demonstrated psychotic symptoms in association with anabolic steroid use
     c. The data suggested that major psychiatric symptoms are commonly associated with anabolic steroid use.
     d. However, a well-designed study of current anabolic steroid users, previous users, and nonusers demonstrated that while perceived or actual psychological changes may occur, the use of several standardized inventories did not reveal these changes.[37]
  4. **Male reproductive effects**—oligospermia, azoospermia, decreased testicular size,[26] gynecomastia.[38] A case of adenocarcinoma of the prostate has also been reported.[39]
  5. **Female effects**—reduced luteinizing hormone (LH), follicle-stimulating hormone (FSH), estrogens, and progesterone; menstrual irregularities; male pattern alopecia; hirsutism; clitoromegaly; and deepening of the voice.[26] These last three are likely irreversible.
  6. **Youths**—irreversible, premature closure of the epiphyses[26]
  7. **Additional drug use**—several studies have found that anabolic steroid users are likely to use other drugs.[5,40]
  8. **Miscellaneous**
     a. Spontaneous tendon rupture[41,42]
     b. Increase in sebaceous glands and acne[43]
     c. Infectious complications, including acquired immunodeficiency syndrome (AIDS), resulting from the sharing of contaminated needles used with injectable anabolic steroids.[44] Also report of intramuscular abscess.[45]

d. Worsening of tic symptoms in patients with Gilles de la Tourette's syndrome[46]
e. Anabolic steroids were found to suppress humoral immunity and lower immunoglobulin levels.[47]

I. **Detection.** The increasing availability of steroids has led to their widespread use beyond the traditional "power" sports. Clinical suspicion should be aroused by the presence of the aforementioned adverse effects. Drug testing, which is discussed later, can detect anabolic steroids with a high degree of accuracy.

V. Human Growth Hormone

A. **Definition:** hGH is a polypeptide hormone composed of 191 amino acids with a molecular weight of 21,500. Normally, 5–10 mg are stored in the anterior pituitary, and men have a production rate of 0.4–1.0 mg/day.[48]

B. **History**
1. 1930s—Animal breeders discover that animals given crude extract of species-specific pituitary glands develop increased muscle mass, decreased body fat, accelerated growth rate.
2. 1950s—It is found that hGH stimulates production of somatomedins, which increase growth.
3. 1961—hGH concentrations first measured in the plasma via radioimmunoassay
4. 1985—First synthetic hGH preparation is sold in the United States. Currently three products are available: somatrem and two formulations of somatropin.

C. **Prevalence.** With the growing effectiveness of gas chromatography and mass spectrometry in detecting anabolic steroids and testosterone, many athletes have turned to hGH. The prevalence of use is difficult to estimate because there is no reliable method currently available for detecting exogenous hGH. Evidence of hGH use was reportedly found in urine specimens tested at the World Track and Field Championships in Helsinki in 1983, and it is thought to be widely used in football players and bodybuilders.[48]

D. **Mechanism.** Most of the work on the mechanism of action of hGH has been done on children with hypopituitarism; the scientific literature contains no documented reports of its use or effects on athletes.[48]
1. **Function:** Administration of hGH to growth hormone–deficient children results in a positive nitrogen balance and a stimulation of skeletal and soft tissue growth.[48]
2. **Metabolic effects:** Growth hormone reduces glucose and protein metabolism and has a net anti-insulin effect by inhibiting the cellular uptake of glucose.[48] hGH also stimulates the mobilization of lipids from adipose tissue, and protein synthesis is greatly increased in hypophysectomized animals.[48]
3. **Effects on muscle:** Several studies have been done that lead to conflicting data on the effect of hGH on muscle.[49–51] A series of animal experiments by Goldberg[52] concluded that hGH increased the basal metabolic rate of protein synthesis, but that this was also determined by the amount of muscular work. It is difficult to predict the ability of hGH to increase contractile elements and improve the performance of normal muscle in normal humans.[48]
4. hGH treatment of adults with acquired growth hormone deficiency increased lean body mass, decreased fat mass, and increased basal metabolic rate. Study concluded that hGH can regulate body composition through anabolic and lipolytic actions.[53]

E. **Therapeutic uses**
1. hGH is effective in increasing the stature of growth hormone–deficient children[54] and can also increase the rate of growth in some short-statured children who are not hGH deficient.[55,56]
2. hGH is approved for the treatment of growth failure in children with chronic renal failure.
3. Other countries are using hGH to promote growth in Turner's syndrome.

4. hGH may accelerate wound healing in children with large cutaneous burns, in growth hormone–deficient adults, and in the elderly.
5. hGH increases lean body mass and decreases fat in patients postoperatively.[57]

F. **Dosage.** Although little information exists concerning athletes' usage of hGH, there have been reports of athletes consuming 20 times the dosage recommended for therapeutic purposes. The therapeutic dose in deficiency states is 0.3 mg/kg/week divided into doses given either daily or three times a week by the intramuscular route. At this dose, the wholesale cost to the pharmacist for one year's treatment of a 30-kg child would be $19,656, or about $35 per milligram.[57] Cost alone may discourage athletes from abusing hGH.

G. **Adverse reactions**
1. Acromegaly is a potential serious side effect in those abusing megadoses of hGH. It is estimated that acromegalic patients with hGH concentrations of 5–30 ng/ml have production rates of 1.5–9 mg/day.[58] **As little as a twofold increase in the recommended dose may result in acromegaly, leaving a narrow therapeutic window.** With athletes consuming up to 20 mg/day, the risk of acromegaly is significant. Complications of acromegaly include diabetes; arthritis; myopathies; and the characteristic coarsening of the bones of the face, hands, and feet.[48]
2. Side effects reported in growth hormone–deficient patients are generally few. Reported adverse reactions include intracranial hypertension, hyperglycemia, and glycosuria.[57]
3. Adult patients using hGH have described fluid retention, arthralgias, gynecomastia, and possibly carpal tunnel syndrome.[57]
4. The use of hGH in adults who are not deficient in growth hormone has not been established.
5. **Creutzfeldt-Jakob disease has occurred from the use of hGH derived from cadaveric pituitary glands.**[59] Although the use of synthetic hGH eliminates this problem, athletes often obtain substances from black market sources, thereby increasing their risk for this catastrophic neurologic disorder.

H. **Detection.** hGH is banned by the IOC; however, there currently exists no reliable method of detecting hGH. Team physicians should rely on clinical suspicion based on the possible adverse effects and educate athletes about the risks of exogenous growth hormone.

VI. Amphetamines

A. **Definition:** Amphetamines are stimulants that can be classified as indirect-acting sympathomimetic amines that have central and peripheral effects.[60]

B. **History.** Amphetamines were first used in the 1930s in the treatment of nasal congestion, narcolepsy, and obesity.[60] Experiments describing the effects on human performance were conducted in the 1950s, and the popularity of the drug increased. As previously noted, the Danish cyclist Jensen died during the 1960 Summer Olympics from an overdose of amphetamine.

C. **Prevalence**
1. Anderson and colleagues[5] found that among intercollegiate athletes who had used amphetamines in the previous year, one third used amphetamines at least six times.
2. Mandell[61] described the "Sunday syndrome" in professional football players who abuse these drugs.
3. Although the use of amphetamines as an ergogenic aid has decreased, there has been concern about the increasing use of methamphetamine as a recreational stimulant.[62]

D. **Mechanism of action.** Several theories have been proposed to explain the central and peripheral effects of amphetamines:[60]
1. Increased liberation of endogenous catecholamines
2. Displacement of bound catecholamines

3. Inhibition of monoamine oxidase
4. Interference with catecholamine reuptake
5. Production of false neurotransmitters
6. All probably contribute to observed physiologic responses, including:
   a. Increases in blood pressure and heart rate
   b. Bronchodilation
   c. Increased metabolic rate
   d. Increased free fatty acid production

E. **Relationship to athletic performance:** the literature contains contradicting data.
1. Smith and Beecher[63] reported that 75% of trained swimmers, weight throwers, and runners had improved performance after taking amphetamines.
2. Chandler and Blair[64] demonstrated no substantial improvement in athletic performance.
3. The explanation for this may be that tasks that were simple and repetitive would be predicted to result in enhanced performance with amphetamines, whereas more complicated maneuvers would not.

F. **Therapeutic uses.** Amphetamines have been used legitimately to treat many conditions, including:[60]
1. Refractory obesity
2. Narcolepsy
3. Attention deficit disorder
4. Severe depression
5. The high abuse potential of these drugs has limited their utility in these conditions.

G. **Dosage.** When taken orally, amphetamines exert their effects within 30 minutes of ingestion; however, their actions can last 12–24 hours.[60] Dosages are variable depending on the athlete and type of preparation.

H. **Adverse reactions**
1. Central nervous system
   a. Restlessness
   b. Insomnia
   c. Psychological addiction
   d. Psychosis
   e. Tremor
   f. Anxiety
   g. Dizziness
   h. Cerebral hemorrhage
2. Cardiovascular—lowered threshold for arrhythmias and provocation of angina
3. Miscellaneous
   a. Disruptions in thermoregulation
   b. Predisposition to heat illness

I. **Detection.** Amphetamines are readily detected by urine drug testing because both unchanged amphetamines and metabolites appear in the urine.[60]

VII. Cocaine

A. **Definition:** Cocaine is a naturally occurring alkaloid that is derived from the leaves of the *Erythroxylon coca* plant.[65] Although it is a topical anesthetic, it also acts as a central nervous system stimulant. This has led to its use by athletes as an ergogenic aid.

B. **History.** Archaeologists have discovered definitive evidence that cocaine use dates back to at least 3000 B.C.[66] Cocaine was referred to as the "divine plant of the Incas,"[67] and many scientific treatises were written on the subject in the late nineteenth century. Cocaine has enjoyed cyclical peaks since that time, with the current epidemic being one further episode. National attention was captured by the deaths of athletes Len Bias and Don Rogers and the revelations of cocaine use by basketball player Gary McClain.

C. **Prevalence**
1. 30 million Americans have tried cocaine, and there are 5 million regular users.[68]
2. Anderson and colleagues[5] found that 17% of the athletes in their 1985 survey had used cocaine in the previous 12 months; however, this figure had declined to 1% by 1993.

3. The *New York Times* in 1987 stated: "Cocaine has probably joined rotator-cuff injuries, torn ligaments, and broken bones as a potential occupational hazard for athletes."[69]

D. **Mechanism**

1. Cocaine acts by increasing the release and blocking the reuptake of norepinephrine from neurons in the nervous system.
2. Increased availability of epinephrine causes euphoria, increased blood pressure, tachycardia, lowered threshold for seizures, and ventricular arrhythmias.
3. Cocaine may cause hyperglycemia, hyperthermia, and increased peripheral reflex speed.[70]
4. Cocaine stabilizes axonal membranes and blocks nerve impulse initiation and conduction.[71] Combined with its properties as a vasoconstrictor, cocaine is an excellent topical anesthetic.

E. **Therapeutic uses.** Although scientists of the nineteenth century hailed cocaine as a cure for a variety of ailments from hemorrhoids to broken bones, its legitimate use is now limited to its properties as a topical anesthetic.

F. **Dosage.** Cocaine is readily absorbed by the intravenous, intranasal, and pulmonary routes. Recreational users of intranasal cocaine may use 1 to 3 g per week.[70] To mimic the intense high associated with intravenous use, but without the complications of needles, cocaine users have turned to smoking the substance. This began with the smoking of the free alkaloid form, known as "free base." The availability of ready-to-smoke, low-priced free base ("crack") cocaine has led to epidemic smoking in urban areas.[72] The effect of crack is rapid and lasts only 5–10 minutes. The half life of cocaine is 2–6 hours and can be detected in the urine for 3–5 days.

G. **Adverse reactions**

1. **Cardiovascular**—increased levels of catecholamines associated with cocaine use can directly induce ventricular dysrhythmia, coronary vasospasm with thrombosis, and myocardial infarction,[70,73] all of which can lead to **sudden death, even in those patients without underlying heart disease.** Aortic rupture has also been reported, as well as cerebrovascular accidents.[70]
2. **Central nervous system**—chronic use can result in agitation, insomnia, and tremulousness. Toxic psychosis, severe depression, paranoia, and dysphorias have been reported[70] as well as rapid addiction.
3. **Respiratory system**—taken intranasally, cocaine can cause swelling of the nasal mucosa, rhinitis, sinusitis, epistaxis, and nasal septal necrosis. Bronchitis and bronchiolitis obliterans with organizing pneumonia has been reported.[74]
4. **Considerations in athletes**—cocaine has direct effects on central thermoregulation, and an athlete exercising in the heat is thus susceptible to hyperthermia. It has been proposed that the elite sprint-trained athlete may be at greater risk for severe lactic acidosis and cocaine-induced seizures because of the higher percentage of glycolytic muscle fibers.[75] Studies have demonstrated that chronic cocaine-conditioned animals have an exaggerated catecholamine response to cocaine and exercise together.[76]

H. **Detection.** Cocaine is readily detectable by most drug testing. According to the data from Anderson and colleagues,[5] most cocaine users do not participate in drug use with teammates. It may be difficult for coaches, trainers, or team physicians to detect patterns of cocaine usage.

VIII. Caffeine

A. **Definition:** Caffeine is a naturally occurring plant alkaloid derived from aqueous extracts of *Coffea arabica* and *Cola acuminata*.[60] It is classified as a central nervous system stimulant and is found in coffee, tea, and cola drinks. Caffeine is a methylxanthine and chemically related to theobromine and theophylline. It has been used by athletes for its stimulant properties and potential for increased work and power.

B. **History.** The discovery of caffeine-containing plants that could be made into beverages was probably by paleolithic humans.[77] Caffeine has been touted throughout history for its stimulant and antisoporific effects.

C. **Prevalence**
   1. Coffee is consumed in 98% of American homes, and the average annual consumption is 16 pounds per person.[60]
   2. Although 68% of athletes in Anderson and colleagues' study[5] used caffeine, 82% of the users consumed caffeine three times or fewer per day.
   3. Significant amounts of caffeine were found in large numbers of athletes competing in the 1976 Summer Olympic Games in Montreal.[78]

D. **Mechanism of action.** Caffeine is rapidly absorbed, and peak levels are achieved in 30–60 minutes with a half-life of 3.5 hours.[60] Caffeine exerts its effects in several ways.[79]
   1. Adenosine antagonism—caffeine acts as a competitive antagonist of adenosine and causes vasoconstriction (except renal afferent artery), increased diuresis and natriuresis, central nervous system stimulation, increased lipolysis in adipocytes, and increased gastric secretion.
   2. Calcium release channel—caffeine probably acts by potentiating calcium release from skeletal muscle sarcoplasmic reticulum. This increases the force of muscle contraction at lower frequencies of stimulation with sparing of muscle glycogen.

E. **Performance**
   1. The increased work and power probably results from:
      a. Increased mobilization of free fatty acids
      b. Increased rate of lipid metabolism[80]
      c. Direct effects on muscle contraction secondary to increases in calcium permeability of the sarcoplasmic reticulum[81]
   2. Overall, there has been controversy about the ability of caffeine to enhance or prolong work output, and recent studies cast doubts on its effectiveness.[82,83] If there is a benefit in athletic performance, it is limited to endurance activities.[60]

F. **Therapeutic uses.** Caffeine has been used as a stimulant in fatigue states, in combination with analgesic compounds and in diet pills.[60] Table 7 provides information concerning the caffeine content of certain over-the-counter medications.

G. **Dosage.** The IOC has set the maximum urinary concentration of caffeine at 12 μg/ml. One study found that to exceed that threshold, an individual needed to consume almost 1000 mg of caffeine within 3 hours of testing.[84] This is far greater than the average daily consumption of 200 mg of caffeine per day.[77] Athletes concerned about testing should be aware that caffeine excretion is variable and can be affected by many factors, including exercise.[85] Caffeine concentration as it relates to urinary levels is provided in Table 7.

H. **Adverse reactions**
   1. Central nervous system[60]
      a. Anxiety
      b. Hypochondriasis
      c. Insomnia
      d. Headache
      e. Tremors
      f. Depression
      g. Scotomata
      h. Addiction with withdrawal states
   2. Cardiovascular—tachyarrhythmias, especially paroxysmal atrial tachycardia[60]
   3. Renal—diuretic effect, which is of significance in athletes at risk of dehydration

I. **Detection.** Caffeine can be detected by drug screening and is banned by the IOC at concentrations above 12 μg/ml. The NCAA allows a maximum level of 15 μg/ml.

IX. Sympathomimetic Amines

A. **Definition:** Sympathomimetic amines are synthetic congeners of naturally occurring catecholamines.[86] In addition to amphetamines, there are several other weaker sympathomimetic amines that have the potential to be abused by athletes. Examples include:

TABLE 7. Caffeine Content of Commonly Used Substances

Substance	Caffeine Concentration (mg/ml)	Caffeine Level (μg/ml)*
Coffee	55–85	1.5–3 (1 cup)
Tea	55–85	1.5–3 (1 cup)
Cola	10–15	0.75–1.5 (1 cup)
Medications	(mg/tablet)	
Cafergot	100	3–6
NoDoz	100	3–6
Anacin	32	2–3
Midol	32	2–3

* Level dependent on size of athlete and rate of metabolism. These figures represent general estimates based on average size and rate of metabolism.

1. Phenylpropanolamine
2. Phenylephrine
3. Ephedrine
4. Pseudoephedrine

B. **History.** The discovery of epinephrine in 1899 led Barger and Dale to the study of synthetic amines in 1910 that were termed sympathomimetic.[77] Their research suggested that these compounds had an indirect effect on nerve endings.

C. **Prevalence.** Sympathomimetic amines appear in a variety of cold remedies, common nasal and ophthalmologic decongestants, and most asthma preparations. The previously mentioned case of Rick DeMont's disqualification for ephedrine focused attention on the potential use of sympathomimetic amines by athletes.

D. **Mechanism of action**

1. The response of sympathomimetic amines depends on the relative selectivity of the drug, e.g., alpha-, $beta_1$-, or $beta_2$-agonists.
   a. Alpha effects—smooth muscle contraction, primarily vasoconstriction
   b. $Beta_1$ effects:[86]
      i. Production of intracellular cAMP
      ii. Increased heart rate and strength of contraction
   c. $Beta_2$ effects:
      i. Smooth muscle relaxation
      ii. Bronchodilation
      iii. Stimulation of skeletal muscle
2. Although earlier scientific studies demonstrated that the use of ephedrine improved athletic performance, three studies have shown no significant increases in performance.[80,87,88]

E. **Therapeutic uses**[60]

1. Nonemergent treatment of allergic reactions
2. Asthma
3. Hypotension during spinal anesthesia
4. Atrioventricular block
5. Nasal congestion

F. **Dosage.** The many types of drugs in this category have varying potencies and durations of action.

G. **Adverse reactions with increasing doses**

1. Anxiety
2. Epigastric distress
3. Palpitations
4. Tremulousness
5. Insomnia
6. Drowsiness

H. **Detection**

1. Sympathomimetic amines are banned by the IOC and can be detected by drug testing. The IOC allows the use of:

a. Inhaled selective beta$_2$-agonists
b. Terbutaline
c. Albuterol
d. Bitolterol
e. Orciprenaline
f. Rimiterol

2. Sympathomimetic amines have been removed from the NCAA's list of banned-drug classes.

I. **Clenbuterol—the special case of a beta$_2$-agonist that has garnered a great deal of attention for its potential as an anabolic substance**

1. **Definition:** Clenbuterol is a beta$_2$-agonist, similar to albuterol, that has been used as a bronchodilator. It has recently been considered an anabolic drug or a "repartitioning" agent. Anabolic effects of the drug have been purported to occur only with the oral forms, not via the inhalation route.
2. **History.** Clenbuterol has been available in Europe and Mexico since 1977 in the form of tablets, solution, drops, and syrup.[89] It is not approved by the Food and Drug Administration for use in the United States.
3. **Prevalence.** There is little information on prevalence; most of it is derived from the increasing numbers of athletes who are disqualified by positive drug tests. Six Olympians were disqualified in 1992: two Americans, two Germans, and two British. In one study, 25% of anabolic steroid users admitted to use of clenbuterol.[5]
4. **Mechanism of action.** Most of the data on the anabolic effects of clenbuterol are derived from animal studies. No studies to date have examined the effects of oral clenbuterol on nonasthmatic athletes.
   a. Livestock treated with clenbuterol demonstrated increased muscle mass and decreased fatty deposits.[90]
   b. Denervated rat hindlimbs demonstrated reduced muscle wasting when treated with clenbuterol[91] as well as a decreased net bone loss.[92]
   c. Clenbuterol did not show any changes in muscle cross-sectional area in a randomized study of patients undergoing medial meniscectomy. Although not statistically significant, the authors asserted that the clenbuterol group regained strength more rapidly.[93]
   d. The exact mechanism of clenbuterol's anabolic effects has not been determined; however, it has been previously shown that catecholamines attenuate amino acid release from muscle by a beta-mediated depression of protein catabolism. Clenbuterol may also act by increasing contractile tension.[92]
5. **Therapeutic uses.** Clenbuterol is used as a bronchodilator for the treatment of asthma.
6. **Dosage.** The recommended dosage for asthma is 0.02–0.03 mg given twice a day. The anabolic dosage is not known; however, extrapolation from animal data translates into 0.001–0.01 mg/kg or 0.07–0.7 mg in a 70-kg person.[91] Maltin and associates[93] used the lower asthma dose, 0.02 mg twice a day, in their study of orthopedic patients.
7. **Adverse reactions**—typical beta$_2$ effects[89]
   a. Muscle tremor
   b. Palpitations
   c. Muscle cramps
   d. Tachycardia
   e. Tenseness
   f. Headaches
   g. Peripheral vasodilation
8. **Detection.** The use of clenbuterol is prohibited by the IOC and the NCAA. It is also banned by the Association of Official Racing Chemists for its ergogenic effects on thoroughbred racehorses. It can be determined in the urine by gas chromatography-mass spectroscopy.[94]
9. **Other beta$_2$-agonists:** The debate about clenbuterol has opened the door as to whether other beta$_2$-agonists might have anabolic effects and should also be banned. This could be controversial because most studies of athletes reveal that 10% suffer

from exercise-induced asthma and depend on beta$_2$-agonists to compete. Studies have been inconclusive about the ergogenic effects of other inhaled beta$_2$-agonists, and further research is warranted in this area. It would be extremely difficult to deny asthmatics the use of inhaled beta$_2$-agonists.

X. Nonsteroidal Anti-inflammatory Drugs

A. **Definition:** Nonsteroidal anti-inflammatory drugs (NSAIDs) are a class of drugs that have analgesic and anti-inflammatory properties by virtue of their inhibition of prostaglandin synthesis.[95]

B. **History.** NSAIDs are synthetic derivatives of salicylates, which were first isolated from the willow bark in 1829.[77] Although salicylates possess antipyretic properties, the introduction of indomethacin in the 1960s was the first drug of its class to be marketed for anti-inflammatory effects.

C. **Prevalence.** More than 30 billion tablets of NSAIDs are consumed annually in the United States, including aspirin and over-the-counter NSAIDs.[96] Given their use in soft-tissue injuries, it is not surprising that Anderson and colleagues[5] found that 30% of their sample used these drugs.

D. **Mechanism of action**
   1. Although the exact mechanism is uncertain, NSAID inhibition of the synthesis of prostaglandins have several effects.[95]
      a. Inhibition of superoxide generation
      b. Competition with prostaglandins for binding at receptor sites
      c. Inhibition of leukocyte migration
      d. Inhibition of the release of lysosomal enzymes from leukocytes
      e. Interactions with the adenylate cyclase system
   2. The effect of these actions is to ameliorate soft tissue inflammation. In addition, NSAIDs have been shown to uncouple oxidative phosphorylation in skeletal muscle.[97]

E. **Therapeutic uses.** NSAIDs are useful as an adjunct to the treatment of tendinitis, sprains, strains, and other soft tissue derangements. In addition, they are used in the treatment of rheumatoid arthritis, other rheumatologic conditions, degenerative joint disease, acute and chronic pain, and dysmenorrhea.[95]

F. **Dosage.** The United States offers a wider variety of NSAIDs than any other country. In addition to the many prescription NSAIDS, there are over-the-counter medications: aspirin, ibuprofen, and naproxen. Variable half-lives can allow for once-daily dosing. Outside of the United States, NSAIDs are also available in topical formulations.

G. **Adverse reactions**
   1. **Gastrointestinal**—upset that causes the discontinuation of NSAIDs has been reported in 2–10% of patients with rheumatoid arthritis.[98] Effects include nausea, dyspepsia, gastritis, ulceration, bleeding, and hepatotoxicity. NSAIDs have also been noted to cause small intestinal enteropathy.[99]
   2. **Renal**
      a. Increased serum creatinine
      b. Sodium and water retention
      c. Hyperkalemia
      d. Papillary necrosis
      e. Interstitial nephritis
      f. Proteinuria
      g. Acute renal failure
      h. Of note is that renal pathology appears more frequently in those patients who take NSAIDs while they are hypovolemic. A potentially troublesome study of NSAIDs and exercise demonstrated that indomethacin can compromise renal function and potentiate the risk of developing acute renal failure.[100]

3. **Hematologic**
    a. Bone marrow suppression
    b. Reversible inhibition of platelet aggregation
    c. Possible decreased coagulation
4. **Central nervous system**[95]
    a. Headache
    b. Tinnitus
    c. Dizziness
    d. Sedation
5. **Considerations in athletes**—uncoupling oxidative phosphorylation can affect oxygen consumption and directly stimulate ventilation, promote sweating and dehydration, and lead to heat illness.[97]

H. **Detection.** All NSAIDs are allowed by both the NCAA and IOC.

XI. Alcohol

A. **Definition:** Ethanol is the most abused recreational drug in the United States and is classified as a depressant.

B. **History.** The fermenting and imbibing of alcohol have been known since ancient times. In the Middle Ages, alcohol was thought to be the elixir of life.[77]

C. **Prevalence.** Approximately 70% of adult Americans drink alcohol, and the per capita consumption is estimated to be 2.7 gallons per year. Perhaps 5–10% of these drinkers are, or will become, alcoholics, and there are 200,000 annual alcohol-related deaths.[101] Anderson and colleagues[5] demonstrated that alcohol was the most used drug among intercollegiate athletes.

D. **Mechanism of action.** The physiologic effects of alcohol are well-known and are not reviewed here.

E. **Therapeutic uses.** There are currently no therapeutic uses indicated for ethanol.

F. **Adverse reactions.** Physicians are familiar with the many adverse consequences of alcohol abuse.

1. **Following a review of the literature, the American College of Sports Medicine issued a statement regarding the use of alcohol as it relates to athletic performance.**[102]
    a. The acute ingestion of alcohol has a deleterious effect on many psychomotor skills, including:
        i. Reaction times
        ii. Hand-eye coordination
        iii. Accuracy
        iv. Balance
        v. Complex coordination
    b. Alcohol consumption does not substantially influence physiologic functions crucial to physical performance ($\dot{V}O_2max$, respiratory dynamics, cardiac function).
    c. Alcohol ingestion does not improve muscular work capacity and may decrease performance levels.
    d. Alcohol may impair temperature regulation during prolonged exercise in a cold environment.
2. A study has also concluded that alcohol is toxic to striated muscle in a dose-dependent manner.[103]
3. Arrests for driving while impaired substantially increase the risk of eventual death in an alcohol-related crash.[104]

G. **Detection.** Except for shooting events (including the modern pentathlon), neither the NCAA nor the IOC specifically tests for the presence of alcohol. Breath or blood levels may be determined, however, at the request of an International Federation.

H. **Identification**

1. The American Medical Association defines **alcoholism** as "an illness characterized by significant impairment that is directly associated with persistent and excessive use of alcohol. Impairment may involve physiological, psychological, or social dysfunction."[101]

2. Because the effects of alcoholism may take 5–20 years to develop and usually occur after age 30, early identification of those athletes with alcohol problems is imperative. There have been several measures designed to help assess alcohol problems, including the Perceived-Benefit-of-Drinking Scale (PBDS), the Children of Alcoholics Test (CAST), and the Michigan Alcoholism Screening Test (MAST). Perhaps the easiest test to administer is the **CAGE questionnaire.**[105]
   a. Have you ever felt you should *Cut down* on your drinking?
   b. Have people *Annoyed* you by criticizing your drinking?
   c. Have you ever felt bad or *Guilty* about your drinking?
   d. Have you ever had a drink first thing in the morning (*Eye-opener*) to steady your nerves or to get rid of a hangover?
3. A CAGE score of 2 or more is associated with alcohol abuse or dependence. Two additional questions that are helpful are:
   a. Is there a positive family history of alcoholism?
   b. Have you had any driving while intoxicated arrests?
   c. What is your regular consumption? (3 drinks/day for men and 2 drinks/day for women suggests alcohol abuse problem)
4. Education and identification are the keys to prevent this problem in athletes.

XII. Nicotine

A. **Definition:** Nicotine is a volatile alkaloid derived from tobacco and responsible for many of the effects of tobacco. It first stimulates (small doses) then depresses (large doses) autonomic ganglia and myoneural junctions.[106] Methods of consumption:
   1. Cigarettes
   2. Smokeless
      a. Loose leaf tobacco ("chewing")
      b. Moist or dry powdered tobacco ("snuff" or "dipping")
      c. Compressed tobacco ("plug")[107]

B. **History**[107]
   1. 1492—Smokeless tobacco introduced to Christopher Columbus by Native Americans and brought to Europe
   2. 1600s, 1700s—Popularity increases as tobacco touted for medicinal properties
   3. 1800s—Plug tobacco or snuff becomes popular in the United States
   4. 1880—Cigarette-rolling machine patented and cigarette smoking quickly replaces smokeless tobacco
   5. 1969—Public Health Cigarette Smoking Act bans cigarette advertising on television. Tobacco companies circumvent this through the use of billboards and logos at sporting events that are televised. For example, during one 93-minute broadcast of a Marlboro Grand Prix race car event, the Marlboro logo or name was mentioned 5933 times, and this occurred during 46 minutes of the broadcast.[108]

C. **Prevalence of use.** Athletes are aware of the health risks associated with cigarette smoking, and studies indicate fewer than 2% of athletes regularly smoke cigarettes.[5,6] Unfortunately, athletes have turned to smokeless tobacco as an alternative.
   1. Anderson and coworkers[5] found 27% of intercollegiate athletes had used smokeless tobacco in the previous year, and half of this group were regular users.
   2. 34% rate of regular use among professional baseball players[109]
   3. 30% usage rate among Alabama high school football players[109]

D. **Mechanism of action.** Nicotine has a variety of actions depending on receptor binding and dose. Nicotine readily crosses the blood-brain barrier.[110]
   1. Binds to acetylcholine receptors at autonomic ganglia, adrenal medulla, neuromuscular junction, and in the central nervous system

2. Stimulation of central nicotinic receptors activates central nervous system neurohumoral pathways to release:
   a. Acetylcholine
   b. Norepinephrine
   c. Dopamine
   d. Serotonin
   e. Vasopressin
   f. Growth hormone
   g. ACTH
3. Nicotine affects sympathetic nerves by release of catecholamines.
4. At low doses, ganglionic stimulation and sympathetic discharge with increase in heart rate and blood pressure mediated through central nervous system
5. At moderate doses, direct peripheral nervous system effects with ganglionic stimulation and adrenal catecholamine release
6. At high doses, ganglionic blockade with hypotension and bradycardia
7. Pharmacodynamic tolerance develops to subjective and hemodynamic effects.

E. **Therapeutic uses.** As an aid to smoking cessation, nicotine gum and transdermal patches have been developed. These have been somewhat effective in reducing the withdrawal symptoms of physical nicotine dependence in those smokers trying to quit.

F. **Dosage.** Smokeless tobacco users have blood nicotine levels equivalent to nicotine-dependent smokers.[111]
1. Snuff—normal single dose of snuff contains 1.5–2.5 g of tobacco; each gram has 14 mg of nicotine. Ten percent of nicotine is absorbed leading to 2.0–3.5 mg nicotine in bloodstream. This is two to three times the dose of standard 1-mg cigarette.[111]
2. Chew—average single dose is 7 g with a nicotine content of 7.8 mg per gram with 8% available to be absorbed. Eight to 10 chews per day results in the nicotine dose equivalent to 30–40 cigarettes per day.[111]

G. **Adverse reactions.** The long-term effects of cigarette smoking are well known and are not reviewed here. Studies on the effects of **smokeless tobacco** have demonstrated:
1. Oropharynx[107]
   a. 50-fold increase in oral carcinomas
   b. 2.4 times the incidence in dental caries
   c. Increases in gingival disease and leukoplakia
2. Hemodynamics (cigarette smoking compared with smokeless tobacco)[110]
   a. Similar levels of nicotine throughout the day
   b. Equivalent increases in heart rate and myocardial oxygen demand
   c. Increased sodium (added for flavoring) absorption from smokeless tobacco may lead to increases in blood pressure.
3. Reaction time and concentration—smokeless tobacco has long been touted for its ability to improve reaction time and concentration. A study of athletes and nonathletes demonstrated:[112]
   a. No neuromuscular performance enhancement as a result of smokeless tobacco use
   b. No changes in reaction time, movement time, or total response time
   c. Significant elevation in heart rate among users of smokeless tobacco
   d. A survey of major league baseball players who used smokeless tobacco found that only 10% believed that it improved concentration, and none felt it sharpened reflexes.[111]
4. **Addiction.** As noted with the levels of nicotine achieved, smokeless tobacco can be as addictive as cigarette smoking. The National Cancer Institute, in conjunction with major league baseball, has prepared "Beat the Smokeless Habit: Game Plan for Success" to help athletes quit smokeless tobacco.[113]

H. **Detection.** Nicotine is not currently tested for by international organizations or the NCAA.

XIII. Marijuana

A. **Definition:** Marijuana is a naturally occurring cannabinoid containing the active ingredient δ9-tetrahydrocannabinol (THC). It is currently an illegal drug that is used recreationally as a euphoriant.

B. **History.** Marijuana has been used by many cultures for centuries for its mind-altering properties.[114] In the United States, marijuana has enjoyed popularity over the past 25 years.

C. **Prevalence.** It is estimated that 43 million Americans have tried marijuana, and at least 17 million are regular users.[115] Of the 21% of athletes who had used marijuana in the study by Anderson and colleagues,[5] 62% stated that they used marijuana for recreational or social reasons.

D. **Mechanism of action.** THC exerts its effects on a variety of tissues, with the central nervous system and cardiovascular system being most prominent. Effects depend on the route, dose, setting, and prior experience of the user.

1. Cardiovascular[77]
   a. Tachycardia is dose related and can be blocked by propranolol.
   b. Increased systolic blood pressure while supine and decreased standing blood pressure
2. Central nervous system
   a. Impaired motor coordination
   b. Decreased short-term memory
   c. Difficulty concentrating
   d. Decline in work performance
3. Male reproductive system[116]
   a. Decreased plasma testosterone
   b. Gynecomastia
   c. Oligospermia

E. **Therapeutic uses.** THC has been used as an antiemetic agent in conjunction with chemotherapy for cancer patients and lowering the intraocular pressure in glaucoma.[77]

F. **Dosage.** The THC content of marijuana in the United States can range from 0.5–11%, and the serum concentration depends on the smoking technique employed by the user.[77]

G. **Adverse reactions.** There have been well-publicized studies on the side effects associated with marijuana use.

1. Renaud and Cormier[117] studied the effects on exercise performance.
   a. Reduction of maximal exercise performance with premature achievement of $\dot{V}O_2max$
   b. No effects on tidal volume, arterial blood pressure, or carboxyhemoglobin as compared to controls
2. In addition, marijuana causes inhibition of sweating that can lead to an increase in core body temperature.[77]

H. **Detection.** Marijuana is not banned by the IOC, but is considered a street drug by the NCAA and is prohibited. Because of its high lipid solubility, marijuana can be detected for as long as 2–4 weeks by drug testing. Depending on the minimum threshold of the assay, passive inhalation could result in a positive test.

XIV. Blood Doping

A. **Definition:** Blood is removed from an athlete and stored in a frozen state and the athlete's red cell mass is allowed to reequilibrate. Following this, the donated red cells are reinfused with a resultant increase in red cell mass. Also known as blood boosting or blood packing.

B. **History.** The earliest report in the medical literature described the infusion of 2000 ml of freshly transfused blood from matched donors to armed forces personnel in 1947.[118] Although a 34% increase in endurance over controls was demonstrated, subsequent studies using refrigerated blood failed to reproduce their results. Later researchers were able to show more impressive results when the blood was frozen at –80°C.

C. **Prevalence.** The actual extent of blood doping is unknown; however, there have been widespread rumors of this practice for the past 20 years.
   1. 1984—The U. S. Olympic Committee admits that seven U.S. cyclists engaged in blood doping at the 1984 Summer Olympic Games.
   2. 1990—A study of 1018 Italian athletes reveals that 7% have tried blood doping.[119]

D. **Mechanism of action.** Transfusion increases the oxygen delivery to exercising muscle, and studies confirm that red cell mass and $\dot{V}O_2max$ are well correlated.[120] Studies of blood doping in elite runners as compared to controls demonstrated:[121]
   1. Improvement in maximal oxygen consumption
   2. Increased total exercise time
   3. Increased hemoglobin concentration

E. **Therapeutic uses.** Red cell transfusions are limited to patients with symptomatic anemia.

F. **Dosage.** Most studies have used 2000 ml of homologous blood or 900 to 1800 ml of cryopreserved autologous blood.[122]

G. **Adverse reactions.** Improperly matched donor blood can result in transfusion reactions that can be fatal. Immune side effects are reported in 3% of all transfusions.[121] Using donor blood has the attendant risks of infectious complications. There is substantially lower risk with the use of autologous blood.

H. **Detection.** The IOC bans blood doping, but enforcement of this policy is limited by the lack of an effective technique for its detection. Berglund and coworkers[123] developed **an experimental algorithm based on an increase in hemoglobin and a decrease in serum erythropoietin that may eventually be useful in detecting blood transfusion with autologous freezer-stored red blood cells.**

XV. Erythropoietin

A. **Definition:** a sialic acid–containing hormone that enhances erythropoiesis by stimulating the formation of proerythroblasts and release of reticulocytes from the bone marrow. It is mainly secreted by the kidneys, and the level of erythropoietin is inversely related to the number of circulating red cells.[124]

B. **History**
   1. 1878—Paul Bert postulates existence of feedback loop between erythropoietic marrow and tissues[125]
   2. 1906—Carnot and DeFlandre postulate a humoral agent that adjusts erythropoiesis[124]
   3. 1953—Erslev demonstrates existence of erythropoietin
   4. 1957—Jacobson pinpoints the kidney as the source of erythropoietin
   5. 1987—Winearls and Eschbach demonstrate the efficacy of recombinant human erythropoietin (r-HuEPO)

C. **Prevalence.** With the increased attention (and attendant risks) given to blood doping, r-HuEPO has become a potential avenue of abuse for athletes.[126]
   1. The unexplained deaths of 18 Dutch and Belgian cyclists between 1987 and 1990 raised the specter of r-HuEPO abuse.[127]
   2. 1993—Anderson and coworkers[5] find that 7.6% of college athletes using anabolic steroids also admitted to using erythropoietin.

D. **Mechanism of action**
   1. Intravenous use of r-HuEPO stimulates red cell production within days, and effects can be seen for as long as 3–4 weeks.[126]
   2. Using data from red cell reinfusion studies, r-HuEPO can theoretically increase $\dot{V}O_2max$ by 10%.[126]

3. An uncontrolled study demonstrated increase in mean maximal oxygen uptake and run time to exhaustion using r-HuEPO.[128]

E. **Therapeutic uses**
   1. In patients suffering from anemia secondary to end-stage renal disease, studies demonstrate that r-HuEPO:
      a. Eliminates the need for transfusions and restores the hematocrit to normal in many patients[129]
      b. Can partially correct the renal anemia and results in a significant increase of both exercise capacity and maximum work[130]
      c. Can maintain normal hemoglobin concentration in uremic patients over time[131]
   2. r-HuEPO was found to be useful in the treatment of anemias secondary to prematurity,[132] multiple myeloma,[133] cancer, and in patients with AIDs treated with zidovudine.[134]
   3. r-HuEPO increases the yield of autologous blood donors in a safe and efficacious manner over a 21-day period[135] and can reduce the need for transfusions in patients undergoing hip replacement.[136]

F. **Dosage.** In a study of autologous blood donors with initially normal hemoglobin levels, 600 U/kg of r-HuEPO was given intravenously six times over the course of 21 days. Doses in chronic renal patients have ranged between 15 and 500 U/kg, three times per week.

G. **Adverse reactions**
   1. Observed side effects in renal anemia patients[131]
      a. Hypertensive patients required additional antihypertensive medication.
      b. Increases in serum potassium and bilirubin
      c. 20% of patients developed flu-like syndrome.
      d. 14% of patients developed thrombosis of arteriovenous fistulas and veins.
      e. 11 patients reported visual hallucinations.[137]
   2. Potential risks for athletes with normal hemoglobin using r-HuEPO[126]
      a. Increases in hemoglobin and blood viscosity accentuated with dehydration may lead to cerebral or cardiovascular ischemia, vascular thrombosis, hypotension, hyperkalemia, and iron deficiency.
      b. Attendant risks of intravenous medication, e.g. infection with hepatitis, human immunodeficiency virus (HIV), endocarditis

H. **Detection.** There does not appear to be any method of detecting the use of r-HuEPO. The worrisome deaths of the Dutch and Belgian cyclists have signaled an alarm to the sports medicine community about a potential danger to athletes.[138]

XVI. Gamma-hydroxybutyrate

A. **Definition:** Gamma-hydroxybutyrate (GHB) is an endogenous neurotransmitter produced through the metabolism of gamma-aminobutyric acid (GABA) that increases cerebral dopamine levels and acts on the endogenous opioid system.[139] It is structurally similar to GABA and is found under the names sodium oxybate, sodium oxybutyrate, gamma-hydroxybutyrate sodium, Gamm-OH, 4-hydroxybutyrate, gamma hydrate, and Somatomax PM.

B. **History.** GHB has been studied as an inhibitory neurotransmitter and has been marketed illicitly in the United States at least since 1990.[140] It has been available in Europe since the 1970s.

C. **Prevalence.** There are no surveys to date regarding the prevalence of use; however, anecdotal reports seem to indicate that it is widely used. In 1992, Daniel Duchaine, the self-styled “Steroid Guru” and author of the “Underground Steroid Handbook,” was convicted of selling at least 180 pounds of GHB.[141]

D. **Mechanism of action**[142]
   1. GHB crosses the blood-brain barrier and has been shown to double brain dopamine and dynorphin levels.
   2. Hippocampal receptors for GHB have been isolated, and synaptic transmission and regulation have been shown.
   3. GHB facilitates slow wave sleep, which is associated with growth hormone release. It is postulated that this may increase muscle mass.

E. **Potential therapeutic uses**
   1. Because of the ability of GHB to increase cerebral dopamine levels, it has been used experimentally to treat the myoclonus and cataplexy associated with narcolepsy. This is the only indication for use in the United States.
   2. GHB has been used in other countries as an anesthetic agent (especially in children), for ethanol withdrawal, and as a treatment for ischemic conditions.[143]
   3. GHB has been illegally marketed in the United States as a muscle building drug and as a sleeping aid.

F. **Dosage.** The usual directions are 1 tablet or $^1/_2$ to 3 teaspoons of the powder dissolved in water. It is unclear how much athletes are consuming.
   1. 10 mg/kg orally can cause amnesia and hypotonia.
   2. 20–30 mg/kg produces somnolence within 15 minutes.
   3. Greater than 50 mg/kg can cause unconsciousness and coma.[139]

G. **Adverse reactions**
   1. Multiple cases of poisonings secondary to GHB have been reported with patients complaining of gastrointestinal symptoms, central nervous system and respiratory depression, and uncontrolled movements.
   2. At least 11 patients have been hospitalized, and 9 required ventilator support.
   3. In 1991, the FDA issued a report that GHB was unsafe and illicit, and use should be discontinued because of potentially dangerous adverse effects.

H. **Detection.** There are no current tests for GHB.

XVII. Drug Testing

A. **Purpose.** Drug testing has been the major means of attempting to enforce compliance with a banned substance list. Public awareness has been heightened by positive tests in elite athletes. To date, most drug testing has been of the "announced" variety at championship or Olympic events.

B. **Cost.** Organized athletics has devoted great expense toward the testing of athletes.
   1. $3 million on equipping the drug testing laboratory in Montreal in 1976
   2. $1.8 million to fund the UCLA Olympic Analytic Laboratory in Los Angeles for the 1984 Games
   3. $1 million annually for the NCAA to test athletes

C. **Reliability.** Several types of tests are available that vary regarding specificity, sensitivity, and expense.
   1. **Thin-layer chromatography:** This is the least expensive screening test but has less specificity and cannot provide positive identification of a substance. The Centers for Disease Control reviewed 13 laboratories using thin-layer chromatography and found that the laboratories were often unable to detect drugs at concentrations called for by their contracts.[144]
   2. **Radioimmunoassay and enzyme-multiplied immunoassay:** These are the two most commonly used screening methods. During the 1984 Olympic Games, radioimmunoassay was used as a screening test for amphetamines, morphine, and benzoylecgonine.[145] Although manufacturers claim a 97–99% accuracy rate, such is not usually the case. To avoid false-positive tests when an athlete's career may be at stake, a second, highly sensitive and specific test is required.

3. **Gas chromatography/mass spectroscopy (GC/MS)** provides the gold standard and is the only drug test that is legally admissible in court. All state-of-the-art laboratories must use GC/MS as a confirmatory test because it provides a "fingerprint" of the detected substance. At the 1984 Olympics, GC alone was used as a screen for volatile and nonvolatile agents, GC/MS screened for anabolic steroids, and all athletes with positive results underwent a confirmatory GC/MS.[145] Unfortunately, the high cost of both the equipment and the test prohibits most smaller laboratories from using GC/MS.

D. **Testing for anabolic steroids/testosterone**

1. To combat the use of exogenous testosterone, the ratio of testosterone to epitestosterone (T:E) has been quantified. The normal ratio of testosterone to its isomer epitestosterone is 1:1. When exogenous testosterone is administered, however, serum testosterone is elevated out of proportion to epitestosterone. A positive test is considered to be a ratio of greater than 6:1.
2. Athletes have begun taking epitestosterone in conjunction with testosterone to maintain a "normal" T:E ratio. Anderson and colleagues[5] found that in 1993, 21% of anabolic steroid users also used epitestosterone.
3. Athletes using testosterone are also using human chorionic gonadotropin (hCG) to help reduce the T:E ratio. Testing is available for hCG, and hCG is banned by the IOC.[146]

E. **Circumvention by athletes.** Although the GC/MS may approach 100% accuracy, athletes have attempted numerous methods of avoiding detection.

1. **Masking agents:** diuretics and tubular blocking agents such as probenecid have been used to mask the presence of banned substances in the urine. Most drug tests use a minimum urinary specific gravity to combat this, and probenecid and the diuretics have been specifically banned by the IOC.
2. **Determination of drug half-life:** with announced drug testing, athletes can determine how long a drug can be detected in the urine. Table 8 lists some elimination times.[147] This problem can be addressed with random, unannounced testing.
3. **Substitution of urine:** athletes have developed numerous methods to substitute "clean" urine, including self-catheterization and innovative "delivery systems." To eliminate this problem, collection of the urine sample is conducted under constant supervision and close observation.

F. **Extent of testing.**[148] Most athletic organizations, professional and amateur, have developed drug testing programs. These policies are subject to frequent change depending on the law, collective bargaining, and contemporary issues. It is best to check with the respective organizations when specific questions arise.

TABLE 8. Drug Clearance Times

Drug	Approximate Elimination Time
Stimulants, eg., amphetamines	1–7 days
Cocaine	
Occasonal use	6–12 hr
Repeated use	3–5 days
Codeine and narcotics in cough medicine	24–48 hr
Tranquilizers	4–8 days
Marijuana	3–5 weeks
Anabolic steroids	
Fat-soluble injectable	6–12 months
Water-soluble oral	1–6 weeks
Over-the-counter cold preparations containing ephedrine	48–72 hr

1. Olympic level—IOC and the U.S. Olympic Committee conduct formal drug testing at sanctioned events, such as the Olympics, Olympic Trials, and Olympic Festivals. Some nations have begun random testing programs of their elite athletes.
2. Collegiate level—NCAA began testing in 1986 at postseason football games and championship events at the Division I, II, and III levels. The NCAA also conducts random year-round testing of student-athletes competing in Division I-A, I-AA, or II football or Division I indoor or outdoor track. All positive tests result in a loss of eligibility.[149]
3. Major league baseball—random tests for cocaine, marijuana, heroin, and morphine among players with specified drug testing clauses and among owners, managers, executives, umpires
4. National Basketball Association—individual players tested with "reasonable cause" for cocaine and heroin without prior notice
5. National Football League—currently tests at all preseason camps and scouting sessions in announced fashion for "street drugs," anabolic steroids, amphetamines; may also test with "reasonable cause"

G. **Effectiveness.** The effectiveness of drug testing in preventing drug abuse by athletes is difficult to evaluate. A 1987 survey of 500 collegiate athletes revealed that 62% agreed with the statement: "Drug testing is an effective way to prevent drug use."[150] It is difficult to reconcile the disparity between positive drug tests (0.72% at the 1984 Olympics and 2.5% by the NCAA) and the presumed larger prevalence of drug use by athletes. There are still many moral and ethical questions to be answered concerning drug testing, especially for college athletes.[151]

H. **Legal issues.** This is an evolving aspect of the law that varies according to state, and many issues have yet to be fully resolved. It is prudent to consult local legal experts before embarking on a testing program. There have been several landmark cases involving drug testing.
   1. 1987—As a result of a suit by Stanford athletes, it is ruled that drug testing violates student-athletes' right to privacy. This was overturned in 1994 by the U.S. Supreme Court.
   2. 1994—The U.S. Supreme Court rules that random drug tests violate the privacy rights of University of Colorado athletes, trainers, and cheerleaders.[152]
   3. 1995—The U.S. Supreme Court rules that urine drug screening of junior high and high school student athletes is allowable. The Court states that minors are not protected by the Fourth Amendment rights to privacy as adults, and "individualized suspicion" is not necessary to conduct drug testing of athletes.[153]

I. **Guidelines for drug testing.** The NCAA has developed suggested guidelines for member institutions considering adopting a drug testing protocol.[149] Although not obligated to institute a separate program, a university must follow its own guidelines once a drug testing program has begun.

XVIII. Drug Education

The education of athletes is certainly one additional tool that can be used to deter drug abuse. To be effective, however, education needs to be started at a young age. This was emphasized by the data of Anderson and coworkers,[5] which demonstrated that most patterns of drug use are established in junior high and high school. Education begun at the collegiate level is probably too late. Educational intervention is probably best suited for deterring recreational drug use because these substances usually have a negative impact on performance. Although education may be useful in alerting athletes to the risks involved with the use of performance-enhancing substances, the positive benefits of improved performance make drug testing a necessary component of deterrence. Substance abuse patterns of athletes are constantly changing depending on current social practices and technologic advances. It is incumbent on the sport medicine professional to keep abreast of these changes.

Recommended Reading

1. Memorandum of Agreement between the United States Olympic Committee and the National Governing Boards, 1985.
2. Barnes L: Olympic drug testing: Improvements without progress. Phys Sports Med 8:21–24, 1980.
3. Duda M: Drug testing challenges: College and pro athletes. Phys Sports Med 11:64–67, 1983.
4. Clement DB: Drug use survey: Results and conclusions. Phys Sports Med 11:64–67, 1983.
5. Anderson WA, Albrecht RR, McKeag DB: Second replication of a national study of the substance use and abuse habits of college student-athletes. Report to NCAA, Mission, KS, 1993.
6. Nattiv A, Puffer JC: Lifestyles and health risks of collegiate athletes. J Fam Pract 33:585–590, 1991.
7. Loughton SV, Ruhline RO: Human strength and endurance responses to anabolic steroids and training. J Sports Med Phys Fitness 17:285–296, 1977.
8. Cowart V: Steroids in sports: After four decades, time to return these genies to bottle? JAMA 257:421–427, 1987.
9. Wilson JD: Androgen abuse by athletes. Endocr Rev 9(2):181–199, 1988.
10. Buckley WE, et al: Estimated prevalence of anabolic steroid use among male high school seniors. JAMA 260:3441-3445, 1988.
11. Marshall E: The drug of champions. Science 242:183–184, 1988.
12. Tricker R, O'Neill MR, Cook D: The incidence of anabolic steroid use among competitive bodybuilders. J Drug Educ 19:313–325, 1989.
13. Lindstrom M, Nilsson AL, Katzman PL, et al: Use of anabolic-androgenic steroids among bodybuilders—frequency and attitudes. J Intern Med 227:407–411, 1990.
14. Los Angeles Times, November 23, 1992, p C8.
15. Windsor RE, Dumitru D: Anabolic steroid use by athletes. Postgrad Med 84(4):37–49, 1988.
16. Haupt HA: Anabolic steroids and growth hormone. Am J Sports Med 21(3):468–474, 1993.
17. Ariel G: The effect of anabolic steroid upon skeletal muscle contractile force. J Sports Med Phys Fitness 13:187–190, 1973.
18. Berg A, Keul J: Der Einfluss von anabolen Substanzen auf das Verhalten der freien Serumanimosauren von Normalperson und Scwerathleten in Rule and bei Korperarbeit. Oester Z Sportsmed 4:11–18, 1974.
19. Hervey GR, Knibbs AV, Burkinshaw L, et al: Effects of methandienone on the performance and body composition of men undergoing athletic training. Clin Sci 60:457–461, 1981.
20. Stamford BA, Moffatt R: Anabolic steroid effectiveness as an ergogenic aid to experienced weight trainers. J Sports Med Phys Fitness 14:191–197, 1974.
21. Ward P: The effect of an anabolic steroid on strength and lean body mass. Med Sci Sports Exerc 5:227–282, 1973.
22. Hervey GR: Are athletes wrong about anabolic steroids? Br J Sports Med 9:74–77, 1975.
23. Johnson LD, et al: Effects of anabolic steroid treatment on endurance. Med Sci Sports Exerc 7:287–289, 1975.
24. Loughton SV, Ruhline RO: Human strength and endurance responses to anabolic steroids and training. J Sports Med Phys Fitness 17:285–296, 1977.
25. Stromme SB, Meen HD, Aakvaag A: Effects of an androgenic-anabolic steroid on strength development and plasma testosterone levels in normal males. Med Sci Sports Exerc 6:203–208, 1974.
26. American College of Sports Medicine: Stand on the use of anabolic-androgenic steroids in sports. Indianapolis, American College of Sports Medicine, 1984.
27. Elashoff JD, Jacknow AD, Shain SG, Braunstein GD: Effects of anabolic-androgenic steroids on muscular strength. Ann Intern Med 115:387–393, 1991.
28. Council on Scientific Affairs of the AMA: Medical and nonmedical uses of anabolic-androgenic steroids. JAMA 264:2923–2927, 1990.
29. Burkett LN, Falduto MT: Steroid use by athletes in a metropolitan area. Phys Sportsmed 12:69–74, 1984.
30. Tennant F, Black DL, Voy RO: Anabolic steroid dependence with opioid-type features. N Engl J Med 319:578, 1988.
31. Overly WL, et al: Androgens and hepatocellular carcinoma in an athlete. Ann Intern Med 100:158, 1984.
32. McNutt RA, et al: Acute myocardial infarction in a 22 year old world class weight lifter using anabolic steroids. Am J Cardiol 62:164, 1988.
33. Huie MJ: An acute myocardial infarction occurring in an anabolic steroid user. Med Sci Sports Exerc 26(4):408–413, 1994.
34. Frankle MA, et al: Anabolic androgenic steroids and a stroke in an athlete: Case report. Arch Phys Med Rehabil 69:632–633, 1988.
35. Brower KJ, et al: Anabolic-androgenic steroid dependence. J Clin Psychiatry 50(1):31–33, 1989.
36. Pope HG, Katz DL: Affective and psychotic symptoms associated with anabolic steroid use. Am J Psychiatry 145(4):487–490, 1988.
37. Bahrke MS, Wright JE, Strauss RH, Catlin DH: Psychological moods and subjectively perceived behavioral and somatic changes accompanying anabolic-androgenic steroid use. Am J Sports Med 20:717–724, 1992.

38. Aiache AE: Surgical treatment of gynecomastia in the body builder. Plast Reconstr Surg 83(1):61-66, 1989.
39. Roberts JT, Essenhigh DM: Adenocarcinoma of prostate in a 40 year old body-builder. Lancet 2(8509): 742, 1986.
40. DuRant RH, et al: Use of multiple drugs among adolescents who use anabolic steroids. N Engl J Med 328:922–926, 1993.
41. Kramhoft M, Solgaard S: Spontaneous rupture of the extensor pollicis longus tendon after anabolic steroids. J Hand Surg 11(1):87, 1986.
42. Back BR, et al: Triceps rupture: A case report and literature review. Am J Sports Med 15(3):285-289, 1987.
43. Kiraly CL, et al: Effect of testosterone and anabolic steroids on the size of sebaceous glands in power athletes. Am J Dermatopathol 96(6):515–519, 1987.
44. Sklarek H, et al: AIDS in a bodybuilder using anabolic steroids [correspondence]. N Engl J Med 311:1701. 1984.
45. Maropis C, Yesalis CE: Intramuscular abscess—another anabolic steroid danger. Phys Sportsmed 22(10):105–108, 1994.
46. Leckman JF, Scahill L: Possible exacerbation of tics by androgenic steroids [letter]. N Engl J Med 322: 1674, 1990.
47. Calabrese LH, Kleiner SM, Lombardo JA: The effect of anabolic steroids on the immune response in male body builders. Med Sci Sports Exerc 19(suppl):S52, 1987.
48. Macintyre JG: Growth hormone and athletes. Sports Med 4:129–142, 1987.
49. Ahren K, et al: Cellular mechanisms of the acute stimulatory effect of growth hormone. In Pecile, Muller (eds): Growth Hormone and Related Polypeptides. Proceedings of the 3rd International Symposium, Milan, 1975. Amsterdam, Excerpta Medica, 1975.
50. Goldberg AL: Work induced growth of skeletal muscle in normal and hypophysectomized rats. Am J Physiol 213(5):1193–1198, 1967.
51. Kostyo JL, Reagan CR: The biology of growth hormone. Pharmacol Therap 2:591–604, 1976.
52. Goldberg AL: Relationship between growth hormone and muscle work in determining muscle size. J Physiol 216:655–666, 1969.
53. Salomon F, Cuneo RC, Hesp R, et al: The effects of treatment with recombinant human growth hormone on body composition and metabolism with growth hormone deficiency. N Engl J Med 321:1797–1803, 1989.
54. Underwood LE: Report of the conference on uses and possible abuses of biosynthetic human growth hormone. N Engl J Med 311:606–608, 1984.
55. Spilotis BE, et al: Growth hormone neurosecretory dysfunction: A treatable cause of short stature. JAMA 251:2223–2330, 1984.
56. VanVliet G, et al: Growth hormone treatment for short stature. N Engl J Med 309:1016–1022, 1983.
57. Recombinant human growth hormone. Med Lett 36(930):77–78, 1994.
58. Ad Hoc Committee on Growth Hormone Usage, the Lawson Wilkins Pediatric Endocrine Society, and the Committee on Drugs: Growth hormone in the treatment of children with short stature. Pediatrics 72: 891–894, 1983.
59. Koch TK, et al: Creutzfeldt-Jakob disease in a young adult with idiopathic hypopituitarism: Possible relation to the administration of cadaveric human growth hormone. N Engl J Med 313:731–733, 1985.
60. Lombardo JA: Stimulants and athletic performance: Amphetamines and caffeine. Phys Sportsmed 14(11): 128–139, 1986.
61. Mandell AJ: The Sunday syndrome: A unique pattern of amphetamine use indigenous to American professional football. Clin Toxicol 15(2):225–232, 1979.
62. Derlet RW, Beischober B: Methamphetamine: Stimulant of the 1990's? West J Med 153:625, 1990.
63. Smith GM, Beecher HK: Amphetamine sulfate and athletic performance. JAMA 170:542–557, 1959.
64. Chandler JV, Blair SN: The effects of amphetamines on selected physiological components related to athletic success. Med Sci Sports Exerc 12:65–69, 1980.
65. Cantwell JD, Rose FD: Cocaine and cardiovascular events. Phys Sportsmed 14(11):77–82, 1986.
66. Warner EA: Cocaine abuse. Ann Intern Med 119:226–235, 1993.
67. Kunkel DB: Cocaine then and now: Part 1. Emerg Med June 15, 1986, pp 125–138.
68. Roth D, et al: Acute rhabdomyolysis associated with cocaine intoxication. N Engl J Med 319:673–677, 1988.
69. Goodwin M: In sport, cocaine's here to stay. New York Times, May 3, 1987, (sect. 5), p 1.
70. Cregler L, Mark H: Special report: Medical complications of cocaine abuse. N Engl J Med 315: 1495–1500, 1986.
71. Kunkel DB: Cocaine then and now: Part II. Emerg Med July 15, 1986, pp 168–173.
72. Gawin FH, Ellinwood EH: Cocaine and other stimulants. N Engl J Med 318:1173–1182, 1988.
73. Isner JM, et al: Acute cardiac events temporally related to cocaine abuse. N Engl J Med 315:1438–1443, 1986.
74. Patel RC, et al: Free-base cocaine use associated with bronchiolitis obliterans organizing pneumonia. Ann Intern Med 107(2):186–187, 1987.

75. Giammarco RA: The athlete, cocaine, and lactic acidosis: A hypothesis. Am J Med Sci 294(6): 412–414, 1987.
76. Kelly KP, et al: Cocaine and exercise: physiological responses of cocaine-conditioned rats. Med Sci Sports Exerc 27(1):65–72, 1995.
77. Gilman AG, Goodman LS, Rall TW, Murad F (eds): Goodman and Gilman's The Pharmacologic Basis of Therapeutics, 7th ed. New York, Macmillan, 1985.
78. Laurin CA, Letorneau G: Medical report on the Montreal olympic games. Am J Sports Med 6:54–61, 1978.
79. Tarnopolsky MA: Caffeine and endurance performance. Sports Med 18(2):109–125, 1994.
80. Ivy JL, et al: Role of caffeine and glucose ingestion on metabolism during exercise. Med Sci Sports Exerc 10:66, 1978.
81. Welch JM, et al: Effect of caffeine on skeletal muscle function before and after fatigue. J Applied Physiol 54:1303–1305, 1983.
82. Butts NK, Crowell D: Effects of caffeine ingestion on cardiorespiratory endurance in men and women. Res Q Exerc Sport 56(4): 301–305, 1985.
83. Casal DC, Leon AS: Failure of caffeine to affect substrate utilization during prolonged running. Med Sci Sports Exerc 17:174–179, 1985.
84. Van Der Merwe PJ, et al: Caffeine in sport: Urinary excretion of caffeine in healthy volunteers after intake of common caffeine-containing beverages. South Afr Med J 74:163–164, 1988.
85. Duthel JM, et al: Caffeine and sport: role of physical exercise upon elimination. Med Sci Sports Exerc 23(8):980–985, 1991.
86. De Meersman R, et al: The effects of a sympathomimetic drug on maximal aerrobic activity. J Sports Med 26:251–257, 1986.
87. Sidney KH, Lefoe NM: The effects of Tedral upon athletic performance: A double blind cross-over study. Quebec City International Congress of Physical Activity Sciences, 1976.
88. DeMeersman R, Getty D, Schaefer DC: Sympathomimetics and exercise enhancement: All in the mind? Pharmacol Biochem Behav 28:361–365, 1987.
89. Schlesser JL (ed): Drugs Available Abroad. London, Derwent Publications Ltd., 1991.
90. Spann C, Winter ME: Effect of Clenbuterol on athletic performance. Ann Pharmacother 29:75–78, 1995.
91. Maltin CA, Delday MI, Hay SM, Baillie GS. Denervation increases clenbuterol sensitivity in muscle from young rats. Muscle Nerve 14:188–192, 1992.
92. Zeman RJ, et al: Clenbuterol, a beta 2 receptor agonist, reduces net bone loss in denervated hindlimbs. Am J Physiol 261:E285–289, 1991.
93. Maltin CA, et al: Clenbuterol, a beta adrenoceptor agonist, increases relative muscle strength in orthopedic patients. Clin Sci 84:651–654, 1993.
94. Polettini A, Ricossa MC, Groppi A, Montagna M: Determination of clenbuterol in urine as its cyclic boronate derivative by gas chromatography-mass spectrometry. J Chromatogr 564:529–535, 1991.
95. Amadio P, Cummings DM: Nonsteroidal anti-inflammatory agents: An update. Am Fam Phys 34(4):147–154, 1986.
96. Loeb DS, Ahlquist DA, Tally NJ: Management of gastroduodenopathy associated with use of nonsteroidal anti-inflammatory drugs. Mayo Clin Proc 67:354–364, 1992.
97. Day RO: Effects of exercise performance on drugs used in musculoskeletal disorders. Med Sci Sports Exerc 13:272–275, 1981.
98. Butt JH, Barthel JS, Moore RA: Clinical spectrum of upper gastrointestinal effects of nonsteroidal anti-inflammatory drugs. Am J Med 84(suppl 2A):5–14, 1988.
99. Tremaine WJ, Kwo PY: Nonsteroidal anti-inflammatory drug-induced enteropathy: Case discussion and review of the literature. Mayo Clin Proc 70:55–61, 1995.
100. Walker RJ, Fawcett JP, Flannery EM, Gerrard DF: Indomethacin potentiates exercise-induced reduction in renal hemodynamics in athletes. Med Sci Sports Exerc 26(11):1302–1306, 1994.
101. Millhorn HT: The diagnosis of alcoholism. Am Fam Phys 37(6):175–183, 1988.
102. American College of Sports Medicine: Position statement on the use of alcohol in sports. Med Sci Sports Exerc 14:ix–x, 1982.
103. Urbano-Marquez A, et al: The effects of alcoholism on skeletal and cardiac muscle. N Engl J Med 320:409–415, 1989.
104. Brewer RD, et al: The risk of dying in alcohol-related automobile crashes among habitual drunk drivers. N Engl J Med 331:513–517, 1994.
105. Buchsbaum DG, et al: Screening for alcohol abuse using the CAGE scores and likelihood ratios. Ann Intern Med 115:774–777, 1991.
106. Stedman's Medical Dictionary, 26th ed. Baltimore, Williams & Wilkins Company, 1995.
107. Glover ED, Edmundson EW, Edwards SW, Schroeder KL: Implications of smokeless tobacco use among athletes. Phys Sports Med 14(12):95–105, 1986.
108. Barry M. Sounding Board: The Marlboro Grand Prix. N Engl J Med 324(13):913–919, 1991.
109. Bergert N: The dangers of smokeless tobacco. Sports Med Digest 11(6):1–8, 1989
110. Benowitz NL: Pharmacologic aspects of cigarette smoking and nicotine addiction. N Engl J Med 319(20): 1318–1330, 1988.

111. Connolly GN, Orleans CT, Kogan M: Use of smokeless tobacco in major-league baseball. N Engl J Med 318(19):1281–1284, 1988.
112. Edwards SW, Glover ED, Schroeder KL: The effects of smokeless tobacco on heart rate and neuromuscular reactivity in athletes and nonathletes. Phys Sports Med 15(7):141–146, 1987.
113. National Cancer Institute: Beat the smokeless habit: Game plan for success. Washington, DC, U.S. Department of Health and Human Services, 1991.
114. Tashkin DP, Gong H, Fligiel SEG: How the lungs are affected by marijuana smoke. J Respir Dis 8(11): 87–107, 1987.
115. Powell DR: Does marijuana smoke cause lung cancer? Primary Care Cancer October, 1987, p 15.
116. Biron S, Wells J: Marijuana and its effects on the athlete. Athlet Train 18:295–303, 1983.
117. Renaud AM, Cormier Y: Acute effects of marihuana smoking on maximal exercise performance. Med Sci Sports Exerc 18(6):685–689, 1986.
118. Pace N, Lozner EL, Consolazio WV, et al: The increase in hypoxia tolerance of normal men accompanying the polycythemia induced by transfusion of erythrocytes. Am J Physiol 148:152–163, 1947.
119. Scarpino V, Arrigo A, Benzi G, et al: Evaluation of prevalence of "doping" among Italian athletes. Lancet 336:1048–1050, 1990.
120. Klein HG: Sounding board: Blood transfusion and athletics. N Engl J Med 312:854–856, 1985.
121. Buick FJ, et al: Effect of induced erythrocythemia on aerobic work capacity. J Appl Physiol 48:636–642, 1980.
122. American College of Sports Medicine Position Stand: Blood doping as an eregogenic aid. Phys Sportsmed 16(1):131–134, 1988.
123. Berglund B, Birgegard G, Wide L, Pihlstedt P: Effects of blood transfusions on some hematological variables in endurance athletes. Med Sci Sports Exerc 21(6):637–642, 1989.
124. Erslev AJ, et al: The biogenesis of rrythropoietin. Exp Hematol 8(suppl 8):1–13, 1980.
125. Beck WS (ed): Hematology, 3rd ed. Cambridge, MA, M.I.T. Press, 1981.
126. Goldingay R: Potential for abuse of recombinant erythropoietin. Sports Med Dig 11(11):5, 1989.
127. Adamson JW, Vapnek D: Recombinant erythropoietin to improve athletic performance. N Engl J Med 324:698–699, 1991.
128. Ekblom B, Berglund B: Effect of erythropoietin administration on maximal aerobic power. Scand J Med Sci Sports 1:88–93, 1991.
129. Eschbach JW, et al: Correction of the anemia of end-stage renal disease with recombinant human erythropoietin. N Engl J Med 316:73–78, 1987.
130. Mayer G, et al: Working capacity is increased following recombinant human erythropoietin treatment. Kidney Int 34:525–528, 1988.
131. Casati S, Passerini P, Campise MR, et al: Benefits and risks of protracted treatment with human recombinant erythropoietin in patients having hemodialysis. BMJ 295:1017–1020, 1987.
132. Erslev AJ. Erythropoietin. N Engl J Med 324:1339–1344, 1991.
133. Ludwig H, et al: Erythropoietin treatment of anemia associated with multiple myeloma. N Engl J Med 322:1693–1699, 1990.
134. Fischl M, et al: Recombinant human erythropoietin for patients with AIDS treated with zidovudine. N Engl J Med 322:1488–1493, 1990.
135. Goodnough LT, Rudnick S, Price T, et al: Erythropoietin therapy in autologous blood donors. Blood 72(suppl 1):118a, 1988.
136. Canadian Orthopedic Perioperative Erythropoietin Study Group: Effectiveness of perioperative recombinant erythropoietin in elective hip replacement. Lancet 341:1227–1232, 1993.
137. Steinberg H, Stead RB: Erythropoietin and visual hallucinations [letters]. N Engl J Med 325:285, 1991.
138. American College of Sports Medicine: Drugs and sport: Is a level playing field possible? Panel Discussion at American College of Sports Medicine Annual Meeting, Dallas, 1991.
139. Gamma hydroxy butyrate poisoning. Med Lett 33(836):8, 1991.
140. MMWR: Multistate outbreak of poisonings associated with illicit use of GHB. JAMA 25:447–478, 1991.
141. Self-proclaimed 'Steroid Guru' of Venice guilty. The Evening Outlook, Venice, CA, April 18, 1992.
142. Chin MY, Kreutzer RA: Acute poisoning from GHB in California. West J Med 156:380–384, 1992.
143. Lane RB, Auerbach SB, Noji EK, Falk H: Gamma hydroxy butyrate [letter]. JAMA 265:2959, 1991.
144. Hansen HJ, et al: Crisis in drug testing: Results of CDC blind study. JAMA 253:2382–2387, 1985.
145. Catlin DH, et al: Analytical chemistry at the games of the XXIIIrd olympiad in Los Angeles, 1984. Clin Chem 33(2):319–327, 1987.
146. de Boer D, De Jong EG, van Rossum JM, Maes RAA: Doping control of testosterone and human chorionic gonadotrophin: A case study. Int J Sports Med 12:46–51, 1991.
147. USOC Drug Education Program: Questions and answers: Committee on Substance Abuse Research and Education, USOC, 1988.
148. Gall SL, Duda M, Giel D, Rogers CC: Who tests which athletes for what drugs? Phys Sportsmed 16(2): 155–161, 1988.

149. 1994–95 NCAA Drug Testing Education Programs. Overland Park, KS, NCAA Publishing, 1994.
150. Coombs RH, Ryan FJ: Drug testing effectiveness in identifying and preventing drug use. Am J Drug Alcohol Abuse 16:173–184, 1990.
151. Albrecht RR, Anderson WA, McKeag DB: Drug testing of college athletes: The issues. Sports Med 14(6):349–352, 1992.
152. Sports Notes. Los Angeles Times, May 3, 1994, p C6.
153. High court OKs routine testing of students for drugs. Los Angeles Times, June 27, 1995, p A1.

23

Eating Disorders

Amanda D. Randall, MSW, LCSW

I. Anorexia Nervosa

A. Essential features and diagnostic criteria

1. **Refusal to maintain body weight** at or above a minimally normal weight for age and height, e.g., weight loss leading to maintenance of body weight less than 85% of that expected, or failure to make expected weight gain during a period of growth leading to body weight less than 85% of that expected
2. **Intense fear of gaining weight** or becoming fat, even though underweight
3. **Disturbance in the way in which one's body weight or shape is experienced,** or undue influence of body weight or shape on self-evaluation, or denial of the seriousness of the current low body weight
4. In postmenarcheal women, **amenorrhea**, i.e., the absence of at least three consecutive menstrual cycles. A woman is considered to have amenorrhea if her periods occur only following hormone, e.g., estrogen, administration.
5. **Subtypes:**
   a. **Restricting type**—during the current episode of anorexia nervosa, the person has not regularly engaged in binge-eating or purging behavior (i.e., self-induced vomiting or the misuse of laxatives, diuretics, or enemas).
   b. **Binge-eating/purging type**—during the current episode of anorexia nervosa, the person has regularly engaged in binge-eating or purging behavior (i.e., self-induced vomiting or the misuse of laxatives, diuretics, or enemas).

B. Medical symptoms

1. Emaciation
2. Constipation, abdominal pain
3. Hypothermia
4. Hypotension
5. Peripheral edema
6. Osteoporosis
7. Lanugo (neonatal-like hair on face or body)
8. Metabolic changes
9. Amenorrhea

C. Associated features

1. Preoccupation with food—discuss food, recipes, issues of nutrition excessively; prepare elaborate meals for others yet limit own intake severely; restrict food categories, such as all fats
2. May conceal, hide, crumble, or throw away food to avoid eating it
3. May engage in purging behavior (self-induced vomiting, use of laxatives or diuretics) following ingestion of small amounts of food
4. Obsessive-compulsive features, both related and unrelated to food, often prominent
5. Minimization of the severity of the illness or body condition
6. Delayed psychosexual development in adolescents and adults; markedly decreased interest in sex
7. Feelings of ineffectiveness, inflexible thinking, a strong need to control one's environment, limited social spontaneity

D. **Age at onset:** early to late adolescence (mean age of onset is 17); can range from prepuberty to over age 40 (rare)
E. **Sex ratio:** predominantly in females (95%)
F. **Prevalence:** among female adolescents and young adults, rates of 0.5–1.0% for anorexia nervosa; individuals with subthreshold for the disorder are more commonly encountered. Limited data on prevalence rates in males.
G. **Course:** may be unremitting until death, episodic, or consist of a single episode
H. **Impairment:** Severe weight loss often necessitates hospitalization to prevent death by starvation.
I. **Mortality rate is greater than 10%.** Death most commonly results from starvation, suicide, or electrolyte imbalance.

II. Bulimia Nervosa

A. **Diagnostic criteria and essential features**
   1. **Recurrent episodes of binge-eating.** An episode is characterized by eating a large amount of food in a discrete period of time (e.g., within any 2-hour period), and by a sense of a lack of control over the eating episode (e.g., an inability to control what or how much is eaten or to stop eating).
   2. **Recurrent inappropriate compensatory behavior to prevent weight gain,** such as self-induced vomiting; misuse of laxatives, diuretics, enemas, or other medications; fasting; or excessive exercise
   3. The **binge-eating and inappropriate compensatory behaviors both occur,** on average, at least twice a week for 3 months.
   4. **Self-evaluation is unduly influenced by body shape and weight.**
   5. **Subtypes:**
      a. **Purging type**—during the current episode of bulimia nervosa, the person has regularly engaged in self-induced vomiting or the misuse of laxatives, diuretics, or enemas.
      b. **Nonpurging type**—during the current episode of bulimia nervosa, the person has used other inappropriate compensatory behaviors, such as fasting or excessive exercise, but has not regularly engaged in self-induced vomiting or the misuse of laxatives, diuretics, or enemas.

B. **Associated features**
   1. Normal weight range—individuals may range from severely underweight to obese, but weight is typically normal.
   2. Increased frequency of mood disorders (anxiety and depression) and substance-abuse disorders, most frequently involving amphetamines, cocaine, alcohol, and sedatives
   3. Excessive exercise is often used to compensate for binge-eating. Exercise is excessive when it interferes with important activities, when it occurs at inappropriate times or in inappropriate settings, or when an individual continues to exercise despite injury or other medical complication.
   4. Eating binges may be planned or spontaneous, with the binge being characterized most by the abnormality in the amount, not the type, of food eaten. Binge-eating usually occurs in secret or as inconspicuously as possible; the binge continues until the individual is uncomfortably or painfully full. Binges may be triggered by dysphoric mood states; interpersonal stressors;, intense hunger following dietary restriction; or feelings related to body weight, shape, and food.
   5. Binge-eating episodes are accompanied by feelings of loss of control and are followed by compensatory behaviors to rid the body of calories.

C. **Age at onset:** adolescence or early adulthood
D. **Course:** may be chronic or intermittent, with periods of remission alternating with recurrences of binge-eating. The long-term outcome is not known.

E. **Impairment and complications**
   1. Significant and severe loss of dental enamel; increased frequency of dental cavities
   2. Electrolyte imbalance with dehydration, which can lead to severe physical complications (cardiac arrhythmia, sudden death). Rare complications include esophageal tears and gastric rupture.

III. Complications of Eating Disorders for Athletes

Anorexia nervosa and bulimia cause the body to feel the **effects of starvation and dehydration**, with the following conditions possible:

A. Loss of muscle strength and endurance
B. Loss of speed and coordination
C. Decreased aerobic power with decreased oxygen utilization
D. Electrolyte loss
E. Impaired judgment
F. Reduced blood volume (with reduced blood flow to the kidneys)
G. Loss of muscle glycogen
H. Inability to regulate body temperature
I. Reduced heart function
J. Increased heart rate
K. Amenorrhea
L. Loss of bone mass during adolescence
M. Increased susceptibility to injury
N. Impaired brain function with irritability, depression, and withdrawal

IV. Common Behaviors Associated with Anorexia Nervosa and Bulimia

Many athletes engage in weight maintenance or reducing behaviors that are time-limited and appropriate to their performance. Not all thin athletes have an eating disorder, just as being at ideal body weight does not indicate that an athlete is necessarily healthy. **However, certain behaviors do merit attention and are often associated with an eating disorder.**

A. Constant preoccupation with and discussion of weight-related and diet-related issues (repetitive comments about "feeling fat")
B. Weight loss below the ideal competitive weight set for that athlete, which continues even off-season
C. Purposeless, excessive physical activity that is not a part of the training program
D. Extreme or frequent weight fluctuations
E. Secretive eating or evidence of secretive eating (candy or food wrappers in inappropriate places; sneaking or stealing food)
F. Avoidance of situations in which the athlete would be observed eating or refusal to eat with or around others
G. Intense concern with nutrition information or the eating patterns of others
H. Vomitus or odor of vomit in restroom, shower, or wastebasket areas
I. Bloodshot or watery eyes, especially after using the restroom or areas where vomiting could have occurred
J. Complaints or evidence of bloating or edema not explained by medical cause or premenstrual water retention
K. Frequent constipation or diarrhea
L. Lightheadedness, disequilibrium (loss of balance), and mood swings not attributed to any medical cause

V. Treatment for Eating Disorders

A. **An eating disorder is a complex psychological and physiologic problem that should be diagnosed and treated by a physician, psychologist, and nutritionist**

trained in the field. However, coaches and trainers need to be aware of the behaviors that suggest the athlete has an eating disorder and be informed of the resources for treatment. Athletes who exhibit behaviors associated with an eating disorder need to be confronted with the specific observations relating to their behaviors. **Referral to an appropriate treatment program is essential for recovery of the athlete.**

B. **Treatment generally consists of a thorough physical, psychological, and nutritional assessment process. Individual, group, and family psychotherapy and nutritional education therapy are required for effective treatment of an eating disorder.** Treatment is often provided on an outpatient basis.

C. **For athletes in serious physical condition (severe symptoms of chemical imbalances, dangerously low body weight, or a severe binging/purging cycle), inpatient hospitalization and treatment may be necessary.** Periods of inpatient hospitalization may be followed by outpatient aftercare treatment; multiple episodes of hospitalization are not uncommon because of the long-term nature of the disorders.

VI. Prevention

An eating disorder is associated with underlying emotional distress and is not caused by athletic training or participation. Young athletes with an intense desire to succeed and please the coach and trainer can be strongly influenced by comments or behaviors directed toward weight or dieting. Eating disorders in athletes can be reduced by using the following general guidelines:

A. Emphasize the role of overall, long-term good nutrition and weight control in optimizing athletic performance.

B. Do not overly focus on the effect of lower body weight on athletic performance.

C. Set realistic goals that address methods of dieting, rate of weight change, and a *reasonable* target weight for the athlete.

D. **Never suggest or encourage the use of laxatives, diuretics, or purging behavior to reduce or maintain weight.**

E. Be aware of the behaviors associated with eating disorders, and refer athletes for professional help when appropriate.

24

Overtraining

J. B. Ketner, M.D.

Overtraining is a well-documented but poorly understood syndrome in which the athlete's training program exceeds the body's ability to adapt. The result is a symptom complex including decreased performance, generalized fatigue, frequent illness and injuries, and a decline in overall sense of well-being. Complete resolution may take weeks to months.

I. Training Principles and Overtraining

A. **Supercompensation**
   1. Overload stimulus is applied to improve strength or endurance.
   2. Fatigue temporarily reduces functional capacity.
   3. After recovery and regeneration, performance is enhanced.

B. **Genesis of overtraining**
   1. Overload stimulus is excessive.
   2. Recovery time is insufficient.
   3. Large training loads are applied while the athlete is still fatigued or inadequately recovered.
   4. In this setting, overtraining with decreased performance results rather than supercompensation and increased performance.
   5. A delicate balance exists between supercompensation and overtraining.

C. **Variability of athlete response**
   1. Individuals vary greatly in their ability to tolerate training loads.
   2. Outside stressors and life events play a role.
   3. Broad application of rigid overload stimuli is likely to be beneficial for some athletes and detrimental for others.
   4. Career prevalence in elite distance runners may be as high as 60%.

II. Terminology and Definitions

A. **Overload training** is the process of stressing an individual to provide a stimulus for adaptation and supercompensation. This includes increasing training volume and/or intensity beyond that to which the athlete is accustomed.

B. **Training fatigue**, or acute fatigue, is the normal response experienced following 1 or several days of heavy training associated with an overload stimulus.

C. **Overtraining** is the process of training at abnormally high levels of volume or intensity. According to some authorities, this term also includes performance decrements accompanying this stressful training process.

D. **Overreaching** is a form of overtraining that follows short-term intensive training. It is often a planned phase of a periodized training program. Symptoms of overreaching can be reversed by a longer than normal regeneration period.

E. **Overtraining syndrome** or "staleness" refers to the final stage in a proposed continuum of increasingly severe chronic fatigue states that develop as a result of overtraining (Fig. 1). Symptoms associated with overtraining include decreased performance.

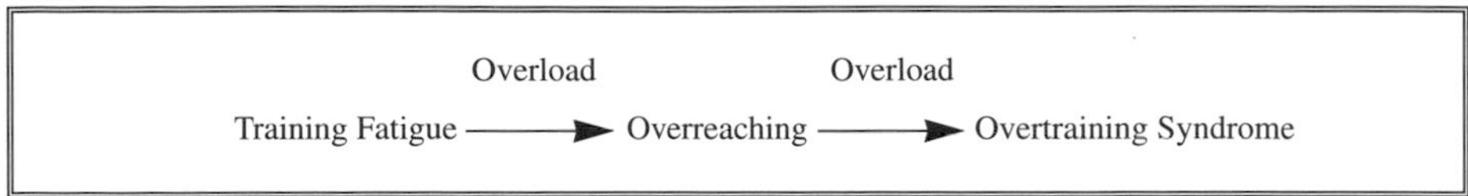

FIGURE 1. Overtraining continuum. (Modified from Van Borselen F, Vos NH, Fry AL, Kraemer WJ: The role of anaerobic exercise in overtraining. NSCA J 14:74–79, 1992.)

F. **Muscular overstrain** is acute tissue damage induced by a single intensive training session that exceeds the athlete's muscular stress tolerance. This generally occurs after single or repeated bouts of excessive exercise that result in damage to muscle fibers. Muscular overstrain does not always accompany overreaching or overtraining.

III. Sympathetic and Parasympathetic Overtraining

The German literature has historically categorized overtraining based on the predominant symptoms exhibited. Many athletes display features of both types of overtraining, and this categorization appears somewhat artificial.

A. **Sympathetic overtraining**
   1. Associated with symptoms of restlessness, excitation, poor sleep, weight loss, tachycardia, hypertension, poor appetite, and irritability
   2. Found in anaerobic sports in which speed, strength, and coordination are stressed

B. **Parasympathetic overtraining**
   1. Associated with depression, bradycardia, hypotension, poor appetite, somnolence, fatigue, and decreased hypoglycemic counterregulatory capacity
   2. Found in aerobic sports and high-volume training

C. **Modern overtraining**
   1. Represents an amalgam of sympathetic and parasympathetic overtraining
   2. Most athletes have predominantly parasympathetic-type symptoms.

IV. Clinical Features of Overtraining

A. Many symptoms are attributed to overtraining. Invariably the athlete is fatigued and performance declines. **Resting heart rate** and heart rate recovery following exercise often **increase**. Severe muscle soreness is common. Illness and injuries occur with increased frequency (Table 1).

B. Because of **individual variation**, few if any overtrained athletes exhibit all of the symptoms and signs associated with overtraining.

C. No laboratory test has been found to diagnose or predict overtraining reliably.

D. Highly motivated athletes appear more susceptible and frequently respond to poor performance by increasing their training loads, thus initiating a vicious cycle of training imbalance.

TABLE 1. Common Problems in Overtrained Athletes

Psychological	Physiologic	Performance
Fatigue	Increased basal heart rate	Decreased maximum work output
Loss of motivation	Increased resting blood pressure	Prolonged reaction time
Poor sleep	Weight loss	Increased perceived exertion at a given workload
Poor appetite	Chronic muscle soreness	Decreased coordination
Depression	"Heavy-legged" feeling	
Loss of confidence	Frequent illnesses and injuries	
	Excessive thirst	
	Postural hypotension	

V. Pathophysiology of Overtraining

A. **Cardiovascular aspects.** Most studies of overtrained athletes have demonstrated increased resting heart rates relative to the athlete's baseline.
  1. **Left ventricular fatigue** may play a role. Studies have shown decreased stroke volume and altered contractility in ultraendurance athletes.
  2. **Decreased plasma volume** and dehydration may account for cardiovascular changes in a subset of overtraining athletes.

B. **Hormonal aspects of overtraining**
  1. **Hypothalamic dysfunction**
    a. Barron and colleagues[1] demonstrated impaired plasma cortisol, ACTH, growth hormone, and prolactin responses to insulin-induced hypoglycemia when compared to controls.
    b. Intense, prolonged exercise produces a luteinizing hormone secretion pattern similar to that found in hypothalamic amenorrhea.
    c. GnRH secretion is decreased in some overtrained athletes.
  2. **Testosterone and cortisol**
    a. Testosterone levels decrease as athletes become overtrained.
    b. Often, cortisol levels increase as testosterone levels fall.
    c. **Testosterone-to-cortisol ratio** may reflect anabolic/catabolic hormone balance. A decrease in this ratio may signal catabolic excess and herald the onset of overtraining.
  3. **Catecholamines**
    a. Many athletes show decreased nocturnal catecholamine release as they become overtrained, possibly indicating reduced sympathetic nervous system activity.
    b. Exercise-related catecholamines often **increase** from baseline values in contrast to nocturnal levels.
    c. It is speculated that central hypothalamic dopamine inhibition may play a role in reducing intrinsic sympathetic activity in overtraining.

C. **Muscular aspects of overtraining**
  1. **Muscle fatigue**—overtrained athletes complain of fatigue at previously tolerated exercise levels. Several studies have shown increased submaximal and maximal lactate values in underperforming overtrained competitors.
    a. Suboptimal carbohydrate intake may lead to decreased muscle glycogen and premature fatigue.
    b. Decreased sympathetic drive may alter glycogenolysis.
  2. **Delayed-onset muscle soreness (DOMS)** is a syndrome that clearly overlaps with overtraining syndrome.
    a. **Syndrome characteristics:**
      i. Severe muscle soreness and swelling
      ii. Increased creatinine kinase levels
      iii. Soreness peaks 2–3 days after inciting bout of exercise
      iv. Common in athletes initiating unaccustomed exercise and high-performance athletes
    b. **Mechanisms:**
      i. **Eccentric movements** (simultaneous elongation and contraction of muscle fibers), such as downhill running, are particularly damaging.
      ii. Damage leads to inflammatory response.
    c. **Adaptation and DOMS:**
      i. Repeated bouts of eccentric exercise provide a protective effect against subsequent episodes of DOMS.
      ii. Planned, intermittent, sport-specific eccentric exercise may reduce disability associated with DOMS.

d. **Importance of DOMS in the overtraining syndrome**
   i. Athletes, coaches, and physicians need to recognize DOMS when it occurs.
   ii. Adequate regeneration can alleviate discomfort and possibly reduce the athlete's risk of injury.
   iii. The adaptive phenomenon can be used prophylactically in training programs.
   iv. Fatigue, decreased muscle glycogen, and propensity for injury are prominent features of both DOMS and the overtraining syndrome.

D. **Psychological aspects of overtraining**
1. Numerous studies have demonstrated that dramatic increases in training volume lead to undesirable **mood changes**.
   a. Increases in fatigue, depression, anger, and global mood disturbance are common as measured by the Profile of Mood States.
   b. Depression can reach clinical significance.
   c. Mood changes increase in direct proportion to training loads and regress with rest.
2. **Tryptophan** may cause central fatigue in overtrained athletes.
   a. Strenuous exercise causes increases in the plasma free tryptophan-to-branched chain amino acid ratio, which, in turn, may give rise to an increase in central nervous system 5-hydroxytryptamine (serotonin) synthesis.
   b. Serotonin is the neurotransmitter responsible for sleep and has been implicated in endogenous depression.

E. **Overtraining and immunity**
1. Highly stressed and overtrained athletes demonstrate increased susceptibility to infectious disease.
2. **Glutamine hypothesis**
   a. Cells of the immune system rely on glutamine for energy.
   b. Muscle tissue is the body's main glutamine source.
   c. One study has shown that overtrained athletes demonstrate decreased plasma glutamine compared to controls.
   d. Specific amino acid supplementation may prevent this glutamine depletion; however, further research is needed in this area.

VI. Detection and Prevention

A. As athletes continue to test the limits of human performance, overtraining and its attendant complications will continue to be a problem.

B. **Proper coaching and training techniques can help prevent overtraining.**
1. **Balance** and **individualization** of workouts is critical.
2. Outside sources of stress should be considered (i.e., finances, scholastics, relationships).
3. Many athletes respond to performance slumps with dramatic increases in training volume or intensity, when in reality they may need rest.
4. Monotony of training and the practice of performing extra workouts when the athlete "feels good" should be avoided.
5. Periodized training that counters heavy work periods with adequate periods of rest appears to reduce the incidence of overtraining.
6. Resistance training should be increased by no more then 5% per week.

C. **Monitoring**
1. Detailed personal logs, with both subjective and objective measurements, are recommended.
2. Data should be compared to previous **individual** measurements rather than group norms.

3. **Parameters used in detection**
   a. Decreased performance
   b. Weight loss
   c. Increased resting heart rate
   d. Decline in general health
   e. Increased thirst and evening fluid intake
   f. Poor sleep or later time to bed
   g. Decrease in mood as measured by the Profile of Mood States
   h. Increased resting heart rate, poor sleep, later time to bed may be most sensitive indicators

VII. Treatment

A. **Overtraining syndrome**
   1. Training should stop for a period of several weeks to months.
   2. Absolute rest period may vary based on severity.
   3. Detraining studies have shown that major cuts can be made in frequency and duration of exercise while maintaining performance. One study of overtrained athletes found that performance actually improved following 3 to 5 weeks of complete rest.

B. **Overreaching or short-term overtraining.** Relative rest with judicious use of noncompetitive exercise may be appropriate.

Recommended Reading

1. Barron JL, Noakes TD, Levy W, et al: Hypothalamic dysfunction in overtrained athletes. J Clin Endocrinol Metab 60:803–806, 1985.
2. Brown RL, Frederick EC, Falsetti HL, et al: Overtraining of athletes. Phys Sportsmed 11:93–110, 1983.
3. Budgett R: Overtraining syndrome. Br J Sports Med 24:231–236, 1990.
4. Costill DL, Flynn MG, Kirwan JP, et al: Effects of repeated days of intensified training on muscle glycogen and swimming performance. Med Sci Sports Exerc 20:249–254, 1988.
5. Fry RW, Morton AR, Keast D: Periodisation and the prevention of overtraining. Can J Sport Sci 17:241–248, 1992.
6. Ketner JB, Mellion MB: The overtraining syndrome: A review of presentation, pathophysiology, and treatment Med Exerc Nutr Health 4:138–147, 1995.
7. Koutedakis Y, Budgett R, Faulmann L: Rest in underperforming elite competitors. Br J Sports Med 24:248–252, 1990.
8. Lehmann M, Foster C, Keul J: Overtraining in endurance athletes: A brief review. Med Sci Sports Exerc 25:854–862, 1993.
9. Lehmann M, Gastmann U, Petersen KG, et al: Training–overtraining: Performance, and hormone levels, after a defined increase in training volume versus intensity in experienced middle- and long-distance runners. Br J Sports Med 26:233–242, 1992.
10. Lehmann M, Schnee W, Scheu R, et al: Decreased nocturnal catecholamine excretion: Parameter for an overtraining syndrome in athletes? Int J Sports Med 13:236–242, 1992.
11. Morgan WP, Brown DR, Raglin JS, et al: Psychological monitoring of overtraining and staleness. Br J Sports Med 21:107–114, 1987.
12. Parry-Billings M, Blomstrand E, McAndrew N, Newsholme EA: A communicational link between skeletal muscle, brain, and cells of the immune system. Int J Sports Med 11:S122–S128, 1990.
13. Parry-Billings M. Budgett R, Koutedakis Y, et al: Plasma amino acid concentrations in the overtraining syndrome: possible effects on the immune system. Med Sci Sports Exerc 24:1353–1358, 1992.
14. Raglin JS, Morgan WP, O'Connor PJ: Changes in mood states during training in female and male college swimmers. Int J Sports Med 12:585–589, 1991.
15. Sharp NCC, Koutedakis Y: Sport and the overtraining syndrome: Immunological aspects. Br Med Bull 48:518–533, 1992.
16. Smith LL: Causes of delayed onset muscle soreness and the impact on athletic performance: a review. J Appl Sport Sci Res 6:135–141, 1992.
17. Stone MH, Keith RE, Kearney JT, et al: Overtraining: A review of the signs, symptoms and possible causes. J Appl Sport Sci Res 5:35–50, 1991.
18. Van Borselen F, Vos NH, Fry AC, Kraemer WJ: The role of anaerobic exercise in overtraining. NSCA J 14:74–79, 1992.

25

Exercise Addiction

Morris B. Mellion, M.D., and Melinda D. Burst, B.S.

An emaciated 45-year-old man runs 210 miles a week. He runs in gale winds, sleet, or lightning. Each evening he consumes an 8000-calorie carbohydrate load and sleeps for a few hours. At 1:30 A.M., he awakens to run 15 miles on a course that is always the same. He reaches each milepost on schedule, checking his time by clocks in the windows of all-night bars and diners along the way. He has previously broken bones from stumbling on rocks in the dark. On one occasion, he was hit by a car. On another, he was struck by a bottle as he was passing a bar fight. He has been harassed by passing motorists and the police. He completes his run at 4:30 A.M. and goes to work at 8 o'clock. He avoids parties and relationships because they might interfere with his running. His life clearly revolves around the run. When asked he proclaims, "I never felt better in my life."

Yates A: Understanding and helping the compulsive athlete.
J Musculoskeletal Med 9(3):45–59, 1992.

I. Exercise and the Criteria for an Addictive Substance

A. **Exercise can produce pleasurable emotions that lead to continued administration.**

1. **General affective benefits**
   a. Joy of motion
   b. Increased sense of control
   c. Improved mental outlook and self-image
   d. Satisfaction with improved appearance and fitness level
   e. Increased energy
   f. Relief of tension
   g. Relief of depression
2. **Runner's high**
   a. **Definition:** a euphoria or state of general relaxation experienced late in a long, slow distance run or sometimes after the run. Described by Wagemaker and Goldstein as "a lifting of spirits and a feeling of harmony with one's surroundings."
      i. Occurs almost exclusively in well-conditioned runners
      ii. Weekly mileage generally 20 or more miles
      iii. Usually starts after many months of running
   b. **Theoretical basis.** Although there are no well-proven explanations for runner's high, there are several hypotheses, which also may apply to the affective benefits of vigorous exercise. Morgan has provided three and Wagemaker and Goldstein a fourth.
      i. **Distraction hypothesis:** proposes that distraction from stressful stimuli produces the affective changes associated with exercise. The exercise itself merely serves as a distraction from the stressors in the runner's life.
      ii. **Monoamine hypothesis:** based on the observation that exercise stimulates increased production of norepinephrine and increased brain uptake of this neurotransmitter, thereby producing an elevated effect. Well-conditioned athletes may be doubly sensitive to this process because they may produce

proportionately more norepinephrine than epinephrine and may have increased receptor sensitivity.

iii. **Endorphin hypothesis:** suggests that the endogenous morphine-like compounds beta-endorphin, met-enkephalin, and leu-enkephalin, known as endorphins, elevate mood and reduce pain. Exercise stimulates central and peripheral endorphin release.

iv. **Right brain/left brain hypothesis:**

(a) The left brain ordinarily performs verbal thinking, which is analytical, and the right brain performs image thinking, which is much more free-form.

(b) Wagemaker and Goldstein noted that in mentally fatigued or emotionally upset individuals, most electroencephalographic (EEG) activity takes place on the right side of the brain. When tired or stressed, individuals may find it difficult to perform verbal or analytical thinking using the left side of the brain. Called right-left confusion, this phenomenon represents "the inability to change from image thinking on the right side to verbal thinking on the left side of the brain."

(c) 25–35 minutes of jogging reversed right-left confusion in an EEG study permitting an appropriate switch from image to verbal thinking.

B. **Tolerance develops**

1. **Definition** (Stedman's Medical Dictionary): "The ability to endure or be less responsive to a stimulus, especially over a period of continued exposure."
2. Tolerance develops to running and other exercise when used as a means of feeling good. Over time, it takes more and more exercise to feel good.
3. Ultimately, it may take even more exercise to prevent feeling bad.
4. **Exercise may become an end in itself.** Endurance exercise, particularly running, may start as a means of improving health, controlling weight, reducing depression, or obtaining social benefit. The habitual exerciser who fails to exercise may experience a level of depression far worse than any negative affect present before starting the exercise program.

C. **Withdrawal**

1. Habitual runners and other habitual endurance athletes who stop exercising may experience a broad range of symptoms.
   a. Anxiety
   b. Restlessness
   c. Depression
   d. Sleep disturbance
   e. Irritability
   f. Nervousness
   g. Guilt
   h. Muscle twitching
   i. Bloated feeling
2. These symptoms can be relieved by reinstituting the exercise activity at the same or increased level.

II. Exercise—Positive or Negative Addiction?

A. **Positive addiction**

1. Glasser was the first to associate addiction with exercise, in 1976. He proposed running and meditation as forms of attainable positive addiction.
   a. Resulting in increased **energy, enthusiasm,** and even mystical **self-transcendence** that may strengthen and make one's life more satisfying. Long distance runners and exercise addicts tend to have an increased hypnotic susceptibility and can easily dissociate themselves from cognitive sensations such as bodily pain and temperature.
   b. Replacing dysfunctional or self-defeating behaviors
2. Exercise addiction viewed as an **extension of normal behavior**

B. **Negative addiction**
  1. In 1979, Morgan demonstrated that for many runners the positive addiction evolved into a **distortion of normal behavior**, which he called a negative addiction.
  2. At first, the formerly sedentary runner enjoys many positive psychological changes. **With time, however, daily exercise is no longer a matter of choice but necessity.** It is "as much a part of the jogger's life as cigarettes for the pack-a-day smoker, alcohol for the alcoholic, and heroin for the mainliner." It becomes the dominant force.
  3. **Three signals of negative addiction**
    a. Less attention to family and other personal relationships
    b. Less concern with external issues, such as work
    c. "Feeling good becomes more important than anything else"
  4. **Ultimate test of addiction to exercise: How does the individual respond when advised to stop exercising because of significant illness or injury?**

C. **The obligatory runner: an insightful model**
  1. In 1983, Yates and coworkers described "obligatory runners" and compared them to anorexics. Although the comparison raises more questions than it answers, it provides many useful insights.
  2. Obligatory runner is "a person who is **not** able to **not** run"
    a. Became committed to running at a time of anxiety, depression, or identity crisis
    b. Lack of exercise produces anger and depression
    c. Ritualistic preoccupation with running
    d. Minimizes or denies pain and injury and continues to run
  3. Shared characteristics with anorexics
    a. Upper middle class
    b. High achievers and competitors
    c. Personality characteristics:
      i. Discomfort with anger
      ii. Restlessness
      iii. Tolerance of physical discomfort
      iv. Introversion
      v. Social isolationism
      vi. Obsessive rumination
      vii. Tendency to depression
    d. "The leaner the better" mentality
    e. Denial of emaciation
    f. Meticulous dieting
  4. **Semistarvation: a proposed physiologic-psychological connection.** Yates suggests that the obligatory runner exhibits some psychological sequelae of a semistarvation state resulting from prolonged caloric restriction combined with increased energy expenditure. Citing the work of Keyes on the biology of starvation, he notes that "when normal persons are starved, they become seclusive, somber, constricted, and compulsive."

III. Diagnosis

A. **Risk factors**
  1. Exercising 7 days weekly
  2. Exercising twice daily
  3. Participating in sports that place a high value on leanness, muscularity, or graceful movement, such as:
    a. Running
    b. Dance
    c. Gymnastics
    d. Figure skating
    e. Swimming and diving

B. **Diagnostic criteria:** none generally accepted. Therefore, information available is often confusing. See Table 1.

TABLE 1. Proposed Diagnostic Criteria for Exercise Addiction

Criteria (Modified from De Coverley Veale)
Restriction of activities to follow a daily or even more frequent exercise schedule
Promotion of exercise to an increasingly higher priority over other activities
Increased exercise tolerance
Withdrawal symptoms following the cessation of exercise, relieved by reinstitution of exercise
Compulsion to exercise
Associated Features (Modified from De Coverley Veale and Morgan)
Less attention to family and other personal relationships
Less attention to work, often with resultant difficulties
Purposeful weight loss (often extreme) to improve performance
Refusal to stop exercising despite serious injury or illness

De Coverley Veale DM: Exercise dependence. Br J Addict 82:735–740, 1987.
Morgan WP: Negative addiction in runners. Phys Sportsmed 7(2):56–70, 1979.

C. **Common comorbidity and sequelae**
   1. Eating disorders
   2. Depression, mild to severe
   3. Marital and family problems
   4. Work problems
   5. Exercise-associated amenorrhea—secondary osteoporosis
   6. Multiple overuse injuries—delayed healing
   7. Overtraining syndrome

D. **Interviewing** the athlete suspected of exercise addiction
   1. Yates provides a series of interview questions that are useful when evaluating an injured athlete who may be addicted to exercise (Table 2).
   2. Sachs and Pargman provide a depth interview approach to evaluating any runner suspected of exercise addiction (Table 3).

IV. Management

A. **Confrontation techniques.** Because denial is as prevalent in exercise addiction as it is in other addictive disorders, confrontational techniques developed for use in alcoholics are often necessary to initiate therapy.

B. **Combination of therapies**
   1. Individual psychotherapy
   2. Group therapy
   3. Support group
   4. Nutritional counseling
   5. Medical management of injuries and illness

TABLE 2. What to Ask the Injured Athlete Suspected of Compulsive Behavior

How do you feel about being inactive while your injury repairs?
What would it take for you not to engage in your sport?
What else in life is as gratifying as your sport?
How much time do you spend thinking about the sport compared with work and family?
How much time do you spend alone?
How exacting is your training schedule?
How strictly do you manage your diet?
After you eat more than you should, do you exercise to get rid of calories?
What other diet methods do you use (diet pills, diuretics, vomiting, laxatives)?
Are you satisfied with your performance?
How are you trying to improve it?

From Yates A: Understanding and helping the compulsive athlete. J Musculoskel Med 9(3):45–49, 1992, with permission.

TABLE 3. Running Addiction: A Depth Interview

How and why did you get into running in the first place?

How many years have you been running? What sort of successes and failures have you had? What sort of injury problems have you had to deal with?

Why do you run?

How do you view your role as a runner? Is it separated from or integrated with the other roles you assume? What is the significance of the running role with respect to the other roles in your life?

What is your estimate of the importance of running in your life? How important is it to you?

What are your basic feelings while you run? What are your basic feelings when you finish running? What sort of feelings do you have when you don't or can't run?

What are the motivational considerations behind your running? What do you see as your future involvement in running?

How would you define the concept of exercise addiction? Do you see yourself as an exercise addict? How long did it take before you got the feeling of being an exercise addict?

From Sachs ML, Pargman D: Running addiction: A depth interview examination. J Sports Behav 2:143–155, 1979, with permission.

V. Anorexia Athletica

A. **Poorly defined entity.** Anorexia athletica is a relatively new term used broadly to describe an anorexia nervosa–like syndrome in which the primary means of reducing weight is compulsive exercise, often coupled with reduced nutritional intake. **No general agreement exists on diagnostic criteria.**

1. Although there are some proposed criteria for anorexia athletica in the nutrition literature, they lack emphasis on the intense exercise which typifies general usage of the term.
2. Some characteristics are presented in Figure 1 on the next page.
3. More research is warranted to determine whether anorexia athletica is a valid clinical entity distinct from exercise addiction and anorexia nervosa.

B. **Characteristics**

1. Compulsive exercise
2. Weight loss
3. Absence of illness or affective disorder explaining the weight loss
4. Distorted body image and/or fear of becoming obese
5. Food restriction common
6. Exercise-induced amenorrhea extremely common

Physical and Behavioral Characteristics of Elite Athletes and Individuals with Exercise Addiction and Eating Disorders

	Elite Endurance Athletes	Exercise Addiction	Anorexia Athletica	Anorexia Nervosa	Bulimia Nervosa
Weight	Variable	Usually below normal	Below normal	Much below normal	Variable, often above normal
Weight loss	None to moderate	Moderate to severe	Moderate to severe	Severe	None to severe
Calorie restriction	None to moderate	Mild to severe	Moderate to severe	Severe	Frequent binging and purging
Specific food avoidance patterns	Variable	Yes	Variable	Yes	Yes
Body image	Rarely distorted	Variably distorted	Severely distorted	Severely distorted	Variably distorted
Fear of obesity	Occasionally	Variable	Severe to overwhelming	Overwhelming	Severe
Binge eating	Rare	Variable	Common	Common	Always (diagnostic criterion)
Purging methods	Rarely	Exercise as purging method	Exercise and others	Common, varied	Multiple and severe
Exercise level	Intense	Overly intense	Intense to overly intense	None to overly intense	None to intense
Workout logs	Common	Often extensive	Often extensive	Variable	Variable
Response to proposed exercise cutbacks	Variable	Refusal	Resistance; often refusal	Variable	Variable
Overuse injuries	Somewhat common	Very common, heal poorly	Common, heal poorly	Common, heal poorly	Common, may heal poorly
Level of denial	Variable	Severe to complete	Severe to complete	Often complete	Variable
Depression	Uncommon	Common	Common	Common	Common
Anemia	Occasional	Occasional	Variable	Common	Occasional
Bradycardia	Almost always	Very common	Very common	Very common	Variable
Low resting blood pressure	Very common	Very common	Very common	Very common	Variable
Menstrual irregularities	Common	Very common	Very common	Always (diagnostic criterion)	Common
Gastrointestinal problems	Occasional	Common	Variable	Very common	Common

FIGURE 1. Exercise addiction, anorexia athletica, anorexia nervosa, and bulimia nervosa share many physical and behavioral characteristics, as evident in this chart. Because clear diagnostic criteria are available only for the two eating disorders, it is much less useful as an analytic or diagnostic tool.

Recommended Reading

1. Blumenthal JA, O'Toole LC, Chang JL: Is running an analogue to anorexia nervosa? An empirical study of obligatory running and anorexia nervosa. JAMA 252:520–523, 1984.
2. Blumenthal JA, Rose S, Chang JL: Anorexia nervosa and exercise: Implications from recent findings. Sports Med 2:237–247, 1985.
3. Callen KE: Mental and emotional aspects of long-distance running. Psychosomatics 24:133–151, 1983.
4. Chan DW, Lai B: Psychological aspects of long-distance running among Chinese male runners in Hong Kong. Int J Psychosomatics 37(1–4):30–34, 1990.
5. DeCoverley Veale DM: Exercise dependence. Br J Addict 82:735–740, 1987.
6. Glasser W: Positive Addiction. New York, Harper & Row, 1976.
7. Lyons HA, Cromey R: Compulsive jogging: Exercise dependence and associated disorder of eating. Ulster Med J 58:100–102, 1989.
8. Mandell AJ: The second second wind. In Sachs MH, Sachs ML (eds): Psychology of Running. Champaign, IL, Human Kinetics, 1981, pp 211–223.
9. Masters KS: Hypnotic susceptibility, cognitive dissociation, and runner's high in a sample of marathon runners. Am J Clin Hypn 34:193–201, 1992.
10. Morgan WP: Affective beneficence of vigorous physical activity. Med Sci Sports Exerc 17:94–100, 1985.
11. Morgan WP: Negative addiction in runners. Phys Sportsmed 7(2):56–70, 1979.
12. Ogles BM: Running addiction: In search of construct validity. Med Sci Sports Exerc 26(suppl 5):S155.
13. Roberts WO, Elliot DL: Malnutrition in a compulsive runner: A case conference. Med Sci Sports Exerc 23:513–516, 1991.
14. Sachs ML, Pargman D: Running addiction: A depth interview examination. J Sports Behav 2:143–155, 1979.
15. Sundgot-Borgen J: Nutrient intake of female elite athletes suffering from eating disorders. Int J Sport Nutr 3:431–442, 1993.
16. Sundgot-Borgen J: Prevalence of eating disorders in female elite athletes. Int J Sport Nutr 3:29–40, 1993.
17. Wagemaker Jr. H, Goldstein L: The runner's high. J Sports Med 20:227–229, 1980.
18. Yates A: Understanding and helping the compulsive athlete. J Musculoskel Med 9(3):45–59, 1992.
19. Yates A, Leehey K, Shisslak CM: Running—an analogue of anorexia? N Engl J Med 308:251–255, 1983.
20. Yates A, Shisslak C, Crago M, Allender J: Overcommitment to sport: Is there a relationship to the eating disorders? Clin J Sport Med 4:39–46, 1994.

PART VI
GENERAL MEDICAL PROBLEMS

26: Infections in Athletes

Morris B. Mellion, M.D.

I. General Issues

A. **Exercise and the immune system**

1. Athletes' lore—"Physical exercise promotes resistance to infection."
   a. Anecdotal evidence only that conditioning reduces respiratory illness. Not verified by epidemiologic study.
   b. Respiratory infections may increase in winter.
      i. May be due to close daily indoor contact
      ii. No evidence that cold exposure increases viral transmission
   c. Overtraining increases susceptibility to infection.
      i. Incidence of upper respiratory infections increases with training mileage in runners.
      ii. Risk of upper respiratory tract infection increases with unusually intense, acute or chronic exercise.
2. **Laboratory studies** support potentially important alterations in the immune system with strenuous exercise, but results are often contradictory and clinical significance is often unclear.
   a. **Granulocytes**
      i. Increase transiently after acute exercise due to demargination from vascular endothelium. Triggered by increased cardiac output and epinephrine surge.
      ii. Secondary increase of granulocytes 2–4 hours post-exercise
         (a) Cortisol surge stimulates release of young granulocytes from marrow
         (b) May last much longer after prolonged, intense exercise
      iii. No significant change in total granulocyte count in highly trained athletes versus sedentary individuals
   b. **Lymphocytes**
      i. Transient rise during exercise stimulated by epinephrine
      ii. After exercise, lymphocyte count falls
      iii. Natural killer (NK) lymphocytes follow same pattern but may fall below baseline level after exercise. Data on how exercise affects NK function are inconsistent.
   c. **Antibodies**
      i. Decreased IgA level found in saliva in a study of Nordic ski racers. Possible etiologies: cold exposure, exercise level, overtraining.
      ii. Other studies show decreased salivary IgA due to exercise in cyclists and swimmers, but not runners.
   d. **Interleukin-1**

i. An immunostimulant
ii. Increases acutely with exercise
iii. Increased T cell/B cell activity
e. **Interferon**
i. Transient increase 2 hours post-exercise
ii. Increase modest compared to increase with viral infection
3. **Conclusions**
a. Clinical significance of laboratory abnormalities unclear
b. Results of clinical trials varied
c. Increased risk of infection in overtrained athlete may be result of exercise and immune system response
d. Acute exercise effects different from chronic exercise effects

B. **Effects of fever on exercise capacity and performance**
1. **Performance**
a. Decreased strength
b. Decreased aerobic power ($\dot{V}O_2max$)
c. Decreased endurance
d. Decreased coordination
e. Decreased concentration
f. All can lead to injury
2. **Physiologic effects**
a. **Cardiovascular**—increased cardiopulmonary effort with reduced peak exercise capacity
i. Cardiac output ↑ at submaximal levels of activity
(a) Heart rate rises
(b) O_2 consumption ↑ at low levels of activity
(c) Ventilation ↑
ii. Maximal cardiac output is ↓
(a) Maximal workload is ↓
(b) Blood pressure ↓
(c) Peripheral resistance ↓
b. **Temperature regulation abnormal**
i. Increased set point in hypothalamus
ii. Danger may be magnified by dehydration
c. **Pulmonary function** abnormal in all but mildest acute respiratory infection
i. Increased airway resistance
ii. Decreased diffusion capacity
iii. Decreased alveolar ventilation to pulmonary capillary gas exchange ratio
iv. All magnified by increased demands of exercise
d. **Musculoskeletal**
i. Isometric muscle strength reduced
ii. Early fatigue
e. **Psychological**—desire to complete exercise (conditioning) decreased
3. **Recommendations**
a. **Avoid strenuous conditioning and competition during febrile state.** Flushing occurs with fever > 38°C (100.4°F) and may be a helpful guide.
b. **Avoid strenuous conditioning and competition in the presence of marked generalized symptoms including severe malaise and myalgias, weakness, shortness of breath, deep cough, vomiting, and diarrhea.**
c. Level of exercise on return to participation varies with time away and severity of illness.

II. Common Respiratory Illnesses

A. **Acute**

1. **Upper respiratory infections**
   a. Symptoms
      i. Fever
      ii. Chills
      iii. Myalgias
      iv. Nasal congestion
      v. Sore throat
      vi. Fatigue
      vii. Cough
   b. Etiology—viral
   c. Treatment
      i. Supportive
         (a) Fluids
         (b) Rest
         (c) Antipyretic (aspirin or acetaminophen)
      ii. Medical
         (a) Decongestants
         (b) Antihistamines
         (c) Cough suppressants (e.g,. 15 mg dextromethorphan/5 cc, 5–10 cc every 4–6 hours)
         (d) Caution about using prescribed or over-the-counter banned substances in NCAA and international competition
      iii. Prevention—good hand washing to decrease spread since transmission is person to person
   d. **Factors for return to athletics**
      i. Afebrile
      ii. Myalgias improved
      iii. Gradual reconditioning
   e. **Complete reconditioning may take longer than expected.** Occasionally, seemingly mild viral respiratory illnesses may cause a 4–6 week delay in return to normal performance. Possibly due to occult pulmonary damage.
2. **Streptococcal pharyngitis**
   a. Symptoms and signs
      i. Fever
      ii. Sore throat
      iii. Swollen, exudative tonsils
      iv. Anterior cervical lymphadenopathy (tender)
   b. Etiology—**group A beta-hemolytic streptococcus**
   c. Diagnosis
      i. Signs and symptoms
      ii. Rapid strep tests (10–30 minutes, office procedure)
         (a) Enzyme-linked immunosorbent assay (ELISA)
         (b) Latex-agglutination test
         (c) Both 85–90% accurate
      iii. Throat culture—incubator required
         (a) 95% accurate
         (b) 24–48 hr delay for results
   d. Treatment
      i. Antibiotic
         (a) Penicillin first choice

(b) Penicillin allergic
- Erythromycin, clarithromycin, azithromycin
- Clindamycin

ii. Supportive
(a) Antipyretics, analgesics
(b) Warm saline gargles, lozenges
(c) Fluids
(d) Rest
(e) Discuss contagious nature

e. Factors for return to athletics
i. Afebrile
ii. Antibiotics started

f. Complications
i. Peritonsillar abscess
ii. Scarlet fever
iii. Rheumatic fever
iv. Acute glomerulonephritis

3. **Infectious mononucleosis:** an acute, generally self-limited, viral lymphoproliferative disease with autoimmune features

a. **Etiology: Epstein-Barr Virus (EBV)**
i. Communicable transmission; excreted in saliva. Many cases with no known prior contact.
ii. **30–50 day incubation period.**

b. **Epidemiology**
i. Attack rate highest from ages 15–25, with 25–50% of those infected developing classic syndrome
ii. Ninety percent of U.S. citizens are infected with EBV by age 30.
iii. In lower socioeconomic classes, infection generally occurs at early age with subclinical disease

c. **Classic infectious mononucleosis syndrome**
i. **Prodrome: 3–5 days**
(a) Headache
(b) Fatigue
(c) Loss of appetite
(d) Malaise
(e) Myalgias

ii. **Classic signs and symptoms: days 5–15**
(a) Moderate to severe sore throat with tonsillar enlargement. One-third of patients have tonsillar exudates.
(b) Moderate fever, possibly sweats
(c) Enlarged tender anterior and posterior cervical lymph nodes. Lymphadenopathy often generalized.
(d) Petechiae of palate
(e) Swollen eye lids
(f) Palpable enlarged spleen by second week in 50–70%
(g) Jaundice in 10–15%
(h) Mild morbilliform rash in 5–15%

iii. **Laboratory findings**
(a) **Serological diagnosis (I_gM)** with rapid slide test based on the classic heterophil antibody absorption test
- Sensitive and accurate in children and teenagers, but up to 15% of adults don't produce heterophil antibody

- If negative in suspected infectious mononucleosis, repeat at weekly intervals

(b) **Complete blood count (CBC)**
- White blood cell count (WBC) moderately elevated: 10,000–20,000 WBC/mm^3
- Marked lymphocytosis: ≥ 50% of WBC
- Atypical lymphocytes: 10–20% of WBC

(c) Liver functions tests reflect mild hepatitis in a great majority of cases.

d. **Septic pattern of infectious mononucleosis** occurs in 10%.
   i. High fever and chills
   ii. Severe pharyngitis
   iii. Protracted acute phase

e. **Common complications**
   i. **Airway obstruction due to massive enlargement of tonsils and adenoids**
      (a) **May require emergency nasotracheal intubation**
      (b) **Definitive treatment is high-dose intravenous corticosteroids.** Tonsils and adenoids shrink within 2–4 hours.
   ii. **Concurrent Group A beta-hemolytic streptococcal pharyngitis (5–30%)**
      (a) Treat with penicillin or erythromycin.
      (b) **Avoid ampicillin, which causes a florid erythematous maculopapular rash due to an antibody present in infectious mononucleosis.**
   iii. **Ruptured spleen (0.1–0.2%)**
      (a) **Occurs only in enlarged spleens, but many are not palpable**
      (b) Occurs on days 4–21 of symptomatic illness
      (c) May be **spontaneous or trauma related**
         - Collision sports are well-documented sources of trauma and strain leading to rupture.
         - May rupture during gentle activities or while straining at stool
      (d) Left upper quadrant pain with radiation to tip of left shoulder
         - Exacerbated by deep inspiration
         - Generalized to entire abdomen
         - Clinical hypovolemia develops
      (e) **Usually marked WBC elevation:** 15,000–30,000/mm^3
      (f) **Medical emergency requiring immediate surgery** to salvage or remove the spleen
   iv. **Neurological complications:** variety of rare CNS and peripheral diseases, including encephalitis and Gullain-Barré syndrome
   v. **Probably increased susceptibility to head trauma.** Brain tissue may be less compliant in some patients with infectious mononucleosis. **Relatively minor blows to the head may cause significant head injury**.

f. **Treatment**
   i. **Supportive therapy**
      (a) Acetaminophen for headache, fever, myalgias
      (b) Stool softeners to prevent straining at stool
   ii. **Corticosteroid therapy**
      (a) **Reserve for patients with specific indications:**
         - Imminent airway obstruction
         - Severe mono-hepatitis
         - Neurologic complications
         - Hematologic complications
         - Myocarditis
         - Septic pattern with high fever and severe pharyngitis

(b) Dose: 40–80 mg prednisone or prednisone equivalents on first day, tapering over 6–12 days

g. **Return to athletics**
   i. **Resume easy training 3 weeks after onset of illness if:**
      (a) Spleen not markedly enlarged or painful
      (b) Afebrile
      (c) Liver functions normal—measure only if hepatomegaly, hepatic tenderness, or jaundice has been present
      (d) Pharyngitis and any complications resolved
   ii. **Resume strenuous exercise and contact sports 1 month after onset of illness if above conditions are met and there is no measurable splenomegaly.**
      (a) **Consider ultrasound measurement** (normal < 14 cm in length)
      (b) **Consider use of "flack jacket" for football**

4. **Pneumonia**
   a. Symptoms
      i. Fever
      ii. Chills
      iii. Productive cough
      iv. Shortness of breath
      v. Chest pain
      vi. Fatigue
   b. **Common etiologic agents—adolescents and young adults**
      i. Viral
      ii. Mycoplasma pneumoniae
      iii. Streptococcus pneumoniae
   c. Evaluation
      i. Clinical exam
      ii. White blood cell count
      iii. Sputum smear and culture
      iv. Chest x-ray
   d. Treatment
      i. Empirical
         (a) Erythromycin, clarithromycin, azithromycin
         (b) Parenteral procaine penicillin G
         (c) Follow-up in 24–48 hours
      ii. Supportive
         (a) Antipyretic
         (b) Fluids
         (c) Rest
         (d) Antitussive optional
   e. Factors for return to athletics
      i. Afebrile
      ii. Resolved shortness of breath

5. **Otitis media**
   a. Symptoms
      i. Ear pain and/or congestion
      ii. Fever
      iii. Hearing difficulties
   b. Etiologic agents
      i. Viral 30%
      ii. Streptococcus pneumoniae 50%
      iii. Hemophilus influenzae 20%

c. Treatment
   i. Antibiotics
      (a) Ampicillin or amoxicillin
      (b) Cefaclor, cefuroxime, axetil, cefixime, amoxicillin/clavulanate and other beta-lactamase resistant agents
      (c) Penicillin allergic: trimethoprim, sulfamethoxazole double strength or erythromycin-sulfisoxazole
   ii. Antipyretics: aspirin or acetaminophen
   iii. Analgesics: nonsteroidal anti-inflammatory drugs (NSAIDs)
d. Factors for the athlete to return to athletics
   i. Afebrile
   ii. Nondraining, intact tympanic membrane for swimmers/divers

6. **Otitis externa** ("swimmer's ear")
   a. Symptoms and signs
      i. Otalgia (ear pain)
      ii. Drainage from ear canal
      iii. Swollen ear canal
      iv. Hearing difficulties
      v. Dizziness
   b. Etiologic agents
      i. Bacterial (*Pseudomonas aeruginosa*) major cause
      ii. Fungus
   c. Treatment
      i. Cleanse ear canal with H_20 or H_2O_2
      ii. Evaluate for tympanic membrane rupture
      iii. Antibiotic/anti-inflammatory ear drops
         (a) Polymyxin b/hydrocortisone, i.e., Cortisporin
         (b) 2% acetic acid/hydrocortisone: VoSol HC
      iv. May need ear canal wick to resolve inflammation/infection
      v. Avoidance of excessive exposure to water (showering, swimming may clinically prolong course)
      vi. May need ear plugs once resolved
   d. Factors for return to athletics
      i. Dependent on sport
      ii. Absence of balance problems

7. **Acute labrynthitis**
   a. Signs and symptoms
      i. Sudden onset
      ii. Marked vertigo
      iii. Accompanying nausea/vomiting
      iv. Tinnitus (ringing in ears)
      v. Unilateral nystagmus is typical
      vi. Hearing loss
   b. Viral etiology
      i. Resolves spontaneously in 1–2 weeks (more severe 4–6 weeks). Re-examine during this time to rule out central etiology, i.e., acoustic neuroma.
      ii. Return to participation based on subjective (how one feels) and objective (clinical exam for sport specific activities)
      iii. Treatment
         (a) Supportive—emotions
         (b) Bed rest
         (c) Meclizine (Antivert)

8. **Sinusitis—bacterial infection of paranasal sinuses**
   a. Signs and symptoms
      i. Facial pain
      ii. Purulent nasal drainage
      iii. Facial edema
      iv. Fever
      v. Fatigue
   b. Diagnosis
      i. Clinical exam
         (a) Transillumination of sinuses
         (b) Percussion of sinuses
      ii. X-ray exam (4 views) or CT scan—generally unnecessary
      iii. Culture—questionable accuracy since nasal flora often contaminate specimen
   c. Etiologic agents
      i. ***Streptococcus pneumoniae and Hemophilus influenzae*** = 60%
      ii. Anaerobes, *Streptococcus pyogenes, Branhamella catarrhalis*, and other = 40%
   d. Treatment
      i. Antibiotics—oral
         (a) Amoxicillin
         (b) Cephalosporins, amoxicillin/clavulanate
         (c) Trimethoprim/sulfamethoxazole (double strength)
         (d) Doxycycline/minocycline
      ii. Decongestants
      iii. Hot packs
      iv. Antipyretic/anti-inflammatory (aspirin or NSAIDs)
   e. Effect on athletic performance is related to decreased air exchange, effects of fever, body fatigue
   f. Return to participation when
      i. Afebrile
      ii. Therapy initiated

B. **Chronic noninfectious respiratory problems**
1. **Cystic fibrosis**
   a. Longer survival secondary to improved antibiotic therapy for pulmonary disease. Increased likelihood of athletic participation.
   b. Effects of exercise conditioning seen in cystic fibrosis:
      i. Increased exercise tolerance
      ii. Increased peak O_2 consumption
      iii. Lower heart rate
   c. Improved feeling of well-being
   d. Symptom-appropriate activities and physical training
   e. Exerciser needs free access to salt or salty foods due to excess sweat electrolyte losses
   f. Limit free water unless accompanied by increased salt intake.
2. **Rhinitis—noninfectious**
   a. Common causes (not limited to athletes)
      i. Allergy
      ii. Noninfectious, nonallergic
         (a) Rhinitis medicamentosa
            • Antihypertensive medication
            • Aspirin sensitivity

- Topical decongestant abuse (rebound rhinitis)
- Cocaine abuse

(b) Endocrine
- Hypothyroidism
- Pregnancy
- Oral contraceptives

(c) Anatomic
- Nasal polyp—most common cause is aspirin allergy
- Deviated nasal septum
- Nasal tumor

(d) Vasomotor rhinitis

b. **Symptoms of noninfectious rhinitis**
   i. Obstruction of nasal airflow
   ii. Clear nasal discharge
   iii. Nasal itching
   iv. Sneezing
   v. Associated itching and puffiness of eyes

c. Treatment
   i. Allergic rhinitis
      (a) Avoidance/environmental control
      (b) Pharmacologic
      - Antihistamine for discharge, sneezing
      - Decongestant for obstruction
      - Antihistamine/decongestant combination
      - Topical cromolyn sodium
      - Topical corticosteroid—beclomethasone, flunisolide
      - Systemic corticosteroid—methylprednisolone dosepak
      - **Caution** when any of above used with athletes, since any agent may be on banned drug list for competition, particularly at high levels of competition
      - Hyposensitization with immunotherapy
   ii. Noninfectious/nonallergic
      (a) Treat underlying cause
      (b) Review medication
   iii. **Asthma** (see Chapter 33, "Exercise-induced Bronchospasm, Anaphylaxis, and Urticaria")

III. Immunizations

A. **Tetanus**
   1. Booster every 10 years after primary series
   2. Booster every 5 years for dirty wound
   3. Tetanus immunoglobulin (250 units) and booster if immunization is not maintained.

B. **Measles (rubeola)**
   1. Recent campus outbreaks
   2. Risk population—vaccination recommended
      a. Born after 1957 with no history of immunization
      b. Immunized prior to 12 months of age
      c. Immunized between 12–15 months of age, with a direct exposure to clinically diagnosed measles
   3. Screening
      a. Document natural infection by history
      b. Proven immunity with rubeola titer-hemagglutination inhibition (HI) testing

4. Revaccination
    a. To all or to nonimmune?
        i. No ill effects of vaccine in previously immunized testing positive (HI)
        ii. Measles-mumps-rubella vaccine may be given without increased risk.
    b. Revaccination recommended for all prior to entering middle school
    c. Reimmunization cost may become a public health issue.

C. **Influenza**
1. Athletes are *not* in recommended group to receive yearly vaccine by standard guidelines.
2. *May* consider vaccination for fall and winter team sports
    a. Close contact increases risk.
    b. Rapid spread may significantly disrupt season.
    c. Advisable if supply of vaccine is sufficient to meet needs of the elderly and chronically ill first

D. **Rubella**—indications
1. All children over age 12 months
2. Susceptible prepubertal, adolescent, and adult females of child-bearing age
3. Susceptibility status is determined by serologic testing. Adequate hemagglutination inhibition. Titer for rubella = protects.

E. **Hepatitis B**
1. No guidelines for athletes in sports with frequent bleeding wounds
2. Guidelines
    a. All infants—three immunizations between 2 and 18 months
    b. All preteens
    c. Health care personnel exposed to blood—includes athletic trainers
3. Teenagers and college students—no consensus. American College Health Association recommends immunization for all college students.

IV. Bloodborne Pathogens

A. **Human Immunodeficiency Virus (HIV)**
1. > 1,000,000 infections in United States (1 in every 250 adults)
2. **Transmission**
    a. **Routes**
        i. Sexual activities
            (a) Semen
            (b) Vaginal secretion
        ii. Parenteral inoculation
            (a) Blood/blood component transfusion
            (b) Needle borne transmission
        iii. Perinatal transmission from infected mother to fetus or newborn
        iv. Contamination of infected blood into open wounds or mucus membranes
    b. **Body Fluids**
        i. **Implicated**
            (a) Blood
            (b) Semen
            (c) Vaginal/cervical secretions
            (d) Amniotic fluid
            (e) Breast milk
        ii. **Not implicated**
            (a) Tears
            (b) Sweat
            (c) Urine

(d) Sputum
(e) Saliva
(f) Respiratory droplets
(g) Vomitus

c. **Transmission in Sports**
   i. **Risk is extremely low**
   ii. Only one case of possible blood-borne transmission has been reported. Case poorly documented: the player who developed HIV infection was not tested for preexisting HIV after a collision with an HIV-infected player caused both of them to develop open wounds.

3. **Participation in sports—HIV infection alone is not sufficient basis to prohibit athletic competition.** This position is supported by most major medical and sports medicine organizations and by most national sports organizations and leaders.
   a. **Boxing is major exception.** Many state boxing commissions require mandatory HIV testing and ban HIV-positive boxers from competition.
   b. Symptomatic athletes may not tolerate competition safely
   c. There is no evidence that moderately intense exercise is harmful to HIV-infected athletes. Data is lacking for intense exercise.
   d. **Mandatory requirements for preparticipation blood-borne pathogen screening is not medically justified**
   e. **Voluntary testing** in situations of possible exposure is warranted.
      i. Pretest and posttest medical counselling important
      ii. Informed consent

4. **Precautions**
   a. **Taken by athletic trainers and other health care professionals**
      i. Gloves
      ii. Wound management
      iii. Management of contaminated bandages, needles, surgical tools, and supplies
      iv. Disinfecting contaminated surfaces
      v. All are "universal precautions" promulgated by the Center for Disease Control and Prevention and by the Occupational Safety and Health Administration
   b. **Sports-related precautions**
      i. **Bleeding wounds**
         (a) Interrupt competition and remove player(s).
         (b) Treat bleeding player, cover wound with occlusive dressing, and change saturated uniform.
         (c) Remove from play other players who have blood on them, until blood is cleaned up and saturated uniforms are changed.
         (d) Disinfect equipment and surfaces with household bleach diluted 1:10 with water.
      ii. **Small cuts or abrasions**
         (a) Do not require interrupting play or removing from competition
         (b) Cleanse and cover
         (c) Small blood stains do not necessitate uniform change.

5. **Education**
   a. Importance of preventive education
   b. Methods of transmission, especially by sexual contact, and preventive strategies
   c. Minimal risk of transmission in sports
   d. Hygienic measures as part of first aid process

6. **Confidentiality**
   a. HIV reportable in most states. Physicians must comply.

b. Otherwise, confidentiality must be preserved. Laws regarding confidentiality vary from state to state.

c. **Legally, the responsibility for sexual transmission rests with the HIV-infected person.** Although there is not yet similar case law in athletics, the analogy is likely to hold. Therefore, the physician is not responsible for notifying opponents, officials, other physicians, teammates, athletic trainers, etc.

B. **Hepatitis B**

1. > 1 million carriers of hepatitis B in U.S.
2. **Hepatitis B more transmissible than HIV**
   a. More concentrated in blood
   b. Appears to be less fragile than HIV
   c. One documented case of transmission in sports
   d. May be transmitted by sexual contact
3. Therefore, the same precautions used for HIV should be used to prevent hepatitis B transmission.
4. Next generation of athletes may be immunized as children.
   a. Current guidelines call for immunizing infants with 3 doses of vaccine from age 2 to 18 months and for immunization of preteens
   b. No clear guidelines for older athletes, but many authorities recommend immunization for all teenagers and college students
   c. Athletic trainers should be immunized

V. Skin Infections (see Chapter 36, "Skin Problems in Athletes")

Recommended Reading

1. American Academy of Pediatrics Committee on Sports Medicine and Fitness: Human immunodeficiency virus [acquired immunodeficiency syndromes (AIDS) virus] in the athletic setting. Pediatrics 88:640–641, 1991.
2. American College Health Association Task Force on Vaccine Preventable Disease: Institutional statement on hepatitis B vaccination, Baltimore, 1993.
3. American Medical Society for Sports Medicine and American Academy of Sports Medicine: Human immunodeficiency virus (HIV) and other blood-borne pathogens in sports: Joint position statement. Am J Sports Med 23:510–514, 1995.
4. Bailey RE: Diagnosis and treatment of infectious mononucleosis. Am Fam Physician 99:879–885, 1994.
5. Brown LS, Phillips RY, Brown CL, et al: HIV/AIDS policies and sports: The National Football League. Med Sci Sport Exerc 26:403–407, 1994.
6. Canadian Academy of Sports Medicine Task Force on Infectious Diseases in Sports: HIV as it relates to sport. Clin J Sports Med 3:63–65, 1993.
7. Centers for Disease Control: Update: Recommendations for prevention of HIV transmission in health-care settings. MMWR 36(suppl 1):1–18, 1987.
8. Centers for Disease Control: Update: Universal precautions for prevention of transmission of human immunodeficiency virus, hepatitis B virus, and other blood-borne pathogens in health-care settings. MMWR 37:377–388, 1988.
9. Eichner ER: Infections, immunity, and exercise: What to tell patients? Phys Sportsmed 21(1):125–135, 1993.
10. Eichner ER: Infectious mononucleosis: Recognizing the condition, "reactivating" the patient. Phys Sportsmed 24(4):49–54, 1996.
11. Haller KH, McKeag DB: Rethinking infectious mononucleosis in active people. Your Patient Fitness 9(1):23–26, 1995.
12. Heath GW, Ford ES, Craven TE, et al: Exercise and the incidence of upper respiratory tract infections. Med Sci Sports Exerc 23:152–157, 1991.
13. Macarthur RD, Levine SD, Birk TJ: Supervised exercise training improves cardiopulmonary fitness in HIV-infected persons. Med Sci Sports Exerc 25:684–688, 1993.
14. McGrew CA, Dick RW, Schniedwind K, Gikas P: Survey of NCAA institutions concerning HIV/AIDS policies and universal precautions. Med Sci Sports Exerc 25:917–921, 1993.
15. National Collegiate Athletic Association: Guideline 2-H: AIDS and intercollegiate athletics. In NCAA Sports Medicine Handbook. Overland Park, Kansas, NCAA, 1995, pp 24–28.

16. Rigsby LW, Dishman RK, Jackson AW, et al: Effects of exercise training on men seropositive for the human immunodeficiency virus-1. Med Sci Sports Exerc 24:6–12, 1992.
17. Seltzer DG: Educating athletes on HIV disease and AIDS: The team physician's role. Phys Sportsmed 21(1):109–116, 1993.
18. Shephard RJ, Verde TJ, Thomas SG, Shek P: Physical activity and the immune system. Can J Spt Sci 16:3, 163–185, 1991.
19. Shields CE: How I manage infectious mononucleosis. Phys Sportsmed 11(1):57–59, 107–110, 1988.
20. Simon HB: Exercise and infection. Phys Sportsmed 15(10):135–141, 1987.
21. Smith JA: Guidelines, standards, and perspectives in exercise immunology. Med Sci Sports Exerc 27:497–506, 1995.
22. Torre D, Sampletro C, Ferrar G, et al: Transmission of HIV-1 infection via sports injury (letter). Lancet 335(8697):1105, 1990.
23. U.S. Department of Labor, Occupational Safety and Health Administration: Occupational exposure to bloodborne pathogens. OSHA 3127, 1992.
24. World Health Organization, International Federation of Sports Medicine: Consensus statement on AIDS in sports. JAMA 267:1312, 1992.

27

Gastrointestinal Problems

Joseph L. Torres, M.D., and Morris B. Mellion, M.D.

Competitive athletes frequently experience gastrointestinal problems, many of which are related to training or competition. Surveys of serious runners have shown that 80% have experienced gastrointestinal symptoms, mostly in the lower tract, before, during, or after competition. The problems are more common, and perhaps more severe, at higher levels of training and competition.

I. Problems Not Unique to Athletes

A. **Anxiety and stress reaction**
   1. Performance anxiety
   2. Inhibitory effect on upper gastrointestinal function activity
      a. Decreased acid secretion in stomach
      b. Motor activity slowed
      c. Blood flow reduced
   3. Continued anxiety may result in acid hypersecretion.
   4. Stimulant effect on lower gastrointestinal activity
      a. Increased motility
      b. Decreased transit time
   5. **Symptoms**
      a. Dry mouth
      b. Dyspepsia ("knot in stomach")
      c. Heartburn
      d. Reflux
      e. Abdominal cramping
      f. Diarrhea
   6. **Treatment**
      a. Reassurance and education
      b. Behavior modification
      c. Relaxation exercises

B. **Acute gastroenteritis**
   1. Incidence second only to upper respiratory tract infections in adolescents and young adults
   2. Etiologic agents
      a. Viral—most common:
         i. Rotavirus
         ii. Norwalk agent
      b. Bacterial
      c. Protozoan (*Giardia lamblia*)
   3. Peak incidence:
      a. Winter in cities
      b. Summer in rural or outdoor sports

4. **Symptoms**
   a. Nausea
   b. Vomiting
   c. Abdominal cramps
   d. Diarrhea
   e. Fever
   f. Myalgia
5. **Treatment**
   a. Usually self-limited, 2–3 days
   b. Clear fluids, electrolyte-containing fluids (e.g., sport drinks) are cornerstone; replace fluid loss liter for liter
   c. Assess degree of dehydration (body weight, urine output, blood pressure) before strenuous practice or game
   d. Antimotility drugs may be effective for abdominal cramps but also may prolong carrier state of some organisms:
      i. Loperamide (Imodium)
      ii. Nonfibrous attapulgite (Diasorb)
      iii. Diphenoxylate hydrochloride with atropine (Lomotil)
   e. **"Traveler's diarrhea"** may respond to:
      i. Trimethoprim/sulfamethoxazole, double-strength, twice a day
      ii. Pepto-Bismol, 1 oz every hour, until symptoms abate or 8 oz consumed
6. Return to competition limited only by hydration status, infective nature of problems, symptom complex (i.e., frequent diarrhea), and reconditioning

II. Hypoperfusion of Gastrointestinal Tract During Intense Exercise

A. **Physiologic arterial shunting during exercise**
   1. During the first few minutes of exercise, 15% of central blood volume is shunted to the working muscles.
   2. As core temperature rises during exercise, 20% of central blood volume is shunted to the skin for cooling.
   3. Central blood volume is maintained by redirecting blood away from other organs, especially the splanchnic bed. For example, normal intestinal blood flow may be reduced by up to 80% to maintain an adequate central blood volume.

B. **Possible etiology of exercise-induced shunting**
   1. Decreased esophageal motility
   2. Erosive hemorrhagic gastritis
   3. Delayed gastric emptying
   4. Diarrhea
   5. Intestinal bleeding

C. **Factors exacerbating hypoperfusion of gastrointestinal tract**
   1. Dehydration
   2. High ambient temperature
   3. Lack of acclimation to exercise in the heat

III. Upper Gastrointestinal Problems

A. **Pain syndromes.** Upper gastrointestinal pain related to training and competition often presents a diagnostic dilemma. "Heartburn" may be even more difficult to diagnose in an athlete because the physical demands of the sport add to the list of potential causes.
   1. **Gastroesophageal reflux**
      a. Vigorous exercise has been shown to cause gastroesophageal reflux in normal subjects. The effect is most severe in runners, but also is substantial in bicyclists and individuals performing a moderate weight-training program.
      b. The frequency, amplitude, and duration of esophageal contractions decline with increasing exercise intensity.

c. Hypoperfusion resulting from physiologic arterial shunting to muscles and skin may cause reduced esophageal motility.
d. There may be some protective effect from increases in lower esophageal sphincter tone that have been demonstrated with moderate exercise.
e. Treatment:
   i. H_2 blockers 4 hours before exercise
   ii. Standard medical management for reflux

2. **Gastritis**
   a. Erosive gastritis:
      i. May be induced by exercise-related hypoperfusion
      ii. Nonsteroidal anti-inflammatory drug-induced
      iii. Anxiety-induced
   b. Often hemorrhagic
   c. Treatment:
      i. H_2 blockers
      ii. Antacids
3. **Peptic ulcer disease**
   a. No more or less common in runners than in general population
   b. Use standard medical management
4. **Delayed gastric emptying**
   a. May be bloating, reflux, or both
   b. May be caused by hypoperfusion due to arterial shunting away from the splanchnic bed
5. **Dyspepsia**
   a. Upper gastrointestinal pain with no identified etiology
   b. Treat empirically with H_2 blockers 4 hours before practice or competition
6. **Angina or cardiac ischemia** must be considered in older athletes

B. **Upper gastrointestinal bleeding**
   1. Hemorrhagic gastritis (see "Gastritis" above)
   2. Peptic ulcer disease (see "Gastritis" above)
   3. A mechanical etiology is proposed in some cases. Shearing forces of the diaphragm on the gastric fundus may induce bleeding.

C. Evaluate and treat with standard upper gastrointestinal methodology

D. Improve hydration before and during performance. Increased plasma volume may not reduce ischemia.

IV. Exercise-induced Diarrhea and Lower Gastrointestinal Bleeding

A. **Runner's diarrhea ("runner's trots")**—stimulated by intense endurance running, with or without accompanying gastrointestinal bleeding
   1. **Descriptive data** from a study of 425 runners in a 10K race[19]
      a. **Incidence**—30% of runners in race
      b. Characteristics of syndrome:
         i. 85% passed semiformed or watery stools
         ii. 60% low abdominal pain or rectal urgency, generally relieved by defecation
         iii. 15% multiple stools
         iv. 13% large-volume stools
         v. **12% frank blood in stool**
   2. Other data
      a. 30–42% of serious runners have urge to defecate
      b. 14–30% report running-induced diarrhea
      c. Direct relationship between severity of symptoms and level of physical exertion
      d. Diarrhea more common in running than in other sports

B. **Lower gastrointestinal bleeding**
   1. **Grossly bloody diarrhea stimulated by intense performance**
      a. May be large amounts of red, maroon, or clotted blood
      b. Often accompanied by severe abdominal pain
   2. Incidence of microscopic increases in fecal hemoglobin after intense running even more common
      a. Also noted in endurance bicyclists
      b. May be due to upper or lower gastrointestinal bleeding
C. **Proposed etiologies**
   1. **Diarrhea only**
      a. **Anxiety-induced diarrhea** (see "Anxiety and stress reaction," page 268)
      b. **Increased gastrointestinal motility:**
         i. Exercise increases secretion of gastrin, motilin, other hormones affecting motility
         ii. Irritable bowel syndrome
      c. **Dietary factors:**
         i. High-fiber diet may cause exercise-induced diarrhea in a small subset of runners.
         ii. Lactose intolerance—higher incidence found with exercise-induced diarrhea than in the general population. Symptoms may occur only when exercising.
         iii. Sorbitol or fructose intolerance with fruit intensive diets
         iv. Large doses of caffeine or vitamin C
      d. **Possible immune system etiology:**
         i. A variant of exercise-induced anaphylaxis
         ii. Generalized urticaria including urticarial lesions in the intestines
   2. **Intestinal bleeding with or without diarrhea**
      a. **Intestinal ischemia:**
         i. Hypoperfusion caused by shunting blood flow from the mesentery to the muscles and skin. Mild exercise decreases intestinal perfusion 40%; strenuous exercise may decrease 80% (may be magnified by dehydration).
         ii. Relative gut ischemia causes focal areas of necrosis and ulceration.
         iii. Ischemia may also cause intestinal malabsorption and, thereby, diarrhea.
      b. **Cecal slap syndrome**—mechanical trauma from running reported to cause hemorrhagic cecal lesions and diarrhea
   3. **Evaluation**
      a. **Detailed history and physical examination:**
         i. Standard procedure, with close review of symptoms and family history of gastrointestinal disease
         ii. Intensity, type, and duration of exercise
         iii. Dietary history
         iv. Travel history focusing on potential food and water pathogens
      b. **Laboratory work** based on history and physical examination
         i. Stool evaluation—culture, ova and parasites, occult blood, white blood cells
         ii. Enterotest for giardiasis
         iii. Complete blood count, erythrocyte sedimentation rate
         iv. Electrolytes
      c. **Endoscopy for frank lower gastrointestinal bleeding** should be performed within 1–2 days of bleeding; otherwise, ischemic lesions may resolve before endoscopy.
   4. **Prevention and therapy**
      a. Encourage bowel movement—have a light meal a few hours before competition and then jog to stimulate the gastrocolic reflex.

b. **Improve hydration before and during performance**—increased plasma volume may decrease ischemia.
c. **Dietary manipulations:**
   i. Athletes on a low-fiber diet may improve by adding fiber to absorb intraluminal fluid.
   ii. Athletes on a high-fiber diet may improve by reducing fiber to decrease stimulation of intestinal motility. Many athletes prefer a high-fiber diet because it stimulates intestinal motility, thus reducing intraluminal contents.
   iii. Eliminate foods that trigger bowel symptoms in the individual athlete—lactose, fructose, sorbitol, caffeine.
d. **Antimotility medications** may be helpful in cases of diarrhea that appear to be a form of functional bowel syndrome and in those that remain undiagnosed:
   i. Imodium
   ii. Lomotil
   iii. Diasorb
e. **Decrease training and competition level 20% to 40% in both mileage and intensity, then build back up slowly.** May be able to cross train.

Recommended Reading

1. Baska RS, Moses FM, Deuster PA: Cimetidine reduces running-associated gastrointestinal bleeding: A prospective observation. Dig Dis Sci 35:956–960, 1990.
2. Baska RS, Moses FM, Graeber G, Kearney G: Gastrointestinal bleeding during an ultramarathon. Dig Dis Sci 35:276–279, 1990.
3. Bingham SA, Cummings JH: Effect of exercise and physical fitness on large intestinal function. Gastroenterology 97:1389–1399, 1989.
4. Butcher JD: Runner's diarrhea and other intestinal problems of athletes. Am Fam Phys 48:623–627, 1993.
5. Clark CS, Kraus BB, Sinclair J, Castello DO: Gastroesophageal reflux induced by exercise in healthy volunteers. JAMA 24:3599–3601, 1989.
6. Cooper BT, Douglas SA, Firth LA, et al: Erosive gastritis and gastrointestinal bleeding in a female runner: Prevention of the bleeding and healing of the gastritis with H_2-receptor antagonists. Gastroenterology 92:2019–2023, 1987.
7. Dobbs TW, Atkins M, Ratliff R, Eichner ER: Gastrointestinal bleeding in competitive cyclists. Med Sci Sport Exerc 20(suppl):S78, 1988.
8. Eichner ER: Gastrointestinal bleeding in athletes. Phys Sportsmed 17(5):128–140, 1989.
9. Fogoros RN: "Runner's trots": Gastrointestinal disturbances in runners. JAMA 243:1743–1744, 1980.
10. Heer M, Repond F, Hany A, et al: Acute ischemic colitis in a female long distance runner. Gut 28:896–899, 1987.
11. Keeffe EB, Lower DK, Goss JR, Wayne R: Gastrointestinal symptoms of marathon runners. West J Med 141:481–484, 1984.
12. Keeling WF, Martin BJ: Gastrointestinal transit during mild exercise. J Appl Physiol 63(3):978–981, 1987.
13. Larson DC, Fisher R: Management of exercise-induced gastrointestinal problems. Phys Sportsmed 15(9):112–126, 1987.
14. McCabe ME, Peura DA, Kadakia SC, et al: Gastrointestinal blood loss associated with running a marathon. Dig Dis Sci 31:1229–1232, 1986.
15. McMahon LF, Ryan MJ, Larson D, Fisher RL: Occult gastrointestinal blood loss in marathon runners. Ann Intern Med 100:846–847, 1984.
16. Mellion MB: Medical syndromes unique to athletes. In Mellion MG (ed): Office Sports Medicine, 2nd ed. Philadelphia, Hanley & Belfus, 1995, pp 150–174.
17. Moses FM, Brewer TG, Peura DA: Running-associated proximal hemorrhagic colitis. Ann Intern Med 108:385–386, 1988.
18. Moses F: The effect of exercise on the gastrointestinal tract. Sports Med 9:159–172, 1990.
19. Priebe WM, Priebe JA: Runner's diarrhea—prevalence and clinical symptomatology. Am J Gastroenterol 79:827–828, 1984.
20. Rehrer NJ, Beckers EJ, Brouns F, et al: Effects of dehydration on gastric emptying and gastrointestinal distress while running. Med Sci Sports Exerc 22:790–795, 1990.
21. Rehrer NJ, Janssen GM, Brouns F, et al: Fluid intake and gastrointestinal problems in runners competing in a 25-km race and a marathon. Int J Sports Med 10(suppl 1):S22–S25, 1989.

22. Rehrer NJ, Meijer GA: Biomechanical vibration of the abdominal region during running and bicycling. J Sports Med Phys Fitness 31:231–234, 1991.
23. Riddoch C, Trinick T: Gastrointestinal disturbances in marathon runners. Br J Sports Med 22:71–74, 1988.
24. Soffer EE, Merchant RK, Duethman G, et al: Effect of graded exercise on esophageal motility and gastroesophageal reflux in trained athletes. Dig Dis Sci 38:220–224, 1993.
25. Stewart JG, Ahlquist DA, McGill DB, et al: Gastrointestinal blood loss and anemia in runners. Ann Intern Med 100:843–845, 1984.
26. Sullivan SN: Overcoming runner's diarrhea. Phys Sportsmed 20(10):63–68, 1992.
27. Sullivan SN, Champion MC, Chrisofides ND, et al: Gastrointestinal regulatory peptide responses in long-distance runners. Phys Sportsmed 12(7):77–82, 1984.
28. Sullivan SN, Wong C: Runner's diarrhea: Different patterns and associated factors. J Clin Gastroenterol 14:101–104, 1992.
29. Schwartz AE, Vaagunas A, Kamel PL: Endoscopy to evaluate gastrointestinal bleeding in marathon runners. Ann Intern Med 113:632–633, 1990.
30. Wilhite J, Mellion MB: Occult gastrointestinal bleeding in endurance cyclists. Phys Sportsmed 18(8):75–78, 1990.

28

Anemia in Athletes

Karl B. Fields, M.D.

I. General Considerations

Although certain anemias are more common in athletes, any of the anemias seen in the general population can occur in the athletic population.

A. Anemia is defined as a reduced number of circulating red blood cells or a reduced hemoglobin concentration.
B. A low red blood cell (RBC) mass can occur from inadequate production, blood loss, or excessive destruction of RBCs.
C. Hemoglobin or hematocrit levels do not indicate the RBC mass and cannot be used as the only measure of anemia.
D. Anemia reduces the oxygen carrying capacity of blood and hinders performance.

II. Basics of Blood Formation

A. A pluripotent stem cell in the bone marrow leads to the formation of colony-forming units that ultimately produce the entire line of RBCs.
B. This cell line is directly stimulated by erythropoietin (EPO), which is produced in the kidneys.
C. Ferroglobulin is proportional to hemoglobin.
D. Hemoglobin is inversely proportional to EPO levels.
E. Whether higher RBC mass in athletes develops from higher EPO levels is unclear.
F. Iron + porphyrin = heme; heme + ferroglobulin = hemoglobin
G. Pyridoxine (vitamin B_6) catalyzes an essential step in hemoglobin formation.
H. Folic acid and vitamin B_{12} play a major role in RNA and DNA production for the nucleus of precursor cells in the marrow.

III. Classification of Anemias

A. Anemia is generally classified by RBC morphology (Table 1).
B. Chronic disease can also cause a microcytic anemia.
C. Leukemias and other malignancies may lead to normocytic or macrocytic anemias.
D. Liver disease typically causes a megaloblastic anemia.
E. A number of problems can cause a variable blood morphology.
   1. Aplastic anemia
   2. Any conditions that increase reticulocytes
   3. Chronic bleeding conditions
   4. Mixed anemias with more than one cause
   5. Hemoglobinopathies

IV. Conditions Common in Athletes

A. **Sports anemia—dilutional pseudoanemia**
   1. Yoshimura coined the term "sports anemia" in 1970.

TABLE 1. Major Causes of Anemia

Microcytic	Macrocytic	Normocytic
Iron deficiency	Folate deficiency	Chronic disease
Thalassemia minor	B_{12} deficiency	Hemolysis
Lead poisoning	Hypothyroidism	Rapid bleeding
Sideroblastic anemia	Drugs	Aplastic anemia

Adapted from American Board of Pediatrics: Program for Renewal of Certification in Pediatrics: Guides for Record Review—Anemia. Pediatric Rev (suppl), 1994.

2. This referred to the common association of lower than expected hemoglobin levels with a number of sports, including running and swimming.
3. Hemoglobin levels in competitive endurance athletes average 0.5 g lower and in elite athletes 1 g lower than sedentary counterparts.
4. However, these athletes actually have an increase in total RBCs and RBC mass, as well as normal mean corpuscular volumes.
5. The explanation for this is an increase in plasma volume in these competitors leading to dilution of the measured hemoglobin level.
6. Several studies have looked at blood volume after exercise and all show an increase. The increase in blood volume occurs because of an increase in plasma with minimal change in RBC mass.
7. During exercise, plasma volume decreases as fluid is pushed into soft tissue by muscle contraction, diffuses into tissue because of osmotic pressure changes from production of metabolites such as lactic acid, and is lost in sweat.
8. The resultant loss in plasma volume means that hemoglobin levels during the actual exercise normalize.
9. Several teleologic explanations have been suggested to explain this finding.
   a. Increased plasma lowers viscosity.
   b. Larger blood volume increases cardiac output and may increase oxygen delivery.
   c. Increased sweating potential reduces risk of hyperthermia with exercise.
10. **Dilutional pseudoanemia does not appear to be pathologic but rather an adaptation to endurance training.** In support of the evidence that this is not a true anemia are several studies that showed an increase in RBC mass in elite distance runners who still had low hemoglobin levels.
11. **No treatment is necessary.**

B. **Iron deficiency anemia**
1. The **most common** true anemia found in athletes
2. As noted above, iron must be incorporated into the formation of hemoglobin.
3. Inadequate intake, inadequate absorption, and excessive loss are all causes for iron deficiency.
4. A concern in adolescent athletes is that rapid growth, particularly in Tanner 3 stage, requires greater quantities of iron. Adolescence is also a time when dietary intake is often inconsistent.
5. Iron deficiency anemia may be asymptomatic. **Symptoms** when they occur include:
   a. Weakness
   b. Lassitude
   c. Palpitations
   d. Shortness of breath
   e. An unexplained symptom is pica—the craving for starch, ice, or clay.
6. **Signs** include:
   a. Paleness
   b. Glossitis
   c. Angular cheilitis
   d. Koilonychia (spoon-shaped nails)

7. **Laboratory confirmation**
   a. Low hemoglobin level in adults:
      i. < 12 grams women
      ii. < 14 grams men
   b. Mean corpuscular volume < 75 fL^3
   c. Peripheral smear—hypochromic, microcytic
   d. Serum iron low with high total iron binding capacity
   e. Serum ferritin < 12 µg/L
   f. Bone marrow—decreased iron staining
8. In practice, most physicians rely on a complete blood count, differential, and serum ferritin to confirm the diagnosis.
9. Clinically, iron deficiency is the most common nutritional deficiency in the United States and in many other countries.
   a. As many as 20% of menstruating women may have low ferritin levels.
   b. The significance of iron deficiency without anemia is unclear.
10. Differential diagnosis (see Table 1)
11. Iron deficiency in long distance runners
   a. Studies that report extremely high levels (40–82% of women; 17–29% of men) based this on ferritin levels of < 25 µg/L, which are borderline and probably lowered by dilutional effects of increased plasma volume.
   b. Studies show declining ferritin levels with the progression of a cross country season but were not controlled for increasing plasma volume.
   c. Low staining for iron occurs in the bone marrow of long distance athletes.
12. Studies do not suggest that athletes are at greater risk of iron deficiency anemia.
   a. Study of athletes in three sports found no difference in male and female distance runners, male triathletes, or female ballet dancers versus controls in percent of true anemia (1.7–3.3% in the three groups).
   b. Iron deficiency without anemia was only slightly more common in athletes (3–5%).
13. **Causes** of iron loss in athletes include gastrointestinal, genitourinary, sweat, and foot strike hemolysis.
   a. Of these, gastrointestinal loss is of the greatest importance.
   b. Genitourinary, sweat, and foot strike hemolysis are not of the magnitude that they should cause athletes to have a significantly higher rate of iron deficiency anemia.
14. Menstruation in women, athletic or not, is the major cause of blood loss and leads to development of iron deficiency anemia in as many as 20% of women followed throughout their menstrual lifetime.
15. Inadequate dietary intake of iron is the number one cause of iron deficiency in women and must particularly be suspected in sports with emphasis on thinness.
16. **Treatment** of iron deficiency anemia
   a. Elemental iron 50 mg three times a day as ferrous gluconate, sulfate, or lactate
   b. Absorption best between meals
   c. Orange juice or ascorbic acid increases absorption
   d. Diet rich in red meat, poultry, fish, and heme sources of iron
   e. Avoid foods high in tannins, phytates, or phosphates
17. Treatment of iron deficiency in the absence of anemia has not clearly been shown to improve performance.
18. In a borderline case, an empiric treatment trial of iron is warranted for approximately 2 months looking for a 1-g increase in hemoglobin.
19. Women with a history of recurrent, documented iron deficiency should be given either daily or every-other-day doses of iron prophylactically.

C. **Foot strike hemolysis in athletes**
   1. Experiments show that foot strike hemolysis occurs.
   2. Magnitude is low and overt hemoglobinuria is rare.
   3. Fleischer in 1881 described "march hemoglobinuria" in soldiers after vigorous activity.
   4. A number of reports have described this condition particularly in marathoners.
   5. Reports regarding role of foot strike hemolysis in hematologic changes of runners are not strong enough to suggest this is a true cause of anemia.
   6. Interestingly, hemolysis occurs in swimmers and rowers, who theoretically do not have the same impact problems.
   7. Thus, other possible associations, such as increased body temperature and flow dynamics in vigorous sport, may be causes for the hemolysis that occurs.
   8. Clinically significant hemolysis in athletes should trigger **a search for problems that traditionally cause hemolytic anemia**.
   9. Foot strike hemolysis from athletic participation should remain a diagnosis of exclusion.
   10. **Treatment**
      a. Changes in shoes or foot support
      b. Changes in running surface
      c. Modification of training program

D. **Hemoglobinopathies and sickle cell trait**
   1. **Thalassemia**
      a. Occurs from a defect in synthesis of one or more hemoglobin subunits
      b. Beta-thalassemia is caused by complex variations in beta globulin synthesis, and this leads to a range of clinical presentations, including thalassemia minor, which is common, and thalassemia major, which is rare but severe.
      c. **Laboratory testing** differentiates the two:
         i. Alpha group shows a decrease in hemoglobin A_2
         ii. Beta group shows an increase in hemoglobin A_2 and an increase in hemoglobin F
      d. Clinical problems are rarer with alpha-thalassemia.
      e. Hemolytic anemia with Heinz bodies can occur.
      f. Mediterraneans, Africans, and Middle Eastern patients commonly have alpha-thalassemia.
      g. About 2% of African-Americans have alpha-thalassemia without symptoms.
      h. Beta-thalassemia occurs in 1% of population of southern Italy and commonly in Central Africa, Middle East, Southeast Asia, and the South Pacific.
      i. Beta-thalassemia minor causes mild anemia characterized by slight icterus, modest splenomegaly, and basophilic stippling on peripheral smear. Thalassemia minor frequently mimics iron deficiency.
      j. **Differentiating features** include:
         i. Normal iron studies
         ii. An extremely low mean corpuscular volume (may be 60 or below in many cases of thalassemia minor)
         iii. A peripheral smear with basophilic stippling
      k. More study in athletes is needed, but currently no treatment is recommended for mild anemia associated with thalassemia.
   2. **Sickle cell trait**
      a. Severity of sickle cell trait varies by individual, with most having about 40% hemoglobin S.
      b. Exercise poses special risks in sickle trait that are incompletely understood.
      c. Well-trained hemoglobin AS individuals (those with sickle cell trait) perform similarly to hemoglobin AA athletes (those with homozygous hemoglobin A) in both anaerobic and aerobic training.

d. No complications were noted for athletes with hemoglobin AS in competition at the Mexico City Olympics, where the altitude was 2135 meters.
e. **Effects of exercise** including dehydration, increased body temperature, hypoxia, and acidosis all increase the likelihood of sickling.
f. Exercise to exhaustion usually produces small numbers of reversibly sickled cells in hemoglobin AS athletes.
g. Clinical syndromes common to SS disease (sickle cell anemia) have not been the problem in AS athletes, although tissue infarction does occur in the renal medulla.
h. Severe hypoxia at high altitudes (> 10,000 feet) has led to splenic infarction.
i. Unexpected death is the major potential complication of AS disease and is most often associated with severe exertional rhabdomyolysis.
j. Military data are alarming in that soldiers with AS have 20–30 times the risk of exertional death compared with African-American soldiers without hemoglobin S. Specific military reports show that all exercise-related deaths at Fort Bliss from 1965 through 1981 were associated with hemoglobin S (five with AS and one with SC).
k. Deaths from exercise in SS have not been reported, perhaps because the severity of the anemia may limit exercise tolerance.
l. The same increased risk pattern may account for the increase in sports deaths in high school and college athletes.
m. Sudden death statistics found sickle cell trait as the cause in 7 of 136.
n. Sickle trait usually does not cause anemia.
o. Currently no special treatment is recommended except for advising caution about exercise at altitude or following illness.

E. **Macrocytic anemias noted in athletes**
1. Vitamin B_{12} deficiency and pernicious anemia are uncommon.
2. Folic acid deficiency is rare in normally nourished individuals.
   a. African populations have been noted with dietary deficiency of folic acid.
   b. Extreme diets or eating disorder behavior can lead to folate deficiency.
3. Drugs should always be suspected when a megaloblastic anemia is noted.
   a. Triamterene
   b. Sulfasalazine
   c. Sulfamethoxazole-trimethoprim
   d. Oral contraceptives
   e. Anticonvulsants:
      i. Phenytoin
      ii. Primidone
      iii. Phenobarbital
4. Hypothyroidism has been reported in athletes and causes a macrocytic anemia.

F. **Hemolytic anemias in athletes**
1. In general, these are uncommon but can be triggered by a number of common illnesses and medications.
2. Drug-induced
   a. Penicillins
   b. Quinidine and quinine
   c. Sulfonamides
   d. Isoniazid
   e. Phenacetin
3. Illnesses
   a. Mycoplasma pneumonia
   b. Infectious mononucleosis
   c. Malarial infections
   d. Sepsis from a variety of bacteria
   e. Certain idiopathic types are suspected to be viral mediated
4. Collagen vascular disease, with lupus erythematosus the most common disorder identified in athletes.
5. Glucose-6-phosphate dehydrogenase deficiency is common worldwide.
   a. Hemolysis following bacterial or viral infection
   b. Triggered by sulfa drugs, antimalarials, and other specific agents such as nitrofurantoin or nalidixic acid
   c. Fava beans

d. African-American and African men are high risk.
e. A different variety affects Mediterranean and Asian populations.

6. Congenital RBC anomalies, such as hereditary spherocytosis and hereditary elliptocytosis, are uncommon and often diagnosed before the age of most sports participation.
7. Hemoglobinopathies

V. Special Anemia Considerations in Athletes

A. Certain situations should alert the clinician to problems that trigger a careful evaluation of all possible causes for anemia.
   1. Iron deficiency anemia in a nonmenstruating female athlete
   2. Anemia in male wrestlers
   3. Normochromic and normocytic anemia in any athlete
   4. Anemia in a weight control or appearance sport, particularly when the sport is not endurance-oriented
   5. Anemia in a patient on medications
   6. Anemia in a population subgroup with more frequent hemoglobinopathies
   7. Anemia in association with decreases in granulocyte cells

B. General rules to follow in an athlete with anemia
   1. All anemias in athletes are considered medical conditions until pathologic causes have been excluded. Careful medical evaluation, nutritional assessment, and sometimes psychological referral may be needed to delineate particularly difficult diagnostic cases involving anemia.
   2. Several nonsteroidal anti-inflammatory drugs have been reported to cause **aplastic anemia** and varying degrees of bone marrow suppression. Keep this in mind for athletes without a clear history to explain recent onset of an anemia.
   3. Iron deficiency anemia in athletes probably relates more closely to diet and menstruation than to any specific loss from sports activity.

Recommended Reading

1. American Board of Pediatrics: Program for Renewal of Certification in Pediatrics: Guides for Record Review—Anemia. Pediatr Rev (suppl), 1994.
2. Balaban EP: Sports anemia. ClinSports Med 11(2):313–325, 1992.
3. Bridges KR, Bunn HF. Anemias with disturbed iron metabolism. In Isselbacher KJ, Braunwald E, Wilson JD, et al (eds): Harrison's Principles of Internal Medicine. New York, McGraw-Hill, 1994, 1721–1726.
4. Bunn HF: Pathophysiology of the anemias. In Isselbacher KJ, Braunwald E, Wilson JD, et al (eds): Harrison's Principles of Internal Medicine. New York, McGraw-Hill, 1994, pp 1717–1721.
5. Colon-Otero G, Menke D, Hook CC: A practical approach to the differential diagnosis and evaluation of the adult patient with macrocytic anemia. Med Clin North Am 76(3):581–597, 1992.
6. Eichner ER: Sports anemia, iron supplements, and blood doping. Med Sci Sports Exerc 24(9):s315–318, 1992.
7. Eichner ER: Hematologic problems. In Grana WA, Kalenak A (eds): Clinical Sports Medicine. Philadelphia, W.B. Saunders, 1991, pp 209–216.
8. Gozal D, Thieiet P, Mbala E, et al: Effect of different modalities of exercise and recovery on exercise performance in subjects with sickle cell trait. Med Sci Sports Exerc 24(12):1325–1331, 1992.
9. Kark JA, Ward FT: Exercise and hemoglobin S. Semin Hematol 31(3):181–225, 1994.
10. Selby GB, Eichner ER: Hematocrit and performance: The effect of endurance training on blood volume. Semin Hematol 31(2):122–127, 1994.
11. Tabbara IA: Hemolytic anemias. Med Clin North Am 76(3):649–668, 1992.
12. Van Camp SP, Bloor CM, Mueller FO, et al: Nontraumatic sports death in high school and college athletes. Med Sci Sports Exerc 27(5):641–647, 1995.
13. Weight LM, Klein M, Noakes TD, Jacobs P: Sports anemia: A real or apparent phenomenon in endurance-trained athletes? Int J Sports Med 13(4):344–347, 1992.

29

Renal and Genitourinary Problems

James M. Lynch, M.D.

I. Anatomy

- A. Genitourinary system composed of internal and external organs of the urinary system and genital organs
  1. Both systems contained in lower abdomen and pelvic region
  2. Urinary system comprised of kidneys, ureters, urinary bladder, and urethra
- B. **Kidneys** located in retroperitoneal upper lumbar area of abdomen
  1. Upper third of right and upper half of left located under 12th rib
  2. Posteriorly are protected by psoas, paravertebral, and latissimus dorsi muscles
  3. Kidneys contained in cushion of pericapsular fat
  4. Ureters run along posterior peritoneal wall
     - a. Protected by muscles of posterior abdominal wall
     - b. Are most vulnerable where they cross bony brim of pelvis
  5. Bladder lies within pelvis and is most vulnerable when full
- C. **Female reproductive system** situated within the pelvis consists of:
  1. Ovaries
  2. Fallopian tubes
  3. Uterus
  4. Vagina
  5. Vulva
- D. **Prostate** and **internal portion of male urethra** located within pelvis. The penis, scrotum, and testes are located externally and are most vulnerable in men.

II. Physiology

The major function of the kidney is to maintain a constant extracellular environment.

- A. Regulates the excretion of fluid and electrolytes
- B. Daily urine volume may vary from 500 mL to 15 L.
- C. Renal blood flow at rest is approximately 1100 mL/minute. Renal blood flow is approximately 20% of cardiac output.
- D. Oxygen consumption of kidneys at rest is 26 mL/minute. Consumption is 10% of resting metabolism.
- E. Volume of urine determined primarily by antidiuretic hormone (ADH)
  1. Regulates water reabsorption by increasing permeability of distal tubule of nephron and collecting duct
  2. ADH released from posterior lobe of pituitary
  3. Response to signals from supraoptic nucleus of hypothalmus
  4. Main stimuli for release
     - a. Increased signals from osmoreceptors in hypothalamus
     - b. Decreased blood volume
     - c. Increased plasma angiotensin concentration

F. At rest, 15–20% of renal plasma flow is continuously filtered by glomeruli.
   1. Results in 170 L of filtrate per day
   2. 99% is reabsorbed in tubular system

G. During maximal exercise, renal blood flow is reduced to 250 mL per minute, which is approximately 1% of the cardiac exercise output.

H. Renal blood flow decreases as blood is shunted to exercising muscle.
   1. Decreases even more if individual is dehydrated
   2. Usually returns to preexercise levels in 60 minutes

I. **Mechanism for decreased renal blood flow** is due to increased levels of epinephrine and norepinephrine and constriction of afferent and efferent arterioles.
   1. Drop in renal blood flow proportionate to intensity of exercise
   2. Glomerular filtration usually well maintained but may decrease
   3. Free water clearance decreases even in short exercise periods.
   4. Transient proteinuria may develop.
   5. Significant reduction in sodium excretion with increased tubular resorption
   6. ADH release may increase threefold in heavy exercise.
   7. Increased exertion of white blood cells, red blood cells, hyalin, and granular casts

J. Damage to renal parenchyma does not occur during heavy exercise. Renal changes are related to constriction of renal vasculature.

III. Injuries

A. **Injuries to kidney**
   1. **Hematuria**
      a. Most common urinary symptom after exercise. Commonly accepted upper limit of normal is three red blood cells per high-power field.
      b. Distance swimmers and runners have greatest incidence; hematuria has been found in many sports.
      c. Usually clears within 48 hours
      d. Issue is **to distinguish transient benign hematuria from organic disease**
         i. Microscopic hematuria may occur in 15% of asymptomatic adults and 4% of children
         ii. Lower urinary tract is most common source after prolonged exercise:
            (a) Can have bladder contusion from repeated impact of flaccid posterior bladder wall against bladder base
            (b) Incidence may be decreased if bladder partially filled
      e. Timing of hematuria is important to consider:
         i. Initial hematuria often urethral in origin
         ii. Terminal hematuria may originate in bladder or posterior urethral
         iii. Continuous hematuria may originate in upper urinary tract (kidney, ureter, bladder)
      f. Dark brown urine may be from upper tract, whereas salmon, pink, or red urine may be from lower tract.
      g. May be caused by:
         i. Direct kidney injury
         ii. Renal vein kinking
         iii. Bladder contusion
         iv. Preexisting pathology
         v. Nephrolithiasis
         vi. Urinary tract infection
         vii. Drug or medication use
      h. Follow-up urinalysis at 24–48 hours is fundamental branching point of evaluation
         i. If gross or microscopic hematuria persists, need:

(a) Culture
(b) Serum creatinine, blood urea nitrogen (BUN), sickle cell preparation (in African-Americans)
(c) Intravenous pyelogram (IVP)

ii. If normal, should consider excretory urogram and cystography to exclude bladder lesions, especially if patient is over 40 years old
iii. If testing remains normal and hematuria persists, must consider intrinsic renal disease:
(a) Creatinine clearance and protein excretion should be measured.
(b) Ultrasound, retrograde pyelography, and computed tomography scan may be useful.
(c) Indications for renal angiography and renal biopsy are controversial.

i. Athletes with benign hematuria secondary to exercise may continue to be active:
i. Should be encouraged to drink quantities of fluids before exercise
ii. Should avoid dehydration

2. **Proteinuria**
a. Occurs in many sports, more often with strenuous, prolonged exercise
b. Normal protein excretion is 30–45 mg/day
c. Exertional proteinuria usually 2+ to 3+ by dipstick measurement
d. Quantitative measurement shows range of 100–300 mg in 24 hours
e. Caused by alterations in renal hemodynamics with vigorous exercise:
i. Have acute decrease in renal blood flow with maintenance of glomerular filtration rate
ii. Caused by elevations in renin, angiotensin II, and ADH
f. Usually occurs within 30 minutes of exercise and clears in 24–48 hours
g. Direct relationship between intensity of exercise and amount of proteinuria
h. If proteinuria does not clear by 48 hours, evaluation is indicated.
i. History should be taken. Personal or family history of:
(a) Renal disease
(b) Anemia
(c) Hypertension
(d) Medication use, e.g., protein powder supplements
ii. Overnight or supine urine sample should be collected
iii. Should also obtain upright sample to exclude benign orthostatic proteinuria
iv. If proteinuria persists in supine position, should consider:
(a) Serum creatinine, BUN, fasting blood glucose
(b) Complete blood count
(c) 24-hour urine collection for creatinine and protein
(d) Urinary protein electrophoresis
(e) IVP

3. **Decreased renal blood flow**
a. Acute renal failure may occur with renal ischemia during heat injury or dehydration.
b. Rhabdomyolysis is most common cause of acute renal failure in sports.
i. Injury to skeletal muscle allows contents to escape to extracellular environment:
(a) Increases in:
(i) Creatine phosphokinase
(ii) Aldolase
(iii) Glutamic-oxaloacetic transaminase
(iv) Myoglobin
(v) Potassium
(vi) Phosphorus
(b) Severe muscle damage may produce myoglobinemia—nephrotoxins may be excreted.
ii. Large number of disorders may lead to rhabdomyolysis:
(a) Exercise stress, heat illness
(b) Ethanol and many drugs
(c) McArdle's syndrome—familial lack of muscle phosphorylase

c. Acute renal failure with rhabdomyolysis may also be associated with:
   i. Disseminated intravascular coagulation
   ii. Hyperkalemia, hyperphosphatemia, hyperuricemia
   iii. Hypocalcemia—caused by precipitation of calcium phosphate in muscle from hyperphosphatemia
d. Acute renal failure should follow normal guidelines for treatment.
e. Prevention is primarily related to proper hydration before and during exercise.

4. **Nephrolithiasis**
   a. Occurs in 0.5% of general population
   b. Peak incidence of first stone formation is in the 4th and 5th decade of life
   c. Most stones are calcium:
      i. 85% in men
      ii. 65% in women
   d. Remainder in men often uric acid stones
   e. Remainder in women often infection-related struvite stones
   f. Composition of every stone should be analyzed:
      i. Greatly affects treatment against recurrence
      ii. Recurrence rate about 10% per year
   g. Renal colic begins suddenly and intensifies over 15–30 minutes:
      i. Steady, unbearable pain that can cause nausea and vomiting
      ii. Pain often passes downward from flank anteriorly toward groin
   h. Stones less than 5 mm usually pass spontaneously; 7 mm or larger have a poor chance of passing spontaneously.
   i. Stone formation is the result of numerous physiologic causes:
      i. Hypercalciuria, primary hyperparathyroidism
      ii. Hyperuricosuria, cystinuria
      iii. Deficient urinary inhibitors
      iv. Urea-splitting organisms in infections
5. **Medication side effects**
   a. Nonsteroidal anti-inflammatory drugs may have deleterious effects because of ability to inhibit cyclooxygenase within kidney
   b. Cyclooxygenase is rate-limiting enzyme for synthesis of prostaglandins (PG) from arachidonic acid:
      i. Prostaglandins are ubiquitous group of 20-carbon fatty acids—influence numerous physiologic processes
      ii. Vasodilatory PGE_2 and PGI_2 play protective role in kidney by modulating renal vasoconstriction caused by:
         (a) Increased renal sympathetic activity
         (b) Circulating catecholamines
         (c) Renin-angiotensin II
   c. In healthy unstressed subjects, renal vasoconstriction is low.
   d. Renal function can become prostaglandin-dependent in:
      i. Hypohydration, sodium depletion
      ii. Heart failure, hypertension, atherosclerosis
      iii. Cirrhosis, diabetes, renal disease
      iv. Aging
   e. Strenuous exercise also increases renal sympathetic activity, circulating catecholamines and renin-angiotensin II:
      i. Not been shown to affect renal function adversely if healthy
      ii. May be problem if coupled with one of the other renal prostaglandin-dependent states, e.g., hypohydrated, sodium-depleted from heat stress
6. **Direct trauma**
   a. May be by direct blow or contrecoup injury from high-speed collision

b. May have pain, tenderness, ecchymosis, and hematuria:
   i. Weak correlation between amount of hematuria and degree of injury
   ii. Hypovolemic shock may result from extensive bleeding
c. **Five classes of renal injury**
   i. Contusion:
      (a) Majority of sports-related renal injuries
      (b) Hematuria usually present but IVP negative
      (c) Treatment usually observation, bed rest, and repeat urinalysis
   ii. Cortical laceration:
      (a) IVP shows extravasation of dye
      (b) X-ray may have loss of psoas shadow
      (c) Treatment often observation, bed rest, and repeat urinalysis
   iii. Caliceal laceration:
      (a) IVP shows intact capsule with intrarenal extravasation and disruption of pelvicaliceal system
      (b) treatment involves observation; surgery in more severe cases
   iv. Complete renal fracture:
      (a) Rare sports injury
      (b) IVP shows separation of pelvicaliceal system with intrarenal and extrarenal dye extravasation
   v. Vascular pedicle injury:
      (a) Will present in hypovolemic shock
      (b) Rare in sports
      (c) Kidneys usually not visualized on IVP
      (d) Selective renal arteriogram shows renal vascular damage
      (e) Treatment always involves surgery.
   vi. Renal trauma in sport usually contusions or intracapsular injuries
d. Athlete who develops hematuria after blow to flank should undergo IVP. If IVP shows nonfunctioning kidney or major injury with extravasation, renal arteriogram should be considered.
e. Examining physician should check for injury to other abdominal organs.
f. Ureter injury usually associated with major renal damage:
   i. Rare in sports
   ii. Must consider pelvic and lumbar vertebrae fracture
g. Bladder injuries most often related to blunt trauma on distended bladder.
   i. Two types of bladder injury are common
   ii. May require urinalysis, cystogram, and retrograde pyelogram for diagnosis
   iii. Contusion:
      (a) May have suprapubic pain and guarding
      (b) May pass small clots and have dysuria and hematuria
      (c) Degree of hematuria does not correlate well with severity of injury.
      (d) Severe contusions require use of indwelling catheter 7–10 days with antibiotics.
   iv. Bladder rupture:
      (a) Rare in sports
      (b) Usually associated with pelvic fracture
      (c) May be intraperitoneal or extraperitoneal
      (d) Requires immediate surgery
   v. Bladder injury present in 10–15% of pelvic fractures

7. **Stress incontinence**
   a. Involuntary loss of urine during physical exertion:
      i. Viewed as bladder outlet incompetence

ii. Women twice as likely to have difficulty as men
iii. Denial is common and the average person waits 7–9 years to seek help.

b. 28–47% of regularly exercising women report some degree of incontinence.

c. Urethral sphincters:
i. Proximal or internal sphincter at bladder neck composed of smooth muscle and innervated by sympathetic system
ii. Intrinsic urethral sphincter composed of type I (slow-twitch) muscle fibers innervated by pudendal and sympathetic nerves
iii. External urethral sphincter composed of type II striated muscle innervated by perineal branches of pudendal nerve

d. Treatment options
i. Behavioral—emphasis on establishing proper pelvic muscle function:
(a) Kegel's exercises; other pelvic floor exercises
(b) Pelvic floor exercises with biofeedback
(c) Vaginal cones (available at Femina)
ii. Pharmacologic:
(a) Internal urethral sphincter under alpha-adrenergic control
(b) Alpha-adrenergic agents such as phenylpropanolamine often effective
iii. Surgical—effective treatment but should be considered *after* other options

B. **Genital injuries**

1. Trauma to unprotected perineal area of either gender may cause hematoma formation.
2. **Testes** are paired organs that descend into scrotum in eighth fetal month.

a. Subject to contusion, torsion, or epididymitis

b. **Direct trauma** to scrotum may cause testicular contusion:
i. Can cause pain, pallor, nausea, and anxiety
ii. Ice and elevate to control bleeding and swelling for 12–24 hours. If pain persists, must consider torsion.
iii. If expanding mass cannot be transilluminated or if epididymis cannot be palpably separated from testicle, consider fracture of testicle or epididymis.
iv. Testicular ultrasound should be performed to assess need for surgery.

c. **Preexisting scrotal abnormalities** may increase risk of testicular injury; evaluation in preparticipation exam is therefore important.
i. Unilateral anorchia found in 5% of boys presenting for surgical exploration—thought to be most commonly due to torsion and infarct before birth
ii. Retractile and undescended testes:
(a) Most commonly reside permanently within inguinal canal and cannot be pulled into scrotum
(b) Require surgical repair
(c) At increased risk for testicular cancer and decreased fertility

d. **Torsion of spermatic cord**
i. Mobility of testis limited by tunica vaginalis, a single ligament that attaches lower end of spermatic cord and epididymis to scrotal lining
ii. Extravaginal torsion occurs if tunica vaginalis is loosely attached to scrotal lining:
(a) Allows spermatic cord to rotate above testis
(b) Not common
(c) Occurs almost exclusively in neonates
iii. Intravaginal torsion occurs if tunica vaginalis is attached unusually high on spermatic cord, allowing motion of testis below. More common in pubertal and prepubertal boys but can occur in any age group.

iv. Torsion should be considered whenever scrotal pain and swelling occur:
    (a) Is a true emergency warranting prompt urologic evaluation
    (b) Develops increasing abdominal or groin pain
    (c) Often develops excruciating testicular pain
    (d) Should be questioned about history of mobile testis
v. Physical examination may reveal:
    (a) Localized tenderness, edema, and hyperemia of scrotal skin
    (b) Vas deferens may be inseparable from swollen cord
    (c) High-riding testicle and abnormal position of epididymis
vi. Epididymitis is other major consideration in differential diagnosis:
    (a) Elevation of scrotum often relieves pain of epididymitis.
    (b) Elevation of scrotum often increases pain of torsion.
vii. If patient presents within 4–6 hours after torsion occurs:
    (a) Cooling of scrotal skin, lidocaine (Xylocaine) cord block, and manual derotation may be attempted. Should not delay surgical exploration and repair.
    (b) Radionuclide scan may distinguish torsion from epididymitis:
        (i) Clinical suspicion should override negative scan.
        (ii) Surgical intervention should not be delayed for scan.
    (c) Torsion can often be reduced through external manipulation.

e. **Epididymitis**
i. Tender indurated epididymis may be palpable early in course.
ii. Subsequently may become hard and fixed to skin with swollen spermatic cord
iii. May develop fever and elevated white blood cell count
iv. Elevation of scrotum may reduce pain—must be distinguished from torsion of spermatic cord.
v. Urinalysis usually positive for leukocytes.
vi. Etiologic agent often chlamydia in men under 35 years and *E. coli* in men over 35. Requires appropriate antibiotic intervention.
vii. Cultures should be obtained, including gonorrhea.

f. **Scrotal masses**
i. Varicocele present in 9–19% of males:
    (a) Varicosities of internal spermatic veins
    (b) Surgical correction may be needed for:
        • Pain control
        • Diminished ipsilateral testicular size
        • Infertility
ii. Spermatoceles are cystic masses:
    (a) Within epididymis or adjacent to testicle
    (b) Caused by extravasation of sperm from trauma or infection
    (c) Require treatment if large or painful
iii. Hydrocele is cystic mass surrounding testicle and epididymis:
    (a) Caused by decreased absorption of tunica vaginalis secretion
    (b) Due to trauma, infection, or tumor
    (c) Acute hydrocele may contain a malignancy and should be investigated by ultrasound or surgery.
iv. Hematocele is blood accumulation in tunica vaginalis:
    (a) Does not transilluminate
    (b) Treatment:
        • Ice
        • Elevation
        • Bed rest
    (c) Rapidly expanding hematoma may need surgical exploration.

v. Testicular cancer is the most common malignancy in 16- to 35-year-old men.
vi. Presence of mass in testicle separate from cord and epididymis demands prompt evaluation.
vii. A mass separate from testicle should be transilluminated; if cannot be transilluminated, ultrasound should be considered.

3. **Penile injuries**
   a. Not a common injury in sports
   b. **Direct blow** may cause vascular injuries and potential impotency:
      i. Caused by straddle injuries or direct blow to pubis
      ii. Mechanism could lead to partial or complete urethral rupture:
         (a) Complete rupture not been described during sports activities
         (b) Immediate pain, swelling, and perineal ecchymosis
         (c) Diagnostic retrograde urethrogram may be needed
      iii. Erect penis susceptible to fracture of tunica albuginea:
         (a) Area of fracture swollen and ecchymotic
         (b) Penis bent to affected side
         (c) Urologic emergency—requires hematoma evacuation and tunica repair
   c. **Penile frostbite** described in runners wearing inadequate clothing in cold weather
   d. **Traumatic irritation** of pudendal nerve may occur:
      i. Particularly in bicycle racers or touring cyclists
      ii. May cause priapism or ischemic neuropathy
4. **Female injuries**
   a. Vulva is quite vascular—trauma can result in hematoma formation.
   b. Fall while water skiing may force water into vagina.

IV. Genitourinary Infections

A. Numerous infections with various causative agents

B. **Urinary tract infection**
   1. Five categories of adult patients
      a. Young women with uncomplicated cystitis
      b. Young women with recurrent cystitis
      c. Young women with acute uncomplicated pyelonephritis
      d. All adults with complicated urinary infection
      e. All adults with asymptomatic bacteriuria
   2. Most common is bacterial cystitis, usually with:
      a. Pyuria
      b. Hematuria
      c. Colony count of > 100,000 per mL
   3. Numerous treatments

C. **Prostatic disease**
   1. Prostatitis
      a. Acute bacterial prostatis uncommon:
         i. Sudden onset of chill, fever, and pain in back and perineum
         ii. Dysuria and obstruction with voiding
      b. Chronic bacterial prostatitis common cause of recurrent urinary tract infection
      c. Need to examine both urine and prostatic fluid
   2. Benign prostatic hypertrophy
      a. Symptoms primarily related to bladder outlet obstruction
      b. Frequent cause of hematuria in men—may have leakage of blood from enlarged veins in benign hypertrophy
   3. Prostatic cancer—current recommendations are annual digital exam, serum prostate-specific antigen determination after age 50

D. **Sexually transmitted diseases (STDs)**
   1. Diagnosis of STD should be sentinel event indicating high-risk behavior
   2. Infections of epithelial surfaces
      a. Chlamydia
      b. Gonorrhea
      c. Genital warts
   3. Bacterial syndromes—nonspecific urethritis and epididymitis
   4. Diseases with genital ulcers or inguinal lymphadenopathy
      a. Syphilis
      b. Chancroid
      c. Herpes simplex
      d. Lymphogranuloma venereum
   5. Control of STD based on four major concepts
      a. Education of persons at risk for disease transmission
      b. Detection of infection in asymptomatic individuals
      c. Effective diagnosis and treatment of current infections
      d. Evaluation, counseling, and treatment of sexual contacts

V. Wheelchair Athletes

A. Neurologic control of urinary tract often lost after spinal cord injury
   1. Paraplegics and quadriplegics at significant risk for:
      a. Bladder and kidney infections
      b. Kidney stones
      c. Bladder distention
      d. Urethral fistula
   2. Kidney damage secondary to infection main cause of death in people with spinal cord injury

B. Wheelchair athletes have demonstrated lower incidence and frequency of urinary tract complications when compared with sedentary wheelchair users.

Recommended Reading

1. Abarbanel J, Benet AE, Lask D, Kimche D: Sports hematuria. J Urol 143:887–890, 1990.
2. Brothers LR: Blunt scrotal trauma: A review. Hosp Med 6:61–80, June 1985.
3. Coe FL, Parks JH, Asplin JR: The pathogenesis and treatment of kidney stones. N Engl J Med 327(16): 1141–1152, 1992.
4. Jacobsen EJ, Fuchs G: Nephrolithiasis. Am Fam Phys 39(3):233–245, 1989.
5. O'Brien WM, Lynch, JH: The acute scrotum. Am Fam Phys 37(3):239–247, 1988.
6. Patrono C, Dunn MJ: The clinical significance of inhibition of renal prostaglandin synthesis. Kidney Int 32: 1–12, 1987.
7. Peattie AB, Plevnik S, Stanton SL: Vaginal cones: A conservative method of treating genuine stress incontinence. Br J Obstet Gynaecol 95:1049–1053, 1988.
8. Stamm WE, Hooton TM: Management of urinary tract infections in adults. N Engl J Med 329(18): 1328–1334, 1993.
9. Thompson C: Hematuria: A clinical approach. Am Fam Phys 30(2):194–200, 1986.
10. Wallace K: Female pelvic floor functions, dysfunctions and behavioral approaches to treatment. Clin Sports Med 13(2):459–482, April 1994.

30

The Diabetic Athlete

Kris Berg, Ed.D.

I. General Considerations

A. Exercise was not typically emphasized in management of diabetes until recently, although it has been a component of overall treatment since the 1920s. Position statement of American Diabetes Association supports exercise for diabetics.

B. **Short-term effects of exercise in both types of diabetes are well understood, but long-term effects are not, particularly in type I patients.**
   1. Anecdotal (e.g., diabetic athletes) and research evidence clearly suggests numerous long-term benefits.
      a. Weight loss
      b. Reduced risk of cardiovascular disease
      c. Increased insulin sensitivity
      d. Improved regulation of blood glucose
   2. Data show type I diabetics who were high school athletes have significantly **lower incidence of cardiovascular disease** as adults than type I diabetics who were not.

C. **Diabetics are as trainable as nondiabetics if under reasonable metabolic control.**
   1. Blood glucose
   2. Ketone levels

II. Key Traits of Type I and II Diabetics Pertinent to Exercise

A. **Type I and type II diabetics using insulin or oral hypoglycemic medication are prone to hypoglycemia, particularly those on multiple daily insulin injections.**

B. **Type I patients are prone to ketoacidosis, whereas type II patients rarely experience this problem.**

C. Hypoglycemia and ketoacidosis can be minimized with appropriate monitoring of blood glucose and ketones.

III. Benefits of Exercise

A. **Motivation to improve as an athlete may enhance diabetic management.**
   1. More frequent blood glucose assessment
   2. Closer attention to diet

B. **Consistent, good control of blood glucose minimizes typical diabetic sequelae** by 30–70% (based on 7-year longitudinal study of more than 1000 type I patients).
   1. Retinopathy
   2. Microangiography
   3. Neuropathy
   4. Some degree of reversal of these conditions occurs with prolonged tight blood glucose control

C. **Physical trainability and performance are probably optimized when blood glucose is consistently good.**

1. More normal substrate utilization
2. Reduced protein degradation
    a. Greater muscle hypertrophy
    b. Possibly greater mitochondrial enzymes
3. Greater muscle and liver glycogen
4. Increased body water—increased heat tolerance

D. **Psychological effects of exercise**
1. Improved self-esteem
2. Improved self-confidence

E. **Reduction in cardiovascular disease risk factors**
1. Reduced total cholesterol and low-density lipoprotein cholesterol
2. Increased high-density lipoprotein cholesterol
3. Reduced triglyceride level
4. Reduced blood pressure
5. Increased fibrinolysis
6. Reduced stress

F. **Increased insulin sensitivity:** reduced insulin or oral hypoglycemic medication doses often result. Some type II patients may be taken off medication.

IV. Contraindications for Exercise

A. An exercise electrocardiogram is warranted if:
1. Over age 40
2. Duration of diabetes exceeds 25 years
3. A primary risk factor for cardiovascular disease exists

B. **If peripheral neuropathy or microangiopathy exist, avoid exercise that traumatizes the feet.**
1. Swimming and cycling are good alternatives to walking and jogging.
2. **Examine the feet daily and keep them well lubricated.**
    a. Trim nails carefully.
    b. Avoid blisters, corns, and calluses. Wear properly fitting shoes and socks.
3. **Treat foot injuries immediately to prevent complications.**
4. Prevent thick callus formation by periodic filing with a pumice stone.

C. **Proliferative retinopathy precludes:**
1. **Strenuous or jarring activity**
    a. Weight lifting and training
    b. Contact sports
    c. Gymnastics
    d. Running
2. Activity that raises the heart rate dramatically and systolic blood pressure beyond 180 mmHg
3. Scuba diving because of increased water pressure
4. Exercise while inverted
    a. Some yoga positions
    b. Standing on head
    c. Hanging upside-down

V. Exercise Guidelines

A. **Good blood glucose control should be established before starting an exercise program.**

B. **Blood glucose should be measured before and after exercise.**
1. Allows patient and physician to study blood glucose response to various exercise conditions
    a. Consecutive hard days of training
    b. Tournaments
    c. Reduced training days before competition

2. **The drop in blood glucose during exercise is greater the higher it is at the onset of activity.**
3. **If blood glucose exceeds 250–300 mg/dl at the start of exercise, blood glucose tends to rise, rather than fall, during exercise.**
   a. **If ketosis exists before exercise, ketone production rises.**
   b. These effects are due to the influence of counterregulatory hormones (catecholamines, cortisol, and growth hormone)
4. **Pregame anxiety mimics hypoglycemia, leading many diabetic athletes to overeat before competition.**
   a. They may treat what is perceived to be an insulin reaction.
   b. They may exaggerate the reduction in dosage of insulin or oral hypoglycemic medication peaking during the contest to avoid hypoglycemia and possibly become hyperglycemic.
   c. These inappropriate steps may lead to accentuated ketoacidosis and poor performance because of limited use of muscle glycogen and reduced blood pH.
5. **Endurance training**
   a. Increases fat utilization because of an increase in mitochondrial density and associated enzymes
   b. Increases muscle and liver glycogen stores, allowing athlete to be active for a much longer time before needing supplemental carbohydrate
   c. Reduces uptake of blood glucose, which reduces likelihood of hypoglycemia
6. **Hypoglycemia is more likely to occur during exercise in the evening and least likely to occur in the morning because of a diurnal variation in growth hormone level.**
   a. If exercising in the evening, the amount of insulin taken that peaks after eating and during the rest of the evening should be reduced, or more food should be consumed before and possibly after exercise.
   b. Before actual competition in the evening, alteration in insulin or food intake should be experimented with several times to mimic the conditions (e.g,. same time and similar energy expenditure) existing during evening competition.
   c. Because insulin sensitivity is affected for at least 4 hours and as long as 24 hours after exercise, hypoglycemia may occur during sleep. Blood glucose may have to be assessed in the middle of the night to prevent insulin reaction.
7. **Exercise performed within 1 hour of injection of regular insulin speeds its absorption and time to peak effect. The same effect occurs for about 2.5 hours after injection of intermediate-acting insulin.**
   a. Type I diabetics typically inject insulin into the thigh, gluteal area, abdomen, triceps, or shoulder. The injection site can be altered depending on the activity to prevent this effect.
   b. If exercise commonly is done soon after the injection of regular insulin, no alteration may be needed because the athlete has probably learned to deal with the effect.
   c. **Elevation of body temperature also increases the rate of insulin absorption.** The duration of warm-up and the amount of clothing worn during warm-up should be reasonably consistent if exercise occurs within the first hour of injecting regular insulin.
8. **Consistent daily energy expenditure facilitates blood glucose control.**
   a. Extra medication or lower food intake may be needed on days of reduced activity, whereas less medication or greater food intake may be needed for days of increased training duration or intensity.
   b. **When exercise lasts for several hours** (e.g., triathlons, mountaineering, cycling, tournament play), **the basal dose of insulin should be reduced in type I diabetics**

by as much as 50%. Supplemental food (about one carbohydrate exchange or 60 kcal) can be consumed every 30–45 minutes. Blood glucose monitoring during the event has proven helpful to diabetics in such sports.

C. **Medication requirements are reduced in the early months of training** (30–40% is typical) and remain lower as long as training occurs.
   1. Mature diabetic athletes usually take about 0.5–0.6 unit of insulin/kg body weight or even less, whereas the typical dosage is 0.5–1.0 unit/kg.
   2. **Some type II patients may eventually need no oral hypoglycemic medication** due to the combined effect of fat loss and exercise on insulin sensitivity

D. Achievement of good blood glucose control facilitates development of muscle mass.
   1. Adequate insulin enhances normal uptake and utilization of amino acids.
   2. Inadequate insulin promotes protein degradation and water loss.

E. **Good blood glucose control facilitates glycogen storage in skeletal muscle.**
   1. This reduces the likelihood of glycogen depletion occurring after consecutive days of vigorous training as well as during a prolonged endurance event.
   2. Evidence suggests that the amount of water stored with skeletal muscle glycogen has a strong effect on exercise capacity in the heat.
   3. Many marginally controlled diabetics have particular difficulty exercising in warm environments, partly because of reduced muscle glycogen and water.

VI. Guidelines for Avoiding Hypoglycemia Associated with Exercise

A. **Hypoglycemia is a fear many diabetics have regarding exercise. Measure blood glucose before exercise.**
   1. If < 130 mg/dl, consume two carbohydrate exchanges per 30–45 minutes of light to moderate exercise (< 60% $\dot{V}O_2max$) and three exchanges if heavy exercise (> 70% $\dot{V}O_2max$).
   2. If 130–180 mg/dl, consume one carbohydrate exchange per 30–45 minutes of light to moderate exercise and two exchanges per 30–45 minutes of heavy exercise.
   3. If 180–240 mg/dl, take no food before exercise. If the exercise is heavy and the duration exceeds 30 minutes, take a second blood glucose reading and use the criteria stated in nos. 1 and 2 above.
   4. If 250 mg/dl or higher, do not exercise because the action of counterregulatory hormones may cause blood glucose to rise during exercise as well as increase the ketone level.

B. **Food should be readily available for supplemental feeding.**
   1. Athletic trainer or coach
   2. Locker
   3. Bus
   4. On person (e.g., carry in pocket of running shorts, in a pack on bicycle)

C. **Decrease dosage of insulin that peaks during exercise.** Short-acting insulin normally taken before a meal might not be needed.

D. **Hypoglycemia occurs during and after exercise more frequently and severely in those who have been type I diabetics for more than 10 years. Those on tight management regimens using multiple daily insulin injections suffer hypoglycemia about three times as frequently as others. The frequent exposure to hypoglycemia seems to reduce awareness of the symptoms, so coaches and trainers need to know the symptoms and steps for treatment.**

E. Avoid exercise in the evening or develop a plan to meet the reduced insulin needed if exercise cannot be avoided at this time of day.

F. After expending an unusually large amount of energy or if exercise is done in the evening, expect possible hypoglycemia at night and the next day. Extra blood glucose monitoring is advisable.

G. Avoid exercising the muscles in the region where short-acting insulin was injected for 1 hour.

Recommended Reading

1. American Diabetic Association: Physician's Guide to Insulin-Dependent (Type I) Diabetes: Diagnosis and Treatment. Alexandria, VA, American Diabetic Association, 1988.
2. American Diabetic Association: Physician's Guide to Non-Insulin–Dependent (Type I) Diabetes: Diagnosis and Treatment, 2nd ed. Alexandria, VA, American Diabetic Association, 1988.
3. A Round Table: Diabetes and exercise. Phys Sportsmed 7:49–64, 1979.
4. Berg K: Blood glucose regulation in an insulin-dependent diabetic backpacker. Phys Sportsmed 11:101–104, 1983.
5. Berger M, Berchtold P, Cuppers JJ, et al: Metabolic and hormonal effects of muscular exercise in juvenile type diabetics. Diabetologica 13:355–365, 1977.
6. Costill DL, Cleary P, Fink WJ, et al: Training adaptations in skeletal muscle of juvenile diabetics. Diabetes 28:812–822, 1979.
7. Felig P, Wahren J: Amino acid metabolism in exercising man. J Clin Invest 50:2703–2714, 1971.
8. Frantz MJ, Norstrom J: Your Game Plan for Diabetes and Exercise: Diabetics Actively Staying Healthy. Minneapolis, DCI Publishing, 1990.
9. Krall LP, Beaser RS: Joslin Diabetes Manual, 12th ed. Philadelphia, Lea & Febiger, 1989.
10. Landt KW, Campaigne BN, James FW, Sperling MA: Effects of exercise training on insulin insensitivity in adolescents with type I diabetes. Diabetes Care 8:461–465, 1985.
11. Larsson Y, Persson B, Sterky G, Thoren C: Functional adaptation to vigorous training and exercise in diabetic and nondiabetic adolescents. J Appl Physiol 19:629–635, 1964.
12. Skyler J, Skyler D, O'Sullivan M: Algorithms for adjustment of insulin dosage by patients who monitor blood glucose. Diabetes Care 4:311–318, 1981.
13. Vranic M, Wasserman D: Exercise, fitness, diabetes. In Bouchard C, Shepherd RJ, Stephens T, et al (eds): Exercise, Fitness, and Health: A Consensus of Current Knowledge. Champaign, IL, Human Kinetics, 1990, pp 467–495.
14. Wasserman DH, Vranic M: Exercise and diabetes. Diabetes Annual 3:527–559, 1987.

31

The Athlete's Heart

Loren A. Crown, M.D., Jerry W. Hizon, M.D., FAAFP and Wm. MacMillan Rodney, M.D.

Athletes can have cardiac changes secondary to chronic exercise. When evaluating an athlete, these changes must be considered as well as certain diseases that may predispose the athlete to sudden death (Tables 1 and 2). A rational approach to the evaluation of the athlete at risk for sudden cardiac death (SCD) may reduce the probability of such events.

I. Types of Cardiac Conditioning

The heart's response to conditioning is a result of the demand required or the stress applied. There can be a need for greater $\dot{V}O_2$max (work capability), which is proportional to cardiac output (CO), which is the product of stroke volume (SV) and heart rate (HR). There can be a stress resulting from increased hydrostatic pressure loads, which are directly transmitted to the structural elements of the cardiac wall.

A. **Increased volume load**
   1. **In exercise that requires an increase in CO, the heart compensates with a significant increase in the size of the ventricular cavity** (left ventricular end-diastolic diameter [LVEDD]), **whereas the wall thickness remains relatively normal.** This allows the SV to increase, which proportionally raises the CO (CO = SV × HR).
   2. Typical exercises that produce an increased SV on the heart are **isotonic, dynamic** exercises, such as running, swimming, bicycling, and cross country skiing. **This occurs in the "aerobic" athlete's heart.**

B. **Increased pressure load**
   1. **When an increased pressure load is intermittently applied to the athlete's heart, the ventricular wall thickens without any significant change in LV volume. The wall thickness must increase proportionally** to the intraventricular pressure to maintain an acceptable wall stress or tension. **This occurs in the "anaerobic" athlete's heart.**
   2. These **isometric** or **static** conditioned athletes (e.g., weight lifters and shot putters) have hearts that must sustain great pressure loads, which may lead to blood pressures in excess of 320/250 at times. However, there is no need in this case to alter CO; thus, there is no increase in SV.

C. **Combination**
   1. **Practically speaking, most anaerobic athletes engage in aerobic training,** and, **conversely, many dynamic athletes do some static training.** Hence the clinician often sees a spectrum of changes rather than a strict dichotomy.
   2. Furthermore, many intermittent exercisers (so-called "weekend warriors") of various ages may be engaging in exercise to comply with prescribed aerobic conditioning. They may also demonstrate cardiac compensations consistent with the **Athletic Heart Syndrome.**

TABLE 1. Cardiac Conditions Contraindicating Participation in Competitive Athletics

Obstructive hypertropic cardiomyopathy
Congenital coronary artery abnormalities
Cystic medical necrosis of the aorta (Marfan's syndrome)
Pulmonic stenosis with right ventricular pressure > 75 mmHg
Aortic stenosis with a gradient > 40 mmHg across the valve

From Hara JH, Puffer JC: The preparticipation physical examination. In Mellion MB (ed): Office Management of Sports Injuries and Athletic Problems. Philadelphia, Hanley & Belfus, 1988.

II. History

A. **Regimen and problems.** Initially, it is helpful to note the type, length, and intensity of the athlete's workout or training regimen. Specifically, ask if there have been any reasons that the athlete has had to interrupt or stop an exercise program. Especially ask if he or she has ever had **syncope, chest pain,** or **dyspnea on exertion.** Does the athlete tire much more quickly than his or her friends during exercise? Has the athlete ever been told not to exercise or been refused medical clearance to participate in athletics? Does the athlete have any reservation about exercising to maximal level for fear of some adverse health consequence? **Premonitory symptoms occur in the majority of SCD events.**

B. **Family history**. Any family history of **sudden death** while exercising or early coronary artery disease **(CAD) before age 50** is important information. CAD in this context may be functionally considered to be any angina, myocardial infarction, or any conditions requiring coronary artery bypass grafting (CABG) or percutaneous transluminal coronary angioplasty (PTCA). Some team physicians include unexplained sudden death before 40 years of age as a significant marker.

C. **General medical history.** Also noteworthy is any history in the athlete of general medical conditions that may increase the risk of sudden death, such as hyperlipidemia; diabetes mellitus; hypertension; smoking; or recreational **drug use**, especially cocaine, amphetamines, or anabolic steroids. Current treatments, medications, and recent hospitalizations should be noted.

III. Cardiovascular Examination

The cardiac examination is most frequently normal in athletes. However, there are numerous common findings that in other contexts signal ill health but in the examination of a conditioned athlete have only benign portent.

A. The **HR commonly is bradycardic** (< 60 beats/min), and rates as low as 25 beats/min have been noted in certain highly trained athletes.

B. **Blood pressures in athletes may be low compared with nonathletes.** It is not uncommon for diastolic blood pressures to be zero in well-conditioned athletes. Use of

TABLE 2. Cardiac Conditions That Would Not Specifically Contraindicate Participation

Mitral valve prolapse in absence of significant ventricular arrhythmias or severe mitral regurgitation
Small shunts associated with atrial septal defect, ventricular septal defect, or patent ductus arteriosus
Wolff-Parkinson-White syndrome in absence of documented atrial fibrillation with rapid ventricular response
Primary ventricular arrhythmias, most commonly unifocal premature ventricular contractions, in the absence of underlying coronary, myocardial, or valvular disease

From Hara JH, Puffer JC: The preparticipation physical examination. In Mellion MB (ed): Office Management of Sports Injuries and Athletic Problems. Philadelphia, Hanley & Belfus, 1988.

phase 4 Korotkoff sounds as the diastolic end point eliminates many of these pseudo-low diastolic readings. Borderline hypertension that is exacerbated with exercise probably indicates labile hypertension, which may respond beneficially to an exercise program. Finally, ensure that **appropriately large cuffs** are used on muscular athletes; the bladder in the cuff should cover two thirds of the arm circumference to avoid false elevations.

C. **During auscultation, ventricular gallops and soft systolic murmurs are commonly heard.** Most pediatric patients have murmurs at some point in their lives; serendipitous athletic examinations may coincide with these times. Additionally, young people in general and athletes in particular may have emergence of benign murmurs during the stress of an examination; try to examine when the HR is slower. Finally, there is high interobserver variability in studies on auscultation of well-trained athletes, and this corresponds to the subjective nature of this aspect of the cardiac exam. **Midsystolic murmurs have been noted in 30–85% of dynamic athletes. Generally, these murmurs are graded I or II/VI. Athletes with cardiac murmurs that are III/VI or greater in intensity should be referred for echocardiograms as should athletes with holosystolic and diastolic murmurs. Also, murmurs that become louder on Valsalva, squatting, or hand grip** (which decrease preload in the early phase of the maneuver) should be investigated; benign murmurs tend to soften. Similarly, **third and fourth heart sounds are common**, being heard in up to 50% of the aerobically conditioned. A mid to late systolic click or a late systolic murmur (which increases on Valsalva) is consistent with **mitral valve prolapse.**

D. On **palpation** of the precordium, cardiomegaly may be noted but usually does not simulate cardiac illness. In the aerobic athlete, a large pulse amplitude and a diffuse left ventricular precordial impulse may also be noted.

E. The **chest x-ray** occasionally shows modest cardiomegaly (cardiothoracic ratio of 0.5:0.6) with or without a globular appearance. There is usually no evidence of specific chamber enlargement. Pulmonary venous engorgement may even accompany some of these cases.

F. **Electrocardiogram (ECG) changes**

1. **Rhythm disturbances seem to be limited to aerobic dynamic athletes** (Table 3). **They typically disappear on exertion.**

   a. The most common abnormality is **sinus bradycardia**, with the prevalence frequently exceeding 50% in several large studies. The degree of bradycardia may correlate with the intensity of the training. It is not yet resolved if this is due

TABLE 3. Frequencies of Rhythm Disturbances on Resting Electrocardiograms of the General Population and Athletes

Arrhythmia	General Population (%)	Athletes (%)
Sinus bradycardia	23.7	50–85
Sinus arrhythmia	2.4–20	13.5–6.9
Wandering atrial pacemaker	—	7.4–19
First-degree block	0.65	6–33
Mobitz I	0.003	0.125–10
Mobitz II	0.003	Not reported
Third-degree block	0.0002	0.017
Nodal rhythm	0.06	0.031–7.0
Ventricular preexcitation	0.1–0.15	0.15–2.5
Atrial fibrillation	0.004	0–0.63

From Huston TP, Puffer JC, Rodney WM: The athletic heart syndrome. N Engl J Med 313:24–32, 1985, with permission.

purely to **vagotonia** or if it is partially due to decreased sympathetic tone or to intrinsic cardiac factors as well.

b. **Sinus arrhythmia** is commonly seen in athletes, ranging from 13.5–69% in dynamic athletes. A wandering atrial pacemaker can be found in up to 20% of conditioned athletes.
c. **Atrioventricular (AV) blocks** are the third most common rhythm abnormalities seen. Given the vagal influence on AV node conduction, this is not surprising. A prolonged conduction time has been observed in controlled studies and has been shown to develop de novo as athletes embark on training programs. Cessation of training results in disappearance of the AV block.
    i. Most common is the **first-degree block**, detected in 6–33% of resting and ambulatory ECGs.
    ii. **Second-degree block (Mobitz I)** is clearly related to training. Long-term follow-up of these patients reveals no association with evolving cardiac disease.
    iii. **Mobitz type II and third-degree heart block** are rare.
    iv. **Junctional rhythms** might also be anticipated from the theory of excess vagal tone. Several studies have revealed a prevalence of 7–20% seen in athletes. These may include atrial and junctional escape rhythms.
d. Isolated **premature supraventricular and ventricular contractions** (PVCs) are seen in athletes probably no more frequently than in nonathletes. **Higher-grade forms of ventricular rhythm abnormalities, such as multifocal PVCs and ventricular tachycardia, suggest further workup.** There are data to suggest that otherwise healthy, asymptomatic young adults probably have a normal range of unifocal PVCs; some use 100 PVCs in a 24-hour period as the upper limit of normal for athletes. If all of the risk factors are negative, exercise testing may be the most helpful single test to demonstrate the beneficial effect of exercise on ventricular ectopy. If other risk factors exist, echocardiography, electrophysiologic studies, Holter monitoring, or cardiac consultation may be considered.
e. Other reported abnormalities include minor conduction abnormalities, usually of the **right bundle-branch block** type, which may be found in up to 50% of combined athletes. Such entities as **tachyarrhythmias, supraventricular tachycardias, and atrial fibrillation** are such uncommon occurrences that further evaluation is indicated.

2. **Alterations in repolarization are a prominent manifestation of the training effect.** ST segment and T wave changes are seen most frequently, but not exclusively, in dynamic athletes. **In general, the more highly trained the athlete, the more likely one will find ST and T wave changes,** which increase in direct relation to training intensity. As with the rhythm changes, they normalize with exertion and are thought to be due to a change of autonomic input to the heart. Table 4 summarizes these repolarization changes. There are four primary patterns of altered repolarization (U waves are also common):
    a. **ST segment elevation with peaked T waves**
    b. **ST segment depression with depressed J points**
    c. **Juvenile T wave pattern** (right precordial J point elevation with inverted T waves)
    d. **T wave inversion in the lateral precordium**
    e. A less common T wave change is a biphasic T wave with terminal negativity in leads V3 to V6.
3. **Typical ECGs of athletes show large voltages, which are a manifestation of the physiologic enlargement that occurs with conditioning.** Increased P wave amplitude as well as evidence of right ventricular hypertrophy **(RVH)** and left ventricular

TABLE 4. Electrocardiographic Changes in the Athletic Heart Syndrome

Voltages seen in athletic heart syndrome
Increased P-wave amplitude
LVH (85% in various surveys)
RVH (less frequent than LVH)
Repolarization
ST segment elevation with peaked T waves
ST segment depression with depressed J points
Juvenile T-wave pattern (right precordial J point elevation with inverted T waves)
T wave inversion most commonly in V1, V2, and V3

LVH = Left ventricular hypertrophy; RVH = right ventricular hypertrophy.

hypertrophy **(LVH)** is found. The prevalence of LVH has reached up to 85% in various surveys. RVH is slightly less frequent. Ventricular hypertrophy of either chamber occurs less frequently in static athletes when compared with dynamically conditioned athletes. The amplitude of the voltages has been observed to increase as training progresses. A 25% increase in voltage amplitude was observed during the 11 weeks of training in one prospective study. As with the repolarization changes, the effect **disappears with cessation of training.** Table 4 summarizes the voltage changes found in athletic hearts.

G. **Morphologic adaptations.** Conditioned dynamic athletes frequently have morphologic changes in their hearts that are needed for maximum efficiency. There is debate whether static isometric exercise alone also causes these changes, but clearly these adaptations in both types of athletes are usually not pathologic. As summarized in Table 5, there are several changes found typically in conditioned athletes; some are also found in pathologic states, such as congestive heart failure or hypertrophic cardiomyopathy. In such cases, however, other parameters easily seen during echocardiographic study readily

TABLE 5. Echocardiographic Changes in Isotonic (Aerobic) and Isometric (Anaerobic) Athletes

Measurement	Isotonic	Isometric
Left ventricular end-diastolic diameter	↑	↑, no Δ
Left ventricular end-diastolic diameter per square meter or kilogram	↑	no Δ
Left ventricular end-systolic diameter	↑, ↓, no Δ	↑, ↓, no Δ
Left ventricular end-diastolic volume	↑	no Δ
Left ventricular posterior wall thickness	↑	↑
Left ventricular mass	↑	↑
Left ventricular mass per square meter or per kilogram	↑	no Δ
Interventricular septal thickness	↑	↑
Interventricular septum-to-posterior wall ratio	↑, no Δ	↑, no Δ
Right ventricular diameter	↑	—
Left atrial diameter	↑	—
Ejection fraction	no Δ	no Δ
Cardiac output (resting)	no Δ	no Δ
Stroke volume	↑	↑, no Δ
Velocity of circumferential fiber shortening	↑, ↓, no Δ	no Δ

↑ denotes increase, ↓ denotes decrease, and no Δ = no change.
From Huston TP, Puffer JC, Rodney WM: The athletic heart syndrome. N Engl J Med 313:24–32, 1985, with permission.

TABLE 6. Ventricular Dimensions in Athletes and Nonathletes as Assessed by Echocardiography in Published Studies

	Nonathlete Controls		Athletes		
Echocardiographic Variable	***Mean Value***	***No. of Subjects***	***Mean Value***	***No. of Subjects***	**Percent Difference**
Ventricular septal thickness (mm)	9.1	313	10.4	461	+14.3
Posterior free wall thickness (mm)	9.0	439	10.7	740	+18.9
LV end-diastolic diameter	49.1	394	53.9	701	+ 9.8
Estimated LV mass (g)	175	252	256	381	+46.3
RV internal transverse diameter (mm)	17.7	146	22.0	147	+24.3

LV = left ventricular; RV = right ventricular.
From Maron BJ: Structural features of the athletic heart as defined by echocardiography. J Am Coll Cardiol 7:190–302, 1986; reprinted with permission from the American College of Cardiology.

discriminate the ill from the athletic heart, and further invasive testing usually is not indicated. **Echocardiograms are not routinely ordered for the asymptomatic athlete.**

1. **Left ventricular end-diastolic diameter** is usually increased and can be observed to change as training progresses, an average of 9.8% with training (Table 6). This increase results directly in an increase in SV, which produces greater CO, thus culminating in an increase in maximal myocardial $\dot{V}O_2max$ and, ultimately, athletic performancc.
2. **Right ventricular end-diastolic diameter** is generally increased in dynamic athletes. If it were not, this rate limiting factor would prevent an increase in $\dot{V}O_2max$.
3. **Left atrial enlargement** of a mild degree occurred in more than half of all studies surveyed. In conditioned athletes, the **right atrial** transverse axis has been increased by up to 22% when compared with nonathletes.
4. **The left ventricular free wall and the septum undergo hypertrophy in response to both static and dynamic exercise.** Average wall thickness increases from 14% to 19% in athletes. These dimensions usually remain within normal limits (< 14 mm), but a thickness of up to 15 mm occasionally has been reported. Either of these changes may begin to revert with deconditioning in as little as 4 days. Overall, the aerobic heart develops eccentric hypertrophy, whereas the anaerobic pattern is one of concentric or uniform enlargement. Stress echocardiography is believed to be a sensitive technique for uncovering ventricular wall motion abnormalities, which may aid in evaluation of difficult situations.

H. **Exercise testing in athletes**

1. Treadmill or bicycle ergometry exercise testing **can be helpful** in specified circumstances to determine how an athlete responds to the stress of dynamic exercise. The desirability of universal exercise ECG screening varies from one community to another.[6] When indicated and if there are no contraindications, athletes may undergo symptom-limited maximal exercise testing. Because there is a wide scatter around age-predicted maximal HRs, subjects should be allowed to exercise to a maximal perceived exertion as outlined by the Borg scale (i.e., exercising to a 20 on a scale of 6 to 20). **Many of the rhythm and electrocardiographic changes seen in dynamic athletes at rest resolve during exercise.** Thallium imaging can elucidate problem cases.
2. Conditioned athletes have a work capacity much higher than nonathletes. $\dot{V}O_2max$ near 70 ml/kg/min can sometimes be attained in world-class performers; the average active 20-year-old attains closer to 40 ml/kg/min. **If athletes can exercise to maximal effort without difficulty, then the clinician can conclude that abnormal ECG changes are likely to represent the Athletic Heart Syndrome.** This is helpful to

clear certain athletes for maximal training. **Routine screening for CAD in asymptomatic athletes is not recommended.** The high rate of false-positive results in such a low-risk population would incorrectly label many healthy athletes as having pathology and lead to additional, expensive, often invasive and usually unnecessary testing. Finally, no screening examination detects all individuals with heart disease or other disorders predisposing to disability or death.

IV. Other Conditions Related to the Athletic Heart and to Exercise-associated Events and Sudden Death in Athletes

A. **Congenital abnormalities of the coronary arteries**, especially **anomalous origin of the coronary artery, valvular stenosis**, and **CAD**, are entities that the team physician seeks to bring to the forefront during the examination. In studies by Maron and associates, 97% of young athletes who died unexpectedly while exercising had structural cardiovascular abnormalities, of which anomalies of the coronary artery were the most common, followed by hypertrophic cardiomyopathy and CAD. Short of angiographic study of vast numbers of athletes, and perhaps even *if* it is done, not all cases of sudden cardiac morbidity and mortality can be avoided. A report of an intussusception of a coronary artery serves as a reminder that clinicians are currently unable to screen for every potentially lethal condition. The previously described screening evaluation consisting of the personal **history**, review of symptoms (**syncope, dyspnea,** and **chest pain**) and **physical** examination is the most practical means of evaluation presently available.

B. **Hypertrophic cardiomyopathy** is another structural cardiovascular abnormality that is often uncovered by the personal history and physical examination: the review of symptoms (especially **syncope**), the family history (**early death**), and the cardiac examination with attention to **murmurs that increase on Valsalva** or other maneuvers that decrease preload, such as sudden standing after squatting. Additional evaluation using echocardiography is an excellent means of confirming this entity if it is suspected. A pattern of pronounced asymmetrically-increased thickening is found particularly in the outflow tract along with the other distinctive features that are diagnostic of the condition.

C. The distinction between a basketball coach's dream and an individual with **Marfan's syndrome** is not necessarily manifestly obvious. It is noteworthy that perhaps 80% of those with Marfan's syndrome have a similarly affected relative. Thus, although no single feature is pathognomonic and clinical features vary, a positive **family history**, presence of a **murmur**, and **physical inspection** and measurements (Table 7) offer appropriate opportunities for uncovering the condition. Confirmation can occur through use of echocardiography or arteriography.

TABLE 7. Suggested Screening Format for Marfan's Syndrome

Screen all men over 6 feet and all women over 5 feet 10 inches in height with electrocardiogram and slit-lamp examination when any two of the following are found:

- Family history of Marfan's syndrome*
- Cardiac murmur or midsystolic click
- Kyphoscoliosis
- Anterior thoracic deformity (i.e., pectus excavatum)
- Arm span greater than height
- Upper-to-lower body ratio more than 1 standard deviation below the mean
- Myopia
- Ectopic lens

* This finding alone should prompt further investigation.

From Hara JH, Puffer JC: The preparticipation physical examination. In Mellion MB (ed): Office Management of Sports Injuries and Athletic Problems. Philadelphia, Hanley & Belfus, 1988.

D. **Mitral valve prolapse** is clinically detectable in about 5% of athletes and is the most common valvular disorder; in suspected groups, i.e., females, those with sickle cell anemia, those with Marfan's syndrome, and those with scoliosis, it is higher. In non-screened echocardiography studies, elements of prolapse may be found in 15–20% of the general population. Most of those individuals are asymptomatic. In those reporting problems, chest pain, unexplained syncope, fatigue, inappropriate dyspnea, and/or palpitations predominate. There is frequently a large autonomic nervous system component involved. **Symptomatic patients are said to have mitral valve prolapse syndrome**, and probably further evaluation is prudent. The ECG usually reveals repolarization abnormalities (commonly biphasic or inverted T waves in the inferior leads), and the echocardiogram illustrates the extent of prolapse. **Asymptomatic patients require no further evaluation or restrictions.**

E. **Myocardial bridging** is a condition in which the coronary arteries at various points in their course become covered by myocardial contractile tissue and are thus compressed and occluded during systole. Because intramural arteries can be found in up to 27% of unselected autopsies, however, and are seen in 12% of cardiac catheterizations, the **significance remains uncertain.**

F. **Neurogenic syncope,** also known as **neurocardiogenic, vasovagal**, or **vasodepressor syncope**, is thought by some to be the **most common disorder responsible for exercise-associated syncope.**

1. A rare but potentially life-threatening manifestation of this entity may be exercise-associated cardiac asystole. Numerous reports of syncope following activity indicate this is a neurally mediated response.
2. A **tilt test** is the primary diagnostic method used following conventional evaluation for athletes without structural cardiac pathology who report syncope during or immediately after exertion.
   a. The patient is placed on a tilt table supine then gradually elevated through intermediate angles until nearly upright; this reduces orthostatic effects.
   b. **A positive test results when bradycardia or hypotension occurs** after several minutes; if no symptoms occur within 30–60 minutes, the test is negative.
3. The syncope possibly results from **vagotonia**, transient increases in amount of or sensitivity to **circulating catecholamines**, and inappropriate vasodilatation.
4. It is also possible that in the athlete additional triggers exist, including:
   a. Diminished absolute blood volume due to sweating
   b. Diminished relative volume due to peripheral cutaneous shunting and vasodilatation, which occurs for cooling purposes
   c. Required increase in skeletal muscle perfusion
5. Treatment modalities are in nascent form.
   a. Drugs, primarily beta-blockers, disopyramide, vasolytics, and pacemakers, are available for both the bradycardiac and the vasodilatation components but are difficult to evaluate because many of the athletes do not have persistent symptoms over time, even after initial positive tilt tests.
   b. Many believe that the indications for such interventions are not present for what is usually a benign condition.
   c. Finally, athletes are not always eager to take drugs or other measures that may lead to negative enhancement of their functional ability.

V. Management Strategy

A. In managing athletes, the clinician encounters changes that in the context of the non-conditioned individual might signal cardiac pathology. **The findings described in the Athletic Heart Syndrome in the absence of symptoms require no evaluation.** Alternatively, it is recognized that the ability to engage in athletics does not necessarily protect against morbidity even in a marathoner (see Pheidippides 490 B.C.). **Further evaluation is needed** in the individual who:

1. Mentions **exertional chest pain, unexplained syncope**, or **inappropriate dyspnea**
2. Reports familial risk factors, especially **early cardiac** or **unexplained sudden death**
3. Demonstrates critical physical findings, i.e., the screening **criteria for Marfan's syndrome or murmurs other than a low-grade midsystolic that does not decrease on Valsalva maneuver**.

B. **SCD is a rare occurrence**, estimated at 10 to 25 events yearly in the under-30 age group. To prevent one event of SCD requires identifying and protecting one specific individual out of a group of approximately 250,000 athletes. It is additionally true that **conditioning is protective** for the population in general, and this may also include those at high cardiovascular risk. It is the place of the team physician to encourage activity whenever appropriate, and **a focused history and appropriate cardiac screening examination is the best way to distinguish those at risk** from those in whom a high probability of health exists. In individuals with physical signs or mild ECG abnormalities attributable to the conditioned myocardium, it is recommended to state categorically that the athlete is absolutely "supernormal" unless one has convincing evidence of possible organic heart disease. Although it is certainly recognized that the American medical profession is in an extremely cautious posture regarding the underdiagnosis of disease, nonetheless, the aforementioned strategy appropriately stratifies those that need further investigation while avoiding unnecessary curtailment of activity, cardiac neurosis, or financial strain in those demonstrating changes commonly encountered in the **Athletic Heart Syndrome**.

Recommended Reading

1. Ades PA: Preventing sudden death. Phys Sportsmed 20:75, 1992.
2. Blake JB, Laaraba RC: Observations upon long distance runners. Boston Med J Surg J 148:95, 1903.
3. Buttrick PM, Scheuer J: Exercise and the heart. In Schlant RC, Alexander RW (eds): The Heart, 8th ed. New York, McGraw-Hill, 1992, pp 2063–2065.
4. Cohen JL, Gupta PK, Lichstein E, Chadda KD: The heart of a dancer: Noninvasive cardiac assessment. J Appl Physiol 51:881–886, 1981.
5. DeMaria AN, Newmann A, Lee G, et al: Alterations in ventricular mass and performance induced by exercise training in man evaluated by echocardiography. Circulation 57:2370–2374, 1978.
6. Detrano R, Lyons KP, Marcondas G, et al: Methodologic problems in exercise testing research: Are we solving them? Arch Intern Med 148:1289–1295, 1988.
7. Erbe RW: Medical genetics. In Dale DC, Federman DD (eds): Scientific American Medicine. New York, Scientific American, 1978–95, 9:IV-29.
8. Fenici R, Caselli G, Zeppilli P, Piovano G: High degree A-V block in 17 well-trained endurance athletes. In Lubich T, Venerando A (eds): Sports Cardiology. Bologna, Aulo Gaggi, 1980, pp 523–537.
9. Gersony WM, Pruett AW: Cardiovascular system: Mitral valve prolapse. In Behrman RE, Kleigman RM, Nelson WE, Vaughn VC (eds): Nelson Textbook of Pediatrics, 14th ed. Philadelphia, W.B. Saunders, 1992, p 1182.
10. Grauer K, Gums J: Ventricular arrhythmias: Part I. Prevalence, significance, and indications for treatment. J Am Board Fam Physicians 1:135–142, 1988.
11. Haidet GC, Mitchell JH: Athlete's heart. In Hurst JW (ed): Medicine for the Practicing Physician, 3rd ed. Stoneham, MA, Butterworth, 1992, pp 1166–1168.
12. Hancock EW: Syncope. In Dale DC, Federman DD (eds): Scientific American Medicine. New York, Scientific American, 1978–95, 1:IV-1.
13. Hauser AM, Dressendorfer RH, Von M, et al: Symmetric cardiac enlargement in highly trained endurance athletes: A two dimensional echocardiographic study. Am Heart J 109:1038–1044, 1985.
14. Herbert WG, Froelicher VF, Cantwell JD: Exercise tests for coronary and asymptomatic patients. Phys Sportsmed 19:55–62, 1991.
15. Huston TP, Puffer JC, Rodney WM: The athletic heart syndrome. N Engl J Med 313:24–32, 1985.
16. Isner JM: Cardiovascular screening of competitive and noncompetitive athletes. In Harrington JT (ed): Consultation in Internal Medicine. Philadelphia, B.C. Decker, 1990, p 99.

17. Lembo NJ, Dell'Italia LJ, Crawford MH, O'Rourke RA: Bedside diagnosis of systolic murmurs. N Engl J Med 1572–1578, 1988.
18. MacDougall JD, Tuxen D, Sale DG, et al: Arterial blood pressure response to heavy resistance exercise. J Appl Physiol 58:785–790, 1985.
19. Maron BJ: Structural features of the athlete heart as defined by echocardiography. J Am Coll Cardiol 7:190–203, 1986.
20. Maron BJ, Roberts WC, McAllister HA, et al: Sudden death in young athletes. Circulation 62:218–229, 1980.
21. Minamitani K, Miyagawa M, Konco M, Kiamura K: The electrocardiogram of professional cyclists. In Lubich T, Venerando A (eds): Sports Cardiology. Bologna, Aulo Gaggi, 1980, pp 315–325.
22. Parker BM, Londeree BR, Cupp GV, Dubiel JP: The noninvasive cardiac evaluation of long distance runners. Chest 73:376–381, 1978.
23. Paulsen W, Boughner D, Ko P, et al: Left ventricular function in marathon runner: Echocardiographic assessment. J Appl Physiol 51:881–886, 1981.
24. Puffer JC: Case of the winded jogger. Fam Pract News Sept 15, 1993.
25. Roeske WR, O'Rourke RA, Klein A, et al: Noninvasive evaluation of ventricular hypertrophy in professional athletes. Circulation 53:286–292, 1976.
26. Rogers CC: Strong statements on kids and sports. Phys Sportsmed 13(8):32, 1985.
27. Sakaguchi S, Shultz JJ, Remole SC, et al: Syncope associated with exercise: Dept of Med, University of MN. Am J Cardiol 75(7):476–481, 1995.
28. Simon HB: Exercise, health, and sports medicine. In Dale DC, Federman DD (eds): Scientific American Medicine. New York, Scientific American, 1978–95, CTM:I-17, 3, 17.
29. Snoechke LHEH, Abelling HFM, Lambregts JAC, et al: Echocardiographic dimensions in athletes in relation to their training programs. Med Sci Sports Exerc 14:428–434, 1982.
30. Tanji JL: Medical problems of the athlete. In Taylor RB (ed): Family Medicine, 4th ed. New York, Springer-Verlag, 1994, pp 383–384.
31. Tse HP, Lau CP: Exercise-associated cardiac asystolic in persons without structural heart disease. Chest 107(20):572–576, 1995.
32. VanCamp SP: Sudden death. Clin Sports Med 11:273, 1992.
33. Zeppilli P, Fenici R, Sassara M, et al: Wenckebach second-degree A-V block in top-ranking athletes: An old problem revisited. Am Heart J 100:281–294, 1980.
34. Zeppilli P, Pirrami MM, Sassara M, Fenici R: Ventricular repolarization disturbances in athletes: Standardization of terminology, ethiopathogenic spectrum and pathophysiological mechanism. J Sports Med Phys Fitness 21:322–335, 1981.
35. Zeppitti S, Sandric S, Cecchetti F, et al: Echocardiographic assessments of cardiac arrangements in different sports activities. In Lubich T, Venerando A (eds): Sports Cardiology. Bologna, Aulo Gaggi, 1980, pp 723–724.

32

The Hypertensive Athlete

Thomas R. Sachtleben, M.D., and Morris B. Mellion, M.D.

I. Hemodynamics and Cardiovascular Anatomy

A. **Hemodynamics of hypertension**

1. Blood pressure (BP) is the result of two factors: **cardiac output (CO)** × **total peripheral resistance (TPR)**
2. Severity of hypertension is classified into six stages (Table 1). Higher stages are associated with a higher risk of nonfatal and fatal cardiovascular disease as well as progressive renal disease.
3. The development of hypertension progresses through various stages, each marked by hemodynamic abnormalities (Fig. 1).
   a. **High normal BP**
      i. Earliest stage of hypertension
      ii. Also known as latent or labile hypertension
      iii. Associated with increased CO and "normal" TPR. TPR is normal when compared with resting levels in normotensives, but is inappropriately high in the face of elevated CO:
         (a) In the nonhypertensive, TPR falls to compensate for rise in CO, thereby maintaining normal BP.
         (b) Lack of TPR decrease is due to impaired baroreceptor function.
         (c) Baroreceptors are "reset" to maintain an elevated rather than a normal BP over time.
      iv. Accompanied by increased serum catecholamine levels, renin levels, and renal blood flow
      v. Individuals with high normal hypertension are hypersensitive to catecholamine secretion and mental stress and have a hyperkinetic circulatory state.
   b. **Stage I (mild) hypertension**
      i. If high normal BPs do not "resolve," they develop into stage I hypertension.
      ii. Most common form of hypertension
      iii. Associated with increased CO and decreased TPR
      iv. Decreased arterial lumen and disturbed autoregulation of blood flow in the periphery
      v. Often the first stage that is detected in a medical setting
   c. **Stage II (moderate) hypertension**
      i. Associated with decreased CO and increased TPR
      ii. Increased afterload leads to left ventricular hypertrophy (LVH)
   d. **Stage III (severe) hypertension**—development of diastolic dysfunction
   e. **Stage IV (very severe) hypertension**
      i. CO can no longer increase in response to exercise or other physiologic demands.
      ii. Marked LVH exists.

TABLE 1. Classification of Hypertension

	Systolic (mmHg)	Diastolic (mmHg)
Normal	< 130	< 85
High normal	130–139	85–89
Hypertension		
Stage 1 (mild)	140–159	90–99
Stage 2 (moderate)	160–179	100–109
Stage 3 (severe)	180–209	110–119
Stage 4 (very severe)	> 210	> 120

For adults aged 18 and older. This categorization applies to individuals not taking antihypertensives and not acutely ill. When systolic and diastolic pressures fall into different categories, the higher category should be selected to classify the athlete's blood pressure status.

Adapted from the Fifth Report of the Joint National Committee on Detection, Evaluation, and Treatment of High Blood Pressure (JNC V). Arch Intern Med 153:154–183, 1993.

iii. Loss of contractility leads to inability to clear fluid:
   (a) Congestive heart failure develops.
   (b) Peripheral edema and cardiac edema are threats to cardiovascular function and electrolyte balance.

B. **Hemodynamics and cardiovascular effects of exercise**
  1. **Isotonic (dynamic) exercise**
    a. **Acute effects**
      i. $\uparrow\dot{V}O_2 = \uparrow CO \times \uparrow A - \dot{V}O_2$ (arterio-venous oxygen difference)
        (a) $\uparrow$CO = $\uparrow$SV (stroke volume) × $\uparrow$HR (heart rate). SV increases with higher workloads up to an exercise intensity between 40% and 60% of maximal capacity, then reaches a plateau.
        (b) $\uparrow A - \dot{V}O_2$ difference = increased oxygen utilization by active muscles. The $A - \dot{V}O_2$ difference can increase threefold from resting levels to maximal intensity exercise because of decreases in venous O_2 content.
      ii. BP = $\uparrow\uparrow$CO × $\downarrow$TPR (normotensive):
        (a) $\uparrow$systolic BP and $\uparrow$mean arterial pressure in direct proportion to increases in exercise intensity

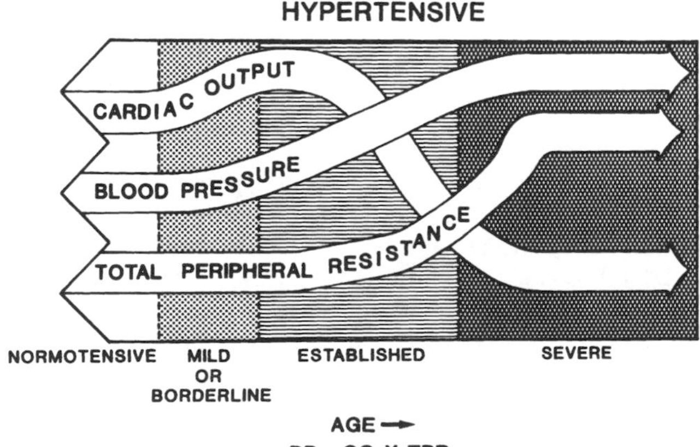

FIGURE 1. The development of hypertension progresses through various stages, each marked by hemodynamic abnormalities. Depicted are the changes in cardiac output, total peripheral resistance, and blood pressure over time in the untreated patient.

(b) ↓TPR, with small decrease in diastolic BP
(c) Eventual ↓ in systolic BP with prolonged exercise due to arteriole dilation in active muscles (normal response)

b. **Chronic effects**
   i. Reduced resting BPs:
      (a) ↓systolic BP average of 11 mmHg
      (b) ↓diastolic BP average of 6 mmHg
   ii. LV size increases:
      (a) Marked increase in LV diameter and lumen produces increased LV mass
      (b) Slight thickening of ventricular walls
   iii. Higher $\dot{V}O_2$max associated with reduced arterial stiffness
   iv. Training effects, including increased SV and LVH, disappear after as little as 2 months of inactivity.

2. **Isometric (static) exercise**
   a. **Acute effects**
      i. ↑↑↑BP dramatically and rapidly with high-intensity training
         (a) Systolic BP increases to 200–300 mmHg have been observed during weightlifting.
         (b) Associated use of the Valsalva maneuver creates a tremendous increase in intrathoracic pressure and subsequent increase in arterial pressure.
         (c) **Exclusive upper body exercise results in greater BP responses compared with lower body exercise at equal rates of energy expenditure.**
         (d) Peak BPs occur at or near exhaustion and during maximal lifts.
      ii. ↑HR
      iii. ↑TPR
   b. **Chronic effects**
      i. Repetitive isometric exercise can lead to thickened LV walls (septal and posterior) and decreased lumen:
         (a) **Concentric LVH can eventually result.**
         (b) Diastolic function is preserved.
         (c) **Anatomic changes may be more prevalent in African-American athletes.**
      ii. Even in normal athletes, **prolonged high-intensity isometric exercise leads to decreased CO.** Adolescent and young adult athletes have a higher resting level of CO, but continued isometric exercise may lead to CO decrease.
      iii. Reduced BPs occur during exercise.
      iv. Chronic exposure to high BPs with resistance training does *not* result in higher resting BPs.

3. **Hypertensive athletes and exercisers**
   a. TPR is increased during dynamic exercise in hypertensives of all classes.
   b. **BP should be controlled before allowing the athlete or exerciser to participate in vigorous sports because both dynamic and isometric exercise cause marked BP increases.**
   c. Caution should be observed in those with cardiovascular disease because of high BP responses during both isotonic and isometric exercise.
   d. Low-intensity warm-up is important before vigorous exercise.
   e. In resistance training, minimize sets to exhaustion.
   f. **Hypertensive athletes or exercisers do not shunt blood to the skin as effectively as normotensives:**
      i. Core temperatures can rise precipitously.
      ii. This makes exercise in the heat particularly dangerous for a hypertensive. The fluid loss that accompanies exercise in the heat may also cause potas-

sium loss, which can be especially dangerous for the hypertensive athlete or exerciser.

g. **Sports participation clearance**
   i. **Stage 1, 2 hypertension:**
      (a) Allow to play if BP is well controlled and there is no target organ damage or heart disease.
      (b) Recheck BP every 2–4 months.
   ii. **Stage 3, 4 hypertension.** Restrict from play, especially from sports with a high static component (wrestling, gymnastics, weightlifting, rock climbing, rowing) until hypertension is well controlled.

II. Diagnosis of Hypertension

A. **Resting BP**
   1. Hypertension is defined as BP above 140/90 on a consistent basis.
   2. **Early, or labile, hypertension is usually marked by an increase in systolic BP.** Primarily caused by ↑CO.
   3. **As hypertension progresses, diastolic BP begins to increase.**
      a. **Primarily caused by ↑ TPR.**
      b. **Diastolic BP above 120 should be treated immediately and aggressively.**
      c. **Elevated diastolic BP places the patient at risk for coronary heart disease, cerebral hemorrhage, and renal damage.**

B. **Progressive hypertension is accompanied by target organ disease.**
   1. Electrocardiogram (ECG) changes suggest LVH or coronary artery disease.
   2. Early renal damage may not be indicated by changes in serum creatinine or blood urea nitrogen.
   3. Microalbuminuria and mild proteinuria may be indicators of early renal damage. May be hard to diagnose in athletes participating in contact sports.
   4. Retinopathy is indicated by retinal hemorrhages or exudates, with or without papilledema.

C. **BP during exercise**
   1. **Exercise stress testing can be used to predict and differentiate types of hypertension.**
      a. **Differentiating stages of hypertension**
         i. Individuals with high normal BP (see Table 1) start at higher resting levels than normotensives but do not show abnormally high BP levels during maximal exercise.
         ii. Some research suggests that labile hypertensives show less increase in pulse pressure than normotensives. This may be due to less compliant vascular beds.
         iii. Rapid elevation in systolic BP indicates established hypertension.
         iv. **Hypertensives tend to increase their diastolic BP** during and after exercise.
      b. **Predicting future hypertension**
         i. **Exaggerated systolic BPs (> 85th percentile) during treadmill testing are associated with a higher risk of developing future hypertension:**
            (a) Systolic BPs greatly amplified during exercise may suggest LVH in normotensive individuals.
            (b) Bicycle ergometry allows more accurate BP measurements than treadmill testing.
            (c) Field testing is more reliable than laboratory monitoring.
         ii. Exercise blood pressure may be a significant predictor of adverse cardiovascular events in high-risk patients.
         iii. Individual differences in cardiovascular reactivity—hyperreactivity may predict future cardiovascular sequelae.

D. **"White coat" hypertension and other stress phenomena**
   1. Initial resting BP may not accurately estimate true BP.
      a. Anxiety provoked by a medical examination can lead to artificially elevated BP, known as "white coat" hypertension.
      b. Other sources of mental stress can lead to elevated BP.
   2. An average of several readings is a better estimate of true BP.
      a. If initial BP is high, have athlete rest for 5 minutes and repeat BP check.
      b. If BP remains elevated, check BP at least once per week for at least 4 weeks before making the diagnosis of hypertension.
   3. Averaged daily BP is a better predictor of later end organ damage than random office BP.
      a. Ambulatory 24-hour BP monitoring remains difficult and expensive.
      b. Athletes/exercisers can take their own BP as an alternative:
         i. The athlete/exerciser must be well trained in the measurement of BP.
         ii. Emphasize the importance of *accurate* readings.

III. Approaches to Management of Hypertension

A. Although there are many diverse approaches to the management of hypertension, management of the hypertensive athlete (or the exercising adult with hypertension) generally involves a combination of several nonpharmacologic therapies, often with one or more antihypertensive medications.

B. **Nonpharmacologic strategies** may provide a safe, effective foundation for any good antihypertensive regimen. Their strength lies in the fact that **risk of side effects is low** to nonexistent, but their weakness is that for success **they depend on long-term compliance with major changes in deeply ingrained lifestyle behaviors.**
   1. Nonpharmacologic approaches used without concurrent antihypertensive medications are most appropriate for the control of high normal or stage 1 hypertension, but they may be useful as adjunctive therapies for all levels of hypertension.
   2. **Dietary modification**
      a. **Altering electrolyte intakes**
         i. **Decreasing sodium intake:**
            (a) Goal—2.3 g dietary sodium (6 g NaCl)/day
            (b) Especially important in "salt-sensitive" hypertensives (two thirds of African-American hypertensives are "salt-sensitive")
         ii. **Increasing potassium intake:**
            (a) Hypokalemia may increase BP and induce ventricular ectopy.
            (b) High dietary potassium may be protective against the development of hypertension and may reduce the incidence of stroke.
            (c) No additional benefit of potassium exists in patients already sodium restricted.
         iii. **Increasing calcium intake:**
            (a) Many hypertensives, especially women, may be calcium deficient.
            (b) 800–1200 mg/day (recommended daily allowance) of elemental calcium supplementation may reduce BP in some patients.
         iv. **Increasing magnesium intake (controversial):**
            (a) Magnesium acts as a vasodilator.
            (b) Possible benefit exists, but conflicting research offers no current role in the management of hypertension.
      b. **Weight reduction**
         i. Obesity defined as body mass index (BMI = kg/m^2) > 30
         ii. **Obesity increases both preload and afterload on heart, resulting in hypertensive effect.**

(a) **Elevated preload** (pattern common in normal to stage 1 hypertensives) due to:
(i) ↑intravascular volume
(ii) ↑total peripheral resistance
(iii) ↑left ventricular preload
(b) **Elevated afterload** due to:
(i) ↑central norepinephrine production
(ii) ↑total peripheral resistance
(iii) ↑left ventricular afterload
(c) Hypertensives with combined elevation of both preload and afterload are at high risk for accelerated LVH and congestive heart failure.
(d) Weight reduction may alter both preload and afterload.

iii. Obese hypertensives have **hyperinsulinemia** associated with increased insulin resistance. Insulin levels correlate directly with BP.
iv. Weight reduction diminishes need for concomitant antihypertensive agents.
v. **Weight reduction is the most effective nonpharmacologic measure for BP reduction.** Average reduction in systolic BP of 15 mmHg and diastolic BP of 10 mmHg with 10-kg weight loss.

c. **Elimination or moderation of alcohol consumption**
i. Alcohol use is directly related to hypertension.
ii. Daily consumption should be limited to 1 ounce (2 beers)of alcohol/day.

d. **High-fiber diet**—no significant effect on BP despite some earlier suggestions that dietary fiber may play a role in reducing hypertension.
e. **Dietary fats**—low saturated fat diets have minimal effect on BP.
f. **Caffeine**—acutely raises BP, but avoidance is unnecessary because of the rapid development of tolerance.

3. **Relaxation therapies**—although some individuals may have a good response as adjunct therapy, relaxation techniques have not been proven beneficial in the control of hypertension.
a. Biofeedback can be used directly for BP change or for general relaxation effects through change in other systems, such as muscle tension.
b. Stress management
c. Progressive relaxation, which employs tensing and releasing muscle groups, needs to be used with care in severe hypertensives.
d. Meditation

4. **Exercise therapy**
a. Documented evidence of benefit
i. **Epidemiologic evidence** demonstrates that vigorous exercise correlates with lower risk of developing hypertension.
ii. **Clinical trials** demonstrate:
(a) Aerobic exercise conditioning lowers resting systolic BP an average of 11 mmHg and diastolic BP an average of 6 mmHg in hypertensives:
- Benefit more marked in high normal and stage 1 hypertensives
- Degree of reduction depends on initial systolic BP and increase in work capacity
- Multiple research studies, but most are uncontrolled or poorly designed

(b) Difficult to differentiate the direct effect of exercise on BP from the effect of weight loss that often accompanies exercise conditioning.

iii. Endurance exercise causes an even greater BP reduction in patients with secondary hypertension caused by renal dysfunction.

b. **Prescribing exercise—"FITT"**
i. **Frequency:** five to six sessions/week
ii. **Intensity:** 55–70% of predicted maximum heart rate (MHR)

(a) Moderate intensity (55–70% MHR) exercise lowers BP more effectively than higher intensities (80–85% MHR):
- Moderate intensity exercise also considered 40–70% $\dot{V}O_2max$ by some authorities.
- Higher intensity exercise may actually increase resting BPs.

(b) In older or less fit patients, start at 55–60% MHR; in more fit patients start at 65–70% MHR.

(c) Predicted MHR:
Men: 225 – Age Women: 220 – Age

iii. **Time** (duration): initially 15–20 minutes; eventually 30–40 minutes/session

iv. **Type of exercise:** "dynamic isotonic exercise" or moving body through space:

(a) Walking (d) Cycling
(b) Jogging (e) Cross country skiing
(c) Swimming (f) Aerobic dance

c. **Avoid intense isometric exercise.**

i. **Massive BP elevation is associated with resistance training involving heavy loads and low repetitions.**

ii. Low-weight (40–50% of maximum repetition), high-repetition resistance training, i.e., circuit training, does not lead to hypertension.

iii. There are no good research data about the safety of isometric exercise in well-controlled hypertensives.

iv. Hypertensives should avoid inversion therapy (i.e., hanging in an inverted position).

C. **Pharmacotherapy**

1. **General principles**

a. **All current antihypertensives permit an essentially normal exercise response except beta-blockers and diuretics.**

i. Some do so better than others.

ii. There is still a role for beta-blockers, especially cardioselective types.

b. The choice of agent may depend on other considerations:

i. Athletes with a history of electrolyte disturbances or heat illness

ii. Certain drugs, such as beta-blockers, may be banned from particular levels of competition.

c. Consider eliminating common causes of drug-induced hypertension:

i. Nonsteroidal anti-inflammatory drugs (including aspirin and ibuprofen) may decrease BP control:

(a) Reduce effects of beta-blockers and angiotensin-converting enzyme (ACE) inhibitors

(b) Antagonize effects of diuretics

ii. Sympathomimetics (decongestants)

iii. Oral contraceptives

iv. Appetite suppressants

d. **Classes of antihypertensives that reduce TPR have less effect on exercise capacity.**

2. **Best choices for endurance athletes**

a. **ACE inhibitors** (captopril, enalapril, lisinopril, benzapril, fosinopril, quinapril, and ramipril)

i. Block conversion of angiotensin I to angiotensin II:

(a) Block vasoconstriction caused by angiotensin II; therefore ↓TPR

(b) Block sodium and water retention stimulated by aldosterone, which is secreted in response to angiotensin II

(c) ↑bradykinin and vasodilatory prostaglandins

ii. Hemodynamic effects during exercise:
    (a) ↑SV
    (b) ↓HR (slightly)
    (c) ↓TPR
iii. Decrease "exaggerated" BP effect during exercise
iv. Decrease hypertension without an associated decrease in $\dot{V}O_2$max or increase in rate of perceived exertion
v. Anecdotal reports of postural hypotension in athletes stopping abruptly following intense endurance exercise. Emphasize need for cooling down following exercise to prevent venous pooling.
vi. **Drug of choice for many athletes owing to low incidence of side effects:**
    (a) Concomitant use of nonsteroidal anti-inflammatory drugs may cause hyperkalemia because of potassium-sparing effect of ACE inhibitors.
    (b) Caution with additional potassium in fluid replacement drinks

b. **Alpha$_1$-receptor blockers** (prazosin, terazosin, and doxazosin)
   i. Competitively block the postsynaptic alpha$_1$ arteriolar smooth muscle receptors; thus ↓TPR
   ii. Normalize central hemodynamics at rest and during exercise
   iii. Rarely cause an exaggerated hypotensive response to the first dose. Response to first dose should be monitored.

c. **Central alpha-agonists** (clonidine, guanabenz, guanfacine, methyldopa)
   i. Act on alpha$_2$-receptors in brain stem to block central sympathetic stimulation; thus, ↓HR and ↓TPR at rest. Also block sympathetically mediated sodium retention.
   ii. Normal hemodynamic response to exercise
   iii. Clonidine available in a transdermal system (patch replaced once per week)

d. **Calcium antagonists** (diltiazem, nicardipine, nifedipine, felodipine, amlodipine, isradipine, verapamil)
   i. Lower BP by reducing calcium concentration in vascular smooth muscle cells; thus ↓TPR
   ii. No decrease in maximal aerobic capacity
   iii. Normal physiologic hemodynamics at rest and during exercise
   iv. Additive effect with exercise in further reducing BP during postexercise period
   v. Many physicians have found this class of drugs useful as first-step therapy in athletes. Concerns that warrant caution in exercising hypertensives:
      (a) HR suppression—verapamil and diltiazem. CO unchanged, however, because SV↑
      (b) Hemoconcentration during exercise—verapamil
      (c) Reflex tachycardia—nifedipine, nicardipine, and other dihydropyridine derivatives
      (d) ↓LV contractility—verapamil and diltiazem
      (e) Intransigent pedal edema—nifedipine, nicardipine

3. **Beta-blockers** (Table 2)
   a. **Useful in certain groups:**
      i. Intermittent exertion sports
      ii. Untrained or partially trained athlete
      iii. Arteriosclerotic heart disease patients
      iv. Hypertensives with excessive rise in systolic BP during exercise
   b. **General effects of beta-blockers**
      i. **Acute:**
         (a) ↓myocardial contractility and ↓HR
         (b) ↑diastole

TABLE 2. Beta-blocking Agents Arranged by Cardioselectivity and Intrinsic Sympathomimetic Activity (ISA)

	No ISA	ISA
Cardioselective	Atenolol (Tenormin) Metoprolol (Lopressor) Carteolol (Cartrol) Penbutolol (Levatol) Betaxolol (Kerlone) Bisoprolol (Zebeta)	Acebutolol (Sectral)
Noncardioselective	Nadolol (Corgard) Propranolol (Inderal) Sotalol (Sotacor) Timolol (Blocadren)	Alprenolol (Aptin) Oxprenolol (Trasicor) Pindolol (Visken)

(c) ↑coronary perfusion
(d) ↑exercise tolerance in coronary artery disease

ii. **Hemodynamic effects during exercise:**

(a) ↓↓HR with compensatory increase in oxygen extraction (A - $\dot{V}O_2$ diff) and possible compensatory SV (more common with cardioselective agents)

$$\dot{V}O_2 = (HR \times SV)\ (A - \dot{V}O_2 diff)$$
$$\downarrow \quad \downarrow\downarrow\downarrow \quad \uparrow \quad \uparrow$$

- Performance effect: **Well-trained subjects experience a greater drop in $\dot{V}O_2$max than untrained subjects taking beta-blockers.** More potential in the untrained for compensatory ↑A - $\dot{V}O_2$diff and ↑SV. Significant reduction in submaximal endurance exercise performance.
- Beta-blockers increase diastolic BP at all levels of workload.

(b) **↑TPR**

- Peripheral sympathetic effects:
  Alpha cause vasoconstriction
  $Beta_2$ cause vasodilatation
- Beta-blockers (especially noncardioselective) may block peripheral vasodilatation and result in unopposed vasoconstriction. Chronically, this effect may be blunted. **"Readjustment phenomenon"**—TPR returns to normal functional levels over several years.

c. **Metabolic effects of beta-blockers**

i. Block mobilization and utilization of free fatty acids

ii. **Noncardioselective agents block glycogenolysis:**

(a) **Hypoglycemia may occur, especially during or after intense exercise.**
(b) Masks symptoms of hypoglycemia
(c) Decreases insulin secretion from pancreas

iii. Can increase serum cholesterol, low-density lipoproteins, and triglyceride levels

d. Other effects of beta-blockers:

i. **Contraindicated in athletes with asthma**
ii. Associated with a higher incidence of impaired thermoregulation (hyperthermia)
iii. Increased incidence of hyperkalemia
iv. Reduce blood flow to muscles and cause muscle fatigue (more pronounced during first several weeks of therapy)

e. **Beta-blockers increase perceived exertion in working muscles,** thus causing reduced endurance:

i. Probably as a result of metabolic effects
ii. **No increase in cardiovascular perceived exertion**

f. Beta-blockers decrease performance more in individuals with a high percentage of slow-twitch muscle fibers. This effect is more pronounced on propranolol (noncardioselective) than on atenolol (cardioselective).
g. Effect of **intrinsic sympathomimetic activity** in beta-blockers on heart rate and cardiac output during intense exercise is unclear. Intrinsic sympathomimetic activity may prove helpful, but presently there are only a few studies with conflicting results.
h. Nonselective beta-blockers are contraindicated for athletes. Nonselective beta-blockers can significantly diminish maximal aerobic capacity.

4. **Combined alpha- and beta-blocker** (labetalol)
   a. Three effects
      i. **Beta blockade:**
         (a) ↓HR leading to ↓CO
         (b) ↓renin
      ii. **Alpha$_1$-blockade:** ↓vasoconstriction leading to ↓TPR
      iii. **Beta$_2$-agonist:** ↓TPR
      iv. Beta effects are greater than alpha effects (3:1 for oral formulations).
   b. ↓CO 10–14% at rest and during exercise after 1 year of therapy:
      i. CO gradually returns to baseline over next 5 years because of ↑SV.
      ii. TPR remains ↓15–20%.
5. **Diuretics** (chlorthalidone, hydrochlorothiazide, furosemide, spironolactone)
   a. **Acute effect** (< 30 days):
      i. ↓plasma volume
      ii. ↓SV
      iii. ↓CO
      iv. ↓BP
      v. Little to no change in TPR
   b. **Long-term effects, normal dose range:**
      i. **Small decrease in CO but generally not during exercise**
      ii. **Larger doses may produce a larger decrease in CO,** which may persist during exercise.
   c. Small doses of diuretics (12.5 mg hydrochlorothiazide) may be useful as second-step therapy in exercising patients:
      i. Reduce LV mass as effectively as other antihypertensives (beta-blockers, alpha-antagonists, calcium antagonists, or ACE inhibitors) when used in conjunction with nonpharmacologic means
      ii. Particularly important consideration in African-American athletes, who are more likely to be salt-sensitive hypertensives
      iii. ↓TPR
      iv. ↓BP
   d. Performance effects:
      i. Short-term use reduces maximal exercise capacity and submaximal endurance exercise.
      ii. Diuretics may produce cramping in athletes despite normal serum potassium.
      iii. Exercise in the heat may produce potassium and magnesium depletion as well as rhabdomyolysis.
      iv. Diuretics are not recommended for athletes prone to dehydration (i.e., endurance athletes) because of further reductions in intravascular volume.
6. **Direct vasodilators** (hydralazine, minoxidil)
   a. Direct smooth muscle vasodilation in arterioles

   b. Should be used in conjunction with a diuretic and a beta-blocker because of reflex tachycardia and excess fluid retention
7. **Peripheral acting adrenergic antagonists** (guanadrel, guanethidine, reserpine)
   a. Inhibit catecholamine release
   b. **May cause serious orthostatic and exercise-induced hypotension**

Recommended Reading

1. Alderman MH: Non-pharmacological treatment of hypertension. Lancet 344:307–311, 1994.
2. American College of Sports Medicine: Physical activity, physical fitness and hypertension, position stand. Med Sci Sports Exerc 25:i–x, 1993.
3. Blake GH: Primary hypertension: The role of individualized therapy. Am Fam Phys 50:138–146, 1994.
4. Cleroux J, Yardley C, Marshall A, et al: Antihypertensive and hemodynamic effects of calcium channel blockade with isradipine after acute exercise. Am J Hypertens 5:84–87, 1992.
5. Fifth Report of the Joint National Committee on Detection, Evaluation, and Treatment of High Blood Pressure (JNC V). Arch Intern Med 153:154–183, 1993.
6. Folsom AR: Exercise and hypertension. In Torg JS, Shephard RJ (eds): Current Therapy in Sports Medicine, 3rd ed. St. Louis, Mosby, 1995, pp 650–652.
7. Houston MC: Exercise and hypertension. Postgrad Med 92:139–144, 150, 1992.
8. Kaiser P, Hylander B, Eliasson K, Kaiser L: Effect of beta-1-selective and nonselective beta blockade on blood pressure relative to physical performance in men with systemic hypertension. Am J Cardiol 55:79D–84D, 1985.
9. Kaplan NM, Deveraux RB, Miller HS: Systemic hypertension. Med Sci Sports Exerc 26(suppl):S268–S270, 1994.
10. Liebson PR, Grandits GA, Dianzumba S, et al: Comparison of five antihypertensive monotherapies and placebo for change in left ventricular mass in patients receiving nutritional-hygienic therapy in the treatment of mild hypertension study (TOMHS). Circulation 91:698–706, 1995.
11. Lund-Johansen P, Omvik P, Nordrehaug JE: Long-term hemodynamic effects of antihypertensive treatment. Clin Invest 70:S58–S64, 1992.
12. Lund-Johansen P: Exercise and antihypertensive therapy. Am J Cardiol 59:98A–107A, 1987.
13. Lund-Johansen P: Short- and long-term (six year) hemodynamic effects of labetalol in essential hypertension. Am J Med 75:24–31, 1983.
14. Manolio TA, Burke GL, Savage PJ, et al: Exercise blood pressure response and 5-year risk of elevated blood pressure in a cohort of young adults: The CARDIA study. Am J Hypertens 7:234–241, 1994.
15. McKinney ME, Mellion MB: Office Management of Sports Injuries and Athletic Problems. Philadelphia, Hanley & Belfus, 1988, pp 98–109.
16. Shepherd JT, Blomqvist CG, Lind AR, et al: Static (isometric exercise): Retrospection and introspection. Circ Res 48:I179–I188, 1981.
17. Stone MH, Fleck SJ, Triplett NT, Kraemer WJ: Health- and performance-related potential of resistance training. Sports Med 11:210–231, 1991.
18. Tanji JL: Exercise and the hypertensive athlete. Clin Sports Med 11:291–302, 1992.
19. Tanji JL, Batt ME: Management of hypertension: Adapting new guidelines for active patients. Phys Sportsmed 23:47–55, 1995.
20. Tipton CM: Exercise, training, and hypertension: An update. Exerc Sports Sci Rev 19:447–505, 1991.
21. Vaitkevicius PV, Fleg JL, Engel JH, et al: Effects of age and aerobic capacity on arterial stiffness in healthy adults. Circulation 88:1456–1462, 1993.
22. Virmani R, Robinowitz M, McAllister HA Jr: Exercise and the heart: A review of cardiac pathology associated with physical activity. Pathol Annu 20(part 2):431–462, 1985.
23. Wilmore JH, Costill DL: Physiology of Sport and Exercise. Champaign, IL, Human Kinetics, 1994.

33

Exercise-Induced Bronchospasm, Anaphylaxis, and Urticaria

Roger H. Kobayashi, M.D., and Ai Lan D. Kobayashi, M.D.

I. General Considerations

Exercise-induced bronchospasm (EIB) is a common and troublesome affliction of the pulmonary system, impairing optimal athletic performance. It is frequently underdiagnosed by the physician and underrecognized by the athlete. EIB was first described in the second century A.D. by Aretaeus the Cappadocian, but was written about by the Chinese more than 3000 years ago. Only recently have efforts toward prevention and treatment been made.

A. **Epidemiology** (Table 1)
   1. 12% of the total population experiences EIB.
   2. EIB can be detected in 41% of those with a history of allergic rhinitis.
   3. 70–90% of all asthmatics have EIB.
   4. It can occur at any age and is equally distributed among the sexes.

B. **Definition**
   1. **Clinical features.** EIB typically occurs after strenuous exercise. Following a near maximum (80%) exercise load of ≥ 5 minutes, the athlete experiences difficulty breathing, manifested by shortness of breath, coughing, chest tightness, and/or wheezing.
   2. **Pulmonary function criteria**
      a. ≥ 15% fall of FEV_1 (forced expiratory volume in one second) from baseline after exercise. Normal subjects may have ≤ 10% fall.
      b. ≥ 35% fall of forced expiratory flow, FEF_{25-75}
      c. ≥ 10% fall of peak expiratory flow rate (PEFR)
      d. Increased functional reserve capacity (increase in residual volume [RV] and total lung capacity [TLC]), reflecting air trapping
   3. **Severity**
      a. Mild — 15–20% decrease in FEV_1
      b. Moderate — 20–40% decrease in FEV_1
      c. Severe — > 40% decrease in FEV_1

C. **Factors influencing EIB**
   1. **Type of exercise**
      a. **Sports activities more likely to cause EIB:**
         i. Running
         ii. Cycling
         iii. Soccer or basketball
         iv. Cross country skiing
      b. **Sports activities less likely to cause EIB:**
         i. Kayaking
         ii. Swimming
         iii. Aerobic exercise
         iv. Dancing
         v. Gymnastics
         vi. Downhill skiing
         vii. Playing goalie in soccer
         viii. Playing defense in team sport

TABLE 1. Athletes at Risk for Exercise-Induced Bronchospasm

Those known to have asthma
Those with allergic rhinitis (hay fever)
Those with a family history of asthma
Those with frequent chest symptoms, i.e., coughing, congestion
Those with viral bronchitis
One out of every 10 members of a team

2. **Duration of exercise**
   a. Maximal fall of pulmonary function tests occurs after 5–8 minutes of vigorous exercise.
   b. If activity is extended, generally no further increase of bronchospasm is noted.
3. **Intensity of exercise**
   a. Very strenuous continuous exercise is more likely to induce EIB.
   b. Activity with frequent pauses, e.g., baseball or football, is less likely to cause EIB.
   c. Low-intensity sports are unlikely to cause EIB.
4. **Conditions affecting EIB**
   a. **Increase EIB:**
      i. Cold air
      ii. Dry air
      iii. Air pollution
      iv. Allergens
      v. Viral infections
      vi. Symptomatic asthma
   b. **Decrease EIB:**
      i. Warm air
      ii. Humid air

II. Possible Mechanisms

A. **Historical theories**
1. **Hyperventilation** results in airway heat and water loss, thereby triggering EIB.
2. **CO_2 loss** through hyperventilation may cause EIB. This is prevented by rebreathing expired air, replacing CO_2 with 7% CO_2 inhalation, or breathing slowly and deeply.
3. **Mast cell mediators**—histamine, eosinophilic chemotactic factor of anaphylaxis, and neutrophil chemotactic factor (NCF)—are released. They act on smooth muscles, thus causing bronchospasm.

B. **Current theories** (Table 2)
1. Increased ventilation results in **water loss**. This increases the osmolarity of the epithelial fluid, resulting in bronchospasm by cholinergic or inflammatory mediator release mechanisms.

TABLE 2. Mechanisms of Exercise-Induced Asthma

Early reactions
Respiratory water loss resulting in local changes in respiratory epithelial cell osmolarity
Temperature change; airway cooling and airway-ambient temperature gradients
Airway hyperemia resulting from sudden rewarming that may be mediated by neurotransmitters
Cholinergic response: neurologic, inflammatory stimuli
Late reaction: mast cell and basal cell degranulation
Neutrophil chemotactic factor
Eosinophil chemotactic factor
Leukotrienes (LTC_4, LTD_4, LTE_4)

From Kobayashi RH, Mellion MB: Exercise-induced asthma and related problems. In Mellion MB (ed): Office Sports Medicine, 2nd ed. Philadelphia, Hanley & Belfus, 1996, p 118, with permission.

TABLE 3. Signs and Symptoms of Exercise-Induced Bronchospasm

Shortness of breath
Coughing
Chest "tightness"
Chest pain (in children)
Feeling "out of shape"
Wheezing
Lack of energy (especially in children)

2. **Mediators** (histamine, NCF, platelet-activating factor, leukotrienes) are released after exposure to antigens and exercise.
3. **Mouth breathing** causes cooling of airways, thus triggering EIB.
4. **Airway hyperemia** results from sudden rewarming.

III. Diagnosis and Testing

A. **Clinical signs and symptoms** (Table 3)
   1. Similar to an acute asthma attack but of shorter duration
   2. Common among known asthmatics (70–90% have EIB)
   3. Prior chest disease, such as bronchitis, emphysema, and bronchopulmonary dysplasia, can exacerbate EIB.
   4. Athletes suffering from allergies or sinus disease may have an increased incidence of EIB.
   5. Late phase responses may occur 4–8 hours after initial EIB, manifested by chest tightening and dyspnea (Fig. 1).

B. **Testing**
   1. In typical patients with mild to moderate symptoms and in patients with a classic history, testing may be unnecessary and a trial of prophylactic medication may suffice.
   2. **Equipment**
      a. **For general purposes**, simple equipment such as a peak flow meter is adequate and inexpensive in assessing lung status before and after exercise.
         i. Obtain baseline peak flow readings.

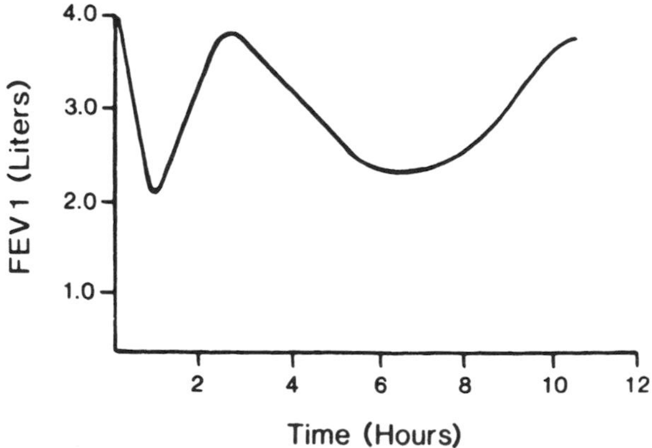

FIGURE 1. Patterns of bronchospasm in early phase (10 min to 2 hrs) and late phase (4–8 hours) exercise-induced bronchospasm. (From Kobayashi RH, Mellion MB: Exercise-induced asthma and related problems. In Mellion MB (ed): Office Sports Medicine, 2nd edition. Philadelphia, Hanley & Belfus, 1996, with permission.)

ii. Important to sustain vigorous exercise, i.e., sprinting for at least 6–8 minutes continuously
iii. Heart rate should exceed 140 beats/min (heart rate ≥ 90% of maximum predicted heart rate [220 – age])

b. **Standardized tests.** Pulmonary function tests (FEV_1, FEF_{25-75}, and PEFR) are measured before and after exercise at 1-, 3-, 5-, 10-, and 15-minute intervals.
   i. **Equipment:** simple spirometer (e.g., Breon spirometer, multispirometer)
   ii. **Free running**
      (a) **Advantages:**
         - Most asthmogenic
         - Requires minimal cardiovascular monitoring devices
      (b) **Disadvantages:**
         - Difficult to maintain constant humidity, ambient temperature, and workload
         - Although inexpensive and simple to perform, may not always detect EIB in every patient
   iii. **Treadmill**
      (a) **Advantages:**
         - Cardiovascular monitoring and pulmonary function can be measured during exercise.
         - Workload can be standardized.
      (b) **Disadvantages:**
         - Less asthmogenic
         - Requires a laboratory with expensive equipment
   iv. **Bicycle ergometer**
      (a) **Advantages:**
         - Workload can be easily maintained.
         - Cardiopulmonary monitoring can be easily accomplished.
         - Other physiologic parameters can be simultaneously monitored.
      (b) **Disadvantages:**
         - Least asthmogenic
         - Requires a laboratory with expensive equipment

3. **Medications to avoid before pulmonary testing**
   a. **Aerosols** containing beta-agonists or anticholinergic agents are to be avoided at least **6 hours** before testing. Newer medications such as bitolterol (**8 hours**), salmeterol (**12 hours**), procaterol or formoterol (**12 hours**) should be stopped for a longer period of time.
   b. **Oral medications** (theophylline, sustained-release beta-agonists) are to be avoided at least **24 hours** before testing.
   c. **Cromolyn sodium or nedocromil sodium** should be withheld for **24 hours**.
   d. **Steroid** preparations may be used unless the patient is also being evaluated for late phase asthma.
   e. **Antihistamines (loratadine, astemizole)** and **decongestants** with antibronchospastic properties are probably best avoided.

4. **Precautions**
   a. Wait at least **3 hours** between testing episodes.
   b. Test no more than twice in 1 day because refractoriness may affect results.
   c. Some athletes experience significant bronchospasm that is difficult to reverse.
   d. Test with caution patients with heart disease, patients with seizures, and patients taking beta-blockers.
   e. Use albuterol or terbutaline inhaler after testing to reverse bronchospasms (2 to 4 puffs).

TABLE 4. Medications Used to Treat Exercise-Induced Bronchospasm

Drugs	Dose	Comments
Beta-agonists		
Albuterol (Proventil, Ventolin)	2–4 puffs	Highly effective, long duration, easy to use
Terbutaline (Brethaire)	2–3 puffs	Highly effective, long duration, easy to use
Bitolterol (Tornalate)*	1–2 puffs	Highly effective, long duration, inconvenient to use
Pirbuterol acetate (Maxair)*	2 puffs	Highly effective, long duration, easy to use
Salmeterol (Serevent)*	2 puffs	Highly effective, very long duration. Slow onset of action. Should be taken at least 1 hour before vigorous exercise
Metaproterenol (Metaprel*, Alupent)	2–3 puffs	Effective, moderate duration, easy to use
Isoetharine (Bronkosol)*	2–3 puffs	Effective, short duration, inconvenient to use
Cromolyn sodium (Intal)	2–4 puffs	Effective, short duration, easy to use, blocks late phase asthma
Nedocromil sodium (Tilade)	2–4 puffs	Effective, blocks both early and late phase EIB. Very safe
Theophylline (sustained release)	5–8 mg/kg, every 12 hr	Effective; regular use may be more effective than occasional use before exercise
Steroids (inhaled)	2–4 puffs	Marginal effect on EIB
Ipratropium bromide (Atrovent)	2 puffs	Limited use in EIB

* Not approved for use by the International Olympic Committee.
EIB = Exercise-induced bronchospasm.

IV. Therapy

A. **Drugs** (Table 4)

1. **Beta-agonists**
   a. Albuterol (Proventil, Ventolin) is highly effective, of long duration, and easy to use.
   b. Terbutaline (Brethaire) is highly effective, of long duration, and easy to use.
   c. Bitolterol (Tornalate) is highly effective, of long duration, but somewhat inconvenient to use.
   d. Pirbuterol acetate (Maxair) is highly effective and of long duration.
   e. Salmeterol (Serevent) is highly effective and of long duration (8–12 hours).
   f. Metaproterenol (Metaprel, Alupent) is effective with moderate duration.
   g. Isoetharine (Bronkosol) is effective but with short duration and is rarely used now.
2. **Cromolyn sodium** (Intal) is effective but of short duration; it blocks late phase asthma and has no bronchodilatory effect.
3. **Nedocromil sodium** (Tilade) is effective and attenuates both immediate and late phase EIB.
4. **Theophylline** is effective. Actions of sustained-release forms may be enhanced if used regularly.
5. Inhaled **steroids** (Vanceril, Beclovent, Azmacort, Aerobid, budesonide) may be used but have only marginal effect on EIB.
6. **Ipratropium bromide** (Atrovent) may have limited usefulness in preventing EIB.
7. **New and experimental drugs**
   a. Antihistamines/anti-inflammatory agents, e.g., ketotifen, loratadine, and astemizole, have mild protective effects.
   b. Calcium channel blockers, e.g., nifedipine, have limited beneficial effects; others have no effect.

c. Leukotriene inhibitors/antagonists—numerous agents are being studied (Ziluton; ICI204, 219; Ly171, 883; SKF104, 353). Some have beneficial effects, but results are preliminary.

B. **General considerations**

1. For mild to moderate symptoms, inhaled albuterol or pirbuterol 2–4 puffs before exercise is helpful. Protective effects are typically 1–3 hours. Cromolyn (less effective) or nedocromil can also be used; duration of protection is typically 1–3 hours.
2. For individuals in whom time of exercise cannot be predicated or use of medication(s) is inconvenient, a longer-acting inhaled beta-agonist such as salmeterol (duration of action 6–9 hours) or bitolterol (duration of action up to 6 hours) can be substituted. Salmeterol may take as long as 2 hours for onset of action, so the patient should be so advised.
3. In individuals who are busy and find swallowing a pill easier, a long-acting oral beta-agonist such as albuterol tablets (Volmax, 4 and 8 mg, or Proventil Repetabs, 4 mg) can be used. Similar to the long-acting inhaled beta-agonist, onset of action may take up to 2 hours. Tremors may be a consideration, so this side effect needs to be considered when fine motor skills are required.
4. In patients with chronic asthma, the regular prophylactic use of inhaled steroids or other anti-inflammatory agents (cromolyn, nedocromil) is necessary to decrease airway reactivity.

C. **Banned drugs**

1. **National Collegiate Athletic Association** (NCAA). Before the 1993–1994 school year, the NCAA maintained a long list of banned substances contained in common medications used to treat asthma and allergic rhinitis. Since that time, any legitimate medication prescribed by a physician for asthma and allergic rhinitis has been permitted, with the exception that beta$_2$-agonists are permitted by aerosol only.
2. **International Olympic Committee**
   a. Approved drugs for asthma (Table 5):
      i. Only two beta$_2$ specific sympathomimetic amine aerosols are approved:
         (a) Albuterol
         (b) Terbutaline
      ii. No sympathomimetic tablets are allowed.
   b. Banned antiasthmatic drugs (Table 6)

D. **Nonpharmacologic**

1. **Conditioning** may reduce the severity of EIB, but it does not prevent it.
2. **Short bursts of vigorous exercise** within a period of time may extinguish EIB and induce short-term refractoriness, e.g., seven 30-second periods of running ("wind sprints") separated by short intervals.
3. **Warming up** before activity induces bronchodilation and refractoriness to EIB.
4. **Cooling down** after strenuous exercise decreases EIB.

TABLE 5. Therapeutic Agents for Exercise-Induced Asthma Acceptable to the International Olympic Committee Medical Commission

Atropine sulfate	Methylxanthines—theophylline
Caffeine*	Sympathomimetic amine aerosols
Corticosteroids†	Albuterol†
Cromolyn sodium	Terbutaline†

* Caffeine is a *weak* bronchodilator, which is banned if urinary concentrations > 15 μg/mL for NCAA and > 12 μg/mL for Olympic competition.

† Requires letter from team physician.

TABLE 6. Sympathomimetic Amines Banned or Permitted in Olympic Competition

Banned	**Permitted** (with a letter from team physician)
Adrenaline	Albuterol (aerosol only)
Ephedrine	Terbutaline (aerosol only)
Isoetharine	
Isoproterenol	
Metaproterenol	
Bitolterol	
Salmeterol	
Fenoterol*	
Rimiterol*	

* Not currently available in the United States. The NCAA allows any legitimately approved asthma medication, provided that it is prescribed by a licensed physician.

5. **Miscellaneous maneuvers**
   a. **"Running through"** EIB
   b. **Avoid hyperventilation.**
   c. **Nasal breathing** humidifies, warms, and cleans the air.
   d. **Cold weather**—wearing a mask or scarf around the nose and mouth creates warm, moist air and may diminish EIB.
   e. Avoid strenuous exercise during periods when air pollution is high or if significant viral infection is present.

V. Exercise-Induced Anaphylaxis

A. **Epidemiology.** There have been more than 500 reported cases of exercise-induced anaphylaxis. Attacks range in frequency from once a year to as often as monthly. Numerous attacks may occur before medical care is sought or the diagnosis is made. Most of the cases occur in accomplished athletes who exercise regularly.

B. **Definition.** Exercise-induced anaphylaxis is characterized by a sensation of warmth, pruritus, cutaneous erythema, urticaria (> 10 mm in diameter), upper respiratory obstructive symptoms, and occasionally vascular collapse. Exercise-induced anaphylaxis is distinct from exercise-induced asthma, cholinergic urticaria, angioedema, and cardiac arrhythmia, which are all recognized as exertion-related phenomena.

C. **Risk factors**
   1. Previous **history of atopy** (50% of all cases)
   2. Family history of atopy (67% of all cases)
   3. **Food ingestion**—certain foods, such as shellfish, nuts, and celery, have been associated with exercise-induced anaphylaxis.
   4. **Weather conditions** (heat, high humidity)

D. **Signs and symptoms** (four stages)
   1. **Prodromal stage**
      a. Fatigue
      b. Generalized warmth
      c. Itchiness
      d. Erythema
   2. **Early stage**
      a. Confluent urticaria
      b. Rash
      c. Angioedema
   3. **Established stage**
      a. Choking
      b. Stridor
      c. Colic
      d. Nausea
      e. Vomiting
      f. Hypotension
   4. **Late stage**—headache

E. **Complications** can be life-threatening.

F. **Mechanisms.** During an exercise-induced anaphylaxis attack, serum histamine levels have been shown to increase from baseline values, thus suggesting mast cell involvement.

G. **Prevention** through modification of exercise program
1. Decrease intensity of exertion.
2. Avoid exercising during warm, humid days.
3. Interrupt exercise at the earliest sign of itching.
4. Avoid meals at least 4 hours before exercise. Avoid certain foods that may be associated with exercise-induced anaphylaxis.
5. Pretreatment with antihistamine may attenuate exercise-induced anaphylaxis; pretreatment with beta-agonists or theophylline does not.
6. Do not exercise alone.

H. **Treatment**
1. Epinephrine, fluid replacement, and antihistamines are commonly used.
2. Patient must have an EpiPen or Ana-Kit immediately available. A companion should also be familiar with its use.
3. Antihistamines and steroids can be given immediately after administration of epinephrine. The liquid form, clemastine fumarate (Tavist Liquid), 1–4 tsps, and prednisolone syrup (Prelone), 1–3 tsps, may be preferable because it does not require the availability of water to swallow and may be easier to ingest in the face of impending laryngospasm.
4. In cases in which life-threatening reactions have occurred, the athlete may have to switch to a less strenuous sport or, in some instances, abandon athletics altogether.

VI. Cholinergic Urticaria

A. **Definition**: generalized small urticarial papules occurring after a warm bath, shower, exercise, or fever. Also known as generalized heat urticaria.

B. **Signs and symptoms**
1. Urticaria is usually small papules that appear first in the upper thorax and neck, spreading caudally to involve the entire body.
2. Systemic reactions, such as abdominal pain, syncope, or wheezing, are **rare**.
3. Cholinergic reactions (lacrimation, salivation, diarrhea) may be observed.

C. **Risk factors**
1. Heat
2. Humidity

D. **Mechanisms**
1. Neurogenic reflex
2. Mediator release (histamine, NCF)

E. **Prevention**
1. Avoid heat and humidity.
2. Antihistamine may prevent or decrease incidence.

F. **Therapy**. Antihistamines are generally used.
1. Hydroxyzine (at a dose of 25–200 mg per day) is the drug of choice.
2. Cyproheptadine may be substituted (at a dose of 4–20 mg per day).
3. Either medication may be supplemented by daily loratadine (10 mg per day).

VII. Summary

A. **Exercise-induced bronchospasm**
1. Common
2. Diagnosis often overlooked
3. Preventable and treatable

B. **Exercise-induced anaphylaxis**
   1. Rare
   2. Potentially fatal
   3. Extreme caution

C. **Cholinergic urticaria**
   1. Not uncommon
   2. Bothersome to patient

Acknowledgment: The author would like to thank Lucinda Gillette for her secretarial assistance.

Recommended Reading

General Review Articles

1. Bierman C: Exercise-induced asthma. NER Allergy Proc 9:193–197, 1988.
2. Eggleston PA: Exercise-induced asthma. Clin Rev Allergy 1:19–37, 1983.
3. Katz R: Exercise-induced asthma. Am J Asthma Allergy Pediatricians 1:71–74, 1988.
4. Kobayashi R, Mellion M: Exercise-induced asthma, anaphylaxis and urticaria. Clin Prim Care 18:809–831, 1991.
5. McFadden ER, Gilbert IA: Exercise-induced asthma. N Engl J Med 330:1362–1367, 1994.
6. National Asthma Education Program, Expert Panel Report: Guidelines for the diagnosis and management of asthma. National Heart, Lung, and Blood Institute, National Institutes of Health, Bethesda, MD. J Allergy Clin Immunol 88:425–534, 1991.

Mechanisms

7. Anderson SD, Daviskas E: The airway microvasculature and exercise-induced asthma. Thorax 47:748–758, 1992.
8. Anderson SD, Daviskas E, Smith CM: Exercise-induced asthma: A difference in opinion regarding stimulus. Allergy Proc 10:215–221, 1984.
9. Anderson SD, Schoeffel RE, Follet R: Sensitivity to heat and water loss at rest during exercise in asthma patients. Eur J Respir Dis 63:459–471, 1982.
10. Bar-Yishay E, Godfrey S: Mechanisms of exercise-induced asthma. Lung 162:195–204, 1984.
11. Finnerty JP, Ward-Baker R, Thompson H, et al: Role of leukotrienes in exercise-induced asthma. Am Rev Respir Dis 145:746–753, 1992.
12. McFadden ER: Hypothesis: Exercise-induced asthma as a vascular phenomenon. Lancet 1:880–881, 1990.
13. McFadden ER, Gilbert IA: Asthma. N Engl J Med 327:1928–1933, 1992.

Testing

14. Backer V, Ulrik CS: Bronchial responsiveness to exercise in a random sample of 494 children and adolescents from Copenhagen. Clin Exp Allergy 22:741–747, 1992.
15. Eggleston PA: Methods of exercise challenge. J Allergy Clin Immunol 73: 666–669, 1984.
16. Haynes RL, Ingram RH Jr, McFadden ER Jr: An assessment of pulmonary response to exercise in asthma and analysis of factors influencing it. Am Rev Respir Dis 114:739–752, 1976.
17. Jones RS, Buston MH, Wharton MJ: The effect of exercise on ventilatory function in the child with asthma. Br J Dis Chest 56:78–86, 1962.
18. Rupp NT, Brudno DS, Guill MF: The value of screening for risk of exercise-induced asthma in high school athlete. Ann Allergy 70(4):339–342, 1993.
19. Silverman M, Anderson S: Standardization of exercise tests in asthmatic children. Arch Dis Child 47:882–889, 1972.

Pharmacology

20. Anderson S, Seale JP, Ferris L, et al: An evaluation of pharmacotherapy for exercise-induced asthma. J Allergy Clin Immunol 64:612–624, 1979.
21. Broulet L, Turcotte H, Tennino S: Comparison of the effectiveness of salmeterol, ipratropium and cromolyn in the prevention of bronchospasm induced by exercise and hyperosmolar challenge. J Allergy Clin Immunol 83:882–887, 1989.
22. Executive Committee, American Academy of Allergy and Immunology: Position statement: Inhaled $beta_2$-adrenergic agonists in asthma. J Allergy Clin Immunol 91:1234–1237, 1993.
23. Green CP, Price JF: Prevention of exercised-induced asthma by inhaled salmeterol zinofolate. Arch Dis Child 67:1014–1016, 1992.
24. Halton JR, Strunk RC: Pathogenesis of exercise-induced asthma: Implications for treatment. Am Rev Med 37:143–154, 1986.
25. Konig P, Horovak NL, Kruetz C: The preventive effect and duration of action of nedocromil sodium and cromolyn sodium on exercise-induced asthma in adults. J Allergy Clin Immunol 79:64–70, 1987.

26. Pearlman DS, Chervinsky P, LaForse C, et al: A comparison of salmeterol with albuterol in the treatment of mild-to-moderate asthma. N Engl J Med 1327:1420–1425, 1992.
27. Rohr AS, Siegel SC, Katz RM, et al: A comparison of inhaled albuterol and cromolyn in the prophylaxis of exercise-induced bronchospasm. Ann Allergy 59:107–109, 1987.
28. Sly, RM: ß-adrenergic drugs in the management of asthma in athletes. J Allergy Clin Immunol 73:680–685, 1984.

Exercise-Induced Anaphylaxis
29. Horan RF, Sheffer AL: Exercise-induced anaphylaxis. Immunol Allergy Clin North Am 12(3):559–570, 1992.
30. Kidd JM, Cohen SH, Sosman AJ, Fink JN: Food dependent exercise-induced anaphylaxis. J Allergy Clin Immunol 71:407–411, 1983.
31. Sheffer AL, Austen KF: Exercise-induced anaphylaxis. J Allergy Clin Immunol 73:699–703, 1984.

Cholinergic Urticaria
32. Daman L, Lieberman P, Ganier M, Hashimoto K: Localized heat urticaria. J Allergy Clin Immunol 61:273–278, 1978.
33. Grant JA, Findlay SR, Theuson DO, et al: Local heat urticaria/angioedema: Evidence for histamine release without complement activation. J Allergy Clin Immunol 67:75–77, 1981.

34

Epilepsy and the Athlete

Barry D. Jordan, M.D.

I. General Comments

A. **Classification of seizures**

1. **Generalized seizures**
   a. Tonic-clonic (grand mal):
      i. Intermittent
      ii. Status epilepticus (convulsive status epilepticus)
   b. Absence:
      i. Typical (petit mal)
      ii. Atypical
      iii. Absence status epilepticus (nonconvulsive status epilepticus)
   c. Myoclonic epilepsy
   d. Febrile seizures
2. **Partial (focal)**
   a. Simple (consciousness not impaired):
      i. Motor
      ii. Sensory
      iii. Autonomic
   b. Complex (with impairment of consciousness):
      i. Automatism
      ii. Psychic
   c. Partial with secondary generalization

B. **Causes of seizures**

1. **Unprovoked (idiopathic)**—no cause of the seizure is identified.
2. **Provoked**
   a. **Posttraumatic:**
      i. Skull fracture
      ii. Intracranial hematoma
      iii. Other
   b. **Metabolic:**
      i. Hyponatremia
      ii. Hypoglycemia
      iii. Hypomagnesemia
      iv. Hypocalcemia
      v. Dehydration
   c. **Drugs and drug withdrawal:**
      i. Alcohol
      ii. Cocaine
   d. **Infections:**
      i. Meningitis
      ii. Encephalitis
      iii. Brain abscess
   e. **Anoxia and hypoxia**
   f. **Cerebrovascular:**
      i. Stroke (thrombolic or embolic)
      ii. Subarachnoid hemorrhage

iii. Intracerebral hemorrhage
iv. Sinus thrombosis

g. **Hyperthermia** (i.e., heatstroke)
h. **Sleep deprivation**
i. **Febrile seizures**
j. **Neoplasm:**
   i. Primary intracranial
   ii. Metastatic
   iii. Carcinomatous meningitis
   iv. Lymphoma, leukemia
k. **Perinatal or hereditary:**
   i. Congenital anomalies
   ii. Genetic and hereditary disorders
   iii. Perinatal trauma or insults

C. **Injuries that occur during seizures (generalized tonic-clonic)**
1. Fractures
   a. Humeral neck
   b. Femoral trochanter
   c. Clavicle
   d. Ankle
   e. Vertebral body compression
2. Dislocations
   a. Shoulders
   b. Hips
3. Head and neck injuries

II. Common Seizure Disorders That May Be Encountered in the Athlete

A. **Intermittent tonic-clonic seizure**
1. May be tonic, clonic, or both
2. Associated with loss of consciousness
3. Typically associated with a postictal period characterized by disorientation, confusion, or lethargy
4. Individual seizure episodes are short-lived, self-limited, and rarely require the use of benzodiazepines.
5. May be associated with tongue biting or incontinence
6. A generalized seizure that is preceded by an aura is suggestive of focal seizure with secondary generalization.

B. **Continuous tonic-clonic seizure (status epilepticus)**
1. Represents a medical emergency
2. Definition
   a. Continuous generalized tonic-clonic convulsions lasting 30 minutes or longer

   or

   b. Recurrent generalized tonic-clonic convulsions without regaining full consciousness between attacks (i.e., each seizure begins before the postictal period of the preceding seizure ends)
3. If lasts longer than 60 minutes, may be irreversible neuronal damage
4. Requires prompt treatment with anticonvulsants (Tables 1 and 2)
5. Monitor airways, breathing, circulation
6. Must also monitor metabolic parameters
   a. Hypoxia
   b. Acidosis
   c. Hypoglycemia

C. **Typical absence (petit mal)**
1. Characterized by brief attacks of loss of consciousness. The attacks last 3–15 seconds in duration and are not associated with loss of body tone or falling.
2. Usually begin between the ages of 4 and 8

TABLE 1. Treatment of Status Epilepticus

Administer a bolus of benzodiazepines (e.g, diazepam, lorazepam, midazolam) while loading with phenytoin intravenously (1 g over 20 min in adults). *Note:* Not to be given faster than 50 mg/min
While administering phenytoin, athlete should be on a cardiac monitor with vital signs monitored.
If no result with phenytoin, may load with intravenous phenobarbital (maximum 1000 mg in adults)
May administer additional boluses of benzodiazepines during the administration of phenobarbital, provided that blood pressure and respiratory function are being closely monitored to avoid hypotension and respiratory depression
If no response with the above sequence, general anesthesia should be induced within 60 min
Correct any metabolic derangements

TABLE 2. Common Anticonvulsants

Generic Name	Trade Name	Indication	Adverse Effects	Comments
Phenytoin	Dilantin	Generalized, partial	Nystagmus, ataxia, megaloblastic anemia, bone marrow suppression, lethargy, gingival hyperplasia, hepatotoxicity, cardiac arrhythmias (intravenous administration)	Therapeutic range (10–20 mg/mL)
Phenobarbital	Luminal	Generalized tonic-clonic, partial	Central nervous system depression, lethargy, ataxia, behavioral changes, allergic dermatitis, cognitive effects	Therapeutic range (20–40 mg/mL)
Carbamazepine	Tegretol	Generalized tonic-clonic, partial, trigeminal neuralgia	Agranulocytosis, aplastic anemia, vertigo, nausea, vomiting	Therapeutic range (4–12 mg/mL)
Primidone	Mysoline	Generalized tonic-clonic, partial	Ataxia, vertigo, nausea, vomiting, sedation, cognitive effects	Therapeutic range (5–12 mg/mL)
Valproic acid	Depakote	Absence, myoclonic, generalized tonic-clonic	Hepatoxicity, thrombocytopenia	Therapeutic range (40–150 mg/mL)
Ethosuximide	Zarontin	Absence, myoclonic	Fatigue, headache, nausea	Therapeutic range (40–100 mg/mL)
Clonazepam	Klonopin	Absence, myoclonic	Sedation, ataxia	Therapeutic range (0.013–0.72 mg/mL)
Diazepam	Valium	Status epilecticus (alternative to lorazepam or midazolam)	Sedation, respiratory depression, hypotension, ataxia	
Lorazepam	Ativan	Status epilecticus (alternative to diazepam or midazolam)	Sedation, respiratory depression	Therapeutic range (30–100 mg/mL)
Midazolam	Versed	Status epilecticus (alternative to diazepam or lorazepam)	Sedation, respiratory depression	
Gabapentin	Neurontin	Partial	Sedation, ataxia, dizziness	
Felbamate	Felbatol	Partial (no longer recommended)	Aplastic anemia	Removed from market because of aplastic anemia
Vigabatrin		Partial	Sedation, behavioral disturbances, gastrointestinal disturbances	Not yet released in U.S.
Lamotrigine	Lamictal	Partial	Dizziness, sedation, nausea, ataxia, blurred vision, headache	

3. Usually tend to resolve spontaneously by the third decade of life
4. Electroencephalogram (EEG) demonstrates a 3 per second generalized spike and wave activity.
5. May be associated with automatisms such as lip smacking or facial twitching. However, automatisms are more commonly associated with complex partial seizures.
6. There is no aura or postictal state, and the attacks begin and end abruptly.

D. **Simple partial seizures**
1. Represents a relatively common type of seizure
2. Characterized by neurologic symptoms that correspond to the area of the cerebral cortex that is affected
3. Examples of focal seizures
   a. Motor activity that involves involuntary movements of the face, limbs, or head
   b. Speech arrest
   c. Somatosensory attacks described as tingling numbness, pins and needles sensation, or loss of feeling
   d. Special sensory attacks—olfactory, gustatory, visual or auditory
   e. Autonomic attacks such as diaphoresis
4. Focal motor seizures may be followed by focal weakness or paralysis in the corresponding body part in which the seizure occurs. This may last for minutes or hours and is called Todd's paralysis.
5. Focal seizures may spread locally along adjoining areas of the cerebral cortex (i.e., jacksonian march).
6. There is no impairment in consciousness.
7. Focal seizures may become generalized to tonic-clonic seizures.

E. **Complex partial seizures**
1. Also referred to as temporal lobe epilepsy or psychomotor seizures
2. Characterized by attacks of integrated purposeful movements or experiences followed by impairment in consciousness
3. These integrated purposeful activities and experiences may include:
   a. Emotions (e.g., depression, fear, paranoia)
   b. Simple automatisms (e.g., chewing, swallowing, lip smacking)
   c. Complex automatisms (e.g., walking into a room, undressing, arranging objects)
   d. Psychic experiences (e.g., déjà vu, jamais vu, forced thinking)
   e. Hallucinations (auditory, visual, gustatory, olfactory)
4. Most cases start between ages 10 and 30.
5. During the activities or experiences, the athlete is unresponsive to verbal stimuli or may exhibit confusion.
6. There is typically amnesia for the attack.

F. **Posttraumatic seizures.** Seizures that are provoked by head trauma may be encountered in sports and are classified as follows:
1. **Impact:** occur immediately at the time of trauma and are considered to be the result of electrochemical changes induced by the trauma
2. **Immediate:** occur within the first 24 hours of head trauma
3. **Early:** occur within the first week of head trauma
   a. Risk factors for early seizures:
      i. Prolonged posttraumatic amnesia (lasting > 24 hours)
      ii. Depressed skull fracture
      iii. Acute intracranial hematoma
   b. Prophylactic phenytoin may be preventive during the first week.
4. **Late:** occur after the first week of head trauma
   a. Risk factors for late seizures:
      i. Early epilepsy

ii. Depressed skull fracture
iii. Acute intracranial hematoma
b. The majority of late seizures occur within the first year.

III. Evaluation of the Athlete With Seizures

A. **History**

1. **Documentation and description of the seizure** (obtained from the athlete and any observers)
   a. Loss of consciousness
   b. Focality (i.e., generalized or partial)
   c. Warning signs (i.e., aura)
   d. Incontinence
   e. Tongue biting
   f. Psychic phenomena:
      i. Déjà vu (familiarity with an unfamiliar environment)
      ii. Jamais vu (unfamiliarity with a familiar environment)
      iii. Paranoid feelings
      iv. Hostile feelings
      v. Gustatory hallucinations
      vi. Olfactory hallucinations
      vii. Forced thinking
   g. Postictal state (drowsiness, confusion)
2. **Precipitating factors**
   a. Head trauma (recent or remote)
   b. Alcohol or drug ingestion
   c. Alcohol withdrawal
   d. Activity (i.e., physical exertion)
   e. Sleep deprivation
   f. Infection or fever
3. **Past medical history**
   a. History of stroke
   b. Remote history of central nervous system infection (e.g, meningitis, encephalitis)
   c. Remote history of head trauma
   d. Previous use of anticonvulsants
   e. Drug allergies
   f. Disease associated with epilepsy
4. **Family history**
   a. Epilepsy
   b. Other diseases associated with epilepsy

B. **Physical and neurologic evaluation**

1. **General physical examination**
   a. Vital signs
   b. Check hydration status
   c. Check for signs of head trauma
2. **Neurologic examination**
   a. Mental status (higher integrative function)
   b. Cranial nerves
   c. Motor function
   d. Coordination
   e. Sensory examination
   f. Reflexes
   g. Gait and station

C. **Laboratory evaluation**

1. Complete blood cell count
2. Biochemistry profile including glucose, blood urea nitrogen, calcium, magnesium, and electrolytes
3. Urinalysis

D. **Neurodiagnostic evaluation**
   1. EEG
   2. Magnetic resonance imaging or computed tomography
   3. Lumbar puncture if meningitis is suspected
   4. Positron-emission tomography

IV. General Principles of Management

A. **Establish the seizure type.**
B. **Select the appropriate therapy.**
   1. Increase dose of a single agent until the therapeutic effect is achieved or until toxicity develops.
   2. Follow serum levels of anticonvulsants.
   3. Monitor appropriate chemistries.
      a. Complete blood count
      b. Liver function tests
      c. Biochemistry profile
   4. Add a second drug if:
      a. The athlete is experiencing dose-related side effects from the first drug.
      b. One drug alone does not adequately control seizures.

V. Exercise-Induced Seizures

A. Seizures occurring during exercise or in the immediate postexercise period are infrequent.
B. Seizures that occur during prolonged exercise such as marathons or triathlons may be associated with metabolic disturbances.
   1. Hyponatremia
   2. Hypomagnesemia
   3. Hypoglycemia
C. **Any athlete that experiences a new-onset seizure during exercise, especially a partial seizure, should undergo a detailed neurologic evaluation.**
D. Athletes with exercise-induced seizures may exhibit baseline EEGs that are normal. Therefore **athletes suspected of exercise-induced seizures should have an EEG performed during exercise.**
E. Increase in epileptiform abnormalities on EEG after exercise may be related to decreasing pH.
F. Exercise-induced seizures should be considered in any athlete that experiences exercise-induced syncope.

VI. Participation Guidelines for the Athlete with a Seizure Disorder

A. **The decision as to whether an athlete should participate in a sport or physical activity should be governed by the following:**
   1. Type of sport (i.e., contact or collision versus noncontact)
   2. Risk of death or severe injury if athlete has a seizure during sports participation
   3. Preexisting brain injury and neurologic dysfunction
   4. Risk of potential brain injury from participation in the sport (e.g., concussion, intracranial hematoma)
   5. Seizure control
   6. Potential effects of anticonvulsants on athlete performance (e.g., impaired judgment, delayed reaction times)
B. The decision as to whether an athlete with a history of seizures should participate should be determined on an individual basis. There are certain high-risk sports (Table 3), however, in which athletic participation by an epileptic should be cautioned.

TABLE 3. Potential HIgh-Risk Sports for Athletes with Seizures

Boxing	Football	Cycling
Auto racing	Rugby	Gymnastics
Motorcycling	Diving	Wrestling
Mountaineering	Equestrian sports	Martial arts
Ski jumping	Rodeo	Sky diving
Scuba diving	Ice hockey	Swimming

C. **Any athlete with a history of seizure should be prohibited from boxing regardless of seizure control.**

D. An athlete who is seizure free for 1 year while on anticonvulsants or seizure free 2 years while off of anticonvulsants may be considered at lower risk. However, participation in contact or collision and other high-risk sports should be approached with caution.

Recommended Reading

1. Bennett DR: Epilepsy in the athlete. In Jordan BD, Tsainis PT, Warren RF (eds): Sports Neurology. Rockville, MD, Aspen Press, 1989, pp 116–126.
2. Ogunyemi A, Gomex MR, Klass DW: Seizures induced by exercise. Neurology 38:633–634, 1988.
3. Temkin NR, Dikman SS, Wilensky AJ, et al: A randomized, double-blind study of phenytoin for the prevention of posttraumatic seizures. N Engl J Med 323:497–502, 1990.

35

Headache in the Athlete

Barry D. Jordan, M.D.

I. General Comments

A. Chronic or recurrent headaches tend to be benign and are mostly tension, migraine, or cluster headaches.

B. **Acute severe or explosive headaches may be associated with more serious neuropathology, such as intracranial hemorrhage or mass lesions.**

C. An athlete who experiences a headache should have **a detailed evaluation if he or she exhibits any of the following characteristics:**

1. Prolonged headache after trauma
2. Severe, acute-onset headache with stiff neck
3. Headache, stiff neck, and fever
4. Headache with focal neurologic deficits
5. Persistent headaches in an individual who is typically not prone to headaches

II. Evaluation of the Athlete With Headache

A. **History**

1. **Location of headache**
   a. Unilateral versus bilateral
   b. Region:
      i. Occipital
      ii. Frontal
      iii. Temporal
      iv. Vertex
      v. Face
      vi. Retroorbital
      vii. Auricular or postauricular
2. **Quality of pain**
   a. Dull
   b. Throbbing or pounding
   c. Pressure
   d. Vice-like
   e. Sharp
3. **Duration, frequency, and intensity of pain headache**
4. **Onset**
   a. Sudden
   b. Gradual
5. **Associated physical symptoms**
   a. Fevers, chills, sweats
   b. Nausea and vomiting or other gastrointestinal disturbances
   c. Cardiopulmonary symptoms

d. Fatigue
e. Bleeding

6. **Associated neurologic symptoms**
   a. Mental status changes:
      i. Altered level of consciousness
      ii. Disorientation, confusion
      iii. Changes in speech
      iv. Memory problems
   b. Visual changes
      i. Blurred vision or visual loss
      ii. Scintillating scotoma
      iii. Diplopia
   c. Dizziness, vertigo
   d. Weakness or paralysis
   e. Sensory loss or paresthesias
   f. Difficulty with coordination
   g. Gait disturbance or difficulty with balance
7. **Precipitating conditions**
   a. Head trauma
   b. Physical activity or exertion
   c. Environmental stresses:
      i. Heat
      ii. Cold
      iii. Altitude
      iv. Humidity
      v. Other
   d. Diet and nutrition
      i. Cheeses
      ii. Chocolate
      iii. Caffeine withdrawal
      iv. Chinese food
      v. Other foods
8. **Past medical history**
   a. Previous history of headache
   b. Medications (including birth control pills)
   c. Systemic illnesses
9. Family history of headache

B. **General physical examination**
   1. Vital signs
   2. Head, eyes, ears, nose, and throat examination. Note any evidence of head trauma or infection.
   3. Check nuchal rigidity, and evaluate cervical range of motion.
   4. Evaluate the skin, checking for hydration or trauma.
   5. Cardiopulmonary examination

C. **Neurologic examination**
   1. **Mental status** (high integrative function) testing
      a. Alertness and level of arousal
      b. Orientation to person, time, and place
      c. Memory
      d. Speech
      e. Calculations
   2. **Cranial nerve examination**
      a. Visual acuity and visual fields
      b. Pupillary reaction
      c. Extraocular movements (note any nystagmus)
      d. Facial symmetry

3. **Motor function testing**
   a. Strength
   b. Bulk or atrophy
   c. Tone
   d. Involuntary movements
4. **Sensory function**
   a. Pinprick
   b. Light touch
   c. Vibration
   d. Temperature
5. **Reflexes**
   a. Deep tendon reflexes
   b. Babinski's reflex
6. **Coordination**
   a. Rapid alternative movements of upper and lower extremities
   b. Finger-to-nose
   c. Heel-to-shin
7. **Gait and station**

D. **Laboratory and radiologic investigations (as indicated)**
   1. Computed tomography (CT) or magnetic resonance imaging (MRI)
   2. Complete blood count
   3. Biochemistry profile

III. Common Headaches (Table 1)

A. **Tension headaches**
   1. The most common type of headache encountered in the general population
   2. Tend to get worse as the day progresses
   3. Typically respond to acetaminophen, nonsteroidal anti-inflammatory drugs, or butalbital

B. **Common migraine**
   1. More common in females
   2. First headache tends to appear between the ages of 10 and 30
   3. Treatment of migraine
      a. Abortive
         i. Ergotamine
         ii. Sumatriptan (Imitrex)

TABLE 1. Common Non–Exercise-Induced Headaches

	Tension (Muscle Contraction)	Common Migraine	Classic Migraine
Location	Bilateral (occipital, frontal, or temporal)	Unilateral or bilateral	Unilateral
Quality	Dull, aching or pressure sensation, nonthrobbing	Throbbing	Throbbing
Duration	Constant, unremitting	Hours–days	Hours
Associated Symptoms	Anxiety, depression	Nausea, vomiting, photophobia, phonophobia	Visual aura, nausea, vomiting, photophobia, phonophobia
Risk Factors	Stress	Smoking, lack of sleep, stress, tyramine-containing cheeses	Smoking, lack of sleep, stress, chocolate, tyramine-containing cheeses
Treatment	Acetaminophen NSAIDs Butalbital Tricyclics	Ergotamine Sumatriptan Tricyclics Beta-blockers Butalbital	Ergotamine Sumatriptan Tricyclics Beta-blockers Butalbital

NSAIDs = Nonsteroidal anti-inflammatory drugs.

iii. Dihydroergotamine (DHE)
iv. Butalbital
v. Ketorolac
vi. Narcotic analgesics
vii. NSAIDs

b. Preventive
i. Beta-blockers
ii. Tricyclic antidepressants
iii. Anit-inflammatories (e.g., aspirin, NSAIDs)
iv. Methysergide (Sansert)
v. Calcium channel blockers

C. **Classic migraine**
1. Differs from common migraine in that a visual aura precedes the headache. This aura may include scintillating scotoma or other visual changes.
2. Treatment is identical to that of common migraine.

D. **Comments**
1. Some patients with migraines develop chronic daily headaches. These headaches are the result of the overuse of medications. Therapy is directed toward weaning the athlete off of medications.
2. **Migraine variants**
a. **Migraine associee:** headache is associated with a transient neurologic deficit.
b. **Migraine dissociee:** neurologic deficit occurs in the absence of the headache.
c. **Complicated migraine:** neurologic deficit persists because of a cerebral infarction.

IV. Headaches Associated With Exercise (Table 2)

A. **Benign exertional headache**
1. Also referred to as **weight lifter's cephalgia**
2. Not associated with aura
3. Tend to resolve over time

TABLE 2. Headaches Associated With Exercise

	Benign Exertional Headache	Exercise-Induced (Effort) Migraine	Vascular Headache with Prolonged Exercise
Location	Bilateral (occipital or frontal)	Retro-orbital or unilateral	Diffuse
Quality	Throbbing	Throbbing	Throbbing
Onset	Rapid onset near the initiation of exercise (associated with maximal activity)	At the end of activity	After prolonged exercise
Duration	Short duration (usually < 5 min), but may be associated with dull pain for 24 h	May last for 1 h	May last up to 24 h after exercise
Associated Symptoms	Usually none	Visual aura, nausea, vomiting	Transient or persistent neurologic deficits
Risk Factors	Sports that require a brief sudden expenditure of maximum energy (e.g., weightlifting), more common in men	Previous history of migraine, high altitude	Poor conditioning, heat stress, hypoglycemia, dehydration
Treatment	NSAIDs	Usually self-limited NSAIDs Tricyclics Butalbital	NSAIDs If associated with cerebral ischemia, should be treated as a stroke

NSAIDs = Nonsteroidal anti-inflammatory drugs.

4. **Two descriptions of exertional headache in the clinical literature**
   a. The first, outlined in Table 2, is characterized by a headache that occurs with maximal activity at the initiation of exercise. The duration of the headache is usually brief, lasting less than 5 minutes. These headaches are believed to be secondary to an increased intrathoracic pressure from a Valsalva maneuver resulting in a transient increase in intracranial pressure or distention of intracranial venous structures.
   b. The second type of exertional headache is an exercise-associated headache that lasts for a longer duration of time. This type of headache has been described in weight lifters and is believed to be due to a stretching of cervical ligaments and tendons causing a tension-type headache.
5. **Approximately 10% of individuals with exertional headache have serious intracranial pathology. Accordingly, all athletes with exertional headaches should be evaluated.** The differential diagnosis of benign exertional headache includes:
   a. Arnold-Chiari malformation
   b. Platybasia
   c. Basilar impression
   d. Subdural hematoma
   e. Brain tumor
6. Subarachnoid hemorrhage should also be considered in the differential diagnosis of benign exertional headache. In this scenario, the athlete exhibits an acute explosive headache associated with a stiff neck.

B. **Exercise-induced migraine (effort migraine)** can be prevented by using a graded warm-up period.

C. **Vascular headache with prolonged exercise** appears to occur in the presence of cerebral ischemia.

D. **Comments**
1. **A delayed postexertional headache associated with intracranial hypotension** has been described in racquet sports. Two athletes presented with severe and continuous headaches 6–12 hours after vigorous exercise. Both athletes devloped a postural headache that was associated with a low cerebrospinal fluid pressure and normal neuroimaging (CT and MRI) of the brain. It was believed that the pathophysiologic mechanism of this headache was repeated traction on the brachial plexus and disruption of a nerve root sleeve that could cause a transient cerebrospinal fluid leak and resultant intracranial hypotension. This condition tends to be benign.
2. Exercise-related headache has been reported in **pheochromocytoma** with associated paroxysmal hypertension.

V. Headaches Associated With Facial Pain (Table 3)

A. **Trigeminal neuralgia (tic douloureux)**
1. More commonly involves the second and third divisions of the trigeminal nerve
2. May be associated with other neurologic disorders (e.g., multiple sclerosis, brain tumor)

B. **Cluster headache**
1. More common in men than women
2. Alcohol can exacerbate
3. Occurs in clusters, lasting weeks to months

C. **Temporomandibular joint dysfunction:** direct trauma to the temporomandibular joint can be associated with boxing and other contact and collision sports.

D. **Sinus**

E. **Comments**

TABLE 3. Headaches Associated with Facial Pain

	Trigeminal Neuralgia	Cluster Headache	TMJ Dysfunction	Sinus Headaches
Location	Distribution of cranial nerve V	Unilateral, usually retro-orbital	TMJ or temporal region	Localized over involved sinus
Quality	Lacinating, stabbing	Constant, severe, sharp, boring	Dull	Dull but can be pulsatile
Duration	Seconds–minutes	Minutes–hours	Variable	Variable
Associated Symptoms	Trigger zones on lips, gums, or just below nose	Lacrimation, nasal stuffiness, miosis, ptosis, flush and edema of cheek	TMJ noise with movement (e.g., clicking), pain with opening and closing mouth	Fever, concurrent respiratory infection or seasonal allergy; local tenderness over sinus
Risk Factors	Mutliple sclerosis; posterior fossa tumor	More common in men	Stress, malocclusions, improper mouth guard, trauma	Barometric pressure changes
Treatment	Carbamazepine Phenytoin Baclofen	Ergotamine Narcotics NSAIDs	Mouthpiece Oral surgeon Stress management	Antibiotics Decongestants

NSAIDs = Nonsteroidal anti-inflammatory drugs; TMJ = temporomandibular joint.

1. **Facial pain associated with headaches has been noted in scuba divers wearing tight goggles or tightly gripping their mouthpiece with their teeth.**
2. **Other causes of facial pain**
   a. Acute angle-closure glaucoma
   b. Dental caries

VI. Headaches Associated With Head Trauma (Table 4)

A. **Tension (muscle-contraction):** similar in quality and location as the typical muscle contraction–type headache

TABLE 4. Headaches Associated With Head Trauma

	Tension (Muscle Contraction)	Posttraumatic Migraine	Dysautonomic Cephalgia
Location	Bilateral, frontal/occipital	Unilateral	Unilateral
Quality	Constant, nonthrobbing, dull	Throbbing	Throbbing
Onset	Within minutes or post-trauma	Follows a symptom-free interval	May be delayed after a history of neck pain
Associated Symptoms	Postconcussion syndrome (e.g., dizziness, fatigue, decreased concentration, impaired memory)	Visual aura, vomiting, and postconcussion syndrome	Partial Horner's syndrome between attacks; during attacks can have pupillary dilatation and excessive sweating (unilateral)
Risk Factors	More common after milder head trauma	Previous history of migraine; family history of migraine	Injury to sympathetic fibers that run parallel with the carotid vessels
Treatment	Acetaminophen NSAIDs Butalbital	Same as regular migraine	Beta-blocker (propranolol)

NSAIDs = Nonsteroidal anti-inflammatory drugs.

B. **Posttraumatic migraine:** also referred to as **footballer's migraine**. Has been reported in soccer players who experience migraines after repetitive heading of the ball. Condition may be amenable to prophylactic migraine therapy.

C. **Dysautonomic cephalgia** is associated with anterior neck trauma.

D. **Comments**

1. **Any athlete sustaining head trauma should have a detailed neurologic evaluation before returning to play (especially in contact sports).**
2. **Posttraumatic headache is usually a component of the postconcussion syndrome, which may be associated with:**
   a. Irritability
   b. Memory loss
   c. Fatigability
   d. Dizziness or vertigo
   e. Impaired concentration
3. **Any athlete who is experiencing a postconcussion syndrome should not be allowed to return to contact sports until asymptomatic.**
4. An athlete who is exhibiting a postconcussion syndrome and is allowed to return to participate in a contact sport is at risk of the second impact syndrome.
5. **The second impact syndrome is** a catastrophic event in which an athlete sustains a first concussion and has a postconcussion syndrome and then sustains a second minor concussion while still symptomatic from the first. As a result, the athlete has an exaggerated response to the second trauma that can result in coma or death.
6. Posttraumatic headaches can also present as a mixed tension-migraine type of headache.
7. Posttraumatic headache that localizes to the site of scalp injury may also be encountered.

VIII. Headaches Associated With Intracranial Hemorrhage (Table 5)

A. **Epidural hematoma:** classic presentation is the athlete sustaining head trauma, followed by a brief loss of consciousness, followed by a lucid period, then progressive neurologic deterioration.

B. **Subdural hematoma**

1. Three types
   a. Acute: < 3 days
   b. Subacute: 3–20 days
   c. Chronic: 21 days or more
2. Should be considered in the differential diagnosis of exertional headache

C. **Subarachnoid hemorrhage** should also be considered in the differential diagnosis of exertional headache.

D. **Intracerebral hematoma**

TABLE 5. Headaches Associated With Intracranial Hemorrhage

	Epidural Hematoma	Subdural Hematoma	Subarachnoid Hemorrhage	Intracerebral Hematoma
Location	Variable	Variable	Generalized or diffuse	Variable
Quality	Severe, progressive	Variable	Severe, explosive	Severe, explosive
Associated Symptoms	Altered level of consciousness, focal neurologic deficits	Altered level of consciousness, focal neurologic deficits	Nuchal rigidity, altered level of consciousness, focal neurologic deficits	Altered level of consciousness, focal neurologic deficits
Risk Factors	Trauma, skull fracture	Trauma	Trauma, aneurysm, arteriovenous malformation	Trauma, hypertension
Treatment	Neurosurgical consultation	Neurosurgical consultation	Neurosurgical consultation	Neurosurgical consultation

TABLE 6. Headaches Associated With Systemic Conditions

	Systemic Infections (Nonneurologic)	Hypertension
Location	Diffuse	Occipital
Quality	Mild, constant, or throbbing	Pounding
Onset	Gradual	Gradual
Duration	Depending on underlying infection	Days
Associated Symptoms	Elevated white cell count, fever, myalgias, evidence of underlying infection (e.g., cough, diarrhea)	Malignant hypertension (diastolic blood pressure > 130), exudates and hemorrhages on endoscopic examination, focal neurologic findings, intracranial hemorrhage
Risk Factors	Systemic infection (e.g., respiratory or gastrointestinal	More common in African-Americans, essential hypertension
Treatment	Treat underlying infection	Antihypertensive medication

IX. Headaches Associated With Systemic Conditions (Table 6)

A. **Systemic infections**
B. **Hypertension**

X. Environment-Induced Headaches (Table 7)

A. **High altitude**
B. **Hyperthermia**
C. **Hypercapnea**
D. Changes in barometric pressure can also cause headaches.
   1. **Low barometric pressures** have been noted to trigger headaches in migraine patients.
   2. A migrainelike headache has been observed after **decompression from a hyperbaric environment** and return to normal atmosphere pressures.

XI. Drug Therapy for Headaches

A. Common medications used in the treatment of headache and potential adverse side effects are listed in Table 8.
B. Once the proper diagnosis is established, treatment of the athlete with headache should be based on the following considerations:
   1. Efficacy of treatment
   2. Potential side effects
   3. Effects on athletic performance

TABLE 7. Environment-Induced Headache

	High Altitude	Hyperthermia
Location	Generalized	Generalized
Quality	Throbbing	Throbbing
Onset	6–96 h after rapid ascent to altitudes > 8000 feet	Gradual when core temperature > 41° C
Associated Symptoms	May show signs of acute mountain sickness	Elevated rectal temperature, tachycardia, hyperventilation
Risk Factors	Poorly acclimated athlete	Cardiovascular disease, diabetes mellitus, malnutrition, alcoholism, cystic fibrosis

TABLE 8. Drug Therapy for Headaches in the Athlete

Medication	Type of Headache	Adverse Effects
NSAIDs	Most headaches except posttraumatic and those associated with hemorrhage	Gastrointestinal upset, antiplatelet actions
Beta-blockers	Prophylactics for migraine	Bradycardia, exercise intolerance, fatigue
Tricyclic antidepressants	Tension, migraine	Dry mouth, constipation
Calcium channel blockers	Prophylaxis for migraine, cluster	Constipation, muscle aches, fatigue
Methysergide	Cluster	Muscle cramps, retroperitoneal fibrosis, pleural fibrosis, cardiac fibrosis
Ergotamine	Migraine (abortive)	Intermittent claudication, arterial occlusion
Corticosteroids	Cluster, high altitude	Water retention, sodium retention, peptic ulcers
Anticonvulsants	Trigeminal neuralgia	Lethargy, ataxia, liver toxicity, bone marrow suppression
Acetazolamide	High altitude	Diuresis, electrolyte imbalance
Sumatriptan	Migraine	Injection site reaction, flushing, chest discomfort, dizziness, tingling

Recommended Reading

1. Atkinson R, Appenzeller O: Headache in sports. Semin Neurol 1:334–344, 1981.
2. Diamond S, Solomon GD, Freitag FG: Headache in sports. In Jordan BD, Tsairis P, Warren RF (eds): Sports Neurology. Rockville, MD, Aspen Press, 1989, pp 127–132.
3. Lambert RW, Barnell DL: Prevention of exercise-induced migraine by quantitative warm-up. Headache 25:317–319, 1985.
4. Rooke EO: Benign exertional headaches. Med Clin North Am 52:801–808, 1968.
5. Seelinger DF, Coin GC, Carlow TJ: Effort headache with cerebral infarction. Headache 15:142–145, 1975.
6. Tobin WE: Subarachnoid hemorrhage associated with aerobic exercise. Phys Sportsmed 17:145–148, 1989.
7. Vijayan N: A new post-traumatic headache syndrome: Clinical and therapeutic observations. Headache 17:19–22, 1977.
8. Williams SJ, Nukada H: Sport and exercise headache: Part 1. Prevalence among university students. Br J Sports Med 28:90–95, 1994.
9. Williams SJ, Nukada H: Sport and exercise headache: Part 2. Diagnosis and classification. Br J Sports Med 28:96–100, 1994.

36

Skin Problems in Athletes

Rodney S. W. Basler, M.D.

Functioning as the interface between the athlete and the competitive environment, the integument assumes a unique position by establishing a resilient barrier, protecting the organism from often unnatural and inhospitable surroundings. While most organ systems show positive benefits from increased physical activity, **the skin may develop pathologic conditions directly attributable to sport participation.** Fortunately, the special cutaneous problems of the athlete are, for the most part, easily observable and usually can be recognized early and appropriately treated. With proper care, these dermatoses rarely cause serious interruption of a training or competition schedule.

The athlete's skin often experiences significant trauma producing compensatory changes, such as callus formation and chafing. Specific injuries may be observed, including sunburn, frostnip, friction blisters, subungual hematomas, piezogenic papules, and black heel. The athletic milieu also exposes the skin to a multitude of infective organisms while making it more vulnerable to their invasion. The team physician encounters all of these special cutaneous conditions.

I. Direct Cutaneous Injury

- A. **Friction**
  - 1. **Calluses**
    - a. **History**
      - i. Occur at interface between skin and article of equipment
      - ii. Most commonly seen on feet, especially over areas of anatomic or frictional deformity
      - iii. Observed over hands of serious golfers and in oar and racket sports
      - iv. Compensatory, protective response of skin
      - v. Competitive advantage to gymnasts
    - b. **Diagnosis**
      - i. Thick, hypertrophied stratum corneum
      - ii. Lack punctum of keratin seen with corns
    - c. **Treatment**
      - i. Often unnecessary
      - ii. Mainly treated to prevent blisters
      - iii. Paring
      - iv. Soaking followed by abrasion with pumice stone or file
    - d. **Prevention**
      - i. Often not preventable
      - ii. Use of protective equipment, such as gloves for weight lifters
      - iii. Modification of footwear
  - 2. **Blisters**
    - a. **History**
      - i. Often occur under calluses

ii. Especially common over feet:
(a) Constant friction in nearly all sports
(b) Moisture-laden environment leading to maceration

b. **Diagnosis**
i. Tender vesicle or bulla at site of shearing force
ii. May be filled with clear fluid or blood

c. **Treatment**
i. Allow the epidermal "roof" to remain intact.
ii. Drain fluid three times, at 12-hour intervals, for first 24 hours.
iii. If covering skin has been removed, apply hydrocolloid gel (DuoDERM) for 5–7 days.

d. **Prevention**
i. Paring of calluses
ii. Proper fitting for shoes
iii. Two pair of socks of a different material allowing interface of friction between them
iv. Lubricant such as Aquaphor over pressure points

3. **Chafing**

a. **History**
i. Mechanical friction from opposing areas of body
ii. Usually from long distance sports such as running and bicycling
iii. Aggravated by sweat
iv. More often caused by fabric against skin than skin on skin
v. Aggravated by excess muscle or subcutaneous fat

b. **Diagnosis**
i. Abraded erosion of epidermis
ii. Most common over upper inner thighs
iii. May be seen on neck and axilla

c. **Treatment**
i. Cool compresses
ii. Allowing air to area
iii. Soothing ointments to add lubrication:
(a) Neosporin ointment
(b) Petrolatum
(c) Aquaphor

d. **Prevention**
i. Sports shorts with longer legs of lower friction fabric
ii. "Bun hugger" athletic briefs with leg
iii. Lubricating ointments, as listed above
iv. Friction-reducing powders such as Zeasorb
v. Weight loss

4. **Jogger's nipples**

a. **History**
i. Most common in men
ii. Friction comes from coarse fabric or logo on jersey
iii. More of a problem the greater the running distance

b. **Diagnosis**
i. Denuded erosions of nipple and areola (Fig. 1)
ii. May hemorrhage in severe cases

c. **Treatment**
i. Compress with warm water and antibacterial soap
ii. Antibiotic cream and simple dressing

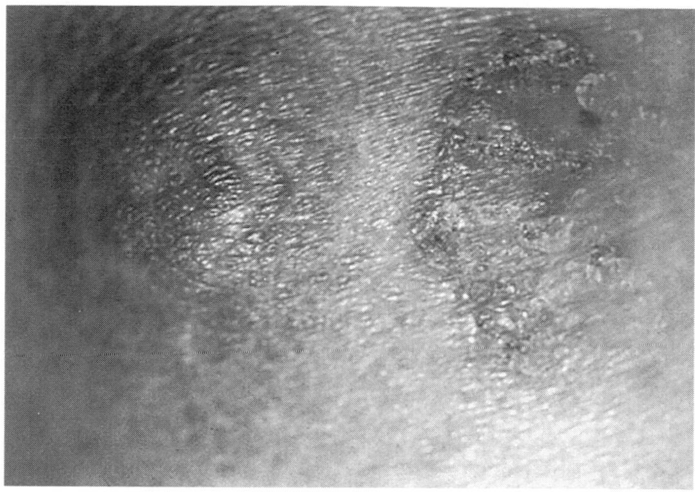

FIGURE 1. Erosion of areola in jogger.

d. **Prevention**
   i. Run without shirt when possible (men only)
   ii. Sports bra (women only)
   iii. Soft, clean fabric in running shirt
   iv. Lubricating ointment such as petrolatum or Aquaphor
   v. Tape with minimal adhesiveness applied directly to nipple and areola:
      (a) Paper tape
      (b) Adhesive part of Band-Aid or circular Band-Aid

5. **Abrasions**
   a. **History**
      i. Acutely applied friction from athletic environment
      ii. Examples include turf burn, mat burn, cinder burn, road rash "raspberry" and "strawberry"
   b. **Diagnosis**
      i. Injury localized to exposed skin in contact with environment
      ii. Denuded epidermis and upper dermis with punctate bleeding and exudate
   c. **Treatment**
      i. Initial cleansing with warm water and antibacterial soap or hydrogen peroxide
      ii. Removal of gravel or other foreign debris
      iii. Hydromembranes such as DuoDERM applied and left on wound for several days especially effective
      iv. In place of DuoDERM, may use antibiotic cream (not ointment) or spray and cover with clean nonadherent dressing, changed daily
   d. **Prevention**
      i. Additional skin protection in areas of potential trauma, especially elbows and knees
      ii. Aggressive early treatment to eliminate secondary infection

6. **Black heel**
   a. **History**
      i. Often referred to as "talon noir"
      ii. Seen almost exclusively in teenagers and young adults
      iii. Especially common in basketball players

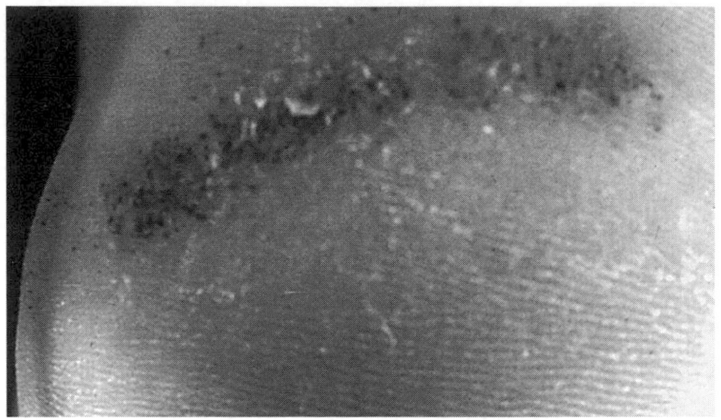

FIGURE 2. Black heel.

b. **Diagnosis**
   i. Asymptomatic
   ii. Blue-black punctate petechiae (Fig. 2)
   iii. Posterolateral aspect of heel
   iv. Palmar equivalent ("black palm") seen in weight lifters, golfers, and tennis players
c. **Treatment**
   i. No treatment required ("intelligent neglect")
   ii. Reassurance it is not malignant melanoma
   iii. Spontaneous resolution at end of activity
d. **Prevention**
   i. Probably not preventable
   ii. Properly fitting shoes
   iii. Gloves for weight lifters and racquet sports enthusiasts

7. **Acne mechanica**
   a. **History**
      i. Causative factors include heat, occlusion, pressure along with friction
      ii. Sometimes referred to as "football acne"
      iii. Flare seen in athletes with preexisting acne
      iv. May be seen in prepubertal boys
      v. Besides football, may be seen in weight lifters from weight bench, golfers from carrying bag, hockey players from stick, and dancers from leotards
   b. **Diagnosis**
      i. Distribution in areas under bulk of equipment:
         (a) Shoulders, forehead, and chin in football players
         (b) Shoulders and lateral back in golfers
         (c) Center of back in weight lifters
      ii. Inflammatory papules and pustules
      iii. Unattended, may become cystic
   c. **Treatment**
      i. Systemic antibiotics less effective than with standard acne vulgaris
      ii. Area of involvement should be cleansed thoroughly after workout with mildly abradant cleanser and back brush or Buf Puf scrub.
      iii. Application of topical astringent or 10% benzoyl peroxide
      iv. Usually greatly improves or resolves after season

d. **Prevention**
   i. Clean absorbent T-shirt under football pads (must stress "clean" to athletes)
   ii. Treat underlying acne vulgaris.
   iii. In severe cases, consider isotretnoin (Accutane) in off-season.
   iv. Remove exercise leotard *immediately* after workout.

8. **Folliculitis keloidalis**
   a. **History**
      i. Mostly seen in African-American athletes
      ii. Precursor is inflammatory folliculitis with more profound cystic component than seen with acne mechanica
   b. **Diagnosis**
      i. Nontender firm fibrous papules
      ii. Appear around edges of football helmet, especially posterior neck and occipital scalp
      iii. Seen under shin and thigh pads in hockey players (rare)
   c. **Treatment**
      i. Serial injection of dilute triamcinolone solution directly into papules
      ii. Delay treatment until season over, causative gear no longer worn
      iii. Surgical excision in worst cases
   d. **Prevention**
      i. Padding over equipment to reduce friction at involved points
      ii. Aggressive antibiotic treatment of underlying folliculitis

B. **Pressure**

1. **Corns**
   a. **History**
      i. Very tender
      ii. Most common on feet:
         (a) Often seen following switch to new competition or formal footwear
         (b) Usually over distal metatarsal heads
         (c) May be underlying anatomic defect
   b. **Diagnosis**
      i. Characteristically over pressure points
      ii. Main differential from plantar warts:
         (a) Pearly central "core"
         (b) Lack punctate vessels ("black dots") of warts
   c. **Treatment**
      i. Consistent regular paring:
         (a) Best done by another person such as trainer
         (b) May use scalpel or pumice stone
      ii. 50% trichloroacetic acid under 40% salicylic acid plaster for 2 days
   d. **Prevention**—modification of footwear to reduce or remove pressure points:
      i. Metatarsal bars
      ii. Widening of the toe box if between toes

2. **Subungual hemorrhage**
   a. **History**
      i. Most commonly seen in racquet sports with repeated forceful contact of anterior nail plate with anterior parts of shoe
      ii. Caused by proximal dyshesion of nail from nail plate by lateral shearing force
      iii. Usually called "tennis toe"
      iv. "Jogger's toe" and "skier's toe" describe same pathologic event
      v. Symptoms usually minimal

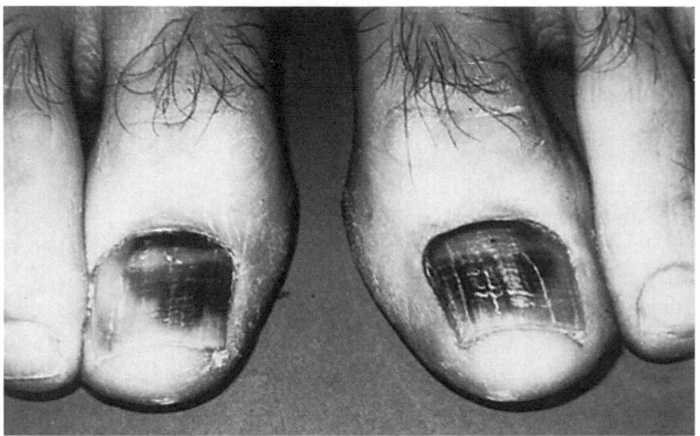

FIGURE 3. Skier's toes.

b. **Diagnosis**
   i. Pooled blood noted under great toenail (Fig. 3)
   ii. Color varies from bright red to dark brown depending on acuteness.
c. **Treatment**
   i. Blood may be drained from under nail plate in acute cases:
      (a) May use cautery or flamed paper clip
      (b) Procedure fairly traumatic and usually not necessary
   ii. Soaking in warm water of palliative benefit
   iii. Elimination of causative footwear or activity
d. **Prevention**
   i. Severe trimming of great toenails in a straight tangential plane to shortest point that does not cause discomfort
   ii. Careful attention to proper fit of shoes:
      (a) Shoes may be too short.
      (b) Toe box may not be high enough to permit unrestricted dorsal flexor of great toes.

3. **Runner's rump**
   a. **History**
      i. Usually seen in serious long distance runners
      ii. Anatomic variant of "high buttock" a predisposing factor
      iii. Similar clinical picture as seen from excessive sit-up–type exercises
      iv. Asymptomatic
      v. Athlete or family concerned about more serious disease
   b. **Diagnosis**
      i. Ecchymosis over sacrum at upper gluteal cleft
      ii. Color varies from blue to deep brown depending on chronicity
   c. **Treatment**
      i. No treatment required
      ii. Reassurance to athlete that finding does not represent serious disease
   d. **Prevention**—spontaneously resolves on cessation of causative activity
4. **Piezogenic papules**
   a. **History**
      i. Most likely in serious long distance runners
      ii. Pain may be of sufficient severity to preclude continuation of activity.

b. **Diagnosis**
   i. Protrusions of fat appear as dome-shaped papules over mediolateral surfaces of midfoot and especially heel
   ii. Condition apparent only when pressure placed on sole of foot from below
   iii. May not be tender in resting state
c. **Treatment**
   i. No medical or surgical intervention shown to be of definitive value
   ii. Usually not symptomatic during normal walking
d. **Prevention**—some sufferers benefit from special orthotics or heel cups.

C. **Miscellaneous external factors**
1. **Sunburn**
   a. **History**
      i. Exposure to sun with no or inadequate protection
      ii. Athlete misinformed about value of cloud cover or self-tanning lotions, which are of limited protective value
      iii. Fair complected with freckles at greatest risk
      iv. Injury worst under midday sun
   b. **Diagnosis**
      i. Erythema varies from light pink to dark purple
      ii. Marginated to area of exposure
      iii. Vesicles may form.
      iv. 24–48 hours before full extent of injury can be evaluated
      v. Systemic illness may accompany worst cases with:
         (a) Fever
         (b) Chills
         (c) Nausea
         (d) Prostration
   c. **Treatment**
      i. Varies according to severity of burn
      ii. Disability and discomfort secondary to dehydration and inflammation of skin
      iii. Immediate and continued systemic use of aspirin or ibuprofen is valuable in all degrees of burn
      iv. Minor burns are treated with over-the-counter hydrocortisone 1% creams or lotions and covered with moisturizing lotion such as Eucerin.
      v. Prescription cortisone sprays are beneficial in more severe burns and preclude application discomfort.
      vi. In disabling cases with vesicle formation, aggressive therapy with systemic steroids may be warranted.
   d. **Prevention**
      i. Most preventable of all injuries by using common sense
      ii. If possible, avoid midday (10:00 A.M. to 3:00 P.M.) exposure to sun.
      iii. Wear protective clothing if possible. Darker colors are more beneficial because they absorb photoenergy.
      iv. Hats with brims are much better than caps or visors, but still only equal to SPF of 2.
      v. Sunscreens of SPF 15 or above are cornerstones of prevention:
         (a) Should be applied 20–30 minutes before exposure
         (b) Reapplied every 2–4 hours, especially if sweating profusely
         (c) Must be applied evenly over all exposed areas to prevent "islands" of sunburn
         (d) Must have high "substantivity" (ability to maintain efficacy when subjected to moisture)
         (e) Must be nonirritating, especially to athlete's eyes
         (f) Sunscreen sprays work well for top of head.
         (g) Sunscreen lip protectants should also be used.

vi. Reflectant photoenergy potentiates direct sunlight, especially in water sports and winter sports.

2. **Erythema ab igne**
   a. **History**
      i. Seen in athletes who regularly apply heat to certain area of body.
      ii. Asymptomatic
   b. **Diagnosis**
      i. Reticulated erythema in acute phase directly over area of applied heat
      ii. Progresses to reticulated dark hyperpigmentation over time
   c. **Treatment**
      i. Reassurance to athlete that this finding does not indicate serious disease
      ii. Cessation of applied heat leads to spontaneous resolution in 3–6 months.
   d. **Prevention**
      i. Avoid application of causative heat.
      ii. Present other therapy options.
3. **Frostnip**
   a. **History**
      i. Most common form of cutaneous injury from hypothermia
      ii. Represents superficial frostbite involving only skin and superficial subcutaneous tissue
   b. **Diagnosis**
      i. Occurs in exposed areas:
         (a) Most commonly seen over nose and ears
         (b) Chin, cheeks, and anterior neck occasionally affected
      ii. Acutely presents as numb, white patches of skin
      iii. Superficial vesication and persistent numbness may result for 48–72 hours.
   c. **Treatment**
      i. Friction by rubbing while in cold environment
      ii. Rapid indoor rewarming recommended
      iii. Application of warm damp compresses or running warm water (shower works well) where possible
   d. **Prevention**
      i. Cover all exposed areas of skin; especially remember anterior neck.
      ii. "Layered look" with multiple lightweight garments:
         (a) Less restrictive
         (b) Air trapped between layers is excellent insulator
         (c) Can lose up to 90% of effectiveness if becomes wet
      iii. Terry cloth towel can be wrapped around neck:
         (a) Less irritating than wool scarf
         (b) More absorbent
      iv. Natural oil on face has insulating effect:
         (a) Postpone shower or washing of face until after exercise outing.
         (b) Postpone shaving until later in day.
      v. Effect potentiated by application of lotion, cream, or ointment:
         (a) Petrolatum nearly as protective as ski mask and much less cumbersome
         (b) Water-free emulsions do not crystalize in subfreezing temperatures.
         (c) Cream-based sunscreens offer two levels of protection simultaneously.
4. **Pernio**
   a. **History**
      i. Old term is "chilblains"
      ii. Young women most commonly affected
      iii. Onset usually coincides with first exposure to lower temperatures.

b. **Diagnosis**
   i. Violaceous to cyanotic areas over distal fingers or, especially, toes
   ii. Painful, often exquisitely tender
c. **Treatment**
   i. Topical steroids helpful:
      (a) Reduce inflammation
      (b) Must be low potency to prevent potentiation of vasoconstriction
   ii. Heavy woolen socks should be worn at all times, indoors and even when sleeping.
   iii. Careful use of topical nitroglycerin or systemic pentoxifylline useful in severe cases
d. **Prevention**
   i. Avoid constricting clothing such as tight-fitting gloves or boots.
   ii. Keep extremities warm at all times.
   iii. Heavy woolen socks (as mentioned above) for those prone to problem

II. Infections

A. Bacterial infections

1. Pyoderma

a. **History**
   i. Hazard of all contact sports
   ii. May reach epidemic proportions among wrestling teams or at large wrestling meets
   iii. Contact with infected opponent, often through superficial abrasion
b. **Diagnosis**
   i. Thin-walled vesicles or bullae usually primary lesions (Fig. 4)
   ii. Progress rapidly to sharply marginated erosions with heavy yellow crust
c. **Treatment**
   i. Application of compress made with warm water and antibacterial soap
   ii. Application of antibacterial cream
   iii. Systemic antibiotics
d. **Prevention**
   i. Prohibition of infected individuals from competition
   ii. Careful and regular sterilization of wrestling mats with appropriate disinfectant
   iii. Showering with antibacterial soap immediately after competition

2. Occlusive folliculitis

a. **History**
   i. Seen under heavy protected padding (see "Acne mechanica," page 344)
   ii. Deeper infection of follicles with furuncle production as opposed to acne mechanica
   iii. Swimmers affected when going long periods of time without getting out of swimsuit
   iv. Often referred to as "bikini bottom" in swimmers
b. **Diagnosis**
   i. Deep, inflamed, pustular papules (Fig. 5)
   ii. Tender to touch
   iii. Area of involvement coincides with overlying equipment
   iv. Inferior gluteal fold especially affected in swimmers
c. **Treatment**
   i. Application of a topical antibiotic solution such as clindamycin phosphate (Cleocin T) or erythromycin (Erygel) to areas of involvement

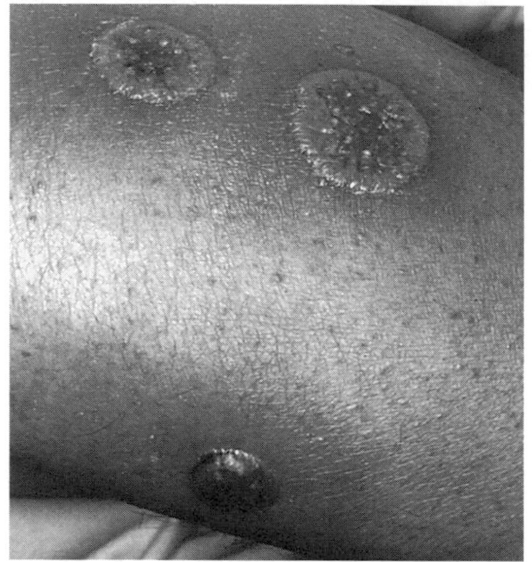

FIGURE 4. Purulent bullae of gram-negative pyoderma.

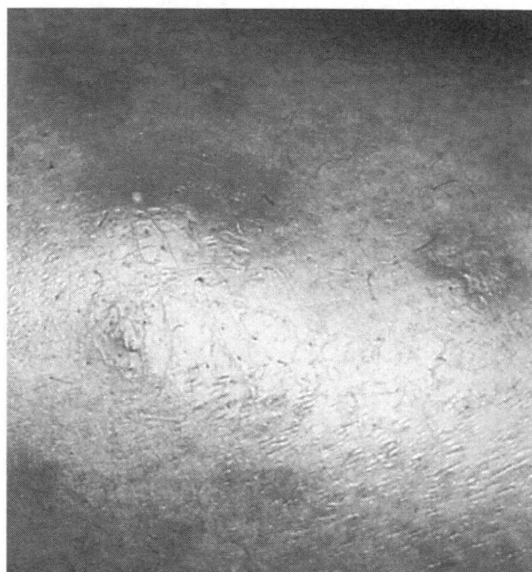

FIGURE 5. Folliculitis under football thigh pad.

ii. Appropriate systemic antibiotics, but may need to be used over long periods of time

d. **Prevention**
   i. Application of absorbent powder such as Zeasorb over areas of involvement
   ii. Removal of causative equipment or swimwear as soon as possible after workout
   iii. Aggressive treatment may preclude appearance of folliculitis keloidalis.

3. **Pitted keratolysis**
   a. **History**
      i. Often history of hyperhidrosis as precursor condition
      ii. Usually described by athlete as strongly malodorous
      iii. Caused by *Corynebacterium* species
      iv. Only mildly symptomatic
   b. **Diagnosis**
      i. Bottom of feet usually affected
      ii. Marginated areas of macerated skin with distinct pits in stratum corneum
      iii. Faint erythema sometimes precedes maceration and may be seen surrounding area of involvement.
   c. **Treatment**
      i. Application of over-the-counter 10% benzoyl peroxide gels
      ii. Topical prescription clindamycin
      iii. Topical prescription erythromycin
   d. **Prevention**
      i. Careful washing of the feet with antibacterial soap
      ii. Air drying of feet after towel drying
      iii. Application of absorbent powder inside of stockings
      iv. Regular application of a 20% aluminum chloride solution (Drysol)
4. **Otitis externa**
   a. **History**
      i. Seen in participants of water sports, especially swimmers
      ii. Caused by a *Pseudomonas* species
      iii. People with anatomic anomalies of the ear canal may be especially predisposed.

iv. Pain and itching most common symptoms; relapsing fever and diminished hearing more serious complications
v. Caused by alkalinization of the ear canal by presence of water

b. **Diagnosis**
i. Prevalent drainage from ear canal usually visible.
ii. Inspection of ear canal reveals deep erythema.
iii. Condition almost always bilateral.

c. **Treatment**
i. Combination antibiotic hydrocortisone drops
ii. Antifungals usually of little value
iii. Aggressive systemic therapy with anti-*Pseudomonas* antibiotics, such as ciprofloxacin, in severe cases

d. **Prevention**
i. Gentle drying of the ear canal after leaving water
ii. Application of 2% acidic acid solution (Vō Sol) into ear canals

B. **Viral infections**

1. **Plantar warts**

a. **History**
i. Relatively common in athletes
ii. Macerating effect of perspiration in athletes contributing factor
iii. Exposure to virus in locker rooms suspected in causation
iv. Symptoms may be disabling when over weight-bearing portions of the foot.

b. **Diagnosis**
i. Any area of the plantar portion of the foot may be involved.
ii. Small black dots representing vessels in capillary tips are usually seen, especially after paring.
iii. Confluence of individual papules may result in mosaic plantar warts (Fig. 6).

FIGURE 6. Mosaic plantar wart.

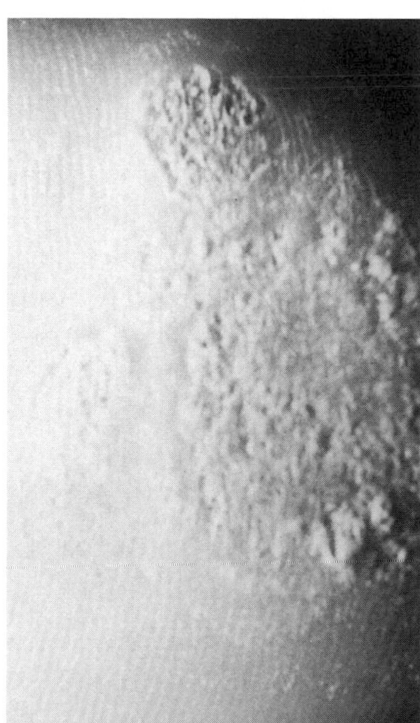

c. **Treatment**
   i. Conservative approach allows for continued competition during treatment.
   ii. Topical application of 40% salicylic acid plaster, left on wart for 3 days, followed by vigorous paring is often effective.
   iii. Over-the-counter salicylic acid preparations (Duoplant) may be applied daily.
   iv. Aggressive ablative therapies, such as excision, electrodesiccation, or laser treatment, carry significant risk of permanent scarring and disability.
   v. Daily application of solution of 5% salicylic acid and 30% formalin in ethanol is noninvasive and especially effective against mosaic variety.

d. **Prevention**
   i. Wearing of shower thongs in locker room
   ii. Foot powders to diminish maceration
   iii. Regular application of 20% aluminum chloride (Drysol) to feet

2. **Molluscum contagiosum**

a. **History**
   i. Commonly seen in wrestlers ("wrestler's warts")
   ii. Less common but often seen in swimmers
   iii. May have nonathletic etiology such as "coed wrestling"

b. **Diagnosis**
   i. Small, grouped waxy papules usually seen (Fig. 7)
   ii. Individual papules often show central dimple or "umbilication"
   iii. Sometimes appear in a linear distribution along line of previous scratch (pseudokoebnerization)

c. **Treatment**
   i. Easily removed with curettage after season but leads to superficial epidermal abrasions
   ii. May be frozen with liquid nitrogen
   iii. "Tape stripping," with high-quality adhesive applied to the affected area and then removed, is a simple, noninvasive treatment.
   iv. Studies have shown systemic griseofulvin to be effective in widespread cases, but it must be taken for 2–3 months.

d. **Prevention**
   i. Prohibition of competition by infected participants
   ii. Removal of individual lesions at first appearance to prevent self-inoculation

3. **Herpes gladiatorum**

a. **History**
   i. As name implies, seen in wrestlers
   ii. Regular, often monthly, recurrences in same site
   iii. Burning and tenderness often symptoms
   iv. Initial outbreak usually seen 1 week after exposure.

b. **Diagnosis**
   i. Head, neck, and upper extremities sites of predilection
   ii. Group vesicles appear on erythematous base
   iii. Dermal edema usually present

c. **Treatment**
   i. Carefully unroofing vesicles and applying benzoin leads to more rapid crusting and drying of lesions. (Extreme care must be taken to prevent herpetic whitlow in caregiver) (Fig. 8).
   ii. Intralesional injection of dilute triamcinolone under infected area also speeds clearing.
   iii. Systemic use of acyclovir in dosage of 400 mg three times a day should be initiated on first symptoms (itching or tingling) during prodrome:

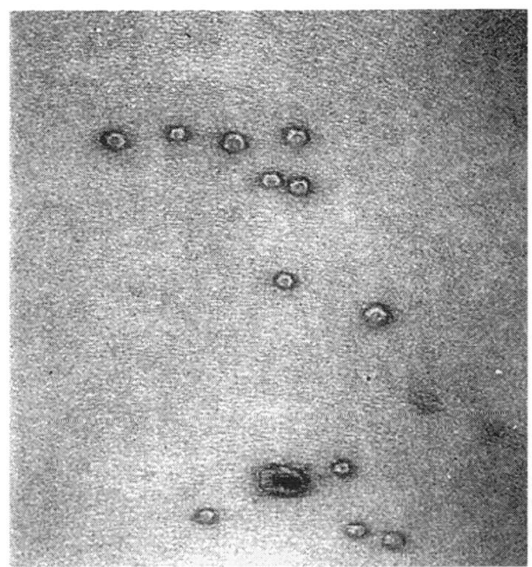

FIGURE 7. Molluscum contagiosum.

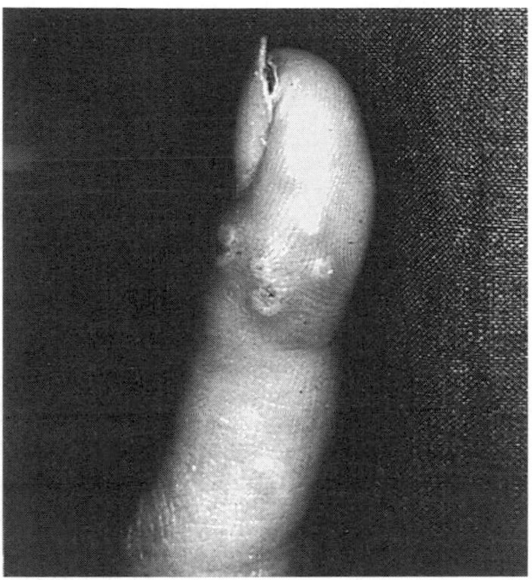

FIGURE 8. Herpetic whitlow in athletic trainer.

(a) 5-day course of therapy for recurrences
(b) 10-day course of therapy for suspected primary or initial infections

d. **Prevention**
   i. Athletes with history of recurrent herpes may greatly benefit from prophylactic acyclovir:
      (a) 1–2 capsules of 400 mg acyclovir (Zovirax) daily
      (b) Started before season and carried out through entire course of competitive schedule
   ii. Any athlete with active herpes must be prohibited from competition.
      (a) Out of contact during stage of intact or draining vesicles
      (b) 4–6 days usually a safe period of time for quarantine

C. **Fungal infections**
1. **Tinea pedis**
a. **History**
   i. Term "athlete's foot" indicates close association with sports
   ii. Macerating effect of perspiration in athletic environment reduces natural barrier of epidermis to invasion by fungal elements.
   iii. Locker room implicated as source of causative microbes
   iv. "Athlete's foot" broad general term—does not rule out contact dermatitis or dyshydrotic eczema
   v. Commensal infection with yeast, fungus, and bacteria causes erosio interdigitalis blastomycetica.

b. **Diagnosis**
   i. Toe webs usually first sight of infection
   ii. Erosio interdigitalis blastomycetica presents as extremely tender, deep erosion sometimes with accompanying lymphangitis (Fig. 9)
   iii. Fourth toe web especially examined when suspicious of tinea pedis
   iv. Erythema and scaling over feet, sometimes with vesicle formation
   v. Chronic form extends over lateral margins—moccasin-type effect

c. **Treatment**
   i. Frustrating in patients with "localized immune defect" to dermatophytes
   ii. Boro soaks help to eliminate maceration.

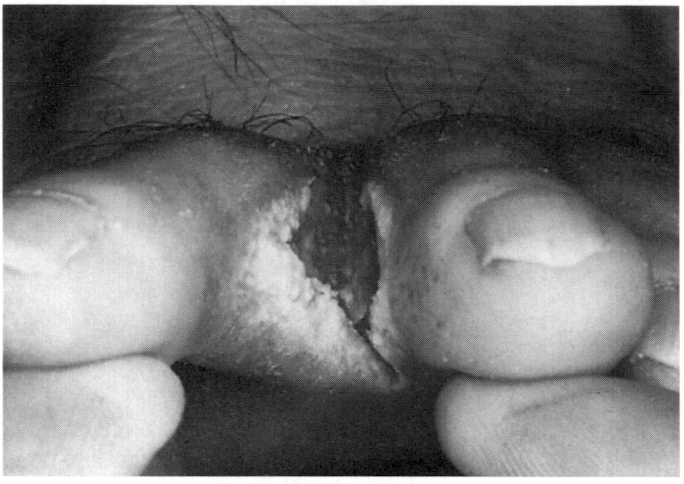

FIGURE 9. Commensal fungal, yeast, and bacterial infection of toe web.

   iii. Topical antifungal creams, such as terbenafine (Lamisil), are effective in some cases.
   iv. Topical antifungal solutions work particularly well in toe webs.
   v. Systemic antifungals, such as griseofulvin, fluconazole, or itraconazole, may be particularly effective for short-term relief of chronic cases during an athletic season.
   vi. Strong, broad-spectrum antibiotics such as ciprofloxacin are especially helpful in erosio interdigitalis blastomycetica.
  d. **Prevention**
   i. Careful attention to drying of feet a necessity:
    (a) Careful towel drying, particularly toe webs
    (b) Regular application of foot powder
    (c) Application of 20% aluminum chloride (Drysol) in patients with maceration
    (d) Antifungal foot powder such as Zeasorb-AF
   ii. Shower thongs may be beneficial to those with chronic recurrent infections.
   iii. Long-term treatment with a systemic antifungal (fluconazole or itraconazole) with dosage as low as 200 mg per month may be highly effective for prophylaxis.
2. **Tinea corporis**
  a. **History**
   i. Often referred to as "jock itch" when occurs in groin
   ii. May be seen in axillae or groin in patients with chronic tinea pedis
   iii. Macerating effect of chronic perspiration in males particular causative factor
   iv. Groin infection by dermatophytes rare in female athletes
  b. **Diagnosis**
   i. Needs to be differentiated from yeast infection of groin:
    (a) Dermatophyte infection erythematous and scaling with sharp margination
    (b) Does not appear on genitalia because of fungistatic effect of scrotal sebum
    (c) Usually marginated at inguinal crease
   ii. Does not develop satellite lesions

c. **Treatment**
   i. Localized ringworm-type patches in groin or axillae often respond to topical antifungals (miconazole, clotrimazole, or terbinafine).
   ii. Oral griseofulvin is the drug of choice for systemic treatment of dermatophytes.

d. **Prevention**
   i. Shower immediately after each exercise session and dry all areas thoroughly.
   ii. Daily change of sports briefs made of absorbent fabric
   iii. Absorbent powder in axillae and groin before workouts

3. **Yeast infections**

a. **History**
   i. More prominent in female athletes
   ii. Often history of long-term wearing of swimsuit or competition uniform

b. **Diagnosis**
   i. Usually seen in skinfolds, such as axillae, groin, and inframammary chest
   ii. Deep, beefy-red color, more striking than with dermatophyte
   iii. Groin involvement expands to include genital area.
   iv. Usually develops satellite lesions

c. **Treatment**
   i. Topical preparations are often effective for localized infection, especially miconazole or clotrimazole.
   ii. Tolnaftate is not effective against yeast organisms.
   iii. Mycostatin powder is especially good for intertriginous areas.
   iv. Systemic ketoconazole, fluconazole, or itraconazole are effective in extensive or chronic cases.
   v. Griseofulvin is of no benefit.

d. **Prevention**
   i. Shower immediately after exercise.
   ii. Daily change of sports briefs made of absorbent fabric
   iii. Absorbent powder in groin and axillae before workouts

4. **Hyperhidrosis**

a. **History**
   i. Common among athletes
   ii. Contributing factor to many infective processes
   iii. May affect performance when present on palms

b. **Diagnosis**
   i. Obvious production of excess sweat over palms
   ii. Axillary and plantar excess sweating more subjective

c. **Treatment**
   i. Application of desiccating agents to palms and soles
   ii. Systemic propantheline bromide (Pro-Banthine) or glycopyrrolate (Robinul)
   iii. "Drionics" equipment in extreme cases

d. **Prevention**—above-mentioned treatment procedures also of preventive value

5. **Bites and stings**

a. **History**
   i. Common for athletes in outdoor sports
   ii. Known history of allergic reaction, especially anaphylaxis, significant
   iii. Order *Hymenoptera* (bees, wasps, and ants) usual culprits:
      (a) Most likely to produce anaphylaxis
      (b) 20% of population have *Hymenoptera* allergy

b. **Diagnosis**
   i. Immediate wheal and flare

ii. Papular erythema with dermal edema over exposed areas, often in pattern
iii. Diaphoresis, lightheadedness, and shortness of breath in early allergic reaction

c. **Treatment**
 i. Must be immediate when highly sensitive athlete has *Hymenoptera* sting:
  (a) Should carry emergency treatment kit
  (b) Stop strenuous exercise immediately on being stung
  (c) Close observation for evidence of anaphylaxis
  (d) Steroids and antihistamines in mild reactions
  (e) Subcutaneous or intravenous epinephrine
 ii. Topical corticosteroids, topical antibiotics, or combination for minor bites
 iii. Systemic antibiotics for infected bites
 iv. Systemic steroids for severe cases

d. **Prevention**
 i. Special preventive measures as listed previously for allergic individuals
 ii. Insect repellent, especially those with "deet"
 iii. Avoidance of brightly colored clothes, shiny jewelry, and scented lotions and perfumes while exercising outdoors

6. **Scabies**

a. **History**
 i. Intense itching is hallmark of disease.
 ii. May have "miniepidemic" in wrestling team.
 iii. May be spread by fomites such as towels, uniforms, or equipment.
 iv. Close friends or family members often also infested.

b. **Diagnosis**
 i. Finger webs nearly always involved.
 ii. Papules or small vesicles in linear distribution following mite burrows.
 iii. Dermal papules on penile shaft essentially pathognomonic.

c. **Treatment**
 i. Must be aggressive and persistent
 ii. Single application therapy often inadequate in active cases
 iii. Lindane (Kwell) lotion over entire body from neck down first night at bedtime; then to affected areas only, every 3 nights until resolved
 iv. May alternate corticosteroid cream in mentholated lotion two times a day with lindane.
 v. All close contacts and family members must be treated with Lindane lotion to entire body at bedtime, two applications 1 week apart, even if asymptomatic.

d. **Prevention**
 i. Any participant with a suspicious rash must be held out of wrestling.
 ii. May compete again after 1 night's treatment with Kwell

7. **Green hair**

a. **History**
 i. Susceptible athlete is swimmer with very light blond or bleached hair
 ii. The problem usually occurs in several individuals in areas with high copper content in water.
 iii. May be from swimming in pool with older-type copper tubing
 iv. Not caused by chlorine

b. **Diagnosis**
 i. Obvious green tint in hair
 ii. Especially apparent when hair is wet

c. **Treatment**
 i. Application of 2–3% hydrogen peroxide removes color.
 ii. Commercial chelating agents (Metolex) are also useful and do not bleach hair.

d. **Prevention**
   i. Can change pools
   ii. Usually not enough of problem to warrant drastic changes in routine

D. **Exacerbation of preexisting dermatoses**
1. **Physical urticarias**
   a. **History**
      i. Cholinergic urticaria most common of this group
      ii. Induced by factors common to athletic endeavor:
         (a) Rapid temperature changes, especially cold to hot
         (b) Emotional stress
         (c) Exertion
      iii. Cold urticaria and aquagenic urticaria nearly disabling to swimmers
      iv. Pressure urticaria may appear under athletic equipment
   b. **Diagnosis**
      i. Papular erythema with dermal edema
      ii. Papules smaller than with standard urticaria and wheal less pronounced
      iii. Inner aspects of arms and legs and lateral flanks common sites
   c. **Treatment**
      i. Cyproheptadine (Periactin) taken regularly at bedtime seems particularly helpful.
      ii. "Combination" therapy with H_1 and H_2 inhibiting antihistamines often works better than a single drug regimen (hydroxyzine plus doxepin).
      iii. Alternate-day steroids may be required in extreme cases.
   d. **Prevention**
      i. Often difficult, short of complete cessation of athletic activity
      ii. Warming or cooling body temperature very slowly
      iii. Biofeedback techniques for stress reduction
      iv. Any of the drugs mentioned under "Treatment" can be taken prophylactically.
2. **Contact dermatitis**
   a. **History**
      i. Any known contact allergen may be an obscure component of athletic equipment.
      ii. Individuals with no known allergens may experience contactants unique to athletic environment.
   b. **Diagnosis**
      i. Sharp margination configuring to athletic equipment is the hallmark finding (Fig. 10).
      ii. Varying degrees of erythema initially, with scaling and exudate later
      iii. Vesicle formation in acute cases, with strong sensitivity (Fig. 11)

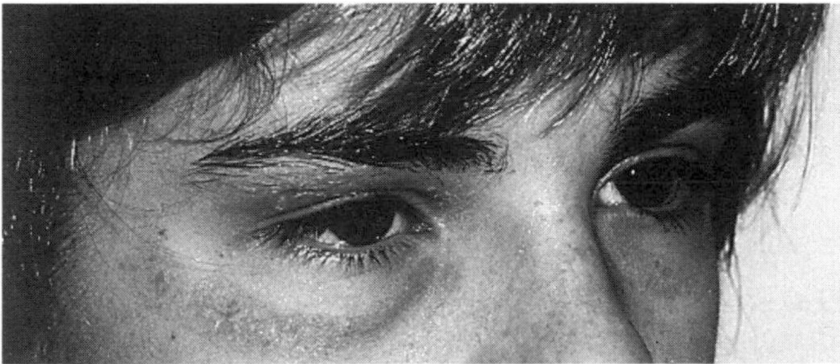

FIGURE 10. Contact allergic reaction to rubber on swim goggles.

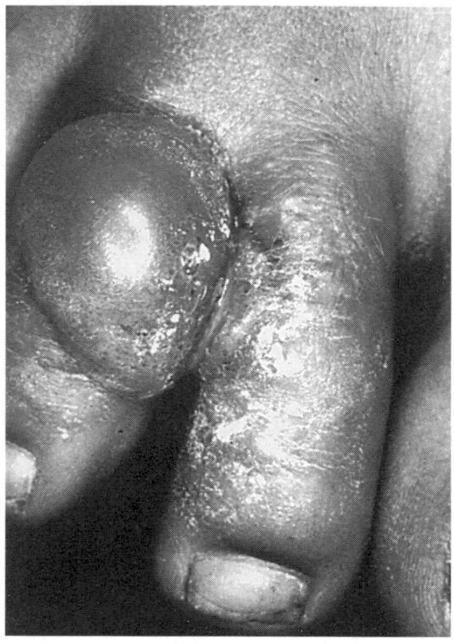

FIGURE 11. Swimmer with poison ivy leaf caught between toes.

c. **Treatment**
   i. Corticosteroids are cornerstone of therapy:
      (a) Gel, lotion, and spray preparations especially effective topically
      (b) Systemic "burst" of prednisone in acute cases
      (c) Parenteral steroids often faster acting and eliminate problems with patient compliance
   ii. Cool compresses of Boro solution are soothing in acute phase.
   iii. Antihistamines diminish reaction and relieve itching.

d. **Prevention**
   i. Identification and elimination of allergen key to resolution
   ii. Barrier between skin and causative factor:
      (a) T-shirt or leggings under pads
      (b) Nail polish over metal surfaces
      (c) Cordran tape for small areas
      (d) Specially constructed equipment such as allergy-free shoes may eliminate the problem but are usually expensive.

3. **Eczema**
   a. **History**
      i. Lifelong problem of skin sensitivity or atopy
      ii. Most forms are aggravated by increase in body heat and perspiration, both inescapable in athletic competition.
   b. **Diagnosis**
      i. Poorly marginated erythema with scaling and often exudate
      ii. Flexural areas and neck most often involved
      iii. Persistent itching with evidence of excoriation
   c. **Treatment**
      i. Topical corticosteroids in emollient cream or ointment base
      ii. Antihistamines for relief of itching and mild sedation
      iii. Systemic corticosteroids during acute flares

d. **Prevention**
   i. Short, tepid showers using oil or cream-based soap (Dove, Lever-2000)
   ii. Application of bath oil after shower (Alpha-Keri Oil)
   iii. Constant lubrication with emollient cream or lotion

III. Conclusion

As is the case with nearly all sports-induced medical problems, skin conditions unique to the athletic environment can be successfully managed with cooperative interaction between the athlete and the sports-medicine professional (physician or athletic trainer). Because of easy accessibility, most of these skin changes are easily diagnosed and with informed care need not detract from athletic participation or performance. The skin can maintain its position as an effective and conditioned interface between the athlete and the sporting environment.

Recommended Reading

1. Amundson LH: Managing skin problems in athletes. In Mellion MB (ed): Team Physicians Handbook. Philadelphia, Hanley & Belfus, 1990, pp 236–250.
2. Amundson LH, Mellion MB: Common skin problems. In Mellion MB (ed): Office Management of Sports Injuries and Athletic Problems. Philadelphia, Hanley & Belfus, 1988, pp 146–159.
3. Basler RSW: Acne-mechanica in athletes. Cutis 50:125–128, 1992.
4. Basler RSW: Skin problems encountered in winter sports. In McCasey MJ, Foster C, Hixon EG (eds): Winter Sports Medicine. Philadelphia, FA Davis, 1989, pp 142–147.
5. Basler RSW: Sports-related skin injuries. In Callen JP, Dahl MV, Golitz LE, et al (eds): Advances in Dermatology, vol 4. Chicago, Year Book Medical Publishers, 1989, pp 29–50.
6. Basler RSW: Skin injuries in sports medicine. J Am Acad Dermatol 21:1257–1262, 1989.
7. Basler RSW: Dermatologic aspects of sports participation. Curr Concepts Skin Dis 6:15–19, 1985.
8. Basler RSW: Skin lesions related to sports activity. Prim Care 10:479–494, 1983.
9. Basler RSW: Damaging effects of sunlight on human skin. Nebr Med J 63:337–340, 1978.
10. Basler RSW, Rheim JE: Sunlight and skin. J Dermatol Allergy 5:23–27, 1982.
11. Bergfeld WF: Dermatologic problems in athletes. Clin Sports Med 1:3, 1982.
12. Cortese TA, Fukuyama K, Edstein WL, et al: Treatment of friction blisters. Arch Dermatol 97:717–721, 1968.
13. Farber GA, Burks JW, Hegre AM, et al: Football acne. Cutis 20:356–360, 1977.
14. Houston SD, Knox JM: Skin problems related to sports and recreational activities. Cutis 19:487–491, 1977.
15. Levine N: Dermatologic aspects of sports medicine. J Am Acad Dermatol 3:415–424, 1980.
16. Levit P: Jogger's nipples. N Engl J Med 297:1127, 1977.
17. Liteplo MG: Sports-related skin problems. In Vinger PF, Hoerner EF (eds): Sports Injuries: The Unthwarted Epidemic. Boston, John Wright, 1982, pp 188–202.
18. Resnick SS, Lewis LA, Cohen BH: The athlete's foot. Cutis 20:351–355, 1977.
19. Sher RK: Jogger's toe. Int J Dermatol 17:719–720, 1978.
20. Wilkinson DS: Black heel: A minor hazard of sport. Cutis 20:393–396, 1977.

PART VII

INJURY PREVENTION, DIAGNOSIS, AND TREATMENT

37: Musculoskeletal Injuries in Sports

W. Michael Walsh, M.D., Ronnie D. Hald, PT, ATC, Laura E. Peter, M.D., and Morris B. Mellion, M.D.

I. General Classification of Musculoskeletal Sports Injuries

Can be broken down into **traumatic** and **overuse** injuries.

A. **Traumatic injuries** result from specific episode(s) of trauma, whether recent (acute) or in the more distant past (subacute or chronic)
   1. **Bone.** Traumatic injury to bone most commonly results in **fracture**, though rarely there can be another process, such as **subperiosteal hematoma**. Various descriptive terms used with fractures include:
      a. **Closed fracture:** fracture that does not produce open wound in skin
      b. **Open fracture:** open wound in skin communicates with fracture site
      c. Descriptive terms for direction of fracture line:
         i. Fracture at right angles to long axis of bone is called **transverse**
         ii. Fracture line at other angle to long axis of bone is called **oblique**
         iii. Bone twisted apart creates **spiral** configuration of fracture
      d. **Comminuted fracture:** bone is broken into three or more pieces
      e. **Avulsion fracture:** a "pull-off" fracture; a piece of bone is pulled off by ligament or tendon attachment
      f. **Greenstick fracture:** incomplete fracture in children. One side of a bone is broken, whereas the other side appears bent.
      g. **Torus fracture:** localized buckling in the cortex of the bone, common in children
      h. **Epiphyseal fracture:** fracture that involves the growth center at the end of a long bone in children
   2. **Joint.** Traumatic injury to joint and supporting structures (capsule, ligaments) often results in an instability episode referred to as **dislocation** or **subluxation**. Rarely, some other process occurs from a direct blow, such as joint contusion or hemarthrosis.
      a. **Dislocation:** complete displacement of joint surfaces so that they no longer make normal contact at all. Important to distinguish **first time** or **recurrent** dislocation.
      b. **Subluxation:** partial displacement of joint surfaces, usually transient in nature. Important to distinguish **first time** or **recurrent** subluxation.
      c. Dislocation or subluxation implies damage to ligaments or other supporting structures of joint. Important to ascertain injury to those tissues; discussed below.
   3. **Ligament.** Traumatic injury to ligament referred to as **sprain**. Sprains are classified as:
      a. **1st degree**—tear of only a few ligament fibers. Mild swelling, pain, disability. No instability of joint created.
      b. **2nd degree**—tear of a moderate number of ligament fibers, but ligament function is still intact. Moderate amount of swelling, pain, disability. Little to no instability of joint.

c. **3rd degree**—complete rupture of ligament. Severe swelling and disability. Definite joint instability. Instability may be classified as:
   - **1+** Joint surfaces normally stabilized by ligament displaced 3–5 mm from their normal position
   - **2+** Joint surfaces separated by 6–10 mm
   - **3+** Joint surfaces separated by more than 10 mm

4. **Muscle-tendon unit**
   a. Traumatic injury to muscle or tendon due to **indirect force** (i.e., contraction of muscle itself) is referred to as **strain**. Strains are classified as:
      i. **1st degree**—tear of only a few muscle or tendon fibers. Mild swelling, pain, disability. Can also be characterized by patient's ability to produce strong, but painful, muscle contraction.
      ii. **2nd degree**—disruption of a moderate number of muscle or tendon fibers, but muscle-tendon unit still intact. Moderate amount of pain, swelling, disability. Characterized by patient's weak and painful attempts at muscle contraction.
      iii. **3rd degree**—complete rupture of muscle-tendon unit. May be at origin, muscular portion, musculotendinous junction, within tendon itself, or at tendon insertion. Characterized by patient's extremely weak but painless attempts at muscle contraction.
   b. Traumatic injury to muscle due to **direct force** may produce **deep muscle contusion**.
      i. Typically, quadriceps or brachialis muscles involved in contact or collision sports
      ii. May lead to **myositis ossificans** and therefore permanent loss of function
   c. **Myositis ossificans** (traumatic myositis ossificans)—heterotopic bone formation caused by deep muscle contusion or strain, especially after marked hematoma formation
      i. **Common sites**
         (a) Quadriceps
         (b) Biceps, triceps, brachialis
         (c) Hip girdle
         (d) Groin
         (e) Lower leg
      ii. **Risk factors** (Reid)
         (a) Severe contusion
         (b) Continuing to play after injury
         (c) Massaging injured area
         (d) Early application of heat
         (e) Passive, forceful stretching
         (f) Overly rapid rehabilitation
         (g) Premature return to sport
         (h) Reinjury of same site
         (i) Individual propensity to heterotopic bone formation
      iii. **Calcification** follows injury by 3–6 weeks
         (a) May continue to develop for 6 weeks or more
         (b) May remodel or reabsorb over 3–12 months, especially if close to musculotendinous junction
      iv. **Treatment**
         (a) Treat strain or contusion with basic athletic first aid (see Chapter 38, "Comprehensive Rehabilitation of the Athlete") represented by the mnemonic "PRICES"

•**P**rotection	• **C**ompression
• **R**est	• **E**levation
• **I**ce	• **S**upport

Followed by progressive symptom-guided rehabilitation.

(b) **Excision rarely necessary**
- Only warranted in cases of persistent weakness or limited range of motion
- Only after calcification matures (6–12 months)
- High rate of recurrence if excised too early

5. Other soft tissues
   a. Traumatic injury to bursa with bursal swelling referred to as **traumatic bursitis**, usually due to bleeding into bursa
   b. Traumatic injuries to other soft tissues include various **contusions** and **hematomas**
   c. Lacerations may involve musculoskeletal tissues
   d. Shearing injuries—avulsions, abrasions, blisters

B. **Overuse injuries** account for more than 50% of injuries seen in primary care practices.

1. **General overuse concepts.** If viewed as a function of Newton's third law of motion, athletic injury can be described as resulting from equal and opposite reactions, which in turn result in macro- or microtrauma.
   a. Macrotrauma—equal and opposite forces exceed the strength of a specific anatomic structure, and therefore the structure fails (See "Traumatic injuries," page 361).
   b. Microtrauma—microscopic subliminal injury from repeated activity. Repetitive microtrauma can be cumulative over time and can result in inflammation, characterized by pain and dysfunction.
2. **Predisposition.** Equally important are intrinsic or extrinsic factors that predispose the athlete to overuse injury.
   a. **Intrinsic**—malalignment of limbs, muscular imbalances, other anatomical factors
   b. **Extrinsic**—training errors, faulty technique, incorrect surfaces and equipment, poor environmental conditions
3. **Degenerative processes** may influence traumatic injuries as well, but more commonly have effect on overuse injuries. Normal degenerative processes occur in many musculoskeletal tissues with aging. May add to likelihood of certain injuries. Common examples are rotator cuff and Achilles' tendon problems.
4. **General classification.** Overuse injuries can be classified as four stages, according to pain:
   a. **Stage 1** Pain after activity only
   b. **Stage 2** Pain during activity, does not restrict performance
   c. **Stage 3** Pain during activity, restricts performance
   d. **Stage 4** Chronic, unremitting pain, even at rest
5. **Bones.** Overuse injury of bone may be **stress fracture** or **apophysitis**.
   a. **Stress fracture:** most often found in lower extremity, but can also be found in the spine (see section on spondylolysis and spondylolisthesis, Chapter 47) and in the upper extremity when it is subjected to weightbearing (e.g., gymnastics, weight training)
   b. **Apophysitis:** in skeletally immature athletes, traction injuries can occur to the apophysis. Appear to result from repeated stress at tendinous insertion into bony growth center, followed by reactive bone formation. Most common apophysitis is Osgood-Schlatter's disease (see Chapter 49).
6. **Joints.** Overuse joint injuries are almost invariably the result of mechanical factors. While they may create a condition that could be called "arthritis," it may be more valid when treating athletes to think of it as a **synovitis**.
   a. Synovitis may be generalized, with swelling, warmth, pain, and occasionally redness.
   b. Some synovitis is more localized, e.g., synovial plica of knee, peripatellar synovitis in extensor mechanism malalignment of knee (see Chapter 49).

7. **Ligament.** There are few examples of pure overuse injuries to ligaments. Theoretically, they may occur whenever a ligament is subjected to repeated stress. Examples include:
   a. **Medial elbow injuries:** part of this spectrum may include overuse injury to the medial collateral ligament of the elbow, resulting from repetitive throwing with valgus loading.
   b. **Breaststroker's knee:** probably the most common example of pure ligament injury through overuse. Typically involves medial collateral ligament of knee at femoral attachment, secondary to breaststroke kick.
   c. **Plantar fasciitis:** technically a ligament connecting bone to bone, the plantar fascia is commonly involved in overuse syndromes of the foot (see Chapter 52).
8. **Muscle-tendon unit.** Overuse injury of muscle-tendon unit may be **myositis, tendinitis,** or **tenosynovitis**.
   a. Myositis overuse injuries of muscle tissue are rather nondescript. Can involve practically any muscle in the body. More distinct syndromes are known when overuse syndromes occur at muscular origin and attachment to bone/periosteum. Those syndromes include:
      i. Lateral epicondylitis of the elbow
      ii. Medial epicondylitis of the elbow
      iii. Chronic groin strain
      iv. Shin splints
   b. Tendinitis: inflammatory reaction within the tendon tissue itself. Closely related to the concept of normal aging and degenerative changes within tendons (tendonosis), which may predispose to microtrauma. Common examples are:
      i. Bicipital tendinitis
      ii. Rotator cuff tendinitis
      iii. Achilles tendinitis
   c. Tenosynovitis (peritendinitis, tenovaginitis): inflammatory change involves tissue surrounding the tendon itself. Classic physical finding is crepitation or "dry leather creaking" sensation over involved tendon as tendon is moved through its sheath. Common locations include:
      i. Extensor tendons of forearm
      ii. Tibialis anterior in the lower leg
9. Other soft tissues. The most common overuse musculoskeletal injury involving other soft tissue is **bursitis**.
   a. Bursae lie between tissue planes and help to reduce frictional stress between those structures.
   b. Common sites for mechanical bursitis in athletes include:
      i. Subacromial bursa
      ii. Greater trochanteric bursa of the hip
      iii. Retrocalcaneal bursa just anterior to the Achilles' tendon insertion

II. General Treatment of Musculoskeletal Injuries

A. Basic athletic first aid—PRICES (see page 362)
B. Other treatment methods
   1. **Oral anti-inflammatory medication.** Non-steroidal anti-inflammatory drugs (NSAIDs) are commonly used in treating musculoskeletal sports injuries. Many different types and brands exist. Their use is usually based on clinician's empiric results rather than on objective scientific studies. Choice should always be tempered by known side effects (e.g., renal damage). Best thought of as adjunctive treatment to other modes.
   2. **Physical modalities.** Cold, heat, ultrasound, iontophoresis, and electrical muscle stimulation are commonly employed. See Chapter 38 for discussion.

3. **Therapeutic exercises.** Most important, but most commonly underutilized means of treating musculoskeletal sports injuries. Important to correct not only deficits that may result from injury, but also those that predispose to injury.
4. **Injection therapy.** Most commonly injected material is corticosteroid, with or without local anesthetic. **Studies have demonstrated direct harmful effect of steroid on articular cartilage and weakening effect on tendon.**
   a. **Should never inject corticosteroid into:**
      i. **Young athletes' joints**
      ii. **Major joint (e.g., knee, shoulder)** in athlete of any age when there is not already objective degenerative change
      iii. **Major load-bearing tendons,** e.g., patellar tendon, Achilles' tendon. **To do so may hasten rupture.**
   b. Acceptable to inject corticosteroid into:
      i. Muscular trigger points
      ii. Bursae
      iii. Small non-weight-bearing joints, e.g., acromioclavicular joint
      iv. **Muscular** attachments to bone, e.g., lateral epicondyle. **Total number** of injections should be limited.
      v. Ligament attachments to bone where subsequent rupture of ligament would not be disastrous, e.g., plantar fascia attachment to calcaneus
      vi. Tendon **sheath**, but not the tendon itself, e.g., for de Quervain's disease at wrist
      vii. Already degenerated joint in older athlete
5. **Braces, supports, and other devices.** A variety of products have been developed to aid in the treatment of athletic injuries. These range from simple compressive sleeves for various joints to expensive custom-made braces. These are discussed in the chapters on anatomical parts and individual sports and in Chapter 53.
6. Calcification excision—rare

III. Selected Musculoskeletal Evaluation Techniques

Certain musculoskeletal parameters are so commonly evaluated in athletic injuries that they are presented here for easy reference when reading other chapters.

A. **Flexibility testing.** Flexibility is limited by the length of a muscle across a joint. Lack of flexibility in two-joint muscles (muscles that cross two joints) is often indicated as a cause of musculoskeletal problems. In testing for flexibility, one must consider whether the restriction seen is due to muscular tightness, or other sources of restriction, such as lack of joint range of motion or pain.
   1. **Heel cord flexibility** (Fig. 1): Athlete sits with knee extended and is asked to actively dorsiflex the ankle. Measurement is made goniometrically. Normal value is considered to be at least 10° beyond plantigrade. This may also be done with the knee flexed to assess tightness within the soleus (normal value is at least 20° beyond plantigrade).
   2. **Hamstrings flexibility** (Fig. 2): Athlete lies supine with hip maintained at 90° flexion and is asked to extend the knee actively without repositioning the hip. Measurement is made goniometrically. Normal value is considered to be less than 10° short of full extension.
   3. **Quadriceps flexibility** (Fig. 3): Athlete lies prone and knee is flexed passively by examiner. Normal value is considered to be full knee flexion without tilting of the pelvis.
   4. **Iliotibial band flexibility** (Fig. 4): Athlete lies on the opposite side, near the edge of the examining table, facing away from the examiner. On the side to be examined, the hip is slightly extended and passively adducted by gravity. Take care not to let iliotibial band slip anterior or posterior to the greater trochanter, or to allow lateral tilting of the pelvis. Normal is considered to be when the knee drops level or below the level of the table. This test is also referred to as the modified Ober's test.

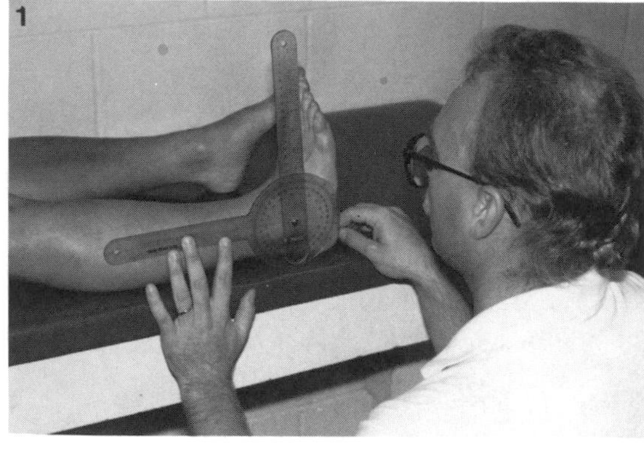

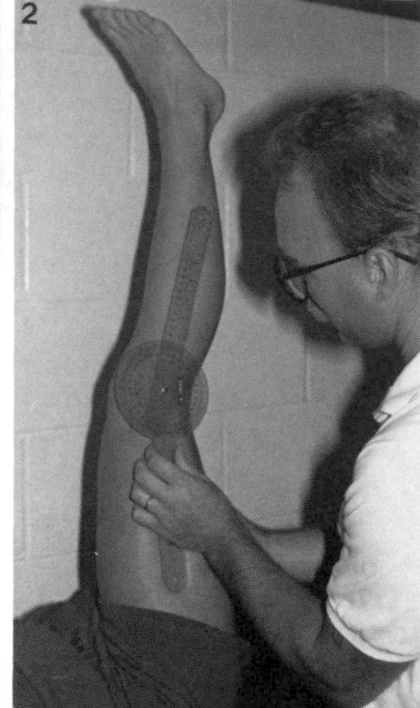

FIGURE 1. Heel cord flexibility.

FIGURE 2. Hamstrings flexibility.

FIGURE 3. Quadriceps flexibility.

FIGURE 4. Iliotibial band flexibility.

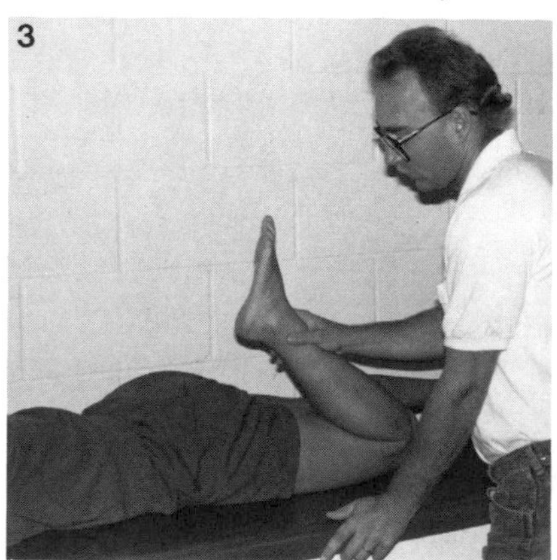

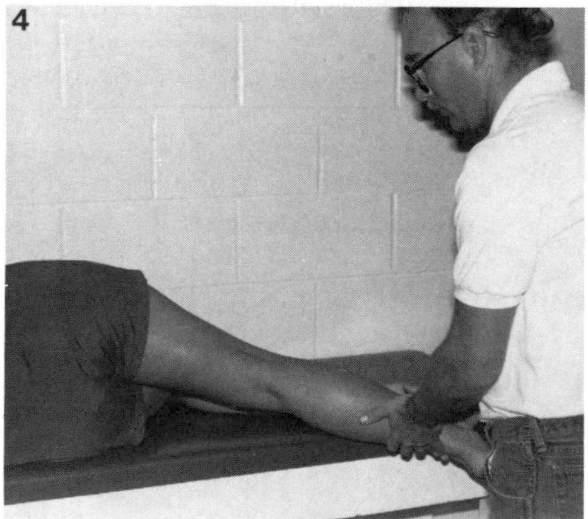

B. **Strength testing.** Although there are many ways to assess strength, the authors prefer the manual muscle "break" test technique. This requires the athlete to generate a maximal contraction of the muscle in the shortened range, and the examiner then applies an opposite force in an attempt to move the athlete from the testing position. A common muscle testing rule is not to apply forces across adjacent joints, but athletes are generally able to support adjacent joints adequately, thus allowing the examiner to apply more force to the area in question. Strength is usually graded on a 0–5 scale (0 = zero, 1 = trace, 2 = poor, 3 = fair, 4 = good, 5 = normal). Most athletic applications of the scale are in the upper range of this scale and are subjective in nature. Although more objective methods are available, the manual muscle test continues to be the most easily administered. The hip flexion, hip abduction, and supraspinatus strength tests are included, since weakness may indicate a new condition or an unrehabilitated condition more distal in the kinetic chain. The ankle dorsiflexion strength test is included because of its relationship to patellofemoral problems.

1. **Hip flexion strength** (Fig. 5): Athlete sits at edge of table with arms crossed. Athlete flexes hip and examiner performs a manual muscle "break" test. If a break occurs, observe whether the weakness identified is located in the hip or the abdominals.
2. **Hip abduction strength** (Fig. 6): Athlete lies on opposite side, facing away from the examiner. Athlete abducts hip and examiner performs a manual muscle "break" test. If a break occurs, observe whether the weakness identified is located in the hip or the abdominal obliques.
3. **Ankle dorsiflexion strength** (Fig. 7): Athlete sits with knee extended and is asked to dorsiflex ankle. Examiner performs a manual muscle "break" test.
4. **Supraspinatus strength** (Fig. 8): Athlete sits or stands with shoulders abducted to 90°, horizontally adducted to 30°, and in a "thumbs down" position (fully internally rotated). Examiner performs a manual muscle "break" test, taking care to eliminate substitution from the trapezius.

IV. Myofascial Pain Syndrome

A. Definitions

1. **Myofascial trigger point:** an intensely irritable spot in muscle and/or adjacent fascia which stimulates and sends distress signals to the central nervous system
   a. Feels like an indurated nodule or "ropey" taut band of muscle
   b. Occurs only in characteristic anatomic sites
   c. Each site has specific **"reference zones"** of radiating/referred pain or paresthesia. Reference zone pain is often presenting complaint.
   d. **May trigger a spasm-pain-spasm cycle** (see page 369)
   e. **Active trigger point**
      i. Symptomatic reference zone pain
      ii. Palpation reproduces both trigger point tenderness and reference zone pain
   f. **Latent trigger point**
      i. Tender on examination
      ii. No reference zone again
2. **Myofascial pain syndrome** (myofascial syndrome): presence of one or more active trigger points with characteristic reference zone pain
3. **Scapulocostal syndrome:** clustering of trigger point spasms in the trapezius, levator scapula, and posterior cervical muscles

B. Diagnosis

1. **Knowledge of precise anatomic sites** of trigger points and reference zones. Common trigger point sites:
   a. Levator scapula, splenius capitis, trapezius, sternocleidomastoid
   b. Infraspinatus, supraspinatus, rhomboids
   c. Quadratus lumborum, gluteus medius, tensor fascia lata
   d. Biceps femoris, vastus lateralis, adductor longus
   e. Gastrocnemius/soleus
2. **Initiating, precipitating, and perpetuating phenomena**
   a. **Physical**
      i. Trauma
         (a) Major/minor
         (b) Old/recent
      ii. Overuse
         (a) Sports/exercise
         (b) Work: repetitive motion
         (c) Muscle cramps
      iii. Inadequate warm-up

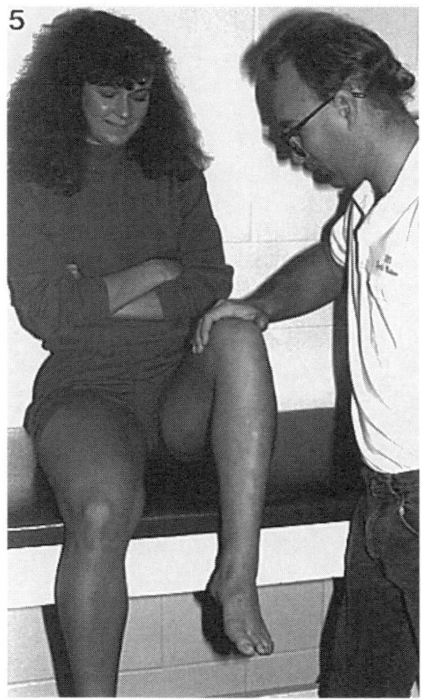

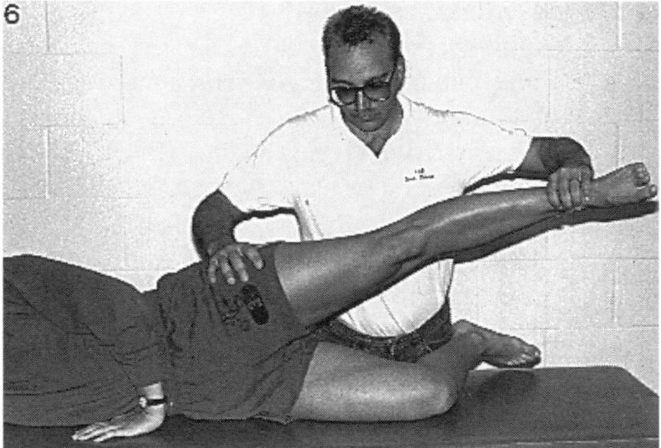

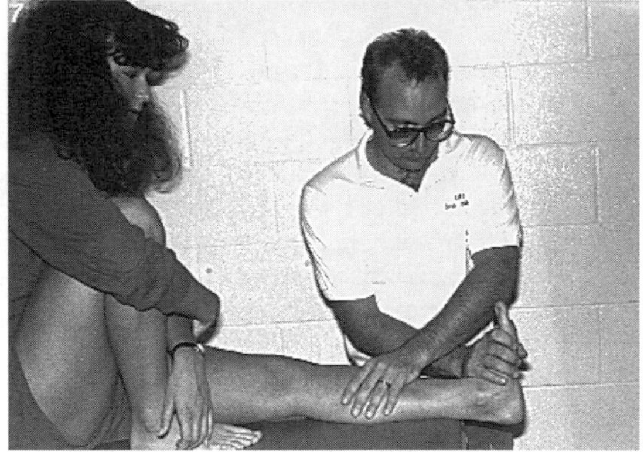

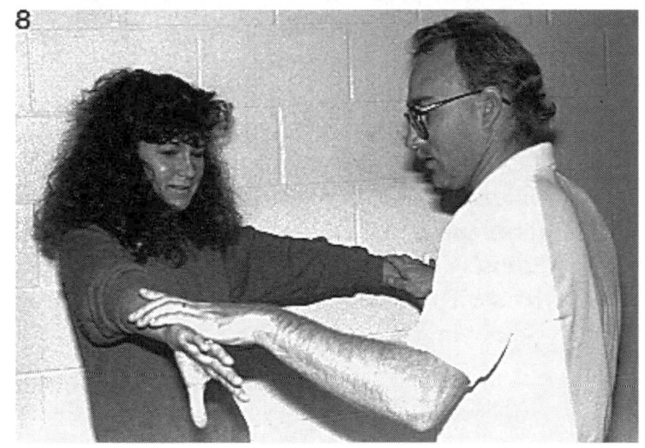

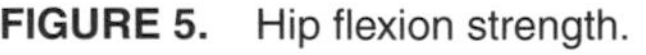

FIGURE 5. Hip flexion strength.

FIGURE 6. Hip abduction strength.

FIGURE 7. Ankle dorsiflexion strength.

FIGURE 8. Supraspinatus strength.

- iv. Cold exercise/work environment
- v. Posture
    - (a) Poor posture
    - (b) Poor body mechanics
    - (c) Anatomic abnormalities
    - (d) Poorly designed or sized workstation (especially computer worksite)
- vi. Disease
    - (a) Rheumatoid arthritis
    - (b) Multiple sclerosis

b. **Mental**

- i. Fatigue

ii. Anxiety/stress
iii. Depression
3. **Palpation of trigger points**
   a. "Rubbery" or "ropey"
   b. Indurated
   c. Tight
   d. Exquisitely tender

C. **Pain-Spasm-Pain Cycle**
1. Trigger point activation
   a. →Pain
   b. →Local muscle activation and fatigue
   c. →↑Pain spreads
   d. →Additional trigger points recruited
   e. →↑Pain spreads further
2. "Key" or "matrix" trigger point recruits "satellite" trigger points

D. **Treatment**
1. **Stretch and spray**—passive stretching using vapocoolant (fluori-methane) for distraction
2. **Massage**—deep friction or pressure (acupressure); manual, elbow, dowel
3. **Trigger point injection**
   a. 0.5% procaine
      i. Other local anesthetics may be myotoxic
      ii. Dilute 2% procaine with 3 parts of normal saline
   b. "Needling" by inserting 18 gauge needle without local anesthetic may inactivate trigger points.
   c. Corticosteroids provide no additional benefits because trigger points contain no inflammatory cells.
4. **Therapeutic exercise**
   a. Improve strength
   b. Improve flexibility
5. **Ice** (heat may exacerbate trigger points)
6. Ultrasound
7. Muscle energy manipulation techniques

E. **Levator scapula syndrome**
1. Strain of levator scapula insertion with trigger point spasm of the muscle body
2. Treat trigger point as above; may also need to treat muscle insertion with corticosteroid injection, iontophoresis or phonophoresis

Recommended Reading

1. Deluca SA: Myositis ossificans. Am Fam Physician 32(3):127–128, 1985.
2. Estwanik JJ, McAlister JA: Contusions and the formation of myositis ossificans. Phys Sportsmed 18(4): 53–64, 1990.
3. Hartley A: Practical Joint Assessment: A sports medicine manual. St. Louis, Mosby-Year Book, Inc., 1990.
4. Jobe FW, Moynes DF: Delineation of diagnostic criteria and a rehabilitation program for rotator cuff injuries. Am J Sports Med 10:336–339, 1982.
5. Kaeding CC, Sanko WA, Fischer RA: Quadriceps strains and contusions: Decisions that promote rapid recovery. Phys Sportsmed 23(1):59–64, 1995.
6. McKeag DB: The concept of overuse: The primary care aspects of overuse syndromes in sports. Primary Care 11:43–59, 1984.
7. Nicholas JA, Strizak AM, Veras G: A study of thigh weakness in different pathological states of the lower extremity. Am J Sports Med 4:241–248, 1976.
8. Pfenniger JL: Injections of joints and soft tissue: Part II. Guidelines for specific joints. Am Fam Physician 44:1196–1202, 1991.

9. Pfenninger JL: Injections of joints and soft tissue: Part II. Guidelines for specific joints. Am Fam Physician 44:1690–1701, 1991.
10. Pfenninger JL, Fowler GC: Procedures for Primary Care Physicians. St. Louis, Mosby-Year Book, Inc., 1994.
11. Puffer JC, Zachazewski JE: Management of overuse injuries. Am Fam Physician 38(3):225–232, 1988.
12. Reid DC: Sports Injury Assessment and Rehabilitation. New York, Churchill Livingstone, Inc., 1992.
13. Ryan JB, Wheeler JH, Hopkinson WJ, et al: Quadriceps contusions: West Point update. Am J Sports Med 19:299–304, 1991.
14. Simons D: Fibrositis/fibromyalgia: A form of myofascial trigger points? Am J Med 81(Suppl 3A):93–98, 1986.
15. Simons D, Travell J: Myofascial pain syndrome. In Wall PD, Melzack R (eds): Textbook of Pain, 2nd ed. New York, Churchill Livingstone, 1989, pp 368–385.
16. Travell J, Simons D: Myofascial Pain and Dysfunction: The Trigger Point Manual, vol. 1. Baltimore, Williams & Wilkins, 1983.
17. Travell J, Simons D: Myofascial Pain and Dysfunction: The Trigger Point Manual, vol 2. Baltimore, Williams & Wilkins, 1991.

38

Comprehensive Rehabilitation of the Athlete

Guy L. Shelton, M.A., PT, ATC

I. Goals of Rehabilitation

A. Return athlete to participation as soon as safely possible.
   1. **Decrease recovery time and promote healing.**
      a. Decrease swelling, congestion, and muscle spasm (pain).
      b. Facilitate nutrient supply for rebuilding injured tissue.
   2. **Decrease morbidity.**
      a. Minimize deconditioning—range of motion (ROM), strength, endurance
      b. Recondition—injured and uninjured areas
   3. **Prevent further injury or reinjury.**
      a. Allow adequate healing time.
      b. Protect

II. Steps in Treatment

A. Common treatment **misconceptions:**
   1. Treat with medication only.
   2. Ice for 24–48 hours, then heat.
   3. Wrap for support, not compression.
   4. Do not use crutches unless pain is intolerable.
   5. Immobilization instead of rehabilitation
   6. Time heals all.
   7. Return to play is based on calendar timetable.

B. **Prevention**
   1. First step in treating injuries
   2. An ounce of prevention is worth a pound of cure.

C. **Triage**
   1. **Evaluate**—within your skill and knowledge level
   2. **Assessment**
      a. On the field "diagnosis"
      b. Not necessarily specific but detailed enough to make the proper initial decision
   3. **Decision**
      a. What next step to take?
         i. Return to play?
         ii. Hold out?
         iii. Refer for further evaluation?
            (a) Urgent?
            (b) Routine?
      b. **Be conservative!**

D. **Basic athletic first aid—PRICES**
   1. ***P*rotection** from further injury
      a. Crutches for any lower extremity injury when the athlete is unable to walk normally (no pain, limping, or buckling)
      b. Splint or sling to immobilize extremity when more serious injury is suspected
      c. Stretcher to move injured athlete if any doubt about the injury
   2. ***R*est** to avoid aggravating injury further
      a. **Absolute rest:**
         i. Complete rest from activity
         ii. Best until serious injury ruled out
      b. **Relative rest:**
         i. Partial participation based on symptoms
         ii. Used only in minor injuries until further evaluation is made
   3. ***I*ce**
      a. Decreases swelling, pain, inflammatory response, nerve conduction velocity, and muscle spasm
      b. Cold applied for **up to 30 minutes**, depending on degree of symptoms
      c. **Ice bag best,** gel packs and cold water immersion good
   4. ***C*ompression**
      a. Circumferential wrap limits swelling in injured area
      b. May also provide some support
   5. ***E*levation—gravity** helps decrease swelling
   6. ***S*upport**
      a. Implies a more **functional type of protection** (taping, bracing)
      b. Used when injury is minor and athlete can return to play

E. **Definitive diagnosis and treatment**
   1. Thorough clinical **examination**
   2. **Special tests** where applicable
   3. **Referral** to appropriate medical specialty
   4. **Diagnosis needs to be specific** so best treatment plan can be determined.
   5. **Treatment**
      a. **Immobilization:**
         i. Used for certain fractures and sprains
         ii. Do not use with a less serious injury just to keep athlete from participating.
         iii. **Always should be followed by functional treatment**
      b. **Surgical:**
         i. Should be used for specific indications
         ii. Sometimes indicated in acute injuries
         iii. Often considered only after failed conservative care
         iv. **Always should be followed by functional treatment**
      c. **Functional (rehabilitative):**
         i. Activity-oriented goals require **active treatment**.
         ii. **Most important** form of treatment
         iii. **Integral part of both immobilization and surgical treatment**

F. **Rehabilitation—functional treatment**
   1. **Pyramid of recovery** (Figs. 1 and 2)
      a. **Building blocks** of therapeutic exercise
      b. **Primary treatment** in most cases
      c. **Total athlete concept:** when an injury occurs, the **entire athlete is affected**. The longer the recovery period, the greater the potential for **systemic deconditioning**. The injured area deserves primary consideration, but the other parts of the athlete cannot be ignored.

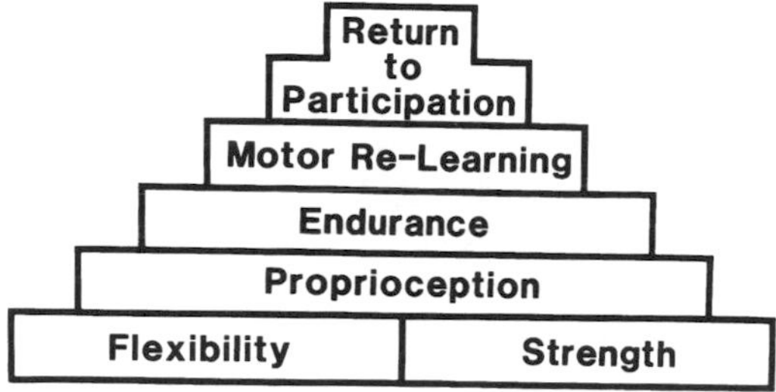

FIGURE 1. Pyramid of recovery (therapeutic exercise).

   i. **Local treatment**—injured area itself
   ii. **Limb treatment**—limb functions as a kinetic chain
   iii. **System treatment:**
      (a) Uninjured limbs
      (b) Cardiovascular system
      (c) Overall agility and timing

2. **Specifics of therapeutic exercise**
   a. **Flexibility** (see Figs. 3 through 11 for selected flexibility exercises)
      i. Joint ROM:
         (a) Respect healing structures.
         (b) Should be regained with **minimal aggravation of symptoms**
      ii. Muscle elasticity:
         (a) Inflexibility decreases muscle function at extreme positions, decreases adaptability of muscle-tendon unit, and increases joint compression forces.
         (b) Repetitions should be **prolonged and static** with moderate tension felt in muscle.

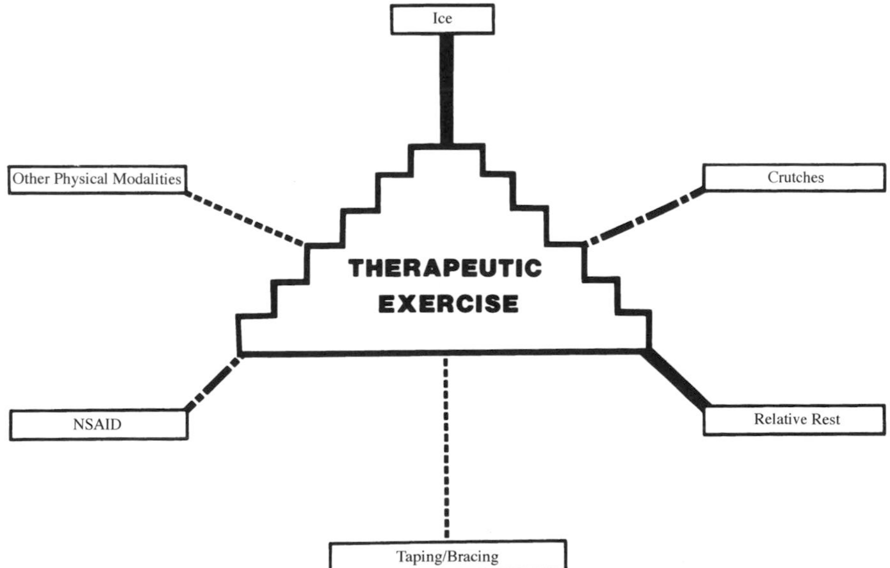

FIGURE 2. Relationship of therapeutic exercise to adjunct treatments.

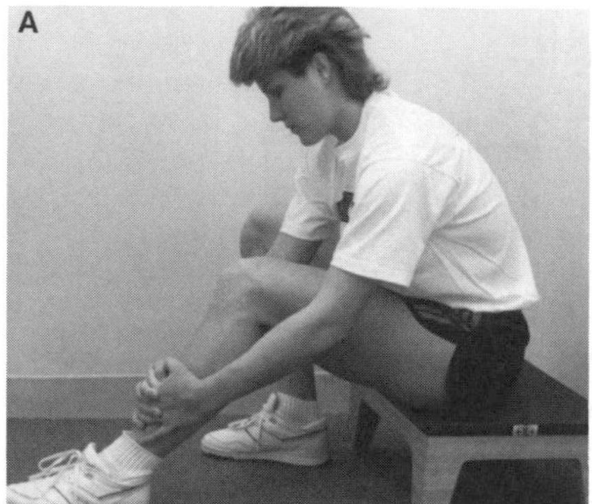

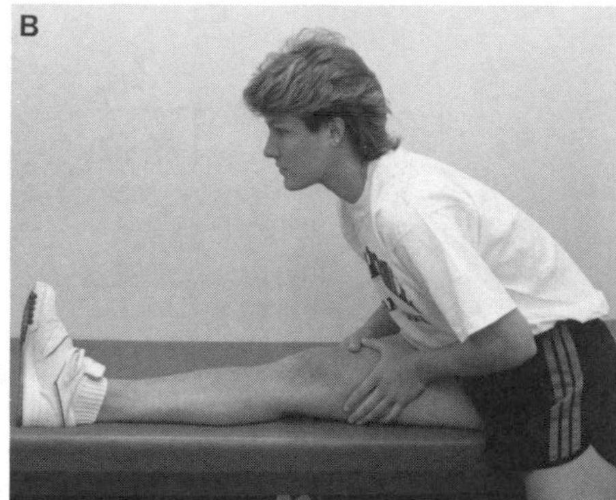

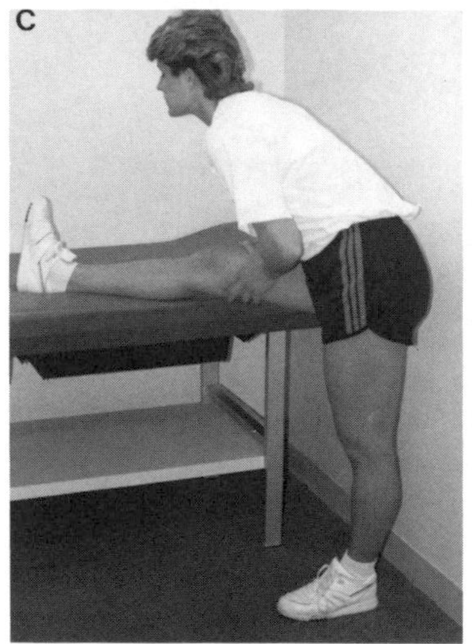

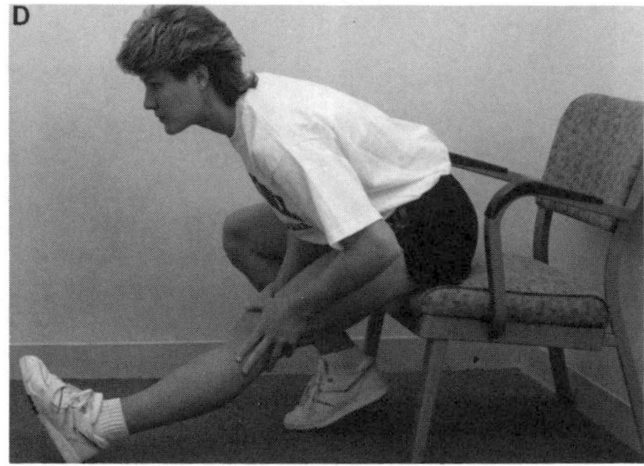

FIGURE 3. A, Assisted knee flexion. Low seat keeps hip lower than knee and minimizes substitute movement of lifting hip instead of flexing knee. **B,** Hamstring stretching sitting at edge of table or couch; **C,** standing; **D,** from chair with foot on floor.

(c) Degree of flexibility varies, so adequate time should be allowed each session **based on individual levels of flexibility**.

b. **Strength** (see Figs. 12 through 20 for selected strength exercises)

i. General considerations:

(a) Muscle must be **overloaded** to facilitate strengthening.

(b) Exercises need to be **specific** with regard to ultimate activity.

(c) Rate of **progression** is determined by initial level of fitness, healing stage of injury, and individual differences.

ii. **Exercise prescription:**

(a) **Intensity**

- Must be adequate to **create overload**
- **Lower intensity during early rehabilitation to avoid symptoms**

(b) **Frequency**

- Number of sessions per day/days per week
- **Higher frequency while intensity is low**

(c) **Duration/repetitions**

- **Higher number of repetitions while intensity is low**
- Watch for fatigue and symptoms.

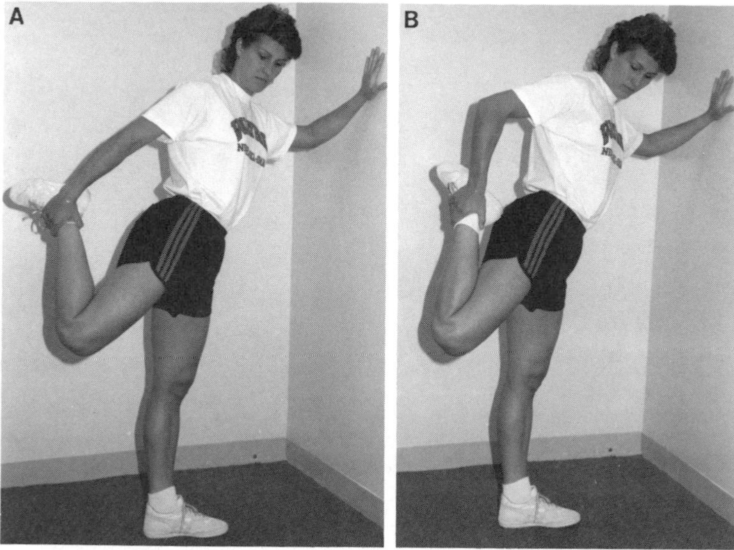

FIGURE 4. Quadriceps stretching. **A,** Keep heel away from buttocks initially. **B,** As flexibility and comfort progress, gradually pull heel to buttocks as long as symptoms do not increase.

(d) **Mode/specific techniques**
- Must be adjusted to **patient's tolerance**
- **Modification** of standard techniques and equipment must be made for certain injuries.

iii. **Types of strengthening exercise:**

(a) **Isometric**
- Muscle contraction against **immovable resistance**
- Muscle contraction **intensity can be varied** from very light to maximum.
- Usually **well tolerated** fairly soon after injury

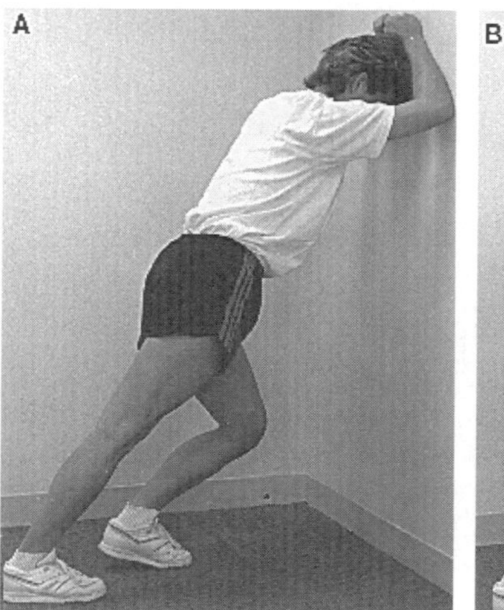

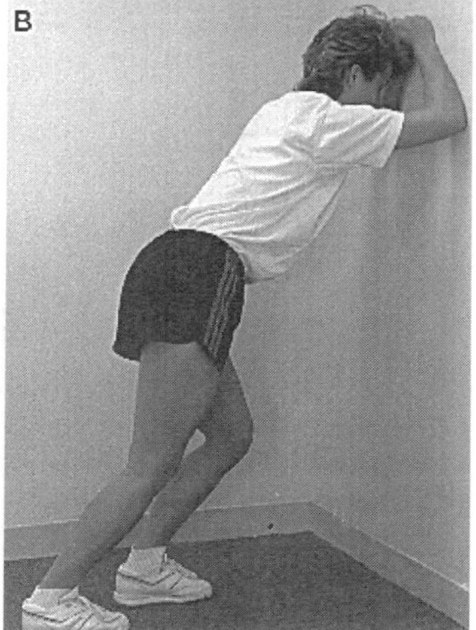

FIGURE 5. Heelcord stretching. **A,** Knee straight to stretch the gastrocnemius muscle. **B,** Knee bent to stretch the soleus muscle and Achilles' tendon.

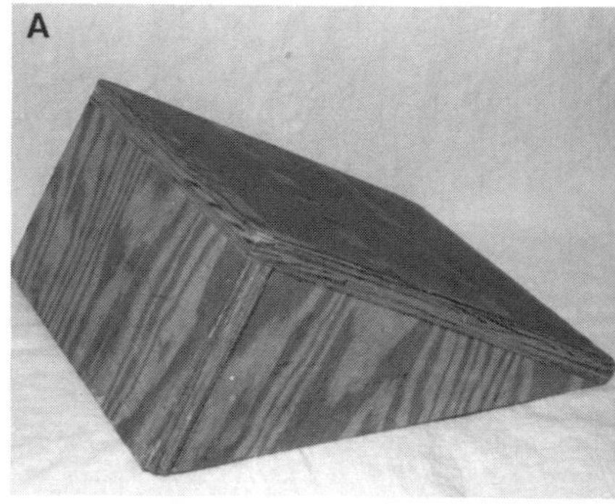

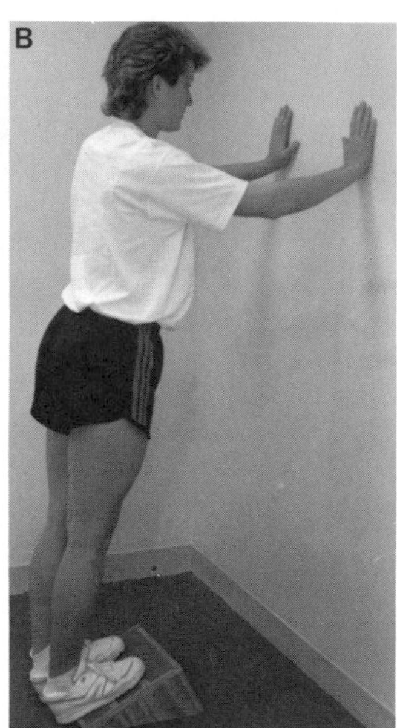

FIGURE 6. A, Slant board (12″ × 12″ × 6″ high) used to increase stretch on calf. **B,** Heelcord stretching using slant board.

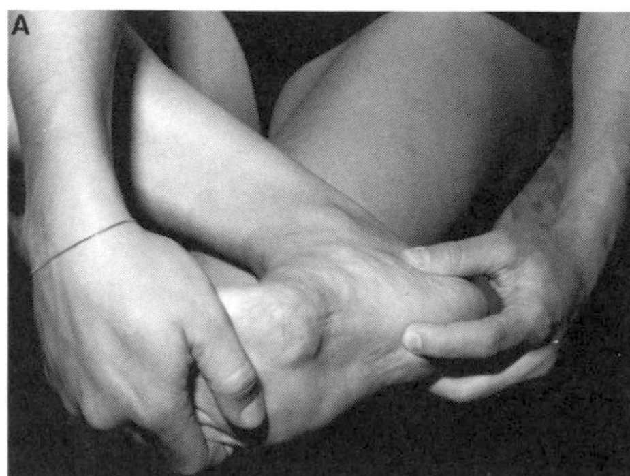

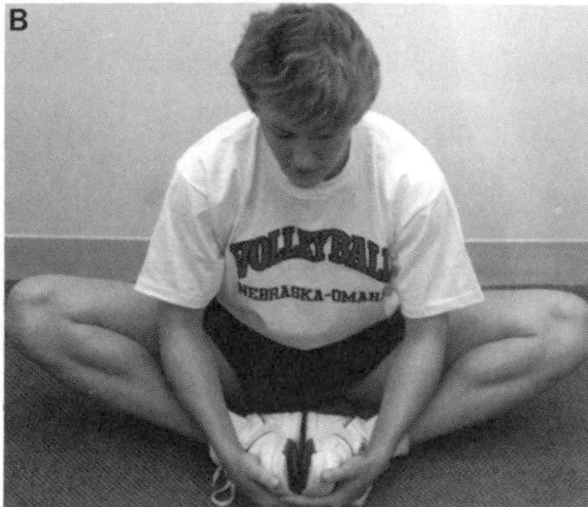

FIGURE 7. A, Plantar fascia stretch. Used as a treatment for plantar fasciitis. **B,** Adductor stretch.

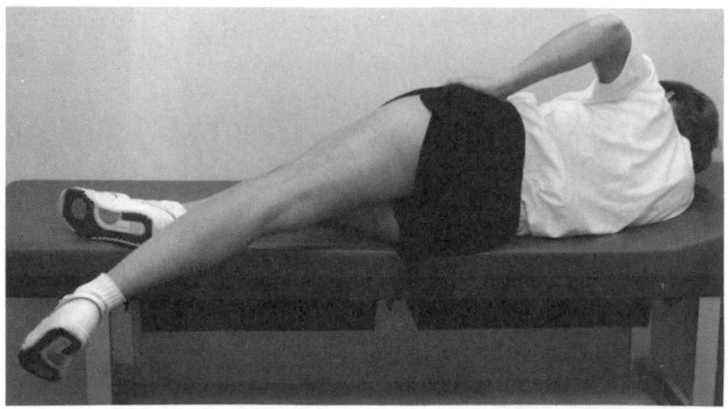

FIGURE 8. Iliotibial band stretch. Used for iliotibial band friction syndrome.

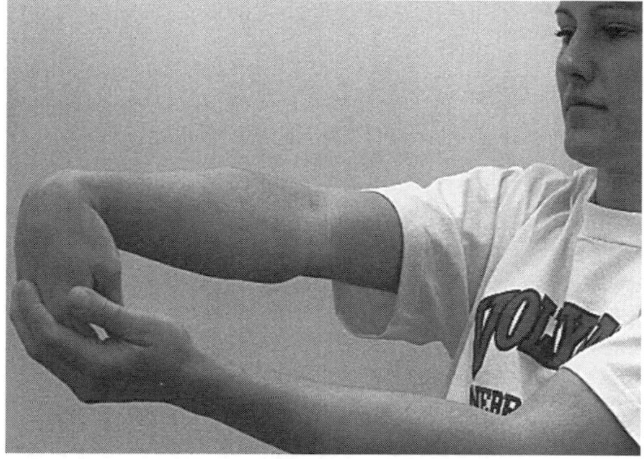

FIGURE 9. Wrist extensor stretch. Used for lateral epicondylitis.

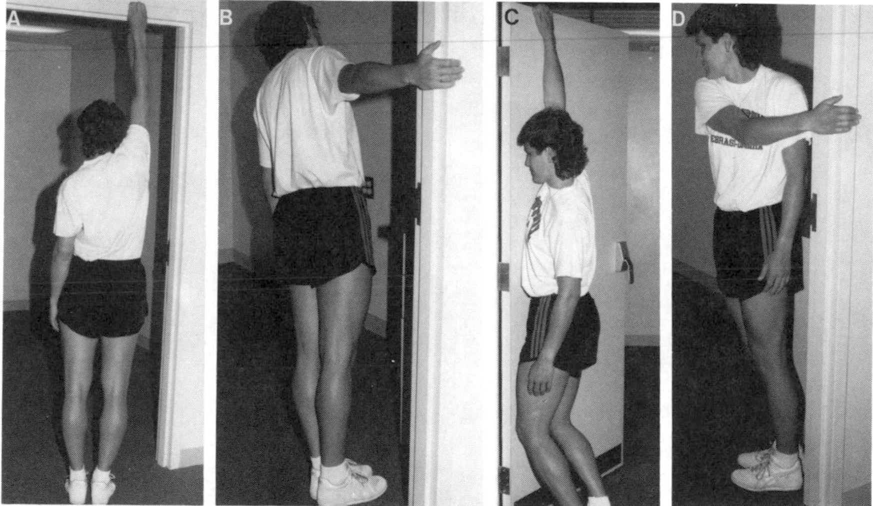

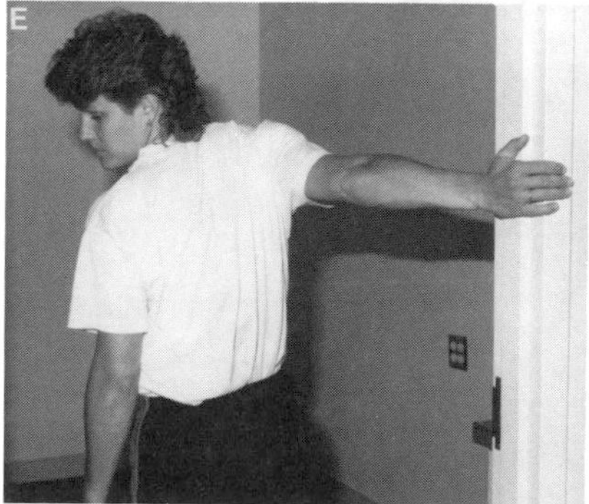

FIGURE 10. A, Shoulder flexion stretch using doorway to anchor hand. **B,** Distraction stretch for glenohumeral joint. Useful as early stretching exercise in impingement syndrome and rotator cuff problems. **C,** Overhead version of distraction stretch. This is a more advanced technique and should be achieved gradually. **D,** Horizontal adduction with distraction. Useful in impingement syndrome as acute symptoms decrease. **E,** Horizontal abduction stretch.

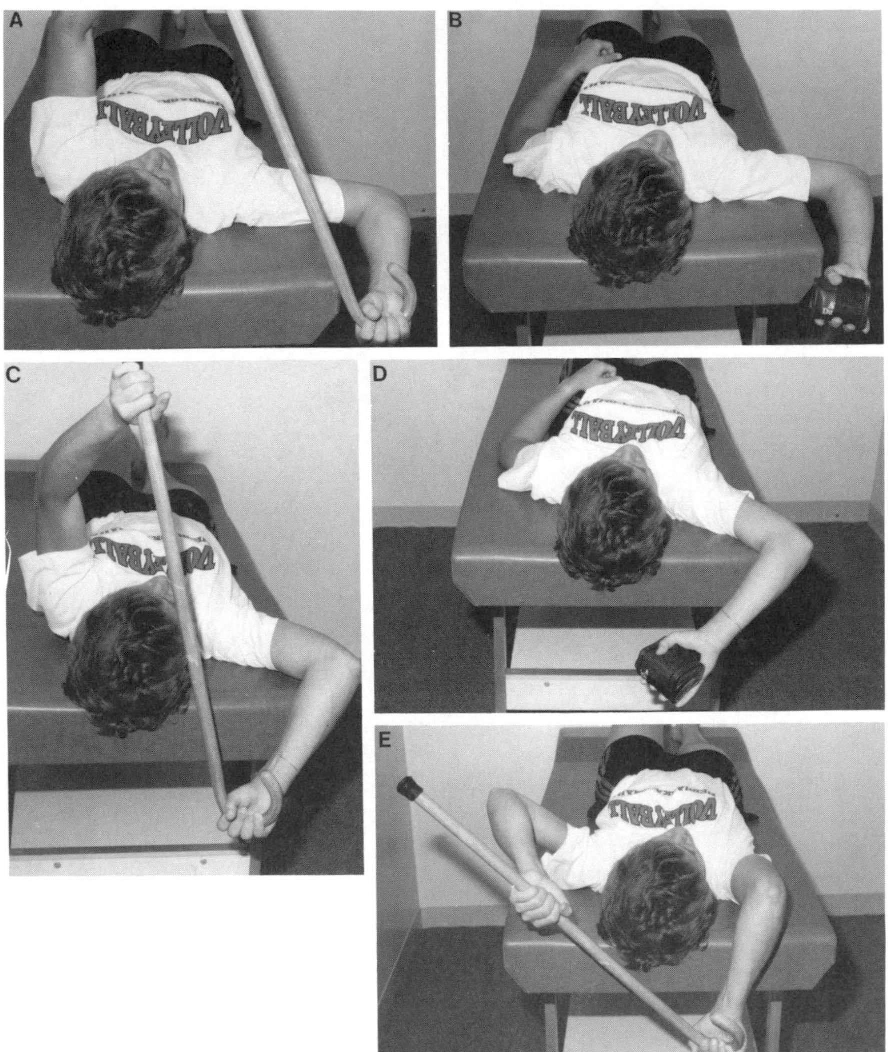

FIGURE 11. **A,** Supine external rotation stretch in 90° abduction using wand to provide stretch. **B,** Supine external rotation stretch in 90° abduction using weight to provide stretch. **C,** Supine external rotation stretch in 135° abduction using wand to provide stretch. Progression of stretch in A. **D,** Supine external rotation stretch in 135° abduction using weight to provide stretch. Progression of stretch in B. **E,** Supine external rotation stretch in 180° abduction. Progression of stretch in D. Helpful with shoulder problems in throwing athletes.

- Strengthening effects are **specific to joint position**.
- Resistance provided manually or against a solid object

(b) **Isotonic** (most common)

- Muscle contraction against **constant resistance** through ROM
- **Speed of movement can vary.**
- With **concentric** contractions, muscle shortens during contraction.
- With **eccentric** contractions, muscle lengthens during contraction.
- **Eccentric contractions are an important component of many sports activities.**

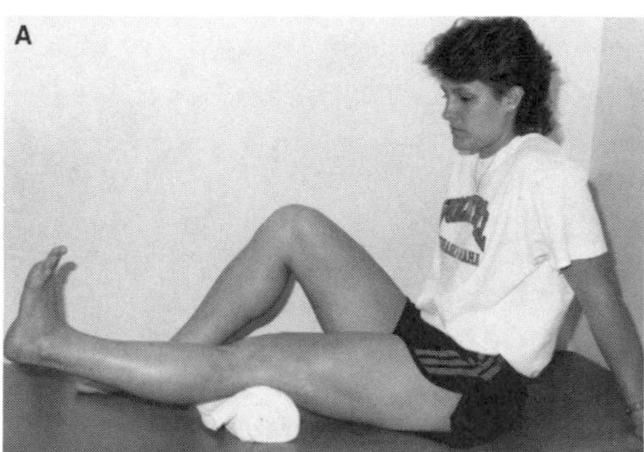

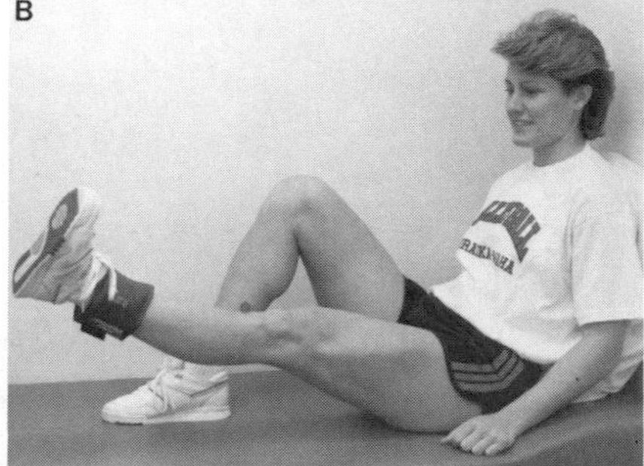

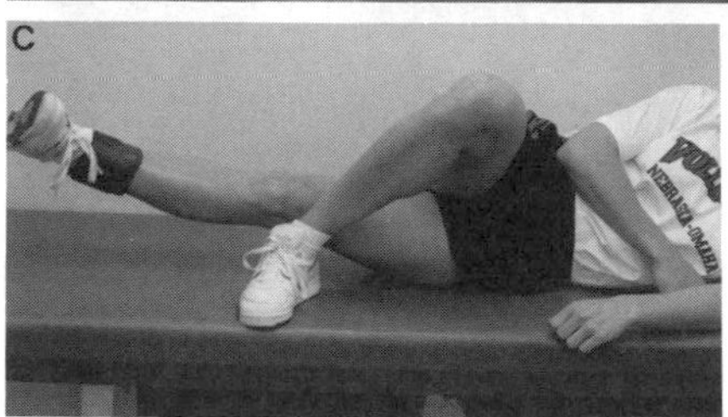

FIGURE 12. **A**, Terminal knee extension. Used in regaining full active knee extension and early quadriceps strengthening. May be done as initial phase of leg raise. **B**, Straight leg raise with external rotation. Used for quadriceps strengthening. External rotation component used for patellofemoral problems. Biases strength toward vastus medialis obliquus (VMO). **C**, Hip adduction sidelying. With quadriceps set at onset, can provide additional stimulus to VMO to improve patellofemoral stability.

- Resistance may be provided by limb weight, strap-on weights, barbells, machines, hydraulics, and elastic bands or tubing.

(c) **Isokinetic**

- Muscle contraction against device that holds **speed of movement constant**
- Resistance **varies according to effort provided by patient (accommodating resistance)**
- Speed-specific exercise program possible
- Helpful in intermediate and advanced rehabilitation programs
- Intensity can be quite high, so **symptoms must be monitored**.
- Equipment cost quite high

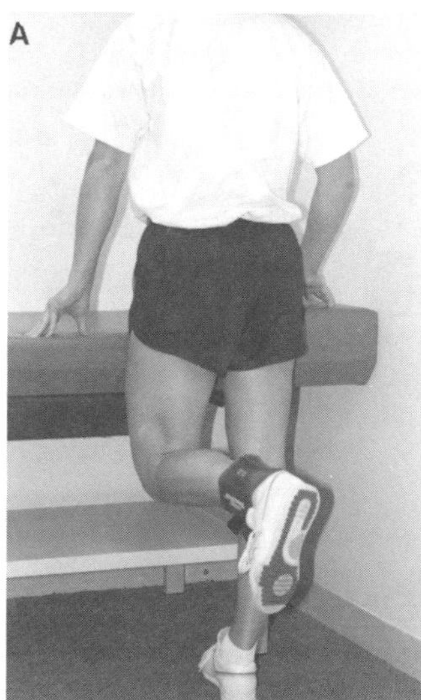

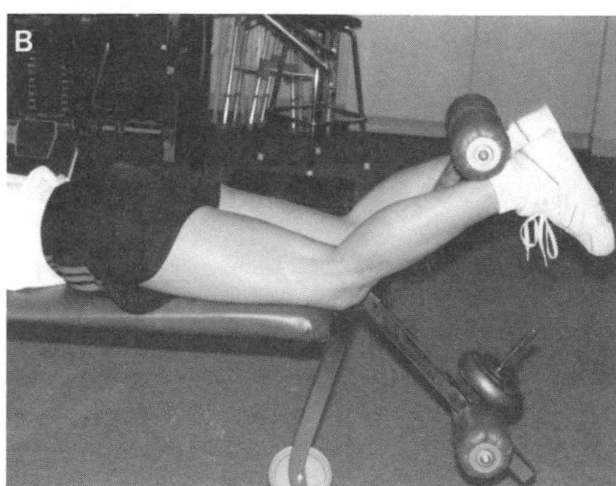

FIGURE 13. Knee curls for hamstring strengthening. **A,** Standing position. **B,** Prone position using curl machine—a more advanced exercise.

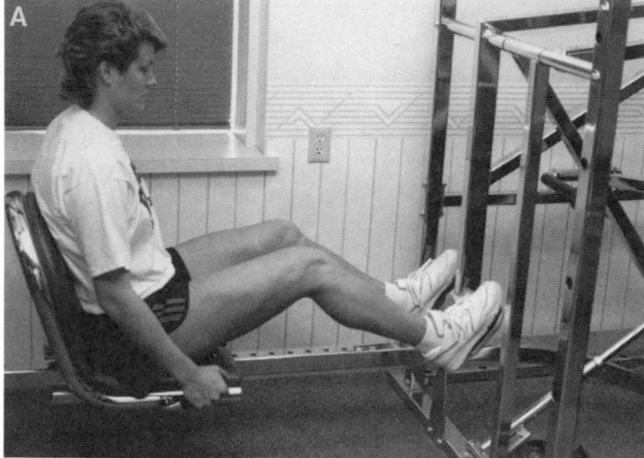

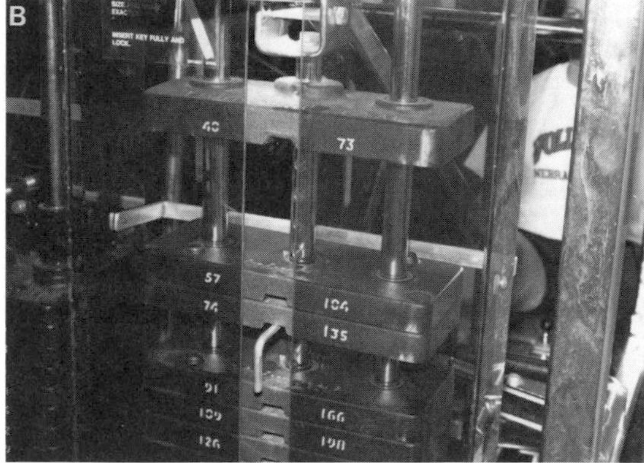

FIGURE 14. **A,** Leg press. Closed kinetic chain strengthening for quadriceps and hip extensors. A more physiologic method than knee extensions for quadriceps strengthening. **B,** Modified weight stack for leg press. Allows less-flexed starting position and thus less patellofemoral stress.

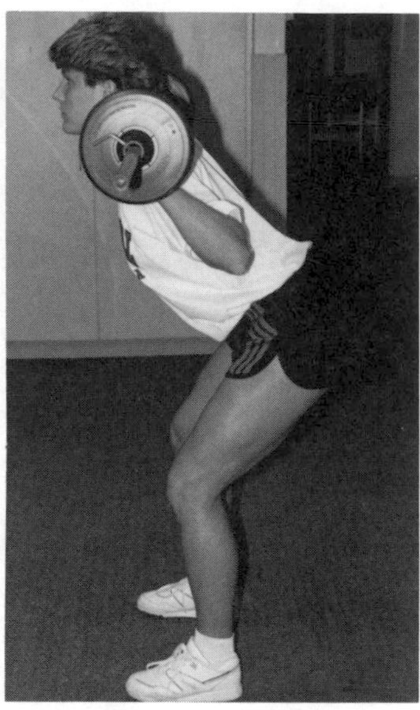

FIGURE 15. Mini-squat. Partial depth is preferred over the traditional parallel squat. Keeping shins vertical lessens shear force at knee. Used in intermediate and advanced phases.

c. **Proprioception** (see Figs. 21 through 23 for selected proprioception exercises)
   i. Synergistic muscle action
   ii. **Reaction time**—quickness
   iii. Balance boards, weighted balls and implements, and basic coordination and agility exercises

d. **Endurance** (see Fig. 24 for selected endurance exercises)
   i. Muscle endurance—repetitions
   ii. Cardiorespiratory fitness—aerobic

e. **Motor relearning**
   i. Advanced coordination and agility drills
   ii. Progressive running drills (Table 1)
   iii. Progressive throwing/racquet drills (Table 2)
   iv. Sports-specific fundamental drills
   v. Progressive return to activity

f. **Evaluation for return to participation**
   i. **Family or referring physician:**
      (a) Provides clearance to begin to workout
      (b) Statement of **adequate healing**
   ii. **Team physician, athletic trainer, coach or combined** must document athlete's **readiness to return and perform**:

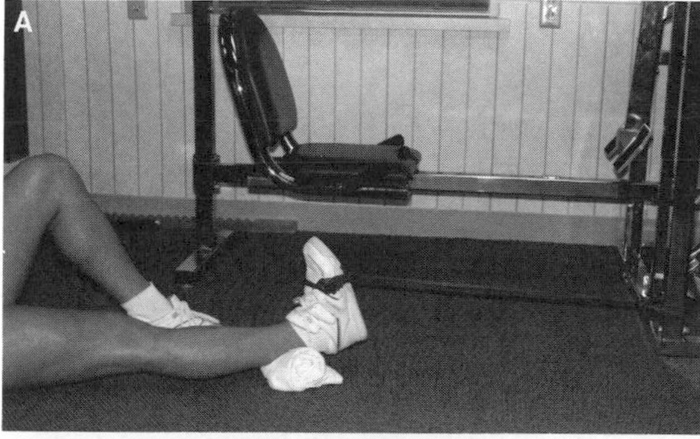

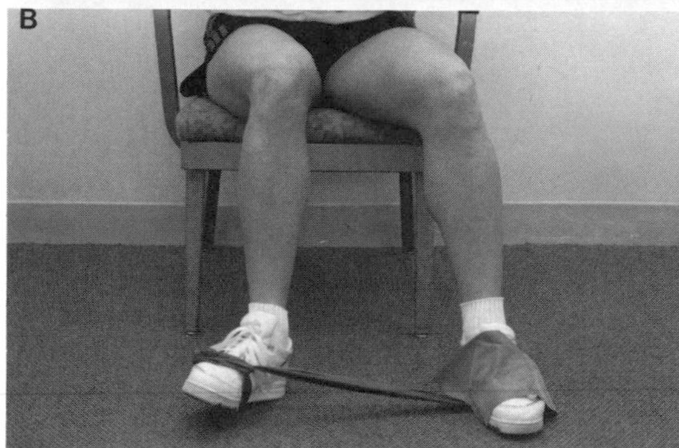

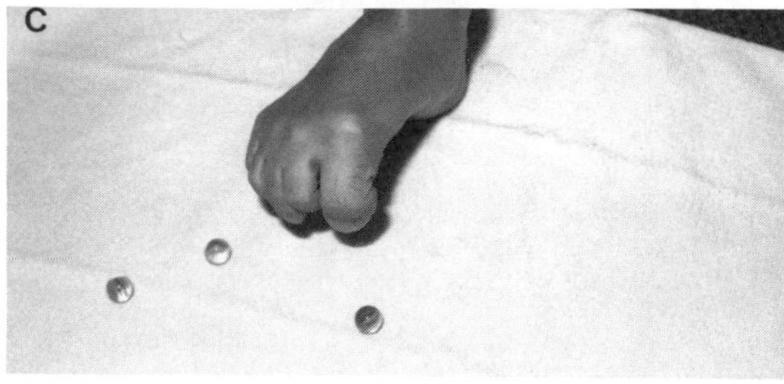

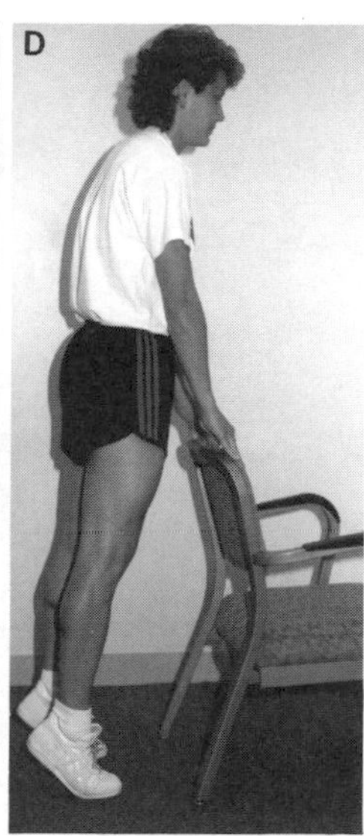

FIGURE 16. **A,** Ankle dorsiflexion. Used for ankle rehabilitation. Also helpful for patellar tendinitis when eccentric phase is emphasized. **B,** Ankle eversion. Used to strengthen dynamic stabilizers with inversion ankle injuries. **C,** Toe curls. Marbles or small, smooth stones are grasped by toes. Used to strengthen foot intrinsic muscles. **D,** Toe raises. Used to strengthen calf. Start on both legs, progress to only one leg.

TABLE 1. Progressive Running Program

Step	Progression Criteria
Bicycle	30–45 min
Walk	2 miles in 30 min or less
Jog	Jog 50 yards, walk 50 yards up to ¼ mile, increase total distance to 1 mile, then increase jogging and decrease walking until jogging 1 mile straight through
Run	Increase jogging to 2–4 miles, then increase pace to preinjury level
Sprint	Take 10–15 yards to build up to ½ speed, sprint at ½ speed for 40 yards, take 15–20 yards to slow down and stop. Gradually work up from ½ to ⅔ to ¾ to full speed. Do 10–20 sprints per session
Figure-eight	Gently jog to a large (20–30 yards) figure-eight. Gradually run the eight faster. Then decrease the size of the eight by 2–3 yards at a time so that the cutting is progressively sharper. Work down to a 4–5 yard eight. Do 10–20 figure-eights at a session
Basic drills	Work into jumping rope, power jumping activities, stairs, backward running, side step running, side crossover running, quick starts and stops, cutting, and other basic drill activities important to the athlete's specific sport
Sports drills	Target these fine-tuning drills to the specific activity the athlete wants to resume

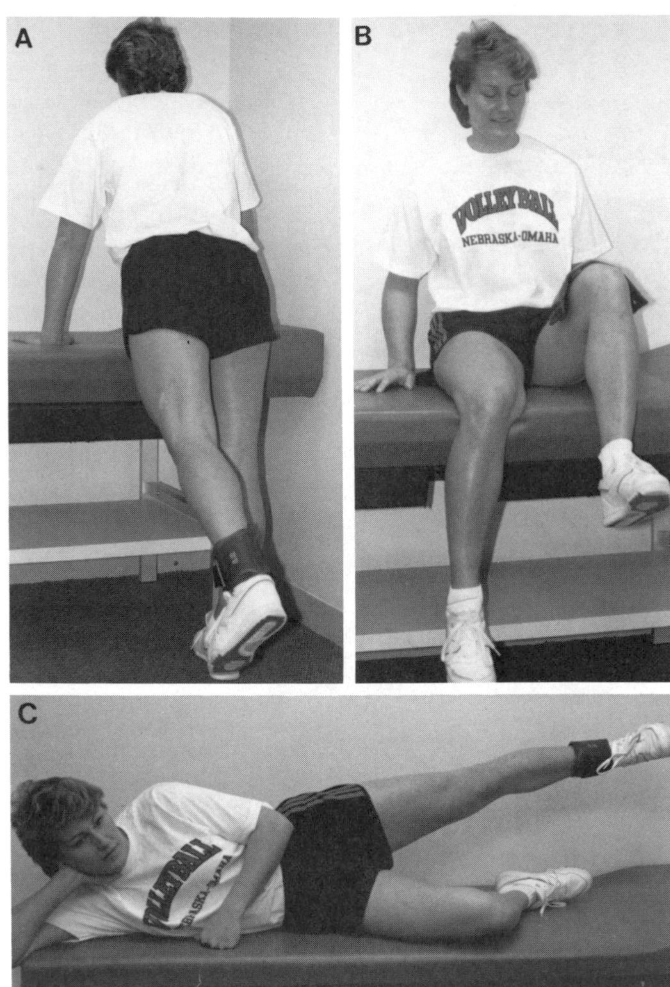

FIGURE 17. **A,** Standing hip extension. **B,** Sitting hip flexion. **C,** Sidelying hip abduction.

TABLE 2. Progressive Pitching Program

Step	Progression Criteria
Short toss	Toss ball 10–15 feet for accuracy using good throwing mechanics
Long toss	Stand in short center field. Throw ball so that it rolls to second base. Then throw so that ball reaches second base in 4 bounces, then 3 bounces, then 2 and finally 1. Use good mechanics and throw for accuracy
Mound toss	From the mound throw at ½ speed toward the plate. Emphasize accuracy and mechanics
Straight throws	Throw straight pitches progressively faster up to ¾ speed
Breaking throws	Throw curve and slider pitches progressively faster up to ¾ speed
Speed	Increase speed on all pitches toward full speed while maintaining good mechanics and accuracy
Special pitches	Add any specialty pitches to program
Fielding	Work on fielding ground balls and throwing to various bases from gradually more awkward positions

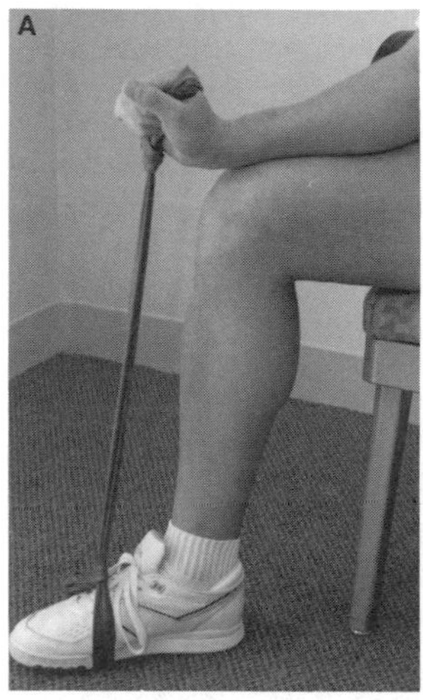

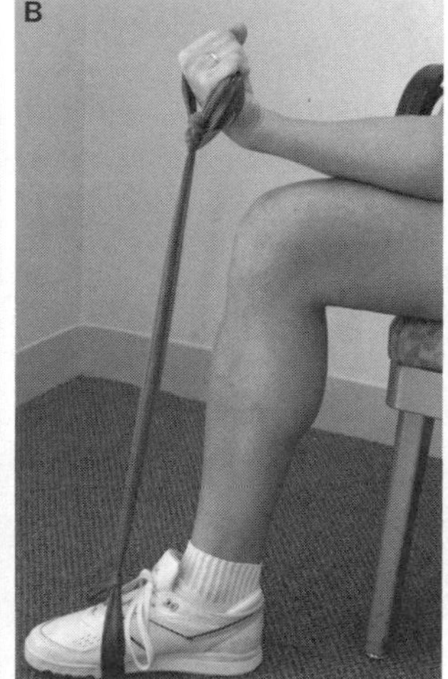

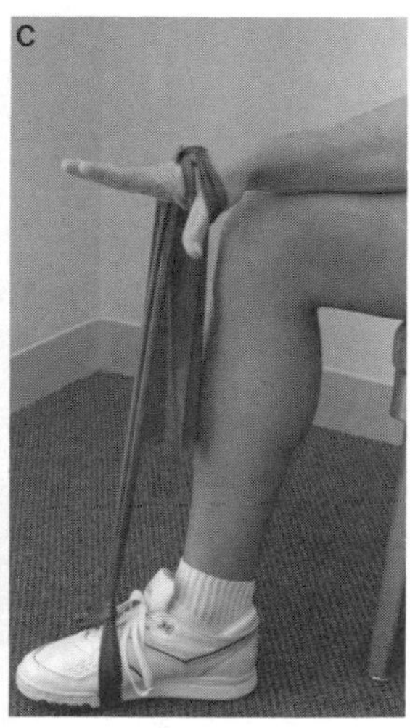

FIGURE 18. Elastic band exercises. **A,** Wrist extension. **B,** Wrist flexion. **C,** Forearm pronation.

(a) **Fully rehabilitated**—strength, flexibility, endurance, coordination, agility
(b) Athlete must **demonstrate full-speed performance** in all phases.
(c) **No symptoms** at any point
(d) **Full confidence**—no favoring or hesitation

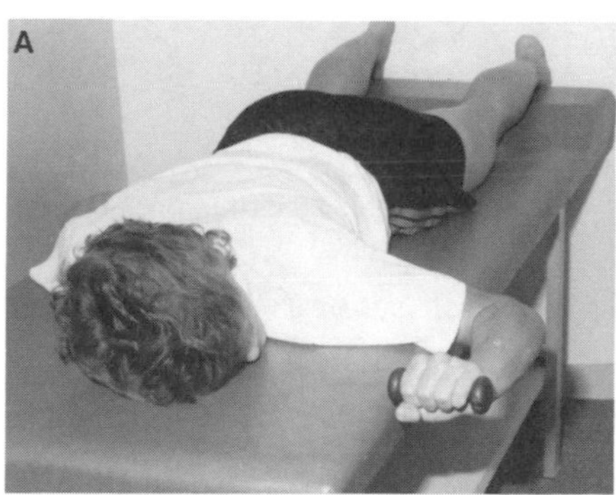

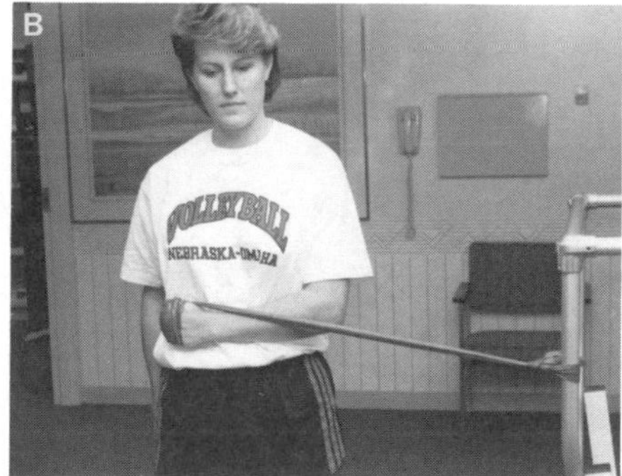

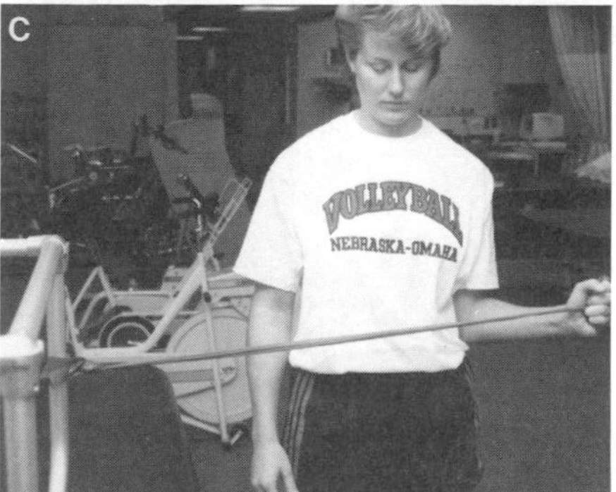

FIGURE 19. A, Shoulder external rotation prone for rotator cuff strengthening. **B,** Standing internal rotation using elastic band. **C,** Standing external rotation using elastic band.

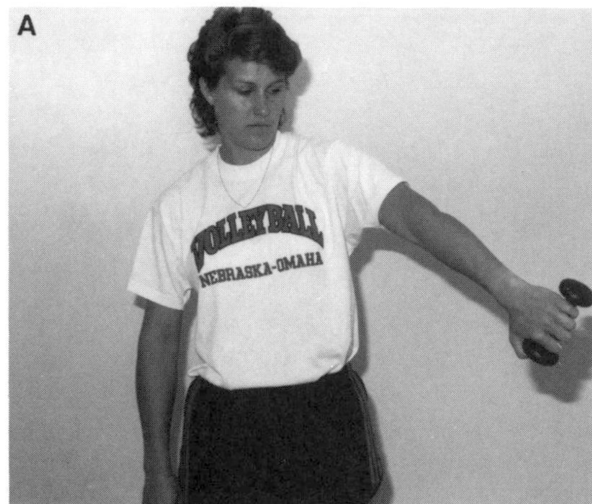

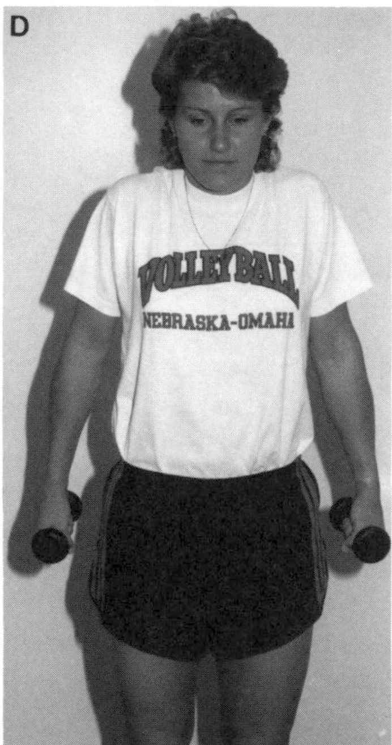

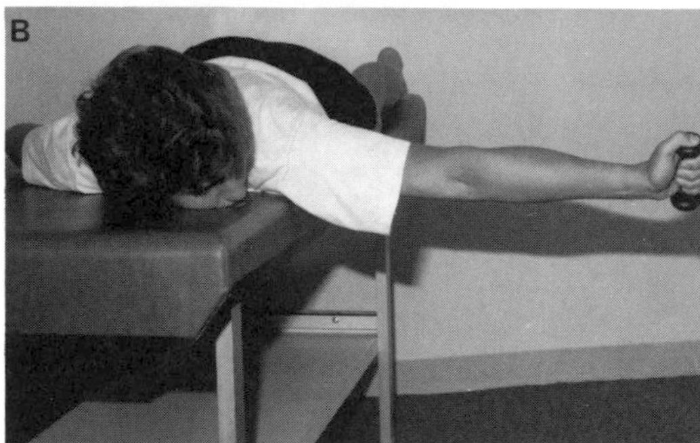

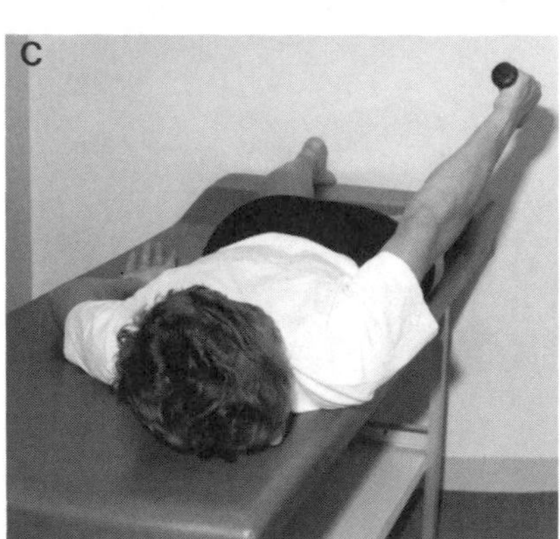

FIGURE 20. A, Isolated position for the supraspinatus muscle for rotator cuff strengthening. **B,** Horizontal abduction prone with arm externally rotated for rotator cuff strengthening. **C,** Shoulder extension prone. **D,** Shoulder shrug/scapular adduction for scapulothoracic stability.

g. **Timetable for return to participation:**
   i. Should be **based on individual's symptoms and tolerance** to progressive activity—"one day at a time"
   ii. A fixed length of time to recover from an injury does not exist and should not be used.

G. **Adjunctive treatment to therapeutic exercise** (see Fig. 2)
   1. **Functional taping and bracing**

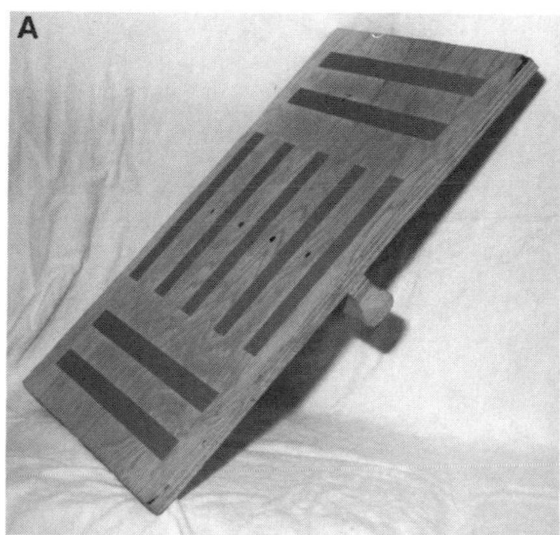

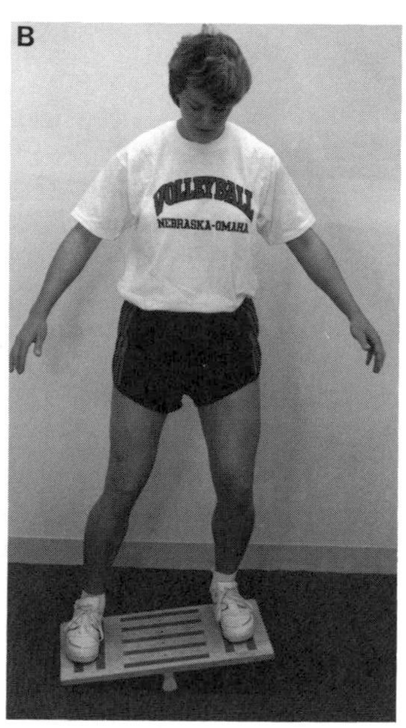

FIGURE 21. A, Uniaxial balance board (16″ × 24″ with 2″ to 2.5″ tall pivot on bottom). **B,** Uniaxial balance board in use. Foot position can be varied to balance side to side or front to back.

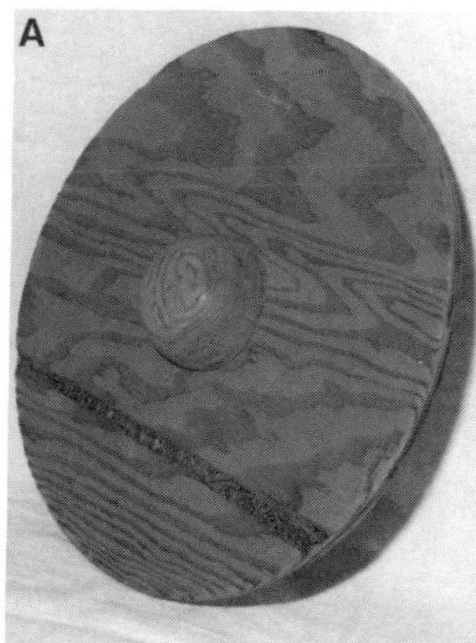

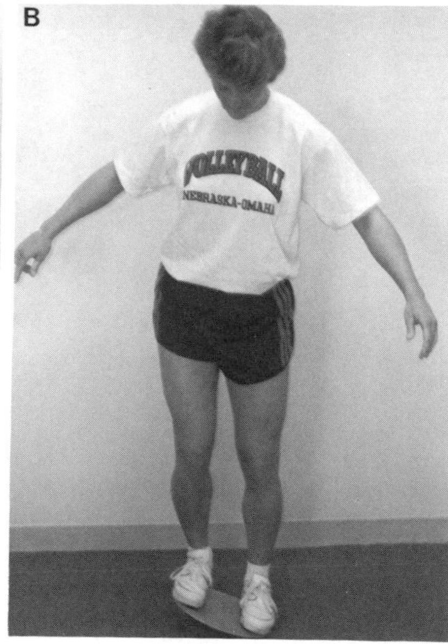

FIGURE 22. A, Multiaxial balance board (15″ diameter with 2″ semisphere on bottom). **B,** Multiaxial balance board in use. As balance ability is achieved, the athlete's attention is diverted by playing catch to make the reactions more automatic.

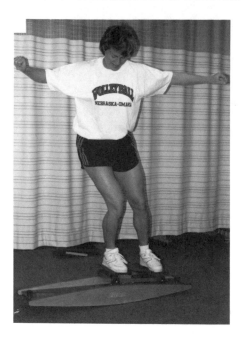

FIGURE 23. Fitter. Used for proprioception training and can be adjusted to various levels of resistance.

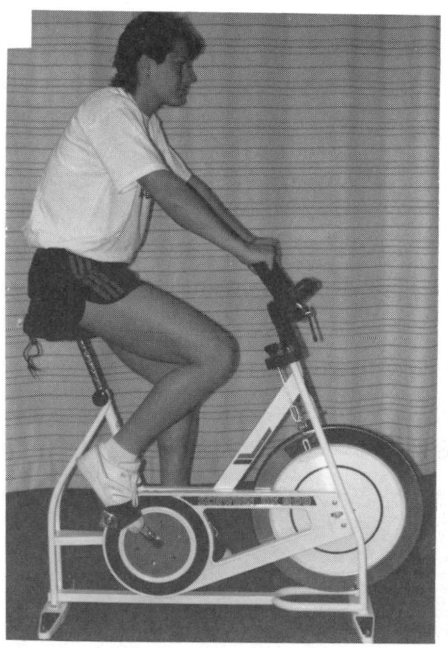

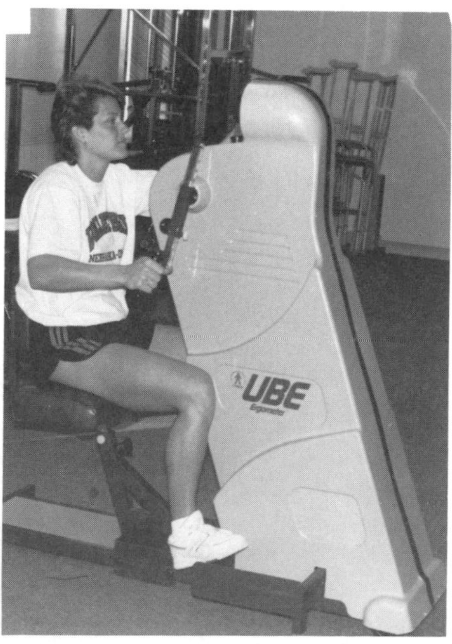

FIGURE 24. **Left,** Stationary bicycle riding. Seat height, pedaling resistance, pedaling speed, and pedaling phase effort can be adjusted for treatment of various injuries. **Right,** Upper Body Exercise (UBE) Ergometer (Cybex, Ronkonkoma, NY). Used for upper extremity endurance training and maintenance of aerobic capacity during rehabilitation.

   a. Taping and bracing are adjuncts to healing and rehabilitation.
   b. They **do not provide a short-cut** to participation.
   c. Tape or brace may **limit extremes of motion** and increase **proprioceptive feedback** to the injured area.
   d. **An unhealed or unrehabilitated injury is more likely to be reinjured, no matter how well taped or braced.**
   e. Patellofemoral taping techniques can help balance patellar tracking, reduce pain, and improve function during rehabilitation of vastus medialis obliquus control, retinacular tightness, and muscular flexibility.
2. **Modalities**
   a. General considerations:
      i. **Adjunctive**, not primary or long-term treatment
      ii. Used to **control symptoms** and facilitate healing
      iii. Helps allow patient to rehabilitate more effectively
      iv. **Should not be used indiscriminately**
   b. **Cold**
      i. Therapeutic effects:
         (a) Vasoconstriction
         (b) Decreased tissue metabolism
         (c) Decreased inflammatory response
         (d) Decreased pain
         (e) Decreased muscle spasm
      ii. **Advantages:**
         (a) Effective to decrease inflammation
         (b) **Relatively safe** for patient self-application
      iii. Disadvantages:
         (a) Possible patient intolerance to cold
         (b) Messy
         (c) Cold injury risk
      iv. Technique of application:
         (a) Ice bags, gel packs, cold water immersion, ice massage, fluid-filled sleeve around injury are all effective; chemical cold packs, freon gas-filled sleeve around injury are much less effective.
         (b) **10–30 minutes treatment time**
         (c) **Followed by at least an equal time off**
         (d) Treatment customized based on method of cooling used, patient's tolerance, and cold intensity
      v. Safety:
         (a) Start with mild cold and progress colder as tolerated.
         (b) Inspect area before, during, and after treatment for signs of cold injury.
         (c) Provide thorough home instructions for patient self-application.
   c. **Heat**
      i. Therapeutic effects:
         (a) Vasodilation
         (b) Increased tissue metabolism
         (c) Decreased pain
         (d) Increased local circulation
         (e) Increased tissue extensibility
      ii. Advantages:
         (a) Increased circulation may promote healing.
         (b) Relatively comfortable for patient
         (c) Relatively safe for patient self-treatment
      iii. Disadvantages:
         (a) Risk of skin injury (burn)
         (b) If applied too soon following injury, may increase swelling and other symptoms.

iv. Technique of application:
(a) Hot pack, heating pad, hot watter bottle, warm soaks, and whirlpool may all be effective.
(b) 20 minutes average treatment time
v. Safety:
(a) Start with mild warmth and progress as tolerated.
(b) Inspect area before, during, and after treatment.
(c) Consider electrical safety when electrical modalities used.

d. **Contrast treatment**
i. Therapeutic effects:
(a) Alternate vasoconstriction and vasodilation.
(b) Creates vascular "exercise" to help reduce swelling
ii. Advantage—benefits of heat with protection of cold
iii. Disadvantage—premature heat can increase swelling.
iv. Technique of application:
(a) Alternate warm and cool.
(b) Warm-to-cool ratio of 1:1 to 4:1
v. Safety—as with heat and cold as listed above

e. **Ultrasound**
i. Therapeutic effects:
(a) Thermal—**deep heating** effects up to 2.5 cm
(b) Mechanical:
(i) Increases **extensibility** of connective tissue
(ii) **Phoresis** of therapeutic medications (cortisone, salicylates)
(c) Analgesic—**decreases nerve conduction velocity**
ii. Technique of application is **best left to professionals** trained in the proper use of, safety with, and contraindications to these techniques.

f. **Electrical stimulation**
i. Transcutaneous electrical nerve stimulation (TENS)—pain control post-injury and postsurgery
ii. Functional electrical stimulation:
(a) **Facilitates** muscle contraction after reeducation
(b) **Supplements** voluntary muscle effort
(c) Helpful with **selective retraining** of muscles
iii. **Iontophoresis:**
(a) Introduce therapeutic medications (usually lidocaine or dexamethasone) into areas for anti-inflammatory and other effects depending on medication used.
(b) Small local burns from direct current a risk
(c) Must check for **allergy** to medications used
iv. Technique of application is **best left to professionals** trained in the proper use of, safety with, and contraindications to these techniques.

g. **EMG biofeedback:**
i. **Facilitates patient's reeducation efforts**
ii. Allows patient to monitor and quantify exercise efforts
iii. Often used after functional electrical stimulation
iv. Technique of application is **best left to professionals** trained in the proper use of, safety with, and contraindications to these techniques.

h. Modality summary:
i. **Therapeutic exercise most important modality**
ii. All others adjunctive
iii. If something is not helping, do something different.

H. **Protective equipment**
   1. **Standard equipment** must fit properly.
   2. **Modified standard equipment** may be adapted for specific injury.
   3. **Special equipment** can be created to provide protection for a specific injury.

I. **Patient education**
   1. Successful rehabilitation cannot be accomplished without the **cooperative efforts of the patient**.
   2. Patient must know how to best help himself or herself.
   3. Patient education is **more than just handing the patient a list of instructions** (not a cookbook).
   4. Patient must be **"sold"** on the idea of the rehabilitation program.
   5. Method of "selling" (teaching method) should be based on patient's **learning style**.
      a. **Demonstration of deficits** that exist
      b. **Explanation of injury** and treatment methods
      c. **Testimonials**
   6. **Initial instruction**
      a. **Instruction and demonstration** of rehabilitation techniques by **clinician**
      b. **Patient** is asked to **demonstrate** newly learned techniques and **echo** other instructions.
      c. Patient's technique and understanding are **fine-tuned** by the clinician.
      d. Patient's **questions are answered; follow-up questions are encouraged.**
      e. **Written handouts** are provided to **supplement, not replace,** instructions and demonstrations.
      f. A **follow-up visit** is scheduled.
   7. **Subsequent follow-up visits**
      a. Open-ended question—"How are you doing?"
      b. Rehabilitation program **echoed and redemonstrated** by patient
      c. What helps? What hurts?
      d. Current **functional level assessed**
      e. Exercise **technique corrected** where necessary
      f. Rehabilitation **program modified** as reevaluation dictates
      g. New and modified techniques are echoed and reviewed and new handouts provided.

J. **This level of care and concern for the patient takes time and effort on the part of the clinician.**
   1. Physician may not have the time or expertise in rehabilitation techniques to deal with these details.
   2. Physical therapist or certified athletic trainer:
      a. **Possesses skills and expertise** in rehabilitation
      b. **Motivates** patients
      c. **Troubleshoots** problems the patient encounters during the rehabilitation process

III. Rehabilitation Principles for Specific Injury Types

A. **Fractures**
   1. **Respect immobilization** or protection.
   2. Exercise involved area based on type of fracture and type of immobilization or protection.
   3. Exercise **uninvolved areas**.
   4. Fully rehabilitate all areas once specific injury is healed.

B. **Sprains**
   1. Flexibility and joint ROM as specific injury dictates
   2. **Dynamic joint stability**—synergistic muscle contraction

3. **Do not disrupt healing** static stabilizers.
4. Consider kinetic chain.

C. **Strains**
1. **Flexibility**—improves muscle's ability to adapt to extremes
2. **Strength**—restores muscle's contractile capabilities
3. Adjacent areas—kinetic chain

D. **Contusions**
1. Treat as strains
2. **Beware of myositis ossificans.**
   a. **Inadequate recognition or suspicion** of initial injury
   b. **Repeated injury** before full healing has occurred
   c. **Overly aggressive physical therapy**—heat, passive stretching

E. **Overuse**
1. **Relative rest**—avoid irritating amounts and types of activity
2. **Control inflammation**
   a. Nonsteroidal anti-inflammatory drugs
   b. Ice massage
   c. Phonophoresis
   d. Iontophoresis
   e. Injection—last resort
3. **Correct contributing and acquired deficits**
   a. Conditioning
   b. Training errors
   c. Mechanical factors

Recommended Reading

1. Anderson B: Stretching. Bolinas, CA, Shelter Publications, 1980.
2. Buschbacher RM, Braddom RL: Sports Medicine and Rehabilitation: A Sport-Specific Approach. Philadelphia, Hanley & Belfus, 1994.
3. Gould JA, Davies GJ: Orthopaedic and Sports Physical Therapy, Vol. 2. St. Louis, Mosby, 1990 (New ed. scheduled for Sept 1996)
4. Mellion MB: Office Sports Medicine. Philadelphia, Hanley & Belfus, 1996.
5. Mellion MB: Sports Medicine Secrets. Philadelphia, Hanley & Belfus, 1994.
6. Saunders HD, Saunders R: Evaluation, Treatment and Prevention of Musculoskeletal Disorders. Vol. 1, Spine. Chaska, MN, Educational Opportunities—A Saunders Group Company, 1993.
7. Saunders HD, Saunders R: Evaluation, Treatment and Prevention of Musculoskeletal Disorders. Vol. 2, Extremities. Chaska, MN, The Saunders Group, 1994.

39

Head Injuries

John M. Henderson, D.O.

I. Spectrum of Injuries

A. **Head injuries** include a wide variety of problems. Focusing on the brain may allow another injury to be missed.

1. **Scalp.** This tough, well-vascularized covering protects the bony skull. When the scalp is found open, a greater and deeper injury should be suspected.
2. **Skull.** The bony calvarium is vulnerable in the preauricular temporal area and at the basilar area. When the skull is violated, vascular as well as brain injuries are suspected. Distant, contralateral brain injuries should be sought. Subtle signs of skull fracture:
   a. Postauricular or periorbital ecchymosis
   b. Clear or blood-tinged rhinorrhea or otorrhea
3. **Facial**
   a. Soft tissue trauma
   b. Cranial nerve end organ trauma
4. **Maxillofacial.** Rich innervation and arterial supply make these injuries complex. Several unrelated systems must be kept in mind.
   a. **Dental**
      i. Tooth avulsion
      ii. Malocclusion injuries
   b. **Eye:** anterior chamber injuries are common; retinal detachment must be remembered. Extraocular muscle entrapment from fracture of the bony orbit is common.
   c. **Ear:** perichondral hematoma of the pinna and concha and avulsed pinna need attention to restore aesthetic shape and function.
   d. **Nose:** fracture of the nasal spine may not be obvious. Septal hematoma must be evacuated to maintain cartilaginous integrity.
   e. **Oral:** buccal and glossal lacerations can accompany dental trauma or occur isolated; they are all exposed to contamination by mouth anaerobes.
5. **Brain injuries** include an array of wounds similar to any other solid organ. The difference is that parts of the brain have a solid consistency (white matter tracts), whereas other parts are rubbery or gelatinous (immature gray matter of children), and part is liquid (cerebrospinal fluid). Brain injuries involve more disability than any other body part.
   a. Laceration by a sharp foreign body
   b. Contusion from a crush injury
   c. Displacement by a hematoma
   d. Concussion from closed, blunt, low-energy trauma
   e. Each lesion can accompany the others.

B. **Neck injuries**. Evaluation of any head injury should include consideration of a neck injury. (See Chapter 40, "Neck Injuries" for detailed information.) Devastating neck injuries can accompany minimal head injuries.

1. **Skin**
   a. Ecchymoses
   b. Abrasions
   c. Split-thickness skin avulsions
2. **Vascular**
   a. Carotid contusion
   b. Vascular compression
3. **Larynx**
   a. Stridor
   b. Hoarseness
   c. Expanding hematoma
4. **Spine**
   a. Immobilization is the most important aspect of care.
   b. Rule out fracture.
5. **Spinal cord.** If the bony spine is protected, then the cord is also.

II. General Considerations

A. **The energy transfer in head injuries** dictates the extent of the injury. The head moves in three planes in response to a force applied to it. Sagittal (cervical flexion-extension), frontal (cervical side-bending), and coronal plane (cervical rotation) motion must be taken into consideration. For every action, there must be a reaction. Coup-contrecoup injuries must be considered.

B. **Open versus closed.** The vast majority of head injuries are closed. Closed injuries can be subtle because the scalp and calvarium are intact and so the brain is presumed, erroneously, uninjured. Other than a brain laceration, any brain injury sustained in an open head injury can also be found in the closed variety.

C. **High-energy versus low-energy transfer.** The vast majority of head injuries involve low-energy transfers. Brain concussions and contusions result. Because the main architecture of the brain remains unchanged, these lesions are difficult to image. Nonetheless, the functional changes can be appreciated through the clinical examination.

III. The Brain Exam

A. The functional brain exam is broken down into its basic elements.

1. **The cerebral cortex**
   a. Motor and sensory areas
   b. Abilities for expression and perception
   c. Sophisticated analysis and interpretation
   d. Intellect
   e. Memory
   f. Orientation
   g. Judgment
   h. Thought content
   i. Thought processing including abstract thinking
   j. Emotion or affect
2. **The midbrain**
   a. Assess
      i. Body temperature
      ii. Pulse
      iii. Blood pressure
      iv. Pupil reflexes
      v. Other cranial nerves
   b. Evaluate
      i. Level of consciousness or alertness
      ii. Appetite
      iii. Sexual function
      iv. Behavior patterns
      v. Sleep patterns
3. **The cerebellum**
   Evaluate
   a. Gait
   b. Coordination
   c. Repetition of fine motor skills
   d. Balance

TABLE 1. Signs of Lower Motor Neuron Disease Versus Upper Motor Neuron Disease

	Lower Motor Neuron	Upper Motor Neuron
Paralysis	Flaccid	Spastic
Deep tendon reflexes	Hyporeflexic	Hyperreflexic
Extensor plantar response	Down	Up
Example	Sciatica	Stroke

B. **Upper versus lower motor neuron injury.** It is important to be able to distinguish between cerebral cortical dysfunction, regardless of cause, and peripheral nerve dysfunction. The classic signs of upper motor neuron disease in contrast to lower motor neuron disease are listed in Table 1.

C. **Mental status.** Rapid evaluation of mental status is promulgated by Advanced Cardiac Life Support proponents. Response to stimulation can include (acronym AVPU):
   1. *A*—Alert and oriented with an appropriate response
   2. *V*—Verbal stimuli elicit a response.
   3. *P*—Painful stimuli elicit a response.
   4. *U*—Unresponsive to all stimuli.

D. **Mini-neurologic exam:** an integrated, yet rapid method to evaluate brain function. These observations are usually followed serially for the purpose of comparison.
   1. **Vital signs:** a rising blood pressure with lower pulse rate is an ominous sign of increased intracranial pressure.
   2. **Eye signs**
      a. Large, unresponsive pupils are seen with ipsilateral brain damage.
      b. Small yet responsive pupils can be seen with midbrain injury.
      c. Extraocular muscle palsy, such as lateral glaze, can be seen with ipsilateral cranial nerve nuclei involvement as well as involvements anywhere along the tract of the nerve.
   3. **Breathing pattern**
      a. Slow deep respirations, Biot breathing, can be seen in midbrain injury.
      b. Crescendo-decrescendo or diamond-shape pattern breathing, Cheyne-Stokes breathing, can be seen in lower central dysfunction.
   4. **Reflexes**
      a. Primitive reflexes such as “rooting” or “snout” reflex and palmomental reflex are a sign of deep brain dysfunction.
      b. Hyperreflexic deep tendon or myotatic stretch reflexes can be seen with cortical dysfunction as well as basal ganglion injury.
   5. **Pathologic posturing**
      a. Decorticate posturing is seen with injury to the motor areas of the cerebral cortex.
      b. Decerebrate posturing is seen with injury to the lower cerebrum and is much more serious. The brain injury is contralateral to the side on which the sign is seen.
   6. **Purposeful movement**
      a. Even the obtunded person is capable of purposeful movement, such as defense against a noxious stimulus.
      b. Inability to defend oneself with a purposeful motor response, or pathologic posturing as a response, is a sign of deep and serious brain dysfunction.
   7. **Extensor plantar response**
      a. An up-going great toe, or fanning of the other toes, indicates contralateral cortical dysfunction but not necessarily irreversible injury.

b. The Babinski reflex can be confirmed using the Chaddock, Oppenheim, or Gordon reflexes:
    i. Chaddock reflex—deep pressure stroking of the anterior tibia
    ii. Oppenheim reflex—stroking the fibular margin of the foot
    iii. Gordon reflex—forcefully squeezing the calf muscles

8. **Subtle changes from head injuries** ("soft signs") can involve a wide array of manifestations.
    a. **Emotional lability:** wide swings in affect ranging from violent behavior to a sedentary, vegetative state
    b. **Sleeping disorders**
        i. Narcolepsy
        ii. Insomnia
    c. **Eating disorders**
        i. Polyphagia
        ii. Bulimia
        iii. Anorexia
    d. **Alcohol intolerance:** behavioral changes after intake of small amounts of alcohol are not uncommon.
    e. **Memory defects** range from peri-incidental amnesia to the loss of distant memory. Usually the athlete with a concussion cannot retain the most recently remembered facts. This results in perseverating ("Tell me again what happened").
    f. **Agnosia:** part of the anorexia is the decreased ability to differentiate smells.
    g. **Vertigo:** subjective or objective spinning and loss of balance can be seen especially with rapid head and neck movements. They are sometimes accompanied by nausea, dyspepsia, and pyrosis.

IV. Cervical Spine Exam

Every head injury can be accompanied by a severe cervical spine and spinal cord injury. **Care of the cervical spine takes precedence over head injuries in the evaluation and treatment of the head-injured athlete.** There is current controversy about prioritizing cervical spine care ahead of securing an effective airway and ventilation. The time it takes to immobilize the cervical spine allows safe management of the airway and even cardiac function. **No head injury warrants helmet removal before stabilizing the cervical spine.** See Chapter 40, "Neck Injuries" for more information on cervical spine injuries.

V. Specific Problems

A. **Intracranial hemorrhage**
1. **Epidural hematoma:** a high-pressure, arterial bleed caused by the jagged edge of a skull fracture, such as the temporal bone, lacerating the temporal artery.
    a. Rapidly deteriorating mental function follows an initial lucid period after the head trauma.
    b. Surgical evacuation is necessary.
2. **Subdural hematoma:** a low-pressure, venous bleed caused by a tear in the venous plexus resulting from blunt trauma. The clinical picture can be variable; behavior changes over months (even years) can be seen contrasted against progressive deterioration in mental function and alertness over several hours.
3. **Subarachnoid hemorrhage:** may be due to an aneurysmal bleed, arteriovenous malformation, hypertensive hemorrhage, or trauma. Heralded by an excruciating headache and incessant nausea with fairly immediate prostration.

B. **Cerebral concussion.** Concussion is characterized by a loss of consciousness or memory defect after closed, blunt head trauma that is usually of the low-energy transfer variety.

1. Several severity grading schemes for concussion are based on the artificial differentiation of alert consciousness and posttraumatic amnesia.
2. There is no scientific basis or broad-based documentation of the natural history of this entity.
3. Treatment is based on:
   a. Protecting the athlete from the near occasion of a second defect
   b. Allowing resolution of not only the memory defect, but also the "soft signs" (see "Subtle changes from head injuries," page 394)
4. Histologic changes after a concussion include:
   a. Interstitial edema
   b. Petechial hemorrhages
   c. Microinfarcts
   d. Axonal shearing

C. **Second-impact syndrome.** After the athlete sustains "minor" head trauma, such as a concussion, a second minor impact may cause a massive brain injury. Massive cerebral edema, interstitial edema caused by increased vascular permeability as a result of the initial injury, can develop rapidly. Rapid deterioration and profound incapacitation result. Only a high index of suspicion can lead to a timely diagnosis and expeditious treatment.
   1. In addition to the usual supportive measures, including guarding the airway and overbreathing, parenteral glucocorticosteroids, such as dexamethasone, and osmotic diuretics, such as mannitol, are given.
   2. Serial imaging studies may be needed to rule out intracranial hemorrhage.

D. **Posttraumatic seizure disorder**
   1. Type of seizure
      a. Generalized—obvious, tonic-clonic type
      b. Partial—subtle, can be localized, can involve only sensory changes
   2. Temporal aspect
      a. Immediately posttraumatic:
         i. Most common but less serious
         ii. Usually a single event with no sequelae
      b. Late in postevent:
         i. Less common but more serious
         ii. May signal a longer, protracted convalescence with recurring ictal events
   3. Occurrence:
      a. Most common in high-velocity trauma (missile injuries)
      b. Most common when dura is violated

E. **Posttraumatic cervical dystonia**
   1. After trauma, the muscles supporting the spine may develop persistent spasm. Consequently, the victim's head is cocked to one side in a combination of side-bending with rotation and slight flexion.
   2. Even though the sternocleidomastoideus, trapezius, and levator scapulae muscles are most obviously involved, deeper muscles play an important role in this problem. The splenius capitis, splenius cervicis, intertransversari rotatores, scalenus anterior and medius, and the strap muscles of the anterior neck may all be involved.
   3. Treatment
      a. Ice massage and stretch routines
      b. Proprioceptive neuromuscular facilitation (reciprocal innervation) exercises
      c. Fatiguing interferential or galvanic stimulation
      d. Botulinum toxin administration
      e. Range-of-motion exercises and shoulder shrug exercises
      f. Trigger point injections
      g. Ethyl chloride spray techniques

4. Prolonged neck bracing and long-term use of muscle relaxants and narcotic analgesics are not beneficial; they may actually prolong disability.

F. **Encephalopathica pugilistica.** A movement disorder similar to paralysis agitans (parkinsonism) can develop after repeated blows to the head. Shuffling gait, resting tremor, poor balance, expressionless face, and inflexibility characterize this condition.

G. **Spastic diplegia.** Contralateral partial spastic paralysis similar to that found in cerebral palsy can be seen after hemorrhage or infarction of the internal capsule. Subtle findings:
1. Increased rigidity and extensor tone
2. Hyperreflexia
3. Poor balance and coordination

VI. Return to Play Considerations

This issue is highly controversial.

A. **The most widely published and accepted guidelines are not based on science** or even longitudinal, outcome-based studies.

B. These guidelines are not followed by the sports medicine community even though they exist in medical literature.

C. This issue attracts litigation.

D. The guidelines presented in Chapter 7, "Injuries and Emergencies on the Field," Table 3 are practical and are useful to the practitioner until a truly scientifically validated approach is developed.

E. Additional considerations that should be weighed in developing an individualized, tailor-made approach:
1. **Is the desired sport collision/contact?** Return participation to a collision/contact sport presents more risk than return to noncontact activities (i.e., if a golfer sustained a concussion in an automobile accident, he may be cleared to play golf).
2. **Is there imminent risk of a repeat injury?** For the athlete with a concussion returning to a collision-based sport, head injury risk is increased when the cervical spine has not regained its normal lordotic curve. Posttraumatic muscle spasm flattens the normal cervical lordosis into a "military straight" posture. When this straightened spine is subjected to axial loading in a subsequent injury, there is greater risk for spinal fracture. Additionally the spine cannot help dissipate the energy of the injury.
3. **Can appropriate precautions be taken?** It is common for the athlete with a concussion to demonstrate a generalized seizure in the immediate posttraumatic period. Later, seizure precautions should be considered, e.g., strict supervision in water sports.
4. **Have the signs of head injury resolved?** The two main signs are defects in alertness and amnesia. These should be resolved for the most part, although peri-incidental memory loss could exist indefinitely.
5. **Have the soft signs resolved?** The soft signs may persist for weeks, months, or years. The issue is whether or not these truly jeopardize the athlete's health and safety.
6. **Can adequate follow-up be arranged?** Follow-up includes observation in the immediate posttraumatic period as well as some form of medical reevaluation. This should involve credible and responsible adults who can be relied on for dependability.
7. **Does the athlete pose any safety or health risk to self or others?** Health and safety issues extend to teammates and competitors. A head-injured athlete with a new-onset seizure disorder needs restriction in marksmanship, swimming, diving, motocross, and other such sports.

VII. Future Considerations

Well-designed, functional outcome clinical studies are being carried out to quantify the results and residual problems of head injuries better.

A. **Practice-based method:** the American Medical Society for Sports Medicine is conducting a Concussion Outcome Study based on the practice of the membership, consisting of family physicians, internists, pediatricians, and emergency physicians who evaluate and provide long-term follow-up to athletes with concussion.

B. **Neurosciences method:** the Johns Hopkins Brain Injury Study and the New York State Athletic Commission Study are based on the long-term follow-up of boxing injuries to the head. These studies are evaluating psychometric tests in conjunction with imaging studies performed periodically to assess anatomic changes.

40

Neck Injuries

Joseph Moore, M.D., and E. Lee Rice, D.O.

Contact sports such as football, rugby, and wrestling put the athlete at risk for cervical trauma. Football accounts for over half of all spinal cord injuries in high school and college athletes. Additionally, recreational use of trampolines still accounts for significant numbers of pediatric neck injuries.

I. Acute Cervical Strain or Sprain

A. **Definition:** injury (tearing) of muscle and ligamentous components of neck

B. **Clinical findings:** acute cervical sprains are frequently seen in contact sports.

1. **Mechanisms of injury**
   a. Flexion
   b. Extension
   c. Compression
   d. Rotation
   e. Combinations of these motions
2. **Symptoms**
   a. Pain
   b. Decreased range of motion of the neck in all planes
   c. Paraspinous muscle tenderness and spasm may be present
   d. Bony tenderness to palpation not evident
   e. Absence of neurologic dysfunction such as numbness or weakness
3. **Differential diagnosis** in acute injuries includes cervical spine instability.
4. **X-ray studies**
   a. Normal or show loss of usual lordotic curve
   b. If instability is suspected, lateral flexion and extension views are indicated. These views are obtained by patient actively flexing and extending to pain tolerance; more easily taken in lateral decubitus position with patient's head resting on a support.

C. **Treatment:** athlete exhibiting less than full pain-free range of motion should be excluded from contact and limited contact sports. Therapy involves:

1. Rest
2. Ice
3. Nonsteroidal anti-inflammatory drugs (NSAIDs)
4. Muscle relaxants
5. Range-of-motion, stretching, and strengthening exercises
6. Advance to contact activities when pain-free

II. Herniated Nucleus Pulposus (ruptured discs, herniated discs, "slipped" disc)

A. **Definition:** extrusion of center of disc (nucleus pulposus) through a tear in fibrous outer coverings of disc (annulus fibrosus), with subsequent nerve root or spinal cord compression

1. Diffuse bulge—circumferential bulging of the disc, sometimes seen incidentally on magnetic resonance imaging (MRI) in asymptomatic patients; of little clinical significance if not impinging on the spinal cord or nerve root.

   2. Protrusion—a focal bulge or herniation, still attached to the host disc and impinging on the sac, cord, or nerve root. May be broad-based or narrow-based.
   3. Extrusion—herniation of a disc fragment that is separated or sequestered from the host disc and impinging on the sac, spinal cord, or nerve root.

B. **Clinical findings**
   1. **Mechanisms of injury**
      a. Cervical compression
      b. Axial loading
      c. Hyperflexion injuries
      d. Predisposing factors may include a history of repetitive minor neck injuries or axial loading forces, as is often seen in competitive divers and down-linemen in football.
   2. **History**
      a. Presenting complaints include sharp neck pain with radiation into the shoulder or upper extremity.
      b. Pain often exacerbated by Valsalva maneuvers (breath-holding, straining, or coughing) and neck movement
      c. May be associated numbness, weakness, and paresthesia in a dermatomal (nerve) distribution into the arm
      d. In severe cases, complete loss of motor function below level of injury
         i. Arm and leg paralysis
         ii. Loss of bladder, bowel, or sexual function
      e. Spurling's maneuver (turning the head with the neck extended) often reproduces sharp radicular pain into affected extremity in distribution of compressed nerve root.
      f. Babinski's signs (up-going toe when plantar surface of foot is stroked) often present if spinal cord is compressed
   3. **Physical examination**
      a. Decreased range of motion of neck
      b. Paraspinous muscle spasms
      c. Neurologic deficits, including weakness, numbness, and reflex changes compatible with nerve root affected (Table 1)
   4. **Differential diagnosis**
      a. Nerve root tumors
      b. Nerve root compression from cervical arthritis or fracture
      c. Brachial plexus injuries
   5. **X-ray studies**
      a. Cervical spine films may reveal disc space narrowing, but are usually normal
      b. MRI, computed tomography (CT) scan, or myelography are often required to demonstrate neural compression by bulging and displaced disc fragment.
      c. Electromyography studies demonstrate nerve root irritation.

C. **Treatment**
   1. Cervical collar and traction in combination with NSAIDs, pain medicines, and muscle relaxants

TABLE 1. Neurologic Deficits with Cervical or Nerve Root Injuries

Disk	Root	Reflex Affected	Muscle Affected	Test
C4–C5	C5	Biceps	Deltoid	Shoulder abduction
C5–C6	C6	Brachioradialis	Biceps	Elbow flexion
C6–C7	C7	Triceps	Triceps	Elbow extension
C7–C8	C8	FDS	FDS	Finger flexion
T1–T2	T1	—	Hand	Abduction and adduction

FDS = flexor digitorum superficialis.

2. Surgery may be indicated when symptoms persist or progress despite conservative measures or in presence of major neurologic defects

III. Spinal Stenosis

A. **Definition:** narrowing of sagittal diameter cervical spinal canal, as a result of a congenital abnormality or an acquired condition, most commonly osteoarthritis. Spinal stenosis may predispose athlete to spinal cord or nerve injury after relatively minor trauma.

B. **Clinical findings**

1. Often asymptomatic until direct blow to forehead (forced hyperextension) or occiput (hyperflexion) produces neurologic signs. Lateral blows causing rapid side-bending with or without rotation can also elicit acute symptoms.
2. Narrowed spinal canal diameter restricts spinal cord's ability to decompress itself. Compression of spinal cord during hyperextension may cause infolding of ligamentum flavum, contributing to a compromised canal diameter.
3. C5 and C6 cord segments are most frequently involved.
4. Athletes may develop immediate quadriparesis, with arm weakness greater than leg weakness, secondary to contusion (bruising) of central portion of spinal cord (central cord syndrome).
5. Milder cases may produce "burning" of one or both arms.
6. **Differential diagnosis:** burners or stingers secondary to brachial plexus stretch may be ruled out by careful history confirming a hyperextension or flexion injury.
7. **X-ray studies**
   a. Plain films may show narrowing of cervical spine canal from congenital or arthritic changes.
   b. Torg ratio of spinal canal diameter to vertebral body diameter is a common measurement to assess adequacy of spinal canal. Ratio of < 0.8 suggests spinal stenosis (Fig. 1).
   c. Torg ratio may be unreliable in well-developed athlete.
   d. Evidence indicates that ratio of spinal cord diameter to canal diameter on MRI is a more reliable indicator for spinal stenosis.

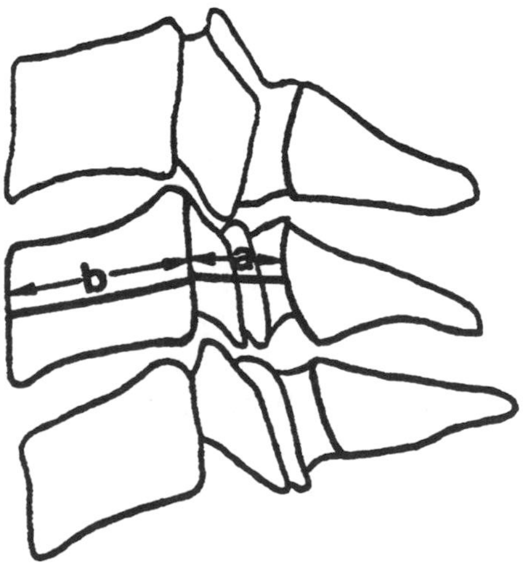

FIGURE 1. The spinal canal-to-vertebral body ratio is the distance from the midpoint of the posterior aspect of the vertebral body to the nearest point on the corresponding spinolaminar line *(a)* divided by the anteroposterior width of the vertebral body *(b)*. Pavlov's ratio is a/b. (From Torg JS, Pavlov H, Genuario S, et al: J Bone Joint Surg [Am] 68-A:1354–1370, 1988, with permission.)

C. **Treatment**
   1. Treatment initially consists of observation because most patients improve without surgery.
   2. Steroids may be beneficial to reduce spinal cord swelling.
   3. Some patients may require anterior cervical fusion and removal of osteophyte or laminectomy to decompress a congenitally narrowed cervical spinal canal.

IV. Cervical Instability

A. **Definition:** injury and disruption of ligaments (anterior and posterior longitudinal ligament, infraspinous ligament) supporting vertebral bodies. May occur with or without associated cervical fractures. May result in dislocations without associated fractures, causing catastrophic neurologic injury.

B. **Clinical findings**
   1. Most common complaint is neck pain, usually exacerbated by neck extension or flexion.
   2. Neurologic examination may initially be normal.
   3. Regardless of presence or absence of fractures, ligamentous injuries can lead to varying degrees of neurologic dysfunction, ranging from mild weakness to complete quadriplegia.
   4. **X-ray studies**
      a. X-rays should be obtained in all athletes with complaints of significant neck pain.
      b. If x-rays do not reveal bony abnormalities, flexion and extension films must be obtained. These are best done by having athlete perform these maneuvers in an active flexion. Pain or paresthesia usually limits neck motion and forewarns of any potential neurologic damage.
      c. Patients with mental status changes may also have ligamentous injuries. In this situation, neck must be immobilized with a cervical collar, with postponement of flexion/extension films until mental status examination has returned to normal.
      d. **Flexion/extension films should never be performed when routine spine films show evidence of severe trauma with subluxation or locked facets.**
      e. Myelography, MRI, and CT scanning are useful in defining extent of injury to spinal cord and nerve roots.

C. **Treatment:** in cases of cervical dislocation or neurologic defect, spine must be reduced and stabilized. Cervical tongs should be applied to distract vertebrae into their normal position.

V. Fractures

A. **Definition:** injury to bony components of spine, usually resulting in compression of vertebral bodies
   1. **Stable fracture**—integrity of spine still preserved
   2. **Unstable fracture**—excess movement between adjacent osseous elements

B. **Clinical findings**
   1. Local tenderness and less often palpable deformity
   2. Pain localized to an injured vertebra
   3. Posterior "step-off" deformity
   4. Prominence of a spinous process
   5. Edema
   6. Ecchymosis or pain with attempted motion
   7. Note the presence or absence of:
      a. Tracheal tenderness or deviation
      b. Head tilt
      c. Oropharyngeal hematoma

C. **X-ray findings**

1. Identify all seven cervical vertebrae.
2. Anatomic assessment
   a. Alignment (congruity of four lordotic curves)
      i. Anterior vertebral body line
      ii. Anterior spinal canal line
      iii. Posterior spinal canal line
      iv. Spinous process tips
   b. Bone
      i. Defects in vertebral body contour
      ii. Lateral bony masses
      iii. Spinous processes
   c. Cartilage
      i. Intervertebral discs
      ii. Posterolateral facet joints
   d. Soft tissue spaces
      i. Prevertebral space
      ii. Fat stripe
      iii. Space between spinous processes
3. Guidelines for abnormalities
   a. Alignment (Fig. 2A–B)
      i. Vertebral malalignment > 3.5 mm—dislocation, vertebral instability
      ii. Anteroposterior spinal canal space < 13 mm—spinal cord compression
      iii. Angulation of intervertebral space > 11°—cervical instability
   b. Bones (Fig. 3A–E)
      i. Vertebral body
         (a) Anterior height < 3 mm posterior height—compression fracture, anterior wedge deformity
         (b) Oblique lucency—teardrop fracture

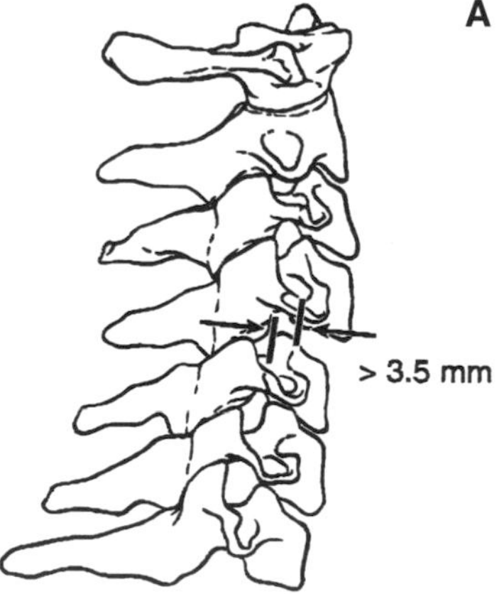

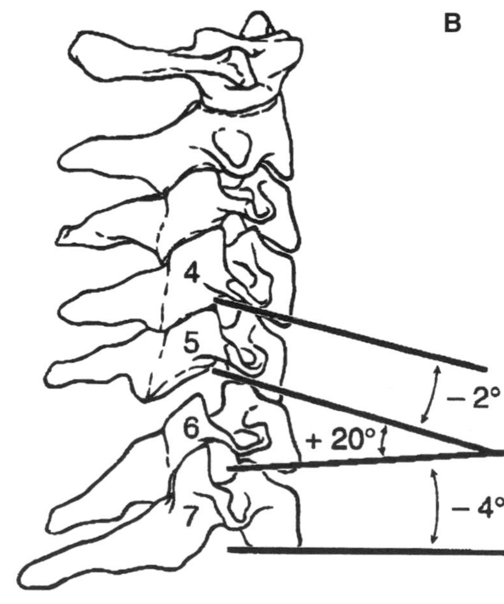

FIGURE 2. **A,** Vertebral body anterior displacement > 3.5 mm. Measurements are taken at the posterior aspects of adjacent bodies. **B,** Angulation of intervertebral space > 11°.

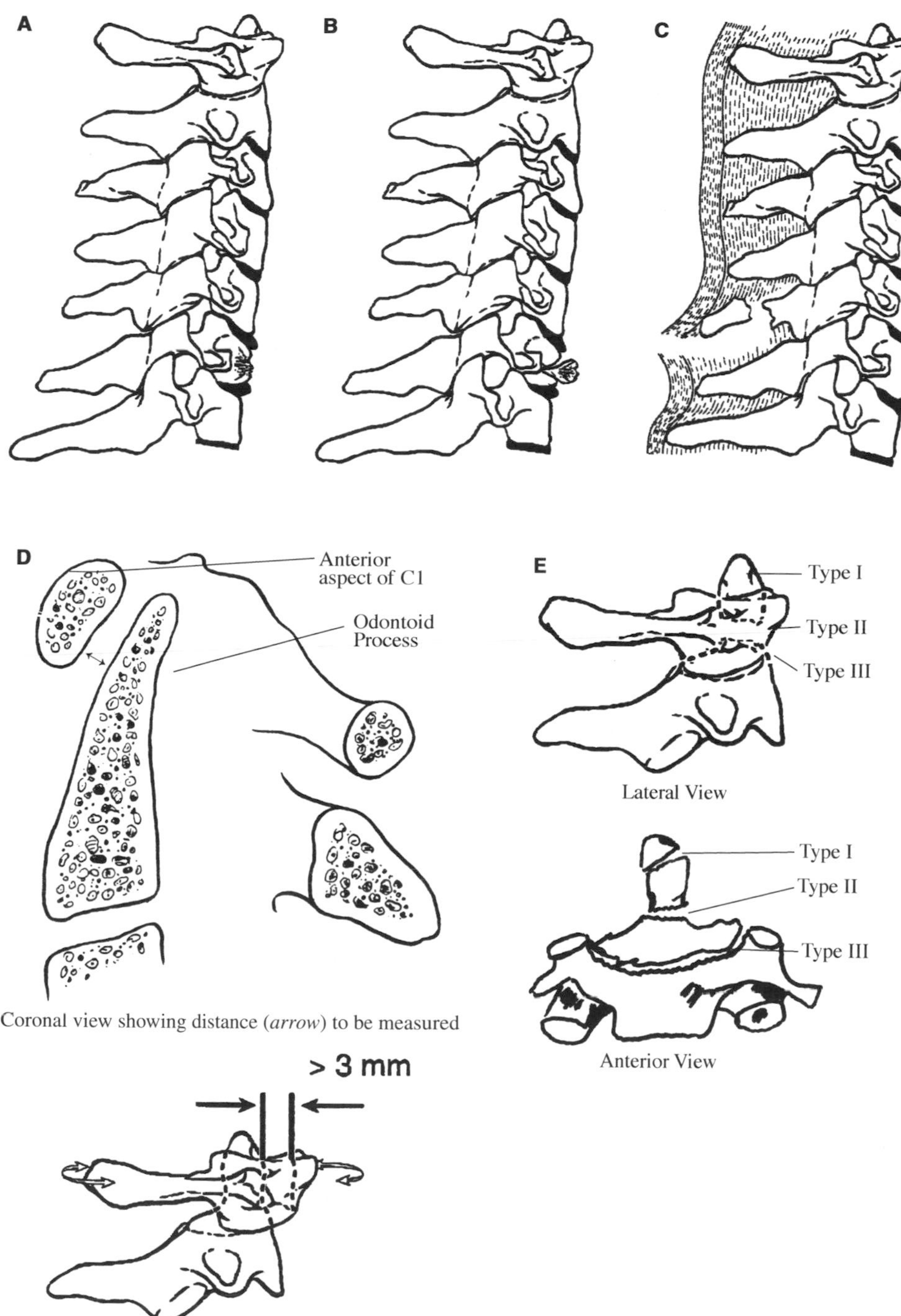

FIGURE 3. **A,** Anterior wedge deformity caused by flexion compression. **B,** Crushed vertebral body with anterior "teardrop" fragment. **C,** Avulsion fracture shows lucency through tip of spinous process. **D,** Distance (*arrow*) between posterior aspect of C1 and anterior border of odontoid process > 3 mm suggests atlanto-axial instability. **E,** Three possible C2 odontoid fracture sites, seen in two views.

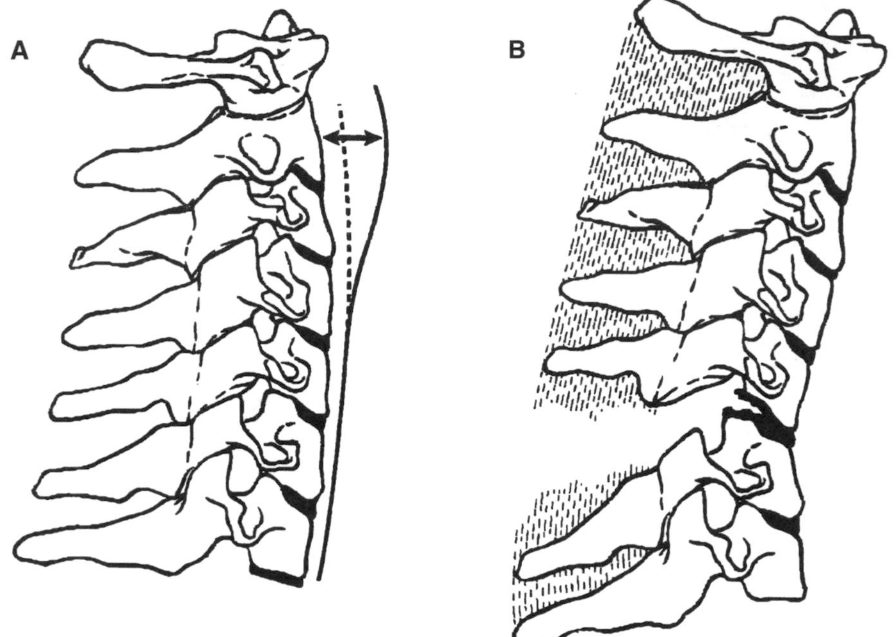

FIGURE 4. **A,** Widening of prevertebral space > 5 mm secondary to hemorrhage signifies adjacent spinal injury. **B,** Torn interspinous ligaments cause widening of interspinous space and suggest anterior spinal canal fracture.

ii. Lack of parallel facets of lateral mass—possible lateral compression fracture

iii. Lucency through tip of spinous process—avulsion fracture

iv. Atlas and axis (C1 and C2)

(a) Distance between posterior aspect of C1 to anterior odontoid process > 3 mm—C1 and/or C2 dislocation, instability

(b) Lucency through the odontoid process—C2 fracture

c. Soft tissue space (Fig. 4A–B)

i. Widening of the prevertebral space > 5 mm—hemorrhage accompanying spinal injury

ii. Obliteration of prevertebral fat stripe—fracture at same level

iii. Widening of space between spinous processes—torn interspinous ligaments and likely spinal canal fracture anteriorly

D. **Treatment:** same as for cervical instability. Should be managed as if potential for spinal cord injury is present.

1. **Acute spinal cord injury management**

a. **A conscious athlete who complains of neck pain, numbness, or weakness should be treated as if he or she harbors an underlying unstable spinal injury. Any unconscious participant should be considered to have a potential spinal cord injury until proved otherwise.**

b. **In moving such an athlete, it is imperative to maintain airway with the cervical spine control** (Fig. 5A–B). If possible, a hard collar should be placed before initial movement. One person in charge should be assigned task of immobilizing head and neck, while at least four others take care of trunk and other

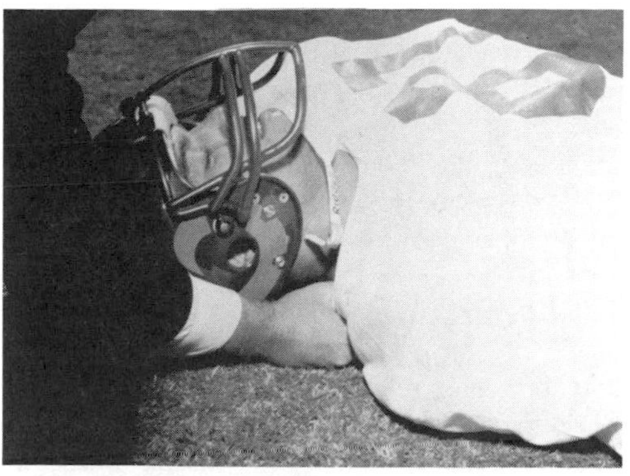

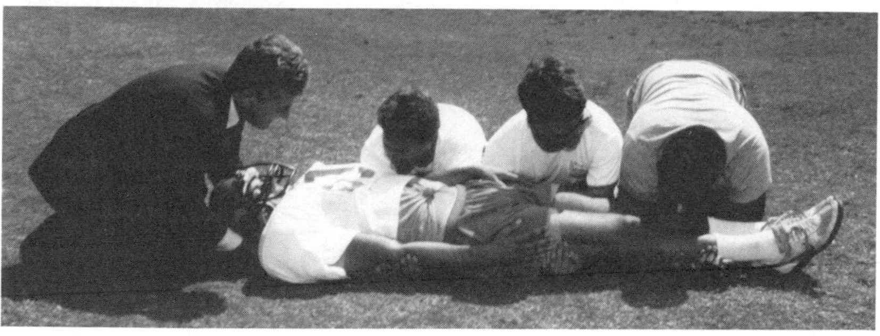

FIGURE 5. A, To immobilize head to trunk, chief of transport team holds trapezius-clavicle-scapula area with hands and holds head with forearms. **B,** Chief calls signals to six transport team members, three on each side of the body (three on near side are not pictured), as they join hands and lift. A back board is introduced underneath. (From Watkins RG, et al: Cervical spine injuries in football players. Spine State Art Rev 4(2): 391–408, 1990, with permission.)

body parts. All obstructive elements to face such as face guards should be removed, but helmet should be left on during transport. Large bolt cutters should be available to cut away all obstructive athletic gear.

i. At least four, but better five or six, people should be assembled for transport team.
ii. One person should be in charge and should be positioned at head of injured athlete to call movers.
iii. The person in charge should control head and shoulders by cradling head between forearms, clasping trapezius, clavicle, and scapula if possible, or inside of shoulder pads and trapezius.
iv. An additional person on transport team can help to support and fix head of chief's forearms during the move.
v. Other members of team should be positioned one on each side of shoulders and one on each side of waist, and if available a member should support legs and feet.
vi. At direction of person in charge, members of team should reach under athlete, clasp hands, and lift injured athlete in unison onto back board.

c. Intubation:
   i. If athlete is seriously injured and requires intubation, care must be taken not to hyperextend the cervical spine.
   ii. Airway and circulatory systems must be stable before athlete can be safely transported.

d. Prone position ("log roll")—if athlete is initially injured in prone position, he or she should be log-rolled and placed in supine position, followed by placement of collar. Rolling onto a long spine board should be done whenever possible, so that immobilization of entire spine may be accomplished.

e. Immobilization:
   i. Most emergency transport teams have spinal boards equipped with cervical head immobilizing units. If none is available, sand bags or other weights may be placed on either side of head.
   ii. After cervical immobilization, athlete should be transferred to an appropriate neurosurgical facility as soon as possible. Haste should never be sought at expense of excellent immobilization.

VI. Brachial Plexus Injuries ("burners," "stingers")

A. **Definition**
1. A spectrum of brachial plexus injuries, primarily related to upper trunk, especially C5–C6, caused by a traction injury to shoulder.
2. Stretch-type injuries to nerves of upper extremity are caused by forceful downward distraction of shoulder while head is distracted to opposite side.
3. Injuries caused by forced side-bending of head to affected side are more worrisome for nerve root compression.

B. **X-ray studies**
1. X-rays are usually normal.
2. Mild unilateral systems not resolving within 1 week should be evaluated with electromyography.

C. **Treatment**
1. No further contact until symptoms resolve. Athletes with compression-type injuries should be disqualified from contact activities until imaging studies resolve question of foraminal stenosis or a herniated disc.
2. Prevention of burners in football involves proper fitting and modifications of shoulder pads.
   a. Lifters
   b. Supplemental pad at base of neck
   c. Modified A-frame shoulder pad with thicker padding at base of neck
   d. A collar roll attached to posterior aspect of shoulder pads

Recommended Reading

1. Herzog RJ, Weins JJ, Dillingham MF, Sontag MJ: Normal cervical spine morphometry and cervical spinal stenosis in asymptomatic professional football players: Plain film radiography, multiplanar computer tomography, and magnetic resonance imaging. Spine 16(suppl):178–186, 1991.
2. Marzo JM, Simmons EH, Whieldon TJ: Neck injuries to high school football players in western New York State. N Y State J Med 91(2):46–49, 1991.
3. Mueller FO, Cantu RC: Eleventh Annual Report, Fall 1982–Spring 1993. Chapel Hill, National Center for Catastrophic Sports Injury Research, University of North Carolina.
4. Ramenofsky ML (ed): Advanced Trauma Life Support Manual. Chicago, American College of Surgeons, 1989, pp 173–176.
5. Taylor JR, Finch PM: Neck sprain. Aust Fam Phys 22(9):1623, 1993.
6. Torg JS: Injuries to the Head, Neck, and Face. Philadelphia, Lea & Febiger, 1982.
7. Torg JS: Cervical spinal stenosis with neurapraxia in transient quadriplegia. Clin Sports Med 9:279–296, 1990.
8. Tysvaer AT, Sortland O, Storli OV, Lochen EA: Head and neck injuries among Norwegian soccer players: A neurological, electroencephalographic, radiologic and neuropsychological evaluation. Tidsskrift for Den Norske Laegeforening 112(10):1268–1271, 1992.
9. Watkins RC: Cervical spine and spinal cord injuries. In Fu FH (ed): Sports Injuries. Baltimore, Williams & Wilkins, 1994, pp 853–877.
10. Watkins RC, Dillin H, Maxwell J: Cervical spine injuries in football players. Spine State Art Rev 4:391–408, 1990.
11. Woodward GA, Furnival R, Schunk JE: Trampolines revisited: A review of 114 pediatric recreational trampoline injuries. Pediatrics 89(5 pt 1):849–854, 1992.

41

Eye Injuries in Sports: Evaluation, Management, and Prevention

Gerald R. Christensen, M.D.

About 1.5% of all sports injuries involve the eye or ocular adnexa, and almost all are preventable. Baseball and basketball accidents are the leading causes of eye injuries. However, as a percentage of total sports injuries, the highest incidence of eye injuries occurs in racquet sports, soccer, swimming, and boxing. Of all sports eye injuries, 30–40% seen by the ophthalmologist are associated with racquet sports.

I. Mechanisms of Sports Eye Injuries

A. **Lacerations** are usually from flying objects and may occur with the shattering of a lens mounting frame.

B. **Blunt injuries** occur with objects that are smaller than the orbital opening whereby all force is transmitted to the globe. With larger objects, some of the force is absorbed by the surrounding tissue.

C. **Head trauma** requires huge forces to cause ocular injury. This risk is generally limited to collision sports.

II. Principles of Protection from Sports Eye Injuries

A. A protective device needs to dissipate the potentially harmful force over time and area. Performance standards require that these force transfer devices must be acceptable to the athlete, not change the appeal of the game, and not generate unacceptable liability. Sometimes it is necessary to make design or style compromises to achieve these goals.

B. Specifically, eye protectors need to shift the impact from the eyes and face to the skull without increasing the risk of injury to the brain.

C. In some cases, it is necessary to integrate helmets with eye and face protectors.

III. Certification of the Athlete for Participation

This involves evaluating the athlete for eye injury risk factors in his or her particular sport.

A. **General considerations.** Ideally, the athlete should have a visual acuity of 20/20 or better in each eye, either unaided or with modest correction.

1. **Visual risk factors**
    a. A best corrected visual acuity of less than 20/40 in either eye or a spectacle correction for myopia or hyperopia that is greater than 6 diopters
    b. Disability from high corrective spectacle lenses can sometimes be mitigated by contact lenses; however, contact lenses themselves can be a risk factor.
    c. **Contact lenses should never be used as a substitute for an eye protective device.**
2. **Anatomic risk factors** include disease, degeneration, or structural weakness of the eye itself.

a. Myopia greater than 6 diopters
b. Thin sclera
c. History of retinal degenerative disease
d. Any history of previous eye surgery that weakens the outer coats of the eye, especially cataract or refractive surgery
e. **Athletes with such risk factors should be evaluated by an ophthalmologist before engaging in high-risk or extremely high-risk sports.**

B. Special considerations are necessary for the one-eyed athlete, who is defined as a person with visual acuity in one eye of 20/200 or less.
1. The American Medical Association classification of sports relative to paired organ loss is based on the risks of bone, muscle, and internal organ injury and forbids all contact and collision sports while allowing unrestricted access to all racquet sports.
2. **These criteria are not relevant to the one-eyed athlete** because many such athletes can safely participate in some collision and contact sports activities when equipped with proper protection. Conversely, in many noncontact sports, eye protection is mandatory for the one-eyed athlete and strongly recommended for others.
3. **The one-eyed athlete should be evaluated by an ophthalmologist before deciding to participate in a particular sport.**

C. **Routine visual testing**
1. Visual acuity should be measured periodically and reported to the team physician.
2. Testing for distance visual acuity is done with a Snellen card or a commercial vision tester with the distance correction in place and each eye measured separately.
3. Anyone testing less than 20/40 in either eye should be referred to an ophthalmologist.

IV. Functional Testing Following Injury

A. **Visual acuity is the single most important test in evaluating eye injuries.**
1. If formal materials for visual acuity testing are not available, vision can be evaluated with any reproducible object, such as printed material, fingers, or lights.
2. **Decreased visual acuity suggests a variety of disorders.**
a. Disruption of the refractive surfaces of the eye such as seen in corneal or lens injury
b. Clouding of the ocular media
c. Injury to the retina and optic nerve

B. **Extraocular muscle balance** is tested with a penlight to determine if the eyes are in parallel alignment. This is determined when the pupillary light reflex falls on corresponding areas of both corneas.
1. Muscle function is tested in both eyes simultaneously, having the patient:
a. Gaze right
b. Gaze left
c. Gaze up and right
d. Gaze up and left
e. Gaze down and right
f. Gaze down and left
2. Any suggestion of restriction of movement or report of diplopia suggests the possibility of an injury to the soft tissue of the orbit or interference of extraocular muscle function from paresis or entrapment.
3. Failure of the eyelids to open or close suggests the possibility of a motor nerve deficit or soft tissue injury.

C. **Sensory nerve testing is especially important in cases of blunt trauma involving the orbit.** Always test the sensory nerve functions throughout the distribution of the maxillary branch of the trigeminal nerve (V2) because orbital floor fractures frequently disrupt this nerve, producing hypesthesia on the surface of the face.

D. **The pupil** should be round and symmetric and react to direct and consensual light.
   1. Pupillary paresis following blunt injury to the globe is not uncommon and frequently presents as a sluggish response to any stimulation.
   2. A pupillary reflex that is reduced to direct but not consensual light is suggestive of an injury involving the retina or optic nerve (Marcus Gunn pupil).

E. **Intraocular pressure** is best tested with the Schiøtz tonometer; however, in the absence of a Shiøtz tonometer, pressure can be estimated by palpating the globe and using the palpated tension in the fellow eye for comparison.
   1. Care should be taken to avoid compression of a ruptured or perforated globe by this test.
   2. Intraocular pressure may be elevated with hemorrhage or swelling of the orbital contents and may be decreased in certain cases of blunt injury to the globe.

F. **The funduscopic examination** can be done with any device that is designed to pass a light beam through the length of the eye and focus on the surface of the retina and optic nerve disc.
   1. **Assessment of the media**
      a. **Clear ocular media are necessary to produce the normal red reflex pattern seen when directing an ophthalmoscope light through the pupil.**
      b. The reflex depends on a normally transparent cornea and lens, with smooth unblemished surfaces and clear aqueous and vitreous humor. Wrinkling of the cornea or defects on its surface or subluxation of the lens interferes with this normal phenomenon.
      c. **Even modest bleeding into the ocular media can alter or obscure the red reflex. Sometimes this may be the only sign of occult rupture of the globe.**
   2. **Fundus anatomy**
      a. The normal image of the posterior pole of the eye, as seen with the ophthalmoscope, consists of the diffuse red choroidal circulation viewed through the normally transparent retinal tissue.
      b. Retinal edema resulting from any interruption of circulatory dynamics produces a loss of retinal transparency and an obscuration of background choroidal circulation. Such changes not only alter the intensity of the red reflex, but also obliterate the image detail of the choroid.
      c. Retinal edema occurs in contusion injuries to the globe and is also seen in retinal detachments from any of a variety of mechanisms.

V. Examination of the Injured Eye

A. **History**
   1. **Types of injury.** The history is a most important means to **determine the exact mechanism of injury.** This information is necessary in evaluating the injury itself and for developing protective gear and gathering statistical data regarding particular sports and their hazards.
   2. **Signs and symptoms.** Inquiry should be made regarding specific ocular complaints that might have particular diagnostic significance relative to eye injury.
      a. Pain
      b. Decreased vision
      c. Diplopia
      d. Flashing lights
      e. Past history of eye disease or surgery

B. **Gross inspection.** Many sports eye injuries are contusions or lacerations, which distort the gross appearance of the normal ocular anatomy.
   1. **Eyelids and orbit**
      a. Evaluate for symmetry between the two sides and especially look for ptosis of the upper eyelid or proptosis of the globe on the injured side.

   b. Ecchymosis of the eyelids and subconjunctival hemorrhage is frequently associated with orbital hemorrhages and proptosis.
2. **Cornea and sclera**
   a. Examine carefully for signs of perforation and rupture indicated by darkly pigmented uveal tissue presenting through a laceration. These injuries can result in distortion of the pupil and other asymmetries of the iris.
   b. Apply fluorescein stain to identify superficial corneal epithelial defects and use the ophthalmoscope to verify the presence of the red reflex.
3. **Anterior chamber**
   a. Look carefully for signs of microscopic bleeding or hyphema.
   b. When present, blood is generally found layered out in the anterior chamber angle inferiorly, forming a crescent of blood at the 6 o'clock position.

VI. Sports Injuries

A. **Corneal abrasion** is the result of a loss of surface epithelium and is most significant. The cornea must maintain a smooth mirrorlike anterior surface, using its epithelial layers, to function as an optical quality refracting surface. Disruption of this smooth surface near the central visual axis interferes with the visual acuity.
1. **Signs and symptoms**
   a. Pain
   b. Photophobia
   c. Conjunctival injection
   d. Tearing (epiphora)
   e. Decreased visual acuity if the central corneal area is involved
2. **Examination**
   a. Fluorescein solution stains denuded and devitalized areas.
   b. In some cases, topical anesthetic may be necessary to facilitate examination.
   c. Additional ocular injury must be ruled out.
3. **Treatment**
   a. Healing is best facilitated by the management of pain and discomfort and controlling lid movement.
   b. Postinjury infection is uncommon; however, topical antibiotics may be useful in some cases.
   c. Patching, if adequate to prevent movement of the eyelids, is generally sufficient to manage the discomfort.
   d. In a large abrasion in which there is significant pain and photophobia, a topical cycloplegic drug such as 2% homatropine is helpful and can be applied before patching.
   e. Generally, avoid topical corticosteroid preparations except in complicated cases.
4. **Prognosis**
   a. Uncomplicated corneal epithelial injuries heal completely within 24 to 48 hours without scarring. Even though frequently contaminated, they rarely become infected.
   b. **Long-term use of topical anesthetics for pain management interferes with corneal reepithelialization and is absolutely contraindicated.**
   c. Topical steroids may enhance corneal fungal and viral infections and consequently should be used with extreme caution.
   d. **Recurrent epithelial erosion** is occasionally a complication from abrasion injuries, and the patient needs to be advised that this difficulty may occur.

B. **Foreign bodies on the eye and eyelid surfaces**
1. **Signs and symptoms** are the same as for abrasions.
2. **Examination**
   a. Tiny foreign bodies may require magnification to be properly visualized and removed.

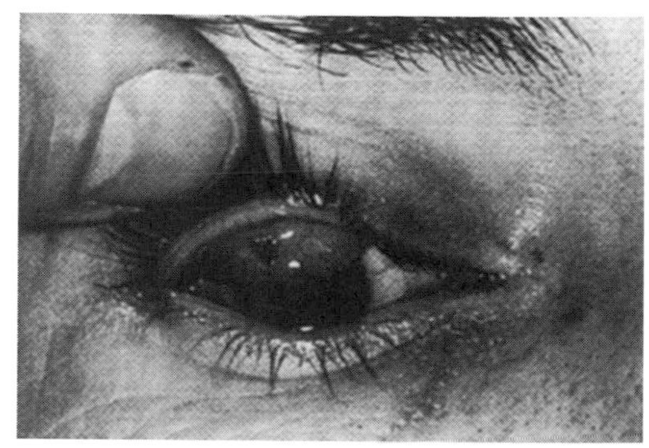

FIGURE 1. Foreign body in the upper tarsal conjunctiva. (From Tucker W: Ophthalmic emergencies. Office Procedures State Art Rev 1(1):106, 1986, with permission.)

b. In the cornea, their localization can be enhanced by fluorescein stain, and the use of topical anesthetic may be necessary to facilitate the examination.
c. Both upper and lower conjunctival fornices should be examined carefully for the presence of foreign body.
d. The upper eyelid should be everted and the conjunctival surface over the tarsal surface specifically inspected for the presence of foreign body (Fig. 1).

3. **Treatment**
    a. For corneal foreign bodies, apply a short-acting topical anesthetic and remove the foreign material with a cotton-tip applicator or disposable hypodermic needle. Rust rings, if present, should be removed as well (Fig. 2).
    b. Successful removal of a foreign body converts the injury into an abrasion, which is then subsequently treated as described for corneal abrasions at left.
4. **Prognosis** is the same as for corneal abrasion. In cases with minimal epithelial defects, patching may not be necessary.

C. **Lacerations** may occur in association with blunt trauma as well as from sharp objects and can result from the propulsion and shattering of eye protection equipment.

1. **Eyelid lacerations**
    a. **Signs and symptoms**
        i. Swelling
        ii. Hemorrhage
        iii. Anatomic disruption of the lids
        iv. Damage may be subtle and the appearance normal
    b. **Examination**
        i. Evaluation of the normal anatomic relationship of the lid margins and front surface of the globe as well as the symmetry with the uninjured side.

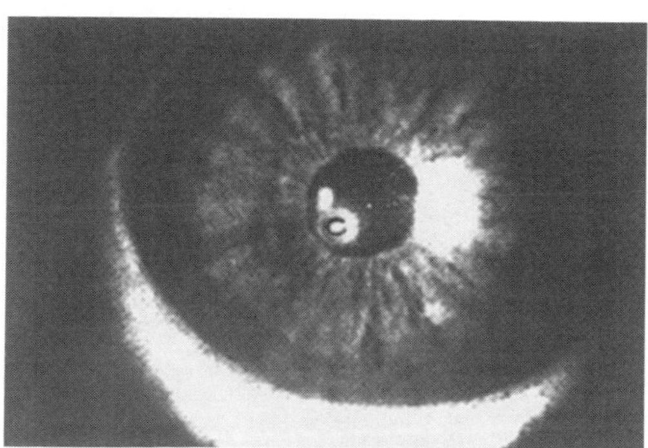

FIGURE 2. Corneal foreign body surrounded by a rust ring. (From Tucker W: Ophthalmic emergencies. Office Procedures State Art Rev 1(1):106, 1986, with permission.)

ii. Opening and closing functions are assessed specifically, especially to verify that the lids can be spontaneously closed.
iii. Attention needs to be directed to rule out the possibility of upper eyelid ptosis or lacerations in the lacrimal drainage system.
iv. Globe must be thoroughly inspected for signs of damage.

c. **Treatment.** Lacerations require individual suturing of the lid tissue layers and additional repairs specific to any injuries involving the integrity of the lacrimal drainage apparatus.

d. **Prognosis.** Because of a rich vascular supply to the eyelids, healing is rapid and deformities are minimal in cases in which there is minimal tissue loss and good anatomic approximation.

2. **Eyeball lacerations**

a. **Signs and symptoms**

i. Decreased visual acuity
ii. Pain
iii. Discomfort
iv. Distortion or displacement of the pupil
v. Loss of the red reflex of the fundus

b. **Examination**

i. Evaluate the anterior segment of the globe for signs of subconjunctival hemorrhage
ii. The pupil should be round, central, and symmetric with the fellow eye.
(a) Lacerations of the cornea frequently incarcerate iris tissue, causing distortion and displacement of the pupil (Fig. 3).
(b) Scleral lacerations also may displace the location of the pupil because of herniations of the uveal tract through the defect.
iii. Prolapsed uveal tissue presents as a dark brown or black mass, even in fair-complected, blue-eyed individuals.
iv. Lacerations of the globe that extend to involve the lens zonules may result in subluxation of the crystalline lens.
v. Intraocular bleeding is also a frequent complication, causing obscuration of the ocular media and loss of the red fundus reflex.
vi. The intraocular pressure may be decreased; however, many lacerations are self-sealing and pressure levels can vary.

c. **Treatment**

i. Once a lacerated globe is suspected, manipulation should be minimized.
ii. The patient needs to be transported to the care of an ophthalmologist, taking care to avoid further injury to the eye. The patient should be moved in either the supine or upright position (avoid a prone or head-down position) with the eye protected by a rigid ocular shield (Fig. 4). If necessary, a makeshift ocular shield can be fashioned from a disposable drinking cup.

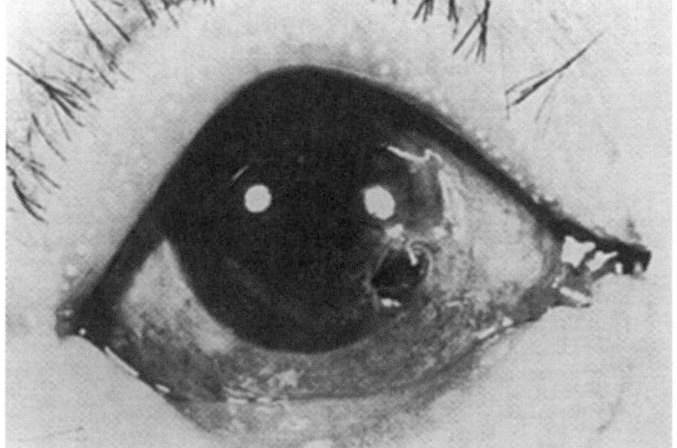

FIGURE 3. Corneal laceration with prolapsed iris and irregular pupil. (From Tucker W: Ophthalmic emergencies. Office procedures State Art Rev 1(1):106, 1986, with permission.)

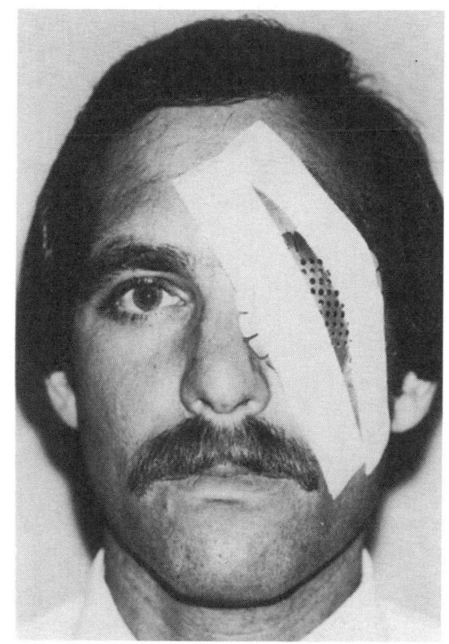

FIGURE 4. Protective metal shield. (From Tucker W: Ophthalmic emergencies. Office Procedures State Art Rev 1(1):106, 1986, with permission.)

iii. Repair is accomplished by approximation of the laceration and surgical clearing of any opacity in the ocular media.

d. **Prognosis** is generally guarded but varies with the location and severity of the injury.

i. Injuries of the cornea and limbus can produce an irregular astigmatism as a result of healing contractures. A loss of corneal transparency may also occur in the area of scarring.

ii. Injuries involving the lens generally produce a cataract, which often can be managed in the usual, surgical fashion.

iii. Lacerations involving areas posterior to the ciliary body have a more guarded prognosis, often necessitating complex surgical procedures and frequently a poor visual result.

D. **Contusion injuries.** Blunt injuries to the globe are the most common sports injury to the eye and may be associated with abrasions and lacerations. They result from facial blows directly to the orbital contents or from sudden pressure increases transmitted to the eye from the surrounding orbital tissue.

1. **Blunt trauma to the orbit**

a. **Orbital hemorrhage** and edema frequently coexist with facial fractures and injuries to the globe.[9] Uncomplicated orbital hemorrhage from blunt trauma is a result of the extensive force necessary to create such an injury. The resulting swelling of the orbital contents increases the tissue pressure surrounding the globe and forces the globe outward into a position of proptosis.

i. **Signs and symptoms**

(a) If the globe has escaped injury, vision may be unaffected.

(b) Restrictions to ocular motility, if present, are frequently associated with diplopia, which can be demonstrated especially in extremes of gaze.

(c) Intraocular pressure may be increased, sometimes to levels that compromise retinal circulation, resulting in pulsation of the retinal arterioles at the optic nerve head. (Pulsation of the venules is not a diagnostic sign and is frequently a normal finding.)

(d) Proptosis, if present, can be associated with upper eyelid retraction and inability to close the lid completely.

ii. **Examination**

(a) Record the visual acuity and conduct an inspection to rule out injury to the eyeball.

(b) Examine the binocular eye movements (versions) by observing both eyes simultaneously moving through the six cardinal positions of gaze (see page 408). This examination is best accomplished with a small penlight. Look for loss of the parallel alignment of the eyes during this maneuver, especially at extremes of gaze, and inquire as to the presence of diplopia.

(c) Test for proptosis (exophthalmos) by measuring the distance from the lateral edge of the orbit to a plane aligned with the apex of the cornea and compare this measurement with the uninjured side.

(d) Conduct appropriate studies to rule out orbital fracture.

iii. **Treatment** is generally symptomatic, except in unusual circumstances of massive hemorrhage that may require surgical drainage or decompression. Rest and analgesics are indicated, and cold compresses may control further edema and bleeding.

iv. **Prognosis** is good.

b. **Orbital fracture (blowout fracture).** See also pages 435–436.

i. **Signs and symptoms**

(a) Fracture injuries to the orbit most commonly involve the floor (roof of the maxillary sinus) (Fig. 5) and the medial wall (wall of the ethmoid sinus), but the floor fracture is the one most likely to be symptomatic.

(b) A triad suggesting orbital floor fractures consists of diplopia, obscured maxillary sinus cavity on x-ray, and hypesthesia of the face.

(c) Large fenestrated fractures of the floor allow the orbital contents to be displaced from the orbit into the maxillary sinus, thereby causing the globe to be displaced posteriorly and downward. These injuries are frequently associated with significant bleeding into the maxillary sinus.

(d) Fractures of the orbital floor can interrupt the second branch of the trigeminal nerve (V^2) leading to hypesthesia that innervates the face.

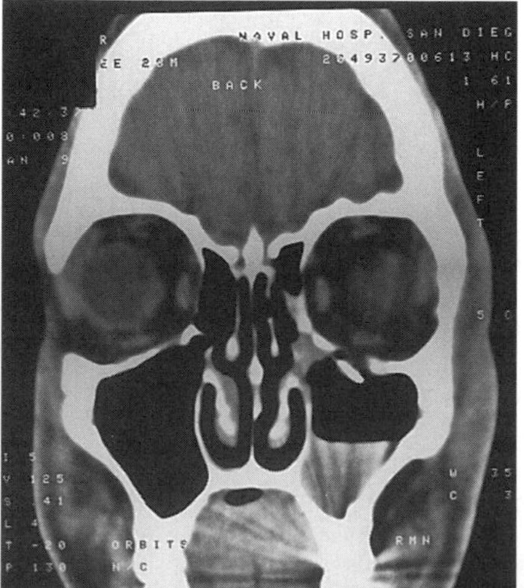

FIGURE 5. Blowout fracture of the floor of the left orbit. Note the air-fluid level in the left maxillary sinus.

(e) Linear nonfenestrated fractures can cause tissue entrapment of orbital contents resulting in restricted motility of the globe, especially in elevation. Such a situation results in a tethering of the globe to the orbital floor.

(f) Version testing elicits diplopia, which becomes worse (farther apart) on upward gaze.

(g) In nonfenestrated fractures, proptosis rather than enophthalmos may be present if there is sufficient contusion with hemorrhage and edema.

ii. **Examination**

(a) The visual acuity is recorded, followed by an examination of extraocular muscle function:

- With the eyes in the primary gaze position, inspect the globe for evidence of retropositioning backward into the orbit and displacement of the posterior pole of the globe inferiorly. This gives the appearance of the globe in a position of enophthalmos with the visual axis directed slightly upward.
- **Attempts to elevate both eyes by directing gaze further upward accentuate the misalignment, especially if there is entrapment of the orbital tissue in a floor fracture.**
- In the presence of enophthalmos of the globe, there is a relative ptosis of the upper lid present.

(b) Maxillary nerve function is tested by comparing the sensation of light touch over the distribution of this nerve on both the normal and the affected side of the face.

(c) Appropriate radiologic studies may reveal clouding of the maxillary sinus cavity as well as actual fracture defects in the orbital floor on the injured side.

iii. **Treatment**

(a) Surgical repair of these injuries is directed toward restoring the normal topography of the orbital floor. This can be accomplished by mobilizing any tissue trapped within the fracture and replacing any defect in the orbital floor either by placing an implant underneath the periosteum of the orbital bones or by stabilizing the periosteum by filling the adjacent sinus cavities with temporary packing material.

(b) Surgical treatment is usually necessary only when there is an actual interruption or herniation of orbital tissue.

(c) Diplopia may be transient following these injuries, so surgical intervention should be deferred until a significant portion of the contusion injury has resolved.

(d) Conversely, in cases with little contusion injury and obvious interruption or herniation of orbital tissue, there is no need to delay definitive repair.

iv. **Prognosis** varies depending on the degree of injury:

(a) Obviously, it is best when there is minimal orbital tissue damage.

(b) Prolonged tissue entrapment and inflammation can result in fibrosis and contractures, which can lead to permanent functional disabilities.

2. **Blunt trauma to the globe** causes a sudden increase of intraocular pressure, which can result in swelling, bleeding, tearing, and displacement of the structures within the eye.[9] Intraocular hemorrhage is an important sign that the eye has sustained significant injury, and there is a high probability that damage to the eye has occurred. Management of intraocular hemorrhage depends on the location and extent of the hemorrhage.

   a. **Hyphema** refers to the presence of blood in the anterior chamber and is an important diagnostic and prognostic sign (Fig. 6). Frequently, it occurs in microscopic

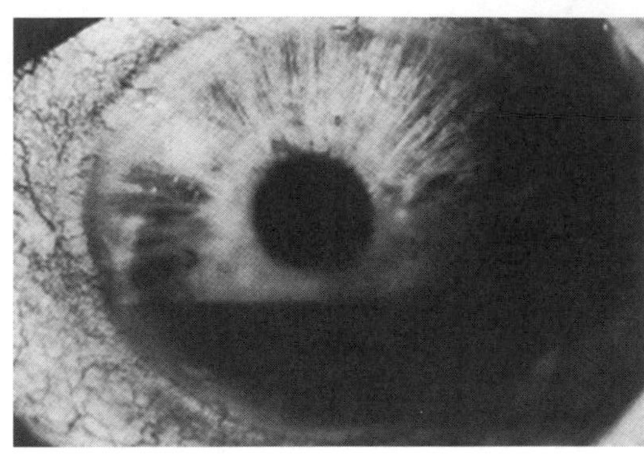

FIGURE 6. Layered hyphema caused by trauma. (From Tucker W: Ophthalmic emergencies. Office Procedures State Art Rev 1(1):106, 1986, with permission.)

quantities and, consequently, can be easily overlooked in a cursory examination. **Such bleeding indicates that there has been an intraocular injury of sufficient intensity to result in a vascular disruption. It is important that this situation be identified, because recurrent bleeding from such injuries can occur, which may be both massive and destructive.** Such rebleeding has been referred to as "eight-ball hemorrhage."

i. **Signs and symptoms**
   (a) Because many hyphema are of small volume, the visual acuity may be unaffected by their presence. There may be only mild injection of the globe with moderate transient discomfort and photophobia. Gradually the blood settles into the inferior chamber angle forming a crescent-shaped precipitate that can easily be overlooked.
   (b) In addition to the hyphema, other damages associated with contusion injuries may also be found:
      - Pupillary paralysis
      - Pupillary contour irregularities
      - Tearing of the uveal tract

ii. **Examination**
   (a) Unless the hyphema is of such quantity to occlude the pupillary axis, the visual acuity may be unaffected.
   (b) Slit-lamp examination is necessary to identify any turbid microscopic hyphema before it has had time to settle out in the chamber angle.

iii. **Treatment**
   (a) The important treatment aspect is the prevention of recurrent bleeding.
   (b) Hemostasis following the initial injury is due to formation of a fibrin clot within the lumen of the damaged vessel.
   (c) Physical activity should be severely restricted and the use of antifibrinolytic drugs considered.
   (d) Recurrent bleeding, if it occurs, is most frequent during the first 4 days following injury.

iv. **Prognosis** is generally excellent, especially if the blood clears rapidly and there is no recurrent bleeding or concurrent ocular damage.

b. **Vitreous hemorrhage**, when it is due to trauma, requires significant force and is generally associated with additional injury to the eye.

i. **Signs and symptoms**
   (a) Vitreous hemorrhage frequently arises from tearing of the retinal arterioles or the choroidal vasculature. The blood obscures the light path through the vitreous cavity of the eye and reduces the visual acuity.

(b) On ophthalmoscopic examination, the fundus detail is blurred or disappears entirely and may be seen only as a "black reflex."
(c) Isolated vitreous bleeding is not associated with other symptoms such as pain or discomfort.

ii. **Examination**
(a) Measurement of the visual acuity
(b) Careful funduscopic examination with emphasis on the red fundus reflex and clarity of fundus detail

iii. **Treatment**
(a) Generally conservative
(b) Severe cases may require surgical removal of the blood and vitreous. Such procedures are often done at the time of repair of associated ocular injuries.

iv. **Prognosis** is guarded.

c. **Retinal hemorrhages and edema** can occur as a result of direct trauma to the eye by transmission of the force to the retinal surface. Occasionally, these same changes can be due to the retinal capillary instability seen in situations of violent exercise performed in conditions of decreased oxygen saturation. Elevated venous pressure from Valsalva maneuvers can also produce retinal edema and hemorrhages. Such findings have been documented in activities such as mountain climbing and weightlifting.

i. **Signs and symptoms**
(a) It is not uncommon to have multiple areas of retinal hemorrhage and edema that are asymptomatic, especially if the affected areas are confined to the peripheral retina.
(b) **Involvement with the macula results in decreased visual acuity or a distortion of the visual perception of form (metamorphopsia).**

ii. **Examination**
(a) This includes visual acuity measurement and testing for metamorphopsia with the Amsler grid.
(b) Ophthalmoscopic examination reveals both flame-shaped hemorrhages typically seen in the superficial retina and round-blot hemorrhages characteristic of those occurring within the deeper retinal layers.
(c) Retinal edema results in a loss of retinal transparency, giving the appearance of an opacity within the retina that blocks the normal red fundus reflex.

iii. **Treatment** is symptomatic.

iv. **Prognosis** varies depending on the location, extent, and severity of the involvement.

d. **Dislocated lens** is the result of tearing of the lens zonules and loss of support for the lens in its normal position. Zonular injury confined to an isolated sector may result in a subluxation or a movement of the lens away from the site of the injury, causing the lens to decenter slightly but otherwise remain in a relatively normal position. More extensive damage may displace the lens entirely, causing it to fall either into the anterior or posterior chamber. Lens dislocation with or without trauma is common in Marfan's syndrome.

i. **Signs and symptoms**
(a) Visual acuity is affected by even the slightest shift in the position of the crystalline lens:
- Lens decentration causes irregular astigmatism.
- Complete dislocation results in the condition of aphakia.

(b) In both cases, a different refractive correction is required to reestablish the visual acuity.

(c) Shifts of lens position, even though slight, can also cause a loss of iris stability and a resulting tremulousness to slight ocular movements or vibrations (iridodonesis).
(d) With significant subluxation, the lens may be displaced to the extent that its edge (equator) may come to lie within the pupillary axis.

ii. **Examination**
(a) The visual acuity may be initially reduced but can frequently be corrected by a change in refraction, which may have changed significantly from the previous correction.
(b) Slit-lamp examination may reveal iris undulations (iridodonesis) at the pupillary margin following rapid eye movements.
(c) Pupillary dilatation can aid in the assessment of the lens position.

iii. **Treatment** is variable and may necessitate surgical removal of the lens.

iv. **Prognosis** varies with the extent of the injury.

e. **Chamber angle recession** describes the appearance of a gross anatomic deepening of the chamber angle as the result of a laceration of the face of the ciliary body, followed by posterior displacement of the ciliary muscles of accommodation. This is generally the result of blunt trauma to the globe causing a sudden increase in pressure within the anterior chamber, which is transmitted to the lens-iris diaphragm, propelling it backward. The dynamics of this injury are similar to that of lens dislocation; however, in angle recession, the lens position is usually normal. Following a blow to the eye, the lens and iris together react in the same fashion as the diaphragm of a drum. The bowing posteriorly results in the angle damage. In a few cases, the force of the injury is sufficient to produce an associated injury to the trabecular meshwork, which may eventually lead to glaucoma.

i. **Signs and symptoms**
(a) In cases in which there is development of glaucoma, the onset is almost invariably delayed from the time of the injury and progresses slowly.
(b) As with other forms of chronic glaucoma, visual loss is insidious, beginning with the peripheral areas of the visual field involved initially.
(c) Angle recession glaucoma should always be suspected in cases of unilateral chronic glaucoma.

ii. **Examination** consists of the usual methods for evaluating chronic glaucoma:
(a) Measurement of intraocular pressure
(b) Visual field examination, with special attention to the classic field defects commonly seen in chronic glaucoma

iii. **Treatment.** Angle recession glaucoma is frequently not responsive to medical therapy and may require surgical treatment.

iv. **Prognosis** varies with:
(a) Extent of the pressure elevation
(b) Length of time it has been present
(c) Responsiveness to treatment

f. **Retinal detachment** is the result of the development of holes or tears within the retinal tissue associated with areas of vitreous body degeneration, liquefaction, and traction. This allows a segment of the retina to separate from the underlying retinal pigment epithelium, producing an immediate loss of visual function within the detached segment. In the absence of treatment, the entire retina eventually becomes involved, and a total retinal detachment develops. Any form of blunt or perforating trauma can produce retinal detachment. Indirect trauma, such as severe head injury, myopia, and vitreous traction, is a risk factor that can affect patients with certain predispositions for detachment.

i. **Signs and symptoms**
   (a) Retinal detachment almost invariably begins at the retinal periphery and results in a positive scotoma (a blind spot perceived by the patient) at the edge of the visual field.
   (b) As the detachment progresses, there may be physical stimulation to the retina, resulting in the visualization of "lightning flashes" or "flying sparks." The enlarging scotoma may be seen as a waving, black curtain encroaching on the central vision.
   (c) If the macular area of the retina becomes involved, the central visual acuity is markedly reduced.

ii. **Examination**
   (a) As areas of detached retina become elevated from the underlying retinal pigment epithelium, the retinal tissue undergoes a loss of transparency (Fig. 7). This results in the inability to visualize the normal underlying choroidal vascular pattern during the ophthalmoscopic examination.
   (b) As the retina becomes more elevated, it is necessary to add additional convex or plus lenses to the ophthalmoscope viewing port to maintain a sharp focus on the internal retinal surface.
   (c) Because detachments begin in the far periphery, it is necessary to dilate the pupil widely to visualize the disorder during its early stages.
   (d) Visual field defects are also present in areas corresponding to the retinal detachment.

iii. **Treatment**
   (a) In cases in which retinal holes or tears exist in the absence of detachment, cryosurgery and laser surgery may be adequate to seal the holes and prevent further progress of the disease.
   (b) Surgical intervention is almost invariably necessary after actual separation of the retina has occurred.

iv. **Prognosis** depends on the extent of the involvement. The chance for recovery of good central vision is generally poor if the retina becomes detached in the area of the macula.

E. **Burns associated with sports injuries** are generally confined to radiation exposure from sunlight. Because of the additive effects of reflection from water surfaces and snow, they are most commonly seen in sports related to this environment. **Ultraviolet radiation burns the conjunctiva and corneal surfaces in the same manner that it does the skin.** The result is necrosis with loss of individual surface epithelial cells and burning injury to the underlying substantia propria (dermis).

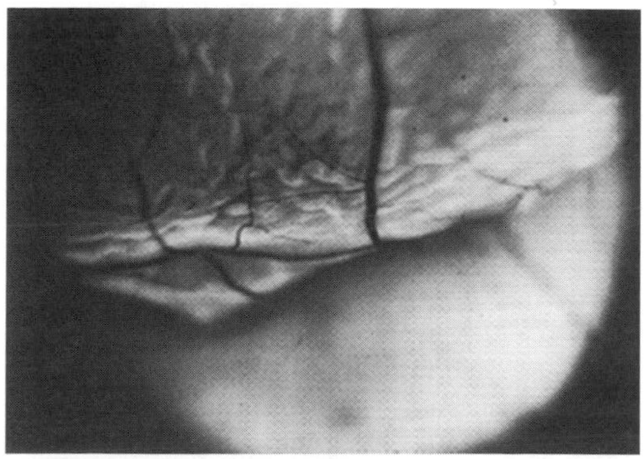

FIGURE 7. Retinal detachment. (From Tucker W: Ophthalmic emergencies. Office Procedures State Art Rev 1(1):106, 1986, with permission.)

1. **Signs and symptoms**
   a. The most prominent signs of ocular burn by ultraviolet light are intense pain and photophobia that develop after a significant delay following exposure.
   b. Visual acuity may be somewhat reduced because of the roughening of the corneal epithelial surface.
   c. Fluorescein stain of the cornea reveals scattered areas of punctate epithelial defects on the surface.
   c. Pain is intense and disproportionately severe in relation to the corneal epithelial involvement.
   e. The relative amount of pain and the delay in the onset of symptoms from the time of exposure are classic signs for ultraviolet burn.
2. **Examination**
   a. Diagnosis confirmed by:
      i. Typical fluorescein staining pattern
      ii. Intense pain
      iii. Photophobia
      iv. History of exposure with delay of onset of symptoms
   b. Because of the severe pain, it may be necessary to use a topical anesthetic to allow the patient to cooperate with the examination.
3. **Treatment**
   a. This is directed toward pain relief and should include:
      i. Systemic analgesics
      ii. Topical corticosteroid preparations
      iii. Cycloplegic drugs
   b. As with other painful corneal disorders secondary to surface damage, the long-term use of topical anesthetic agents is absolutely contraindicated as part of the management plan.
4. **Prognosis** is excellent.

VII. Injury Prevention

A. **Selected excerpts from the International Federation of Sports Medicine Position Statement on Eye Injuries and Eye Protection**
   1. Sports eye injuries are relatively frequent and almost completely preventable.
   2. Loss of sight of any degree has serious financial consequences for both the individual and society.
   3. All athletes should be prescribed eye protection when appropriate to the sport.
   4. One-eyed athletes **must** have a diagnostic evaluation and appropriate eye protection prescribed.
   5. Glass lenses, ordinary plastic lenses, and open eye guards (class III sports eye protectors) **do not** provide adequate protection for those involved in active sports and in some cases may increase the risk for injury both in frequency and in severity.

B. **Classification of eye injury risk in sports when protective eyewear is not used**
   1. **Low risk:** Sports that do not involve a thrown or hit ball, a bat, a stick, or close aggressive play with body contact. Examples:
      a. Track
      b. Field
      c. Swimming
      d. Gymnastics
      e. Rowing
   2. **High risk:** Sports that involve a high-speed ball or puck, use of a bat or stick, or close aggressive play with intentional or unintentional body contact or collision. Adequate eye protective devices are available for these sports.

a. Hockey (ice, field, street)
b. Racquet sports
c. Lacrosse
d. Baseball
e. Football
f. Basketball
g. Handball
h. Soccer
i. Volleyball

3. **Extremely high risk:** Sports that are combative and for which adequate eye protective devices are not available. Functional one-eyed athletes should be discouraged from participation in these sports. Examples:
   a. Boxing
   b. Full-combat karate

C. **Other risk factors for sports eye injuries**
   1. **Physical development and skill level**
      a. Beginners may have an increased risk because of lack of necessary refinement of the skill of the sport.
      b. Advanced players, especially in some high-risk sports, may play more aggressively and be at greater risk for an eye injury.
   2. **Existing visual impairment** increases the risk of injury, especially in activities included in the high-risk and extremely high-risk groups.
   3. **Preexisting eye disease** may present an increased risk factor to athletes in all risk groups.
      a. Conditions that may lead to serious eye disorders or get worse following even minor trauma to the eye include:
         i. Retinal detachment
         ii. Retinal degeneration
         iii. Severe myopia
         iv. Thin sclera
         v. Prior ocular surgery
      b. Systemic eye diseases and previous serious injuries may be risk factors as well.
   4. **The functional one-eyed athlete** is at most serious risk because of the disability that can result from an injury to the remaining eye. Most people with only one normally functioning eye do not appreciate any significant disability in their athletic performance as a result of their vision and thus may not be overly concerned about eye safety. With the exception of extremely high-risk sports, one-eyed athletes should be able to participate safely while using adequate protective eyewear.

D. **Safety aspects of ophthalmic lenses**
   1. All ophthalmic lenses are minimally required by law to withstand the impact of a 5⁄8 inch steel ball dropped from a height of 50 inches
   2. The impact standards differ between dress eyewear and occupational or protective lenses
   3. Occupational and protective lenses additionally require proper frame mounting and radiation absorption protection.

E. **Performance standards for eye protective devices**
   1. Are developed in the following sequence:
      a. A problem is recognized.
      b. The forces are analyzed.
      c. Performance and design standards are set by committee.
      d. Products are widely tested.
      e. Injuries are reduced.
   2. They define the degree of impact resistance as well as the fields and distribution of forces and establish minimal levels of safety for the device.
   3. They result in a device specifically designed for a particular activity. For example, in racquet sports, certain street glasses mounted in a sturdy frame may be adequate for tennis but inadequate for squash or racquetball.

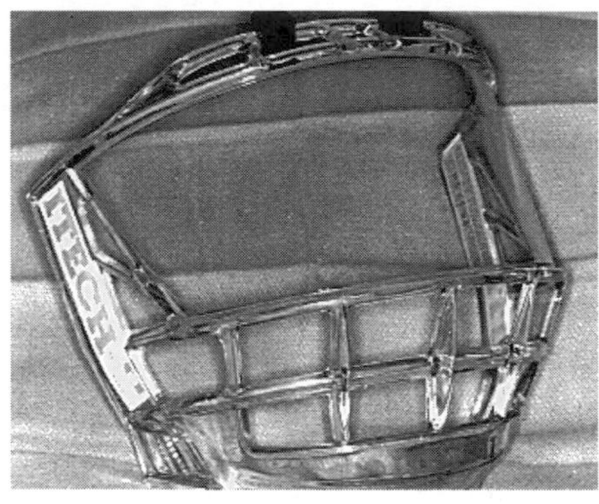

FIGURE 8. Solid face shield with fenestrated mouth guard cast in a single unit. It can be attached to an appropriate helmet and used for goal tending in ice hockey.

F. **Types of eye protectors**

1. **Total head protector**—A combination of helmet and face shield designed to protect the eyes, teeth, jaw, and larynx and transfer forces to the skull. Designed for use in high-risk sports that require total head protection:
   a. Football
   b. Hockey
   c. Lacrosse
2. **Full face protector** (Fig. 8)—Designed for use in conjunction with eye protectors for high-risk sports that do not require protection for the brain:
   a. Fencing
   b. Some positions in baseball and softball
3. **Helmet with separate eye protectors**—For use in sports with low risk for injuries to the lower face and neck:
   a. Cycling
   b. Snowmobiling
   c. Skiing
   d. Automobile racing
   e. Bobsled racing
4. **Helmet only**—These protectors are designed to protect the brain only. They afford little protection to the face or eyes and are used in:
   a. Boxing
   b. Cycling
5. **Sports eye protectors**—Used only to protect the eyes and are recommended in all high-risk sports for which additional head and face protection is impractical:
   a. All racquet sports
   b. Baseball
   c. Soccer
   d. Basketball
   e. Softball
6. **"Sports" sunglasses**—Most are inadequate for both impact resistance and ultraviolet radiation blockage. Adequate eye wear of this type should:
   a. Contain a manufacturer's statement recommending the intended sport
   b. Block light from the sides and below
   c. Protect from glare (transmit < 30% of the light)
   d. Be lightweight, cosmetically acceptable, and aerodynamically designed to prevent drying in the wind

G. **Necessary components for impact safe sports eyewear**

1. Frames that firmly hold and totally encircle the lenses
2. Impact-resistant lenses, made of polycarbonate plastic
3. Strong nose bridge and nose pads firmly attached to the frame

H. **Classification of eye protectors**

1. **Class I:** Face, frame, and lenses are molded as a single unit, with the temples and straps attached separately (Fig. 9)

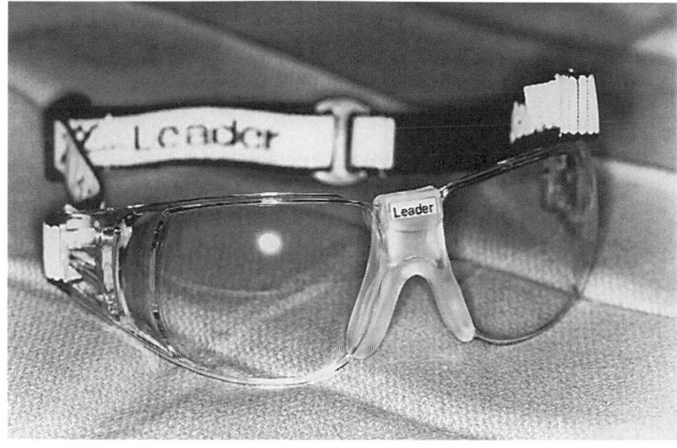

FIGURE 9. Class I eye protector. Frame and lenses are a single unit.

2. **Class II:** The lenses are molded and installed in a frame that is a separate unit (Fig. 10). This presents the risk of the lenses popping out of the frame under certain conditions.
3. **Class III:** Single-unit face frame containing no lenses. This device is **not recommended.**

I. **Classification of spectacles**
1. **Street wear spectacles:** Designed to correct refractive error only and are not recommended for use as sports eye protection
2. **Safety glasses:** When made of polycarbonate plastic and equipped with lear side shields, they generally provide adequate eye protection for high-risk sports.
3. **Sports eye protectors:** Best when designed for a specific sport and made of polycarbonate plastic

J. **Special recommendations for specific sports**
1. **Floor hockey:** When played with a plastic puck or tennis ball, a racquet sports eye protector is probably adequate.

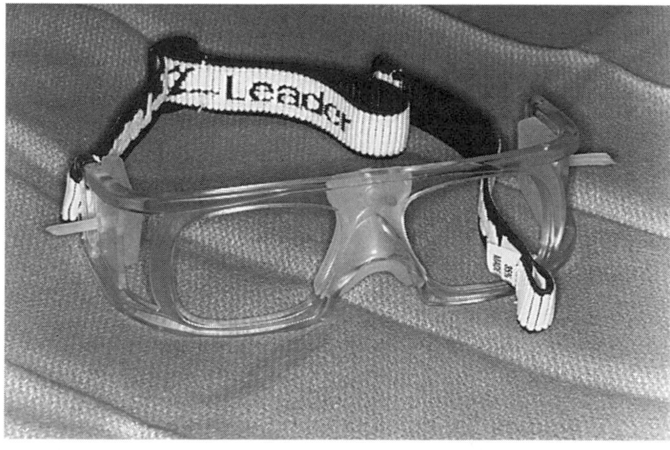

FIGURE 10. Class II eye protector. Lenses are installed into a separate frame.

2. **Soccer:** Contrary to popular belief, balls in excess of 4 inches in diameter *can* cause eye injuries. In fact, most eye injuries that occur with soccer are caused by the ball. Racquet sports eye protection is adequate.
3. **Basketball**: Risk of eye injury is from both the ball and the fingers and elbows. Racquet sports eye protector is adequate.
4. **Baseball:** This is the leading cause of sports eye injuries seen in the emergency department. A racquet sports eye protector is recommended for all players plus a helmet with mouth guard for the batter.
5. **Football:** The standard helmet with face guard is inadequate for eye protection. Racquet sports eye protection worn under the helmet and face mask are strongly recommended for one-eyed players.
6. **Boxing:** There is no adequate method of eye protection. Not recommended for one-eyed athletes.
7. **Karate:** There is no adequate method of eye protection. Not recommended for one-eyed athletes.
8. **Wrestling:** There is no adequate method of eye protection. Not recommended for one-eyed athletes.
9. **Swimming:** "Caution; the eye protector is slippery when wet." There is a risk of blunt injury when adjusting a wet eye protector on the face, so tight elastic bands on these devices should be avoided. In addition, swimmers wearing soft contact lenses have an increased risk of infection. Tight goggles have been reported to elevate the pressure inside the eye.
10. **Sailing:** The predominant risk is reflected solar radiation. Recommend goggles or wraparound ultraviolet-absorbing polycarbonate lenses with or without tint.
11. **Skiing:** The predominant risk is reflected solar radiation. Recommend goggles or wraparound ultraviolet-absorbing polycarbonate lenses with or without tint.
12. **Golf:** Injuries are infrequent but serious. Injuries can be due to impact from the club, impact from the ball, or an explosion of the pressurized liquid center in the ball.
13. **Cycling:** There are a variety of risks from dust, dirt, tree branches, and solar radiation. Recommend a bike helmet and polycarbonate ultraviolet absorbing lenses.
14. **Snowmobile:** Recommend a helmet and full face mask.
15. **Mountain climbing:** There are a variety of risks from solar radiation as well as retinal hemorrhages from hypoxia and increased intravascular pressure. Recommend glasses or goggles that block 90% of the ultraviolet light below 320 nm. It is important that there be adequate protection from the sides and below.

Recommended Reading

1. American Society of Testing and Materials: Eye protectors for use by players of racket sports, standard specification F803-85. Philadelphia, American Society of Testing and Materials, 1983.
2. Bishop PJ: Head protection in sports with particular application to ice hockey. Ergonomics 19:451, 1976.
3. Burke MJ, Sanitato JJ, Vinger PF, et al: Soccer ball induced eye injuries. JAMA 219:2682, 1983.
4. Canadian Standards Association: Racket sports eye protection, preliminary standard P400-M1982. Toronto, Canadian Standards Association, 1982.
5. Hulse WF: Sports equipment standards. In Vinger PF, Hoerner EF (eds): Sports Injuries: The Unthwarted Epidemic. Littleton, MA, PSG, 1981.
6. Joselo MM: Goggles increase eye pressure. Phys Sportsmed 11:16, 1983.
7. Keeney AH: Prevention of eye injuries. In Freeman HM (ed): Ocular Trauma. New York, Appleton-Century-Crofts, 1979, p 337.
8. Legwold G: Pterygium found in Olympic sailors. Phys Sportsmed 11:23, 1983.
9. Leibson J, Burton TC, Scott WE: Orbital floor fractures: A retrospective study. Ann Ophthalmol 8:1057, 1983.
10. Meyer C: Preparticipation health evaluation. In Smith N (ed): Sports Medicine: Health Care for Young Athletes. Evanston IL, American Academy of Pediatrics, 1983, p 75.

11. Millar GT: Golfing eye injuries. Am J Ophthalmol 64:741, 1967.
12. O'Grady R, Shoch D: Golfball granuloma of the eyelids and conjunctiva. Am J Ophthalmol 76:148, 1973.
13. Pashby TJ: Eye injuries in hockey. Int Ophthalmol Clin 21(4):59, 1981.
14. Schneider RC, Antine BE: Visual field impairment related to football headgear and face guards. JAMA 192:120, 1965.
15. Stein H: Swimming with soft contact lenses. Contact Lens J 10:10, 1976.
16. Vinger PF: Preventing ocular injuries. Am Orthop J 32:56, 1982.
17. Vinger PF: The incidence of eye injuries in sports. Ophthalmol Clin 21(4):21, 1981.
18. Vinger PF: Eye injuries. In Vinger PF, Hoerner EF (eds): Sports Injuries: The Unthwarted Epidemic. Littleton, MA, PSG, 1981.
19. Vinger PF, Knuttgen HG, Easterbrook M, et al: International Federation of Sports Medicine position statement: Eye injuries and eye protection in sports. Phys Sportsmed 16:49, 1988.
20. Vinger PF, Tolpin DW: Racket sports: An ocular hazard. JAMA 239:2575, 1978.
21. Wilkerson JA (ed): Medicine for Mountaineering. Seattle, The Mountaineers, 1967.

42

Maxillofacial Injuries

Harold K. Tu, M.D., DMD, Leon F. Davis, M.D., DDS and Thomas A. Nique, M.D., DDS

I. General Considerations

A. Injuries of the maxillofacial region are **common in sports**, especially when protective head and mouth gear are not worn. The injuries may be classified into **three major categories:**
   1. Soft tissue injuries
   2. Dentoalveolar trauma
   3. Facial skeletal trauma

B. Overall treatment objectives are the restoration of function and facial appearance. Treatment priorities should be consistent with:
   1. Maintaining airway
   2. Control of hemorrhage
   3. Treatment of shock
   4. Management of associated injuries (e.g., cervical spine)
   5. Definitive care of facial injuries

C. Rehabilitation after definitive treatment varies with the type of injury as well as the type of sport to be resumed. Rehabilitation time is naturally prolonged in boxing.

II. History

A. Document the history of the injury and all related clinical findings, including the cause of the trauma (e.g., baseball, hockey stick).

B. Take a complete medical history with special attention to medications and allergies.

III. Initial Care

The primary considerations are maintenance of airway, prevention of shock (although rare from facial injuries) through prompt hemorrhage control, and assessment and management of loss of consciousness. Early physical examination and continuous neurologic evaluation are essential.

A. **Airway maintenance**
   1. In the conscious patient, without evidence of neck injury, this can be accomplished by sitting the patient upright and slightly forward.
   2. Blood clots, vomitus, and foreign objects (dentures) may be cleared by sweeping a finger deep into the back of the throat.
   3. Maintaining airway in the unconscious patient or patient with suspected cervical spine injury requires the use of appropriate airway techniques in conjunction with appropriate cervical spine stabilization. These techniques should be performed by those with proper training.
      a. Jaw thrust
      b. Oral airway
      c. Nasoendotracheal tube
      d. Coniotomy or tracheostomy

B. **Hemorrhage** is sometimes difficult to control because of the abundant blood supply in the maxillofacial region. Direct pressure and prevention of airway obstruction is the initial treatment.

C. **Cervical spine injuries** must be suspected in all athletes with significant maxillofacial injuries or who are unconscious. Constant cervical traction or use of sandbags or cervical collar with tape stabilization to a back board to immobilize the neck during any manipulation or transportation is required. Cervical collars should be used by those with proper training.

IV. Physical Assessment of Injuries

A. **Cervical spine injuries.** Check for:
   1. Neck pain
   2. Neurologic deficits (motor or sensory)
   3. Limitation of motion

B. **Laryngeal injuries.** Check for:
   1. Change in voice (usually hoarseness)
   2. Cervical emphysema (subcutaneous air)
   3. Loss of thyroid cartilage prominence (Adam's apple)

C. **Facial injuries**
   1. Signs and symptoms
      a. Laceration
      b. Discomfort
      c. Edema (swelling)
      d. Ecchymosis (bruising)
      e. Gross deformity
   2. Visual inspection
      a. Facial asymmetry
      b. Areas of swelling
      c. Discoloration
      d. Obvious deformity
   3. Assess the occlusion or bite of the teeth.
   4. Bimanual manipulation of the facial bones can show areas of bone discontinuity and mobility.
   5. Suspected upper jaw fracture can be diagnosed by grasping the upper teeth and determining evidence of gross movement of the upper jaw and midface.
   6. Assess jaw opening and determine if it is associated with pain, limitation, or deviation.

D. **Radiographs**
   1. Anteroposterior and lateral cervical spine views should be obtained before other radiographs unless there is a life-threatening injury to determine cervical spine fractures.
   2. Other views
      a. Oblique evaluates:
         i. Mandible
         ii. Lower third of the face
      b. Panoramic evaluates:
         i. Mandible
         ii. Teeth
         iii. Maxillary sinus
         iv. Condyle
      c. Lateral evaluates the nasal bones
      d. Submental evaluates the zygomatic arch
      e. Waters' evaluates:
         i. Maxilla
         ii. Zygoma
         iii. Sinuses
         iv. Orbits
   3. **Special imaging techniques.** Tomograms, computed tomography (CT) scan, and nuclear magnetic resonance may provide additional information at the discretion of the consultant.

V. Soft Tissue Injuries

A. **Incidence.** Injuries to soft tissues of the scalp, forehead, cheeks, nose, lips, and internal structures of the mouth constitute some of the most common sports injuries. Not surprisingly, ice hockey, squash, and racquetball lead in the frequency of facial soft tissue injuries, but no sport is immune, including swimming.

B. **Mechanisms of injury**
   1. Athlete is struck by a wayward projectile
      a. Hockey puck
      b. Baseball
   2. Athlete is struck with other athletic equipment
      a. Hockey sticks
      b. Squash racquets
      c. Face guards or helmets
      d. Shoe cleats
   3. Athlete strikes a stationary object
      a. Diving board
      b. Basketball backboard
      c. Hockey cage
   4. Athlete has contact with another body
      a. Faces
      b. Elbows
      c. Knees
      d. Fingers

C. **Prevention.** Many of these injuries could be prevented with proper protection, such as face masks in hockey or racquetball. The use of mouth guards, primarily designed to prevent injuries to the teeth and jaws, are also effective in minimizing soft tissue injuries around the mouth and tongue.

D. **Classifications**
   1. Contusion
   2. Abrasion
   3. Laceration, including punctures

E. **Examination**
   1. The area of injury is readily apparent, particularly if bleeding is occurring. It is important to remember that **any trauma severe enough to injure the soft tissues may also have injured the underlying bony structure.**
   2. Hemorrhage is controlled with the application of pressure, using sterile gauze 4 × 4s. Once the hemorrhage has been controlled and hemostasis is present, the wound should be inspected.
   3. The wound should be thoroughly cleaned, making sure to remove any debris by irrigation with saline.

F. **Treatment**
   1. Contusions are easily treated by applying an ice pack.
   2. Abrasions are treated by thoroughly cleansing the area, applying an antibiotic ointment, and then a gauze dressing.
   3. As a temporizing measure, minor lacerations may be stabilized with Steri-strips, then protected with an occlusive dressing of gauze and tape.
   4. Because lacerations and abrasions of the facial area are cosmetically serious, appropriate medical attention is needed to minimize disfiguring scarring.
   5. Lacerations of the face must be sutured. Suture no larger than 5–0 is mandatory. Care should be taken that deep wounds are closed in appropriate layers.
   6. Lacerations of the lip that cross the vermilion border and are not repaired appropriately can result in significant disfiguring scars. With the laceration closure, it is extremely important that the vermilion border be properly aligned.
   7. Almost all lacerations can be closed with local anesthesia.
   8. Intraoral lacerations deserve the same attention as facial lacerations.

G. **Athletic restrictions**
   1. If the laceration is minor and can be stabilized well with Steri-strips or temporary sutures, then the athlete may return to competition with definitive treatment delayed until completion of the contest, provided that the wound is completely protected with an occlusive dressing.
   2. Subsequent participation requires similar protection until healing is complete.

3. External lacerations in swimmers require a waterproof dressing if further participation that day is desired.

VI. Dentoalveolar Injuries

A. **Description:** Dentoalveolar injuries involve the teeth and supporting structures.

B. **Mechanism of injury**

1. Anterior teeth usually bear the brunt of most sports-related injuries (e.g., bat, balls, hockey pucks). Individual teeth may be luxated (loosened), partially or totally avulsed (come out), intruded, or fractured.
2. Lacerations of the face, lips, and mucosa are often present; despite their sometimes extensive appearance, careful debridement and meticulous closure achieves anatomic reapproximation and minimal scarring.
3. Panoramic radiograph may be the most useful, but additional dental films can provide more detail. Chest films and lateral neck films, if debris is suspected to be lodged in the throat area, should be obtained if an avulsed tooth cannot be found because aspiration into lungs is possible.

C. **Examination**

1. Regional examination to rule out other facial injuries.
2. Intraoral examination to determine the presence of missing and fractured teeth, lacerations, and foreign objects (e.g., gravel).

D. **Treatment**

1. Most dentoalveolar injuries can be prevented with the use of proper face and mouth guards. Custom mouth guards (preferred) can be fabricated by a dentist, or commercial mouth guards are available in most sport stores.
2. Repair the dentoalveolar damage before management of facial or lip lacerations.
3. **The reimplantation of a recently avulsed tooth should always be attempted.** How an athlete or trainer handles the avulsed tooth can have a significant impact on the overall prognosis.
   a. Handle the tooth by the crown. Do not rub it to remove dirt.
   b. Gently rinse the tooth in saline or tap water to remove blood and dirt.
   c. Replace the tooth in the socket and bite down on a gauze to keep the tooth in place. Refer to a dentist. If a tooth cannot be replaced in the socket quickly, then place in a cup of warm, mild salt water, the patient's saliva, or milk. With an adult, the tooth can be placed under the tongue or in the cheek pouch.
   d. Most alveolar (tooth-bearing bone) fractures can usually be reduced with digital pressure and stabilized by using a splint.
   e. The mouth guard is an excellent splint if it has not been distorted.
   f. Antibiotics are indicated when teeth are avulsed. Penicillin is the antibiotic of choice: Penicillin-VK, 500 mg, orally four times a day for ten days.
   g. Antitetanus prophylaxis should be considered when the tooth has contacted soil and the athlete's immunization has been 5 years or longer. Tetanus toxoid 0.5 ml should be given.

E. **Athletic restrictions**

1. Contact drills or competition should be restricted during the period when the patient is in stabilization splint, generally 2 or 3 weeks.
2. Appropriate face and mouth guards should be worn to prevent further injury.
3. If it is imperative for the athlete to return to competition before complete healing, special protective devices and shields may be custom fabricated.

VII. Nasal Fractures

A. **Description:** Isolated nasal fractures are the most common sports-related facial fracture and may be the most commonly injured structure of the face (Fig. 1).

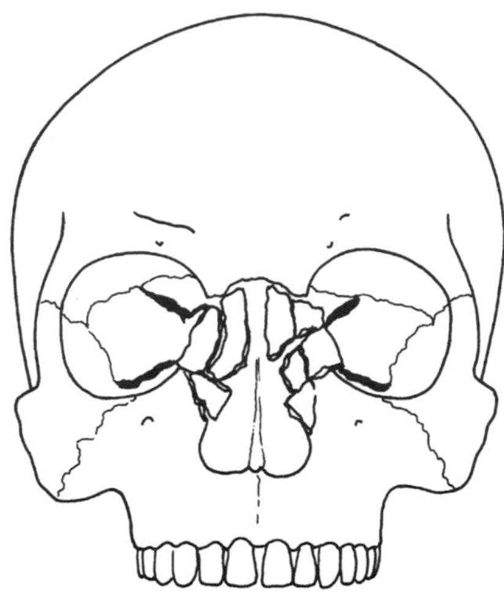

FIGURE 1. Frontal view of the skull showing common isolated nasal fractures.

B. **Mechanism of injury**
   1. The prominence of the nose and its low impact tolerance make it especially susceptible to sports injury.
   2. Nasal injuries are seen particularly in contact sports.
      a. Basketball
      b. Rugby
      c. Football
      d. Boxing
   3. The fracture most commonly seen in sports injuries is lateral displacement of the nasal bones.
   4. The severity may range from slightly depressed greenstick fracture (commonly seen in adolescents and younger children) to displacement or disruption of the bony and cartilaginous components of the nose.

C. **Examination**
   1. **Signs and symptoms**
      a. Epistaxis (nosebleed)
      b. Nasal airway obstruction
      c. Nasal asymmetry
      d. Crepitus (crackling) over nasal bridge
      e. Possible periorbital and subconjunctival ecchymosis
      f. Possible cerebrospinal fluid leak
      g. Septal deformity
      h. Septal hematoma (possible)
   2. **Radiographs**
      a. Waters' view
      b. Posteroanterior and lateral skull
      c. Nasal bone films

D. **Treatment**
   1. Control nasal hemorrhage with pressure or intranasal packing
   2. If septal hematoma present, must be drained
   3. Protect from further injury and refer
   4. Nondisplaced or minimally displaced nasal fractures can be treated with closed reduction and intranasal packing with external splinting. Complex nasal fractures may require open reduction and internal fixation.

E. **Athletic restrictions**
   1. Workouts and strenuous exercises are restricted while the patient has intranasal packing, usually 3 to 4 days.
   2. The athlete should be restricted to noncontact drills and competition for the first 3 to 4 weeks. Protective headgear should be worn for 2 to 3 months and can be custom fabricated.

VIII. Maxillary Fractures

A. **Description:** These fractures, also known as midface fractures, essentially involve the upper jaw and associated bony structures. They are classified as LeFort I, II, and III fractures depending on if the nasal or cheek bones are involved (Fig. 2).

B. **Mechanism of injury**
   1. Usually involves a direct blow to the middle portion of the face. This can occur from:
      a. Hockey stick
      b. Bat
      c. Punch
      d. Projectile such as a ball
      e. Collision
   2. Any sport with these potentials is a risk, although these fractures are uncommon.

C. **Examination**
   1. **Common signs and symptoms**
      a. Lengthening of face
      b. Mobility of maxilla and midface
      c. Open bite deformity—malocclusion (teeth apart in front)
      d. Ecchymosis (bruising) in buccal vestibule
      e. Epistaxis (nosebleed)
      f. Nasal deformity
      g. Flattening and splaying of the naso-orbital region
   2. **Radiographs**
      a. Waters' view
      b. Posteroanterior and lateral skull
      c. CT scan or magnetic resonance imaging (MRI)

D. **Treatment**
   1. **Temporary**
      a. The patency of airway is of primary concern in these injuries, followed by rapid transfer for definitive diagnosis and treatment. The airway in a conscious patient

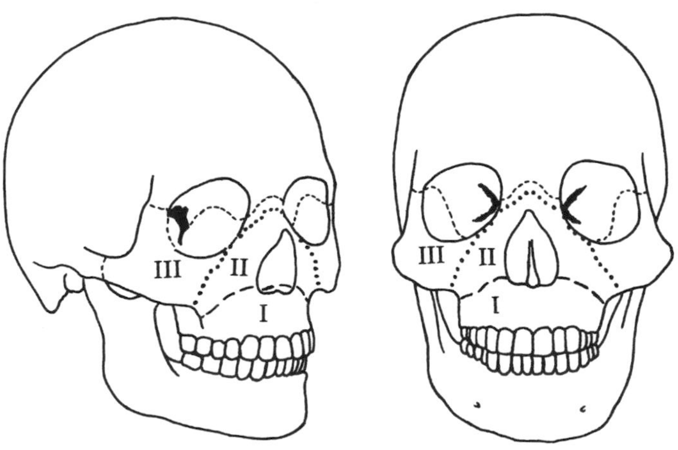

FIGURE 2. Left and frontal views of the skull showing Le Fort I, II, and III fractures of the upper jaw.

may be best managed in a forward-sitting position allowing dependent drainage of saliva and blood to occur externally.

b. A cervical spine injury should be suspected and precautions taken (see page 427).

c. Nasal packing for bleeding is discouraged unless cerebrospinal leakage can be ruled out.

2. **Definitive treatment** involves reduction, fixation, and immobilization of the fractures (see page 433). Complex midface fractures may require extensive surgery and possibly secondary reconstruction.
3. **Rehabilitation** is similar to mandibular fractures (see following).

IX. Mandibular Fractures (lower third of face fractures)

A. **Description:** Mandibular fractures are the third most common facial bone fractures related to sports injury. They involve the lower third of the facial skeleton and are classified by their anatomic location (Fig. 3) and whether they are simple, comminuted, or compounded in nature.

B. **Mechanism of injury**

1. Participants in sports in which the face is exposed or involved are susceptible to injury, especially if protective devices are not worn.
   a. Basketball
   b. Hockey
   c. Boxing
   d. Skiing
   e. Motor sports
   f. Football
2. Mandibular fractures are usually not isolated. More than half of the patients have multiple fractures.
3. The anatomic region of the mandible where fracture is most likely to occur obviously depends on the direction and amount of the force, but most commonly the mandibular angle and condyle are involved.

C. **Examination**

1. **Common signs and symptoms**
   a. Change in the bite
   b. Mobility of mandible in segments
   c. Pain on function
   d. Inability to chew or open mouth widely
   e. Numbness or change in sensation of the lower lip
   f. Bruising of gums and floor of mouth
   g. Deviation of lower jaw on opening
2. **Radiographs**
   a. Panorex
   b. Lateral obliques of mandibular angles

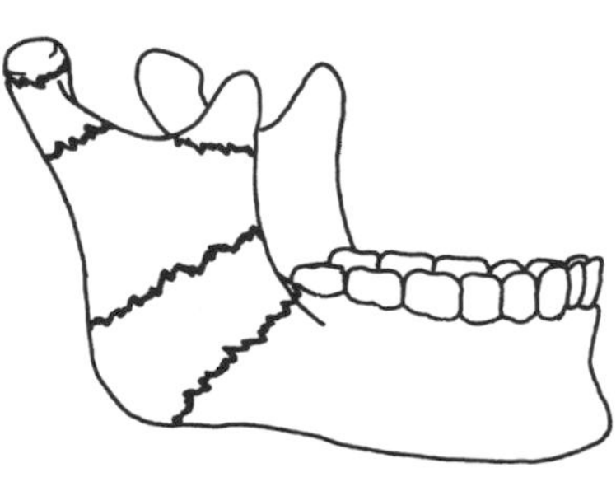
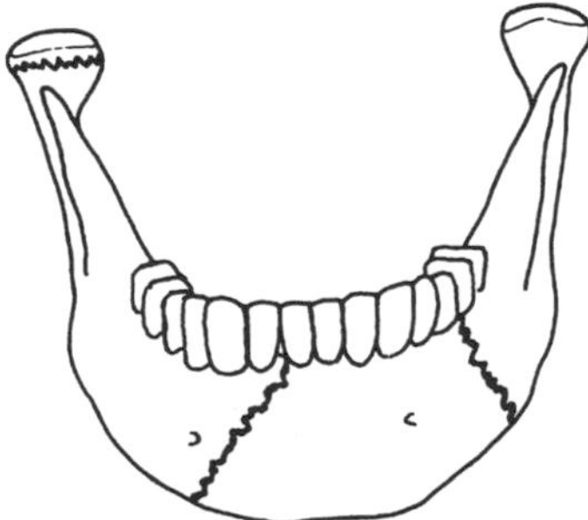

FIGURE 3. Left and frontal views of the mandible showing common mandibular fractures or an injury to the temporomandibular joint.

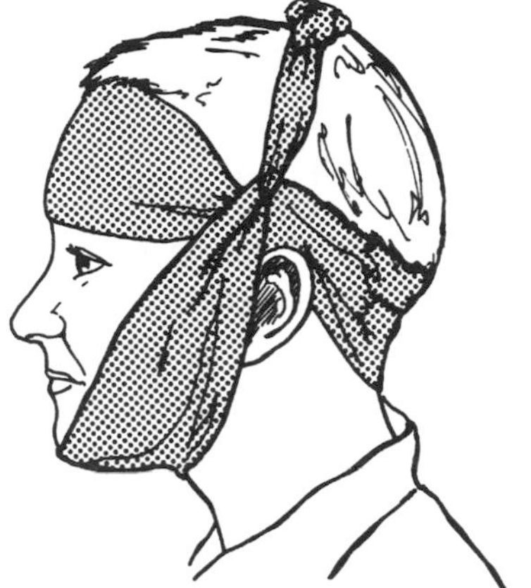

FIGURE 4. Barton (barrel) bandage for temporary immobilization in the treatment of a mandibular fracture or an injury to the temporomandibular joint.

c. Posteroanterior mandible
d. Towne's view

D. **Treatment**

1. **Reduction, fixation, and stabilization** are the principles of fracture management.
   a. Temporary immobilization can be obtained by a Barton (barrel) bandage (Fig. 4) or Ace wrap from under the chin around the occiput. In most cases, this is adequate stabilization until definitive care can be provided.
   b. **Definitive treatment** in most cases involves reduction and appropriate fixation of the fracture. The use of intermaxillary fixation (wiring jaws together) continues to be a common technique. Indicated use of rigid internal fixation (bone plates), however, obviates the need for intermaxillary fixation. This is especially advantageous for those athletes wanting to return to their sport at the earliest opportunity.
2. **Rehabilitation**
   a. May be delayed for 4–6 weeks when the jaws are immobilized
   b. As is true with all patients (mandibular or maxillary) with intermaxillary fixation (wired jaws), during the healing period **a high-protein, carbohydrate liquid diet is required.** Close monitoring of the patient's weight loss is required, and a 5–10% weight loss is commonly seen. Weight loss exceeding 10% requires further nutritional supplementation.
   c. During the period of intermaxillary fixation, activities such as weightlifting, running, and contact workouts should be avoided because it may be difficult to breathe and the fractures may be displaced. **Repetitive mild activities** such as stationary bicycling, swimming, and use of light weights to maintain muscle tone and conditioning are recommended.
   d. Once the jaws are unwired, the athlete can resume training with minimal restrictions. **Resumption of direct contact sports**, e.g., boxing or football, **should be delayed** an additional 1–2 months, with special headgear customized to provide further protection to the athlete.
   e. **Physical therapy** to improve jaw opening is recommended.
   f. The alternative to intermaxillary jaw wiring is the use of direct bone plating. When bone plates are used, rehabilitation may begin as early as 10–14 days after surgery with return to full activity 1 month earlier.

E. **Mandibular condyle fractures (in most cases associated with mandibular fractures)**

1. **Common signs and symptoms**
   a. Tenderness and pain in the preauricular area (front of the ear), especially on mouth opening

   b. Deviation of the jaw
   c. Limitation of jaw motion
   d. Change in the bite
2. **Radiographs**
   a. Panorex
   b. Towne's
   c. Lateral obliques mandible
   d. Tomograms of the condyle
3. **Treatment**—See page 433. The period of intermaxillary fixation (wired jaw) is usually 2–3 weeks.
4. **Rehabilitation**
   a. These patients require a much shorter period of immobilization, approximately 2–3 weeks, and early physical therapy is required to prevent joint ankylosis.
   b. Close follow-up is especially important in children and adolescents because condylar injury may affect their jaw growth (see page 437).

X. Zygomatic Complex Fractures

A. **Description:** Zygomatic complex fractures (cheekbone) occur as the result of a force striking the prominence of the zygomatic bone (Fig. 5).

B. **Mechanism of injury**
1. This is the second most common facial bone fracture seen in sports-related injuries. Injury is caused by a direct blow, such as a hockey stick, bat, baseball, head butt, to the cheekbone.
2. Classification of this type of fracture is based on displacement and severity of the fracture.
3. Because the zygomatic complex is intimately associated with the orbit, evaluate for ocular injuries.

C. **Examination**
1. **Common signs and symptoms**
   a. Flatness of the cheek
   b. Limited mandibular opening
   c. Paresthesia or anesthesia (numbness) of the affected cheek
   d. Periorbital edema (swelling) and ecchymosis (bruising) or emphysema (air in tissue)
   e. Subconjunctival hemorrhage
   f. Enophthalmos (eye sunken in)
   g. Diplopia (double vision)

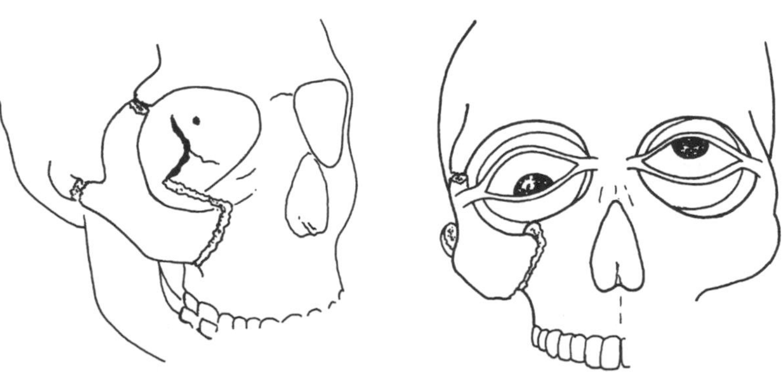

FIGURE 5. Left and frontal views showing zygomatic complex fracture.

h. Step defects (bone discontinuity) at inferior and lateral orbital rims and zygomatic buttress
i. Intraoral buccal (inside cheeks) ecchymosis (bruising)
j. Limitation of ocular movement
k. Pupillary level discrepancy

2. **Radiographs**
   a. Waters' view
   b. Submental vertex
   c. Posteroanterior and lateral skull
   d. CT of head or orbital apex tomograms are indicated when there is suspected ocular injury.

D. **Treatment**
1. Protect from further injury and transfer for definitive care.
2. Fractures of the zygomatic bone are usually reduced readily. The fractured complex is elevated into position through various approaches (intraoral or temporal), and the zygomatic bone reduces into place and remains stable.
3. Healing is usually complete in 6–8 weeks. Special headgear designed to protect the cheekbone should be worn for 3–4 months. Visual problems such as diplopia (double vision) may be a complication of zygomatic fractures. Athletes involved in sports requiring eye-hand coordination such as baseball, tennis, racquetball, or motor sports, may suffer delay in return of their previous skill level. Any visual problems should be evaluated by an ophthalmologist.

XI. Orbital Floor Fracture (blowout fracture). See also pages 414–415.

A. **Description:** This is an isolated fracture of the orbital floor (eye socket). It is a rare fracture involving a segment of orbital floor (bone) and a portion of the periorbita (eye fat) into the maxillary sinus with or without muscle entrapment. The orbital rim is intact in a pure blowout fracture (Fig. 6).

B. **Mechanism of injury**
1. Injury is caused by a rapid increase in intraorbital pressure.
2. The force is usually a blunt object (tennis ball, racquetball) directed at the globe and lids that is only slightly larger than the inlet.
3. The sudden increase in pressure fractures the bony orbit at areas of weakness, usually along the orbital floor.

C. **Examination**
1. **Common signs and symptoms**
   a. Decreased mobility of the globe (ability to look around)
   b. Diplopia (double vision)

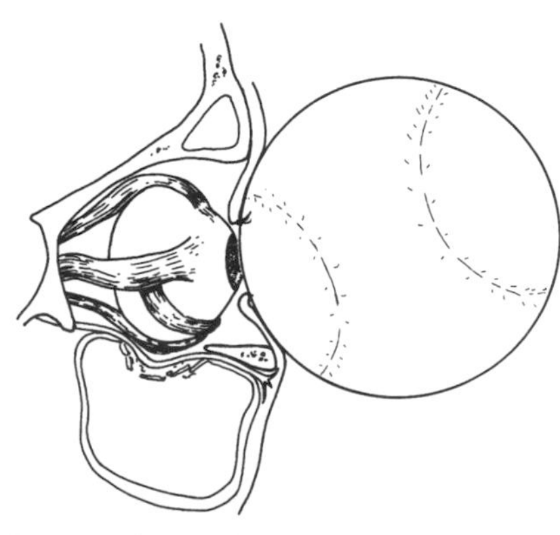

FIGURE 6. Orbital floor fracture (blowout fracture) caused by the force of the baseball striking the eye. The orbital rim is left intact.

c. Periorbital edema, ecchymosis, or emphysema
d. Subconjunctival ecchymosis (bruising)
e. Enophthalmos (eye sunken in)
f. Unilateral epistaxis (nose bleeding)
g. Unequal pupillary level

2. **Radiographs**
   a. Waters' view
   b. CT scanning of the orbit and maxillary sinus

D. **Treatment**
1. **Immediate**—protect from further injury and refer for definitive care.
2. **Definitive care** may require open exploration from a lower lid incision with reconstruction of orbital floor.
3. **Rehabilitation** is similar to zygomatic complex fractures.

XII. Temporomandibular Joint Injuries

A. The **temporomandibular joint** is a sliding hinge joint and articulates the mandibular condyle and temporal bone of the skull. It is functionally associated with the dentition and contralateral joint. The joint is separated into upper and lower compartments by a fibrocartilage meniscus. The joint is stabilized by ligaments.

B. **Mechanism of injury.** Injury can result from any blow to the mandible due to forces being transmitted to the condyle.
1. Hemarthrosis (intracapsular bleeding)
2. Capsulitis (inflammation of the capsular ligaments)
3. Internal derangement (meniscal displacement)
4. Subluxation/dislocation (condylar displacement with or without voluntary reduction)
5. Fracture (see page 433–434)

C. **Examination**
1. **Common signs and symptoms**
   a. Limitation of opening (normal > 40 mm)
   b. Deviation to the side of injury on opening
   c. Pain on opening and biting
   d. Malocclusion (change in bite)
   e. Joint noise (clicking, popping, crepitus)
   f. Unable to close (dislocation and meniscus displacement)
2. **Radiographs**
   a. Panoramic and Towne's view
   b. MRI or temporomandibular joint arthrogram to evaluate meniscal displacement

D. **Treatment**
1. Temporary immobilization can be accomplished with an Ace bandage wrapped around the chin over top of the head (see Fig. 4), although this is generally not needed.
2. Limitation of opening for 7–10 days
3. Soft diet
4. Moist heat to the area
5. Aspirin or acetaminophen, 650 mg, orally every 4 hours for 7–10 days, or ibuprofen, 600 mg, orally four times a day for 7–10 days.
6. Dislocation can be reduced manually by grasping each side of the jaw with the thumb hooked inside the mouth (away from the teeth) and exerting firm downward and posterior force (Fig. 7). In some cases, a local anesthetic injection of the joint, sedation with midazolam (Versed), 3 to 5 mg, or general anesthetic may be required.

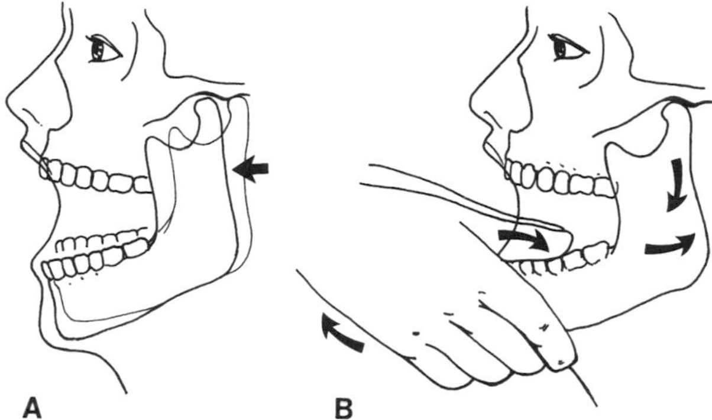

FIGURE 7. A, Temporomandibular joint dislocation. **B,** Manual reduction. Using both hands, hook thumbs inside the mouth, away from the teeth, and exert firm downward and posterior force. Anesthetic may be necessary.

E. **Rehabilitation**
  1. Physiotherapy consists of repetitive, passive opening exercises using tongue blades as an aid. The gradual addition of tongue blades increases the opening and documents the progress.
  2. Thermotherapy, coolant therapy, electrical stimulation, massage, and relaxation therapy can all be useful adjunctive therapy.

F. **Athletic restrictions**
  1. Following acute injury, physical contact activities should be restricted until acute signs and symptoms have diminished, usually in 7–10 days.
  2. Heavy weightlifting should be restricted during the acute period.
  3. Athletes taking muscle relaxants should be restricted from workouts and competition.
  4. Athletes undergoing arthroscopy should follow the same restrictions as those suffering from acute injury.
  5. Athletes undergoing arthroplasty can usually expect 4- to 6-week recovery before returning to contact activities and competition.

Recommended Reading

1. Converse J: Reconstructive Plastic Surgery, vol 2, 2nd ed. Philadelphia, W.B. Saunders, 1964.
2. Hawkins RW, Lyne ED: Skateboarding fractures. Am J Sports Med 9:99, 1981.
3. Kendrick RW: Some "sporting" injuries. Int J Oral Surg 2(suppl 109):245, 1981.
4. Koplik B, Koplik M: Mouthguards prevent most oral injuries in contact sports. N Y J Dent 44:84, 1974.
5. Morton JG, Burton JF: An evaluation of the effectiveness of mouthguards in high-school rugby players. N Z Dent J 75:151, 1979.
6. Rowe NL, Killey HC: Fractures of the Facial Skeleton, 2nd ed. Edinburgh, Churchill-Livingstone, 1968.
7. Rowe NL, Williams JL: Maxillofacial Injuries, vol 1. New York, Churchill-Livingstone, 1985.

43

Shoulder Injuries

Kirk S. Hutton, M.D., and Michele J. Julin, M.S., PAC

I. History

Historical information is invaluable in the investigation of a shoulder problem. A specific diagnosis can be obtained if the examining physician asks the appropriate questions and carefully listens as the patient explains his or her symptoms. The following areas should be queried:

A. Specific sport in which injury occurred
B. Specific activity
C. Chronic (overuse) vs. traumatic (acute)
D. Do symptoms increase with activity and/or improve with rest?
E. Sensation of instability of the shoulder: "Has the shoulder ever slipped out or felt like it could slip out of place?"
F. Weakness
G. Pain—character and location as well as incidence of night pain
H. Crepitation
I. Radicular symptoms

II. Physical Examination

A. **Inspection/observation:** Look for obvious deformities when comparing injured shoulder to normal shoulder.
   1. Note **abnormalities** involving the humeral head position, clavicle alignment, including the AC (acromial clavicular) joint, SC (sternoclavicular) joint, and scapular rhythm and winging of the scapula.
   2. Significant **muscle atrophy** may indicate nerve damage or disuse atrophy secondary to a rotator cuff tear or pain. Atrophy may be identified in deltoid, trapezius, supraspinatus, and infraspinatus muscles.
   3. Overall **appearance of skin** on affected shoulder should be examined for swelling, ecchymosis, color changes, and venous distension.

B. **Palpation:** Palpate shoulder to identify areas of significant pain.
   1. Biceps tendon is directly anterior with arm in approximately 10° of internal rotation.
   2. With arm extended, greater tuberosity is brought anteriorly and is easily palpated.
   3. Lesser tuberosity is just medial to biceps tendon and is palpated as humerus is internally and externally rotated.
   4. Other areas—coracoid, coracoacromial ligament, acromion, and scapula, to include its body, superior and medial borders, and spine
   5. While palpating shoulder during active and passive motion, note crepitation that may originate from the AC joint, glenohumeral joint, subacromial bursa, or subscapular bursa.
   6. Palpate spinous processes of cervical spine for **tenderness** which may indicate cervical spine pathology as a cause of shoulder pain.

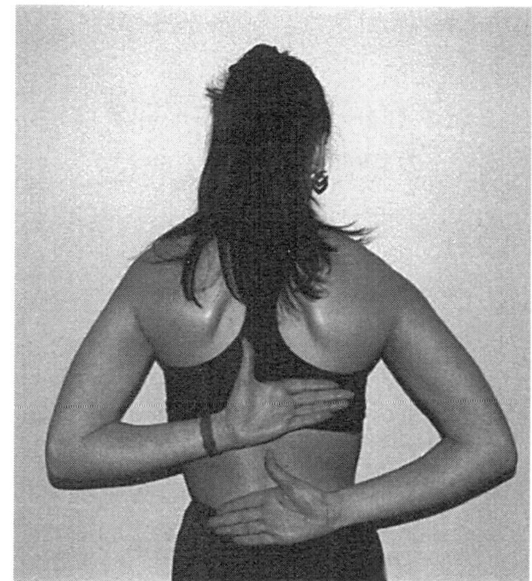

FIGURE 1. Internal rotation of the shoulder is best determined by measuring the height that the thumb reaches on the vertebral body. It is important to compare the right side with the left side.

C. **Movement**
   1. Compare active and passive range of motion of injured shoulder with normal extremity.
   2. Document ranges of forward flexion, extension, abduction, adduction, internal rotation, and external rotation. All motions are determined as degrees from neutral position, except for internal rotation, which is best described by indicating vertebral body level at which thumb reaches up back (Fig. 1).
   3. Note whether motion causes pain or if any signs of apprehension or subluxation are identified.
   4. Motion of cervical spine should be noted in flexion, extension, rotation, and lateral bending.

D. **Manual muscle testing**
   1. **Supraspinatus**—mainly responsible for abduction
      a. Position patient's arm in 70° of abduction, 30° of forward flexion, and internal rotation so that thumb points down (Fig. 2).
      b. Examiner pushes arm downward against resistance.
      c. Pain and weakness are considered positive for supraspinatus tendinitis or tearing. Routinely, severe pain and weakness are associated with complete tears.

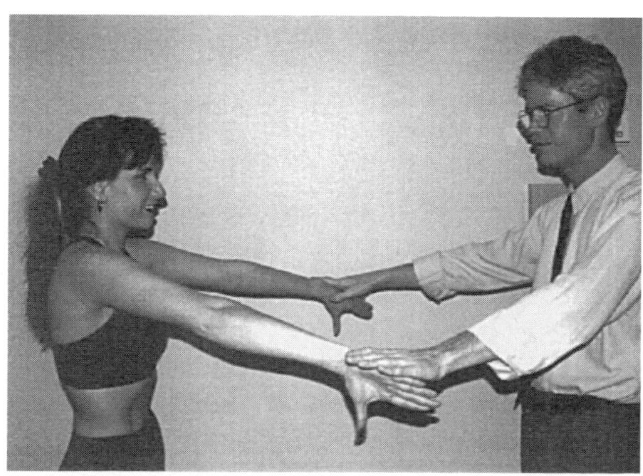

FIGURE 2. Supraspinatus strength is tested by having the patient abduct the arms approximately 70° with slight forward flexion and thumbs pointing down. The patient attempts to elevate the arms against examiner resistance.

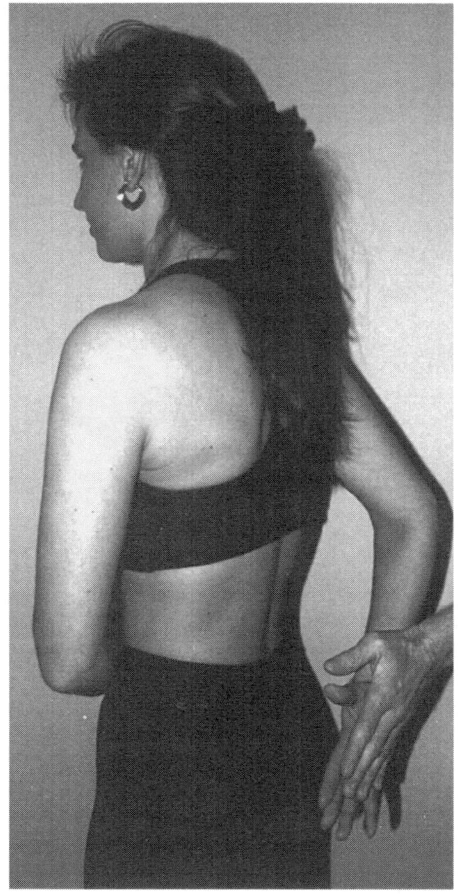

FIGURE 3. In the "lift-off test" of the subscapularis, the patient places the arm on the lower back area and attempts to forcefully internally rotate against the examiner's hand. It is important to document first that the patient has enough passive motion to allow the shoulder to be internally rotated away from the lower back area.

2. **Subscapularis**—mainly responsible for internal rotation
   a. Christian Gerber coined term "lift-off test" to look specifically for abnormalities of subscapularis muscle tendon unit:
      i. Patient rotates arm behind back at approximately mid lumbar level and attempts to push examiner's hand away from the back (Fig. 3).
      ii. Significant weakness with this movement in comparison with opposite side indicates subscapularis pathology.
      iii. **Note:** care must be taken to make sure that patient can normally lift hand away from back without resistance.
   b. Another way of evaluating subscapularis is by testing resisted internal rotation with patient's arm adducted and elbow flexed 90° (Fig. 4A).
3. **Infraspinatus and teres minor**—mainly responsible for external rotation
   a. Patient's arm adducted to body and elbow flexed 90°.
   b. Patient attempts to externally rotate while examiner resists this motion (Fig 4B).

E. **Specific tests**
1. **Glenohumeral joint stability**
   a. **Anterior apprehension/instability test** may be performed in supine, sitting, or standing position:
      i. Arm is abducted 90° and shoulder is slowly externally rotated while patient's response is noted (Fig. 5).

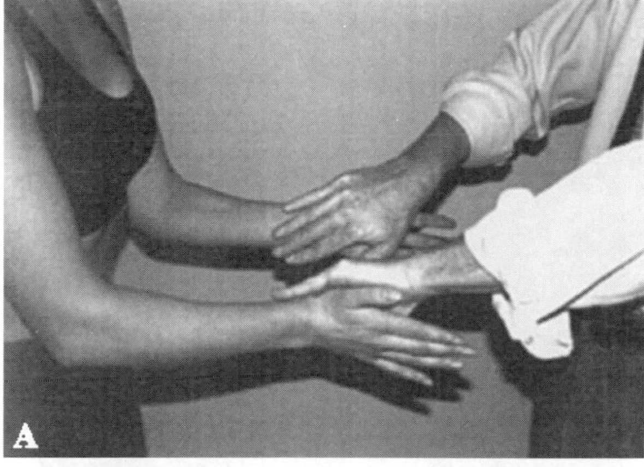

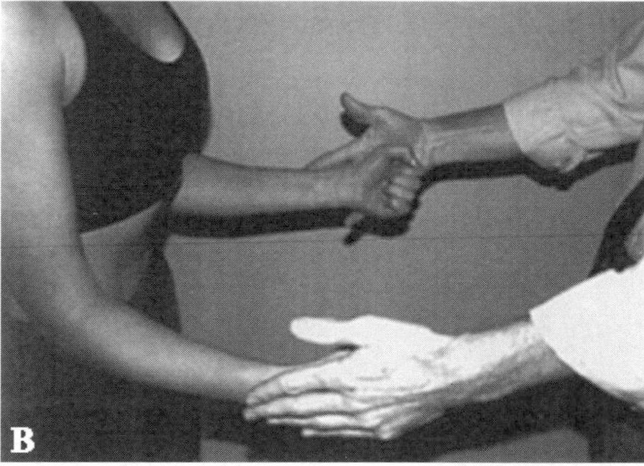

FIGURE 4. A, Internal rotation strength is tested by the patient adducting the arm to the side with the elbow flexed to 90° and forcefully internally rotating, pressing in against the examiner's hands. **B,** External rotation is tested in a similar manner but the patient externally rotates, pushing outward against the examiner's hands.

- ii. Examiner should place his or her fingers anteriorly over the humeral head to prevent complete dislocation during this test.
- iii. Maneuver should be repeated at varying degrees of abduction.
- iv. Patient's apprehension, or a feeling that the shoulder is going to slip out of the joint, may indicate anterior instability. However, sensation of pain only does not necessarily mean anterior instability is present.
- v. Important to compare injured side with uninjured side, as varying degrees of laxity are present in the normal population.

b. **Relocation test** is performed in a similar manner to apprehension test:
- i. While patient is in supine position, with arm abducted 90°, gently externally rotate the humerus (Fig. 6A). Note patient's response as well as degree of external rotation when symptoms appear.
- ii. Apply posteriorly directed force to anterior aspect of humeral head, thus preventing anterior translation (Fig. 6B). Again, externally rotate humerus and note patient's response as well as degree of maximum external rotation.
- iii. If anterior instability, relocation or posterior force should decrease feeling of apprehension as well as increase amount of external rotation obtained.

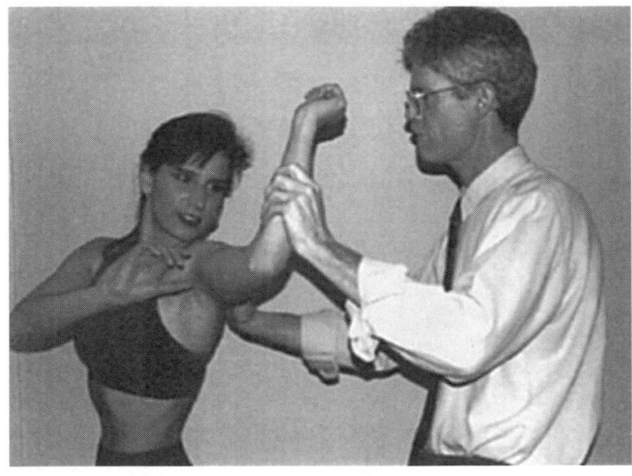

FIGURE 5. In the apprehension test, the arm is abducted to approximately 90° and progressively externally rotated while the patient's response is noted. A positive response is elicited by the patient having a sensation that the shoulder will slip out of joint.

c. **Augmentation test** is essentially reverse of relocation test:
   i. An anteriorly directed force on posterior aspect of humeral head is applied while arm is externally rotated (Fig. 6C).
   ii. This maneuver augments anterior translation of humeral head and should increase symptoms of apprehension as well as limit amount of external rotation in a patient with anterior instability.

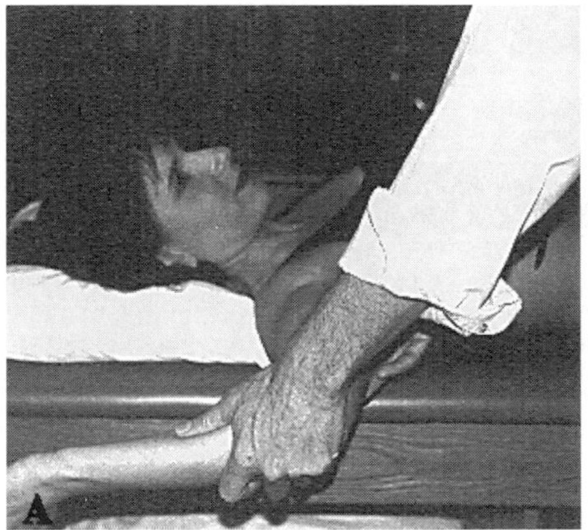

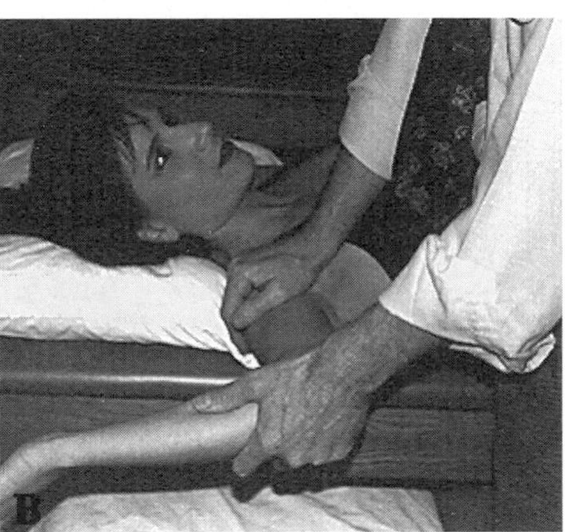

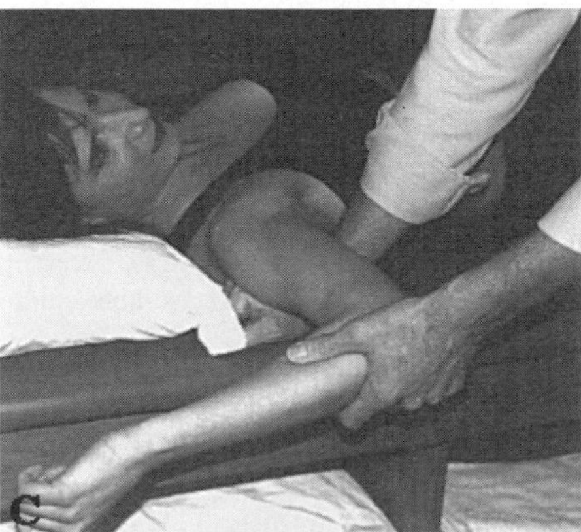

FIGURE 6. **A,** The relocation test is started by documenting the degree of external rotation with the patient's arm abducted to 90°. **B,** The relocation effect is performed by the examiner placing a posteriorly directed force on the humeral head, thus limiting the anterior translation of the humeral head. A positive response is seen when the patient has less pain and is able to obtain more external rotation. **C,** The augmentation effect is performed when the examiner places his hand posterior to the humeral head and directs an anterior pressure, thus increasing the anterior translation, causing more pain and more limitation of external rotation.

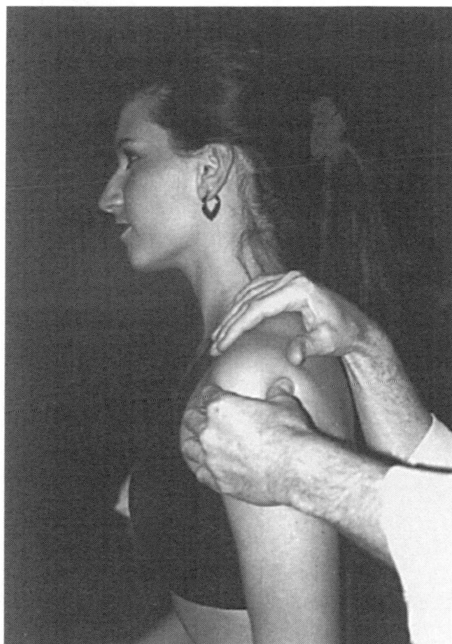

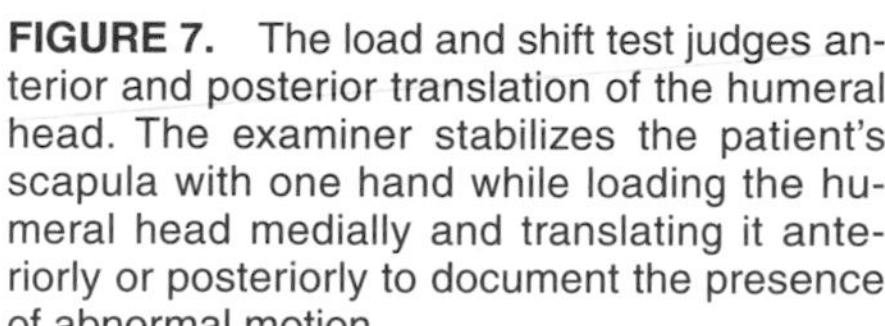

FIGURE 7. The load and shift test judges anterior and posterior translation of the humeral head. The examiner stabilizes the patient's scapula with one hand while loading the humeral head medially and translating it anteriorly or posteriorly to document the presence of abnormal motion.

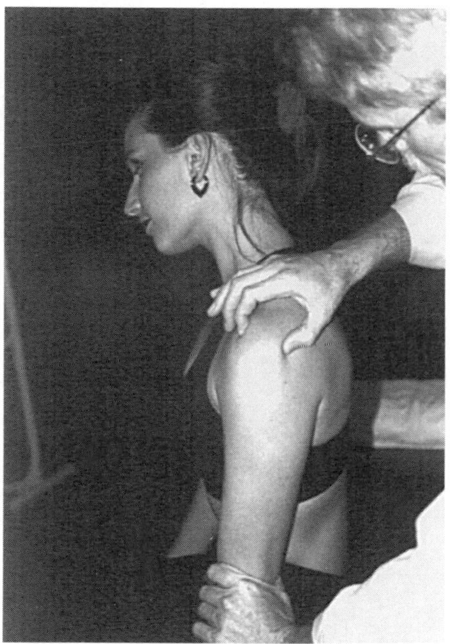

FIGURE 8. The inferior sulcus sign is performed by creating an inferior axial traction on the patient's arm and measuring the sulcus created between the inferior aspect of the acromion and the humeral head.

d. **Load and shift test**
   i. With patient in sitting position, examiner stands adjacent and slightly behind involved shoulder.
   ii. Examiner's hand is placed over scapula and shoulder to stabilize shoulder girdle while opposite hand grasps humeral head between thumb and fingers.
   iii. Humeral head is loaded with a medially directed force to seat it in the glenoid (Fig. 7).
   iv. An anterior and posterior translation stress is then applied while noting amount of translation. Quality of end point should also be considered.

e. **Inferior apprehension/instability test**
   i. With patient sitting, elbow is grasped and entire humerus is pulled inferiorly.
   ii. Look for an **inferior sulcus sign**, indicated by a space created between humeral head and acromion (Fig. 8). A positive inferior sulcus is greater than one centimeter.
   iii. As always, involved side should be compared to normal side.

f. **Posterior apprehension/instability test** can be performed with patient supine or sitting:
   i. Seated—load and shift test to document posterior instability
   ii. Supine—arm in 90° of abduction and 90° of elbow flexion. Apply a posteriorly directed force to mid humerus in attempt to displace humeral head posteriorly.
   iii. Alternatively, arm can be placed at 90° of forward flexion with internal rotation and 90° of elbow flexion. Apply a posteriorly directed force to elbow

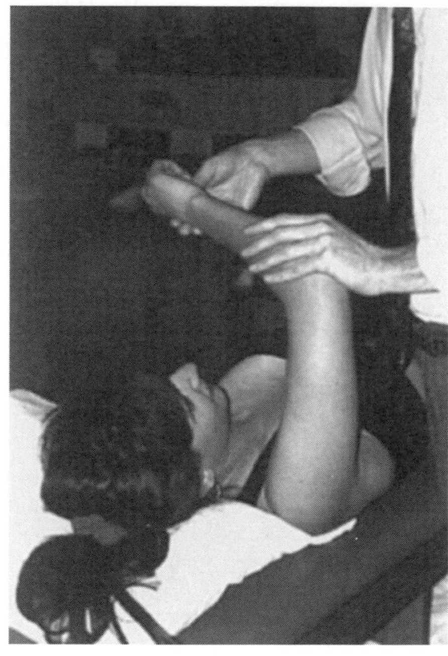

FIGURE 9. Posterior instability can be documented by creating a posterior force on the patient's elbow causing the humeral head to subluxate posteriorly.

in attempt to displace humeral head posteriorly (Fig. 9). Compare with opposite side.

2. **Rotator cuff.** Hawkin's and Neer's signs, positive with pain, can indicate impingement or rotator cuff tendinitis. They create pressure between insertion of supraspinatus and acromion or coracoacromial ligament.
   a. **Neer's sign**—arm fully pronated, bringing shoulder into maximum forward flexion (Fig. 10A)
   b. **Hawkin's sign/impingement reinforcement sign**—arm forward flexed 90° and elbow flexed 90°. Shoulder is then progressively internally rotated (Fig. 10B).
3. **Biceps.** Although not technically part of rotator cuff, close proximity to rotator cuff accounts for biceps tendon's frequent inflammation in conjunction with rotator cuff tendinitis. Yergason's and Speed's tests, positive with pain, can indicate biceps tendinitis. They create tension at proximal insertion of long head of biceps.
   a. **Yergason's test**—elbow flexed 90° with forearm pronated. Hold patient's wrist and direct patient to actively supinate against resistance.
   b. **Speed's test**—elbow flexed 20–30° and forearm supinated. With humerus forward flexed to approximately 60°, patient is asked to actively forward flex arm against resistance (Fig. 11).
4. **Labrum.** The **clunk test** identifies glenoid labrum tears.
   a. With patient supine, place one hand posterior to humeral head while other hand rotates humerus. Maintain elbow flexion at 90°.
   b. Bring arm into full overhead abduction while rotating humerus through varying degrees of internal and external rotation. Apply gentle axial compression to humerus.
   c. Sensation of a clunk, grind, or pop may indicate a glenoid labrum tear. Compare with opposite side.
5. **Acromioclavicular joint.** Direct pressure over AC joint or distal one-third of clavicle may cause pain or abnormal motion about AC joint (Fig. 12A).

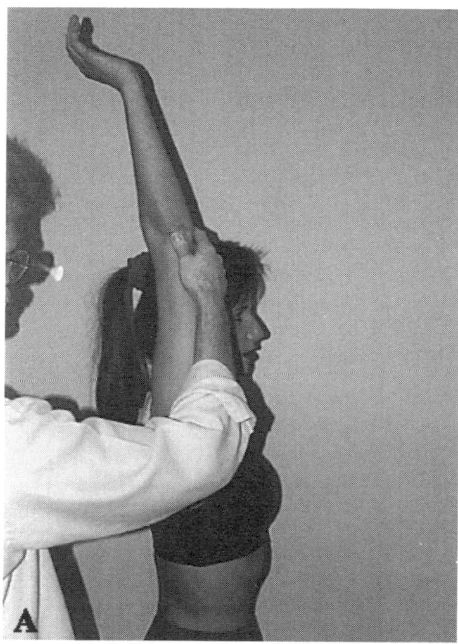

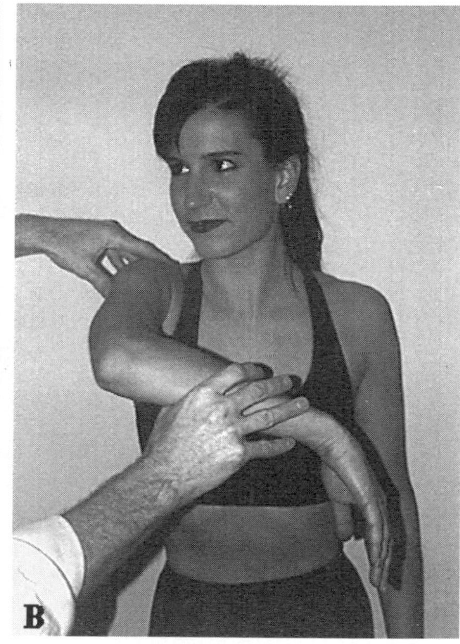

FIGURE 10. **A,** Neer's impingement sign is performed with the arm pronated bringing the shoulder into full overhead elevation. It is important to stabilize the scapula during this maneuver. **B,** Hawkin's sign can also be used to document impingement rotator cuff tendinitis.

a. Examine AC joint for abnormal instability by grasping clavicle between thumb and forefingers and observing any anterior and posterior laxity (Fig. 12B).
b. With shoulder positioned in 90° of forward flexion, pain with resistance to maintain this position may signify AC joint pathology.

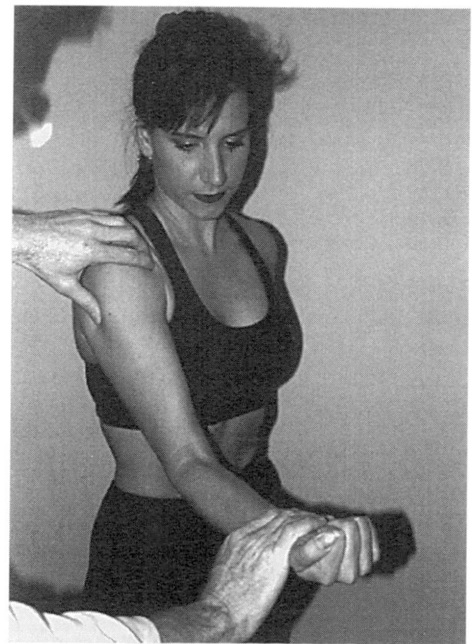

FIGURE 11. Speed's maneuver or test is used to examine the proximal biceps long head tendon. While performing this maneuver, the examiner should palpate the area of the biceps tendon on the anterior aspect of the shoulder.

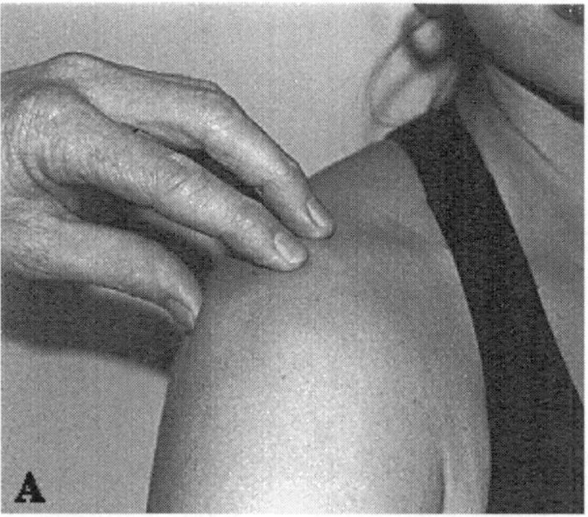

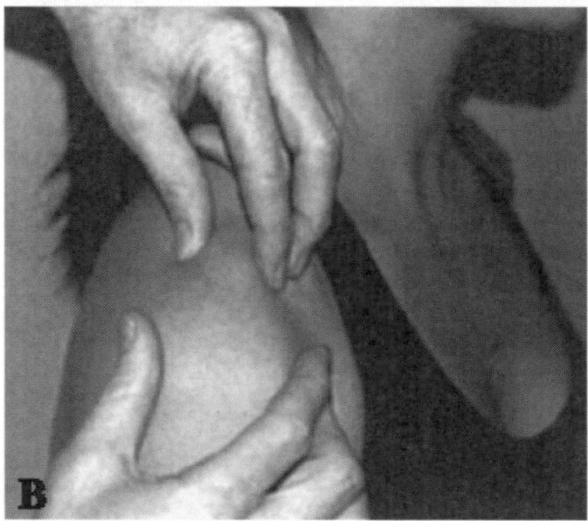

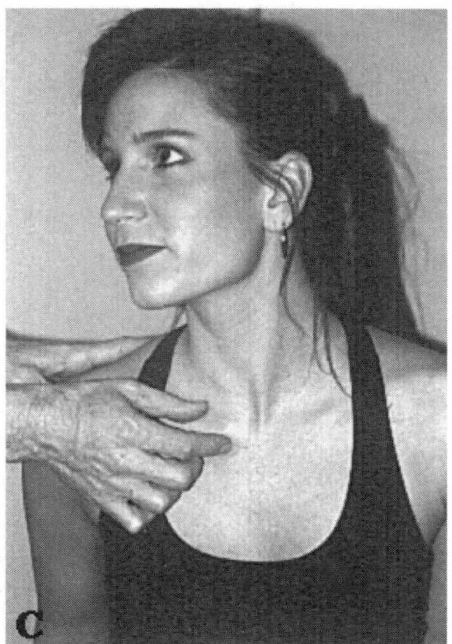

FIGURE 12. **A,** Examination of the clavicle and acromioclavicular (AC) joint should include palpation over the distal clavicle and AC joint. **B,** Instability can be documented by translating the clavicle anteriorly and posteriorly between the examiner's fingers. **C,** Sternoclavicular joint.

   c. Likewise, with arm posterior to coronal plane, resisted abduction may also stress AC joint and increase pain.
      i. **Crossed arm adduction test** (crossover test)—involved arm is brought across body in a horizontal plane so that elbow points towards opposite shoulder.
      ii. Is specific for AC joint; pain at AC joint in this position indicates pathology.
6. **Sternoclavicular (SC) joint** (Fig. 12C)
   a. Pressure or traction on medial clavicle may produce pain and motion at SC joint.
   b. When examining SC joint, it is important to view patient from above while looking down on clavicles to make sure there is no abnormal anterior or posterior alignment.
7. **Scapulothoracic joint** (Fig. 13A–B). Observe motion of scapula in relation to motion of glenohumeral joint. For every 2° of glenohumeral joint motion, there should be 1° of scapulothoracic motion.
8. **Neurologic examination:** It is important to perform a thorough neurologic examination of upper extremities when dealing with shoulder problems.
   a. Look at deep tendon reflexes, including biceps (C5 nerve root), brachioradialis (C6 nerve root), and triceps (C7 nerve root).
   b. Test sensation as well as muscle strength of all muscle groups of upper extremity.
   c. Use the Atlanto-Occipital axial compression test (Fig. 14) and the Spurling's maneuver to look for radicular symptoms from the cervical spine.

III. X-rays

A minimum of two views at right angles to each other are necessary to completely evaluate any significant shoulder injury. **Note:** An AP x-ray with the shoulder in internal and external

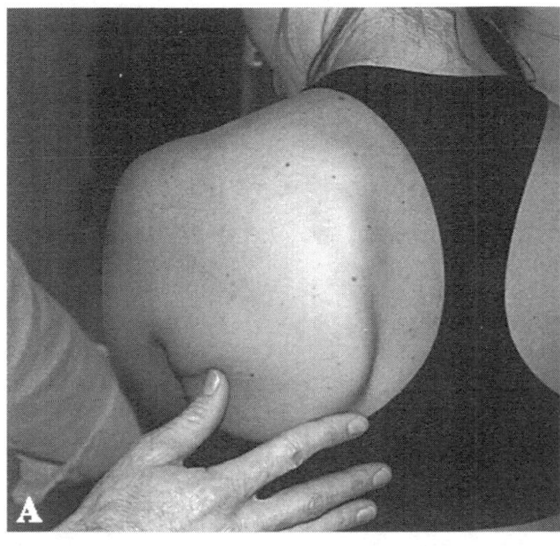

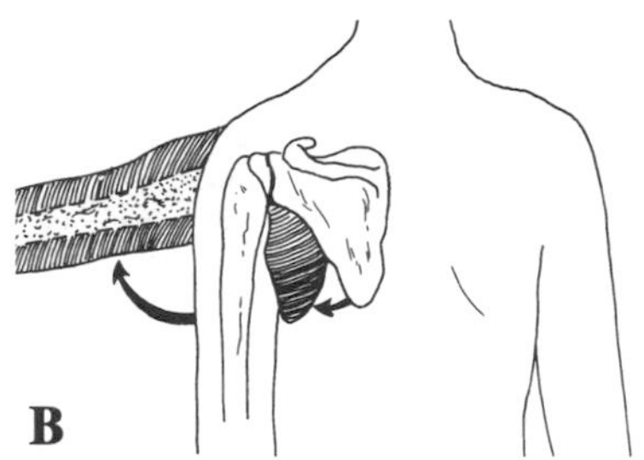

FIGURE 13. **A,** Scapulothoracic motion should be documented during the range of motion examination. The inferior tip of the scapula should be palpated and should also be noted, as in this patient there is significant winging of the medial border of the scapula. **B,** For every 2° of glenohumeral joint motion, there should be 1° of scapulothoracic motion.

rotation is not adequate and should not be considered a complete series. An AP view of the shoulder and either an axillary view or a transscapular lateral view are the minimum views required. Other views for specific injuries are covered elsewhere in this chapter.

IV. Specific Shoulder Injuries

A. **Anterior glenohumeral instability**

1. **Description:** Anterior glenohumeral instability is classified according to degree of instability and translation of humeral head.
   a. **Dislocation** is complete separation of articular surfaces.
   b. **Subluxation** is abnormal translation of humeral head on glenoid without complete separation of articular surfaces.
2. **Mechanism of injury**
   a. Patient usually relates symptoms of a complete dislocation to an event in which the arm was forced into extension, abduction, and external rotation, such as during an open arm tackle or a fall on an abducted arm. A less frequent mechanism may be a direct blow to the posterior or posterolateral shoulder.
   b. Subluxation, on the other hand, may occur after repeated episodes of overuse or may occur following recovery from a complete dislocation.

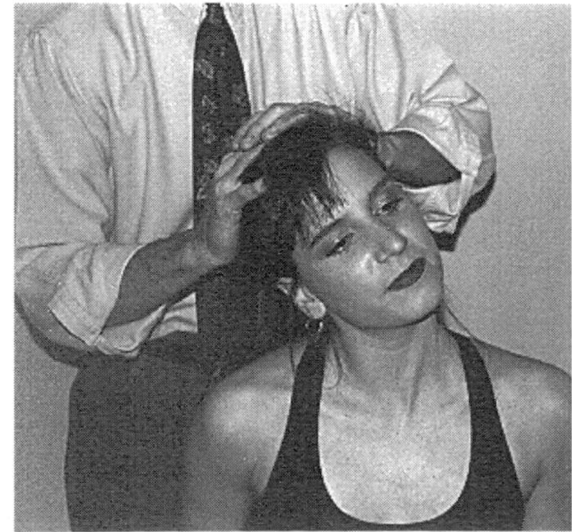

FIGURE 14. In the Atlanto-Occipital axial compression test, the examiner places pressure on the top of the patient's head and looks for resulting radicular signs. The Spurling's maneuver is performed with the patient's neck extended, laterally bent, and rotated to look for additional radicular symptoms.

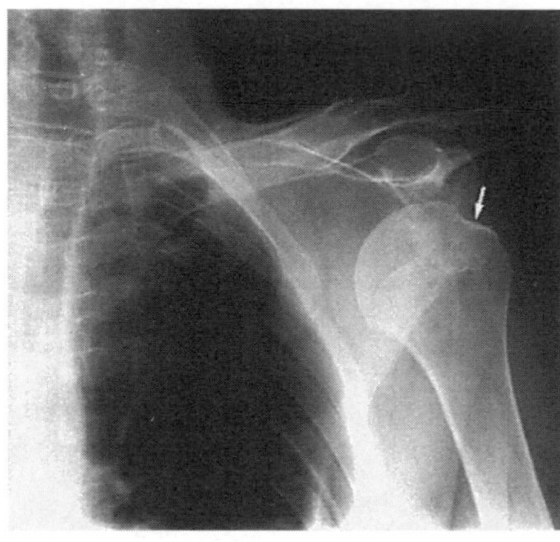

FIGURE 15. Hill-Sachs lesion.

3. **Examination**
   a. Patient with acute anterior dislocation presents with intense pain, holding arm in slight abduction and external rotation.
   b. Examination from behind patient reveals that posterior shoulder has a void beneath the acromion. Contour of dislocated shoulder is obviously different from normal side.
   c. Patient is unable to completely internally rotate or abduct the shoulder.
   d. Perform a thorough neurovascular exam, as there is a frequent association of axillary nerve injuries involved with anterior dislocations.
4. **X-ray studies:** Minimum x-rays required in evaluating an anterior dislocation include an AP as well as axillary or transscapular lateral view.
   a. A West Point view (modified axillary view) may reveal a chip fracture (Bankart lesion) off anterior inferior rim of glenoid.
   b. Fractures of the greater tuberosity are best identified on an external rotation view.
   c. The Hill-Sachs lesion, or a defect of posterior humeral head caused by compression of head against glenoid as humerus subluxates, may also be identified on routine shoulder series (Fig. 15).
   d. An MRI scan may be necessary in patients over 40 or in patients who do not regain strength within three weeks after injury because of high incidence of an associated rotator cuff tear in older individuals.
5. **Differential diagnosis:** Acute dislocation is usually obvious. When not so clear-cut, consider anterior subluxation, glenoid labrum tear, rotator cuff tear, and fracture of the proximal humerus.
6. **Treatment:** Initial treatment for an anterior dislocated shoulder is prompt reduction of the dislocation.
   a. If diagnosis is not certain, x-rays should be obtained prior to reduction. Athlete should lie supine with arm held in 30–45° of abduction.
   b. Intravenous medications may be necessary to relax patient and muscle spasm if shoulder has been dislocated for a long period of time. Gentle traction is applied to arm in its longitudinal axis. Occasionally counter traction is maintained with a sheet around upper thorax.
   c. Once reduced, arm is placed in a sling and post-reduction x-rays made. Most authors recommend treating patient with protected range of motion in "safe zone," using a sling for first week or so for comfort. Safe zone is generally considered within 90° of forward flexion and abduction, limiting external rotation to neutral. Ice and anti-inflammatory medication are used in acute period.

d. When acute pain resolves, patient begins a rotator cuff strengthening program.
e. Return to sport is allowed when normal strength and motion are regained.
f. If athlete experiences recurrent anterior dislocations and/or subluxations, surgery is appropriate.

B. **Posterior glenohumeral instability**
1. **Description**
   a. Subluxation may be more common than true dislocation. In either instance, posterior capsular structures are stretched and/or torn from posterior glenoid, allowing abnormal posterior translation of humeral head.
   b. Particularly in the elderly population, chronic posterior dislocations are often misdiagnosed as adhesive capsulitis.
2. **Mechanism of injury**
   a. An anterior blow to shoulder which forces humeral head posteriorly
   b. A fall on the outstretched hand in which force is transmitted up the humerus
3. **Examination**
   a. **Posterior dislocation** can be difficult to recognize as commonly there is no obvious deformity.
      i. Shoulder is usually held in sling position, i.e., adduction and internal rotation.
      ii. Prominent features include flattening of anterior shoulder when viewed from the side as well as a bulge posteriorly when viewed from above.
      iii. The prominent coracoid may also be noted.
      iv. Important findings are significant limitation of external rotation, often less than 0°, and limited elevation, usually less than 90°.
   b. Patient with **posterior subluxation** will obviously not have above mentioned findings, but will have pain and/or apprehension with a posteriorly directed force on humeral head and in response to relocation-augmentation test and load and shift test.
4. **X-ray studies:** Standard x-rays include an AP and axillary lateral view. Fractures of the lesser tuberosity are not uncommon.
5. **Differential diagnosis:** Posterior subluxation, proximal humerus fracture, glenoid fracture, and adhesive capsulitis in the non-acute setting
6. **Treatment**
   a. In acute setting, prompt reduction is indicated. Performed by applying forward traction with arm in forward flexion, internal rotation, and some adduction. Gradually elevate arm while applying pressure posteriorly to humeral head.
   b. If one or two trials are unsuccessful, closed reduction under a general anesthetic or IV sedation may be indicated.
   c. If all closed reductions are unsuccessful, then open reduction is indicated.
   d. The elderly patient with a chronic posterior dislocation will usually require different treatment. Reduction routinely requires anesthesia. Surgery may be required for reduction or replacement if the joint has been destroyed.
   e. After obtaining anatomic reduction, x-rays are obtained to verify appropriate alignment.
   f. Most authors elect to treat first-time traumatic posterior dislocation with a splint holding the arm in slight abduction and slight external rotation. Immobilization is usually required for 4–6 weeks in a young patient and only 2–3 weeks in an older patient.
   g. After appropriate immobilization, patient begins gentle, protected range of motion and rotator cuff strengthening exercises.
   h. Patient with recurrent posterior instability has option to give up specific sports that cause symptoms or undergo posterior shoulder reconstruction. Posterior reconstruction is significantly less successful than anterior reconstruction.

C. **Multi-directional instability** (MDI)
   1. **Description:** First described by Charles Neer as an abnormal translation of the shoulder, specifically with inferior laxity in conjunction with anterior, posterior, or both directions.
      a. Mild forms of MDI are not uncommon in "overhead" athletes such as throwers and swimmers.
      b. More severe forms may be seen in patients with psychiatric problems who can voluntarily dislocate their shoulder for secondary gains, or in patients with connective tissue disorders such as Ehlers-Danlos where multi-joint hypermobility exists.
   2. **Mechanism of injury**
      a. Often secondary to repetitive "microtrauma," as in the overhead athlete and in people with ligamentous and capsular laxity.
      b. Can also result from severe trauma, subsequently tearing multiple capsular restraints within the shoulder.
   3. **Examination**
      a. A pathognomonic feature of MDI is a positive inferior sulcus sign with anterior or posterior instability or both.
      b. Patient can often dislocate or subluxate shoulder voluntarily.
      c. Patient may also exhibit excessive (> 90°) external rotation.
      d. Important to look for generalized ligamentous laxity such as recurvatum of knees and elbows, hyperextension of fingers at metacarpophalangeal joint, and thumb to forearm sign.
   4. **X-ray studies:** Routine x-ray evaluation including AP and axillary lateral views may demonstrate erosions of anterior or posterior glenoid rim with abnormal version of glenoid. A Hill-Sachs lesion may also be evident.
   5. **Treatment:** MDI is often bilateral and recalcitrant to standard forms of treatment (rehabilitation and strengthening exercises).
      a. Physical therapy emphasizes rotator cuff strengthening. Stretching exercises are not advised, as generally, inflexibility is not a problem.
      b. Six months of rehabilitation is minimum in most cases before considering surgery. Surgical management can be difficult.

D. **Acromioclavicular sprains, separation, and dislocations**
   1. **Description:** Involve stretching or partial tearing of acromioclavicular and coracoclavicular ligaments
   2. **Classification system**
      a. **Type I**—sprain of acromioclavicular ligament. AC joint is essentially intact as are coracoclavicular ligaments.
      b. **Type II**—coracoclavicular ligaments are sprained. AC joint is disrupted and there may be slight vertical separation as well as slight increase in coracoclavicular interspace.
      c. **Type III**—both acromioclavicular and coracoclavicular ligaments are disrupted. Distal clavicle is displaced above acromion and shoulder complex is displaced inferiorly. Coracoclavicular interspace is 25–100% greater than opposite shoulder.
      d. **Type IV**—complete AC dislocation in which clavicle is anatomically displaced posteriorly into trapezius muscle
      e. **Type V**—exaggerated Type III injury with gross disparity between distal clavicle and acromion such that it is displaced 100–300%
      f. **Type VI**—extremely rare dislocation in which clavicle is displaced inferior to acromion or coracoid process
   3. **Mechanism of injury**
      a. Patient usually gives history of falling on point or lateral aspect of shoulder such as an impact with ground or shoulder pads during football.
      b. Some patients fall on an outstretched hand and force is transmitted up arm to AC joint.

4. **Examination**
   a. Even with a mild sprain, patients have pain to palpation about AC joint and pain with movement of shoulder.
   b. **Crossover test**, or crossed arm adduction, increases pain at AC joint.
   c. In Types II, III, and V injuries, clavicle can be seen riding above acromion.
   d. There may be tenderness to palpation along shaft of clavicle, SC joint, and clavicular attachments of trapezius and deltoid.
5. **X-rays:** Routine views of glenohumeral joint do not show AC joint well due to over penetration; therefore, it is necessary to decrease intensity by about 50% for quality views.
   a. Zanca view, an AP view with a 10–15° cephalic tilt, provides good visualization of AC joint.
   b. Standard axillary view helps to determine anterior or posterior displacement of distal clavicle.
   c. Stress x-rays, with 10–15 pounds of weight suspended from arms by loops around wrists, help to further document differences in distal clavicle elevation between injured and normal shoulder.
6. **Differential diagnosis:** Contusion to distal clavicle (shoulder pointer) which has no palpable AC joint tenderness, synovitis or degenerative arthritis of AC joint, osteolysis of distal clavicle, and fractures of distal clavicle or acromion
7. **Treatment**
   a. Grades I and II separations
      i. Ice
      ii. Rest
      iii. Anti-inflammatory medicines
      iv. A sling as necessary for symptom control
      v. Early rehabilitation consisting of range of motion and gentle rotator cuff and scapulothoracic strengthening exercises are begun when pain allows.
   b. Grade III separation
      i. Controversial, but most agree that conservative treatment should be attempted initially unless patient is a throwing athlete or a laborer involved in heavy overhead lifting.
      ii. As with Grades I and II, arm should be placed in a sling for comfort. Most have abandoned use of reduction braces, such as Kenny Howard sling.
      iii. Early range of motion and progressive strengthening exercises when pain allows.
   c. Surgical treatment for reduction of AC joint or for excision of distal clavicle can be considered for Types II and III in patients who continue to have pain or limited function. Types IV, V, and VI may require reconstructive procedures. Surgical treatment may also be considered for cosmetic reasons.

E. **Sternoclavicular dislocations/sprains**
1. **Description:** Involves spraining or tearing of costoclavicular and/or sternoclavicular ligaments or disruption of medial physis of clavicle in immature patients
   a. Most common injury results from an anteriorly directed force resulting in a sprain or anterior dislocation of medial clavicle.
   b. Posterior dislocation is less common, but has increased morbidity with potential injury to underlying vasculature, lung, trachea, and esophagus. **Emergency treatment is indicated for posterior dislocation, especially if airway is obstructed.**
2. **Mechanism of injury**
   a. Most common cause of injury is indirect force applied to SC joint from anterolateral or posterolateral aspect of shoulder. Usually involves an athlete who falls on one side with an opposing force to top of opposite shoulder, such as a pile up in a football game. Generally causes an anterior sprain or dislocation of SC joint.

b. Less commonly, a direct force applied over anteromedial portion of clavicle can displace clavicle posteriorly resulting in a posterior SC dislocation.

3. **Examination**
   a. With anterior SC dislocations, there is prominence of proximal or medial clavicle with tenderness and swelling over SC joint. It is easy to observe anterior displacement when viewing patient from a superior position, looking directly down onto SC joint.
   b. With posterior dislocations, proximal clavicle is located behind sternum. **Posterior dislocations can quickly become a medical emergency due to airway obstruction or vascular compromise.**
      i. Immediate determination of respiratory status is mandatory.
      ii. Patient will usually complain of severe pain, and possibly hoarseness, dysphagia, and dyspnea as proximal clavicle impinges on underlying structures.
      iii. In vascular compromise, there may also be discoloration, swelling, and pulselessness in arm of affected side.
      iv. In addition, look for signs of subcutaneous emphysema and pulmonary problems.
4. **X-ray studies:** Difficult to evaluate SC joint on routine x-rays. "Serendipity" or apical lordotic view as described by Rockwood best shows anterior or posterior dislocations of SC joint. CT scanning may be helpful in difficult cases.
5. **Treatment**
   a. For mild sprains, application of ice for first 12–24 hours and use of a sling
   b. For subluxations, a padded figure of 8 clavicle strap for 4–6 weeks to support joint while healing
   c. For complete anterior dislocation, a gentle reduction maneuver. Then most favor a conservative treatment program involving a figure of 8 brace or a sling, depending on position in which clavicle is most stable.
   d. For posterior dislocations, reduction as soon as possible. Gentle on-site reduction can be attempted by placing athlete supine with a rolled up towel between scapulae. Posterior pressure is then applied on lateral aspect of shoulders. If this maneuver fails, athlete should be transported to hospital for definitive treatment. Routinely, posterior dislocations are stable once they are reduced and rarely need further treatment. Most posterior subluxations in younger patients (less than 24 years old) are actually physeal injuries. These are treated conservatively unless there are persistent symptoms of hoarseness, dysphagia, or dyspnea, in which case surgery (reduction) is indicated.

F. **Glenoid labrum tears**

1. **Description:** Most common pathologic entity involves an anterior inferior labral tear or Bankart lesion that is seen with anterior shoulder dislocations. Stephen Snyder coined the term "SLAP" for lesions involving the *S*uperior *L*abrum *A*nterior and *P*osterior. Common overuse injury in throwing athletes as well as other athletes who have significant impact to upper extremities. Another overuse entity that can be found in pitchers and throwing athletes is fraying and partial tearing of posterior superior glenoid labrum that, in turn, causes an undersurface rotator cuff impingement.
2. **Mechanism of injury:** Multiple mechanisms have been suggested that contribute to various labrum injuries.
   a. During acceleration phase of throwing, horizontal adduction and internal rotation place grinding forces on anterior superior labrum resulting in a SLAP lesion.
   b. Traction on biceps tendon as it tries to depress humeral head causes glenoid labrum tearing.
   c. Rotator cuff tendinitis, asynchrony in firing of rotator cuff, and weakness in posterior portion of cuff allow anterior and superior translation of humeral head which can cause fraying and tearing of glenoid labrum.

d. Posterior superior glenoid labrum tears occur via "internal impingement." With throwing arm in cocked position, rotator cuff is pinched against posterior superior labrum, causing fraying and irritation of undersurface of rotator cuff and posterior superior labrum.

3. **History:** SLAP lesions and other glenoid labrum tears are very common in throwing athletes. Patient presents with a painful shoulder that occasionally clicks or snaps with motion. Patients commonly point to posterior shoulder as location of pain, although pain may not be located in one specific area when a SLAP lesion is present. Patient may notice pain with cocking, release, and follow through phases of throwing. Routinely, patient will not be able to throw as hard or for as long a period of time when a labrum tear is present.
4. **Physical examination**
   a. Patients with large labrum tears occasionally have a positive **clunk test**, especially while in overhead position.
   b. Tenderness to deep palpation about anterior glenohumeral joint and tenderness to palpation posteriorly around teres minor–teres major junction may be present.
   c. Signs of anterior instability such as anterior laxity and apprehension may be present with a Bankart lesion.
5. **X-ray studies:** Routine AP and axillary x-rays are generally normal. MRI scan may be used to delineate rotator cuff or labral pathology. Some recommend a saline MRI to further displace torn labrum and make it easier to view on MRI scan.
6. **Differential diagnosis:** Glenoid labrum tears are difficult to diagnose because typical symptoms are consistent with many other shoulder injuries such as rotator cuff tendinitis, rotator cuff tears, glenohumeral instability, biceps tendon lesions, and AC joint abnormalities.
7. **Treatment**
   a. Initial treatment involves a standard shoulder rehabilitation program with strengthening, stretching, ice, and anti-inflammatory medications.
   b. For patients that do not respond to standard rehabilitation, arthroscopy may be indicated. Small labral tears can be debrided arthroscopically. Small labral tears involving attachment of biceps tendon should be repaired.

G. **Rotator cuff**

1. **Rotator cuff tendinitis/impingement syndrome**
   a. **Description:** Rotator cuff, especially supraspinatus, and biceps tendon may impinge against undersurface of acromion and coracoacromial ligament.
   b. **Mechanism of injury:** Subacromial bursa and rotator cuff tendons become inflamed secondary to friction against undersurface of acromion and coracoacromial ligament. May be result of overuse of shoulder and rotator cuff weakness or mild anterior instability causing a secondary impingement syndrome. Direct trauma to shoulder can cause an acute inflammation and rotator cuff tendinitis.
   c. **Predisposing factors:**
      i. Any activity that requires repetitive motion of shoulder above horizontal plane, e.g., swimming, throwing, tennis, weight lifting, and golf, puts athlete at higher risk. In addition to repetitive nature of these sports, there is a tendency toward mechanical and technical errors.
      ii. Fatigue of rotator cuff may cause abnormal mechanics of shoulder.
      iii. Subtle instability can cause a secondary impingement.
      iv. Other predisposing factors include upper extremity inflexibility and anatomic predisposition with regard to bony anatomy, such as an anterior sloped or hooked acromion and AC joint spurring/hypertrophy.
   d. **History:** Athlete typically presents with pain referred to anterolateral shoulder that occurs during overhead activities. Pain at night is a hallmark of significant rotator cuff disease.

e. **Physical examination**
   i. Athlete has positive impingement signs and varying degrees of rotator cuff and biceps weakness (see "Manual muscle testing," page 439 and "Rotator cuff," page 444).
   ii. A painful arc usually within 70–120° of abduction
   iii. Possibly significant crepitus and a snapping feeling that occurs with external to internal rotation
   iv. May be atrophy of the supra- and infraspinatus muscles. Remember, this important finding will be missed if patient is not observed shirtless or in a tank top.
   v. Typically tenderness to palpation about greater tuberosity and along biceps tendon anteriorly
   vi. May be limited range of motion, especially internal rotation
   vii. A diagnostic test for impingement can be performed in the office by injecting local anesthetic into subacromial space. This reduces pain associated with overhead activity and impingement positions.
f. **X-ray studies**
   i. Standard AP and axillary views are necessary to work up rotator cuff tendinitis and impingement. They may show some undersurface AC joint spurring as well as some early glenohumeral degenerative changes.
   ii. Suprascapular outlet view is important in looking at morphology of acromion.
      (a) A Type II or III acromion that involves a gentle anterior curve or a large spur on undersurface of acromion may predispose a patient to rotator cuff tendinitis and/or tears.
      (b) An enlarged, laterally directed coracoid may impinge against lesser tuberosity of humerus with crossed arm adduction, causing a rare form of coracoid impingement.
g. **Differential diagnosis:** Rotator cuff tear, thoracic outlet syndrome, and primary subtle anterior instability with secondary rotator cuff tendinitis. Occasionally, cervical spine pathology can mimic shoulder pain that is typical of rotator cuff disease.
h. **Treatment**
   i. Temporary avoidance of aggravating activity, usually by restricting motion to below horizontal plane, is generally indicated in symptomatic cases.
   ii. Ice and anti-inflammatory medicines
   iii. Physical therapy to regain strength and motion and modalities such as ultrasound to decrease inflammation
   iv. Corticosteroid injections into subacromial bursa may be indicated if previously described treatment is not helpful.
   v. If all above conservative measures fail, then arthroscopic subacromial decompression may be necessary.

2. **Rotator cuff tears**
   a. **Description:** Full thickness disruption of tendon fibers that make up rotator cuff. Most frequent site of injury is within supraspinatus tendon at its insertion into greater tuberosity of humerus. Larger tears will extend to infraspinatus and even teres minor.
   b. **History**
      i. **Acute rotator cuff tears**
         (a) Indirect force on abducted arm or direct blow to lateral shoulder
         (b) Characterized by acute pain and weakness immediately following traumatic episode
      ii. **Chronic rotator cuff tears**
         (a) Neglected longstanding tendinitis which leads to thinning of rotator cuff and ultimate rupture

(b) Patients usually older than 45 years of age
(c) Long history of shoulder pain that has progressed to significant pain, weakness, and loss of motion. Complaints of significant night pain

c. **Physical examination**
  i. May be painful arc within 70°–120° of abduction
  ii. Manual muscle testing generally reveals marked weakness in supraspinatus and external rotators.
  iii. Usually a positive impingement sign and an impingement reinforcement sign
  iv. Generally pain to palpation about greater tuberosity at rotator cuff insertion
  v. In chronic tears, atrophy is occasionally noted in supraspinatus and infraspinatus muscles.
  vi. Physical findings are more pronounced in a massive rotator cuff tear. There may even be a characteristic "bone-on-bone" crepitation palpable or audible during shoulder motion as humeral head migrates proximally through tear to come in contact with acromion.

d. **X-ray studies**
  i. Early in disease, routine x-rays may be normal.
    (a) Occasionally, AP view shows **sourcil sign** or **"eyebrow sign,"** which demonstrates subacromial sclerosis from chronic loading of undersurface of acromion during impingement process.
    (b) Subchondral cysts may be seen at rotator cuff insertion on greater tuberosity in advanced or chronic instances.
  ii. Large or massive rotator cuff tears may show proximal migration of humeral head on a routine AP view.
  iii. An arthrogram will show obvious dye leakage outside of joint into subacromial space.
  iv. An MRI scan is considered gold standard to evaluate rotator cuff. MRI advantages over arthrogram are many. For example:
    (a) Arthrogram can only determine whether a complete thickness tear is or is not present. MRI can quantify degree of rotator cuff pathology (i.e., tendinitis vs. partial thickness tear vs. complete thickness tear).
    (b) MRI can also indicate size and location of tear and whether there is any medial retraction of tendon.

e. **Differential diagnosis:** Impingement syndrome/rotator cuff tendinitis, suprascapular nerve entrapment, cervical radiculopathy, and adhesive capsulitis

f. **Treatment**
  i. In the older patient, initial treatment involves a conservative program similar to that of rotator cuff tendinitis (see "Treatment," page 454).
  ii. If a young patient has rotator cuff tear from an acute traumatic episode, surgery is indicated sooner.
  iii. If conservative treatment fails, surgery is indicated.
    (a) Arthroscopic subacromial decompression in patients who only desire pain relief, in instances where tears are too massive to be repaired, or in patients whose other health problems preclude open surgery
    (b) In patients whose tear is amenable to repair and who have no other health problems, open repair is indicated.

H. **Biceps tendon pathology**

1. **Biceps tendinitis**
  a. **Description:** Inflammation and irritation of long head of biceps tendon. Generally occurs in area of bicipital groove just as biceps tendon enters intra-articular area. Commonly associated with underlying rotator cuff impingement or tearing.

b. **History:** Patient generally presents with a vague history of anterior shoulder pain of variable duration.

c. **Examination:** Athlete generally has pain to direct palpation along biceps tendon in its groove. Speed's and Yergason's test usually positive.

d. **X-ray studies** are not necessarily helpful in evaluating the biceps tendon.
   i. Occasionally—calcific tendinitis
   ii. Rarely—a narrow bicipital groove on bicipital groove x-ray view

e. **Treatment**
   i. Similar to that of rotator cuff tendinitis (rest, ice, and anti-inflammatory medications)
   ii. Exercises and modalities with a physical therapist
   iii. Corticosteroid injections directly into the biceps tendon generally contraindicated due to increased incidence of biceps tendon rupture
   iv. Subacromial corticosteroid injection may bathe tendon enough to decrease symptoms

2. **Subluxation of long head of biceps tendon**
   a. **Description:** Proximal portion of long head of biceps tendon subluxates out of bicipital groove
   b. **Mechanism of injury:** Biceps tendon subluxation generally occurs secondary to a rotator cuff tear, especially those involving subscapularis and coracohumeral ligament/rotator interval.
   c. **History:** Patient generally presents with shoulder pain and a snapping sensation in anterior aspect of shoulder, occurring with internal and external rotation as well as overhead activity. There are generally symptoms of rotator cuff pathology.
   d. **Examination**
      i. Generally the same as for biceps tendinitis with a positive Speed's and Yergason's test
      ii. Routinely, significant rotator cuff weakness due to an associated rotator cuff tear
      iii. In some instances, biceps tendon may be so unstable that examiner can sublux tendon out of its groove with gentle manual pressure during internal and external rotation of shoulder.
      iv. When tear involves subscapularis as well as coracohumeral ligament, there is generally a positive lift-off test (see "Subscapularis," page 440).
   e. **Differential diagnosis:** Biceps tendinitis, impingement syndrome, rotator cuff tear, and glenoid labral pathology
   f. **Treatment**
      i. Initially, as with many shoulder conditions, icc, anti-inflammatory medications, and physical therapy
      ii. If conservative treatment fails, then surgery is indicated.
         (a) If tendon is in good condition and there is an obvious rotator cuff tear, appropriate procedure is to repair rotator cuff and relocate biceps tendon within groove.
         (b) If biceps tendon is significantly frayed, abnormal portion is resected and a biceps tenodesis onto proximal humerus may be indicated.

3. **Biceps tendon rupture**
   a. **Description:** Complete disruption of proximal longhead of biceps tendon, usually near its position in the bicipital groove
   b. **History:** Generally, a traumatic injury resulting from forceful flexion of elbow against excessive resistance
      i. With acute injury, patient notes significant pain, swelling, and ecchymosis about anterior shoulder.

ii. In elderly patient, can be result of chronic attritional tendinitis.
iii. Many times patient does not even know that biceps tendon is ruptured and it is only discovered during a thorough physical examination.

c. **Examination**
i. Acute injuries generally present with ecchymosis, swelling, and considerable pain about upper arm and anterior shoulder.
ii. There is a "popeye" appearance to upper arm as biceps muscle belly retracts distally, producing a visible hump in mid portion of upper arm.
iii. Muscle testing generally reveals mild weakness with forearm flexion and supination.
iv. A distal biceps rupture results in marked weakness with flexion and supination of forearm.

d. **X-ray studies:** Routine x-rays are generally normal. An MRI scan may be indicated if diagnosis is uncertain.

e. **Differential diagnosis:** Partial tearing of biceps tendon, rotator cuff tear, and proximal humerus fracture

f. **Treatment**
i. Proximal ruptures in **older patients** generally respond well to conservative treatment including ice, anti-inflammatory medicines, and rotator cuff rehabilitation.
ii. **Younger patients** may be best treated surgically with a biceps tenodesis.
iii. **Distal ruptures** of the biceps tendon at the elbow require surgical repair for best results.

I. **Shoulder contusion**

1. **Description:** Contusion and bruising about deltoid and trapezius muscles of shoulder. Can also involve exposed portion of lateral clavicle and acromion resulting in a shoulder pointer. If significant hemorrhaging into muscle, myositis ossificans can develop.
2. **History:** Typically results from a direct blow to shoulder usually seen in contact or collision sports.
3. **Examination:** Tenderness to direct palpation over contused area. Often swelling, but rarely ecchymosis early on. Motion generally restricted due to pain.
4. **X-ray studies:** Initial x-rays are routinely normal. Occasionally, later in the course (2–6 weeks after injury), ectopic bone formation (myositis ossificans and "tackler's exostosis") is visualized in lateral upper arm.
5. **Differential diagnosis:** AC separation, rotator cuff tear, rotator cuff tendinitis, glenohumeral subluxation/dislocation, clavicle fracture, and proximal humerus fracture
6. **Treatment:** Standard athletic first aid including rest, ice, compression, anti-inflammatory medicines, gentle range of motion, and gentle massage

J. **Fracture of the clavicle**

1. **Description:** Most commonly fractured in its middle third where it is most prominent and angulated
2. **History and mechanism of injury:** Generally occurs from a fall on an outstretched arm or a fall on point of shoulder. Less commonly, results from a direct blow to mid portion of clavicle. Displacement occurs due to muscle pull on opposing fragments.
3. **Physical examination**
a. Generally a visible and palpable deformity in grossly displaced fractures.
b. Greenstick type fractures in preadolescents may occur without obvious deformity; therefore, careful physical examination and x-rays are important for a correct diagnosis.
c. Marked swelling and ecchymosis may occur while pain is present. Pain will typically radiate into trapezius and occasionally into neck.

d. In significantly displaced fractures, especially when one portion is displaced inferiorly, it is necessary to auscultate the lungs to rule out a pneumothorax.
e. Neurovascular examination is important to detect any brachioplexus injury.

4. **X-ray studies**
   a. AP and axillary views are generally adequate.
   b. Occasionally, a chest x-ray is needed to rule out pneumothorax.
   c. The scapula should be completely visualized to rule out fracture here as well. If a scapular fracture is suspected based on these x-rays, further views are indicated (see "X-ray studies" below).
5. **Differential diagnosis:** AC separation, SC separation, and shoulder contusion
6. **Treatment:** Generally, a figure of 8 strap is adequate to protect area from further injury. Some patients do not feel comfortable if strap rides directly over fracture and, therefore, are more comfortable in a standard sling. Distal one-third fractures of clavicle are more difficult to treat and may require surgery.

K. **Fracture of scapula**

1. **Description:** Can occur in many places, including body, neck, glenoid articular surface, coracoid process, and scapular spine. Fracture site varies depending on mechanism of injury.
2. **History and mechanism of injury:** Generally occurs with a high-energy injury such as a fall from a height, severe blow in football, or motor vehicle accident. Scapula fractures may also be associated with fractures of rib, sternum, and cervical spine.
3. **Physical examination**
   a. In a patient with a scapula body fracture, tenderness to palpation over scapula posteriorly and pain with shoulder range of motion.
   b. Other scapula fractures involving glenoid neck, articular surface, and coracoid also have pain during shoulder range of motion.
   c. Fractures of acromion may cause impingement type symptoms. If fracture goes through suprascapular notch, do a neurologic exam to document status of suprascapular nerve.
4. **X-ray studies**
   a. An AP view of shoulder to include entire scapula and a transscapular lateral view are minimum requirements.
   b. Other appropriate views may be indicated depending upon pathology of fracture.
   c. Most fractures of scapula that involve glenoid neck and glenoid articular surface are best delineated with CT scan.
5. **Treatment**
   a. Extra-articular fractures of scapula—a sling, protected range of motion, ice, and anti-inflammatory medications
   b. A large displaced fracture of articular surface of glenoid, unstable fracture of glenoid neck, displaced fracture of acromion, non-united fractures of coracoid process—possibly open reduction and internal fixation

L. **Fractures of the proximal humerus**

1. **Description:** Usually arise from a violent force applied to shoulder and should be considered in any athlete with an acute traumatic injury. Less common in young, healthy individuals as opposed to elderly people with osteoporotic bone.
2. **Mechanism of injury:** Generally, caused by a fall on an outstretched hand with elbow extended or a direct impact injury to shoulder. Fractures of greater and lesser tuberosities can occur with anterior or posterior shoulder dislocations respectively.
3. **Physical examination**
   a. Significant pain with any attempted motion of upper extremity.
   b. Usually swelling and ecchymosis about the shoulder.
   c. Typically, patient splints arm against body to increase comfort.

   d. A neurovascular exam is important, as neurovascular injuries are not uncommon with significantly displaced proximal humerus fractures.
4. **X-ray studies:** AP, transthoracic lateral, and axillary views generally delineate fracture lines. CT scans are helpful in a significantly comminuted fracture to plan surgical reduction.
5. **Differential diagnosis:** Glenohumeral dislocation, AC separation, distal clavicle fracture, shoulder contusion, and glenoid neck/scapula fracture
6. **Treatment**
   a. Displaced fractures (> 1 cm) generally require open reduction and internal fixation.
   b. Most fractures displaced < 1 cm can be treated with a sling and progressive range of motion.
   c. Some greater tuberosity fractures displaced < 1 cm may require open reduction and internal fixation, depending on anatomy of fracture and its relationship to rotator cuff insertion.

M. **Adhesive capsulitis (frozen shoulder)**
1. **Description:** Involves adhesions and capsular contractions causing restriction of motion in glenohumeral joint and significant pain
2. **Mechanism of injury**
   a. True etiology is unknown. Some believe it is a vicious cycle starting out with pain and guarding of shoulder and developing into inflammatory capsulitis. Pain increases and patient tries to protect shoulder by not using it; thus, shoulder becomes increasingly stiff and frozen.
   b. Other possible causes include trauma, rotator cuff tendinitis, reflex sympathetic dystrophy, coronary artery disease, diabetes mellitus, and even hormonal imbalance.
3. **History:** Generally, shoulder pain and limited motion that is insidious in onset. Pain progressively increases as motion progressively decreases. Typically, significant pain at night that prevents sleep.
4. **Physical examination:** Hallmark is significant decreased range of motion with a firm end point on motion testing. Internal and external rotation seem to be limited most, with abduction and forward flexion limited to a lesser degree.
5. **X-ray studies:** Routine x-rays are usually normal. It is important, however, to rule out a missed posterior dislocation as a cause of limited shoulder rotation and motion. An arthrogram may demonstrate decreased joint volume.
6. **Differential diagnosis:** Rotator cuff impingement syndrome with rotator cuff tendinitis or tear, fracture about shoulder, cervical radiculopathy, arthritis of shoulder, thoracic outlet syndrome, and missed posterior dislocation
7. **Treatment** is conservative.
   a. All patients should be started on an exercise program that includes gentle range of motion, anti-inflammatory medication, ice, and other physical therapy modalities.
   b. Some recommend intra-articular as well as subacromial corticosteroid injections.
   c. Occasionally, course will be self-limited and if patient can tolerate pain long enough (approximately 1–2 years), range of motion and pain generally improve. Those patients with more recalcitrant symptoms may need to undergo a manipulation under anesthesia or shoulder arthroscopy.
   d. Patients with diabetes mellitus have a more resistant course and generally do not respond well to manipulation under anesthesia; occasionally motion improves, but patient continues to have impingement type pain. In this instance, an arthroscopic lysis of adhesions and subacromial decompression can be helpful.

N. **Trigger point spasms**
1. **Description:** A painful, persistent localized muscle spasm that can occur in any muscle. Most common sites are along medial and superior borders of scapula. Multiple trigger points are common.

2. **Mechanism of injury:** Unknown, but may accompany other injuries such as rotator cuff tendinitis or cervical radiculopathy. Some trigger point spasms may be aggravated by stress and poor posture.
3. **Treatment:** Deep muscle massage or accupressure may help to break muscle spasm and pain cycle. Occasionally, a Lidocaine or cortisone injection may also help. Adjunctive treatments include ice, ultrasound, muscle stimulation, good posture, scapulothoracic strengthening, massage, and evaluation or work place ergonomics.

Recommended Reading

1. Bassett RW, Cofield RH: Acute tears of the rotator cuff. Clin Orthop 175:18–24, 1983.
2. Boublik M, Hawkins RJ: Clinical examination of the shoulder complex. J Orthop Sports Phys Ther 18(1):379–385, 1993.
3. Brems J: Rotator cuff tear: Evaluation and treatment. Orthopedics 11:69–81, 1988.
4. Cofield RH: Current concepts review: Rotator cuff disease of the shoulder. J Bone Joint Surg 67A:974–979, 1985.
5. Gerber C, Krushnell RJ: Isolated rupture of the tendon of the subscapularis muscle. J Bone Joint Surg 73B:389–394, 1991.
6. Hawkins RJ: Musculoskeletal Examination. St. Louis, Mosby Year Book, Inc., 1995.
7. Hawkins RJ: The Rotator Cuff and Biceps Tendon in Surgery of the Musculoskeletal System. New York, Churchill Livingstone, 1983, pp 3, 5–33.
8. Hawkins RJ: Surgical management of rotator cuff tears. In Bateman JE, Welsh RP (eds): Surgery of the Shoulder. Philadelphia, B.C. Decker, 1984, pp 161–166.
9. Hawkins RJ, Abrams JS: Impingement syndrome in the absence of rotator cuff tear (stages 1 and 2). Orthop Clin North Am 18:373–382, 1987.
10. Hawkins RJ, Bell RH, Hawkins RH, et al: Anterior dislocation of the shoulder in the older patient. Clin Orthop 206:192–195, 1986.
11. Hawkins RJ, Hobeika PE: Impingement syndrome in the athletic shoulder. Clin Sports Med 2:391–405, 1983.
12. Hawkins RJ, Mohtadi NG: Clinical evaluation of shoulder instability. Clin J Sports Med 1:59, 1991.
13. Jobe FW: Serious rotator cuff injuries. Clin Sports Med 2:407–412, 1983.
14. Jobe FW, Jobe CM: Painful athletic injuries of the shoulder. Clin Orthop 173:117–124, 1983.
15. Kieft GJ, et al: Rotator cuff impingement syndrome: MR imaging. Radiology 166:211, 1988.
16. Matsen FA, Arntz CT: Subacromial impingement. In Rockwood CA, Matsen FA (eds): The Shoulder. Philadelphia, W.B. Saunders, 1990, pp 623–646.
17. Matsen FA, Arntz CT: Rotator cuff tendon failure. In Rockwood CA, Matsen FA (eds): The Shoulder. Philadelphia, W.B. Saunders, 1990, pp 647–677.
18. Matsen FA, Thomas SC, Rockwood CA: Anterior glenohumeral instability. In Rockwood CA, Matsen FA (eds): The Shoulder. Philadelphia, W.B. Saunders, 1990, pp 526–622.
19. Mirowitz SA: Normal rotator cuff: MR imaging with conventional and fat suppression techniques. Radiology 180:735, 1991.
20. Rockwood CA: Disorders of the sternoclavicular joint. In Rockwood CA, Matsen FA (eds): The Shoulder. Philadelphia, W.B. Saunders, 1990, pp 492–493.
21. Rowe CR: The Shoulder. New York, Churchill Livingstone, 1988, pp 103–155.
22. Silliman JF, Hawkins RJ: Current concepts and recent advances in the athlete's shoulder. Clin Sports Med 10(4):693–706, 1991.
23. Snyder SJ, Karzel RP, Del Pizzo W, et al: SLAP lesions of the shoulder. Arthroscopy 6(4):274–279, 1990.

44

Elbow Injuries

Thomas L. Mehlhoff, M.D., and James B. Bennett, M.D., FACS

I. Diagnosis of Elbow Disorders in the Athlete

A. **History**
   1. Type of injury
   2. Location of pain
   3. Activities that aggravate symptoms
   4. Activities that relieve symptoms
   5. Recent changes in technique or training schedules
   6. Results of previous treatment

B. **Physical examination**
   1. **Inspection**
      a. Look at entire upper body
      b. Compare size (dominance, exercise hypertrophy)
      c. Swelling
      d. Carrying angle (cubitus valgus, cubitus varus)
   2. **Manipulation** (painful movements last)
      a. **Active and passive range of motion (ROM)** (compared with uninjured elbow):
         i. Extension (0°)
         ii. Flexion (150°)
         iii. Pronation (70°)
         iv. Supination (90°)
      b. **Resisted isometric movements**
      c. **Stability**
         i. Valgus-varus stress
         ii. Anterior-posterior stress
   3. **Palpation**
      a. Identify areas of tenderness as anterior, posterior, medial, or lateral.
      b. Differential injection with local anesthetic may more precisely localize pain.
         i. **Anterior elbow pain** (Fig. 1)
            (a) Biceps tendinitis
            (b) Biceps rupture
            (c) Anterior capsule tear
            (d) Median nerve compression syndrome
         ii. **Posterior elbow pain** (Fig. 2)
            (a) Triceps tendinitis
            (b) Triceps rupture/olecranon fracture
            (c) Olecranon impingement syndrome
            (d) Olecranon bursitis
         iii. **Medial elbow pain** (Fig. 3)
            (a) Medial epicondylitis

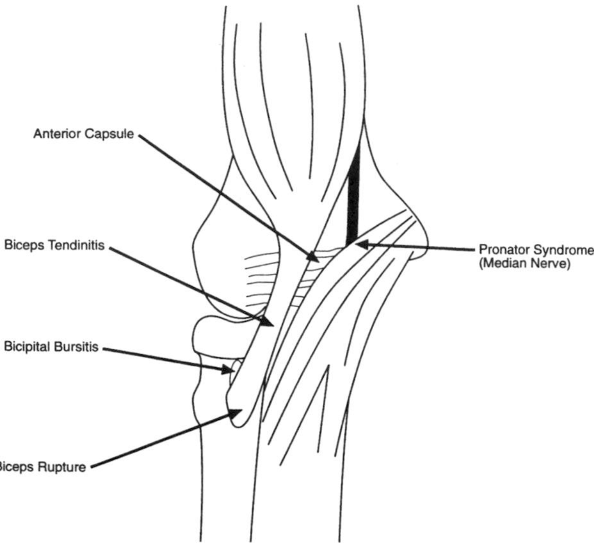

FIGURE 1. Anterior elbow pain.

 (b) Flexor-pronator strain
 (c) Medial collateral ligament sprain
 (d) Ulnar nerve compression syndrome

vi. **Lateral elbow pain** (Fig. 4)
 (a) Lateral epicondylitis
 (b) Radiocapitellar chondromalacia
 (c) Osteochondritis dissecans capitellum
 (d) Radial head fracture
 (e) Posterior interosseous nerve compression syndrome

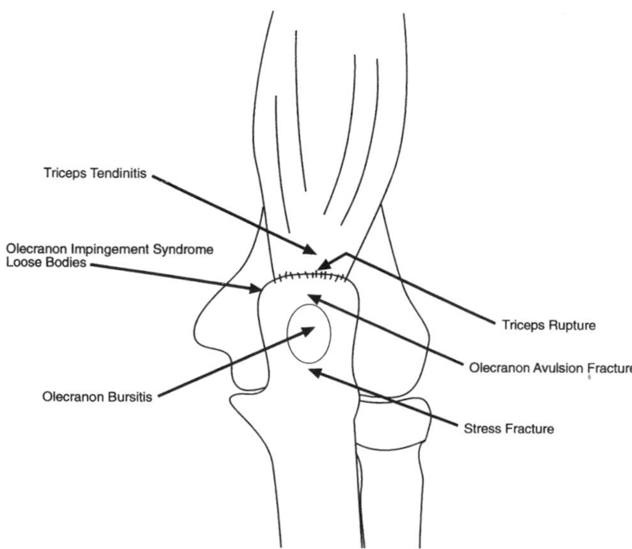

FIGURE 2. Posterior elbow pain.

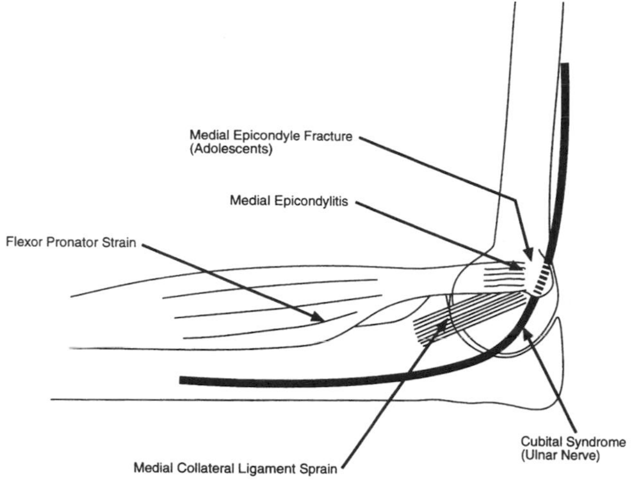

FIGURE 3. Medial elbow pain.

C. **Ancillary tests**
   1. **X-ray**
      a. Anteroposterior and lateral
      b. Special views:
         i. Oblique views (radial head view)
         ii. Axial projections (olecranon fossa)
         iii. Gravity stress view
   2. **Arthrogram/arthrotomogram**
      a. Articular incontinuity
      b. Loose bodies
   3. **Computed tomography (CT) scan**
      a. Fracture-dislocation
      b. Exostosis

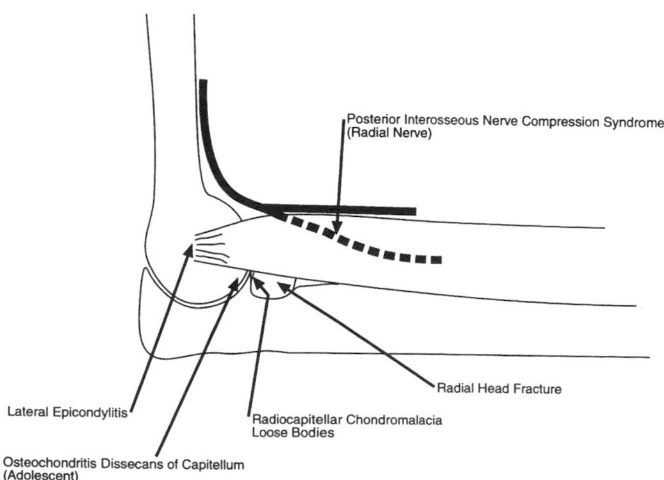

FIGURE 4. Lateral elbow pain.

4. **Magnetic resonance imaging (MRI)**
   a. Soft tissue mass
   b. Ligament rupture
   c. Chondral defects
5. **Arthroscopy**—intra-articular inspection
   a. Loose bodies
   b. Chondral lesions
   c. Synovitis

II. Anterior Elbow Injuries

A. **Biceps tendinitis**
1. Overuse syndrome caused by repetitive overloading of biceps as a result of excessive elbow flexion and supination activities
2. **Symptoms**
   a. Anterior elbow pain with flexion and supination
   b. Weakness secondary to pain
3. **Signs**
   a. Tender biceps tendon to palpation
   b. Increased pain on resisted forearm supination
4. **X-rays**—negative
5. **Differential diagnosis**
   a. Bicipital bursitis
   b. Biceps tendon rupture (partial or complete)
   c. Brachialis muscle tear
   d. Anterior capsule tear
   e. Lateral antebrachial cutaneous nerve compression syndrome
6. **Management**
   a. Rest, ice or heat, nonsteroidal anti-inflammatory drugs (NSAIDs)
   b. Splint or cast
   c. Selected injection (complication is tendon rupture)
   d. Modification of training schedule or technique

B. **Distal biceps rupture**
1. 97% of biceps ruptures are proximal; only 3% of biceps ruptures occur at the elbow.
2. Although a single traumatic event is usually recalled, preexisting degenerative changes in the tendon make it vulnerable to rupture.
3. **Predisposing factors**
   a. Male
   b. Over 30 years of age
   c. Steroid medication
4. **Symptoms**
   a. Pain in the antecubital fossa
   b. Weakness of supination and flexion (decreased 40%)
5. **Signs**
   a. Tenderness, swelling, ecchymosis in antecubital fossa
   b. No palpable biceps tendon
   c. Deformity as muscle belly retracts proximally
   d. Can still flex (brachialis) and supinate (supinator), but these movements are weak when resisted
6. **X-ray**—unusual to see changes, but these may include:
   a. Avulsion fragment from the radial tuberosity
   b. Degenerative changes on volar aspect radial tuberosity

7. **Management**
   a. Treatment of distal rupture is surgical.
   b. Goal is to restore full supination and flexion power.
   c. Repair biceps tendon to the radial tuberosity through two-incision approach of Boyd and Anderson.
   d. Elbow is immobilized at 90° flexion with moderate forearm supination for 8 weeks, followed by gradual active ROM and strengthening.

C. **Anterior capsule strain**
1. Painful microtears of the anterior capsule resulting from a hyperextension injury, not sufficient to cause dislocation
2. **Symptoms and signs**
   a. Anterior elbow pain poorly localized after traumatic event
   b. Deep tenderness of anterior elbow joint to palpation
3. **X-ray**—usually normal, but may reveal:
   a. Capsular fleck avulsions from medial or lateral epicondyle
   b. Heterotopic ossification in capsule or collateral ligaments on later follow-up
4. **Differential diagnosis**
   a. Dislocation (may have spontaneously reduced)
   b. Fracture-dislocation
   c. Coronoid process fracture
5. **Management**
   a. Document neurovascular examination and stability.
   b. Immobilize 3–5 days, then active ROM as pain allows.
   c. Flexion contracture may result from fibrosis due to repeated injury (strain) of the capsule.

D. **Median nerve compression syndrome (pronator syndrome)**
1. Entrapment neuropathy of the median nerve caused by mechanical compression by hypertrophied muscle or aponeurotic fascia
   a. Supracondylar process/ligament of Struthers
   b. Lacertus fibrosus
   c. Pronator teres (most common)
   d. Flexor digitorum superficialis arcade
2. **Symptoms**
   a. Pain in anterior proximal forearm, sometimes cramping
   b. Aggravated by resisted pronation activities
   c. Numbness in volar forearm or radial 3½ digits and thumb
3. **Signs**
   a. Positive Tinel's sign proximal forearm
   b. Negative Tinel's, Phalen's sign at wrist
   c. **May elicit symptoms for each site:**
      i. Supracondylar process by elbow flexion 120–135°
      ii. Lacertus fibrosus by resisted forearm supination
      iii. Pronator teres by resisted forearm pronation
      iv. Flexor digitorum superficialis arcade by resisted flexion long finger
4. **X-ray**—normal (supracondylar process present in 1% of limbs)
5. Confirm with electromyogram/nerve conduction velocity (EMG/NCV) test, although not always reliable
6. **Management**
   a. Rest, modification of training
   b. Graduated flexibility and strengthening of forearm
   c. Surgical decompression in unrelieved cases

III. Posterior Elbow Injuries

A. **Triceps tendinitis**

1. Overuse syndrome due to overloading of triceps by repetitive extension of the elbow
2. **Symptom**—pain posterior elbow
3. **Signs**
   a. Tenderness at or above the insertion of the triceps
   b. Increased pain with resisted extension of the elbow
4. **X-ray**—usually normal, but may reveal:
   a. Degenerative calcification
   b. Hypertrophy of the ulna
   c. Triceps traction spur
5. **Differential diagnosis**
   a. Intratendinous or subtendinous bursitis
   b. Stress fracture of olecranon
   c. Fracture or nonunion of olecranon osteophyte
6. **Management**
   a. Rest, ice or heat, NSAIDs
   b. Injection (complication is rupture)
   c. Rehabilitation with graduated stretching and strengthening

B. **Triceps rupture/olecranon avulsion**

1. An uncoordinated triceps contracture during a fall or a direct blow to the elbow may cause tendon rupture or olecranon avulsion.
2. Spontaneous rupture is associated with systemic disease or steroids.
3. **Symptoms**
   a. Pain and swelling in the posterior elbow, usually severe acutely
   b. Weakness or loss of active elbow extension
4. **Signs**
   a. Tenderness at insertion of extensor mechanism
   b. Palpable defect in the triceps tendon or step-off of olecranon
   c. If complete, no active extension of elbow
5. **X-ray**
   a. Flecks of avulsed bone (80% ruptures)
   b. Large olecranon fragment
6. **Management**
   a. Partial tears may be treated conservatively.
   b. Treatment is surgical:
      i. Reattachment of avulsed triceps tendon to olecranon with nonabsorbable suture through drill holes
      ii. Open reduction and internal fixation of fragment if sufficiently large; otherwise excision and repair of triceps to articular surface
      iii. Immobilize 45° flexion for 4 weeks, allow 0–45° flexion for 4 weeks, then graduated active ROM and strengthening.

C. **Olecranon impingement syndrome (hyperextension valgus overload syndrome, olecranon fossitis, "boxer's elbow")**

1. Overuse syndrome caused by repetitive valgus extension overloading, which causes the olecranon process to be forced against the medial wall of the olecranon fossa.
2. **Symptoms**
   a. Insidious onset of pain while extending the elbow (especially throwing)
   b. Catching or locking of elbow in extension
   c. Loss of pitching velocity or control
3. **Signs**
   a. Tenderness or swelling posteriorly

   b. Lack of full extension
   c. Pain on forced extension with valgus stress
   d. Palpable loose bodies
4. **X-ray** (recommend axial view in addition to anteroposterior and lateral)
   a. Hypertrophy of olecranon
   b. Spurring of olecranon tip and medial wall olecranon fossa
   c. Loose bodies
5. **Management**
   a. Rest, NSAIDs
   b. Correction of poor throwing mechanics
   c. Surgical removal of olecranon tip, osteophytes, and loose bodies via arthroscopy or posterior arthrotomy

D. **Olecranon bursitis ("miner's elbow," "student's elbow")**
1. Repetitive trauma causes irritation to olecranon bursa
2. **Symptom**—relatively painless posterior swelling
3. **Signs**
   a. Fluctuant bursa
   b. No cellulitis
4. **X-ray**—negative
5. **Differential diagnosis**—septic bursitis
6. **Management**
   a. Prevention with protective elbow pads
   b. Aspiration, compression, NSAIDs, and elbow pad
   c. Splinting for protracted cases
   d. Culture if septic bursitis is suspected
   e. If chronic, surgical excision can be recommended, but there is risk of poor wound healing over the olecranon.

IV. Medial Elbow Injuries

A. **Medial epicondylitis ("golfer's elbow")**
1. Repetitive tension overloading of the wrist flexors causes microtears in the tendinous insertion at the epicondyle.
2. **Symptoms**
   a. Painful inflammation over the medial epicondyle
   b. Weakness secondary to pain
3. **Signs**
   a. Tenderness at flexor origin medial epicondyle
   b. Increased pain with resisted wrist flexion and forearm pronation
   c. Negative Tinel's sign at cubital tunnel
4. **X-ray**—usually negative, but small calcific deposits occasionally seen
5. **Differential diagnosis**
   a. Flexor-pronator strain
   b. Medial collateral ligament sprain
   c. Ulnar neuritis
6. **Management**
   a. Conservative management usually successful
      i. Rest
      ii. Splint (wrist in flexion)
      iii. NSAIDs
      iv. Steroid injection (limit to three)
      v. Wrist flexion curl exercises
   b. Surgery for rare patient who does not improve

i. Recession of flexor origin from medial epicondyle
ii. Four weeks immobilization in splint followed by flexibility and strengthening for 12 weeks

B. **Flexor-pronator strain**
1. Repetitive tensile stresses to a vulnerable flexor-pronator mass may result in microruptures of the muscle, especially after inadequate warm-up or after fatigue.
2. **Symptoms**
   a. Medial elbow and proximal forearm pain
   b. Aggravated by wrist flexion (pitching curve balls, curling) and forearm pronation (golfing)
3. **Signs**—tender flexor-pronator muscle bellies distal to medial epicondyle
4. **X-ray**—negative
5. **Management**
   a. Rest, ice, compression
   b. Modification of training schedule
   c. Proper warm-up activity
   d. Brief immobilization may be warranted in acute cases
   e. Flexor-pronator stretching and conditioning

C. **Medial collateral ligament sprain**
1. Repetitive valgus stress (pitching, throwing, racquet sports) causes tensile loading of the medial collateral ligament, resulting in microtears or complete rupture.
2. **Symptoms**
   a. Insidious medial elbow pain
   b. Provoked by valgus stress activities
   c. Relieved by rest
   d. Pain returns when throwing exceeds 70% normal velocity
3. **Signs**
   a. Tenderness below the medial epicondyle over the humeroulnar joint (anterior oblique ligament)
   b. Pain increased by manual valgus stress (elbow 30° flexion)
   c. Signs of ulnar neuritis may be associated because the medial collateral ligament forms the floor of the cubital tunnel.
4. **X-ray**
   a. Heterotopic ossification of the medial collateral ligament
   b. Spurring at sublime tubercle of ulna
   c. Gravity stress view negative unless medial collateral ligament totally incompetent
5. **Management**
   a. Rest, NSAIDs
   b. Strengthening pronator-flexor group
   c. Complete medial collateral ligament insufficiency in chronic cases may require surgical reconstruction with palmaris longus tendon.

D. **Medial epicondyle stress lesions ("Little Leaguer's elbow")**
1. Because the closing growth plate of the medial epicondyle in adolescents is sensitive to tension stress, repetitive or a sudden muscular contraction may result in partial or complete avulsion of the medial epicondyle.
2. **Symptoms and signs**
   a. Acute or insidious pain in medial elbow
   b. Tenderness in medial epicondyle, sometimes with swelling, ecchymosis
3. **X-ray**
   a. Widening of apophyseal line
   b. Partial or complete separation
4. **Management**

a. **Medial epicondylar stress lesion**—no throwing allowed for 6–12 weeks
b. **Medial epicondyle fracture**
   i. May treat closed if minimally displaced (< 5 mm)
   ii. **Must treat open if:**
      (a) Valgus instability present (> 10 mm displacement or positive gravity stress view)
      (b) Medial epicondyle incarcerated within the elbow joint
      (c) Ulnar nerve symptoms present

E. **Ulnar nerve compression syndrome (cubital tunnel syndrome)**
1. Entrapment neuropathy of ulnar nerve at the elbow, incited by trauma, cubitus valgus deformity, or subluxing ulnar nerve
2. **Symptoms**
   a. Aching medial elbow pain, which may migrate proximally or distally
   b. Frequently accompanied by grip weakness
   c. Numbness and occasional shocking into ulnar 1½ digits
   d. No pain; ROM not limited
3. **Signs**
   a. Positive Tinel's cubital tunnel
   b. Pain increased with full-forced elbow flexion
   c. Weakness of thumb–index finger pinch
   d. Intrinsic muscle wasting uncommon unless problem long-term
   e. Negative foraminal compression testing for cervical radiculopathy
4. **EMG/NCV**—slowing of conduction velocity across the elbow
5. **Differential diagnosis**
   a. Cervical radiculopathy
   b. Thoracic outlet syndrome
   c. Ulnar nerve compression at wrist (Guyon's canal)
6. **Management**
   a. Protection with elbow pad
   b. Rest, NSAIDs
   c. Modification of training
      i. Avoidance extreme flexion
      ii. Avoidance valgus stress
   d. Surgical decompression necessary for increasing motor involvement, pain, sensory deficit, or chronic cases
   e. Anterior transposition reserved for neuropathy associated with elbow deformity (cubitus valgus) or subluxation of the ulnar nerve

V. Lateral Elbow Injuries

A. **Lateral epicondylitis ("tennis elbow")**
1. Painful degenerative tears in the extensor carpi radialis brevis (ECRB) caused by repetitive tension overloading of the forearm and wrist extensors (hyperpronation greatly increases the overloading stresses)
2. Lateral epicondylitis is 10 times more frequent than medial epicondylitis.
3. **Predisposing factors**
   a. Age 30–50 years
   b. Faulty mechanics ("leading" elbow, off-center hits in racquet sports)
   c. Poorly fitted equipment (handle too small, string too tight)
4. **Symptoms**
   a. Aching pain over lateral epicondyle radiating proximally into forearm extensors during and after activity
   b. Initially subsides but with repetition becomes more severe

5. **Signs**
   a. Localized tenderness to lateral epicondyle
   b. Pain increased with resisted dorsiflexion of wrist
   c. **"Coffee cup" test**—pain increased with picking up a full cup of coffee
6. **X-ray**—small calcific deposits in extensor aponeurosis (22% of cases)
7. **Differential diagnosis**—posterior interosseous nerve compression (coexistent in 15% of cases)
8. **Management**
   a. **Nonsurgical management successful for most**
      i. Rest:
         (a) No grasping in pronation
         (b) Use supination when lifting
      ii. NSAIDs
      iii. Volar cock-up splint
      iv. Counterforce bracing
      v. Steroid injection (limit to three)
      vi. Wrist extension curls or lifts
      vii. Proper mechanics for the sport
      viii. **Proper equipment**
         (a) Larger racquet head
         (b) Correct grip size = midpalmar crease to tip of ring finger
         (c) Medium tension strings, 50–55 lb
   b. **Surgical treatment for refractory cases**
      i. Debridement of ECRB with repair
      ii. Rehabilitation
         (a) Progressive strengthening with wrist curls
         (b) Daily warm-up
         (c) Postexercise icing
         (d) Counterforce bracing for 3 months
         (e) Return to sports in 6 months

B. **Radiocapitellar chondromalacia**
1. Valgus stress of throwing and racquet sports imparts strong tensile forces to the medial collateral ligament and strong compressive forces to the lateral joint of the elbow.
2. Repeated compressive forces can cause damage to the radial head, capitellum, or both (osteochondral fracture and even loose body may result).
3. **Symptoms**
   a. Lateral elbow pain with activity
   b. Catching and locking
4. **Signs**
   a. Tender radiocapitellar joint, lateral swelling
   b. Crepitus with forearm pronation-supination
5. **X-ray**
   a. Loss of radiocapitellar joint space
   b. Marginal osteophytes
   c. Loose bodies
6. **Management**
   a. Difficult to treat once joint damage established
   b. Mild disorder
      i. Rest, NSAIDs
      ii. Graduated activity dictated by pain, swelling
   c. Severe disorder

   i. Joint debridement through lateral arthrotomy with removal of marginal osteophytes and loose bodies
   ii. Prognosis is proportional to cartilage damage.

C. **Osteochondritis dissecans capitellum**
   1. Focal lesion in young athletes with open growth plates (age 10 to 15 years), attributed to lateral compressive forces
   2. **Symptoms**
      a. Pain with activity
      b. Pain improved with rest
      c. Occasionally clicking or locking of elbow
   3. **Signs**
      a. Tenderness radiocapitellar joint, swelling
      b. Grating with pronation-supination
      c. Lack of full extension
   4. **X-rays**, tomograms, or arthrotomograms
      a. Irregularity or flattening of capitellum
      b. Crater with loose body
   5. **Differential diagnosis**—Panner's osteochondrosis
   6. **Management**
      a. Rest (6–18 months)
      b. If no loose body, no further treatment may be needed
      c. If fragment is displaced, then recommend reattachment of articular fragment if large, but otherwise excision

D. **Radial head fracture**
   1. Compressive axial loading force across the radiocapitellar joint during a fall onto outstretched arm may result in fracture of the radial head.
   2. Mason describes **types** as:
      a. Type I—nondisplaced
      b. Type II—displaced (impaction > 3 mm, angulation > 30°)
      c. Type III—comminuted
   3. **Symptom**—severe lateral elbow pain
   4. **Signs**
      a. Tenderness well localized to radial head
      b. Passive pronation-supination painful
      c. Crepitus may be present, but examiner should not attempt to demonstrate this repeatedly.
      d. May have associated valgus instability of the elbow or axial instability of the forearm (Essix-Lopresti lesion)
   5. **X-ray**
      a. Positive posterior fat-pad sign suggests an intra-articular fracture
      b. Nondisplaced fracture difficult to diagnose unless oblique views are taken
      c. Check capitellum for osteochondral fracture.
   6. **Management**
      a. Type I: Treatment nonoperative, with early ROM
      b. Type II: Controversial but suggest open reductions, internal fixation for large fragments
      c. Type III: Usually requires excision radial head. Beware of associated elbow medial collateral ligament or forearm instability (interosseous membrane).

E. **Posterior interosseous nerve compression syndrome (radial tunnel syndrome)**
   1. Entrapment neuropathy of the posterior interosseous branch of the radial nerve under the fibrous arch of supinator (arcade of Frosche) or more distally in the supinator muscle

2. **Symptoms**
   a. Arching lateral elbow pain radiating into dorsal forearm
   b. Aggravated by pronation-supination activities
   c. Extensor weakness of the wrist and fingers but no numbness
3. **Signs**
   a. Positive Tinel's sign 8 cm (four fingerbreadths) distal to the lateral epicondyle
   b. Weakness of extensor digitorum communis, especially middle finger
   c. No sensory loss
4. **X-ray**—normal
5. **EMG/NCV** rarely confirmatory for posterior interosseous nerve compression
6. **Differential diagnosis**
   a. Lateral epicondylitis
   b. Extensor tendon rupture
   c. Extensor tendon dislocation (hood injury)
7. **Management**
   a. Rest, modification of training schedule
   b. Surgical decompression in recalcitrant cases

VI. Dislocations and Fracture-dislocations

A. Acute injury to the elbow following specific traumatic event, usually a fall onto outstretched arm
B. **Symptom**—severe pain, often too painful to move
C. **Signs**
   1. Acute tenderness and swelling
   2. Deformity of the elbow
   3. Limited motion, possibly with crepitus
   4. Neurologic or vascular compromise
D. **X-ray**
   1. Dislocation
   2. Dislocation with associated fracture
      a. Radial head
      b. Coronoid process
      c. Medial epicondyle
   3. Monteggia fracture
   4. Supracondylar humerus fracture
   5. T-intercondylar humerus fracture
E. **Management**
   1. Document neurovascular examination
   2. Immobilize the injured extremity with splint.
   3. Refer urgently to emergency room for x-ray evaluation and further treatment as indicated:
      a. Closed reduction
      b. Open reduction and internal fixation

Recommended Reading

1. Anderson RL: Traumatic rupture of the triceps tendon. J Trauma 19:134, 1979.
2. Bosworth DM: Surgical treatment of tennis elbow: A follow-up study. J Bone Joint Surg 47:1533–1536, 1965.
3. Boyd HD, Anderson LD: A method for reinsertion of the distal biceps brachii tendon. J Bone Joint Surg 43:1041–1043, 1961.
4. Brogdon BE, Crow WF: Little leaguer's elbow. Am J Roentgenol 8:671, 1960.
5. Buehler MJ, Thayer DT: The elbow flexion test: A clinical test for cubital tunnel syndrome. Clin Orthop 233:213, 1988.

6. Canoso JJ: Idiopathic or traumatic olecranon bursitis: Clinical features and bursal fluid analysis. Arthritis Rheum 20:1213, 1977.
7. Coonrad RW, Hooper WR: Tennis elbow: Its course, natural history, conservative and surgical management. J Bone Joint Surg 55:1177–1182, 1973.
8. Dellon AL: Review of treatment results for ulnar nerve entrapment at the elbow. J Hand Surg 14:688–700, 1987.
9. Froimson AI: Treatment of tennis elbow with forearm support band. J Bone Joint Surg 53:183–184, 1971.
10. Gugenheim JJ, Stanley RF, Woods GW, Tullos HS: Little league survey: The Houston study. Am J Sports Med 4:189, 1976.
11. Jobe FW, Stark H, Lombardo SJ: Reconstruction of the ulnar collateral ligament in athletes. J Bone Joint Surg 68:1158–1163, 1986.
12. King D: Osteochondritis dissecans: A clinical study of twenty-four cases. J Bone Joint Surg 14:535, 1932.
13. Learmouth JR: A Technique for transplanting the ulnar nerves. Surg Gynecol Obstet 75:792–793, 1942.
14. Leffert RD: Anterior submuscular transposition of the ulnar nerves by the Learmouth technique. J Hand Surg 7:147–155, 1982.
15. Lister GD, Belsole RB, Kleinert HE: The radial tunnel syndrome. J Hand Surg 4:52–59, 1979.
15a. Mason MB: Some observations on fractures of the head of the radius with a review of 100 cases. Br J Surg 42:123, 1954.
16. Mehlhoff TL, Noble PC, Bennett JB, Tullos HS: Simple dislocation of the elbow in the adult. J Bone Joint Surg 70:244–249, 1988.
17. Morrey BF, An KN: Articular and ligamentous contribution to the stability of the elbow joint. Am J Sports Med 11:315, 1983.
18. Morrey BF, Askew LJ, An KN, Dobyus JH: Rupture of the distal tendon of the biceps brachii: A biomechanical study. J Bone Joint Surg 67:418–421, 1985.
19. Nirschl RP: The etiology and treatment of tennis elbow. J Sports Med Phys Fit 2:308–323, 1974.
20. Panner HJ: A peculiar affliction of the capitellum lumeri resembling Calve-Perthes disease of the hip. Acta Radiol 8:1617, 1927.
21. Pantazopoulos T, Exarchow E, Stavrou Z, Hartofilakidis-Garofalidis G: Avulsion of the triceps tendon. J Trauma 15:827, 1975.
22. Pappas AM: Osteochondritis dissecans. Clin Orthop 158:59, 1981.
23. Ritts ED, Wood MB, Linscheid RL: Radial tunnel syndrome: A ten year surgical experience. Clin Orthop 279:201–205, 1987.
24. Schwab GH, Bennett JB, Woods GW: Biomechanics of elbow stability. Clin Orthop 146:42, 1980.
25. UnVerforth JL: The effect of local steroid injections on tendons. J Sports Med 11:31–37, 1973.
26. Wilson FD, Andrews JR, Blackburn TA, McClusky G: Valgus extension overload in the pitching elbow. Am J Sports Med 11:83–88, 1983.
27. Zarins B, Andrews R, Carson WG Jr: Injuries to the Throwing Arm. Philadelphia, W.B. Saunders, 1985, pp 191–258.

45

Hand and Wrist Injuries

Jeffrey J. Tiedeman, M.D., and Thomas P. Ferlic, M.D.

I. History and Physical Examination

A. **History.** Evaluation of a patient with a hand or wrist injury begins with an accurate history. Location of injury and duration of symptoms should first be elicited. Any treatment patient may have received and prior history of injury are important factors to note.

B. **Physical examination**
1. A thorough examination of an injured hand or wrist includes inspection as well as palpation of the involved area.
2. Precise localization of tenderness is of great value in determining specific injury to digit.
3. Comparison to opposite side is also helpful in determination of such factors as physiologic laxity.

C. **Diagnostic studies.** Appropriate x-rays or specialized studies are helpful. Radiographs should be obtained whenever there are:
1. Persistent symptoms
2. Swelling
3. Limited joint motion
4. Cases of dislocation

II. Distal Interphalangeal (DIP) Joint Injuries

A. **Mallet finger**
1. **Description:** A flexion deformity of the DIP joint caused by loss of continuity of extensor mechanism to distal phalanx. Injury to extensor mechanism may involve tendon only, or tendon may remain attached to an avulsed piece of bone or fracture fragment.
2. **Mechanism of injury:** Usually caused by sudden forceful flexion of DIP joint. Often seen when a ball hits tip of an extended finger. Consequently, this injury is frequently referred to as a **"baseball finger."**
3. **Diagnosis**
   a. **Examination** reveals pain, swelling, and a variable lack of active extension of the DIP joint.
   b. **X-rays**
      i. May be remarkable only for a flexed DIP joint or show a fracture of proximal portion of distal phalanx (Fig. 1).
      ii. Volar subluxation of distal phalanx may accompany a fracture, particularly if the fragment is large.
4. **Treatment**
   a. Acute mallet fingers treated by splinting DIP joint in complete extension fulltime for 6–8 weeks. This can be accomplished with one of several commercially available splints.
      i. Encourage proximal interphalangeal and metacarpophalangeal joint motion.

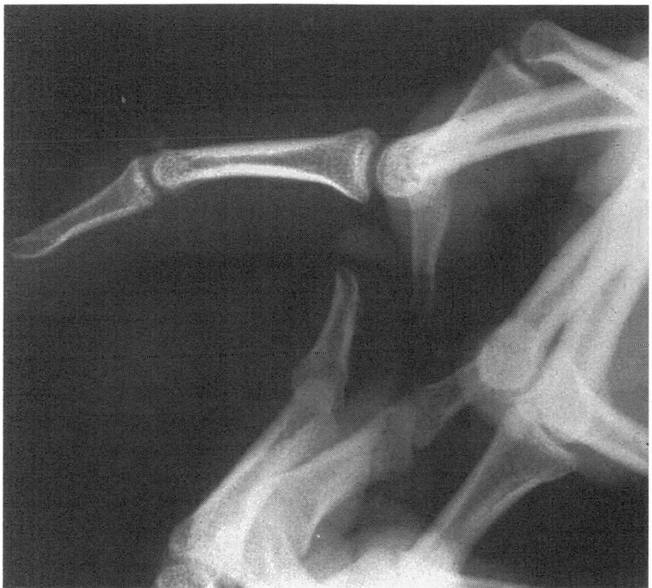

FIGURE 1. X-ray of a mallet finger. Note the flexed posture and the small fracture of the proximal dorsal portion of the distal phalanx.

ii. Night splinting for an additional 2 weeks and serial reevaluation to make sure that extension has been maintained

iii. Soft tissue irritation or ulceration on dorsum of DIP joint may occur secondary to splinting. Patient should frequently inspect this area.

b. Operative treatment may be required in mallet fingers with large fracture fragments, such as those involving more than 30% of articular surface or in cases of volar subluxation of distal phalanx.

B. **Jersey finger**

1. **Description:** Traumatic avulsion of insertion of flexor digitorum profundus (FDP) tendon. Ring finger followed by small finger are most commonly involved.
2. **Mechanism of injury:** Hyperextension of DIP joint on attempted flexion of finger. Commonly happens to football safeties and linebackers who attempt to stop a running back from behind, grab his jersey with their fingers flexed, and apply sudden and forceful power to flexor tendon system. FDP tendon is avulsed from its bony insertion in the distal phalanx.
3. **Diagnosis**

a. **Examination**

i. **Lack of active flexion at the DIP joint**

ii. May be hematoma formation in entire flexor tendon sheath and resultant tenderness to palpation

(a) Specific localization of tenderness should be elicited if possible because this may indicate level of tendon retraction.

(b) If tendon is avulsed with a piece of bone, it may become trapped distal to A4 pulley in middle phalanx or distal to A2 pulley, or it may retract all the way into the palm.

b. **X-rays:** Look for a bony fragment on volar aspect of digit in one of three areas mentioned. A high index of suspicion is often required to identify and localize this fragment correctly if present.

4. **Treatment: Operative intervention is required.** No conservative treatment can be expected to bring flexor tendon back to its normal length. Perform surgery as soon as possible within first few days of injury. Occasionally, this injury is missed, and depending on position or level of flexor tendon retraction, a later repair may be feasible. Surgery involves reattachment of FDP tendon to its insertion in distal phalanx followed by a controlled mobilization program.

C. **Dislocation of DIP joint**
1. **Description:** Rare, but when does occur is almost always dorsal. Is frequently associated with an open wound.
2. **Mechanism of injury:** A forceful, direct blow to the tip of the finger
3. **Diagnosis**
   a. **Examination**
      i. Tenderness to palpation over DIP joint and inability to flex or extend joint
      ii. Distal phalanx usually displaced dorsally or laterally
      iii. An open wound in conjunction with this injury is quite common and should be identified if present.
   b. **X-rays:** Confirm dislocation of joint. Important to look for an associated osteochondral fracture. If present, this injury should be treated aggressively because amount of joint disruption is typically greater than that which can be appreciated on x-rays alone.
4. **Treatment**
   a. Dislocation should be addressed by gentle closed reduction. Key to reducing joints is both pushing and pulling in a controlled and gentle manner.
      i. If dislocation is associated with open soft tissue injury, thorough irrigation and debridement before reduction.
      ii. A digital block may be of benefit before reduction.
   b. After reduction, hyperextension and medial/lateral stress examination, but DIP dislocations are typically stable.
      i. A short period of immobilization (10–14 days) of DIP alone
      ii. Postreduction x-rays to make sure no fractures are present

III. Proximal Interphalangeal (PIP) Joint Injuries

A. **Collateral ligament sprain**
1. **Description:** Collateral ligament sprain implies that supporting structures for radial or ulnar side of PIP joint have been torn.
2. **Mechanism of injury:** Abduction or adduction force applied to the finger, usually in extended position. Often, patient may have had a dislocation that has spontaneously reduced or been reduced. Radial collateral ligament is injured more frequently than ulnar collateral ligament. Collateral ligament injuries are classified as either acute or chronic and as stable or unstable.
3. **Diagnosis**
   a. **Examination**
      i. Point tenderness over specific site of tear is common.
      ii. Ligament failure usually occurs at its attachment to proximal phalanx or, less frequently, in the midportion.
      iii. Stress testing should be performed with joint held both in extension and in 20–30° of flexion (Fig. 2).
      iv. Lack of a discernible end point is diagnostic of a complete tear.
      v. A digital block facilitates examination.
   b. **X-rays**
      i. At least two views of involved finger rather than whole hand
      ii. Stress x-rays with comparison to opposite hand as a reference

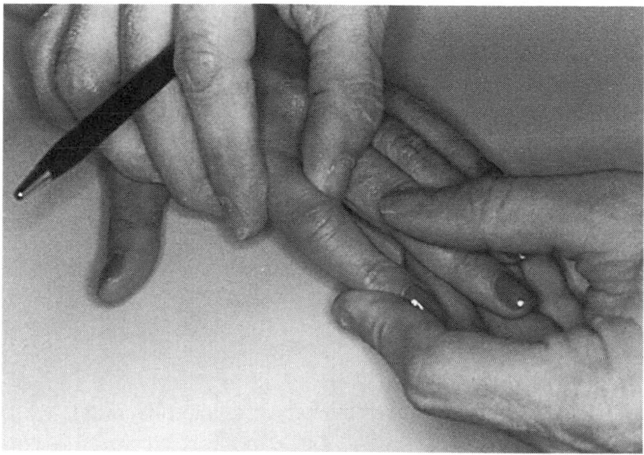

FIGURE 2. Stress applied to radial collateral ligament of index finger.

iii. Angulation > 20° on anteroposterior view is thought to be diagnostic of a complete rupture.

4. **Treatment**
   a. Partial tears (sprains) and some complete tears can be treated with buddy taping to adjacent digit. Tape is worn continuously for 3 weeks and during periods of activity for an additional 3 weeks with active motion encouraged from the outset. Patient should be made aware that there is residual discomfort in joint often for several months and permanent residual enlargement of the joint secondary to underlying scar tissue formation.
   b. Operative repair of a collateral ligament injury may be beneficial in some chronic or acute ruptures depending on finger involved. Radial collateral ligament to index finger is obviously more important in pinch than radial ligament of small finger, and surgery may be a more appropriate choice when the former is injured.

B. **Dorsal PIP dislocation**
1. **Description: Most frequently encountered articular injury in the hand.** A dorsal dislocation implies that middle phalanx has been displaced dorsally relative to proximal phalanx.
2. **Mechanism of injury:** Hyperextension of PIP joint along with simultaneous longitudinal compression. Typically occurs when finger is forcibly bent back, such as in a **"jammed finger."**
3. **Diagnosis**
   a. **Examination**
      i. At time of presentation, joint may still be dislocated with obvious deformity, but more frequently it has spontaneously reduced or been reduced by a bystander or coach.
      ii. **Swelling and localized tenderness over volar plate region, most commonly at its distal insertion into middle phalanx, are hallmark clinical findings.**
      iii. Hyperextension stress testing by examiner helps determine residual instability. Performance of this stress test after digital block and comparison to opposite side allows a more accurate assessment because some individuals have an underlying hyperextension laxity. Test is done by holding pressure over dorsum of proximal phalanx and applying hyperextension force to middle phalanx (Fig. 3).

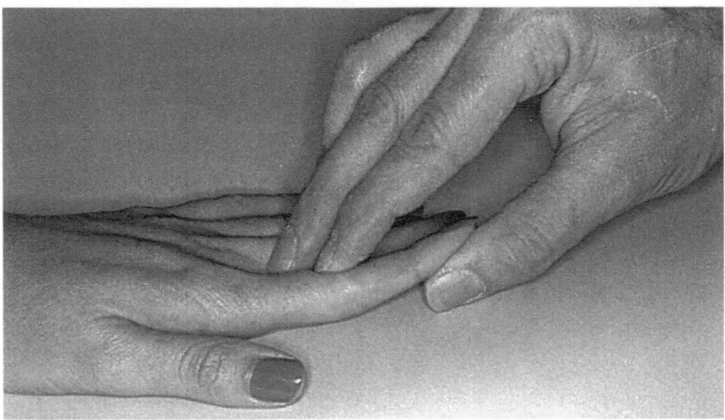

FIGURE 3. Stress applied to volar plate of the proximal interphalangeal joint by attempting to hyperextend it.

iv. Collateral ligaments should also be examined for tenderness or laxity, but in a pure dorsal dislocation these structures are not typically injured.

b. **X-rays**

i. An anteroposterior and lateral x-ray of the finger

ii. **A small fracture of proximal portion on volar aspect of middle phalanx is pathognomonic for a volar plate tear.**

4. **Treatment**

a. Reduction is easily accomplished with longitudinal traction. Most dorsal dislocations with volar plate injuries can be treated with 3–6 weeks of continuous buddy taping, which allows early active motion and prevents hyperextension.

b. More unstable injuries can be protected in a position of flexion with an extension block splint, gradually allowing the joint to regain further extension over 3–4 weeks.

c. Hyperextension instability after a dorsal dislocation is rare. A flexion contracture of PIP joint is actually most frequently observed complication following dorsal dislocation. This flexion contracture results in what is referred to as a pseudoboutonniere deformity. It can be treated with a dynamic extension splint for PIP joint, which can be applied as early as 6 weeks after injury.

d. If fracture fragment contains more than 10–15% of volar surface, concern is that this is actually a fracture dislocation of PIP joint—an entirely different and potentially disabling injury. Operative intervention with surgical stabilization of joint is often required. A true lateral x-ray of finger is required to assess adequacy of joint reduction.

C. **Volar PIP joint dislocation**

1. **Description:** Less common and often associated with massive soft tissue damage that can lead to long-term joint disability. Extensor mechanism insertion into proximal portion of middle phalanx, so-called central slip, is often disrupted in a volar PIP dislocation. Primary function of central slip is to extend PIP joint.

2. **Mechanism of injury:** A blow or direct force applied to the dorsum of the middle phalanx. Central slip can also be damaged by a laceration over dorsum of PIP joint.

3. **Diagnosis**

a. **Examination**

i. If joint remains dislocated, deformity is obvious.

ii. After reduction, point tenderness over middle phalanx on dorsal proximal aspect is diagnostic of a central slip injury (Fig. 4).

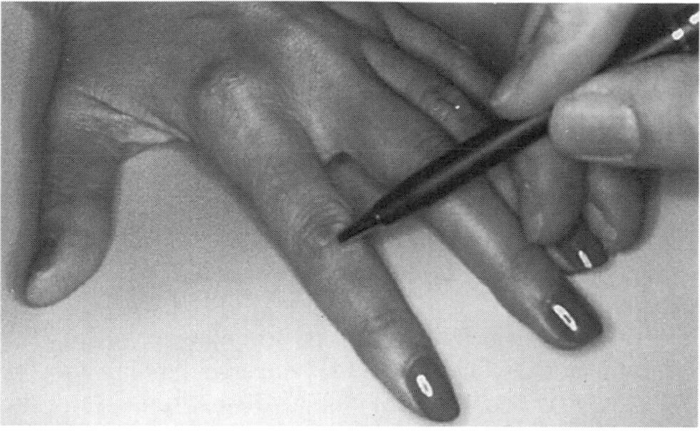

FIGURE 4. Pen points to insertion of central slip.

iii. **Definitive sign of this injury is lack of active extension of middle phalanx against resistance.**

iv. Collateral ligaments should also be inspected for both tenderness and laxity.

b. **X-rays:** Two views of involved digit, including an anteroposterior and lateral. No particular bony abnormality may be evident, or there may be a small avulsion in dorsum of middle phalanx from disrupted central slip insertion.

4. **Treatment**

a. Volar PIP joint dislocations that have been reduced and with suspected central slip injury should have PIP joint splinted in complete extension for 6 full weeks. During this time, active motion of DIP joint is imperative to maintain active pull-through of FDP tendon and extensor mechanism.

b. If fracture fragments are large, operative intervention with internal fixation can be considered.

c. Failure to diagnose a central slip injury and appropriately splint the PIP joint in extension can result in progressive volar subluxation of lateral bands of extensor mechanism. This subsequently results in an extension contracture of DIP joint. **Subsequent deformity in which PIP joint is held in flexion and DIP joint in hyperextension is referred to as a boutonniere deformity.**

IV. Metacarpophalangeal (MCP) Joint Injuries

A. Collateral ligament sprain

1. **Description:** Stability of MCP joint primarily depends on boxlike configuration formed by volar plate and ulnar and radial collateral ligaments. Isolated injury to collateral ligaments of finger MCP joint is relatively uncommon because of its protective position within digital web space as well as protection afforded by adjacent digit. Radial side of index finger is most susceptible to injury.

2. **Mechanism of injury:** Most commonly an ulnarly-directed force on MCP joint. Collateral ligament usually fails at its attachment to metacarpal head and may include avulsed bone.

3. **Diagnosis**

a. **Examination**

i. Local tenderness and subtle swelling in web space between two metacarpal heads directly over involved collateral ligament is most typical.

ii. Lateral stress testing should be applied to MCP joint, both in extension to look for pain and in flexion to look for instability.

b. **X-rays:** Usually demonstrate no abnormality or may reveal a small avulsion fracture fragment from metacarpal head

4. **Treatment**
   a. Conservative treatment of collateral ligament injuries of MCP joint in majority of cases. Either protection with buddy taping or splinting of MCP joint in 50° of flexion for more unstable injuries. Chronic pain and stiffness is a more frequent problem than persistent instability.
   b. Surgical treatment should be considered if there is an avulsion fracture present that is large (> 20% of the articular surface) or that is displaced more than 2 mm.

B. **MCP dislocation**
1. **Description:** MCP dislocations occur most frequently in a dorsal direction, with volar dislocations being quite rare. Index finger and thumb are most commonly involved. **There are two types of dorsal dislocations—simple and complex.** Important to differentiate between because required treatment is often different.
2. **Mechanism of injury:** Both simple and complex dorsal dislocations at MP joint result from hyperextension injuries. In both types volar plate is torn from its proximal insertion to neck of metacarpal.
3. **Diagnosis**
   a. **Examination**
      i. In a simple dislocation, there is noticeable deformity with marked MCP joint hyperextension.
      ii. In a complex dislocation, deformity is not as obvious, with joint only slightly hyperextended and proximal phalanx lying on dorsum of metacarpal head.
      iii. **A common finding in complex dislocation is a skin dimple evident in distal palmar crease.**
   b. **X-rays**
      i. In a simple dislocation, proximal phalanx rests in 60–90° of hyperextension on dorsum of metacarpal head.
      ii. In a complex dislocation, proximal phalanx and metacarpal are nearly parallel with only slight angulation.
      iii. **A pathognomonic radiographic finding of complex dislocation is presence of a sesamoid within a widened joint space.** This indicates that volar plate is trapped in joint.
4. **Treatment**
   a. Simple dislocations are reduced by joint hyperextension and distally directed pressure applied to base of proximal phalanx. Important not to apply just longitudinal traction to digit because this may convert a simple dislocation to a complex one.
   b. In complex dislocations, a single attempt at closed reduction after adequate anesthesia. Be prepared to follow with immediate open reduction if this maneuver is unsuccessful. After reduction MCP joint is typically stable, and no immobilization is required with early active motion encouraged. Protect with buddy taping for 2–3 weeks for activities.

V. Thumb MCP Injuries

A. **Ulnar collateral ligament sprain**
1. **Description:** Tear of ulnar collateral ligament of thumb is often referred to as a **"gamekeeper's thumb"** or **"skier's thumb."** A competent ulnar collateral ligament is critical for effective pinch.
2. **Mechanism of injury:** Usually a fall on an outstretched hand with thumb caught in a position of abduction

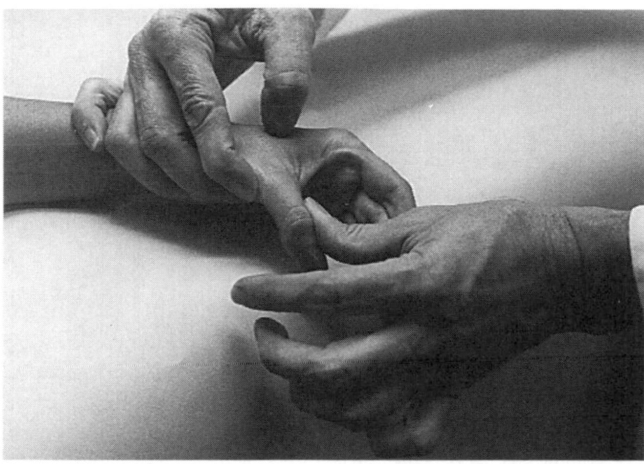

FIGURE 5. Stress applied to ulnar collateral ligament of the thumb.

3. **Diagnosis**
   a. **Examination:** Point tenderness is found over ulnar aspect of joint, specifically at insertion of collateral ligament in ulnar and volar aspect of proximal phalanx.
      i. Important to differentiate a partial from complete tear with stress testing
      ii. A digital or regional block is often required.
      iii. Testing should be performed with MCP joint both in flexion and in extension and comparison made to opposite side (Fig. 5).
   b. **X-rays**
      i. Radiographs of thumb before stress testing to look for any associated fracture
      ii. If after examination degree of injury remains uncertain, obtain stress radiographs. If > 20° of instability compared with opposite side is noted, a complete tear of ligament is likely.
4. **Treatment**
   a. For partial tears of ulnar collateral ligament, cast immobilization or functional bracing with MCP joint held in slight flexion for 4–6 weeks
   b. In complete tears, distal edge of ligament is often held in a displaced position by adductor aponeurosis, a problem known as a **Stener lesion.**
      i. Ligament cannot heal back to its normal anatomic position, and residual instability can occur.
      ii. For complete ruptures, operative intervention with surgical repair of ligament is indicated.

B. **Radial collateral ligament sprain**
1. **Description:** Injury of radial collateral ligament of MCP joint of thumb is far less common. Consequently, diagnosis is often missed and treatment delayed.
2. **Mechanism of injury:** Sudden forceful adduction of thumb MCP joint across hand
3. **Diagnosis**
   a. **Examination:** Localized swelling and tenderness on radial aspect of thumb MCP joint. Stress testing to elicit pain or instability.
   b. **X-rays:** Two views of thumb to evaluate for any associated fracture
4. **Treatment:** Because of anatomic differences on radial aspect of thumb, a Stener lesion does not occur. Therefore, if diagnosed acutely, almost all radial collateral injuries to thumb MCP joint can be treated conservatively with thumb spica cast immobilization or a functional brace for 4–6 weeks.

VI. Penetrating Injuries: Guidelines for Evaluation and Management

A. **Description:** The initial phase of evaluation involves eliciting an accurate history. Questions of when, where, and how injury occurred all need to be answered. Other constitutional factors need to be identified, including drug allergies, medications taken on a regular basis, or history of significant medical illness.

B. **Diagnosis**

1. **Examination:** Many mistakes can be avoided if examination and treatment are done in a systematic fashion. Several factors should be addressed:
   a. Patient as calm and comfortable as possible
   b. All jewelry removed to avoid complications of future swelling
   c. All bandages or dressing removed to allow complete evaluation
   d. Inspection directed at identifying specific location that has been violated. Other structures not directly underneath entry wound may be injured if penetrating object came in at an angle, and injuries to these structures should also be identified.
   e. Testing passive motion of digits is helpful to identify possible tendon injury.
      i. With passive flexion of wrist, extensor tendons naturally bring fingers into extension (Fig. 6). If there is a laceration over dorsum of hand and one finger does not extend, extensor tendon may be lacerated.
      ii. Likewise, with wrist held in dorsiflexion, fingers normally flex (Fig. 7). If one finger fails to flex and stays in extension and there is a laceration in the palm, it is likely a flexor tendon has been lacerated. Use opposite hand to determine typical resting posture of involved digit.
   f. Test active motion of digits. Assess both FDP and flexor digitorum superficialis (FDS) tendon function:
      i. Block motion of FDS tendon by holding PIP joint of affected finger in extension and having patient actively flex DIP joint (Fig. 8A). **Tenderness to resisted motion of the DIP joint is a hallmark finding of a partial tendon laceration.**
      ii. Test FDS tendon function by holding all fingers in extension except for finger to be tested (Fig. 8B). Have patient actively extend DIP joint and PIP joint separately.
   g. Check sensation carefully, remembering great sensory overlap in hand. Usually median nerve provides sensation to volar aspect of radial 3½ digits, whereas ulnar nerve provides sensation to ulnar 1½ fingers. Because of slight cross innervation,

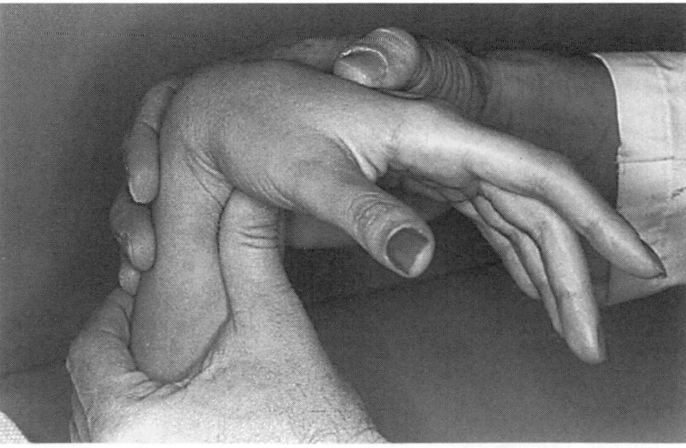

FIGURE 6. Wrist palmar flexed. Note extension of metacarpophalangeal joints.

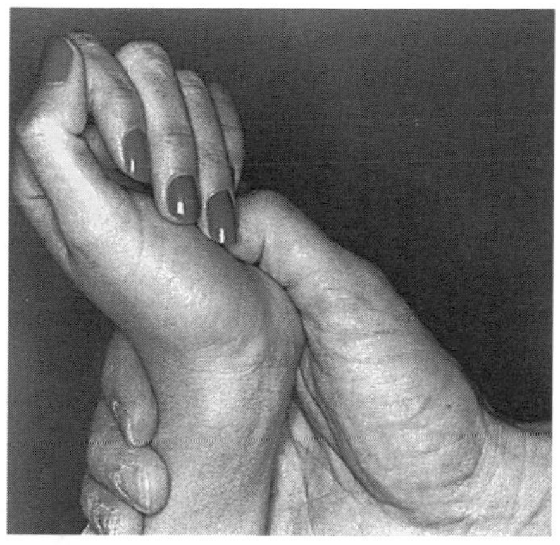

FIGURE 7. Wrist dorsiflexed. Note flexion of fingers.

important to know that volar aspect of index finger is always innervated by median nerve and small finger is always innervated by ulnar nerve.

h. Check vascularity of digit by noting temperature of skin and nail bed blanching or capillary refill. If not sure of vascularity of finger, recheck on several occasions to determine whether referral to a surgeon experienced in reestablishing circulation is necessary.

i. Test motor strength of specific hand muscles to determine median and ulnar nerve function. Median nerve supplies thenar musculature, which is responsible for thumb opposition to remaining digits on hand. Check ulnar nerve by having patient cross fingers and by testing small finger abduction strength against resistance.

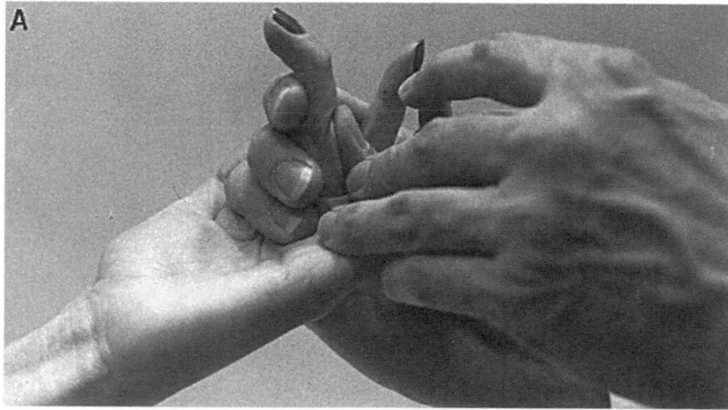

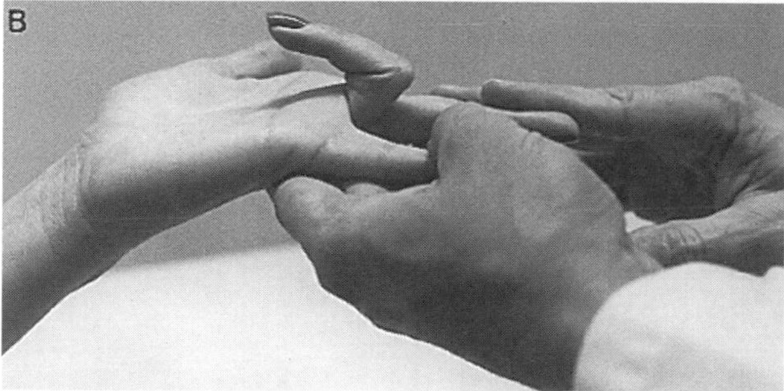

FIGURE 8. **A**, Testing of flexor profundus. **B**, Testing of flexor superficialis.

2. **X-rays:** At least two views of hand to rule out retained foreign body or an underlying unsuspected fracture

C. **Treatment**

1. Give tetanus toxoid based on guidelines from U.S. Centers for Disease Control
2. Thorough wound irrigation and debridement, best done under tourniquet hemostasis. Take care to avoid underlying tendon, nerve, and vascular structures.
3. Achieve meticulous hemostasis after debridement is finished, but avoid blind clamping of vessels to prevent iatrogenic injury to surrounding structures, e.g., a digital nerve.
4. Perform wound closure. However, if a wound is more than 8 hours old, has any crush component, or debridement is believed to be less than adequate, a possible secondary closure at a later date should be considered. Not all hand wounds need to be closed because healing by secondary intention is effective in hand injuries.
5. Lastly, apply a sterile dressing and perform a wound check 24–48 hours later.

VII. Nerve Entrapment Syndromes

A. **Carpal tunnel syndrome**

1. **Description**

a. Caused when median nerve is compressed at level of wrist joint. Median nerve supplies sensation to radial 3½ digits of hand as well as innervation of thenar musculature. Carpal tunnel syndrome can be seen in athletes who use their hands repetitively and develop flexor tenosynovitis within distal forearm and hand.

b. Symptoms:

i. Tingling in finger tips may be intermittent in nature or constant.
ii. Numbness or pain may occur at night and often awakens patient.
iii. Pain can travel retrograde up arm and patient may complain of discomfort as far as shoulder or intrascapular areas.
iv. **Proximal pain is a well-known phenomenon of distal entrapment syndromes of any nature.**

2. **Mechanism of injury:** Carpal tunnel is a fibro-osseus canal that contains nine tendons which flex fingers as well as median nerve. Carpal tunnel syndrome or compression on median nerve results either from an increase in contents of canal, such as secondary to tenosynovial proliferation, or a decrease in size of canal.

3. **Diagnosis**

a. **Examination**

i. Hallmark findings include **Tinel's sign**, which is production of paresthesias in median nerve distribution by percussion or tapping on volar aspect of wrist (Fig. 9), and **Phalen's test**, which is reproduction of tingly sensation by having patient place wrist in maximal flexion for up to 60 seconds (Fig. 10).

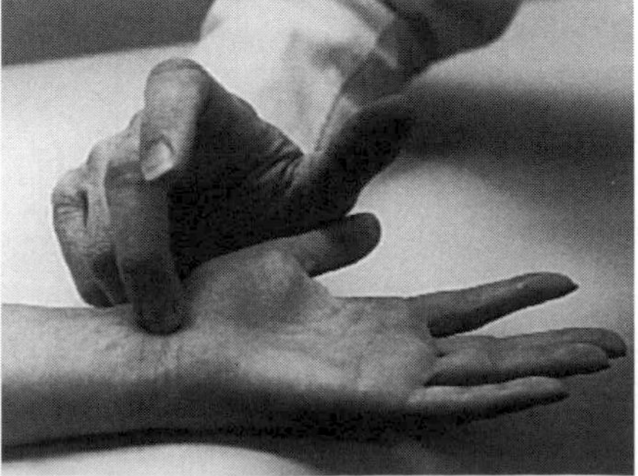

FIGURE 9. Tinel's sign for median nerve at the wrist.

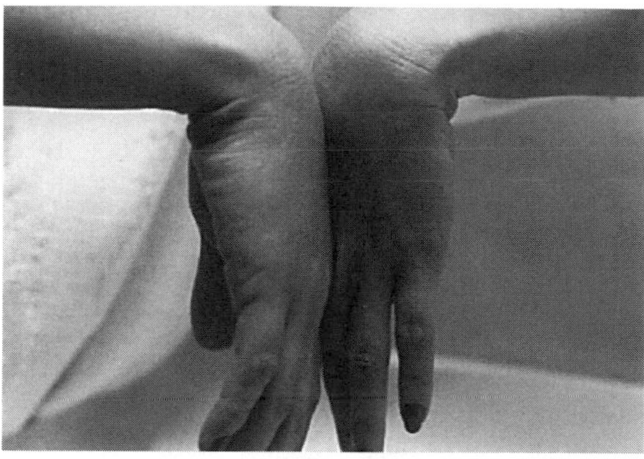

FIGURE 10. Phalen's test.

ii. Late findings include weakness of abductor pollicis brevis muscle with atrophy of thenar musculature or sensory loss in median nerve distribution. Can be elicited by testing a patient's two-point discrimination. Normally a patient can differentiate one from two points at a distance of 5 mm.

b. **Special tests:** Electromyography (EMG) and nerve conduction velocity studies (NCV) are generally diagnostic.

4. **Treatment**
   a. **Splinting wrist in a neutral position is standard initial treatment for carpal tunnel syndrome.**
      i. Night splinting is particularly effective in reducing tendon swelling that contributes to nerve compression.
      ii. Twenty-four-hour splinting may be necessary in some cases.
   b. Nonsteroidal anti-inflammatory drugs can help reduce inflammation and swelling.
   c. A corticosteroid injection in carpal tunnel can help relieve swelling around tendons, but care must be taken at time of injection not to injure median nerve.
   d. Surgical decompression is warranted if symptoms persist and there is electrodiagnostic evidence of median nerve injury.

B. **Pronator syndrome**
1. **Description:** A purely sensory syndrome in which median nerve can become entrapped either between or just distal to two heads of pronator teres muscle in proximal forearm. Patient generally experiences pain, paresthesias, and reduced sensation in median nerve distribution. Impaired pronation and grip are rare.
2. **Mechanism of injury:** Repetitive use of forearm in pronation occasionally responsible, but at other times no mechanism of injury can be elicited. Anomalous anatomic situations or muscles may also be involved in pathogenesis.
3. **Diagnosis**
   a. **Examination**
      i. Forearm pronation against resistance, or resisted flexion of FDS tendon of long finger may reproduce symptoms. Median nerve may be squeezed at arch of FDS origin.
      ii. Important to differentiate this from more common carpal tunnel syndrome. In pronator syndrome, Phalen's test is normally negative.
   b. **Special tests:** An EMG/NCV study should be obtained but is not always positive in this condition because this is a difficult area to assess.

4. **Treatment:** Conservative with modification of activity to relieve offending motion. Splint for 3–6 weeks. If no improvement, consider operative intervention.

C. **Anterior interosseous syndrome**

1. **Description:** Anterior interosseous portion of median nerve innervates flexor digitorum profundus to index finger, flexor pollicis longus, and pronator quadratus muscle. Injury to this nerve may affect one or all of these muscles. There is no sensory cutaneous portion to anterior interosseous nerve.
2. **Mechanism of injury:** Injury may come on after a set of strenuous or repetitive elbow motion exercises. Presentation is usually in one of two ways.
   a. Acute onset in which patient suddenly loses use of flexor pollicis longus and index finger profundus tendons
   b. Slow weakening of these muscles in which patient notes gradual weakness with heavy activity
3. **Diagnosis**
   a. **Examination:** Weakness or loss of flexion of interphalangeal joint of thumb and DIP joint of index finger. **Characteristically, patient is unable to make a circle with index and thumb.** Patient is unable to get thumb or index finger flexed, with distal joints of thumb and index finger remaining in extension (Fig. 11).
   b. **Special tests:** EMG testing is warranted after this injury. To avoid a false-negative test, however, wait 3 weeks after onset of problem before proceeding with electrodiagnostic studies.
4. **Treatment:** Initially, splint extremity and avoid heavy activity. If after 6 months no return of function is noted, consider exploration and possible decompression of nerve.

D. **Cubital tunnel syndrome**

1. **Description:** A fibro-osseous groove in posteromedial aspect of elbow that contains ulnar nerve. Ulnar nerve supplies intrinsic musculature of hand, flexor carpi ulnaris muscle, and FDP muscles to small and ring fingers. It also supplies sensation to ulnar 1½ digits of hand. Patients may complain of lancinating pain in volar medial forearm or numbness in distribution of ulnar nerve.

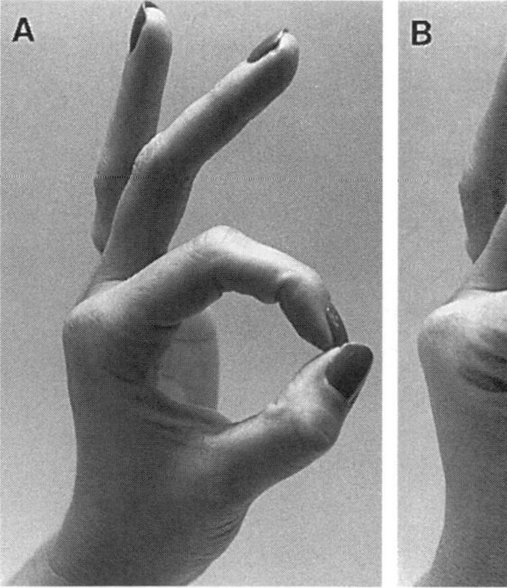

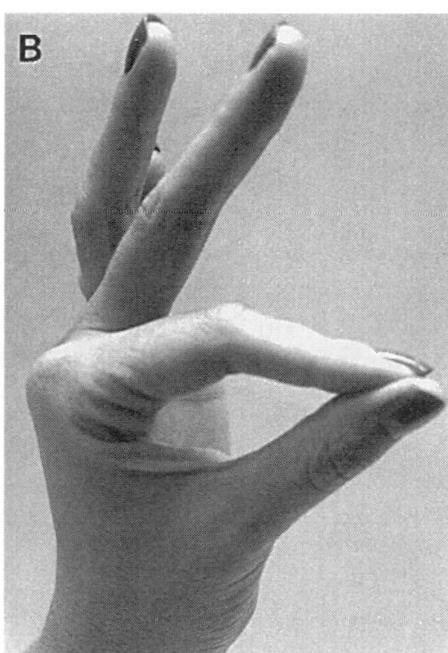

FIGURE 11. Test for anterior interosseus nerve. **A**, Normal attempt at "making a circle." **B**, Abnormal test, with inability to flex distal interphalangeal joint of index and interphalangeal joint of thumb.

2. **Mechanism of injury:** People who engage in repetitive flexion sports are particularly at risk, especially those with any type of abnormal anatomy. Fractures that occurred in childhood or adolescence may give rise to deformity about the elbow, which can cause stretching of ulnar nerve as it travels through cubital tunnel. This injury is also seen in throwing athletes.
3. **Diagnosis**
   a. **Examination**
      i. Tenderness to palpation either above or below elbow in cubital tunnel is a common finding.
      ii. Percussion in area (Tinel's sign) generally reproduces patient's paresthesias in ulnar 1½ digits.
      iii. Perform hyperflexion test by having patient flex elbow for 60 seconds to see if this reproduces symptoms.
      iv. Weakness may be present in intrinsic musculature of hand, but this is a relatively late finding, as is sensory loss.
   b. **X-rays:** Usually of little benefit unless patient has a past history of traumatic injury
   c. **Special testing:** Electrodiagnostic testing can localize an area of compression of ulnar nerve at cubital tunnel.
4. **Treatment:** Primary aim of treatment is to relieve pressure on ulnar nerve.
   a. Avoid repetitive flexion activities.
   b. Splint elbow in 20° of flexion at night and administer nonsteroidal anti-inflammatory drugs.
   c. Operative treatment, usually decompressing ulnar nerve and transposing it anteriorly, is indicated if conservative treatment fails.

E. **Ulnar nerve entrapment at wrist (Guyon's canal)**
1. **Description:** Guyon's canal is an anatomic analog of and lies just medial to carpal tunnel. Guyon's canal is sometimes called the pisohamate tunnel. Entrapment of nerve in this area may cause some weakness in intrinsic musculature as well as numbness in ulnar 1½ digits.
2. **Mechanism of injury:** Repetitive trauma or microtrauma related to athletic events such as bicycling or work situations such as operating a jack-hammer
3. **Diagnosis**
   a. **Examination**
      i. Point tenderness over Guyon's canal is a common finding.
      ii. Check for intrinsic muscle weakness by having patient cross index and long fingers or by testing resisted abduction of small finger.
      iii. A sensory examination should be performed, but actual sensory loss is a relatively late finding.
   b. **X-rays:** Usually of no benefit. However, obtain a carpal tunnel view to rule out any associated problems, such as a hook of hamate fracture.
   c. **Special tests:** Electrodiagnostic studies are appropriate, although not typically as reliable or diagnostic as in carpal tunnel syndrome.
4. **Treatment**
   a. Splinting, nonsteroidal anti-inflammatory drugs, and avoidance of any precipitating activity
   b. If pain and weakness persist, exploration of area and decompression of Guyon's canal

VIII. Tendinitis

A. **De Quervain's tenosynovitis**
1. **Description:** De Quervain's disease is stenosing tenosynovitis of first dorsal compartment of wrist. Abductor pollicis longus and extensor pollicis brevis tendons are

contained within first dorsal compartment and serve to abduct and extend thumb MCP joint.

2. **Mechanism of injury:** Usually repetitive use of thumb for some activity. As tendinitis develops, pain increases with more use. Patient can usually identify activity, which may be as seemingly innocuous as typing.
3. **Diagnosis**
   a. **Examination**
      i. Tenderness to palpation, often marked, located at or just proximal to radial styloid
      ii. **A Finkelstein test is diagnostic, and this is performed by having patient tuck thumb inside other fingers as examiner passively ulnarly deviates wrist.** Pain elicited with this maneuver constitutes a positive test (Fig. 12).
      iii. Swelling and inflammation of first dorsal compartment is occasionally present.

   b. **X-rays:** Typically not indicated but can be helpful in ruling out other possible sources of radial sided wrist pain
4. **Treatment**
   a. Splinting with a thumb spica splint, avoidance of aggravating activity, anti-inflammatory medication, and possibly physical therapy with localized treatment over area
   b. If no response, corticosteroid injection of first dorsal compartment often proves successful.
   c. Lastly, surgical correction with release of first dorsal compartment is a reliable procedure when conservative management fails.

B. **Intersection syndrome**
1. **Description:** Tenosynovitis or friction tendinitis between first and second dorsal compartments, which occurs on dorsum of distal forearm approximately two to three fingerbreadths proximal to wrist joint
2. **Mechanism of injury:** Muscle bellies of extensor pollicis brevis and adductor pollicis longus cross over wrist extensor tendons of second compartment at virtually a 60° angle. With overuse, friction tendinitis develops.
3. **Diagnosis**
   a. Point tenderness on dorsal radial aspect of forearm in intersection region (Fig. 13)
   b. Palpable crepitus with passive or active motion of wrist

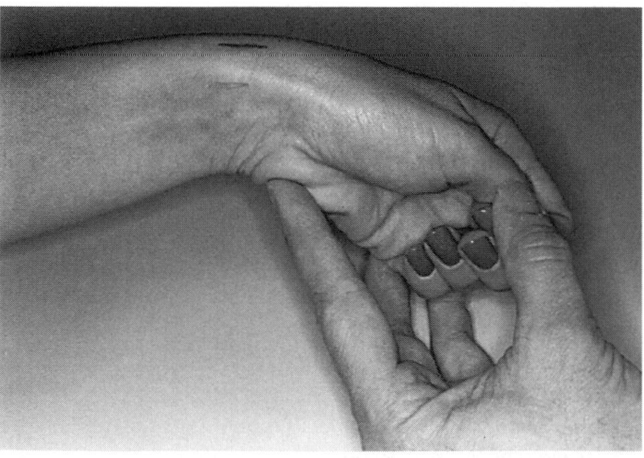

FIGURE 12. Finkelstein's test.

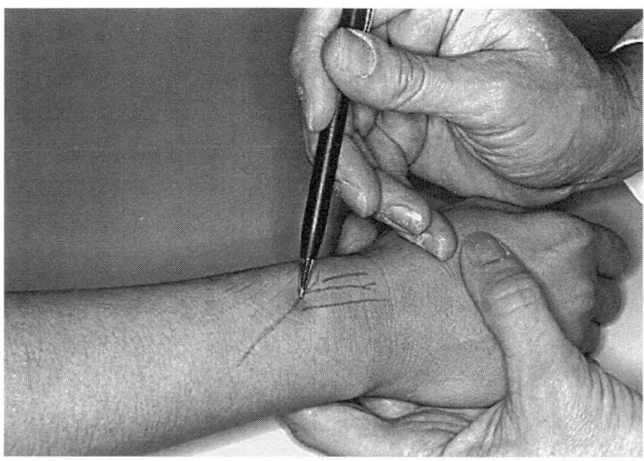

FIGURE 13. Site of swelling and tenderness in intersection syndrome.

4. **Treatment**
   a. Splinting of wrist, anti-inflammatory medication, and avoidance of aggravating activity
   b. Corticosteroid injection avoiding bodies of tendons themselves in persistent cases
   c. Surgical intervention rarely necessary

C. **Ganglion cysts**
1. **Description:** Most commonly seen on dorsum of wrist or on volar aspect near radial artery. Represent a type of degenerative process that originates usually from scapholunate joint or interface. Can usually be traced back to this area surgically.
2. **Mechanism of injury:** Typically, no specific injury associated with ganglion cysts; they are usually spontaneous in onset.
3. **Diagnosis**
   a. A fusiform mass that is freely mobile to palpation and may transilluminate light
      i. Mass is normally over dorsum of wrist and extensor tendons but may also be seen on volar aspect of wrist.
      ii. Mass may be closely opposed to radial artery, and with auscultation a radial artery aneurysm may be differentiated.
   b. Small ganglions on dorsum of wrist also occur that cannot be palpated, and these so-called "occult ganglions" may be cause of obscure dorsal wrist pain.
4. **Treatment:** Goal is to alleviate symptoms associated with ganglia.
   a. Because many ganglia are seen and are asymptomatic, majority of cysts should be treated only with observation.
   b. If a ganglion remains symptomatic, aspiration followed by injection of a corticosteroid
   c. Lastly, if continued pain and dysfunction, then surgical intervention
   d. Splinting usually of no benefit

D. **Gymnast's wrist**
1. **Description:** Gymnasts, especially those who do numerous floor exercises, often present with pain over dorsum of wrists. Most bothersome as wrist is carried into maximum dorsiflexion, such as in vaulting, tumbling, and beam work.
2. **Mechanism of injury:** Appears to be a type of injury in which dorsal capsule is entrapped or repetitively traumatized by hyperdorsiflexion of wrist. Extremely difficult to treat because most gymnast routines involve dorsiflexion of wrist.

3. **Diagnosis**
   a. **Examination**
      i. Diffuse tenderness is typically present over dorsum of midcarpal area. Generally, there is no edema, discoloration, or clinical instability. Pain elicited by extremes of wrist motion is typical.
      ii. Important to rule out other potential causes of dorsal wrist pain, including avascular necrosis of a carpal bone or a possible ligamentous injury to carpus. Differential diagnosis also includes an occult ganglion cyst on dorsum of wrist.
   b. **X-rays** are usually negative.
4. **Treatment**
   a. Hallmark of treatment for obscure wrist pain is judicious wrist splinting and nonsteroidal anti-inflammatory medication.
   b. Evaluate athlete's technique to ensure that arm is being used solely as a functional unit with proper position of hand, wrist, and forearm locked until transferring most of pressure up into shoulder girdle rather than with arm unit in a highly flexed position at elbow and shoulder, giving abnormal stress to wrist.
   c. A dorsal block splint might be beneficial for practice and competition to avoid extremes of wrist extension.

Recommended Reading

1. American Society for Surgery of the Hand: Hand Surgery Update. Englewood, CO, 1994.
2. American Society for Surgery of the Hand: The Hand: Examination and Diagnosis, 2nd ed. New York, Churchill Livingstone, 1983.
3. American Society for Surgery of the Hand: The Hand: Primary Care for Common Problems. New York, Churchill Livingstone, 1985.
4. Barton N: Fractures of the Hand and Wrist. New York, Churchill Livingstone, 1988.
5. Brand PW: Clinical Mechanics of the Hand. St. Louis, C.V. Mosby, 1985.
6. Fess EE: Hand Splinting: Principles and Methods, 2nd ed. St. Louis, C.V. Mosby, 1987.
7. Green DP: Operative Hand Surgery, 3rd ed. New York, Churchill Livingstone, 1988.
8. Hoppenfeld S: Physical Examination of the Spine and Extremities. East Norwalk, CT, Appleton & Lange, 1976.
9. Hunter JM, Schneider LH, Mackin EJ, Callahan AD: Rehabilitation of the Hand, 3rd ed. St. Louis, C.V. Mosby, 1989.
10. Lichtman DM: The Wrist and Its Disorders. Philadelphia, W.B. Saunders, 1988.
11. Milford L: The Hand, 3rd ed. St. Louis, C.V. Mosby, 1988.
12. Morrey BF: The Elbow and Its Disorders. Philadelphia, W.B. Saunders, 1985.
13. Nicholas JA, Hershman EB, Posner MA: The Upper Extremity in Sports Medicine. St. Louis, C.V. Mosby, 1990.
14. Pettrone FA (ed): American Academy of Orthopaedic Surgeons: Symposium on Upper Extremity Injuries in Athletes. St. Louis, C.V. Mosby, 1988.
15. Rockwood CA, Green DP: Fractures, 3rd ed. Philadelphia, J.B. Lippincott, 1984.
16. Spinner M: Injuries to the Major Branches of the Peripheral Nerves of the Forearm, 2nd ed. Philadelphia, W.B. Saunders, 1978.
17. Strickland JW: The Thumb. New York, Churchill Livingstone, 1989.

46

Athletic Injuries of the Thorax and Abdomen

Cindy J. Chang, M.D.

Injuries to the thorax and abdomen can occur with any sport but are more often seen in those involving sudden deceleration and impact, such as football, ice hockey, or skiing. Although these injuries do not occur as often as injuries to the extremities, when they do occur, it is imperative that they are immediately recognized and appropriately managed. Often the situation can be life-threatening, and repeated assessment and a high index of suspicion are essential for accurate evaluation of these injuries. Once a severe thoracic or abdominal injury has been recognized, the fundamentals of stabilization are standard protocol and should be initiated until transfer can be made to a hospital.

Torso injuries often overlap with injuries to the extremities. For example, traction apophysitis of the iliac crest, although anatomically involving the hip and pelvic region, commonly presents as a subjective complaint of lower abdominal pain because of its close proximity. Meanwhile, many shoulder conditions can radiate to the thorax, causing confusion as to the source of the symptoms. Although this chapter focuses primarily on injuries to the thorax and abdominal contents, several important conditions such as thoracic outlet syndrome and effort thrombosis are also discussed.

I. Chest Wall Injuries

A. **Sternal fracture**

1. **Description: Although the fracture itself is not significant, there is a high incidence of associated intrathoracic trauma.**
2. **Mechanism of injury**
   a. High-impact injuries
   b. Acute flexion—upper fragment usually displaced anteriorly over lower fragment
3. **Diagnosis and physical examination**
   a. Localized pain with pressure over sternum
   b. Pain aggravated with deep inspiration
   c. Palpable defect suggesting displacement
4. **Laboratory and radiographic studies**
   a. Lateral chest film is best to evaluate fracture.
   b. Computed tomography (CT) scan
   c. Electrocardiogram (ECG) and chest x-ray if suspect intrathoracic trauma
5. **Associated injuries**
   a. Myocardial contusion
   b. Injury of internal mammary vessels
   c. Pulmonary laceration or contusion
6. **Treatment**
   a. If displaced, reduction possible by lifting both arms above the head and hyperextending the thoracic spine.

b. **Because of the high incidence of associated intrathoracic trauma, observation in the hospital with cardiac monitor is advisable.**
c. Displaced fractures may require open reduction with internal fixation.

B. **Dislocation of the sternoclavicular joint**
1. **Description**
a. Relatively infrequent, constituting < 1% of somatic dislocations
i. Type I—sprain with no ligamentous damage or instability
ii. Type II—stretch or partial rupture of the sternoclavicular and costoclavicular ligaments; joint is partially displaced
iii. Type III—dislocation with gross disruption of capsule and ligaments
b. The sternoclavicular joint is the only articulation between the upper extremity and the axial skeleton, yet has the least amount of osseous stability of any joint in the body.
c. Divided into anterior and posterior disruptions; most common is anterior, with ratio from 2:1 to 20:1
d. Rarely, superior dislocation
2. **Mechanism of injury**
a. Caused by direct or indirect trauma to shoulder girdle
i. Most common causes are vehicular accidents (⅔) and athletic injuries (⅓)
ii. Other causes or risk factors include voluntary or habitual dislocation, congenital dislocation, and dislocations associated with normal process of aging or joint diseases, such as rheumatoid arthritis.
b. A force applied at the lateral aspect of the shoulder or along the abducted arm is transmitted along the clavicle to the sternoclavicular joint, displacing the clavicle.
c. A posterior dislocation can also result from a direct blow on the anterior aspect of the medial end of the clavicle.
3. **Diagnosis**
a. Severe pain, especially with any movement of the arm
b. Increased discomfort when lying in supine position
4. **Physical examination**
a. Bruising, pain, and swelling at the joint
b. Noticeable displacement of the sternoclavicular joint
c. Observe ease of respiration and neurologic and vascular status of upper extremity to rule out pressure on adjacent vital structures.
i. Hoarseness, dysphagia, dyspnea
ii. Claudication, dysthesias, swelling, pulselessness of ipsilateral arm
5. **Radiographic studies**
a. Diagnosis with plain x-rays with cephalic tilt views (Fig. 1). Tube distance for children, 45 inches; for thicker-chested athletes, 60 inches.
b. CT scan (axial CT images)—may need coronal plane paraxial CT reconstruction if suspect superior component of dislocation
6. **Associated injuries**
a. **Posterior dislocations more serious**
b. **30% incidence of injury to the vital structures traversing the thoracic outlet, including major vessels of neck, dome of pleurae, trachea, and esophagus**
7. **Treatment**
a. For type II injuries:
i. Avoid stress to joint for at least 3 weeks for adequate healing.
ii. Goal is to avoid increased symptomatic mobility at joint
b. For type III injuries:
i. Immediate closed reduction for posterior dislocations (Fig. 2)

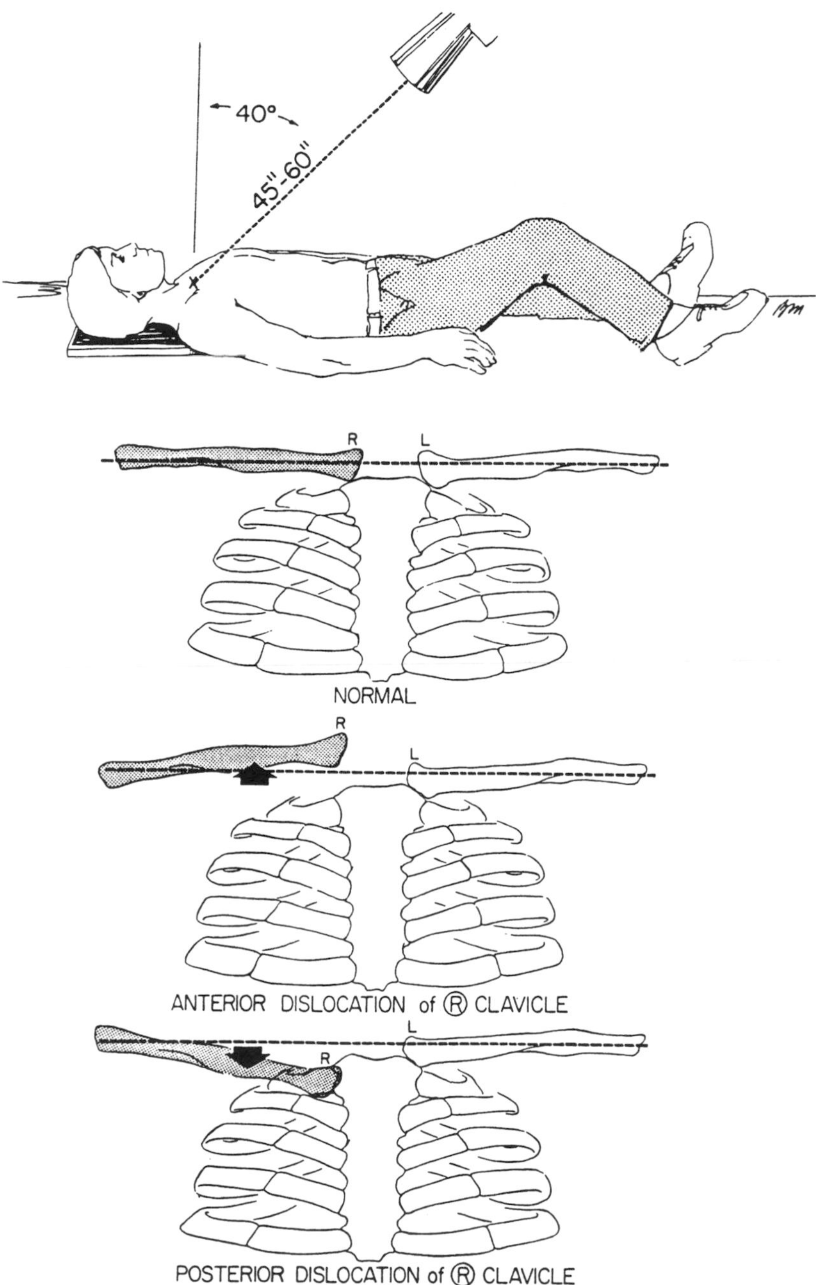

FIGURE 1. Positioning of the athlete and interpretation of the cephalic tilt reontgenogram of the sternoclavicular joints. (Adapted from Rockwood CA, Green DP, Bucholz RW: Injuries of the sternoclavicular joint. In Rockwood CA, Green BP (eds): Fractures in Adults, 4th ed. Philadelphia, J.B. Lippincott, 1996, pp 1415–1471, with permission.)

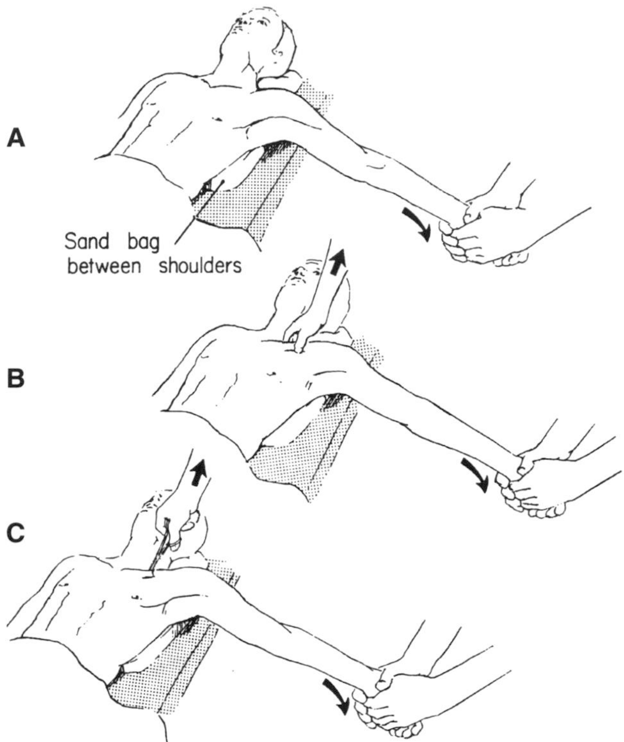

FIGURE 2. Technique of closed reduction of sternoclavicular joint dislocation. **A**, With the thorax elevated, apply traction and extension to the arm. **B**, Obtain additional leverage by grasping the clavicle with the fingers. **C**, If reduction is still unaccomplished, use a sterile towel clip to lift the clavicle anteriorly and laterally. (From Rockwood CA, Green DP, Bucholtz RW: Injuries of the sternoclavicular joint. In Rockwood CA, Green DP (eds): Fractures in Adults, 4th ed. Philadelphia, J.B. Lippincott, 1996, pp 1415–1471, with permission.)

ii. Despite immobilization with sling or figure-of-eight, healing is often inadequate and continued sternoclavicular instability usually exists, with a propensity for recurrent subluxation.
iii. Unfortunately, operative repairs can be difficult with unsatisfactory results.

C. **Rib fractures**
1. **Description**
a. Most common serious injury of the chest
b. Nondisplaced fractures are more common. If displaced, look for other injuries, including laceration of intercostal artery.
c. Uncommon in children because thorax is more elastic and flexible
2. **Mechanism of injury**
a. Blunt trauma
i. Force usually applied in the anteroposterior plane
ii. Fractures located at posterior angles of fifth to ninth ribs
b. Direct force over a small area of chest wall leads to a fracture immediately beneath point of impact.
c. Violent muscle contraction
i. **"Floating rib fractures"** or avulsion fractures of attachments of external oblique muscle to the lower three ribs

ii. Reported in baseball pitchers and batters

d. **Fracture of first rib**

i. Direct external trauma is rare cause, as protected by shoulder girdle

ii. Other causes are indirect trauma from falling on outstretched arm or violent hyperabduction of arm and repetitive stresses.

e. **Stress fractures of the ribs**

i. Caused by excessive forceful muscular traction at the muscular attachments of the ribs

ii. Opposing muscular pulls of the scalene muscles and upper digitations of serratus anterior may fracture the **first rib** at its thinnest segment, where the subclavian artery crosses (subclavian sulcus), e.g., with **weightlifting, pitching** (Fig. 3).

iii. Anterolateral stress fractures of **fourth** and **fifth ribs** are reported in **rowers**, due to excessive action of the serratus anterior muscle.

3. **Diagnosis**

a. History of traumatic event with intense localized pain

b. With stress fractures, insidious onset of pain associated with specific activities

c. If fracture becomes unstable, acute knifelike pain

d. Pain aggravated by deep inspiration or coughing

e. Pain with twisting or side flexion, causing tension on fractured rib

f. Dyspnea

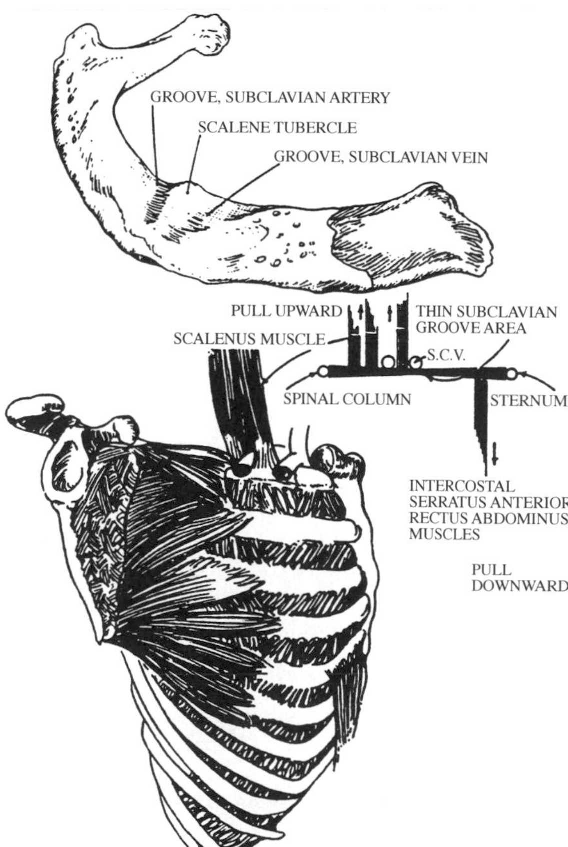

FIGURE 3. The narrow, flat first rib and the attached muscles with their opposing pulls. (From Proffer DS, Patton JJ, Jackson DW: Nonunion of a first rib fracture in a gymnast. Am J Sports Med 19(2):198–201, 1991, with permission.)

4. **Physical examination**
   a. Localized tenderness, ecchymosis, and edema
   b. Crepitus
   c. Shallow, rapid breathing
   d. With anteroposterior and transverse compression of rib cage, pain at site of suspected injury
   e. Subcutaneous emphysema if pleural injury
5. **Radiographic studies**
   a. Chest x-ray
      i. Establishes diagnosis in 90% of cases
      ii. Can also exclude any complication, such as pneumothorax, if high suspicion
   b. Oblique views may detect anterior and lateral fractures.
   c. Bone scan if suspect stress fracture of rib
6. **Differential diagnosis**
   a. Severe rib contusion
   b. Costochondral separation
   c. Muscle strain—occurs with tennis and other racquet sports, e.g., forceful contraction of thoracic muscles during a tennis serve
   d. Pneumothorax
7. **Associated injuries**
   a. The more ribs fractured, the greater incidence of intrathoracic injuries.
   b. **If first rib fracture displaced posteriorly, look for vascular injury**, e.g., subclavian artery.
   c. **Fracture of lower two ribs may damage kidneys, liver, or spleen**; splenic trauma has been reported in up to 20% of left lower rib fractures and liver trauma in up to 10% of right lower rib fractures.
   d. **Flail chest**
      i. Fracture of at least three consecutive ribs, each in two locations, causing a free-floating segment of the chest wall
      ii. More likely result of vehicular trauma and high chance of internal injury
      iii. Paradoxical chest wall movement results in impaired ventilation and respiratory failure.
8. **Treatment**
   a. Pain relief using ice, nonsteroidal anti-inflammatory drugs (NSAIDs), analgesics
   b. Intercostal nerve block with bupivacaine for relief of severe pain (Fig. 4):
      i. Level of fracture along with two ribs above and below are infiltrated with 3 to 5 mL of lidocaine or bupivacaine
      ii. Risk of causing pneumothorax
   c. Encouragement of deep breathing to prevent atelectasis; therefore, best to avoid rib belt or taping
   d. Modification of activities until symptoms resolve, then gradual resumption of training
   e. Changes in technique if thought to contribute to cause of fracture
   f. Improved conditioning
9. **Return to play**
   a. Return to competition if minimal pain with palpation, no use of analgesics, full range of motion of thoracic cage, and ability to sprint and twist without significant discomfort
   b. Usually 3 weeks before return to contact sports:
      i. Early return inadvisable because of danger of pneumothorax caused by fractured rib penetrating pleura

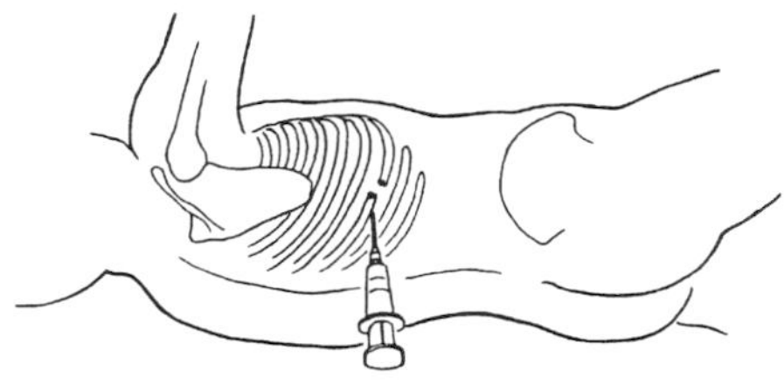

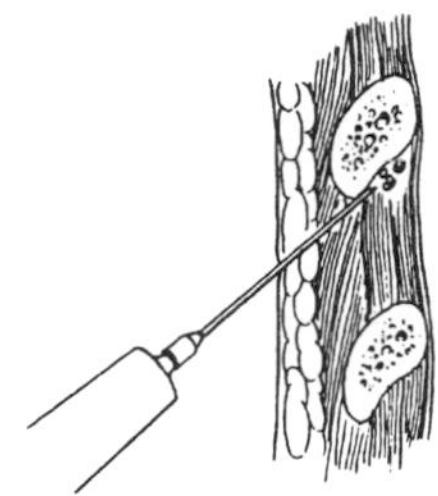

FIGURE 4. Technique of intercostal nerve block. The local anesthesia is infiltrated just below the lower border of the rib, in close approximation to the intercostal vessels and nerve. (From Reid DC: Sports Injury Assessment and Rehabilitation. New York, Churchill Livingstone, 1992, pp 671–738, with permission.)

ii. Timing varies depending on position and level of play of athlete as well as ability to protect the fracture site.
iii. Education of athlete important

c. Protective padding

D. **Costochondral sprain and separation ("rib-tip syndrome" or "slipping rib syndrome")**

1. **Description**
   a. Frequently occurs in contact sports such as football, ice hockey, wrestling, lacrosse, and rugby
   b. Separation of the costal cartilage as it attaches to the sternum
   c. Separation of the anterior margin of the rib from the anterior end of the costal cartilage, putting pressure on the intercostal nerve lying between it and the rib above
   d. More frequently involves the tenth rib, followed by ninth or eighth
2. **Mechanism of injury**
   a. Forced compression of the rib cage, twisting injury, or a stretching injury to the joint when the arm is forcefully pulled to the side
   b. Onset sometimes is insidious, occurring long after the initial trauma.
3. **Diagnosis**
   a. History of feeling a pop
   b. Initial sharp discomfort, with severe pain lasting for several days before slowly decreasing in intensity
   c. Intermittent unilateral pain in anterior ends of the lower costal cartilages
   d. Severe sharp pains during bending maneuvers with a painful click as the cartilage and bone override one another
   e. Pain can radiate toward the epigastric region or spine.
4. **Physical examination**
   a. Localized swelling and tenderness at the involved joint
   b. Possible deformity because of displacement of the cartilage
   c. Reproducible pain and sometimes click by hooking the fingers under the anterior costal margin and pulling the rib cage anteriorly
5. **Radiographic studies:** X-rays if chronic to rule out tumors, Paget's disease, or rheumatoid arthritis

6. **Differential diagnosis**
   a. **Costochondritis or costosternal syndrome:**
      i. Both traumatic and nontraumatic causes and self-limiting
      ii. Multiple sites of tenderness over usually the second to sixth costal cartilages but without swelling
   b. **Tietze's syndrome:**
      i. Traumatic and nontraumatic causes and self-limiting
      ii. Usually only the second or third costochondral junction is involved with localized swelling.
7. **Treatment**
   a. Ice and NSAIDs
   b. Injection of lidocaine with or without corticosteroid at site of separation
   c. Symptoms may take 9–12 weeks to resolve
   d. Slow healing and subject to reinjury
   e. Surgical resection of affected costochondral junction for intractable pain
   f. Return to play with increased padding

E. **Rupture of pectoralis major**
1. **Description**
   a. Pectoralis major is the most important adductor and internal rotator of the shoulder and cosmetically forms the anterior wall of the axilla.
   b. Ruptures can be partial (grades I and II) and complete (grade III)
   c. Excessive tension on the muscle causes tear of the muscle belly itself, at the musculotendinous junction, or at the tendinous insertion on the humerus lateral to bicipital groove.
   d. May be associated with anabolic steroid use because the muscle hypertrophy is not accompanied by increase in tendon size
2. **Mechanism of injury**
   a. Rupture is related to excessive tension on a maximally, eccentrically contracted muscle while the upper arm is externally rotated, extended, or abducted.
   b. Most often seen in weight lifters during bench press when there is sudden exertion against a heavy weight
   c. Also reported during waterskiing, wrestling, and other sudden violent deceleration maneuvers, when there is sudden stretching with co-contraction of the muscle:
      i. Blocking with outstretched arm in football
      ii. Punching in boxing
      iii. Attempting to grasp something to prevent fall
3. **Diagnosis**
   a. History of sudden stress or direct blow applied to shoulder region while arm is abducted and extended
   b. Sudden onset of extreme pain on medial aspect of upper arm or in the chest wall
   c. Snapping or popping sensation at time of injury
   d. Significant swelling and ecchymosis
   e. Painful limitation of motion
   f. Weakness of involved upper extremity
4. **Physical examination**
   a. Swelling and hemorrhage into the arm and across the anterior chest wall
   b. Weakness and pain during resisted internal rotation, flexion, and adduction of the arm on the affected side
   c. Deformity of the chest wall and palpable muscle bulge with resisted adduction
   d. With abduction, defect in the anterior axillary fold if tendon is avulsed at its insertion

5. **Radiographic studies**
   a. Chest x-ray reveals absent pectoralis major muscle shadow.
   b. Magnetic resonance imaging (MRI) to define accurately extent of injury and to aid in surgical planning
6. **Treatment**
   a. Because the extent of tear may be difficult to diagnose immediately after injury due to the ecchymosis, swelling, and extreme pain, serial exams are important.
   b. Partial tear is treated conservatively with ice, analgesia, and activity restriction initially.
      i. Start with early protected range of motion and gentle isometric strengthening.
      ii. Need to regain full range of motion to prevent further injuries, then start to regain full strength
      iii. Activities resumed slowly as pain allows
   c. Complete tear is surgically repaired in competitive athletes, especially those who depend on chest and shoulder strength.
      i. Without surgical repair, a slight weakness can result especially in adduction and flexion.
      ii. Also repaired in bodybuilders for cosmesis
   d. Many do present with delayed diagnosis and thus adhesions, muscle retraction, and atrophy, but late repair is compatible with significant improvement in strength.
   e. After surgery, immobilization in sling for 2–4 weeks, then passive range of motion. Resistive exercises at 12 weeks.

F. **Breast injuries**
1. **Description**
   a. **Breast contusions**
   b. **Runner's nipple/cyclist's nipple**
   c. **Breast pain**
2. **Mechanism of injury and diagnosis**
   a. Contusions are caused by direct trauma with resultant bleeding and swelling; common in softball and basketball.
   b. Nipple chafing, pain, and occasional bleeding from friction and abrasion by clothing during prolonged activity or because of the evaporation of perspiration over the chest
   c. More prevalent in cold weather, when nipple harder and more prominent
   d. Breast pain often experienced during athletic activity, especially involving running, due to strain of Cooper's ligaments (connective tissue that holds and supports the breast on the chest wall)
3. **Treatment**
   a. Prevent excessive movement of breasts with specialized sports brassieres with support from all sides.
   b. Avoid any hooks, fasteners, or seams or ridges in the nipple region.
   c. Proper clothing, such as wind-breaking material, helps to prevent the combination of perspiration and cold that predisposes to nipple problems.
   e. For contusions, ice and NSAIDs and proper support, then heat and added protective padding. Rarely, a hematoma requires aspiration.
   f. Occasionally breast injuries lead to posttraumatic scarring and retraction or thrombophlebitis of the superficial veins (Mondor's disease). These signs must be followed closely to differentiate from breast carcinoma.
   g. Hormonal therapy may help with diminishing the breast tenderness experienced during phases of the menstrual cycle.

II. Lung Injuries

A. **Pulmonary contusion**

1. **Description:** Blood and protein leak into the alveoli and interstitial spaces, leading to atelectasis and consolidation.
2. **Mechanism of injury:** blunt trauma to chest
3. **Diagnosis**
   a. Chest pain
   b. Shortness of breath
   c. Cough
   d. Hemoptysis
4. **Physical examination**
   a. Tachypnea
   b. Rales
   c. Hypoxemia is the hallmark clinical sign.
5. **Laboratory and radiographic studies**
   a. Chest x-ray:
      i. May not initially show severity of injury
      ii. Can show patchy infiltrates or consolidation
   b. CT scan more sensitive
   c. Pulse oximeter or blood gas
6. **Associated injuries:** Flail chest is highly associated with pulmonary contusion and even more so with pneumothorax or hemothorax.
7. **Treatment**
   a. Assisted ventilation including endotracheal intubation if necessary
   b. Watch closely for onset of pneumonia:
      i. Severe thoracic or abdominal trauma represents a major risk factor.
      ii. Mechanical ventilation administered during the first days after trauma seems to reduce the risk of pneumonia; however, ventilatory support lasting more than 5 days is associated with an increased risk of pneumonia.

B. **Pneumothorax**

1. **Description**
   a. Refers to air within the chest cavity in the pleural space, which leads to collapse of the lung
   b. Classified as **spontaneous** versus **traumatic**
   c. Described by the approximate percentage of hemithorax that is occupied by free air, e.g., 10% or 50%
2. **Mechanism of injury**
   a. Blunt trauma is the most common cause, with or without rib fractures or open chest wounds.
   b. Spontaneous, occasionally precipitated by strenuous physical activities, especially in tall, thin, young males
   c. Increased risk if defects in the periphery of the lung present; these bullae usually located in apex
3. **Diagnosis**
   a. Gradual or sudden chest pain and dyspnea, depending on the size and rate of collapse of lung
   b. Pain referred to shoulder tip
4. **Physical examination**
   a. Shallow, rapid respirations
   b. Cyanosis
   c. Tachycardia
   d. Hyperresonance to percussion and decreased breath sounds over affected lung

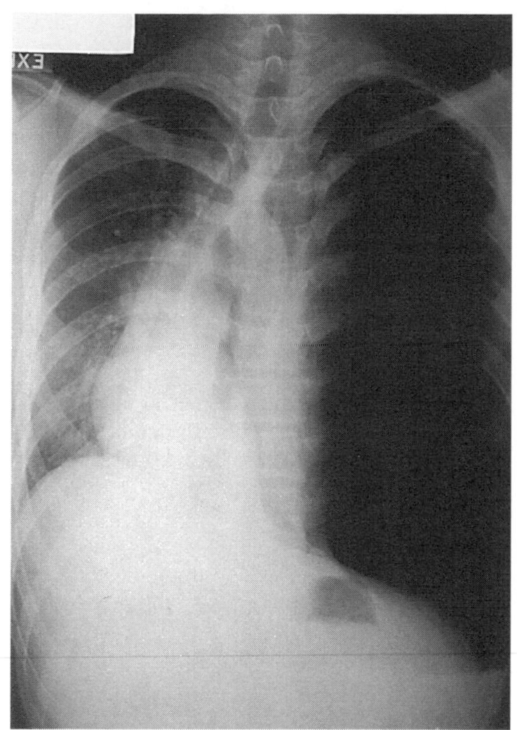

FIGURE 5. Large pneumothorax with a mediastinal shift.

   e. Tracheal shift to contralateral side
   f. Possible subcutaneous emphysema
5. **Radiographic studies**
   a. Chest x-ray shows absence of lung markings in periphery and increased density of collapsed part of lung.
   b. Expiration films may make small pneumothorax more visible.
   c. Mediastinal shift with large pneumothorax (Fig. 5).
6. **Differential diagnosis**
   a. Flail chest—establish ventilation and place athlete on the involved side.
   b. **Hemothorax:**
      i. Blood accumulates in the pleural space as the result of bleeding of thoracic vessels.
      ii. Usually associated pneumothorax
      iii. Dullness to percussion and decreased breath sounds
      iv. Hypotension
7. **Treatment**
   a. If minimal (< 30%), stable, and asymptomatic, observation with serial exams and chest x-ray. Avoid unnecessary physical exertion.
   b. If large enough to cause shortness of breath and discomfort, transport to hospital for possible insertion of chest tube to allow lung to reexpand.
   c. **Open pneumothorax:**
      i. Place foil, cloth, or other item over wound.
      ii. Secure it only on three sides to avoid development of tension pneumothorax.
8. **Return to play**
   a. No vigorous activities for 2–3 weeks after chest tube removed, then slow, monitored return to activity

   b. Education of the athlete regarding risk of further episodes, which have been reported in up to 50% of cases

C. **Tension pneumothorax**
   1. **Description**
      a. Progressive enlargement of a pneumothorax because of a communication between the airways or exterior and the interpleural space. A **flap valve effect** is created so that with each inspiration, air is drawn into the pleural cavity; with each expiration, the air stays trapped.
      b. The positive intrapleural pressure that develops impairs venous return, shifts the mediastinum, and further impairs ventilation of the noninjured lung.
      c. Is an **absolute medical emergency**; progressive hypoxia and hypotension lead to death.
   2. **Diagnosis**
      a. Rapidly increasing shortness of breath
      b. Asymmetry of respiration
   3. **Physical examination**
      a. Distended neck veins
      b. Cyanosis
      c. Hypotension and tachycardia
      d. Dyspnea and tachypnea
      e. Tracheal deviation toward the side opposite the pneumothorax
      f. Absent breath sounds on involved side
      g. Hyperresonance on percussion on involved side
   4. **Laboratory and radiographic studies:** chest x-ray, only if immediately available
   5. **Treatment**
      a. Urgent insertion of large-bore needle (14 to 16 gauge) into the second or third intercostal space along the midclavicular line, just over the superior aspect of the rib to avoid the intercostal vessels
      b. Transport to hospital and chest tube placement for definitive treatment

III. Cardiac and Great Vessel Injuries

Myocardial injury may occur in up to 76% of patients sustaining blunt trauma to the chest, with direct compression of the heart between the anterior chest wall and vertebral column. Motor vehicle accidents are responsible for most of these blunt injuries to the heart and great vessels. Other potentially catastrophic causes of chest pain in athletes include ischemic heart disease and pulmonary embolus, which are not addressed in this chapter. Keep in mind, however, that besides the typical risk factors for coronary artery disease such as hypertension and elevated cholesterol, the use of cocaine in sport has become an established risk factor for myocardial ischemia and infarction, even in teens and young adults.

A. **Myocardial contusion**
   1. **Description**
      a. Blunt trauma causes "bruising" of the cardiac muscle; pathologically, this can range from microscopic changes of hemorrhage and cellular death to gross marked necrosis.
      b. Results in various degrees of myocardial contusion:
         i. Intramyocardial hemorrhage
         ii. Disruption of myocardial fibers
         iii. Myocardial necrosis and rupture of the myocardium, papillary muscle, or valve
      c. Can lead to impaired circulation, arrhythmia, or bleed into the pericardium resulting in cardiac tamponade
      d. Cardiac tamponade can occur at the time of injury or develop as a late complication several weeks after the injury.

e. Of the 51 children ages 4 to 14 who died of baseball-related injury between 1973 and 1983, 23 died as a result of ball impact to the chest.

2. **Mechanism of injury**
   a. Crushing and sudden deceleration injuries mainly from high-impact and motor vehicle accidents
   b. Impact to the anterior chest wall and sternum during boxing or from a thrown baseball, hockey puck, lacrosse ball, field hockey ball, or a kick during martial arts
   c. The sternum is more mobile in a child and can cause impact to the pericardium and cardium, resulting in asystole and death.
3. **Diagnosis**
   a. Difficult to diagnose myocardial contusion because signs vary with the degree of myocardial damage and are typically transient
   b. Athlete can experience minor chest pain or sudden cardiac arrest.
   c. Chest pain is nonpleuritic and relieved by oxygen but not nitroglycerin.
4. **Physical examination**
   a. Tachycardia
   b. Arrhythmias
   c. Signs of decreased cardiac output
   d. Cardiac examination usually normal but may be a friction rub or murmur
   e. May have obvious external chest wall injury
5. **Laboratory and radiographic studies**
   a. ECG:
      i. Findings are nonspecific, but 70–85% show abnormalities.
      ii. 75% of these ECG abnormalities are nonspecific ST segment and T wave changes and sinus tachycardia.
      iii. 10–20% are intraventricular conduction disturbances; right bundle-branch block is most frequent, followed by left bundle-branch block or unifascicular block.
      iv. 3% show partial or complete atrioventricular conduction block.
      v. These findings have been found on initial evaluation and during the first 3 days after injury and are usually transient.
   b. Holter monitor:
      i. If arrhythmias present, majority are premature ventricular contractions; atrial fibrillation and other supraventricular arrhythmias also noted.
      ii. Ventricular tachycardia and fibrillation can occur in the first moments after chest trauma.
   c. Creatine kinase (CK-MB) isoenzymes:
      i. Not specific; misses 40% of contusions when used alone
      ii. Right ventricle, which composes most of the frontal surface of the heart, is usually injured but constitutes little of the total myocardium, thus releasing only a small amount of CK-MB enzyme.
   d. Radionuclide angiogram:
      i. Depressed right or left ventricular ejection fraction and segmental ventricular wall motion abnormalities
      ii. Also nonspecific and not predictive of cardiac complications
   e. Echocardiography:
      i. May help to make initial diagnosis with segmental ventricular wall motion abnormalities, mural thrombi, and dilatation of one or both ventricles
      ii. May be a more effective tool to follow a suspected contusion and manage myocardial decompensation
6. **Associated injuries:** sternal fractures
7. **Treatment**

a. If mild, admit for observation and watch for dysrhythmias, which are more likely to occur in the first 24 hours following injury.
b. If severe contusion and associated with other injuries, may require invasive monitoring and inotropic medications.

9. **Return to play**
   a. Manufacturers are developing softer baseballs to decrease incidence of morbidity and mortality.
   b. Use of a chest protector, especially during batting

B. **Cardiac tamponade**
1. **Description**
   a. Blunt trauma results in an accumulation of blood or edematous exudate into the pericardial sac.
   b. Volume and rate of the accumulation of fluid determine the symptoms.
   c. The tension created within the pericardial sac limits venous inflow and diastolic filling, and cardiac output is diminished.
   d. Shock and death can rapidly evolve without early recognition and treatment.
2. **Physical examination**
   a. **Pulsus paradoxus** (fall in blood pressure of > 10 mmHg on inspiration)
   b. Tachycardia and hypotension
   c. Dyspnea
   d. Weak pulse
   e. Distant heart sounds
   f. Distended neck veins
3. **Laboratory studies:** ECG shows low voltage.
4. **Treatment**
   a. Intravenous fluids if available and urgent transport to hospital
   b. Pericardiocentesis
   c. Emergent thoracotomy

C. **Coronary artery dissection and occlusion**
1. **Description and mechanism of injury**
   a. Uncommon result of blunt trauma, as in high-speed vehicular collisions resulting in rapid deceleration of the body:
      i. Creates enormous shearing forces that may act on the coronary artery near its origin, resulting in an intimal dissection or disruption
      ii. An intraluminal thrombus can form adjacent to the injured arterial wall.
   b. Can be asymptomatic, cause angina or a myocardial infarction, or cause death
   c. The left anterior descending coronary artery is injured in two thirds of reported cases, the right coronary artery in one fourth.
2. **Diagnosis**
   a. Dyspnea
   b. Diaphoresis
   c. Severe chest pain with or without radiation of pain
   d. Nausea
3. **Laboratory and radiographic studies**
   a. ECG may show evidence of myocardial ischemia.
   b. Coronary arteriogram
4. **Treatment**
   a. Conservative, as lesion may heal with medical management:
      i. Intravenous morphine, nitroglycerin
      ii. Anticoagulation with heparin and acetylsalicylic acid
      iii. Beta-blocker, calcium channel blocker, or later angiotensin-converting enzyme inhibitor

b. Watch for postinfarction complications, including complete heart block, ventricular arrhythmias, left ventricular failure, ventricular aneurysm, and pulmonary emboli.
c. Echocardiography to evaluate wall motion abnormality
d. If ongoing ischemia, coronary angiography to confirm diagnosis and assess extent of injury
e. Coronary artery bypass graft surgery

D. **Traumatic aortic rupture**
1. **Description**
a. Approximately 80–90% fatality rate at scene of accident
i. The disruption extends through the full thickness of the aortic wall, allowing rapid exsanguination into the mediastinum and pleural spaces.
ii. In only 20% is the rupture sufficiently contained by the adventitia to allow survival to reach medical attention.
b. Potential higher risk in those athletes with Marfan's syndrome
i. A hereditary disorder of connective tissue involving multiple organs
ii. Causes cystic medial necrosis of the aorta resulting in aortic dilatation
iii. More often the dissection is nontraumatic, but those with the disease are still restricted from contact and high exertion sports.
2. **Mechanism of injury**
a. High-speed deceleration-type injuries seen in motor sports, bicycling, and skiing
b. The tremendous torques that result from the sudden deceleration affect the junction of the fixed and mobile parts of the great vessels, such as between the aortic arch and the fixed descending aorta.
3. **Diagnosis**
a. Nonspecific symptoms
b. Acute onset of sharp interscapular or precordial pain that may migrate
c. Shortness of breath
4. **Physical examination**
a. Hypertension in the upper extremities with widening of the pulse pressure
b. With an **ascending aortic injury**, aortic diastolic murmur radiating to the back due to incompetence of the aortic valve
c. Acute coarctation syndrome in up to 25% of **descending aortic injuries:**
i. Caused by partial obstruction of the aortic lumen
ii. Upper extremity hypertension, diminution of femoral pulses and leg blood pressure, and a systolic murmur
5. **Laboratory and radiographic studies**
a. Chest x-ray: abnormalities present at time of admission in 75–90%:
i. Widening of the superior mediastinum and obscuring of the aortic knob shadow are most consistent findings.
ii. Deviation of trachea to the right, depression of left main stem bronchus, left apical extrapleural density, and left pleural effusion
iii. In ascending or arch injuries, the mediastinal widening may be predominantly to the right of the trachea, resulting in deviation of trachea to the left.
iv. Rib fractures in 50% of cases
b. ECG may show evidence of left ventricular hypertrophy or myocardial ischemia or infarction.
c. Transesophageal echocardiography may be both sensitive and specific enough to plan management without aortogram.
d. CT scan with contrast enhancement or MRI
e. Thoracic aortogram

6. **Treatment**
   a. Medical therapy to avoid sudden rupture, including antihypertensive agents and beta-blockers
   b. Emergent operative repair results in 75–90% survival.

E. **Thoracic outlet syndrome**

1. **Description**
   a. Spectrum of signs and symptoms resulting from compression of the neurovascular bundle (brachial plexus and subclavian and axillary arteries and veins) in the interval between the intervertebral foramina and the axilla
   b. Clinical presentation may differ from patient to patient because of the different degrees of compression that may occur.
   c. Greater incidence in women (4:1); thought to be secondary to lower position of scapula and changing shoulder posture with larger breasts
2. **Areas of compression**
   a. **Supraclavicular region**—interscalene triangle bordered by anterior and middle scalene muscles, which attach to the first rib
      i. Hypertrophy of scalene muscles (Fig. 6A)
      ii. Presence of long transverse process of T-7, cervical ribs, or other rib anomalies (Fig. 6B)
      iii. Presence of fibrous bands (Fig. 6C)
      iv. Changes to alignment and angulation of first rib, such as may occur with age and postural changes
   b. **Subclavicular or costoclavicular region**—between the "mobile" clavicle and "fixed" first rib
      i. Changes in shape and mobility of clavicle, such as callus from a fracture or an alteration in shoulder motion, can narrow the interval.
      ii. Subclavius muscle lies behind the clavicle just anterior to subclavian vein.
   c. **Infraclavicular region**—at coracoid process of scapula
      i. Compression by pectoralis minor, which inserts at the coracoid, during full abduction (Fig. 6D).
      ii. Subcoracoid area has the thickened costocoracoid membrane
   d. Other—any lesion involving the pleura, such as neoplasm
3. **Diagnosis**
   a. Neural compression symptoms:
      i. Pain from root of neck to shoulder and down arm diffusely
      ii. If lower trunk of brachial plexus compressed (most common), paresthesias involving medial aspect of elbow, forearm, and hand, especially little finger and ring finger
      iii. Weakness and occasionally atrophy of affected hand
      iv. Sometimes just vague ache and heaviness in shoulder, upper arm, and upper anterior and posterior chest, including trapezius and suboccipital region
      v. May awaken with symptoms at night if sleep with arms above head
   b. Arterial compression symptoms:
      i. Hand feels cold
      ii. Arm becomes numb and fatigued with rapid overhead movement
   c. Venous compression symptoms:
      i. Swelling and discoloration of arm after exercise
      ii. Prominent superficial venous pattern over ipsilateral shoulder and chest
4. **Physical examination**
   a. Careful examination of neck, cervical spine, shoulder, elbow, and hand
      i. **Diagnosis of thoracic outlet syndrome is one of exclusion.**
      ii. Examination of supraclavicular fossa for masses or bruits

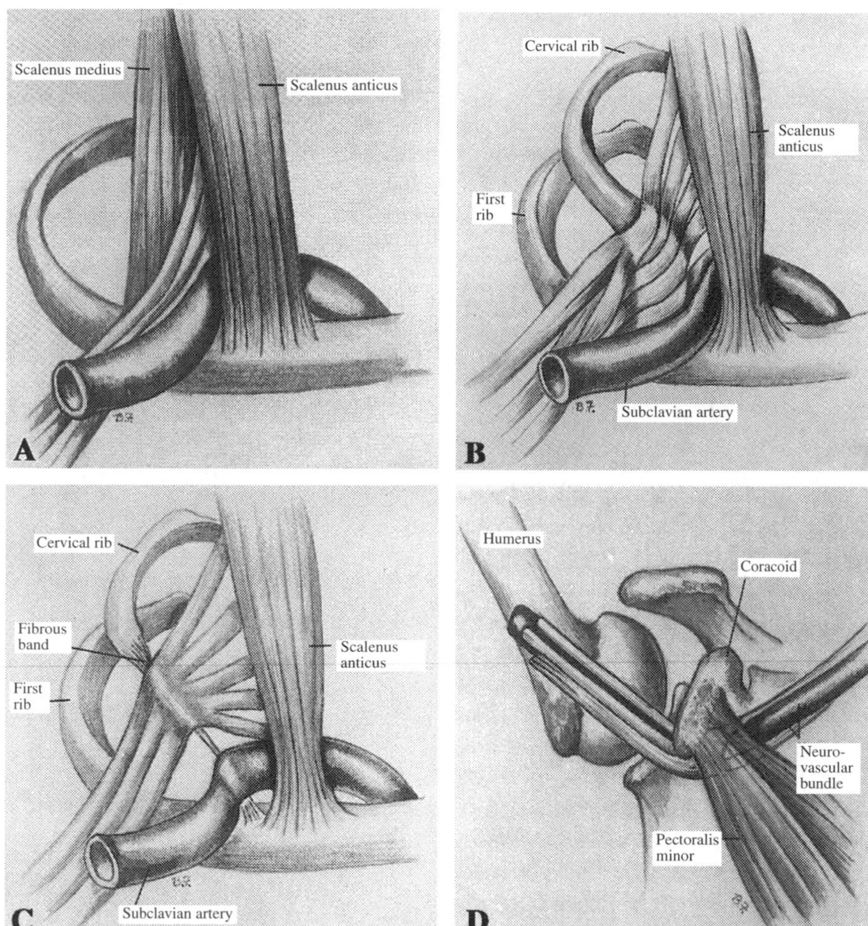

FIGURE 6. Areas of compression of the neurovascular bundle. **A**, Hypertrophy of scalene muscles. **B**, Presence of cervical rib. **C**, Presence of a fibrous band. **D**, Compression by pectoralis minor during hyperabduction. (From DePalma AF: Surgery of the Shoulder, 2nd ed. Philadelphia, J.B. Lippincott, 1973, pp 511–520, with permission.)

iii. Careful neurologic examination

b. **Adson's maneuver:**
   i. Arm abducted and externally rotated, while head is extended and turned to side of lesion
   ii. Radial pulse is monitored while a deep breath is taken and held.
   iii. Positive test if diminution or total loss of pulse; however, this test is positive in up to 30% of asymptomatic population.

c. **Wright's maneuver:** similar to Adson's maneuver except the arm is hyperabducted, with the hand brought over the head with the elbow and arm in the coronal plane

d. **Military brace position or costoclavicular syndrome test:**
   i. Shoulders are retracted and pulled down to narrow the interval between clavicle and first rib and reproduce symptoms, including absence of radial pulse
   ii. Effective test in patients who have symptoms when wearing a backpack

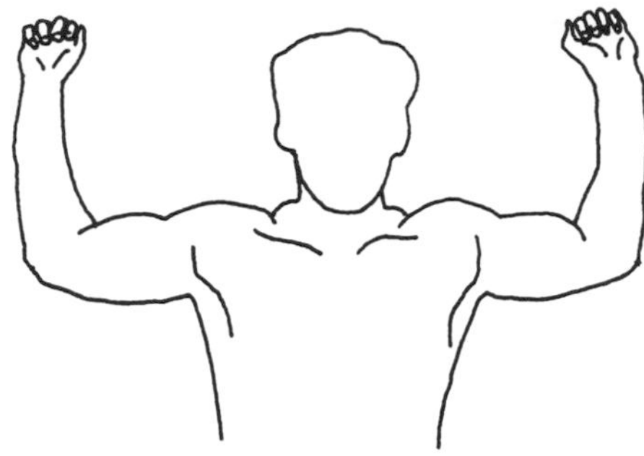

FIGURE 7. The Roos test to evaluate thoracic outlet syndrome.

   e. **Overhead exercise test (Roos test)** (Fig. 7):
      i. Arms are abducted to 90°, shoulders externally rotated, and elbows flexed to 90°
      ii. Hands are opened and closed slowly for 3 minutes to reproduce symptoms of fatigue, cramping, numbness and tingling, or even coolness or paleness of extremity
5. **Laboratory and radiographic studies**
   a. Cervical spine x-rays; myelogram or MRI if necessary
   b. Chest x-ray to evaluate apex of lung
   e. Electrodiagnostic studies:
      i. Difficult to accurately determine nerve conduction velocity at the thoracic outlet
      ii. Should be performed with arm in provocative position
      iii. Helpful in ruling out peripheral entrapment of nerves
   d. Venography or arteriography
   e. Plethysmography
6. **Differential diagnosis**
   a. Shoulder instability and "dead arm syndrome"
   b. Cervical spine pathology
   c. Peripheral neuropathies:
      i. Ulnar neuropathy
      ii. Carpal tunnel syndrome
      iii. Rare to have "double-crush syndrome" (irritation at both sites)
   d. Raynaud's phenomenon can be present with both thoracic outlet syndrome and collagen vascular diseases.
   e. Reflex sympathetic dystrophy:
      i. Similar symptoms of painful swelling, color changes, and other sympathetic dysfunction, but also large element of hypersensitivity
      ii. Dissociation between sensations of touch, pressure, and pain
      iii. Bone scan may be positive.
   f. Pancoast's tumor or other space-occupying lesion in thoracic outlet
   g. **Myofascial syndrome (fibromyalgia or fibrositis syndrome):**
      i. Periscapular region, base of neck, and chest wall are common areas of pain and fatigue.
      ii. Trigger points commonly found in the supraspinous fossa (near rhomboids, levator scapula, and infraspinatus) can cause pain to radiate down arm.
7. **Treatment**
   a. Conservative management results in 50–90% recovery:
      i. Strengthen shoulder girdle suspensory muscles, including trapezius, serratus anterior, deltoid, and erector spinae muscles.
      ii. Stretch the scalenes, lateral neck flexors, and pectoral muscles.

            iii. Weight reduction, posture training (correct the "drooped" shoulder), proper brassiere support
            iv. Avoid hyperabduction of shoulder.
            v. Avoid carrying heavy packages in affected hand.
    b. Consideration of operative treatment only if firm diagnosis and conservative treatment has failed (3–4 months), intractable pain, or major neurologic or vascular complications:
        i. First rib resection has been most dependable procedure.
        ii. Surgical procedure varies depending on the anatomic basis for the symptoms.

F. **Vascular injuries of subclavian and axillary veins**
1. **Description: "Effort thrombosis"** (Paget-Schroetter syndrome), or primary thrombosis, describes the traumatic thrombosis of the subclavian or axillary vein
2. **Mechanism of injury**
    a. May occur after a single traumatic event around the shoulder or clavicle:
        i. Clavicular fracture
        ii. Axillary hematoma
        iii. Injury to axillary or subclavian vein
    b. **More commonly associated with repetitive overhand motions causing trauma to the vessel**, e.g., hyperabduction and external rotation. This primary thrombosis is related to the inherent anatomic structure of the thoracic outlet and axillary region, with compression at various points causing damage to the vein walls.
3. **Diagnosis**
    a. Pain and diffuse swelling in the affected arm
    b. Numbness, heaviness, and easy fatigability
    c. Distention of superficial arm veins with cyanosis (bluish discoloration) of skin
    d. Onset of symptoms commonly within 24–72 hours of activity
4. **Physical examination**
    a. Increase in girth of upper extremity
    b. May be weakness of upper extremity, especially if venous occlusion is long-standing
    c. Symptoms can often be reproduced with an exercise test of the upper extremity or by putting the arms into extreme hyperabduction
5. **Radiographic studies**
    a. Venogram
    b. Chest x-ray to evaluate bony structures
    c. Cervical-spine anteroposterior view
6. **Differential diagnosis**
    a. Rule out secondary causes of thrombosis (sarcoidosis, infection, drug use, hypercoagulable states, metastatic tumor) and poor circulation.
    b. Arterial occlusion, including **aneurysms of subclavian or axillary arteries**, has also been reported in athletes:
        i. Classic symptom also early fatigue during act of throwing
        ii. Other symptoms include absent pulses, cyanosis, decreased skin temperature, and finger ischemia secondary to digital embolization.
7. **Associated conditions:** If upper extremity thrombosis confirmed, watch for signs of pulmonary embolus (incidence approximately 12%).
8. **Treatment**
    a. Thrombolysis with fibrinolytic agents such as streptokinase or urokinase; simultaneous anticoagulation with systemic heparin, then warfarin sodium (Coumadin) for 1–3 months
    b. Thrombectomy and surgical correction of the involved thoracic outlet and axillary structures if documented external compression, e.g., by cervical ribs, medial clavicle, scalenus anticus

c. High incidence of late morbidity, such as swelling, pain, fatigability, and numbness, especially with conservative therapy or anticoagulation alone. Can become asymptomatic if good compensatory collateral veins develop.
d. More promising short-term results seen thus far with thrombolysis alone or in combination with surgery.

9. **Return to play:** No participation in contact sports while on oral anticoagulants.

IV. Abdominal Injuries

Although the abdomen is largely unprotected in most contact sports, the strong and mobile lower ribs as well as the contracted abdominal and back muscles are able to prevent serious injury. **"Getting the wind knocked out"** is a more common occurrence than significant trauma to a visceral organ. This happens when there is an unguarded blow to the epigastric region, or solar plexus. The athlete is unable to breathe freely because of the temporary reflex spasm of the diaphragm and perhaps transient shock of the sympathetic celiac plexus. Usually after loosening of restricting garments and flexion at the knees and abdomen, normal respiration is rapidly restored. Even with the winded athlete, however, there is always some danger of intra-abdominal injury because of the unprotected, unguarded blow to the abdomen. Careful observation and follow-up examination ensure that a significant injury has not been missed (Fig. 8).

A. **Rectus sheath hematoma**

1. **Description:** Major muscle groups of abdominal wall are the two rectus muscles, the external and internal obliques, and the transversus.
2. **Mechanism of injury**
   a. Direct blow to abdominal wall, causing hemorrhage into the muscle
   b. May damage either the epigastric artery or intramuscular vessels causing a hematoma within the sheath, which usually self-tamponades
   c. With violent stretching movements, the inferior epigastric artery can rupture and hemorrhage without associated muscle damage.
3. **Diagnosis**
   a. Sudden abdominal pain
   b. Rapid swelling
   c. Most comfortable in a supported flexed position
   d. May have nausea and vomiting
4. **Physical examination**
   a. Abdomen may be somewhat rigid with guarding.
   b. Increased tenderness over rectus
   c. Fixed (within the rectus sheath) palpable mass most often below the umbilicus when sitting or lying
   d. Bluish discoloration around the periumbilical region 72 hours after injury (Cullen's sign)

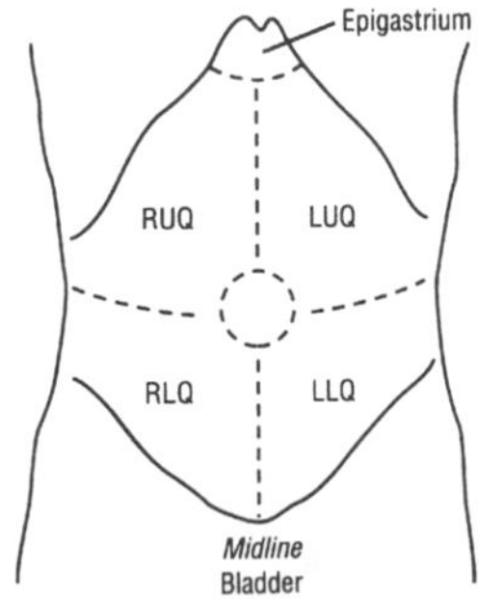

FIGURE 8. The four quadrants of the abdomen with corresponding underlying viscera. (From Reid DC: Sports Injury Assessment and Rehabilitation. New York, Churchill Livingstone, 1992, pp 671–738, with permission.)

e. Pain with resisted trunk or hip flexion
f. Hyperextension of spine causes pain in the anterior abdominal wall.

5. **Radiographic studies**
   a. Ultrasound useful diagnostic tool in hands of experienced ultrasonographer
   b. MRI or CT scan may be used to assist in differentiation between intra-abdominal injury and hematoma if necessary.
6. **Treatment**
   a. Ice, activity modification, and NSAIDs; local heat after 48–72 hours
   b. Avoidance of activities that require rotation, stretching, or flexion of trunk or lower extremities
   c. Rehabilitation concentrating on restoring flexibility, strength, and endurance of all the abdominal muscles
   d. If hemorrhage extensive and superficial epigastric artery is torn, operative evacuation of the hematoma and ligation of the artery may be required.

B. **Rupture of diaphragm**
1. **Description**
   a. Herniation of abdominal contents into the chest
   b. Occurs most commonly on left side with blunt trauma:
      i. Four times more common than on right
      ii. Certain amount of protection from liver on the right
   c. Can be easily overlooked because of delayed onset of symptoms
2. **Mechanism of injury:** blunt chest or abdominal trauma
3. **Diagnosis**
   a. Chest pain
   b. Shortness of breath
   c. Intestinal obstruction
4. **Physical examination**
   a. Decreased breath sounds in affected chest
   b. Excessive percussional tympany in the chest
   c. Bowel sounds in the chest
   d. Scaphoid abdomen
5. **Radiographic studies:** chest x-ray and abdominal films
   a. Dilated stomach in lower chest
   b. Presence of a nasogastric tube terminating in the air space is confirmatory.
6. **Associated injuries:** splenic rupture in 25% of patients with blunt diaphragmatic rupture, liver lacerations in 25%, pelvic fracture in 40%, and thoracic aortic tears in 5%
7. **Treatment**
   a. Immediate surgical repair:
      i. Left-sided injuries explored transabdominally due to high incidence of associated intra-abdominal injuries
      ii. Right-sided injuries explored transthoracically due to location of liver
   b. Watch for complications from pneumonia and abscess.

C. **Splenic rupture**
1. **Description**
   a. Spleen is the organ most commonly injured during blunt abdominal trauma and **is most frequent cause of death due to abdominal injury in sport.**
   b. Although the rib cage offers some protection, rib fractures can leave the spleen even more vulnerable to injury.
   c. Spleen's capacity for encapsulating bleeding delays overt signs and symptoms of rupture; can be days before the condition can suddenly deteriorate.
   d. Spleen can enlarge and weaken during some illnesses, including infectious mononucleosis, making it more susceptible to rupture.

2. **Mechanism of injury:** direct trauma to left lower chest from a fall, sporting injury, or motor vehicle accident
3. **Diagnosis**
   a. Initial sharp pain in left upper abdomen, then continuation of dull, left-sided flank pain
   b. Abdominal distention
   c. Referred pain to either right or more commonly left shoulder (**Kehr's sign**) from free intraperitoneal blood irritating the diaphragm
4. **Physical examination**
   a. Generalized abdominal tenderness; may have rebound tenderness and rigid abdomen
   b. Tachycardia, hypotension, diaphoresis, and rapid respirations suggest internal bleeding
5. **Laboratory and radiographic studies**
   a. Decreased hemoglobin and hematocrit levels
   b. May have markedly elevated white blood count if subcapsular hematoma has developed
   c. Flat-plate abdominal x-rays may show fading splenic outline and growing splenic shadow.
   d. Diagnostic peritoneal lavage is positive unless bleeding is encapsulated (positive is 10 mL of free blood, > 100,000 red blood cells/mm^3, or > 500 white blood cells/mm^3)
   e. CT scan with contrast or MRI
   f. Ultrasound
   g. Spleen scan or arteriogram
6. **Treatment**
   a. If high suspicion, arrange immediate transport to hospital:
      i. If hypotensive, give bolus of intravenous fluids if available.
      ii. Keep athlete lying flat or in modified Trendelenburg position to direct blood flow to the heart.
   b. Nonoperative management of splenic injury in hemodynamically stable patients is safe and is the preferred treatment. Experienced assessment and meticulous observation are necessary.
   c. Exploratory laparoscopy/laparotomy indicated if continuing hemodynamic instability or if require more than 4 units of blood during a 48-hour period:
      i. Repair of capsular lacerations (splenorrhaphy)
      ii. Splenectomy only for extensive injury and uncontrolled hemorrhage
   d. Beware of **"delayed rupture"** of the spleen:
      i. Occurs > 7 days after an initial negative CT scan
      ii. Need high index of suspicion and liberal utilization of other imaging techniques

D. **Liver laceration**
1. **Description**
   a. Relatively rare in contact sports; usually results from high-speed accidents during motor racing and skiing
   b. Capsular hematoma is the most common injury to the liver in athletes.
2. **Mechanism of injury:** blows to the right upper quadrant
3. **Diagnosis:** pain in the right upper quadrant, right shoulder, or neck pain
4. **Physical examination**
   a. Pain and tenderness to palpation over right upper quadrant
   b. Tachycardia and hypotension
   c. May be associated right lower rib fractures
5. **Laboratory and radiographic studies**

a. Ultrasound
b. CT scan with contrast enhancement or MRI
c. Liver scan or arteriogram
d. Liver enzymes—**AST or ALT > 130 IU/L** indicative of liver injury

6. **Treatment**
   a. Rest, observation, and intravenous fluids for those hemodynamically stable with no signs of peritoneal irritation and no other intra-abdominal injuries that might require surgical repair
   b. Laparotomy may be necessary to control bleeding.

E. **Rupture of stomach and intestines**

1. **Description:** Injuries are rare.
2. **Mechanism of injury**
   a. Kicks or blows to the abdomen
   b. Falls off a horse or against equipment, such as in gymnastics
   c. Pile-ons and spearing in football
   d. Handlebar accidents in cycling
3. **Diagnosis**
   a. Persistent abdominal pain with signs of chemical or bacterial peritonitis, including fever, nausea, and vomiting
   b. Referred shoulder pain from irritation of diaphragm
   c. May have blood in stool if intermucosal hemorrhage present
4. **Physical examination**
   a. Localized pain, guarding, rebound tenderness, absence of normal bowel sounds, rigid abdomen
   b. Clammy, sweaty skin
   c. Hypotension and tachycardia
   d. Absence of normal respiratory motion of abdomen
5. **Laboratory and radiographic studies**
   a. Plain x-ray with upright and decubitus abdominal views:
      i. See free air under the diaphragm or along abdominal wall
      ii. Important to have the athlete in those positions at least 3 minutes before the views are taken
   b. Peritoneal lavage—not helpful for duodenal or large intestine injuries because of retroperitoneal position
   c. Nasogastric tube placement to check for blood if suspect damage to stomach
   d. Meglumine diatrizoate (gastrografin) swallow
   e. CT scan
6. **Associated injuries:** Intramural hematoma of the duodenum may manifest as a gastric outlet or high small bowel obstruction.
7. **Treatment**
   a. Urgent transport to hospital if increasing pain, signs of peritonitis, or circulatory collapse develops; if available until transport arrives, infuse intravascular fluid.
   b. Careful serial examinations, nasogastric tube, and intravenous fluids
   c. Abdominal exploration and repair

F. **Hernias**

1. **Description**
   a. Three most common hernias in adults are indirect inguinal (50–70%), direct inguinal (men > 40 years old), and femoral (women).
   b. Hernias involving the anterior abdominal wall include incisional, periumbilical, and linea alba defects.
   c. Potential for **incarceration** (irreducible hernia) and **strangulation** (twisting of the hernia) causing bowel obstruction and toxicity

2. **Mechanism of injury:** repetitive heavy lifting activities
   a. Causes increased intra-abdominal pressure, which can contribute to the development of hernias, especially in those with predisposing weakness of abdominal muscle and fascia
   b. Has been reported secondary to trauma, such as impact from a bicycle handlebar on the abdominal wall
3. **Diagnosis**
   a. Aching sensation and occasionally tender swelling in area of hernia
   b. May be scrotal swelling with indirect hernia, as the sac extends into the inguinal canal
4. **Physical examination**
   a. Indirect and direct inguinal hernias are palpated by invaginating the scrotum with a finger to palpate the external inguinal rings and inguinal canals.
      i. Athlete is asked to Valsalva.
      ii. An elliptic mass descending along the spermatic cord and bulging against the tip of the finger is an **indirect hernia**.
      iii. A globular mass close to the pubis that bulges against the bottom of the finger is a **direct hernia**.
   b. **Femoral hernias** occur below the inguinal ligament, two fingerbreadths medial to the femoral artery.
   c. Hernias more prominent when athlete stands or increases intra-abdominal pressure
5. **Radiographic studies**
   a. **Herniography:**
      i. Intraperitoneal injection of contrast material to diagnose occult hernia sacs
      ii. 84% incidence of inguinal hernia by herniography in soccer players with groin pain; only 8% had hernias detectable by physical examination.
   b. Bone scan—increased uptake in musculature in initial phase
   c. MRI used to examine soft tissues in the groin region
   d. CT scan—contrastographic medium combined with CT scan has been used to study hernias.
6. **Differential diagnosis**
   a. **Iliopectineal/iliopsoas bursitis:**
      i. Groin pain reproduced by passive hip flexion caused by inflammation of bursa between pectineus and psoas muscle
      ii. Pain can be localized over area of lesser trochanter.
      iii. A position of hip flexion and external rotation is most comfortable.
   b. **Osteitis pubis**
   c. **Posterior inguinal wall weakness:**
      i. Presents as gradually worsening, poorly localized groin pain that is aggravated with activity
      ii. Herniography shows bulging, or areas of weakness, of the wall.
   d. Muscular strain
   e. Hydrocele or varicocele
7. **Treatment**
   a. Surgical repair for large or symptomatic hernias
   b. Avoid activities that stretch or pull the abdominal muscles for 2 weeks after repair; then can gradually resume progressive exercise and conditioning. By the fourth week, begin abdominal strengthening.
8. **Return to play**
   a. Can return to noncontact sports by 6–8 weeks and contact sports by 8–10 weeks for indirect hernia repairs
   b. The more extensive repairs of direct inguinal, femoral, and anterior abdominal wall hernias require a longer recovery; contact sports at 12 weeks.

Recommended Reading

1. Abrunzo TJ: Commotio cordis: The single, most common cause of traumatic death in youth baseball. Am J Dis Child 145(11):1279–1282, 1991.
2. Banning AP, Masani ND, Ikram S, et al: Transesophageal echocardiography as the sole diagnostic investigation in patients with suspected thoracic aortic dissection. Br Heart J 72(5):461–465, 1994.
3. Christensen MA, Sutton KR: Myocardial contusion: New concepts in diagnosis and management. Am J Crit Care 2(1):28–34, 1993.
4. DePalma AF: Surgery of the Shoulder, 2nd ed. Philadelphia, J.B. Lippincott, 1973, pp 511–520.
5. Eames NW, Deans GT, Lawson JT, et al: Herniography for occult hernia and groin pain. Br J Surg 81(10):1529–1530, 1994.
6. Grassi CJ, Bettmann MA: Effort thrombosis: Role of interventional therapy. Cardiovasc Intervent Radiol 13(5):317–322, 1990.
7. Holden DL, Jackson DW: Stress fracture of the ribs in female rowers. Am J Sports Med 13(5):342–348, 1985.
8. Jackimczyk K: Blunt chest trauma. Emerg Med Clin North Am 11(1):81–96, 1993.
9. Johnson I, Branfoot T: Sternal fracture—a modern review. Arch Emerg Med 10(1):24–28, 1993.
10. Koury HI, Peschiera JL, Welling RE: Non-operative management of blunt splenic trauma: A 10-year experience. Injury 22(5):349–352, 1991.

10a. Marker LB, Klareskov B: Posterior sternoclavicular dislocation: An American football injury. Br J Sports Med 30(1):71–72, 1996.

11. Micheli LJ: Spine and chest wall. In Johnson RJ, Lombardo J (eds): Current Review of Sports Medicine. Philadelphia, Current Medicine, 1994, pp 8–9.
12. Miles JW, Barrett GR: Rib fractures in athletes. Sports Medicine (12(1):66–69, 1991.
13. Miller MD, Johnson DL, Fu FH, et al: Rupture of the pectoralis major muscle in a collegiate football player: Use of magnetic resonance imaging in early diagnosis. Am J Sports Med 21(3):475–477, 1993.
14. Nuber GW, McCarthy WJ, Yao JST, et al: Arterial abnormalities of the shoulder in athletes. Am J Sports Med 18(5):514–519, 1990.
15. Proffer DS, Patton JJ, Jackson DW: Nonunion of a first rib fracture in a gymnast. Am J Sports Med 19(2):198–201, 1991.
16. Reid DC: Sports Injury Assessment and Rehabilitation. New York, Churchill Livingstone, 1992, pp 671–738.
17. Robertsen K, Kristensen O, Vejen L: Manubrium sterni stress fracture: An unusual complication of noncontact sport. Br J Sports Med 30(2):176–177, 1996.
18. Rockwood CA, Green DP, Bucholz RW: Injuries of the sternoclavicular joint. In Rockwood CA, Green DP (eds): Fractures in Adults, 4th ed. Philadelphia, J.B. Lippincott, 1996, pp 1415–1471.
19. Sahdev P, Garramone RR Jr, Schwartz RJ, et al: Evaluation of liver function tests in screening for intra-abdominal injuries. Ann Emerg Med 20(8):838–841, 1991.
20. St. Louis P, Gandhi S: Cardiac contusion and creatine kinase-MB: A pertinent case history and brief review of the utility of CK-MB. Clin Biochem 27(2):105–111, 1994.
21. Taylor DC, Meyers WC, Moylan JA: Abdominal musculature abnormalities as a cause of groin pain in athletes: Inguinal hernias and pubalgia. Am J Sports Med 19(3):239–242, 1991.
22. Wolfe SW, Wickiewicz TL, Cavanaugh JT: Ruptures of the pectoralis major muscle: An anatomic and clinical analysis. Am J Sports Med 20(5):587–593, 1992.

47

Thoracic and Lumbosacral Spine

John M. Wilhite, M.D.

I. Anatomy

A. **Bony**—lumbar vertebra (Fig. 1)

1. Composed of:
   a. **Vertebral body**, a large anterior weight-bearing structure of each lumbar vertebra
   b. **Vertebral arch**, a horseshoe-shaped structure surrounding the vertebral foramen (through which the spinal cord runs) composed of:
      i. Pedicles—two short, stout, rounded structures projecting from the body, one on each side
      ii. Lamina—broad, flat structures that meet in the midline posteriorly where they are continuous with the posteriorly directed spinous process
   c. Where each pedicle and lamina meet there is a mass of bone from which three processes arise:
      i. Transverse process—projects laterally
      ii. Superior articular process—projects cranially (cephalad)
      iii. Inferior articular process—projects caudally
   d. **Pars interarticularis**, the area between the superior and inferior articular processes on each vertebra. This area is particularly susceptible to sheering forces and stress fracture.
2. Lumbar vertebrae articulate with each other by intervertebral disks and superior and inferior articular processes forming the facet joints. The facet joints have a synovial lining and capsule.

B. **Soft tissues**

1. **Disk** (see Fig. 1)
   a. **Annulus fibrosus**, the outer layer of fibers that functions to hold the nucleus pulposus and limit its displacement during flexion, extension, and load bearing
   b. **Nucleus pulposus**, the gelatinous structure occupying an eccentric position within the annulus fibrosus
2. **Ligaments** (see Fig. 1)
   a. **Anterior longitudinal ligament:**
      i. Runs entire length of spine along the anterior surface of the vertebral bodies
      ii. A broad, strong band of fibrous tissue
   b. **Posterior longitudinal ligament:**
      i. Runs along the posterior surface of the vertebral bodies (anterior surface of spinal canal)
      ii. Slightly weaker and narrower than the anterior longitudinal ligament
   c. **Interspinous ligament**, runs between the posterior spinous processes
   d. **Supraspinous ligament**, connects the spinous processes
   e. Facet capsule

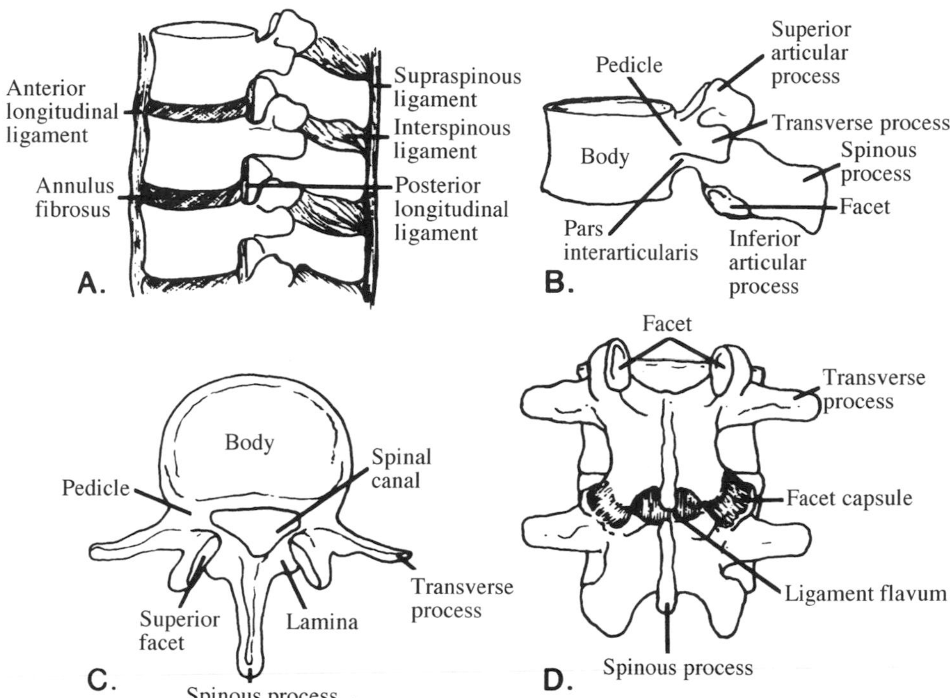

FIGURE 1. Normal lumbar vertebrae anatomy. **A**, Lateral view of three lumbar vertebrae with surrounding ligaments. **B**, Lateral view of one lumbar vertebra. **C**, Looking from above. **D**, Posterior view indicating facet joint and capsule.

3. **Fascia and muscles**
   a. **Thoracolumbar fascia:**
      i. Represents fascia and fused aponeuroses of several muscles
      ii. Lies over the muscles of lower back
   b. **Paraspinal muscles** are composed of the three layers of muscles of which only the superficial layer is palpable—the sacrospinalis.
   c. **Abdominal wall muscles:**
      i. Provide approximately 30% of the lumbar spine support via hydrostatic column effect
      ii. Weakness results in abnormal increase in lumbar lordosis with concomitant stress on soft tissue supporting structures

II. Function

A. Soft tissues act as "guy wires" to maintain alignment and affect the strong, coordinated torso movements.
B. Bony structures and disks provide mobility, support, and protection.
C. Both provide longitudinal support for the abdomen and thorax.
D. Spinal structures permit "universal joint" motion.
E. The spine provides protection for the delicate neurologic structures of the spinal column.

III. Diagnosis

A. **History**
   1. **Pain**

a. **Potential pain-producing structures:**
   i. Supraspinous ligament
   ii. Interspinous ligament
   iii. Longitudinal ligaments
   iv. Ligamentum flavum
   v. Facet joint capsules
   vi. Peripheral fibers of annulus fibrosus
   vii. Back muscles
b. **Pain—local, radicular, or referred?**
c. **Onset**—traumatic or gradual?
d. **Exacerbating factors:**
   i. **Discogenic** usually worse with flexion or prolonged standing or sitting and increased with Valsalva maneuvers (coughing, sneezing, or straining on defecation)
   ii. **Spondylolysis:** worse with hyperextension (i.e., walkovers, tennis serve, golf stroke follow-through)
   iii. **Spinal stenosis:** "pseudoclaudication," worse with ambulation
e. **Relieving factors:**
   i. **Discogenic:** lying with knees flexed improves (by increasing foraminal space)
   ii. **Spinal stenosis:** sitting improves. The room in the lumbar canal enlarges with the spine in flexion, thus decreasing the pain.
f. **Worrisome factors:**
   i. **Unexplained fever** may indicate infection (osteomyelitis or disc space infection).
   ii. **Weight loss and anorexia** may indicate malignancy.
   iii. **Bladder, bowel, or sexual disturbances** may indicate **cauda equina syndromes** or central midline disk herniation.
   iv. **Pain at rest**—suspicious for tumor
g. **Referred pain** may come from abdominal or pelvic disorders (abdominal aortic aneurysm, pelvic tumors or infections, renal disorders, or prostate disease).

2. **Work and social history**—underlying secondary gain?
   a. Financial
   b. Frustration with job or family

B. **Physical examination**
1. **Inspection**
   a. **Stance:**
      i. Listing to one side may be seen in nerve root compression (most often away from side of herniation).
      ii. Flattening of lumbar lordosis seen in more advanced spondylolisthesis
   b. **Gait:** A peculiar short-stride, forward-flexed, rigid gait is seen in disk space infections.
2. **Range of motion**
   a. **Flexion:**
      i. Look for reversal of normal lumbar lordosis.
      ii. **Schober test** for spinal flexibility (Fig. 2):
         (a) Performed by aligning a tape measure vertically along the spine beginning 10 cm above an imaginary line that joins the "dimples of Venus" (small hollows located on either side of the lumbosacral spine)
         (b) Marks are made at 0, 10, and 15 cm, with tape measure held in place
         (c) Patient touches his or her toes and amount of flexibility is measured (normal is 5 cm, i.e., an increase in the total distance from 15 cm to a total of 20 cm between initial reference points)
         (d) A good way to follow patients with **ankylosing spondylitis**

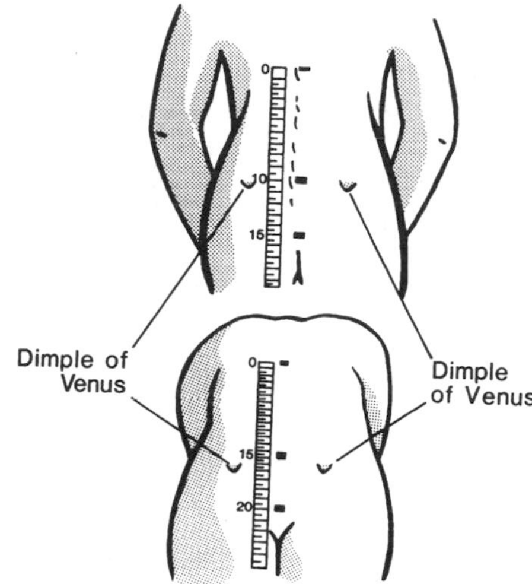

FIGURE 2. Schober test.

b. **Extension**
c. **Lateral flexion** to right and left, unilaterally limited in painful disk
d. **Rotation**
e. Measure **chest expansion:**
    i. Normally approximately 3 inches
    ii. Significant when reduced to 2 inches and may reveal underlying ankylosing spondylitis

3. **Palpation**
    a. Muscle spasm—paraspinal muscles seem prominent and feel more rigid.
    b. Trigger points
    c. Deformities—step-off deformity in spondylolisthesis
    d. Tenderness—in disk herniation with radicular pain, frequently able to elicit tenderness in sciatic notch (midway between ischial tuberosity and greater trochanter)
    e. Palpation of iliac crest levels to check for pelvic obliquity
4. **Percussion over spine** may elicit tenderness in nerve root impingement, tumors, or infections.
5. **Neurologic** (deep tendon reflexes, strength, sensation)
    a. Common nerve root finding (Table 1)
    b. Dermatomes (Fig. 3)
6. **Specific maneuvers:**
    a. **Straight leg raising test (SLR):** aggravates radicular-type pain. Indicative of nerve root impingement or irritation along course of sciatic nerve. Test is considered positive if patient experiences radicular-type pain at < 60–70° of leg elevation.

TABLE 1. Common Nerve Root Findings

Root	Reflexes	Strength	Sensation
L-4	Patellar	Anterior tibialis	Medial leg and foot
L-5	None	Extensor hallucis longus	Lateral leg and dorsum of foot
S-1	Achilles	Peroneus longus and brevis	Lateral foot

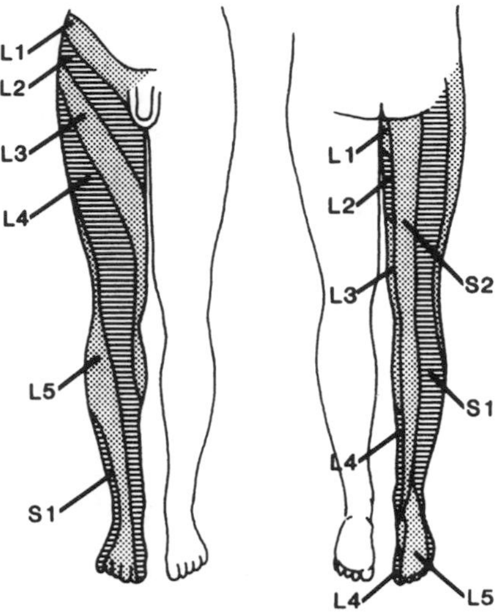

FIGURE 3. Dermatomes of lower extremities.

b. **SLR** with dorsiflexion of the foot (**Lasegue's test**) (Fig. 4): creates additional sciatic stretch. Increased pain on this maneuver is indicative of nerve root compression or involvement of sciatic nerve along its course.
c. **Crossed (or contralateral) SLR:** considered by some to be pathognomonic of herniated disc. With the patient supine, examiner lifts unaffected leg; in the presence of a herniated disk, this maneuver may exacerbate pain in affected leg. A positive crossed SLR often indicates a severe herniation.
d. **SLR while sitting (sitting root test):** positive when extending the knee causes radicular pain or causes the patient to sit back in an effort to relax tension on the sciatic nerve. A strongly positive SLR without complaints on a sitting SLR is inconsistent and should raise suspicion for nonorganic factors. It may be helpful to view this not as malingering, but as a patient's attempt to enlist the physician as an advocate.
e. **One-legged standing hyperextension test** (Fig. 5): when elicits low back pain, is suggestive of spondylolysis, spondylolisthesis, or sacroiliac dysfunction.

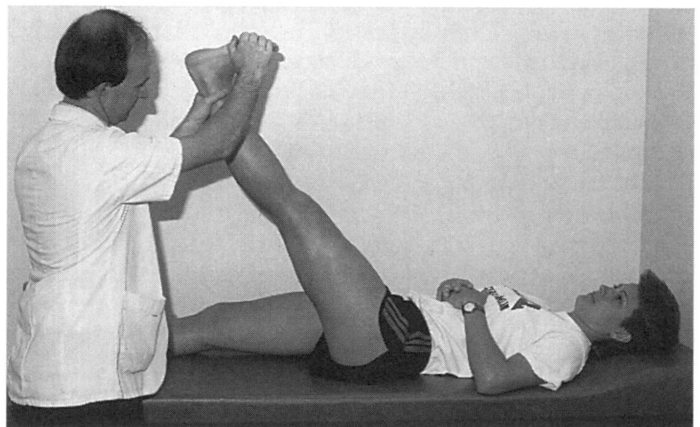

FIGURE 4. Straight leg raising with dorsiflexion of the foot (Lasegue's test) creates additional sciatic stretch and, when pain is increased on this maneuver, is indicative of nerve-root compression or involvement of the sciatic nerve along its course.

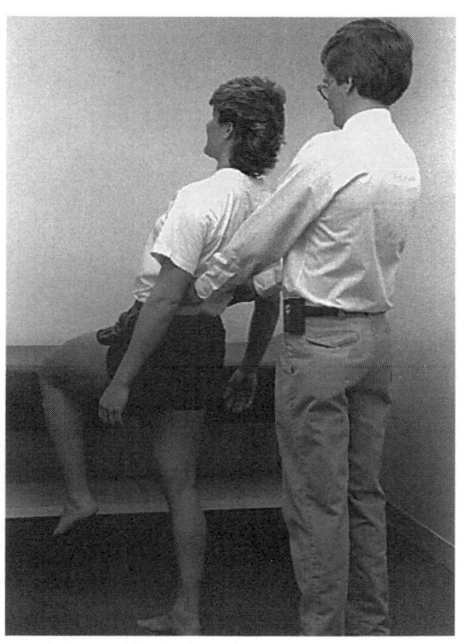

FIGURE 5. One-legged standing hyperextension test aggravates discomfort in the presence of spondylolysis.

f. **Patrick's or FABER test** (Flexion, ABduction, and External Rotation of hip): sacroiliac pain may indicate a sacroiliac joint disorder.
g. **Supine to long sitting test:** examiner checks relative leg length with the patient supine and then with the patient sitting with both legs extended in front by comparing the position of the medial malleoli. Changes of relative leg length 1 cm or greater indicate sacroiliac locking.

C. **Radiologic studies**
1. **Plain films**
a. **Usually unnecessary in acute phase, but collision and strength sports may necessitate earlier x-ray evaluation.**
b. Many argue that x-rays are indicated only when there is:
i. History of serious trauma (possible fracture)
ii. Known cancer (possible pathologic fracture)
iii. Pain at rest (possible tumor)
iv. Unexplained weight loss (possible malignancy)
v. Drug or alcohol abuse (possible disk space infection)
vi. Treatment with corticosteroids (possible pathologic fracture)
vii. Temperature > 38°C (possible infection)
viii. Suspicion of ankylosing spondylitis by history, or neuromotor deficit by physical examination
ix. Unremitting pain of 2–4 week duration
x. Suspicion of pars defect (spondylolysis, spondylolisthesis)
c. **Usually do not provide information about the presence or location of disk herniation, even when narrowed disk space is observed.** In the young population, however, end plate avulsion or a Schmorl's node suggestive of intraosseous herniation may occasionally be seen.
d. **Plain films may reveal:**
i. Spondylolysis—a defect in the pars interarticularis (Fig. 6)
ii. Spondylolisthesis—forward displacement of a superior vertebral body in relation to an inferior vertebral body (Fig. 7)

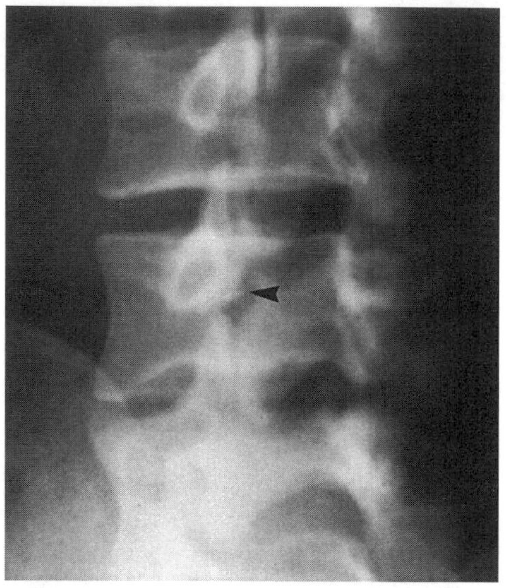

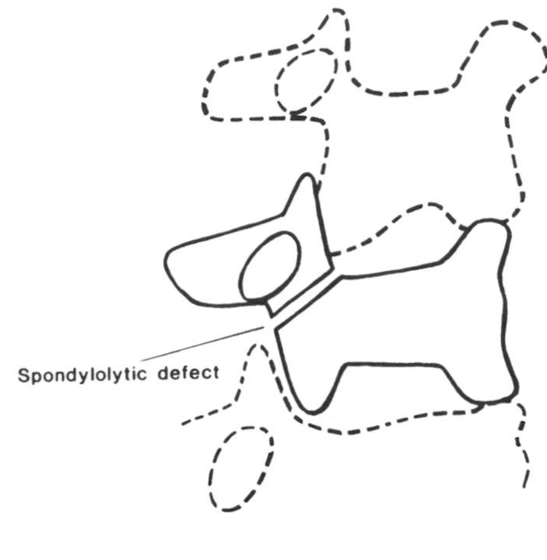

FIGURE 6. The spondylolytic defect is seen as a collar on the Scotty dog's neck (pars interarticularis) on an oblique x-ray of the lumbar spine.

iii. Evidence of disk space infection consisting of narrowing of intervertebral disk space and irregularities and sclerosis of vertebral end plates
iv. Degenerative changes evidenced by disk space narrowing and osteophyte formation

2. **Bone scans**
   a. Useful when locating a lesion that is symptomatic but not yet visible on plain films (i.e., stress fracture of pars interarticularis)
   b. When positive, a scan is indicative of increased bone metabolic activity, which could represent fracture, infection, tumor, or arthritis.
   c. Three-phase study:
      i. When positive in early phase, usually indicative of soft tissue inflammation
      ii. When positive in second and late phases, usually indicative of bone disease
3. **Tomography, computed tomography (CT) scanning, magnetic resonance imaging (MRI) and myelography** are expensive but are of great help in making or confirming a diagnosis and therefore should be used judiciously.
   a. **Tomography of the spine** is helpful in delineating congenital anomalies, fractures, and infections
   b. **CT scan** is used to evaluate the bony spine for fractures and spondylolytic defects, herniated disks, extraspinal soft tissue abnormalities (i.e., hematoma or myositis ossificans), and infections and neoplasms of the spine
   c. **MRI** is helpful in detection of herniated disk, intrinsic spinal cord lesions, and spinal cord and nerve root compression, as well as benign or malignant bony lesions. MRI usually gives more information than CT about far lateral herniations.
   d. **Myelography** remains valuable in evaluation of intrinsic spinal cord and nerve root lesions and compression. More accurate when combined with a postmyelogram CT study.
   e. CT scan most helpful in instances of bone disease (especially cortical bone); MRI most helpful with soft tissue problems and in bone disease involving marrow

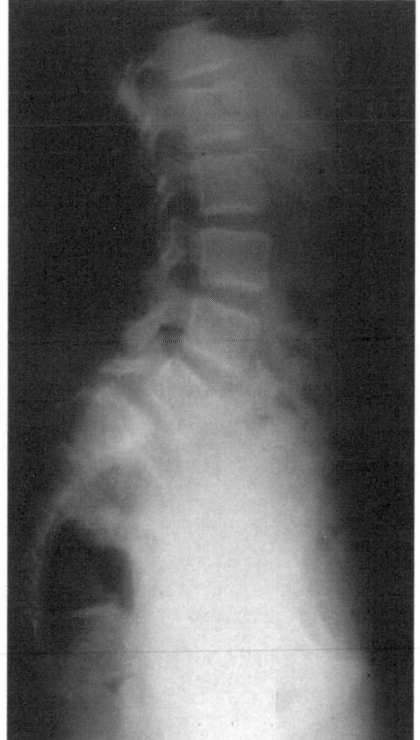

FIGURE 7. Lateral x-ray of lumbosacral spine revealing spondylolisthesis.

f. **Because 30–60% of CT scans and myelograms show disk degeneration or herniation in asymptomatic subjects, a positive study is not diagnostic unless it conforms to the clinical picture.**
   i. Many herniated and degenerated disks are asymptomatic.
   ii. A CT scan not parallel to the disk may give an erroneous impression of disk herniation.

g. The sensitivities of CT, myelography, and electromyography/nerve conduction velocity (EMG/NCV) studies in diagnosing a herniated disk are around 90%. Specificities of CT and myelography are around 88%; specificity of EMG/NCV studies is much less at 38%. MRI is usually the preferred study for diagnosing herniated disk.

4. **Neurologic study—EMG/NCV**
   a. It takes 14–21 days for denervation changes to occur to the degree that they can be picked up on EMG study.
   b. EMG/NCV is helpful in localizing nerve root compression in herniated disk syndromes.

IV. Thoracic Spine

A. **Postural (flexible) roundback**
   1. Most commonly seen in older adolescents
   2. **Presents** with roundback deformity in the form of a long, graceful curve, with or without back pain
   3. **Characterized** by the patient's ability to assume voluntarily a properly erect position (in Scheuermann's disease, the patient cannot correct the kyphosis)
   4. **Radiologic exam**

a. **Lateral** view—the kyphosis measured between the inferior margin of T12 and an upper thoracic vertebra exceeds 40°; no structural abnormalities of the vertebral bodies
b. **Supine** hyperextension film (with bolster under the thoracic spine)—shows correction of the kyphosis to measurably normal degrees

5. **Treatment**
   a. Postural exercises
   b. When severe, treatment similar to that for Scheuermann's disease (see next section)

B. **Classic Scheuermann's disease**
1. Most commonly seen in older adolescents
2. Typically **presents** with round-shouldered appearance, with or without back pain
3. **Etiology** is unknown, but the basic lesion is a **Schmorl's node**, which is a herniation of an intervertebral disk through the anterior end plate of three or more successive vertebrae.
4. **Physical exam:** The patient cannot voluntarily correct the kyphosis (as in postural roundback), and on forward bending the kyphosis is accentuated, showing an area of acute, sharp angulation usually around T7 (whereas postural roundback shows a smooth, symmetric contour).
5. **Radiologic exam:** Lateral view must show three successive thoracic vertebral bodies (each anteriorly wedged more than 5°), slight irregularity of the vertebral end plates, and Schmorl's nodes.
6. **Treatment**
   a. Usually excellent results with Milwaukee brace (Fig. 8) and supervised exercise program
   b. Surgical treatment rarely necessary

C. **Scoliosis**
1. **Definition**—lateral curvature of the spine
2. Present to a minor degree in up 8–10% of population
3. Most common form of scoliosis is **idiopathic** and begins in adolescence
4. **Relatively unrestricted physical activity is desirable for almost all adolescents with scoliosis.** Participation improves strength, flexibility, overall fitness, and self-esteem.
5. Decisions regarding appropriate sports and levels of participation require knowledge about the natural history of scoliosis as well as the particular sport. Each case should be evaluated individually; a routine prohibition from participation is inappropriate.
   a. In general, an otherwise healthy patient with mild-to-moderate scoliosis, even if under treatment with bracing, can safely participate in most levels of sport activity.
   b. Patients with vertebral abnormalities in the cervical spine (or at the cervicothoracic junction) should be counseled against contact or collision sports. (The American Academy of Pediatrics has published useful guidelines on classification of sports by degree of contact and intensity of exertion. See ref. 8.)
   c. **Patients who have had spinal fusion for scoliosis** should be counseled against participating in collision sports and should be warned that even strenuous noncontact sports may increase the risk of degenerative disease in the segments above and below the fusion.
6. **Physical exam:** Look for asymmetry of the back and presence of a rib hump when patient bends forward (Adams' test).
7. **Radiologic exam:** Should include standing posteroanterior and lateral views of the thoracolumbar spine, carefully measuring the curvature.
8. **Treatment of idiopathic adolescent-onset scoliosis**

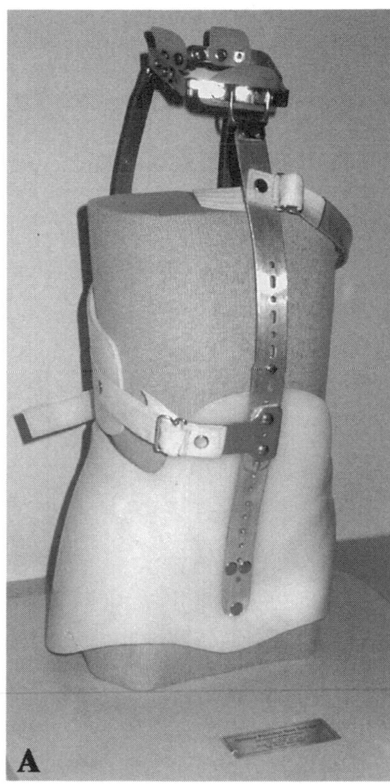

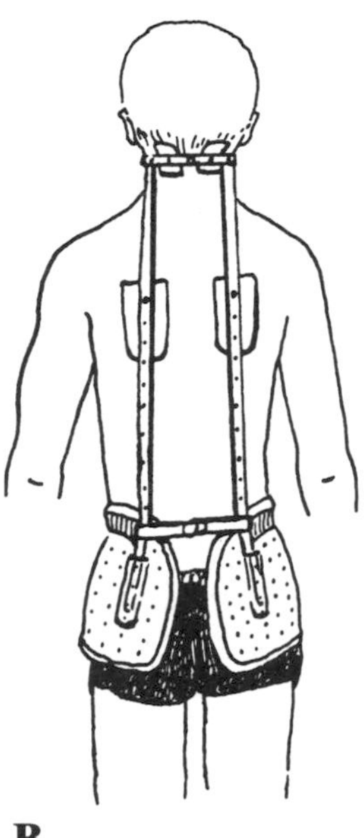

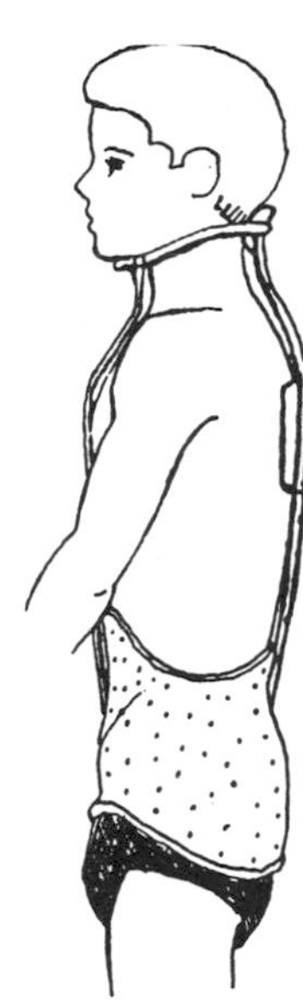

FIGURE 8. **A**, Milwaukee brace used in treatment of Scheuermann's disease. (From Labelle H, Dansereau J: Orthopedic treatment of pediatric spinal disorders and diseases. Spine State Art Rev 4(1):242, 1990.) **B**, Note the pelvic bucket extends posteriorly over the buttocks and holds the patient in a slightly flexed attitude. This helps control the lumbar lordosis so that the dorsal pads can correct the kyphosis. (From Drummond DS: Kyphosis in the growing child. Spine State Art Rev 1(2):347, 1987.)

a. If curvature is mild (< 20°) when first detected, reassessment every 3–4 months during adolescence and until skeletally mature is the usual course of follow-up. Active treatment is not required so long as the curve is nonprogressive.
b. If rib deformity is mild (< 10°), the individual may be followed by scoliometric measurement (Fig. 9), with x-rays only when rotational deformity is progressive.
c. If skeletally immature and the curve is moderate (20–45°) when first detected and is documented to be progressive, bracing is the mainstay of therapy with the goal of arresting progression (not correcting the curve). In many instances, the treatment regimen may safely permit enough time out of the brace for daily participation in sport activity; each case must be individualized and this decision made by a scoliosis specialist.
d. Severe curvature may require surgery (fusion with spinal instrumentation), and discussion is beyond the scope of this text. These patients should be followed by a scoliosis specialist and their activity level adjusted according to the treating physician's established guidelines.

V. Thoracolumbar Spine

A. **Atypical Scheuermann's disease**
   1. **Differs from classic Scheuermann's**
      a. **Thoracolumbar or lumbar spine**

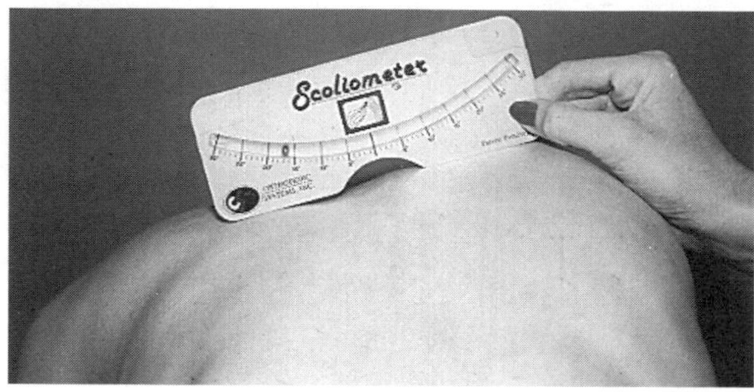

FIGURE 9. Scoliometer. A patient is placed in the forward-bending position, and the Scoliometer is placed on the patient's back. The midportion of the Scoliometer is located directly over the midline of the spine. The Scoliometer is placed over the maximum rib prominence. Note the deflection of the ball within the level. (From Green NE: Adolescent idiopathic scoliosis. Spine State Art Rev 4(1):213, 1990.)

- b. Generally does not involve three successive vertebrae
- c. **Pain** more frequent and more severe
- d. **Seen almost exclusively in adolescent athletes** participating in sports with vigorous spine loading; thus, traumatic (or overuse) etiology suspected.
    - i. Weightlifting
    - ii. Gymnastics
    - iii. Football
    - iv. Wrestling
    - v. Tennis
    - vi. Rowing
    - vii. Bicycle racing

2. **Lesions vary with location**
    - a. **Thoracic lesions** are usually herniation of anterior-inferior end plate into the vertebral body with excavation of the apophyseal region.
    - b. **Lumbar lesions** usually involve anterior-superior end plate; apophysis generally persists and may be enlarged, and excavation may or may not be present.
3. Often, more than one level is affected, but not consecutively.
4. **Associated conditions** (much higher than expected comorbidity)
    - a. Mild scoliosis ≤ 10°
    - b. Spondylolysis ± spondylolisthesis
5. **Treatment**
    - a. Most respond to simple conservative measures (rest and supervised therapeutic exercise)
    - b. **Semirigid thermoplastic brace** if significant vertebral body deformity or if rest and exercise fail to resolve symptoms:
        - i. 15° lordotic brace for thoracolumbar lesion
        - ii. Out of brace 1 hour/day for therapeutic exercise and bathing
        - iii. Bony healing may require 4–6 months

B. **Vertebral apophysitis ("ring apophysitis")**

1. **Presents** with symptoms or findings ranging from vague pain to point tenderness along the spine in adolescents
2. **Symptoms** aggravated by activity, relieved with rest
3. Often seen in athletic individuals (i.e., gymnasts) and believed to be **due to repetitive microfractures of the vertebral end plates**
4. **Radiologic exam:** Changes of vertebral end plate irregularity at one or more anterior vertebral bodies without kyphotic deformity distinguish this from Scheuermann's disease.
5. **Treatment**
    - a. Decreased activity
    - b. Stretching
    - c. Strengthening exercises

C. **Lumbar ring apophyseal fractures**

1. Posterior fracture of the ring apophysis, often with posterior bony protrusion into the spinal canal

2. > 50% of reported cases in athletes and in trauma victims
3. Generally involves inferior apophyseal ring of upper lumbar vertebrae
4. **Treatment: Surgery may be needed to remove a protruding fragment if any significant encroachment on neural structures.**
5. Rare, but growing number of reports

VI. Lumbosacral Spine

A. Acute lumbar strain

1. **Defined** as nonradiating, low back pain associated with mechanical stress to the lumbar spine and its supporting structures
2. **Cause** is not always evident
   a. May be related to a specific traumatic episode
   b. More often may be related to prolonged poor posture, poor physical conditioning, and anterior migration of the center of gravity
3. **Poor sitting posture** may predispose one to develop low back pain.
   a. Relaxed sitting for any length of time usually results in the lumbar spine assuming a fully flexed position, becoming painful due to stretching of the posterior muscles and ligaments.
   b. In sitting, the intradiscal pressure increases as the spine assumes a forward flexed position and decreases as one moves into lordosis.
4. **Improper lifting** may precipitate an episode of low back pain. Lifting with back flexed and knees straight significantly increases the intradiscal pressure as compared to lifting with back straight and flexed hips and knees.
5. **Physical exam**
   a. Local tenderness and muscle spasm may be found over the involved areas.
   b. Usually a limited range of motion (forward and lateral flexion and rotation) is found.
   c. Neurologic exam is entirely normal.
6. **Radiographic evaluation**
   a. In acute low back strain, x-rays are usually not necessary on the initial visit.
   b. Consider x-rays if no improvement occurs within 2–4 weeks.
7. **Treatment**
   a. **Pain control measures:**
      i. Ice packs or ice massage
      ii. Nonsteroidal anti-inflammatory drugs to relieve acute pain and inflammation
      iii. Muscle relaxants in patients with palpable muscle tightness or spasm
      iv. Narcotic analgesics should generally be avoided.
      v. Avoid bed rest but also avoid extremes of motion.
      vi. Transcutaneous electrical nerve stimulator may be helpful in those unresponsive to above measures
   b. The **rehabilitation program** is most important.
      i. The key starting point is finding and then maintaining the **neutral spine position** (NSP).
         (a) Defined as a position of less pain (and less spasm) in which there is also improved mechanics
         (b) Patient can be taught NSP and can practice to form new, improved habits
      ii. Improve **flexibility** with stretching exercises.
         (a) Always maintain the NSP while stretching.
         (b) Stretching exercise should incorporate the upper and lower extremities (i.e., shoulder girdle, trunk, hamstrings, quadriceps, iliopsoas, hip rotators). The more flexibility in the upper and lower extremities, the less motion stress on the spine.

iii. Maintain NSP with **stabilization training**, using muscular control while performing activities of daily living and sports (a **dynamic** process). Emphasis is on maintaining the NSP during all activities.
(a) Starting in the supine position with knees flexed and feet flat on floor and maintaining the NSP, fully extend and lift one extremity and hold. Alternate lifting extremities.
(b) Progress to fully lifting extremities while prone, then kneeling, and then standing.
(c) **Abdominal strengthening** (order of progression):
- Partial sit-ups (no need to perform complete sit-up because abdominal muscles work in the first 45°, and complete sit-ups place greater stress on the lumbar spine)
- Diagonal partial sit-ups
- Partial sit-ups on an inclined bench
- Add resistance by holding a weight across chest

(d) **Quadriceps** strengthening with stationary bicycle and wall slides
(e) **Progressive aerobic conditioning**
- Walking
- Stationary bicycle
- Swimming or cross-country ski machine
- Running on treadmill
- Running on track

(f) **Advanced exercises** incorporate drills on falling, rolling, and sports-specific activities.

8. **Prognosis**
   a. Usual course is gradual improvement over a 2-week period
   b. 90% are well within 2 months

B. **Spondylolysis**

1. Term derived from the Greek **spondylo**, meaning "vertebrae" and **lysis**, meaning "loosening"
2. Occurs at the **pars interarticularis**, the bony segment located between the superior and inferior articulating processes (see Figs. 1 and 10)
3. In sporting activities, is usually due to overuse—repetitive shear forces placed on pars interarticularis (pars is **weakest link** in bony structure of spine)
   a. **Hyperextension** sports (gymnastics, diving, football linemen, tennis, volleyball). Hyperextension is most common contributing factor in development of spondylosis.
   b. **Weight-loading** sports (weight lifters)
   c. **Rotation** sports (golf, tennis)
4. Most commonly seen in the adolescent age group (10–15 years old)
5. **Clinical presentation**
   a. Low back pain near the midline, usually localized
   b. Pain worse at extremes of motion (usually hyperextension)
   c. Pain usually relieved with rest
6. Maintain a high index of suspicion for spondylolysis in an adolescent active in high-risk sport (i.e., gymnastics) who presents with low back pain of more than 2–3 weeks' duration.
7. **Physical examination**
   a. One-legged hyperextension usually aggravates pain (see Fig. 5)
   b. Sciatic tension tests negative
   c. Neurologic exam normal
8. **Radiologic examination:** plain films including anteroposterior, lateral, and oblique views

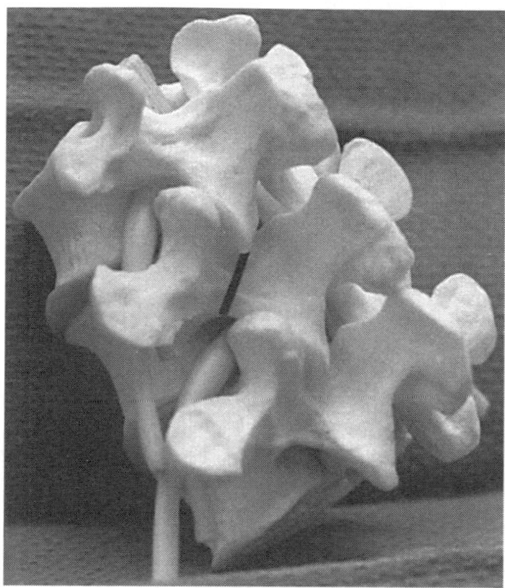

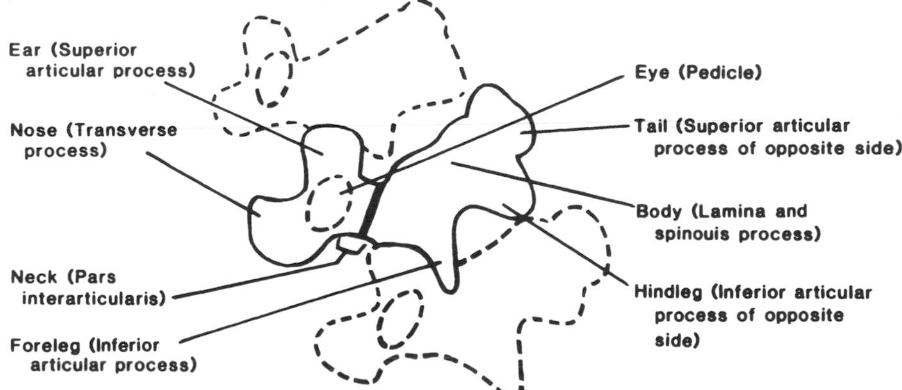

FIGURE 10. Scotty dog outline as seen on the oblique view of lumbar spine. The black line on the neck or pars interarticularis is where the spondylolytic defect occurs and on x-ray is seen as a collar on the Scotty dog's neck.

   a. **The lateral view is best performed standing** (to look for possible accompanying spondylolisthesis).
   b. Plain films may be normal early on in spondylolysis.
   c. If a spondylolytic defect is visible, it is usually seen in the **neck** of the "scotty dog" outline noted on the oblique view (see Fig. 10). At times, the defect may be visible on the lateral view.

9. **Nuclear imaging**
   a. If plain films are normal and one is still suspicious of a possible **occult** (hidden) spondylolysis based on the history and clinical exam, then a **bone scan** (technetium 99m) can be helpful (Fig. 11).
   b. Positive bone scan is indicative of an active process and a potential for bony healing.
10. **Treatment** is usually guided by the plain film and bone scan findings.
    a. Normal plain film and positive bone scan indicate an **acute lesion:**
       i. Limit offending activities (usually hyperextension, rotation, and weight-lifting) for 6–8 weeks.

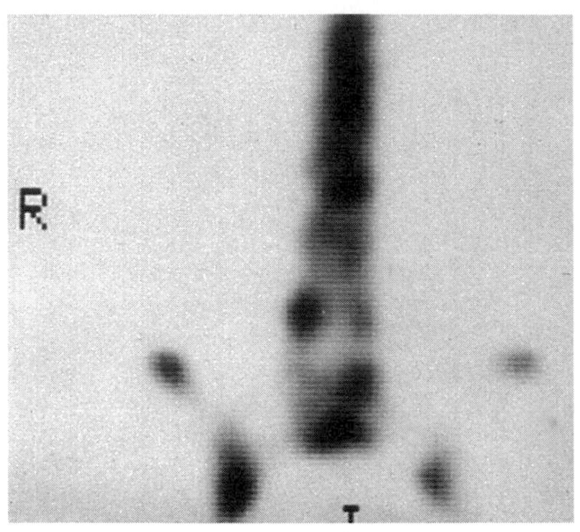

FIGURE 11. Technetium-99m bone scan demonstrates increased uptake in lumbar vertebrae as seen in acute or semiacute spondylolysis.

ii. Rehabilitation exercises may begin when symptoms subside enough to allow comfortable exercise. Rehabilitation centers on strengthening abdominal and trunk musculature.

b. Positive plain film and positive bone scan indicate **semiacute lesions**.

i. Most immobilize with a thermoplastic basic brace (Micheli and associates report success with a zero-degree antilordotic modified Boston brace):

(a) Athlete spends 23 hours each day in the brace and 1 hour each day out of brace for bathing and simple exercises

(b) Brace is usually worn for about 12 weeks (this varies with the clinician's own personal experience, because there are no strict guidelines)

(c) Bracing may be needed for several months depending on clinical response

(d) Athlete should complete course of bracing and be pain free before beginning rehabilitation exercises (increasing strength in the abdominal and trunk musculature)

ii. Follow-up plain films may be helpful in determining if bony healing has occurred following brace treatment. Some cases, however, do not heal with bony callus but rather with a **fibrous union**, in which case the bony defect is still apparent on the plain film.

c. Positive plain film and negative bone scan indicate a **chronic lesion:**

i. Negative bone scan usually indicates poor potential for bony healing.

ii. Most clinicians advocate beginning a rehabilitation program (strengthening abdominal and trunk musculature) when symptoms subside.

iii. **Surgery** is occasionally warranted in resistant cases.

C. **Spondylolisthesis**

1. Term derived from the Greek **spondylo**, meaning "vertebrae" and **olisthesis**, meaning "to slip."
2. Spondylolisthesis is the forward slippage of a vertebra onto the one below it.
3. Usually occurs at the L5–S1 level
4. **Degree of slippage classification** is measured by dividing the distance the superior vertebral body has displaced forward onto the inferior by the anteroposterior dimension of the inferior vertebral body.

a. 0–25% = First Degree (Grade I)

b. 25–50% = Second Degree (Grade II)

c. 50–75% = Third Degree (Grade III)

d. 75–100% = Fourth Degree (Grade IV)

5. Several classification schemes exist in the literature. Spondylolisthesis in athletes usually represents the **isthmic (lytic)** type, in which the lesion responsible for the slippage is in the pars interarticularis either from spondylolytic defects or from an intact but elongated pars that allows forward slippage.
6. High-degree slips are more commonly seen in females.
7. **Clinical presentation**
   a. Grade I and II slips may be asymptomatic; detected incidentally on x-rays for other reason
   b. Localized midline back pain
   c. With high-degree slips, neurologic symptoms may develop.
8. **Physical exam**
   a. As 50% slippage approaches, characteristic findings usually appear:
      i. Flat buttocks (vertical sacrum)
      ii. Tight hamstrings
      iii. Alteration in gait by tight hamstrings and vertical sacrum in which hips do not fully extend
      iv. May be palpable step-off deformity at level of defect
   b. Limitation is forward flexion
   c. Sciatic tension tests are negative but usually limited due to hamstring tightness
   d. Neurologic exam is usually normal
9. **Radiologic exam:** plain films of lumbar spine
   a. **Standing** views in anteroposterior and lateral projections are needed (if these views are taken supine, the spondylolistheses may reduce in some cases and go undetected).
   b. Oblique views may be done lying on the x-ray table.
   c. If spondylolisthesis is detected early, especially below age 10 years, annual x-rays until completion of vertical growth are helpful to look for progression of slippage. Any progression usually occurs during the first few years after the defect appears.
   d. Lateral views reveal the degree of forward slippage of a superior vertebra on an inferior vertebra (see Fig. 7).
   e. In the anteroposterior view, a superior slipped vertebra may overlie an inferior vertebra, creating a "Napoleon's hat" illusion (Fig. 12).
   f. CT and MRI are usually not needed unless evaluating for possible associated nerve root compression or spinal stenosis.
10. **Nuclear imaging** is usually not needed for diagnosis of spondylolisthesis.
11. **Treatment**
    a. Most patients are treated conservatively with restriction of activities until asymptomatic and with strengthening and stretching exercises.
    b. In youngsters with high-degree slips or with a progressive slip, consider surgical fusion.
12. **Possible complications**
    a. **Nerve root compression**
    b. Forward slippage may cause constriction of spinal canal—**spinal stenosis**. Characteristic feature is **neurogenic claudication (pseudoclaudication)** due to bony constriction of the neural structures (spinal cord, cauda equina, or individual nerve roots).
       i. Walking evokes pain.
       ii. Sitting relieves pain.
       iii. **History** rather than objective findings is decisive factor in diagnosis
       iv. CT, MRI, and myelogram are helpful in determining degree and location of stenosis

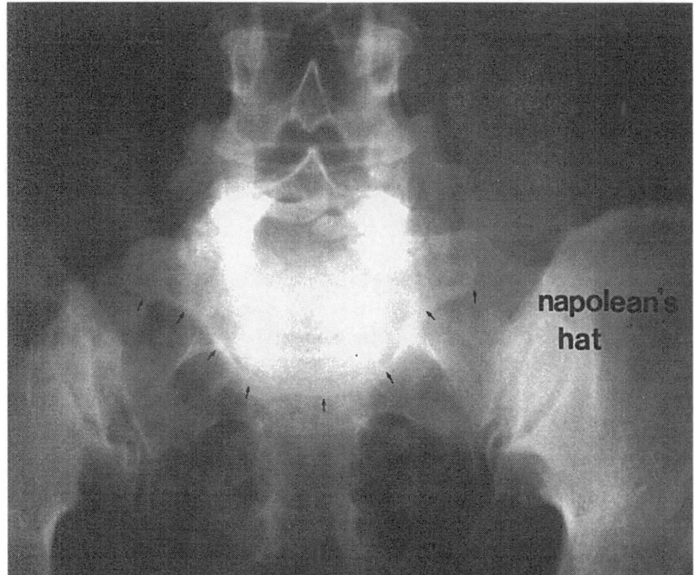

FIGURE 12. Anteroposterior view of lumbosacral spine showing inverted Napoleon's hat sign.

v. **Treatment:** Surgical fusion may be needed for high-degree slips causing spinal stenosis.

D. **Herniated disk disease**

1. Outermost fibers at the annulus fibrosus blend in with the anterior and posterior longitudinal ligaments.
   a. The posterior longitudinal ligament is weaker.
   b. Most herniations occur **posterolateral**, at the weakest link.
2. Highest incidence in third and fourth decades of life
3. Most common sites are L5–S1 and L4–5
4. **Risk factors**
   a. Frequent repetitive heavy lifting and twisting
   b. Prolonged driving
   c. Smoking
5. **Clinical presentation**
   a. May present with back pain, leg pain, or both
   b. Frequently, back pain develops first, then leg pain develops and back pain lessens
   c. Radicular pain and numbness or tingling with nerve root compression usually following the corresponding dermatome
   d. Usually **worsened** with prolonged sitting and with Valsalva maneuvers and usually aggravated by forward flexion
   e. Bladder and bowel disturbances and sexual dysfunction may indicate a large central herniated disk (cauda equina syndrome).
6. **Physical exam**
   a. May present with a **list** (usually away from the side of the herniated disk in an effort to reduce pressure on the nerve root)
   b. Range of motion usually limited
   c. May be associated muscle spasm
   d. Sciatic tension tests are positive if there is nerve root irritation.

   e. Neurologic exam may reveal weakness and decreased deep tendon responses corresponding to the level of the effected nerve root.

7. **Radiologic exam**
   a. **Plain films:**
      i. Usually normal in the younger athlete
      ii. May show narrowing of disk space
   b. **Imaging studies:**
      i. MRI is preferred imaging study for evaluation of possible herniated disk (Fig. 13)
      ii. CT (Fig. 14) and CT-myelography also useful
      iii. MRI with **gadolinium** helpful in distinguishing a recurrent herniated disk from scar tissue in those who have had previous disk surgery
8. **Neurologic study:** EMG is an objective test and may be helpful in localizing the level of nerve root compression. It usually takes 14 to 21 days for denervation changes to occur to the extent that they can be detected on EMG.
9. **Treatment** is usually conservative.
   a. Pain control measures and rehabilitation (as discussed under "Acute lumbar strain" on page 527)
   b. **Bed rest is contraindicated in athletes in all but severe disk disease because of deconditioning effects.**
   c. Surgical consultation may be needed for situations in which there is intractable pain, progressive neurologic deficits, or lack of significant expected improvement after 8 weeks of appropriate treatment measures.
   d. **Cauda equina syndrome** from a large central herniated disk requires urgent surgical consultation and emergency surgical decompression. The syndrome is signaled by loss of bowel or bladder control.

E. **Sacroiliac sprain syndrome**
1. The sacroiliac joints are among the strongest joints in the body.
   a. Possess a synovial membrane
   b. Lined by strong anterior and posterior ligaments
   c. Little movement permitted
2. Sacroiliac joints are a commonly overlooked source of low back pain.

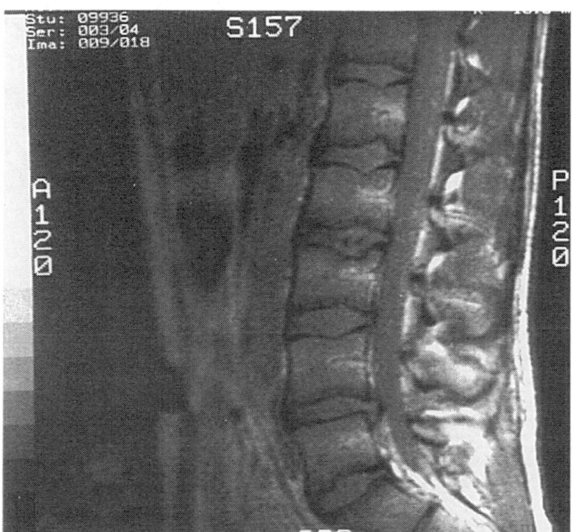

FIGURE 13. MRI of lumbosacral spine (lateral view) shows a herniated disk at the L4–L5 level.

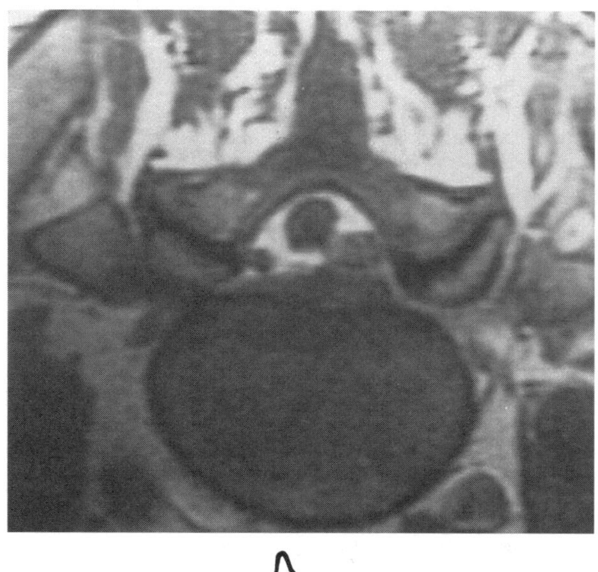

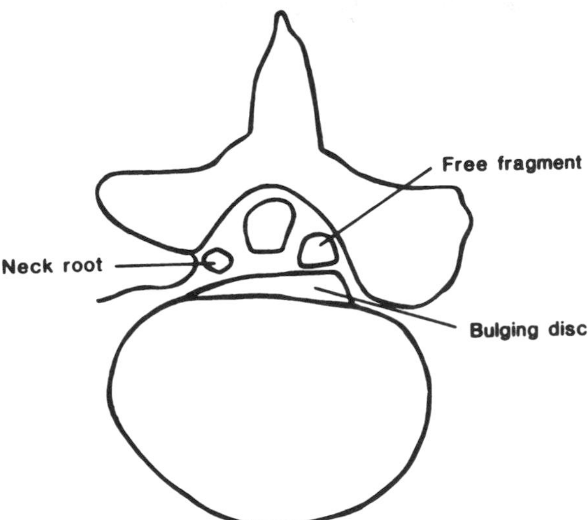

FIGURE 14. CT scan of lumbar spine showing bulging disk and a free fragment.

3. **History**
   a. May be a history of trauma
   b. Pain usually over the sacroiliac joint
   c. Pain also possible in the leg, suggesting a radiculopathy:
      i. Thus, many patients may have already been worked up with negative CT scans and myelograms.
      ii. A spur or inflamed sacroiliac joint could irritate the sciatic nerve due to close proximity.
   d. Pain is usually unilateral.
   e. May be a secondary phenomenon caused by poor low back mechanics due to guarding from other source of low back pain (e.g., lumbar strain or herniated disk)
4. **Physical examination**
   a. Tenderness over sacroiliac joint, posterior superior iliac spine, or buttock

b. Supine to long sitting test indicates sacroiliac locking
c. Painful knee-to-chest maneuver (Fig. 15)
    i. Produces rotary stress on sacroiliac joint increasing pain in sacroiliac joint disorder
    ii. A traditional therapeutic exercise given to many back pain patients that may aggravate symptoms
d. Sacroiliac compression test (patient lies on side and downward pressure is exerted on lateral pelvis) produces pain in majority of patients.
e. Gaenslen's extension test (leg of affected side overhangs side of table, and examiner presses down on thigh to hyperextend hip while performing knee-to-chest maneuver to unaffected side) also produces pain (Fig. 15B).
f. FABER test may elicit pain.
g. Neurologic exam normal

5. **Radiologic evaluation**
    a. Usually is normal
    b. Assists in ruling out other disorders, such as ankylosing spondylitis
6. **Treatment**
    a. Sacroiliac joint mobilization exercises and manipulation
    b. Nonsteroidal anti-inflammatory drugs (NSAIDs) useful
    c. X-ray–guided sacroiliac joint injection with corticosteroid

F. **Facet syndrome**
1. Facet joint is **richly innervated**.
2. Exact pathophysiology is unclear. Theories include possible mechanical irritation of the nearby nerve root or chemical irritation arising from an inflammatory process.

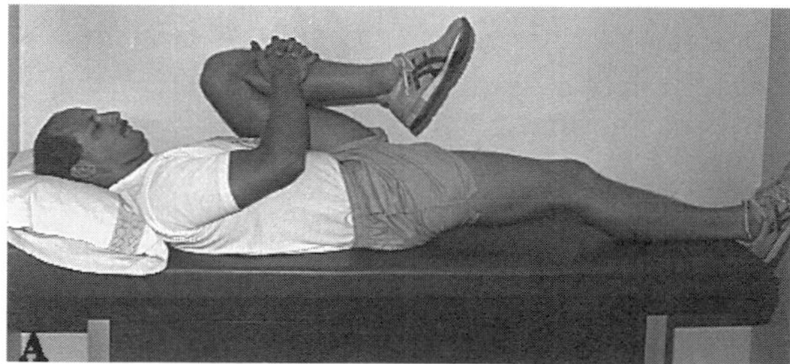

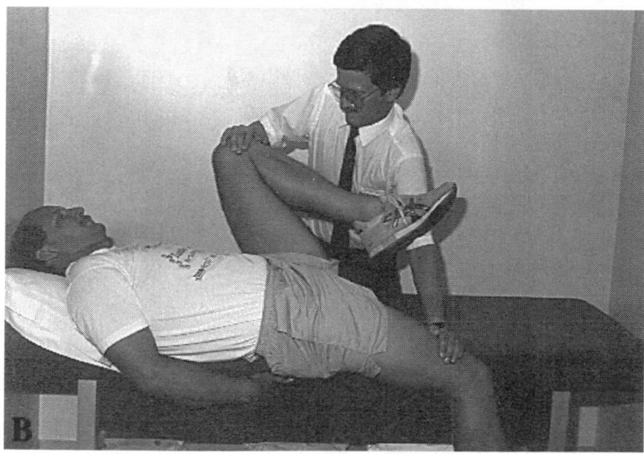

FIGURE 15. Sacroiliac sprain syndrome. **A**, Knee-to-chest maneuver causes pain. **B**, Gaenslen's extension test produces pain.

3. Usually seen in older individuals with degenerative disk disease
4. **Clinical presentation**
   a. Low back, hip, and buttock pain may radiate into posterior thigh and occasionally into calf but rarely into foot
   b. Pain usually worse with extension
   c. Sensory alterations usually absent
5. **Physical exam**
   a. Local paralumbar tenderness
   b. Pain on extension
   c. Sciatic tension tests may elicit low back and buttock pain, rarely leg pain
   d. Neurologic deficits rare
6. **Radiologic exam**
   a. Plain films may show degenerative changes of facet joints and foraminal encroachment.
   b. CT scan may be helpful in demonstrating foraminal encroachment.
7. **Treatment**
   a. Pain control measures:
      i. NSAIDs
      ii. The major role for facet joint steroid injections (performed under fluoroscopic control only by those trained in the procedure) is to attempt to provide pain relief of sufficient duration that an exercise rehabilitation program can be initiated.
   b. The most important part of treatment is an exercise program that incorporates stabilization by strong supportive muscles.
   c. For those who do not respond favorably to an adequate trial of appropriate conservative measures, surgical fusion may be considered.

G. **Ankylosing spondylitis**
1. Clinically oversimplified approach is to think of ankylosing spondylitis as the presence of symptomatic sacroiliitis (low back pain and radiologic evidence of sacroilitis).
2. **Etiology** is unknown but thought to be in the rheumatoid family of autoimmune diseases.
3. **Prevalence** appears to be around 1%.
4. **Clinical presentation**
   a. Age 15–35 years
   b. Insidious onset
   c. Symptoms persisting longer than 3 months
   d. Morning stiffness
   e. Improvement of pain with exercise
5. **Skeletal involvement**
   a. **Spine**—back pain
   b. **Extraspinal**—20% peripheral joint disease
   c. **Insertional tendinitis (enthesopathy):**
      i. Plantar fasciitis
      ii. Achilles tendinitis
      iii. Costochondritis
6. May have **extraskeletal involvement** in eyes, lungs, and heart
7. **Radiographic evaluation**
   a. Sacroiliac joints frequently first involved:
      i. Show blurring of joint margins, irregular erosions, patchy sclerosis, and narrowing (Fig. 16)
      ii. Usually bilateral

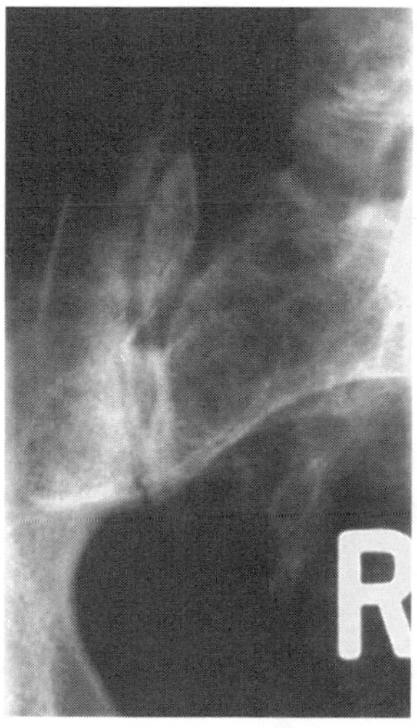

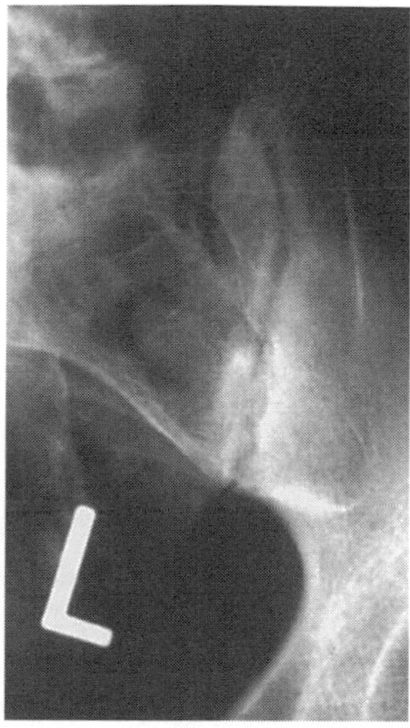

FIGURE 16. Sacroiliac views reveal sclerosis, irregular erosions, and narrowing of the sacroiliac joints in ankylosing spondylitis.

b. Spine:
   i. Initially straightening of lumbar spine and "squaring" of vertebral bodies due to erosion at the corners of the vertebrae where the annulus fibrosus inserts
   ii. With progression of disease, syndesmophytes appear along lateral and anterior surfaces of disk bridging adjacent vertebrae:
      (a) Syndesmophytes extend vertically from vertebrae along outer aspect of disk, differing from osteophytes, which project horizontally before curving to form a bridge
      (b) In advanced disease, widespread formation of syndesmophytes produces "bamboo" spine

8. **Treatment**
   a. Maintaining normal posture and activity key to decreasing progressive deformity (kyphosis)
   b. NSAIDs relieve inflammation and pain.
   c. Surgery may be helpful in correcting extreme flexion deformities.

H. **Piriformis syndrome**

1. **Definition:** Irritation of the sciatic nerve as it passes underneath or through the piriformis muscle, producing a deep localized pain in the posterior aspect of the hip (near the sciatic notch) that often radiates down into the leg
2. **Etiology** is thought to be piriformis muscle spasm or hypertrophy irritating the adjacent sciatic nerve. A history of trauma can be elicited only in about half the cases, and the nature of the trauma is seldom dramatic.
3. **Anatomy:** The piriformis muscle arises from the anterior surface of the sacrum near the sacroiliac joint, then runs laterally through the sciatic notch and inserts as a tendon on the greater trochanter of the femur. In the majority of cases, the sciatic nerve passes underneath the piriformis muscle (Fig. 17).
4. **Function of the piriformis muscle**—external rotation of the hip
5. **Additional historical clue**—dyspareunia in females. Piriformis syndrome occurs about six times more frequently in women than in men.
6. **Physical exam**
   a. May find excellent range of motion of lumbar spine despite severity of symptoms
   b. Almost invariably there is sciatic notch tenderness
   c. Often have positive straight leg raising test indicative of sciatic nerve irritation

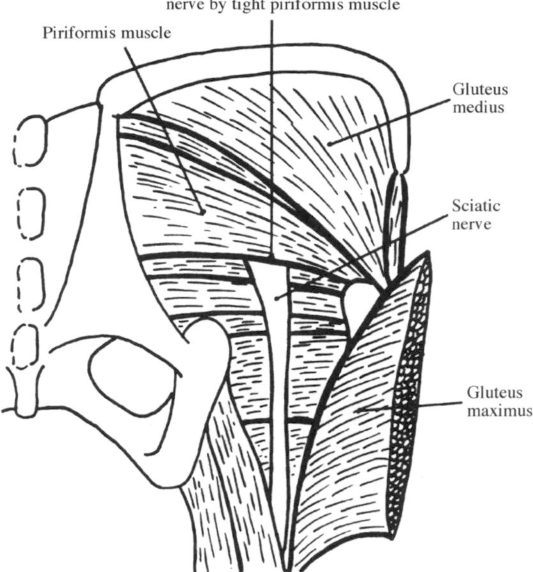

FIGURE 17. Site of compression irritation of the sciatic nerve by piriformis muscle spasm or hypertrophy.

   d. **Most significant finding:** Both active external rotation of the hip against resistance and a passive stretch into internal rotation produce pain.
7. There are no laboratory or radiologic findings in this syndrome.
8. In some cases, **EMG/NCV studies** may show normal activity in the gluteus medius and tensor fascia lata muscles (innervated by the superior gluteal nerve, which arises above the piriformis muscle); however, abnormalities may be present below this level.
9. **Differential diagnosis**
   a. Difficult to diagnose with any certainty and may be diagnosis of exclusion
   b. Most likely to be confused with herniated intervertebral disk:
      i. In herniated disk with sciatica, the pain is usually increased on coughing, sneezing, or straining on defecation, indicating epidural involvement not noted in piriformis syndrome.
      ii. Pain is not aggravated with passive internal rotation of the hip, as it is in piriformis syndrome.
10. **Treatment**
   a. Initially conservative with rest, anti-inflammatory agents, muscle relaxants, and physical therapy consisting of good stretching, range of motion, and isometric exercises to help relieve spasm and pain
   b. Local injection of the muscle belly with lidocaine and corticosteroid by those skilled enough to inject the specific location without injuring the sciatic nerve (not recommended for those who only occasionally make the diagnosis). Can be both diagnostic and therapeutic.
   c. If these measures fail, then, in rare instances, operative dissection of the compressive portion of the piriformis muscle may be necessary.

I. **Infections**
   1. **Disk space infection** and **vertebral osteomyelitis** should be included in the differential diagnosis of back pain.
   2. Usually **present** with back pain aggravated by motion, localized tenderness, limited range of motion, and paravertebral muscle spasm

3. **Pathophysiology**
   a. Hematogenous migration from distant focus via venous plexus
   b. Secondary introduction of bacteria to region (surgery, lumbar puncture) also can be source of inoculation
4. **Temperature** normal or mildly to moderately elevated
5. **Blood culture** positive in < 50% of cases
6. **Sedimentation rate** usually elevated to 40 mm/hr or more, and white blood cell count normal or mildly elevated, with normal differential or slight left shift
7. **Radiologic evaluation**
   a. **Disk space infections:**
      i. **Plain films:** Intervertebral disk space narrowing and irregularity of adjacent vertebral end plates, which may not be visualized for 10–14 days
      ii. **Technetium 99m bone scan** helpful in confirming or localizing diagnosis (positive in both infection and tumor)
      ii. **Gallium/indium-labeled white cell scans** are more specific for infection and are helpful in differentiating other processes, such as tumors, from infection.
   b. **Vertebral osteomyelitis:**
      i. Early on, findings on **plain films** same as in disk space infection; later followed by erosion through the vertebral end plate and destructive and sclerotic changes involving the vertebral bodies
      ii. **Technetium 99m bone scan and gallium/indium-labeled white cell scan** as in disk space infection
      iii. **CT scan** can detect early involvement of vertebral body

J. **Referred pain**
   1. When history suggests possible referred pain, the routine screening exam may need to be tailored to look for specific entities, as discussed below.
   2. **Pelvic disorders** may involve the sacral plexus or its branches, producing low back pain, sciatica, or both. Exam may find positive straight leg raise, but attention to pelvic and rectal areas can reveal underlying pelvic disease (i.e., uterine fibroids, ovarian tumors, pelvic inflammatory disease)
   3. **Prostatitis** may present with low back pain. Rectal exam reveals enlarged, tender, boggy prostate.
   4. **Renal disorders**, such as nephrolithiasis, pyelonephritis, or perinephric abscess, may present with back pain. Abdominal exam, urinalysis, and appropriate radiologic studies reveal these renal disorders.

Recommended Reading

1. Akbarnia BA, Keppler L: Spinal deformities. In Principles of Orthopaedic Practice, vol 2. New York, McGraw-Hill, 1989, pp 889–991.
2. Aprin H, Dee R: Infections of the spine. In Dee R (ed): Principles of Orthopaedic Practice, vol 2. New York, McGraw-Hill, 1989, pp 941–955.
3. Benson DR: The back: Thoracic and lumbar spine. In D'Ambrosia RD (ed): Musculoskeletal Disorders, 2nd ed. Philadelphia, JB Lippincott, 1986, pp 287–365.
4. Bernard TN, et al: Recognizing specific characteristics of nonspecific low back pain. Clin Orthop Rel Res 217:266–280, 1987.
5. Ciullo JV, et al: Pars interarticularis stress reaction, spondylolysis and spondylolisthesis in gymnasts. Clin Sports Med 4(1):95–110, 1985.
6. Degowin EL, DeGowin RL: Bedside Diagnostic Examination, 4th ed. New York, Macmillan, 1981, p 728.
7. Destouet JM, Murphy WA: Lumbar facet block indications and technique. Orthop Rev 14(5):57–65, 1985.
8. Dyment PG, et al: Recommendations for participation in competitive sports. Pediatrics 81(5):737–739, 1988.
9. Epstein JA, Epstein NE: Lumbar spondylosis and spinal stenosis. In Wilkins RH, Rengachary SS (eds): Neurosurgery, vol 3. New York, McGraw-Hill, 1985, pp 2272–2278.

10. Frymoyer JW: Back pain and sciatica. N Engl J Med 318:291–300, 1988.
11. Fu FH, et al: Sports Injuries. Baltimore, Williams & Wilkins, 1994.
12. Gaines RW, Humphreys WG: Spondylolisthesis. In Chapman MW, Madison M (eds): Operative Orthopaedics, vol 3. Philadelphia, JB Lippincott, 1988, pp 2005–2014.
13. Gould JA, Davies GJ: Orthopaedic and Sports Physical Therapy. St. Louis, CV Mosby, 1985, pp 404–406.
14. Green TL, et al: Back pain and vertebral changes simulating Scheuerman's disease. Pediatr Orthop 5:1–7, 1985.
15. Hoppenfeld S: Orthopaedic Neurology. Philadelphia, JB Lippincott, 1977, pp 51–74.
16. Hoppenfeld S: Physical Examination of the Spine and Extremities. East Norwalk, CT, Appleton-Century-Crofts, 1976, pp 237–263.
17. Huurman WW: Spine in sports. In Mellion MB (ed): Office Management of Sports Injuries and Athletic Problems. Philadelphia, Hanley & Belfus, 1988, pp 199–212.
18. Jackson DW, Ciullo JV: Injuries of the spine in the skeletally immature athlete. In Nicholas JA, Hershman EB (eds): The Lower Extremity and Spine in Sports Medicine. St. Louis, CV Mosby, 1986, pp 1350–1352.
19. Johnson RJ: Low back pain in sports. Phys Sportsmed 21(4):53–59, 1993.
20. Lipson SJ: Low back pain. In Kelley WN, et al: Textbook of Rheumatology, 2nd ed. Philadelphia, WB Saunders, 1985, pp 448–465.
21. Micheli LJ, Marotta JJ: Scoliosis and sports. Your Patient and Fitness 2(2):5–11, 1989.
22. Micheli LJ, et al: Use of modified Boston brace for back injuries in athletes. Am J Sports Med 8:351–356, 1980.
23. Micheli LS: Back injuries in gymnastics. Clin Sports Med 4(1):85–93, 1985.
24. Morris JM: Spinal stenosis. In Chapman MW (ed): Operative Orthopaedics, vol 3. Philadelphia, JB Lippincott, 1988, pp 2065–2075.
25. Nachemson A: Towards a better understanding of low back pain: A review of the mechanics of the lumbar disc. Rheumatol Rehabil 14:129–142, 1975.
26. Nakano KK: Sciatic nerve entrapment: The piriformis syndrome. J Musculoskel Med 33–37, 1987.
27. O'Neill DB, Micheli LJ: Recognizing and preventing overuse injuries in young athletes. J Musculoskel Med 106–125, 1989.
28. Pace JB, Nagle D: Piriformis syndrome. West J Med 124:435–439, 1976.
29. Saal JA, et al: Initial stage management of lumbar spine problems. Phys Med Rehabil Clin 2(1):187–203, 1991.
30. Saal JA, et al: Later stage management of lumbar spine problems. Phys Med Rehab Clin 2(1):205–221, 1991.
31. Saal JA: Intervertebral disc herniations: Advances in non-operative treatment. Phys Med Rehab Clin 4(2):175–190, 1990.
32. Schuchmann JA, Cannon CL: Sacroiliac strain syndrome: Diagnosis and treatment. Texas Med 82(June): 33–36, 1986.
33. Weinstein JN, et al: The Lumbar Spine. Philadelphia, WB Saunders, 1990.
34. Wiltse LL, Widell EH, Jackson DW: Fatigue fracture: The basic lesion in isthmic spondylolisthesis. J Bone Joint Surg 57A:17–22, 1975.
35. Winter RB: Spinal problems in pediatric orthopaedics. In Lovell WW, Winter RB (eds): Pediatric Orthopaedics, 2nd ed. Philadelphia, JB Lippincott, 1986, pp 619–631.

48

Pelvis, Hip, and Thigh Injuries

Paul W. Esposito, M.D.

This chapter deals with an anatomic region where injuries result from torsional, tensile, and direct traumatic forces. Overuse syndromes are also quite common in this region. These injuries may become chronic, prevent participation, and, on some occasions, even threaten the life or the long-term function of the athlete. The keys to treatment of problems in this area are primarily prevention, recognition, protection, and appropriate, graded rehabilitation.

I. Physical Exam—Special Considerations

A. **General alignment of spine and pelvis to lower extremities**
   1. Leg length can be best judged by palpating and visualizing the iliac crests from behind with the patient standing with legs straight and knees fully extended.
   2. Check for malrotation of pelvis and spine.
   3. Note skin lesions, dimples, and nevi, especially over the midline of the lower spine and sacrum.

B. **Motor exam and flexibility.** Hamstring tightness:
   1. May indicate spinal pathology (Figs. 1–2)
   2. Lack of flexibility may lead to hamstring tears and patellar problems.
   3. Frequently associated with anterior knee pain

C. **Bursae**—examine iliopsoas, greater trochanter, and ischium.

D. **Sensory exam**
   1. Obturator nerve innervates hips as well as medial thigh and knee.
   2. Medial thigh and knee pain frequently indicates hip problems.

E. **Specific tests for tightness**
   1. **Hip flexion test:** Obligatory external rotation of the hip while flexing the hip, especially in the adolescent or immature athlete, can indicate either slipped capital femoral epiphysis or a significant joint incongruity (Fig. 3).
   2. **Thomas' test for iliopsoas contracture:** Contracture does not allow full extension and may be cause of iliopsoas bursitis and "snapping hip" syndrome (Fig. 4).
   3. **Iliotibial band contracture:** Frequent cause of lateral knee pain iliotibial band friction syndrome (see Chapter 38, Fig. 8).
   4. **Joint motion symmetry:** Asymmetric loss of motion may indicate hip disorder.
   5. **Log roll test** (Fig. 5)
      a. Exquisite pain with gentle to-and-fro motion suggests infection, fracture, or synovitis.
      b. Pain only with extreme internal rotation suggests low-grade synovitis.
   6. **Leg externally rotates when hip is flexed** in patient with slipped capital femoral epiphysis (Fig. 6).
   7. **Flexion, abduction, external rotation test:** Also called Patrick's test. Pain in sacroiliac joint when this joint is involved (Fig. 7).

F. **Radiographs**—taken except with obvious contusions and muscle pulls

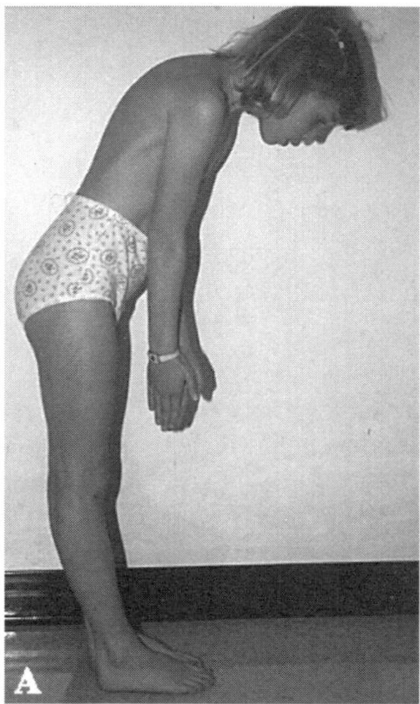

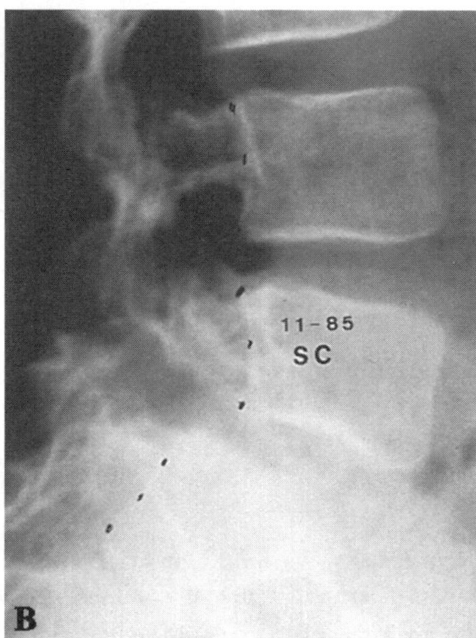

FIGURE 1. Child with acute spondylolisthesis. **A**, Note loss of lumbar lordosis and tight hamstrings. **B**, Radiograph demonstration.

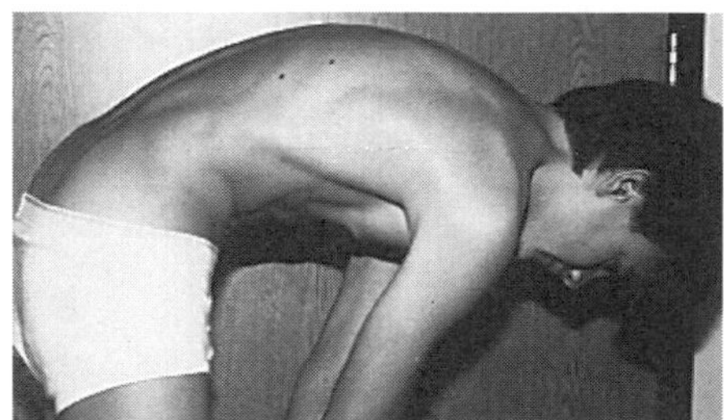

FIGURE 2. More severe listhesis. Note step-off where upper lumbar segments have slipped forward on lower lumbar segments as well as tight hamstrings. There is total loss of lumbar lordosis.

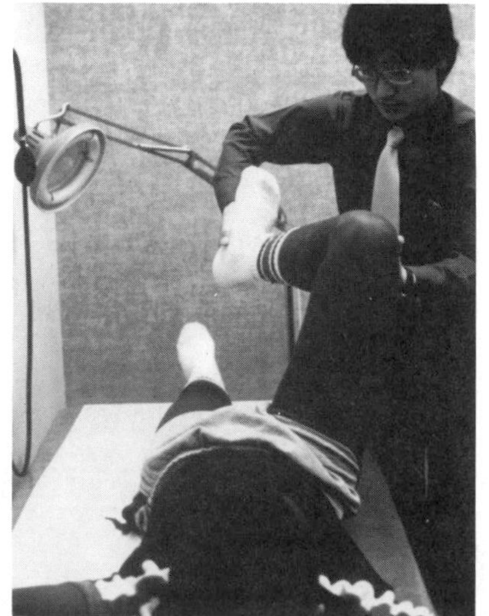

FIGURE 3. Hip flexion test. With slipped capital femoral epiphysis, spontaneous external rotation occurs with hip flexion.

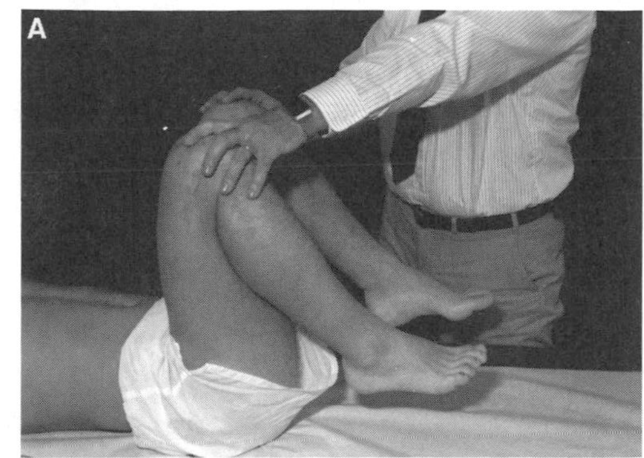

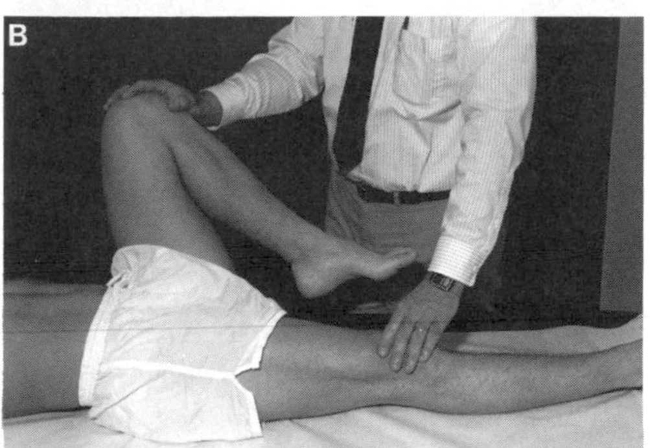

FIGURE 4. Thomas' test. **A**, Flexion of both hips to flatten lumbar lordosis. **B**, Extension of one hip to measure hip flexion contracture and tightness in the iliopsoas.

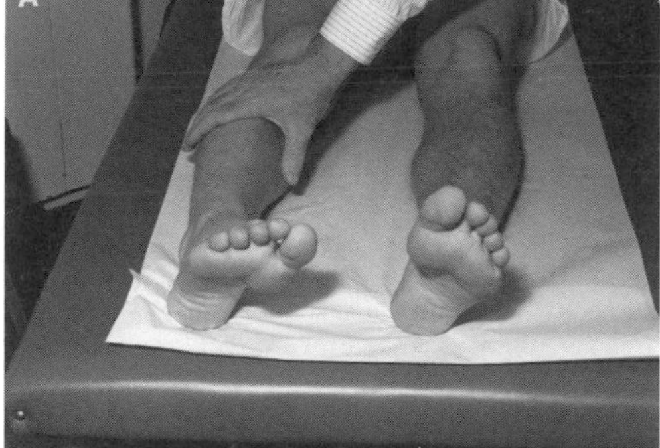

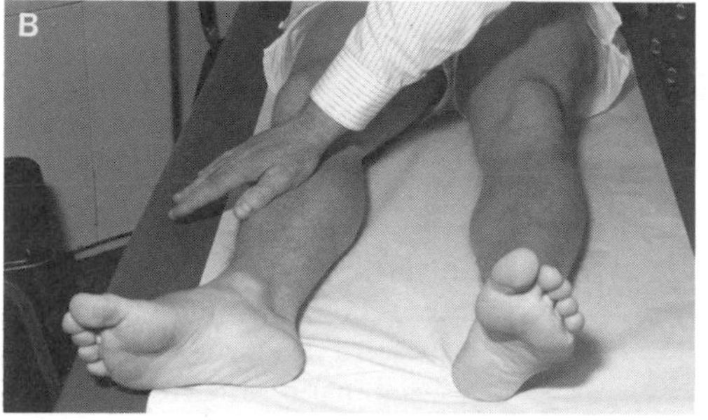

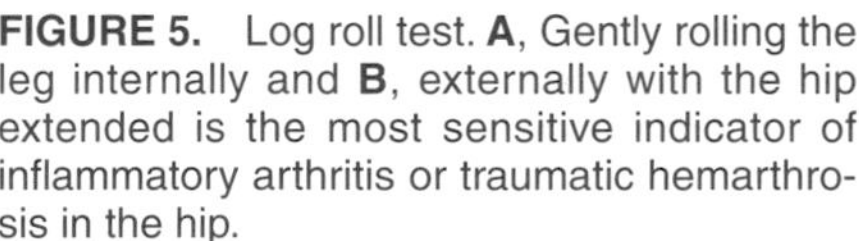

FIGURE 5. Log roll test. **A**, Gently rolling the leg internally and **B**, externally with the hip extended is the most sensitive indicator of inflammatory arthritis or traumatic hemarthrosis in the hip.

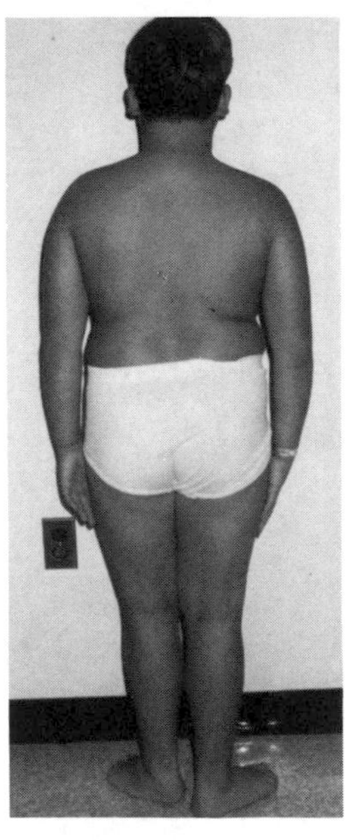

FIGURE 6. External rotation posture and shortening with slipped capital femoral epiphysis. Note patient is standing on his left toes with his heels off the ground to equalize his leg lengths. Also note asymmetric truncal skin folds.

FIGURE 7. Patrick's test (also known as FABER for **F**lexion, **Ab**duction, **E**xternal **R**otation test). Used for sacroiliac joint evaluation and for subtle pelvic trauma.

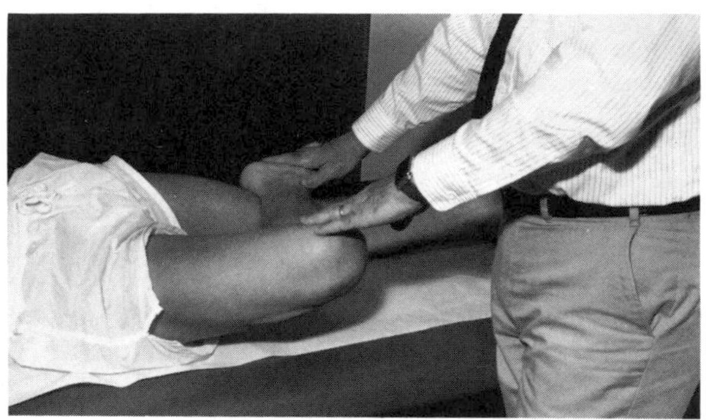

1. Detect fractures, stress fractures, avulsion fractures, and bony problems
2. Reveal pelvic, spine, and lower extremity malalignment
3. Risk of long-term disability and loss of competition if appropriate, timely x-ray studies are not obtained

G. **Bone scan**
1. Positive in stress fractures long before the fracture is revealed on plain x-ray studies—more sensitive than radiographs in stress reaction
2. Extremely helpful in seronegative arthrography (sacroiliac arthritis)
3. Helpful in occult lesions, such as osteoid osteoma

II. Specific Injuries and Problems

A. **Sacroiliac joint**
1. **Seronegative arthropathy**: ankylosing spondylitis and Reiter's syndrome (Fig. 8)
   a. Often confused with sports injuries and overuse
   b. Diagnosed by x-ray, bone scan, and decreased chest wall expansion—generally HLA-B27 positive
   c. May be accompanied by heel pain, urethritis, or other joint and spine involvement
2. **Sacroiliac joint sprain or contracture**
   a. Pelvic rotation
   b. Asymmetric stride or stroke
   c. Leg length inequality
3. **Sacroiliac fracture or dislocation:** usually only with major, high-energy pelvic trauma. May require aggressive treatment.

B. **Avulsion injuries**
1. **Mechanism**
   a. Injuries follow acute muscular contraction against a fixed resistance.
   b. Injuries are a result of inadequate stretching or conditioning.
   c. The combination of overuse and inadequate stretching can lead to chronic apophysitis, which may predispose to avulsion injuries.

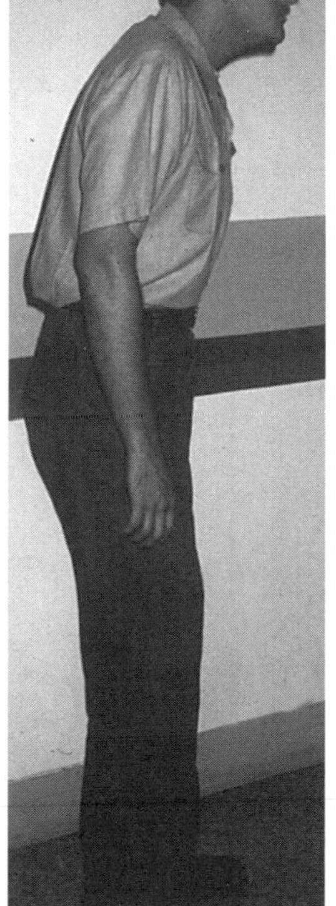

FIGURE 8. Clinical photograph of a young man with sacroiliitis (Reiter's syndrome). Note stiff, forward flexion posture.

   d. Injuries are frequent in sprinters, hurdlers, or others who rely on sudden, forceful acceleration—especially during maximum growth period of puberty, when the physeal plate is thick.
2. **Diagnosis:** palpation of bony prominence and x-ray
   a. **Anterior-superior iliac spine:**
      i. Sartorius avulsion
      ii. Swelling, tenderness, immediate pain over anterior superior pelvis
      iii. Exacerbated with flexion of hip against resistance
      iv. May palpate a gap with avulsion; tenderness only with apophysitis
   b. **Anterior-inferior iliac spine** (Fig. 9A):
      i. Rectus femoris
      ii. Pain, swelling in groin directly over hip capsule just distal to midpoint inguinal ligament
      iii. Follows forceful quadriceps contraction
      iv. Pain increased with flexion of hip against resistance
   c. **Ischium**—hamstring origin avulsion (Fig. 9B)
      i. Especially common in adolescent apophyseal avulsion
      ii. Frequently confused with hamstring tears with pain referred distal to the apophysis
      iii. May rarely require open reduction, fixation, or excision to avoid large, reactive fracture callus—may lead to pain when sitting (sciatic nerve compressed)
   d. **Piriformis**—local tenderness over greater trochanter
   e. **Iliopsoas:**
      i. Tender, medial groin over lesser trochanter
      ii. Pain with flexion, extension, and rotation of hip against resistance

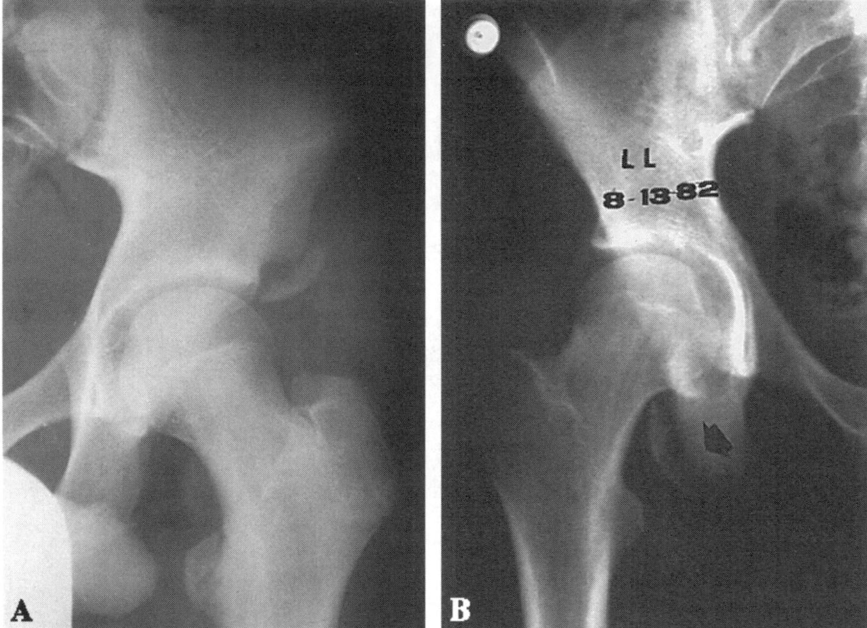

FIGURE 9. Avulsion injuries. **A**, Anterior, inferior iliac spine avulsion by rectus femoris. **B**, Ischial spine avulsion by hamstrings.

3. **Treatment**
   a. **Emphasize prevention** (adequate stretching, conditioning)
   b. **Sartorius (anterior superior iliac spine) rectus iliopsoas (lesser trochanter):**
      i. Ice until pain free, rest, crutches with touch-down weight bearing for up to 4–6 weeks. Too quick a return to vigorous activity may result in formation of bony prominences at the site of the avulsion.
      ii. Surgical reduction or excision if a widely displaced, large cartilaginous or bony fragment
      iii. May rarely require late surgical excision if large bony fragment is symptomatic
      iv. Repeat x-ray studies to assess healing
   c. **Ischium and hamstring avulsion:**
      i. If significantly displaced, rarely surgical repair
      ii. Undisplaced—use ice, crutches for 4–6 weeks

C. **Muscle tears, strains, and contusions**
1. **Mechanism:** similar to avulsion injuries
   a. Inadequate stretching, warm-up, and conditioning
   b. Indirect trauma as opposed to a contusion
2. **Diagnosis:** common in quadriceps, hamstrings, and adductors; forceful, maximal contraction during forced lengthening
   a. Localized tenderness, swelling, and ecchymosis in partial tear
   b. Palpable gap in muscle in complete tear
   c. Pain with gentle passive stretch
   d. More common in rectus than in other quadriceps muscles
3. **Treatment**
   a. Acute—compression from toe to groin with elastic bandage, ice, elevation, crutches, possibly nonsteroidal anti-inflammatory drugs

b. Compression around thigh only may lead to venous thrombosis and/or distal edema
c. Ice, rest, and elevation 48–72 hours for major strains
d. Crutches, touch-down weight bearing. Symptom-guided return to ambulation; may take several days to several weeks

4. **Treatment principles**
   a. Gentle, progressive stretching
   b. Gradual strengthening and reconditioning
   c. Burst-type activities done last
5. **Complications**
   a. If tear occurs near musculotendinous junction (especially quadriceps tendon), surgical repair may be indicated
   b. Retear may occur if inadequate rehabilitation, stretching, or premature return to competition

D. **Contusions**

1. **Mechanism**
   a. Direct blow
   b. Bleeding or swelling into muscle, periosteum, or nerve
2. **Diagnosis**
   a. Immediate pain with normal motion, but weak
   b. **Specific patterns:**
      i. Anterior thigh contusion—most commonly rectus or severity may not be immediately obvious
      ii. **Hip pointer**—direct blow to anterior-superior iliac spine
      iii. **Sciatic nerve involvement:**
         (a) Rarely may be involved with direct blow to buttocks
         (b) Look for appropriate sensory and motor findings.
3. **Treatment**
   a. Toe to groin compression with elastic dressing
   b. Ice, elevation; immobilize knee and hip flexion if rectus involved
   c. Maintain muscle length with **gentle** stretching when pain resolved.
   d. Avoid premature return to competition and reinjury.
   e. Failure to treat appropriately may lead to myositis ossificans only when full strength and motion return.

E. **Myositis ossificans** (Fig. 10)

1. **Mechanism**
   a. Most commonly direct blow or tear to muscle
   b. Metaplasia of muscle to bone
   c. More frequent with repetitive trauma
   d. Common in quadriceps
   e. May be related to severity of trauma
2. **Diagnosis**
   a. Firm mass in muscle after acute hematoma phase
   b. Progressive contracture of muscle
   c. May see decreased passive knee flexion with quadriceps involvement
   d. X-ray findings—early fluctuant calcification in soft tissues later becoming mature, woven bone
3. **Treatment**
   a. **Avoid reinjury.** If significant swelling, muscle tenderness, pain with passive stretch after contusion, avoid competition until pain-free, nontender with normal motion and strength
   b. **Physical therapy**—gentle stretching to maintain muscle length and avoid joint contracture (especially knee)

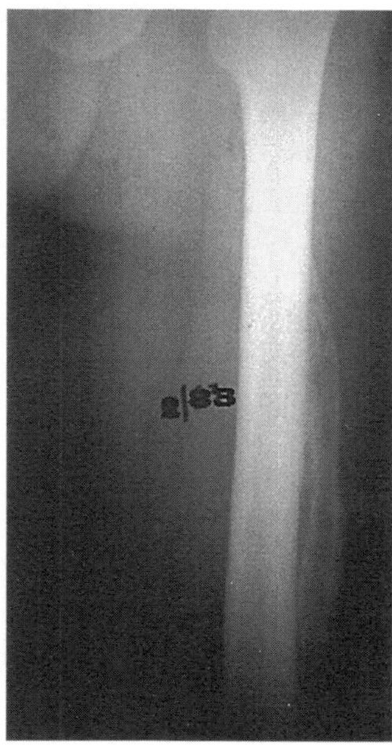

FIGURE 10. Myositis ossificans after football helmet blunt trauma several months previously. Note mature-looking bone in muscular region, superficial to periosteum.

- c. **Crutch ambulation**
- d. **Late treatment:**
  - i. Not always compatible with return to participation
  - ii. Surgical release considered only after myositis is mature (determined by x-ray, clinical exam, and bone scan)
  - iii. Pad involved area

F. **Compartment syndrome**

1. **Mechanism:** may occur after blunt trauma as well as with crush injuries and fractures
2. **Findings:** progressive, severe pain key findings
   - a. Pain with passive motion and tense muscles
   - b. Decreased femoral sensation and motor weakness **late** findings
   - c. Pulse and capillary filling frequently normal
3. **Treatment:** measure compartment pressure if elevated in this setting; emergent surgical debridement indicated with delayed skin closure if pressures elevated

G. **Stress fractures**

1. **Mechanism**
   - a. Excessive and precipitous increase in activity
   - b. Osteoblasts unable to lay down new bone fast enough to remodel completely
2. **Common sites**
   - a. Femoral neck, pubis, femoral shaft—common in distance runners
   - b. Supracondylar femur region
3. **Diagnosis**
   - a. Condition worse before and after activity
   - b. Localized bone tenderness present
   - c. Persistent, increasing pain; may be referred to knee
   - d. X-rays normal for many weeks; bone scan extremely sensitive even in early stage (benchmark of diagnostic tests)
   - e. Late x-rays show periosteal new bone and potentially a faint fracture line

4. **Treatment**
   a. **No alternative to rest when dealing with a femoral fracture**. When diagnosis is made, no participation in running competition until complete healing, then a gradual resumption of activity. Crutch walking until pain free because of the potential significant morbidity if femoral fracture displaces.
   b. **Femoral neck** usually requires prophylactic pin fixation or, at a minimum, prolonged touch-down weight bearing with crutches for many months. Completion of this fracture due to persistent physical activity or inadequate treatment may lead to avascular necrosis of the femoral head with catastrophic results. Stress fractures on the tension (superior) side of the femoral neck at extreme risk for progression to a complete fracture.
   c. **Ischium and pubis**—crutch walking, symptom guided, followed by 2–3 months rest
   d. **Supracondylar femur**—crutches and/or casting to prevent completion of fracture. There is no place for limited treatment and continued activity in stress fractures in this region.
   e. Casting may be indicated in the immature athlete with a distal femoral physeal fracture.

H. **Osteitis pubis (Gracilis syndrome)**
1. **Mechanism**
   a. Mechanical fatigue process of symphysis pubis
   b. Repetitive overpull of adductor longus
2. **Diagnosis**
   a. Tenderness in the symphysis pubis with lysis on both sides of the synchondrosis on plain x-ray, or irregularity on lower aspect of the pubis
   b. Bone scan may be positive—often an incidental finding
3. **Treatment**
   a. Only when symptomatic
   b. Usually responds to rest and anti-inflammatory medications

I. **Bursitis**
1. **Mechanism**
   a. Caused by friction where a tendon passes over bony prominence
   b. Potential space that becomes inflamed and fills with fluid in response to this friction
   c. Usually caused by excessive activity and insufficient stretching of the involved muscle
2. **Diagnosis**
   a. **Greater trochanter:**
      i. Tenderness just posterior to the greater trochanter
      ii. Aggravated by contraction of the tensor fascia lata with the hip abducted against resistance and with patient on his/her side (Fig. 11)
   b. **Iliopsoas:**
      i. Tenderness over lesser trochanter
      ii. Medial groin pain, sometimes with flexion, abduction, external rotation against resistance
   c. **Ischial:**
      i. Tenderness over the ischium
      ii. Aggravated by sitting and contraction of hamstring
   d. **CAUTION: Bursitis is a diagnosis of exclusion**.
      i. Bone scan indicated unless diagnosis is clear-cut
      ii. Femoral neck and ischial stress fractures may mimic bursitis symptoms exactly.

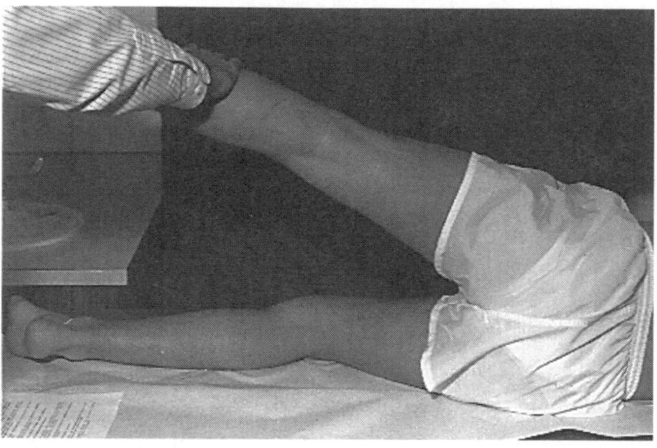

FIGURE 11. Abduction against resistance. Pain seen in trochanteric bursitis and iliotibial band syndrome.

iii. X-ray studies almost universally required to exclude underlying bony pathology, such as tumor, as cause of symptoms

3. **Treatment**
   a. Identifying and developing a stretching and strengthening program for the contracted muscle
   b. Anti-inflammatory medications
   c. Corticosteroid therapy in resistant bursitis:
      i. By injection, iontophoresis, or phonopheresis
      ii. Ice and deep friction massage may be of some benefit.

J. **Snapping hip syndrome**
1. **Mechanism:** Occasionally a communication between the hip joint and the iliopsoas bursa. Usually secondary to tightness in the iliopsoas muscle.
2. **Diagnosis:** Patient complains of snapping in medial groin with flexion of hip.
3. **Treatment**
   a. Frequently requires only reassurance
   b. Sometimes responds to stretching of the hip flexion contracture
   c. May respond to anti-inflammatory agents if persistent and painful
   d. In recalcitrant, severe cases, tendon lengthening may be indicated.

K. **Hernias**
1. **Mechanism**
   a. Musculofascial hernia follows a tear in overlying fascia with herniation of underlying muscle through hole
   b. May strangulate if fascial opening is small or constricting
2. Common sites
   a. Inguinal
   b. Femoral
   c. Tensor
3. **Treatment:** See Chapter 46, "Athletic Injuries of the Thorax and Abdomen."

L. **The immature athlete**
1. Immature athletes are prone to injuries peculiar to their anatomy, especially those related to their physis. There are also diseases and disorders peculiar to specific age groups that may mimic athletic injuries.
2. **Hip**
   a. Obturator nerve innervates both hip and medial thigh

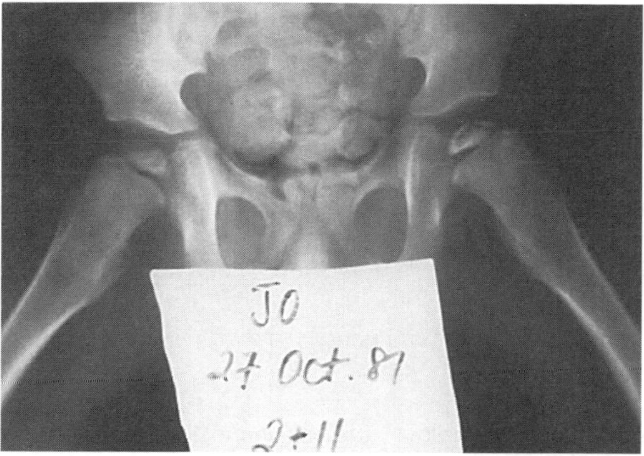

FIGURE 12. Legg-Calvé-Perthes disease. Anteroposterior pelvis x-rays demonstrating subchondral collapse on left (crescent sign) and sclerosis on right.

   b. Children with knee and medial thigh pain should be closely evaluated for hip disorders.
3. **Legg-Calvé-Perthes disease** (Fig. 12)
   a. Presents with irritable hips and medial thigh pain
   b. Most common in children aged 3 to 8
   c. Early x-ray studies normal
   d. Bone scan or magnetic resonance imaging positive
   e. Suspicion with positive log roll, limp, or limited motion in the hip
4. **Toxic synovitis**
   a. Transient inflammatory process of the hip
   b. X-rays universally normal, except for capsular distention
   c. Diagnosed by irritable hip (positive log roll, see Fig. 5). Must be differentiated from septic arthritis.
   d. **Treatment:**
      i. Rest is key.
      ii. Traction for prompt resolution and avoidance of prolonged course
5. **Slipped capital femoral epiphysis**
   a. Usually age 12 to 15
   b. Presents with medial thigh, knee, or groin pain
   c. Limp and limited internal rotation/increased external rotation
   d. Flexion rotation test positive (leg externally rotates with flexion)
   e. Anteroposterior and frog lateral pelvic x-rays mandatory in all hip disease
6. **Severe pelvic, hip, and thigh pain requires immediate radiographic evaluation**. Additionally, any child with leg, medial thigh, or knee pain that does not resolve in 1 week requires, at a minimum, radiographic evaluation and preferably orthopedic consultation to avoid missing diagnoses that may cause lifelong problems and disability. Persistent, unexplained complaints may necessitate extraordinary diagnostic measures before the child can safely return to athletic activity. If a slipped epiphysis is detected, **immediate** hospitalization, bed rest, and surgical fixation are indicated. Radiographs are mandatory in these children also to exclude tumors, bone cysts (which may present with pathologic fractures after activities), and underlying osteochondromas, which may well cause mechanical symptoms similar to bursitis.

M. **Fractures and dislocations**
   1. **Mechanism**
      a. Rarely occur in contact sports
      b. More common in high-energy motor vehicle, skiing, or equestrian sports
      c. Typically severe, direct blows
   2. **Diagnosis**
      a. Localized tenderness with direct pressure or pelvic compression
      b. Radiographs mandatory
      c. Minimal linear fractures may lead to exsanguination; must be treated aggressively in the hospital
      d. Frequent associated visceral injuries and urinary tract injuries
   3. **Dislocations**
      a. **Anterior:**
         i. Occur with direct blow with hips abducted
         ii. Prominence in anterior pelvis with hip lying in abduction
         iii. Frequent associated femoral nerve injury
         iv. Rare arterial injury
         v. Risk of avascular necrosis (increases with length of time before reduction)
      b. **Posterior:**
         i. Usually follows direct blow to knee with hip and knee flexed
         ii. Hip adducted with palpable femoral head in buttocks
         iii. Often posterior acetabular hip fracture associated
         iv. Mandatory in any hip dislocation to obtain x-rays of entire femur as well as pelvis to exclude associated high-energy injuries

III. Summary

The best treatment for pelvic and thigh injuries is prevention. An emphasis on adequate conditioning and adequate stretching before participation prevents many of the injuries to this region. Gentle, protected rehabilitation is vital after adequate assessment of bony and muscular involvement is completed. Premature return to participation can frequently cause reoccurrence and long-term complications.

Recommended Reading

1. Akermark C, Johansson C: Tenotomy of the adductor longus tendon in the treatment of chronic groin pain in athletes. Am J Sports Med 20(6):640–643, 1992.
2. Combs JA: Hip and pelvis avulsion fractures in adolescents. Phys Sportsmed 22(7):41–49, 1994.
3. Crawford AH: Slipped capital femoral epiphysis. J Bone Joint Surg 70A(9):1422–1427, 1988.
4. Estwanik JJ, McAlister JA: Contusions and the formation of myositis ossificans. Phys Sportsmed 18(4):53–64, 1990.
5. Godshall RW, Hansen CA: Incomplete avulsion of a portion of the iliac epiphysis. J Bone Joint Surg 55A(6):1301–1302, 1973.
6. Goldberg B, Pecora C: Stress fractures. Phys Sportsmed 22(3):68–78, 1994.
7. Jackson DL: Stress fracture of the femur. Phys Sportsmed 19(7):39–107, 1991.
8. Jackson DW, Feagin JA: Quadriceps contusions in young athletes. J Bone Joint Surg 55A(1):95–105, 1973.
9. Kaeding CC, Sanko WA, Fischer RA: Myositis ossificans. Phys Sportsmed 23(2):77–82, 1995.
10. Kaeding CC, Sanko WA, Fischer RA: Quadriceps strains and contusions. Phys Sportsmed 23(1):59–64, 1995.
11. Klasson SC, Vander Schilden JL: Acute anterior thigh compartment syndrome complicating quadriceps hematoma. Orthop Rev 19(5):421–427, 1990.
12. Leinberry CF, McShane RB, Stewart WG, et al: A displaced subtrochanteric stress fracture in a young amenorrheic athlete. Am J Sports Med 20(4):485–487, 1992.
13. McKeag DB, Dolan C: Overuse syndromes of the lower extremity. Phys Sportsmed 17(7):108–123, 1989.
14. Micheli LJ: Overuse injuries in children's sports: The growth factor. Orthop Clin North Am 14(2):337–360, 1983.
15. Miller A, Stedman GH, Beisaw NE, et al: Sciatica caused by an avulsion fracture of the ischial tuberosity. J Bone Joint Surg 69A(1):143–145, 1987.

16. Provost RA, Morris JM: Fatigue fracture of the femoral shaft. J Bone Joint Surg 51A(3):487–498, 1969.
17. Swissa A, Milgrom C, Giladi M, et al: The effect of pretraining sports activity on the incidence of stress fractures among military recruits. Clin Orthop Rel Res 245:256–260, 1969.
18. Waters PM, Millis MB: Hip and pelvic injuries in the young athlete. In Stanitski CL, DeLee JC, Drez D(eds): Pediatric and Adolescent Sports Medicine, 3rd ed. Philadelphia, WB Saunders, 1994, pp 279–293.
19. Wiley JJ: Traumatic osteitis pubis: The gracilis syndrome. Am J Sports Med 11(5):360–363, 1983.
20. Winternitz WA, Metheny JA, Wear LC: Acute compartment syndrome of the thigh in sports-related injuries not associated with femoral fractures. Am J Sports Med 20(4):476–478, 1992.
21. Wolfgang GL: Stress fracture of the femoral neck in a patient with open capital femoral epiphyses. J Bone Joint Surg 59A(5):680–681, 1977.

49

Knee Injuries

W. Michael Walsh, M.D.

I. Physical Examination

A. **Observation and measurement**

1. **Standing**
   a. **Alignment** of lower extremities—view patient from front, side, and back. Look for:
      i. **Angular and rotational deformities**—excessive valgus, varus, recurvatum, flexion contracture, femoral or tibial torsion
      ii. **Foot alignment and mechanics**—excessive cavus or pes planus. Heels should invert and arches increase on toe rising.
      iii. **Leg length inequality**—best judged by pelvic levelness on standing
   b. **Other observations**
      i. **Difference in size of legs**—atrophy of one limb vs. hypertrophy of the opposite limb
      ii. **Popliteal masses**—may be seen better in prone position
2. **Sitting**
   a. **Patellar position**—with knees flexed 90°, look from side to judge high or low position. Anterior patellar surface will normally face wall in front of patient sitting with legs over side of exam table. View from front to judge lateral posture. Patella should appear centered in soft tissue outline of knee.
   b. **Osgood-Schlatter's changes**—enlarged and/or tender tibial tuberosity
   c. **Vastus medialis obliquus/vastus lateralis (VMO/VL) relationship**—knees held actively at 45° of flexion. Distal one-third of vastus medialis normally should present as substantial muscle from adductor tubercle inserting into upper one-third to one-half of medial patella. Dysplastic VMO appears hollow in this normal muscular location (Fig. 1). Also observe for apparent hypertrophy of VL.
   d. **Patellar tracking**—observe on active flexion and extension. Watch for excessive displacement of patella.
3. **Lying**
   a. **Supine**
      i. **Range of motion**—both active and passive; compare injured with uninjured side
      ii. **Muscle bulk**—thigh and calf; can measure circumferences, but simple observation may be just as helpful
      iii. **Quadriceps (Q) angle**—with quadriceps **contracted**, angle between the line from anterior superior iliac spine to midpoint of patella, and the line from midpoint of patella to tibial tuberosity (Fig. 2). Normal in males is 10° or less; in females, 15° or less.
      iv. Hamstring and heelcord tightness—see Chapter 37, "Musculoskeletal Injuries in Sports."

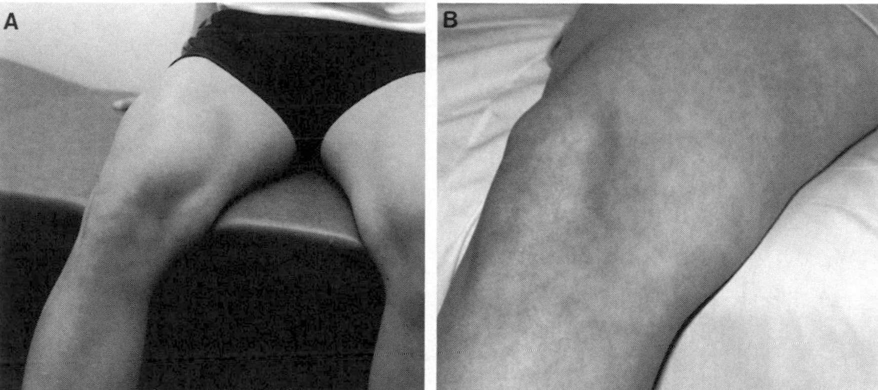

FIGURE 1. Vastus medialis obliquus (VMO) muscle. **A**, With patient holding knee at 45° of flexion, normal VMO bulk is seen. **B**, Patient with marked VMO dysplasia. This is probably most important predisposition to all extensor mechanism syndromes.

b. **Prone**
   i. **Range of motion**—lack of full knee flexion may show quadriceps tightness.
   ii. **Popliteal masses**—compare contours with those of opposite knee.

4. **Walking/running**
   a. **Mechanics of gait**—stance and swing phase from side to side is even. Look for limp, other asymmetry, excessive limb rotation, limb malalignment.
   b. **Patellofemoral tracking**—observe patella closely from front view.

B. **Palpation**
   1. **Joint effusion**—with knee extended, milk fluid from suprapatellar pouch and palpate along medial and lateral sides of patella. Try to distinguish intra-articular effusion that can be moved about from extra-articular swelling that feels more like thick, soft tissues and is not movable.
   2. Significant areas of **tenderness** (Fig. 3) include:
      a. **Menisci**—medial and lateral joint lines

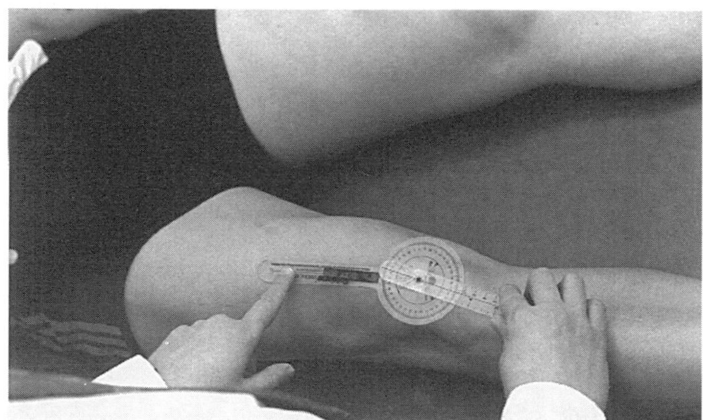

FIGURE 2. Quadriceps (Q) angle measurement. With quadriceps contracted, proximal arm of goniometer is directed toward anterior superior iliac spine, pivot point of goniometer is placed over center of patella, and distal arm of goniometer is placed on tibial tuberosity. Normal in males up to 10°, females 15°.

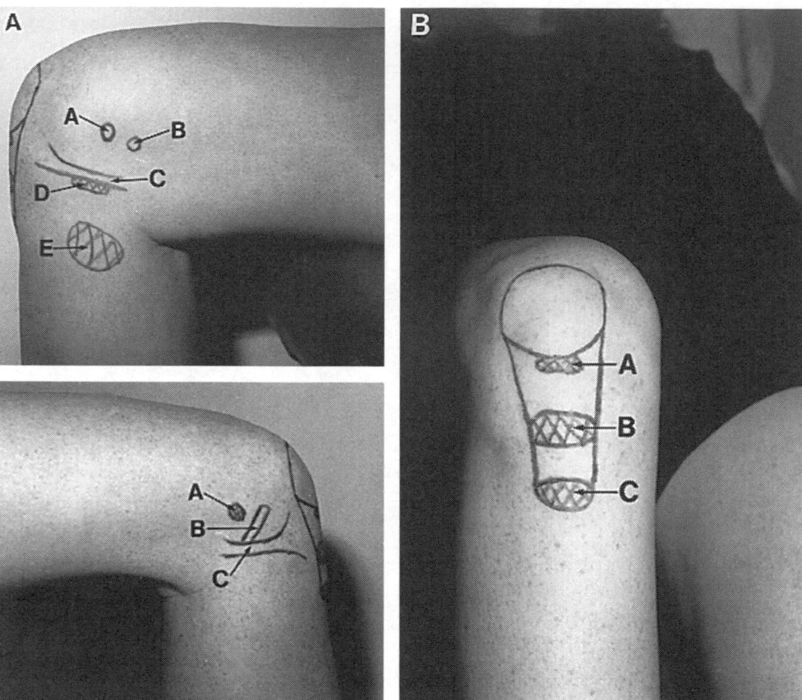

FIGURE 3. Topographical anatomy of knee. **A**, Medial aspect, with medial epicondyle (A), adductor tubercle (B), medial joint line (C), tibial collateral ligament bursa (D), and pes anserinus bursa (E). **B**, Anterior aspect, with areas of tenderness in patellar tendonitis (A), deep infrapatellar bursitis (B), and Osgood-Schlatter's disease (C). **C**, Lateral aspect, with iliotibial band friction area (A), popliteus tendon (B), and lateral joint line (C).

b. **Ligament attachments**—medial femoral epicondyle, adductor tubercle, lateral femoral epicondyle, proximal medial tibia

c. **Tendons**—patellar tendon, quadriceps tendon, popliteus tendon, hamstrings

d. **Bursae**—prepatellar, pes anserinus, tibial collateral ligament, deep infrapatellar

e. **Other**—patellar facets, extensor retinaculum

3. **Crepitation**

a. **During range of motion**—from any rough joint surface (especially patellofemoral joint), fractures, or soft tissue thickness

b. **Patellofemoral compression**—longitudinal and/or transverse compression of patella against femur (Fig. 4). Feel for crepitation or ask about elicited pain.

4. **Muscle tone**—overall turgor of muscle tissue. May be decreased early after injury, even if bulk still measures normal.

C. **Specific tests—perform all tests on uninjured knee first to establish "normal" for that patient**.

1. **Ligaments**

a. **Medial**

i. **Abduction stress test at 30° and 0°:** Patient is supine and relaxed, thigh supported on table. Examiner applies valgus force at foot, while using other hand as fulcrum along lateral side of joint. Watch and feel for medial joint line opening. Perform first with knee flexed 30°, then with maximum possible extension or hyperextension. See Fig. 5.

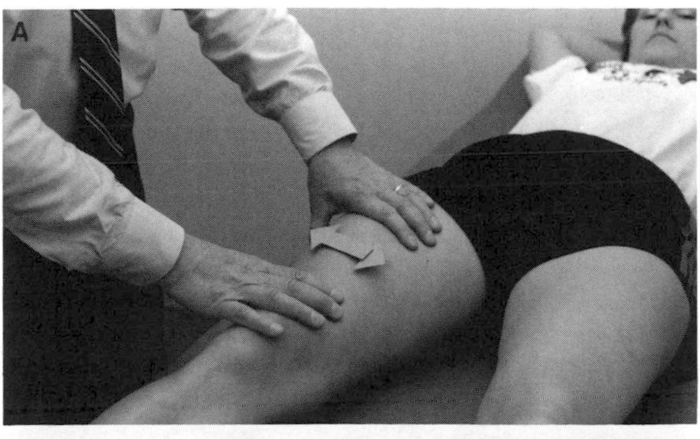

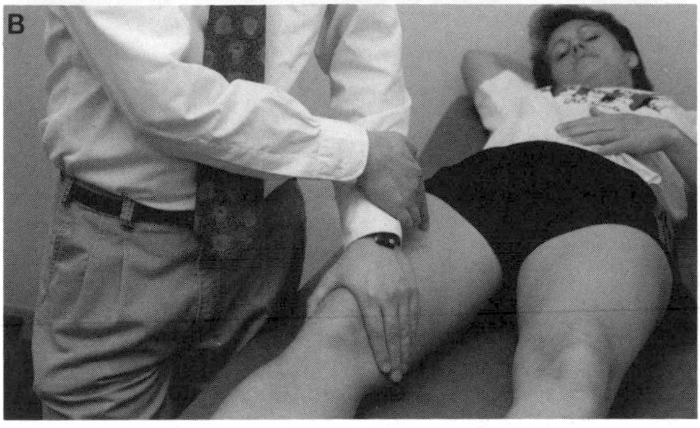

FIGURE 4. Patellofemoral compression. **A**, Compression of patella in transverse direction. Check for crepitation and/or tenderness. **B**, Longitudinal compression of patellofemoral joint. Trap patella distally with hand, then ask patient to maximally contract quadriceps. Check for crepitation and/or tenderness.

ii. **Anterior drawer test with external rotation of tibia:** Patient is supine and relaxed, hip flexed to 45° and knee to 90°. Externally rotate foot 30°, then pin foot to table with examiner's thigh. Grasp proximal tibia with both hands and pull toward examiner. Positive test is excessive anterior rotation of medial tibial condyle. See Fig. 6.

b. **Lateral**

i. **Adduction stress test at 30° and 0°:** Patient is in same position as for abduction stress test (described at left). Reverse hand position so that one hand applies varus stress, while opposite hand acts as fulcrum along medial side of joint. Watch and feel for lateral joint line opening. Perform at 30° of flexion and then at full possible extension or hyperextension. See Fig. 7.

ii. **External rotation recurvatum test:** Patient is supine and relaxed. Lift entire lower extremity by first toe. Observe for excessive recurvatum and external rotation of proximal tibia (tibial tuberosity) and apparent varus deformity of knee. Indicates posterolateral corner injury. See Fig. 8.

iii. **Posterolateral drawer test:** Same position as for anterior drawer test with external rotation of tibia (see above). Examiner's hands push posteriorly on proximal tibia. Positive test is excessive posterior rotation of lateral tibial condyle. See Fig. 9.

iv. **Reverse pivot shift test:** See pivot shift test (page 560). Performed with tibia in external rotation rather than internal rotation. With knee flexed 90°, lateral

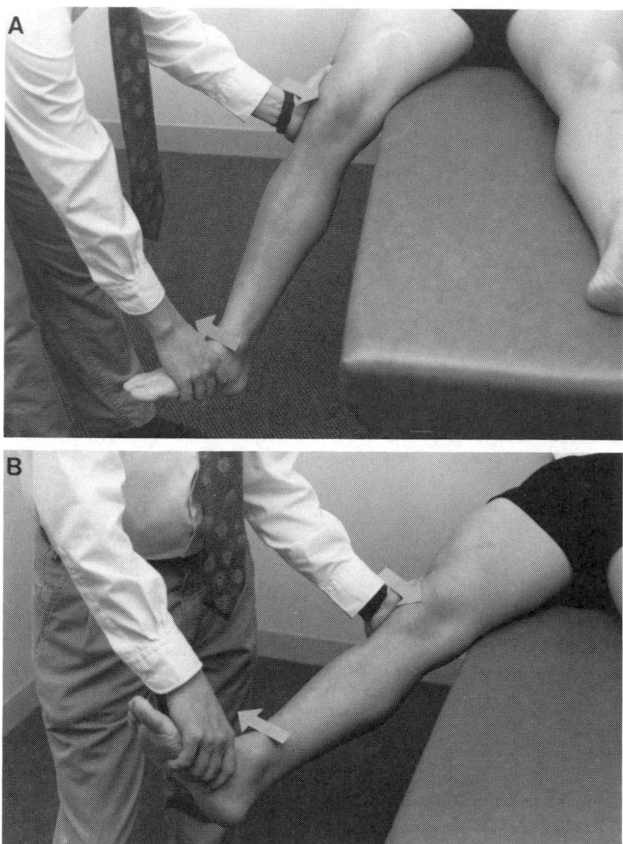

FIGURE 5. Abduction stress test. **A**, Test done at 30° of flexion for medial ligament injury. **B**, Test done in full extension for associated acute posterior cruciate injury.

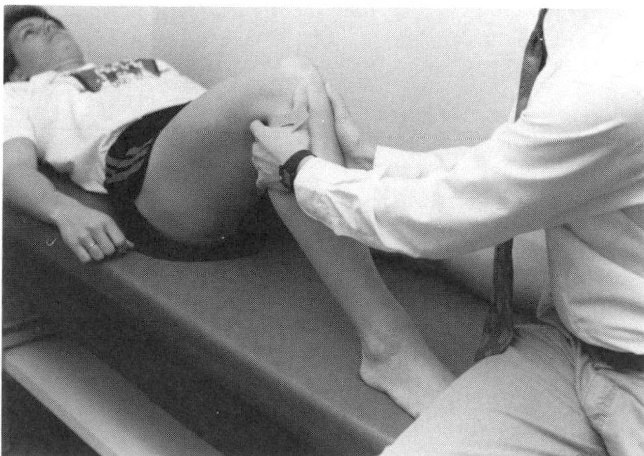

FIGURE 6. Anterior drawer sign with tibia in neutral rotation. Anterior force applied to proximal tibia while index fingers ensure that hamstrings are relaxed. May also be done with external rotation and internal rotation of foot and tibia.

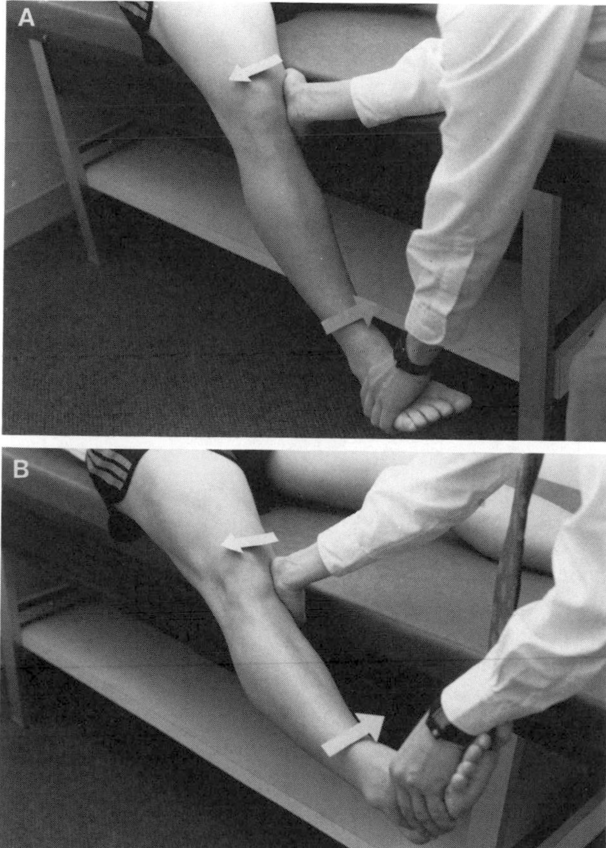

FIGURE 7. Adduction stress test for lateral compartment injury. **A**, Test done at 30° of flexion for lateral compartment rupture. Most knees will have mild instability with this test normally. **B**, Test done in full extension for acute posterior cruciate ligament injury associated with lateral compartment injury.

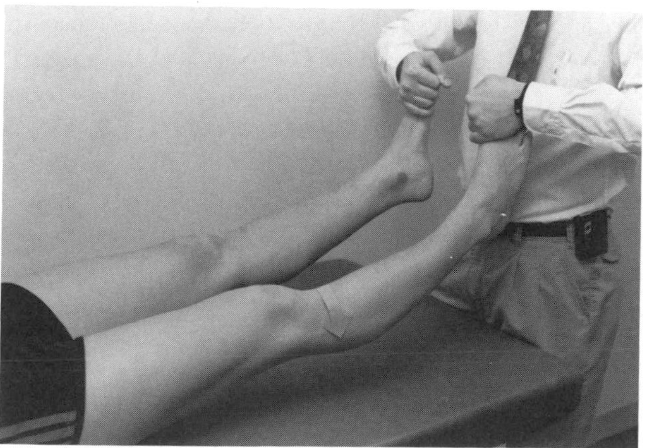

FIGURE 8. External rotation recurvatum test. Both lower limbs are lifted by great toes. Positive test is excessive recurvatum, external tibial rotation proximally, and development of apparent varus at knee. Indicates posterolateral corner injury.

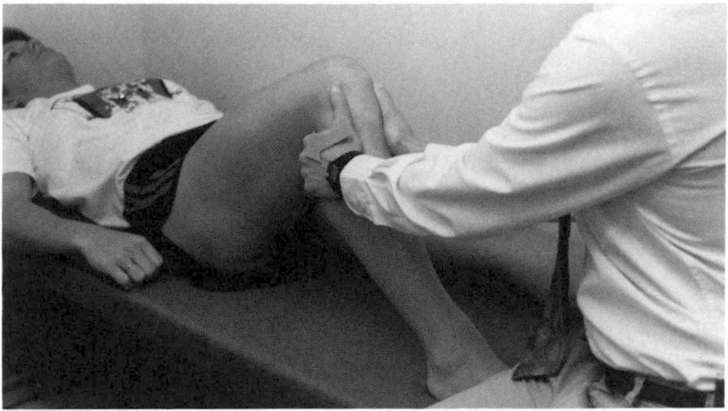

FIGURE 9. Posterior drawer sign. Same position as for anterior drawer sign, but force on proximal tibia is posterior instead of anterior.

tibial condyle is subluxed posteriorly. With further knee extension, tibia reduces with detectable "clunk."

c. **Anterior cruciate ligament (ACL)**

i. **Lachman test:** Patient is supine and relaxed. Examiner grasps distal femur with one hand, while other hand grasps proximal tibia. Knee flexed to approximately 15°–20°. Apply anterior force to proximal tibia. Positive test is excessive anterior translation of tibia beneath femur and lack of firm endpoint. See Fig. 10.

ii. **Anterior drawer test in neutral rotation:** Same position as for anterior drawer with external rotation of tibia (page 557), except that foot and tibia are in neutral rotation. Anterior pull is applied to proximal tibia. Positive test is anterior translation of both tibial condyles from beneath femur. See Fig. 6.

NOTE: This *test is influenced by structures other than the anterior cruciate ligament.* ***Do not*** *rely on this test for diagnosis of ACL tear.*

iii. **Pivot shift test, jerk test:** Patient is supine and relaxed. Begin with knee fully extended (pivot shift) or flexed to 90° (jerk test). Foot and tibia internally rotated. Valgus applied at knee. Knee progressively flexed (pivot shift) or extended (jerk test). At approximately 30°, watch and feel for anterior subluxation of lateral tibial condyle. Tibia suddenly reduces with further flexion (pivot shift) or extension (jerk test). See Fig. 11.

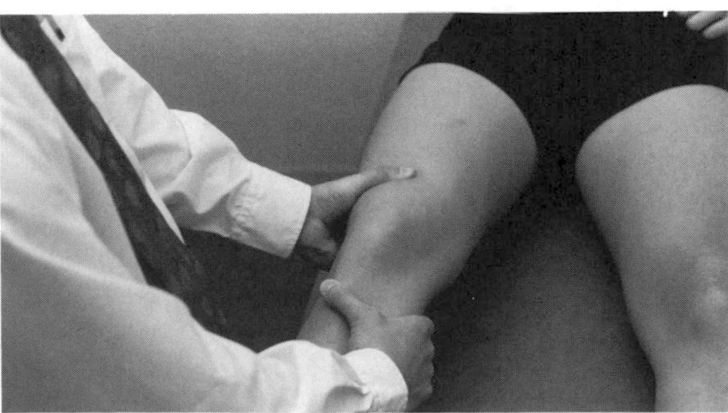

FIGURE 10. Lachman test. Distal femur is stabilized while proximal tibia is pulled anteriorly. Positive test is increased anterior translation of proximal tibia beneath distal femur.

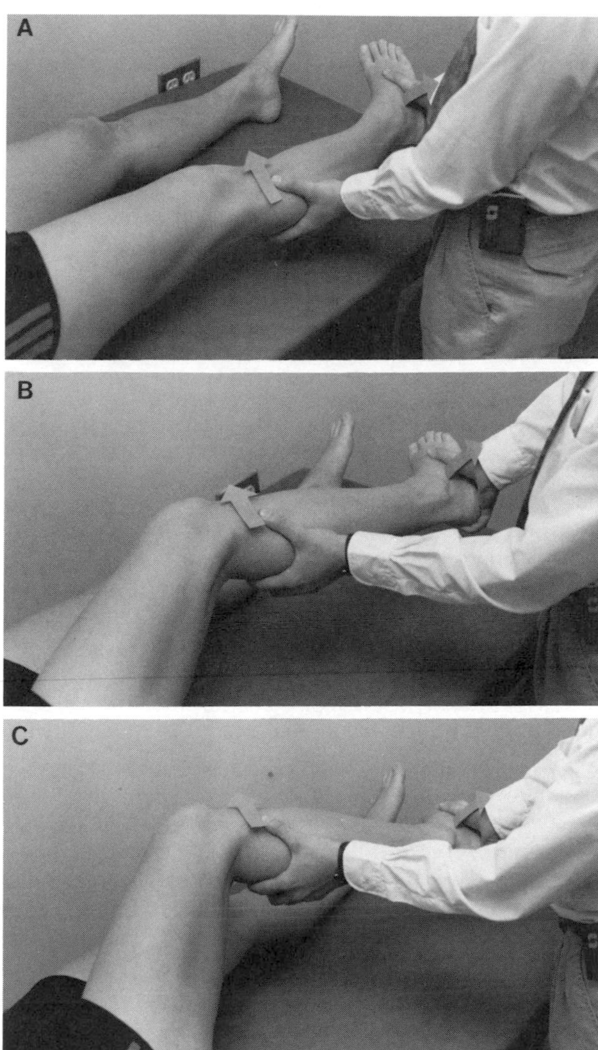

FIGURE 11. Pivot shift/jerk test. **A**, Starting position for pivot shift test. Foot internally rotated and pulled somewhat laterally, creating valgus of knee. Anterior force applied at fibular head. **B**, Position at which anterior subluxation of lateral tibial condyle is seen in positive test. **C**, Ending position for pivot shift test in which reduction of proximal tibia takes place. Jerk test would be reverse of pivot shift, starting at 90° of flexion and ending in full extension.

d. **Posterior cruciate ligament (PCL)**

i. **Posterior drawer test:** Same position as for anterior drawer test in neutral rotation (C.1.c.ii., above). Posterior force is applied to proximal tibia. Positive test is straight posterior displacement of both tibial condyles. See Fig. 9. **CAUTION:** *Make sure of neutral position as starting point. Compare position of tibia relative to femur with normal knee. It is easy to start from posteriorly displaced position and interpret reduction to neutral as positive* <u>*anterior*</u> *drawer sign rather than starting at neutral and interpreting as positive* <u>*posterior*</u> *drawer sign.*

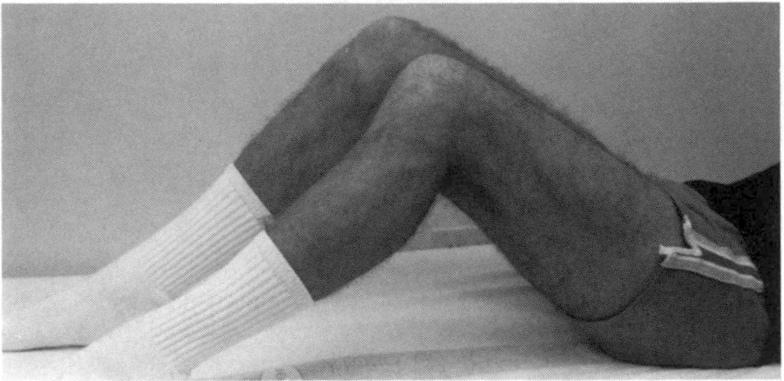

FIGURE 12. Posterior cruciate ligament rupture. Left knee shows positive gravity test with posterior sag of left tibia.

ii. **Gravity or sag test:** Patient is supine and relaxed. Flex hips to 45° and knees to 90° with feet flat on table. With quadriceps relaxed, observe from lateral side for posterior displacement of one tibial tuberosity compared to the other. Then flex hips to 90°, support both legs by ankles and feet, and observe again. See Fig. 12.

iii. **Abduction or adduction stress test at 0°:** As described for abduction and adduction stress tests at 30° and 0° (pages 556–557). Positive test in full extension in acute case is often due to posterior cruciate ligament rupture.

2. **Menisci**
   a. **McMurray's test:** Patient is supine and relaxed. Flex knee maximally with external tibial rotation (medial meniscus) or internal tibial rotation (lateral meniscus). While maintaining rotation, bring knee into full extension. Positive test is painful pop occurring over medial joint line (medial meniscus) or lateral joint line (lateral meniscus). See Fig. 13.
   b. **Apley's compression test:** Patient is in prone position. Knee flexed to 90° with external tibial rotation (medial meniscus) or internal tibial rotation (lateral meniscus). Apply axial compression to tibia while flexing and extending knee. Positive test is painful pop over medial joint line (medial meniscus) or lateral joint line (lateral meniscus). See Fig. 14.
3. **Patella**
   a. **Hypermobility/apprehension test:** Patient is supine and relaxed. Examiner sits on edge of table with patient's knee flexed approximately 30°–45° across examiner's thigh. With quadriceps relaxed, examiner uses both thumbs to forcefully displace patella over lateral femoral condyle. Positive test is increased lateral mobility of patella compared to opposite knee or other patients. More important is discomfort or extreme apprehension that patella is going to dislocate due to lateral displacement. See Fig. 15.
   b. **Plica tests:** Patient is supine and relaxed. With tibia internally rotated, examiner passively flexes and extends knee from 30°–100° of flexion. Examining fingers laid along medial patellofemoral joint may feel tender pop of a pathologic plica. See Fig. 16.

II. Knee Ligament Injuries

A. Medial ligaments

1. **Description:** Injury to medial (tibial) collateral ligament and/or medial capsular ligament
2. **Mechanism of injury:** Valgus force applied to knee with external tibial rotation. May be noncontact twist or a blow to lateral side of joint.

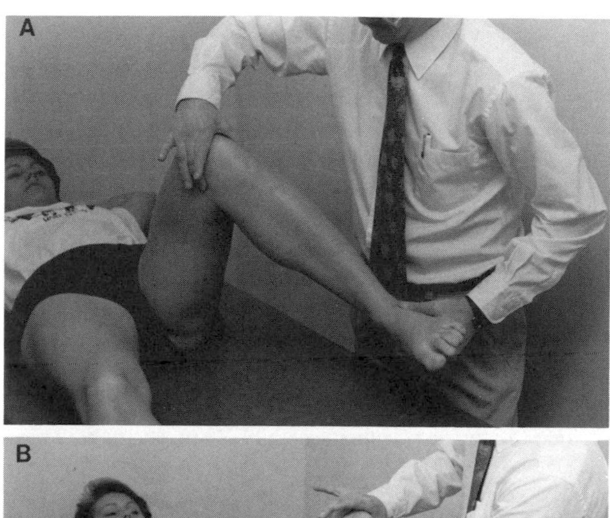

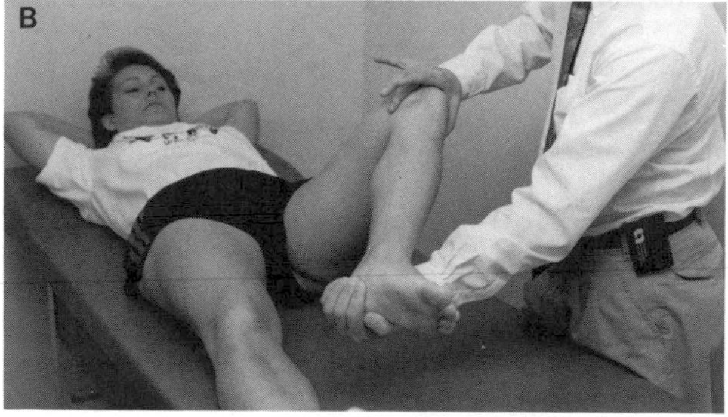

FIGURE 13. McMurray's test. **A**, Position for lateral meniscus. With foot in internal rotation, knee is brought from full flexion to extension while fingers palpate lateral joint line. **B**, Position for medial meniscus. With external tibial rotation, knee is brought from full flexion to extension while fingers palpate medial joint line.

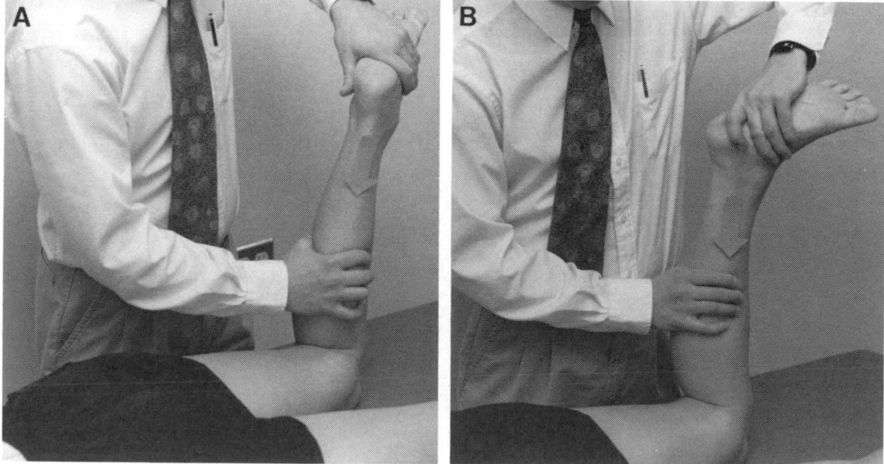

FIGURE 14. Apley's compression test. **A**, Position for medial meniscus. With pressure on sole of foot, tibia is externally rotated while knee is flexed and extended. **B**, For lateral meniscus, foot is internally rotated while knee is flexed and extended.

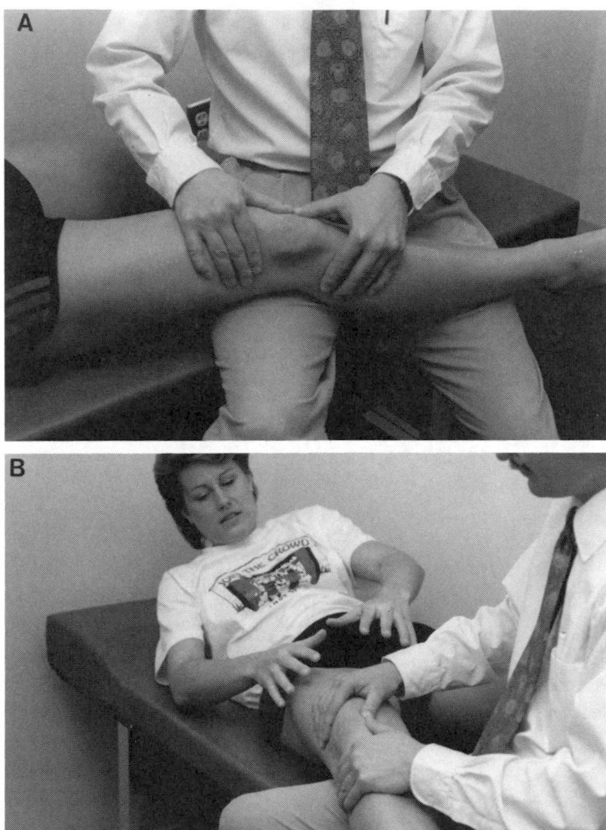

FIGURE 15. Patellar hypermobility/apprehension test. **A**, With knee flexed across examiner's thigh, patella is firmly displaced over lateral edge of femoral trochlea, checking for hypermobility. **B**, Extreme apprehension is created as patient senses impending dislocation or subluxation of patella.

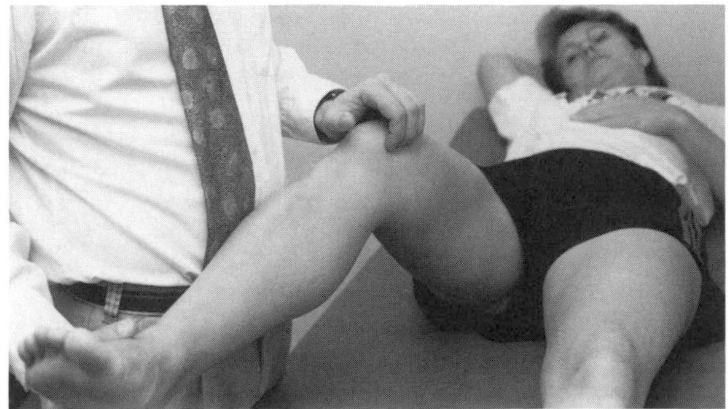

FIGURE 16. Palpation for plica. With tibia internally rotated, knee is passively flexed and extended. Fingers along medial patellofemoral joint feel for tender pop of pathologic synovial plica.

3. **History**
   a. Typical mechanism as described (page 562)
   b. Initial pain on medial side of knee
   c. If complete tear, complaints of knee giving way into valgus
4. **Examination:** Positive abduction stress test at 30° flexion. Compare with opposite knee. If posterior cruciate ligament is intact, will be stable in fullest possible extension or hyperextension. Frequently, but not always, will be a positive anterior drawer sign with tibia in external rotation. Medial tibial condyle rotates anteriorly.
5. **X-rays:** Abduction stress film may be used to distinguish ligament injury from epiphyseal fracture in skeletally immature. Fracture opens at growth plate. Ligament tear opens at joint line. Do in 20°–30° of flexion.
6. **Differential diagnosis**
   a. In the young, epiphyseal fracture of distal femur or proximal tibia
   b. Patellar dislocation (may be associated with medial ligament tear)
   c. Medial meniscus tear (may be associated with medial ligament tear)
7. **Treatment**
   a. Grades I and II sprains—PRICES (see Chapter 38, "Comprehensive Rehabilitation of the Athlete"), crutches, rehabilitation
   b. Grade III sprain (complete ligament tear)
      i. With other associated injuries, surgery may be considered.
      ii. Immobilization has been shown to be effective treatment in **isolated** medial ligament tear.
      iii. With only mild instability, rigid immobilization may not be necessary. PRICES and functional rehabilitation may be adequate treatment.

B. **Lateral ligaments**
1. **Description**
   a. Sprain or tear of lateral (fibular) collateral ligament and/or lateral capsular ligament
   b. May be associated injuries to popliteus tendon, iliotibial band, peroneal nerve
2. **Mechanism of injury**
   a. Varus or twisting injury
   b. May be contact or noncontact
   c. Posterolateral ligaments often injured by hyperextension mechanism, frequently with blow to anteromedial tibia
3. **History**
   a. Typical mechanism, as above
   b. Pain is present over the lateral ligament complex.
   c. Giving way of the knee on twisting, cutting, or pivoting
   d. In chronic case, posterolateral corner injury gives a feeling of giving way into hyperextension when standing, walking, or running backwards.
4. **Examination**
   a. Compare with opposite knee
   b. In acute case, **may** be increased adduction stress test at 30° flexion and positive posterolateral drawer sign
   c. In chronic case, shows positive reverse pivot shift test and external rotation recurvatum test
   d. External rotation recurvatum may also be apparent on standing, giving an increased varus appearance to the knee.
5. **X-rays**
   a. Lateral capsular sign shows avulsion of midportion of lateral capsular ligament with small fragment of proximal lateral tibia. Associated with a high incidence of anterior cruciate tear and indicates anterolateral instability.

b. Arcuate sign shows avulsion of proximal fibula with posterolateral ligament complex. Indicates posterolateral instability.

6. **Differential diagnosis**
   a. Chronic posterolateral injury may be confused with medial compartment arthritis due to progressive varus appearance. Also difficult to differentiate from posterior cruciate injury.
   b. Acute lateral ligament injury may be confused with lateral meniscus tear.
   c. Injury to middle third of lateral capsular ligament, as shown by lateral capsular sign on x-ray, usually associated with anterior cruciate ligament injury
7. **Treatment**
   a. Grade I and II sprains—PRICES (see Chapter 38, "Comprehensive Rehabilitation of the Athlete"), crutches, rehabilitation
   b. Grade III sprain (complete ligament tear)
      i. Surgical repair is usually preferable if the injury involves more than just the lateral (fibular) collateral ligament.
      ii. Immobilization is not really useful by itself.
      iii. Mild instability may be treated by PRICES and functional rehabilitation.

C. **Anterior cruciate ligament (ACL)**

1. **Description**
   a. Tear of part or all of two major bundles (posterolateral, anteromedial) of anterior cruciate ligament
   b. May be associated with tears of the middle one-third of lateral capsular ligament
   c. ACL is torn from the femur or tibia, or torn in its midportion
   d. May avulse the tibial spine in young patients
2. **Mechanism of injury**
   a. May be multiple mechanisms of ACL injury
   b. Hyperextension, varus/internal rotation, and extremes of valgus and external rotation are all possible causes.
3. **History**
   a. Usually a loud pop occurs.
   b. May be followed by autonomic symptoms of dizziness, sweating, faintness, slight nausea
   c. Large swelling usually occurs within the first 2 hours following acute injury (hemarthrosis). Conversely, majority of acute hemarthroses (more than 85%) will be anterior cruciate tears.
   d. In chronic cases, complaints of giving way on twisting, pivoting, cutting
4. **Examination**
   a. **Acute**
      i. Finding of a large hemarthrosis
      ii. Positive Lachman test
   b. **Chronic**
      i. Positive Lachman test
      ii. Positive pivot shift or jerk test
      iii. Perhaps positive anterior drawer sign, but not reliable. **Do not rely on anterior drawer sign**.
5. **X-rays**
   a. Lateral capsular sign (see bottom page 565)
   b. Avulsion of tibial spine may be seen in young patients.
   c. MRI has reported accuracy rates as high as 95% in detecting ACL tears.
6. **Differential diagnosis**
   a. Acute—differentiate from other causes of hemarthrosis (e.g., osteochondral fracture, peripheral meniscus tear, patellar dislocation).

b. Chronic—differentiate from other types of ligamentous laxity and/or meniscal tears.

7. **Treatment**
   a. **Acute**
      i. Various methods to delineate degree of damage and associated injuries
      ii. Knee may be treated symptomatically followed by repeated evaluations over first 2–3 weeks following injury.
      iii. If diagnosis unclear, obtain MRI
      iv. Most active patients engaged in agility sports will require surgical reconstruction.
      v. Reconstruction is now usually delayed at least three weeks post injury to allow decrease in swelling and increase in range of motion.
      vi. For mild laxity with firm end point (partial ACL injury) and no other associated injury, may treat with PRICES, functional rehabilitation, protective bracing
      vii. Apparent partial injury often progresses to more obvious complete tear
   b. **Chronic**
      i. May attempt functional stabilization through rehabilitation, bracing, lifestyle modification
      ii. Often requires surgical reconstruction

D. **Posterior cruciate ligament (PCL)**

1. **Description:** tear of part or all of two major bundles of the posterior cruciate ligament (posteromedial and anterolateral)
2. **Mechanism of injury**
   a. Valgus/varus in full extension
   b. Rarely a severe twist
   c. Direct blow to anterior proximal tibia, as in a fall on artificial turf or other hard playing surface
3. **History**
   a. Usually less swelling than with anterior cruciate ligament
   b. Otherwise, in acute stage, nothing particularly distinguishing
   c. Chronically, a feeling of femur sliding anteriorly off the tibia, especially when rapidly decelerating or descending slopes or stairs
4. **Examination**
   a. **Acute**
      i. If produced by varus or valgus mechanism, may find abduction or adduction stress test positive in full extension.
      ii. If produced by blow to anterior tibia, posterior drawer sign may be positive.
   b. **Chronic:** Rely on posterior drawer sign and gravity test (see pages 561–562).
5. **X-rays**
   a. Cross-table lateral view may show sag of tibia compared to opposite side.
   b. May accentuate by doing posterior drawer sign while taking cross-table lateral view
   c. May see bony avulsion with tibial attachment of the posterior cruciate ligament
   d. MRI shows posterior cruciate well and may help in difficult case.
6. **Differential diagnosis**
   a. Most difficult is distinguishing posterior cruciate injury from posterolateral corner injury.
   b. Posterior drawer sign and posterolateral drawer sign may appear the same.
   c. Both injuries may exist in the same knee.
7. **Treatment**
   a. **Acute**
      i. It is most important to delineate degree of injury.
      ii. May require examination under anesthesia and arthroscopy

iii. For mild laxity (isolated PCL tear), may treat with PRICES, functional rehabilitation, protective bracing
iv. For moderate or severe laxity, surgical repair/reconstruction is usually required.

b. **Chronic**
i. May attempt functional stabilization through rehabilitation and bracing
ii. Often requires surgical reconstruction if instability is more than mild

III. Meniscal Injuries

A. **Medial meniscus**

1. **Description**
a. Disruption of medial semilunar cartilage of the knee
b. May be from single traumatic episode, degenerative processes, or a combination
c. Tears take different forms, such as radial, longitudinal, or horizontal.
d. Most important surgical factor is whether tear is peripheral in vascular zone, or more central in nonvascular zone.

2. **Mechanism of injury**
a. Twisting or squatting
b. May be in association with ligament injuries due to any of their precipitating mechanisms

3. **History**
a. Usually mild swelling and joint line pain
b. In acute setting, important to know whether knee lacked full extension from the time of injury (locked knee from displaced fragment), or knee lacked full extension the next day (pseudolocking from hamstring spasm).
c. In chronic setting, recurrent locking is typical.
d. Otherwise, symptoms may include slipping or catching over the joint line.

4. **Examination**
a. Positive McMurray's test
b. Positive Apley's test
c. Results of these tests may vary considerably from one examination session to the next.
d. Joint line tenderness and mild effusion may be present.
e. Chronically, there is commonly quadriceps atrophy.
f. With a peripheral meniscus detachment and a positive anterior drawer test, a loud "clunk" may be elicited as the meniscus displaces during anterior drawer testing.

5. **X-rays**
a. Plain films are usually normal, unless the meniscal tear has been present for a significant time.
b. After that time, they may show joint line spurring and/or narrowing.
c. MRIs have now supplanted arthrograms for diagnosis of meniscal injury.
d. For medial meniscus, MRI has sensitivity as high as 94%.

6. **Differential diagnosis**
a. Ligamentous injury, causing pain in the same area
b. Patellar problems, which might cause anteromedial joint pain that is confused with pain from a medial meniscus injury
c. Pathologic synovial plicas, which can cause pain, swelling, catching and popping also confused with medial meniscus injuries
d. Loose bodies may cause locking.
e. Medial compartment arthritis may cause medial joint pain similar to that from torn meniscus.

7. **Treatment**
   a. A suspected meniscus tear with no ligamentous instability may be managed initially through symptomatic treatment and functional rehabilitation.
   b. If no improvement, or if time constraints do not allow initial conservative treatment, diagnostic arthroscopy is the most certain way of diagnosing and treating meniscal injury.
   c. Most meniscal tears still require arthroscopic partial meniscectomy.
   d. Vertical tears in the peripheral vascular zone are now routinely treated by meniscal repair rather than removal of the meniscus.
   e. An MRI may help decide whether to proceed with surgical treatment or continue with nonsurgical care.

B. **Lateral meniscus**
1. **Description**
   a. Disruption of lateral semilunar cartilage of the knee
   b. May be from single traumatic episode, degenerative processes, or a combination
   c. With lateral meniscus injury, may also encounter injuries of congenital discoid meniscus
   d. Tears take different forms, such as radial, longitudinal, or horizontal.
   e. Most important surgical factor is whether tear is peripheral in vascular zone, or more central in nonvascular zone
2. **Mechanism of injury** is the same as for medial meniscus injury.
3. **History**
   a. Same as for medial meniscus injury, though often more pain and fewer mechanical symptoms than with medial meniscus tears
   b. May give history of cystic lesion directly over lateral joint line
4. **Examination**
   a. Is much the same as for medial meniscus injury
   b. May palpate localized puffiness or distinct cystic lesion over lateral joint line
5. **X-rays**
   a. Same findings as for medial meniscus injury
   b. In child with congenital discoid lateral meniscus, may see **widening** of lateral joint space
   c. In contrast to medial meniscus, MRI has somewhat less sensitivity (approximately 78%) in detecting lateral meniscus tears.
6. **Differential diagnosis**
   a. Lateral ligamentous injury
   b. Loose bodies
   c. Degenerative arthritis of the lateral compartment
   d. Popliteus tendinitis
   e. Iliotibial band friction syndrome
7. **Treatment**
   a. Same as for medial meniscus injury
   b. Special considerations in youngsters with lateral discoid meniscus include whether to remove or repair and how much meniscus to remove.

IV. Extensor Mechanism Problems

A. **Instability syndromes**
1. **Dislocation**
   a. **Description:** complete, usually lateral displacement of patella from femoral trochlea that persists until reduced, usually by extending knee
   b. **Mechanism of injury:** valgus and/or twisting with strong quadriceps contraction

c. **Predisposing factors:** all of the stigmata indicating congenital **extensor mechanism malalignment**, including VMO dysplasia, VL hypertrophy, high and lateral patellar posture, increased Q-angle, bony deformity, etc. Usually more easily seen in acute case on opposite uninjured side.
d. **History**
   i. May or may not be previous symptoms of instability or patellofemoral pain
   ii. Feeling of patellar dislocation when injury occurred
   iii. Report of lying on ground with knee flexed
   iv. Report of "something coming out" medially, which usually represents uncovered medial femoral condyle rather than patella going medially
   v. Report of something "going back into place" when knee extended
   vi. Swelling that occurs within the first 2 hours
e. **Examination** will depend on whether patella is still dislocated or has been reduced.
   i. Predisposing physical findings seen on opposite knee. If patella is still dislocated, will be located over lateral femoral condyle with prominence of uncovered medial femoral condyle.
   ii. If patella has been reduced, there may be large hemarthrosis with hypermobility and marked apprehension on hypermobility testing.
   iii. May also find associated medial ligamentous instability
f. **X-ray studies**
   i. Unusual to find patella still dislocated on x-ray, since positioning on x-ray table usually reduces dislocation
   ii. Infrapatellar view may show avulsion of medial edge of patella.
   iii. Large osteochondral fracture may be visible.
   iv. Important to take infrapatellar view with knee flexed only 30°–45°, rather than traditional "sunrise" or "skyline" view with knee flexed beyond 90°.
   v. Patella alta can be measured objectively on lateral view.
g. **Differential diagnosis**
   i. In acute case, differentiate from ligamentous tears.
   ii. In chronic recurrent case, distinguish from meniscus disorders.
h. **Treatment**
   i. If patella is still dislocated, knee extension and gentle pressure along lateral patellar edge will usually reduce it easily and without anesthesia.
   ii. Aspiration may be indicated for comfort or to search for fat in blood secondary to osteochondral fracture.
   iii. Thoughts regarding rigid immobilization are changing, even with first time dislocation, due to harmful effect of immobilization on knee joint.
   iv. Immobilize first time dislocation only as needed for symptoms, followed by extensive rehabilitation program and functional patellar bracing
   v. An obvious disruption of VMO insertion into medial patellar edge or a rupture of medial patellofemoral ligament from adductor tubercle does best with early surgical repair.
   vi. If recurrent dislocation treat symptomatically with crutches, followed by functional rehabilitation and bracing

2. **Subluxation**
   a. **Description**
      i. Transient partial displacement of patella from femoral trochlea
      ii. May occur acutely, as in patellar dislocation, or may be intermittent
      iii. There is spontaneous reduction of displacement.
   b. **Mechanism of injury**
      i. Same as for patellar dislocation
      ii. May occur with less severe force or in normal everyday activity

c. **Predisposing factors**—same as for patellar dislocation

d. **History**

   i. May or may not be past history of complete dislocation or patellofemoral pain

   ii. Feeling of slipping when cutting, twisting, or pivoting

   iii. Mild recurrent swelling

e. **Examination**

   i. Predisposing physical findings seen in both knees, but may be more obvious on asymptomatic side, especially if there has been an acute injury on symptomatic side.

   ii. Mild effusion

   iii. Positive hypermobility and apprehension test

f. **X-rays**

   i. Infrapatellar view must be done with proper technique and knee flexed only 30°–45°.

   ii. Infrapatellar views may show lateral tilt and/or lateral subluxation.

   iii. X-rays may all be **normal** in appearance.

   iv. Patellofemoral indices (Merchant, Laurin, Brattstrom) show tendency to patellofemoral problems, but do not give specific diagnosis.

g. **Differential diagnosis**—chronic knee ligament instability, causing giving-way of knee

h. **Treatment**

   i. In acute subluxation, use temporary symptomatic immobilization, followed by functional rehabilitation and bracing of the patella.

   ii. If no acute episode, treat with functional rehabilitation, bracing, and nonsteroidal anti-inflammatory medication.

   iii. If patient is disabled by subluxation, may require arthroscopic lateral release or open extensor mechanism reconstruction

B. **Painful syndromes**

1. **Patellofemoral pain syndrome**

a. **Description**

   i. Any of a variety of syndromes characterized by anterior knee pain as major symptom

   ii. An **imprecise** term in which pain is not explained by a more readily definable cause, such as those discussed below

   iii. Often referred to as "chondromalacia patella," a term that should be reserved for articular cartilage damage actually observed

b. **Mechanism of injury**

   i. May result from extensor mechanism malalignment, with or without an instability syndrome

   ii. May occur as overuse injury with extreme and/or repetitive loading of patellofemoral joint (e.g., knee flexion, running, jumping, etc.)

c. **Predisposing factors**—same as for instability syndromes (see page 569)

d. **History**

   i. Anterior knee pain, often worse with sitting in tight space with knee flexed

   ii. Pain worse on descending stairs or slopes

   iii. Mild swelling (may be bilateral)

   iv. May be snapping and popping around patella

e. **Examination**

   i. Findings predisposing to extensor mechanism problems in both legs

   ii. Pain on patellofemoral compression test

   iii. Crepitation about patella on range of motion

   iv. May be mild effusion

v. Tenderness to palpation around patella
vi. Foot malalignment or leg length inequality may aggravate symptoms.

f. **X-rays**
i. Same as for subluxation
ii. **May be normal**

g. **Differential diagnosis**
i. In preadolescent and young adolescent, consider referred pain from hip disorder (e.g., Legg-Calvé-Perthes disease, slipped capital femoral epiphysis).
ii. Osteochondritis dissecans of femur or patella
iii. Bone tumor, especially in case of unilateral symptoms
iv. In older patient, osteoarthritis or some other inflammatory joint disease

h. **Treatment**
i. Functional rehabilitation program, nonsteroidal anti-inflammatory medication (NSAID), functional bracing of patella, orthotics for foot malalignment
ii. If other treatments are unsuccessful, surgical treatment may be considered—either lateral release or extensor mechanism reconstruction.
iii. Should always look for other more specific cause of anterior knee pain, such as those listed below.

2. **Patellar tendinitis ("jumper's knee")**

a. **Description:** inflammation of patellar tendon, usually at its attachment to inferior pole of patella

b. **Mechanism of injury**
i. Usually excessive jumping or bounding activity or other high patellofemoral stress activity
ii. Less commonly from running

c. **Predisposing factors**
i. Same as for other extensor mechanism disorders
ii. Possibly ankle dorsiflexor muscle weakness, perhaps secondary to ankle injury

d. **History**
i. Participation in activity typically associated with this problem, such as a jumping sport
ii. Complaint of infrapatellar pain, originally after exercise, later during exercise and while at rest

e. **Examination**
i. Tenderness present at inferior pole of patella
ii. Less commonly, tenderness over body of patellar tendon
iii. Other findings of extensor mechanism malalignment
iv. Weakness of ankle dorsiflexors
v. Hamstring, heelcord, and/or quadriceps muscle tightness

f. **X-rays**
i. Occasionally see irregularity at inferior pole of patella
ii. May be findings of extensor mechanism malalignment, including patella alta
iii. MRI may demonstrate degenerative changes in tendon.

g. **Differential diagnosis**
i. Usually firm diagnosis not difficult with this entity
ii. May consider some other soft tissue lesion of patellar tendon or fat pad, such as a tumor
iii. Otherwise, could be any of the other causes of patellofemoral pain

h. **Treatment**
i. Rehabilitative exercise program, concentrating on hamstring, heelcord, and quadriceps flexibility, as well as quadriceps strength
ii. Eccentric strengthening exercises for ankle dorsiflexors are important.

iii. Anti-inflammatory medication
iv. Ultrasound, utilizing hydrocortisone phonophoresis
v. Questionable benefit from infrapatellar strap

3. **Synovial plica**
   a. **Description**
      i. Structurally, a remnant of the embryologic walls that divide the knee into medial, lateral, and suprapatellar pouches
      ii. Appears as a fold of synovium attached to the periphery of the joint and to the underside of quadriceps tendon (suprapatellar plica)
      iii. May also present as a free edge along the medial patellofemoral joint (medial plica), or may be in both locations
      iv. Rarely seen in other configurations
      v. Edge protruding into joint may be of various sizes.
   b. **Mechanism of injury**
      i. Overuse with repetitive flexion and extension, e.g., running
      ii. Direct blow to medial patellofemoral joint, e.g., falling on turf or dashboard injury
   c. **Predisposing factors**
      i. Congenital presence of plica
      ii. Other extensor mechanism malalignment predispositions may increase likelihood of symptoms due to plica.
   d. **History**
      i. Overuse or direct trauma
      ii. Complaints of anterior knee pain
      iii. Pain over suprapatellar or medial peripatellar regions with long periods of knee flexion, especially when accompanied by distinct snap or pop when knee is extended
      iv. Painful catching episodes over medial patellofemoral joint
   e. **Examination**
      i. Often difficult to palpate plica. Best done with passive flexion and extension with tibia held internally rotated. Fingers should lie over medial patellofemoral joint.
      ii. May see other extensor mechanism malalignment stigmata
      iii. Heelcord tightness and hamstring tightness aggravate significantly.
   f. **X-ray studies** are not helpful.
   g. **Differential diagnosis**
      i. Other painful patellofemoral conditions
      ii. Possibly medial meniscus injury or loose body
      iii. Patients often dismissed as "neurotic" because of lack of findings in face of significant symptoms.
   h. **Treatment**
      i. If inflammatory process in synovium is still reversible:
         (a) May improve with hamstring stretching, heelcord stretching, VMO exercises (if VMO is dysplastic)
         (b) NSAIDs, ice, activity modification
         (c) Simple external patellar support may help.
         (d) Phonophoresis to plica area may also be beneficial.
      ii. If inflammatory process is not reversible and plica is fibrotic, persistent symptoms require arthroscopic removal of plica. Promises good relief of symptoms and good future function.
4. **Osgood-Schlatter's "disease"**
   a. **Description**
      i. Painful enlargement of tibial tuberosity at patellar tendon insertion

   ii. Rather than being a disease, condition is due to mechanical stress and excessive tension on growing tibial tuberosity apophysis.
   iii. Occurs in preadolescence and early adolescence, usually during rapid growth period
b. **Mechanism of injury**
   i. Overuse in normal childhood activities, including sports
   ii. Rarely, acute onset of popping and pain over tibial tuberosity
c. **Predisposing factors**
   i. Patella alta
   ii. Other evidence of extensor mechanism malalignment and altered extensor mechanics
   iii. Tight hamstrings, heelcords, quadriceps muscles predispose to symptoms
d. **History:** complaints of painful enlargement of tibial tuberosity
e. **Examination**
   i. Enlarged, tender tibial tuberosity
   ii. Stigmata of extensor mechanism malalignment, especially patella alta
   iii. Tight hamstrings, heelcords, and quadriceps muscles
f. **X-rays**
   i. Enlarged tibial tuberosity
   ii. Irregularity of tibial tuberosity
   iii. Loose ossicle separated from tuberosity
   iv. Patella alta
g. **Differential diagnosis**
   i. Other forms of patellar tendinitis
   ii. In acute episode, avulsion fracture of tibial tuberosity
   iii. Tumorous processes of the tibial tuberosity
h. **Treatment**
   i. Hamstring stretching, heelcord stretching, and quadriceps stretching exercises
   ii. VMO strengthening exercises
   iii. Activity modification as necessitated by symptoms
   iv. Simple modalities
   v. Local padding

5. **Quadriceps tendinitis** (including VL tendinitis and VMO tendinitis)
   a. **Description**
      i. Inflammation of quadriceps tendon at its insertion into superior edge of patella
      ii. May involve only VL insertion into superolateral pole of patella, or VMO insertion into superomedial pole of patella
   b. **Mechanism of injury:** same as for patellar tendinitis (page 572)
   c. **Predisposing factors**—extensor mechanism malalignment
   d. **History**
      i. Involvement in activity consistent with causing this entity
      ii. Complaints of suprapatellar pain
   e. **Examination**
      i. Tenderness at superior pole of patella
      ii. May be over central rectus femoris insertion, superolateral VL insertion, or superomedial VMO insertion
      iii. Other findings of extensor mechanism malalignment
      iv. Hamstring, heelcord, and quadriceps muscle tightness
   f. **X-rays:** Usually there are no findings on x-ray studies.
   g. **Differential diagnosis**
      i. Suprapatellar pain from synovial plica
      ii. Bone tumor of distal femur
   h. **Treatment:** same as for patellar tendinitis (page 572)

V. Miscellaneous Knee Conditions

A. Bursitis

1. **Description**
   a. Inflammation of any of various bursae around the knee, evidenced by swelling and/or pain
   b. Typically prepatellar bursa, pes anserinus bursa, tibial collateral ligament bursa, deep infrapatellar bursa
2. **Mechanism of injury**
   a. Usually overuse
   b. May be secondary to direct blow with bleeding into bursa
3. **Predisposing factors**—for pes anserinus bursitis, tight hamstrings seem to predispose.
4. **History**
   a. Direct blow
   b. Overuse
   c. Complaints of swelling (if prepatellar bursa)
   d. Complaints of pain in prepatellar region (for prepatellar bursitis), in distal patellar tendon region (for deep infrapatellar bursitis), in proximal medial tibia (for pes anserinus bursitis), or over medial joint line (for tibial collateral ligament bursitis)
5. **Examination**
   a. For prepatellar bursa, look for localized swelling and tenderness.
   b. For others, tenderness over described areas.
6. **X-rays** are not helpful for diagnosis.
7. **Differential diagnosis**
   a. For deep infrapatellar bursitis, other causes of patellar tendon pain
   b. For tibial collateral ligament bursitis, medial meniscus tear
   c. For prepatellar bursitis, usually no differential
   d. For pes anserinus bursitis, pain from pes anserinus tendons, tumors, other causes of proximal medial tibial pain
8. **Treatment**
   a. Acute prepatellar bursitis—ice, compression, possible aspiration, padding
   b. Chronic prepatellar bursitis—NSAIDs, compression, hamstring stretching, ultrasound, possible aspiration and corticosteroid injection
   c. Pes anserinus bursitis—hamstring stretching, ultrasound, NSAIDs, corticosteroid injection
   d. Tibial collateral ligament bursitis—injection, both as a diagnostic test as well as treatment
   e. Deep infrapatellar bursitis—hamstring stretching, possible injection **behind** patellar tendon

B. Other tendinitis

1. **Description**
   a. Inflammation of any of the other tendinous structures about the knee, typically the semimembranosus, popliteus, or biceps femoris tendons
   b. Rarely, inflammation of the gastrocnemius tendon
2. **Mechanism of injury**
   a. Usually overuse
   b. Much less commonly, a single episode of strain is the cause
   c. Popliteus tendinitis is usually a running injury.
3. **Predisposing factors:** for semimembranosus, pes anserinus, or biceps femoris tendinitis, hamstring tightness predisposes.
4. **History**
   a. Overuse activity
   b. Occasionally, acute strain

c. Complaints of pain over the appropriate tendon area
d. For popliteus tendinitis, lateral knee pain, especially while running downhill

5. **Examination**
a. Tenderness over appropriate tendon
b. Tight hamstrings
c. For popliteus tendinitis, painful resisted internal rotation of tibia with knee flexed
d. For all, initially pain on stretching tendon, later pain on active contraction of tendon

6. **X-rays**—usually not helpful
7. **Differential diagnosis**
a. Hamstring tendinitis occasionally to be differentiated from sciatica
b. Semimembranosus tendinitis may be confused with medial meniscus disorders.
c. For popliteus tendinitis, lateral meniscus injury, iliotibial band friction syndrome

8. **Treatment**
a. Usual anti-inflammatory methods
b. Hamstring stretching exercises
c. May require corticosteroid injection

C. **Neuromas**
1. **Description**
a. Non-neoplastic enlargement of nerve, usually from direct trauma
b. Typically involves various portions of saphenous nerve around the knee

2. **Mechanism of injury**
a. Direct blow
b. Previous surgery

3. **Predisposing factors**—previous surgical incisions
4. **History**
a. Direct blow
b. Previous surgery
c. Pain, particularly nerve-like quality, i.e., paresthesias, burning, other alterations of sensation

5. **Examination**
a. Tenderness over neuroma
b. Positive Tinel's sign
c. Objective changes in sensation in appropriate distribution

6. **X-rays** are not helpful.
7. **Differential diagnosis**—more central sources of nerve compression
8. **Treatment**
a. Injection
b. Surgical excision

D. **Loose bodies** ("joint mouse," chondral fracture, osteochondral fracture, osteochondritis dissecans)
1. **Description:** Cartilaginous or osteocartilaginous fragments usually free-floating within knee joint (though may be attached to synovium more or less firmly)
2. **Mechanism of injury**
a. Dislocation of patella (see "Instability syndromes," page 569)
b. Other trauma to joint surface
c. May be result of preexisting osteochondritis dissecans
d. Rarely due to synovial osteochondromatosis

3. **Predisposing factors**
a. Predisposition to patellar dislocation
b. Preexisting osteochondritis dissecans

4. **History**
   a. Consistent with previous patellar instability
   b. Other twisting or direct blow injury
   c. Locking episodes
   d. Subcutaneous mass that comes and goes and may be felt in various locations about the knee
5. **Examination**
   a. Patellar findings
   b. May feel movable mass, usually around patellofemoral joint, though it may be at anteromedial or anterolateral joint line
6. **X-rays**
   a. Purely cartilaginous fragments are not visible.
   b. Very small bony loose bodies may be obscured.
   c. Most loose bodies of significance containing bone are visible.
   d. Source (e.g., osteochondritis dissecans) may be seen.
   e. Tomogram, CT scan, or arthrogram may help in delineation.
7. **Differential diagnosis**—meniscal tears as source of locking
8. **Treatment**
   a. Symptomatic loose bodies require surgical removal, usually arthroscopically.
   b. A few loose bodies may require replacement and internal fixation.
   c. Patellofemoral instability may require treatment.
   d. Osteochondritis dissecans may require other treatment.
   e. Large chondral or osteochondral fracture may require surgical debridement of joint surface and prolonged protected weight-bearing.

E. **Cysts** (popliteal cyst, popliteal ganglion, Baker's cyst, meniscus cyst)
1. **Description:** fluid-filled lesion about the knee arising usually as an extension of the synovial space, either into a normal bursal structure or into soft tissue surrounding the knee
2. **Mechanism of injury:** normally, no specific injury is involved.
3. **Predisposing factors**—none
4. **History:** localized swelling in popliteal space or over meniscus
5. **Examination:** cystic swelling in medial popliteal space or over mid-joint line, usually lateral joint line
6. **X-rays**
   a. Plain films are no help.
   b. MRI is very helpful in delineating cysts.
7. **Differential diagnosis**—other tumorous lesions about the knee
8. **Treatment**
   a. May try aspiration and injection with corticosteroid; however, not very likely to give permanent cure
   b. Surgical excision is usually curative.
   c. **Most important** is to understand that presence of cyst is usually secondary to another process in the knee that leads to excessive synovial fluid, in turn causing the cyst. Most likely a meniscal tear causing a popliteal cyst, or lateral meniscus tear causing a lateral meniscus cyst. **Underlying disorders must be treated**.

F. **Iliotibial band friction syndrome**
1. **Description**
   a. Chronic inflammatory process involving soft tissues adjacent to the lateral femoral epicondyle
   b. Presumably due to chronic "friction" of iliotibial band rubbing over bony prominence of this area

2. **Mechanism of injury**
   a. Overuse mechanism
   b. Majority of cases due to running
3. **Predisposing factors**
   a. Varus alignment of knee
   b. Running on sloped surfaces
4. **History**
   a. Lateral knee pain on activity
   b. Occasional popping
5. **Examination**
   a. Tenderness over lateral femoral epicondyle
   b. Tight iliotibial band
   c. Absence of intra-articular findings
6. **X-rays** are no help.
7. **Differential diagnosis**
   a. Other causes of lateral knee pain, especially popliteus tendinitis
   b. Lateral meniscus disorders
   c. Lateral patellofemoral joint sources such as VL tendinitis
8. **Treatment**
   a. Iliotibial band stretching exercises
   b. Anti-inflammatory treatment
   c. Ultrasound to lateral femoral epicondyle
   d. Corticosteroid injection
   e. Rarely, surgery to release area of tightness

50

Ankle and Leg Injuries

David E. Brown, M.D.

I. Physical Examination

A. **Inspection**

1. The goal is to localize the patient's symptoms to a particular anatomic structure.
2. Check for
   a. Localized swelling
   b. Abrasions
   c. Ecchymosis
   d. Deformity

B. **Palpation**

1. Carefully locate specific structures that are tender or swollen.
   a. Bone or soft tissue?
   b. Localized or diffuse?
   c. Intra-articular or extra-articular?
2. Gross crepitus indicates a fracture, whereas fine crepitus can be due to tenosynovitis.
3. Check for hypertrophic spurs over the ankle and thickening of the Achilles tendon.
4. Are all tendons in continuity?
5. Are the compartments of the calf tight?

C. **Ankle range of motion**

1. Assess the total arc of ankle motion in dorsiflexion, plantarflexion, inversion, and eversion. Compare to the opposite side.
2. Marked muscle guarding is usually due to a severe ligament injury, fracture, or sepsis.
3. Determine if active, passive, or resisted motion causes pain.

D. **Neurovascular assessment**

1. Test both manual muscle strength and sensation.
2. Check the dorsalis pedis and posterior tibialis pulses.

E. **Specific tests**

1. **Anterior drawer test**—use to assess anterior-posterior translation of the ankle
   a. Stabilize the distal tibia, grasp the heel with your dominant hand, and apply an anterior force (Fig. 1).
   b. Perform this test with the ankle in neutral position and plantarflexion. Compare to the opposite side.
   c. Significant excursion indicates laxity of the anterior talofibular ligament. Grinding or clicking during translation may indicate an occult fracture or degeneration of the articular surfaces.
2. **Talar tilt**
   a. Position your hands as in the drawer test. Apply an inversion stress to the heel and ankle (Fig. 2).
   b. Excessive tilt with a soft endpoint occurs with injury to the calcaneofibular ligament.

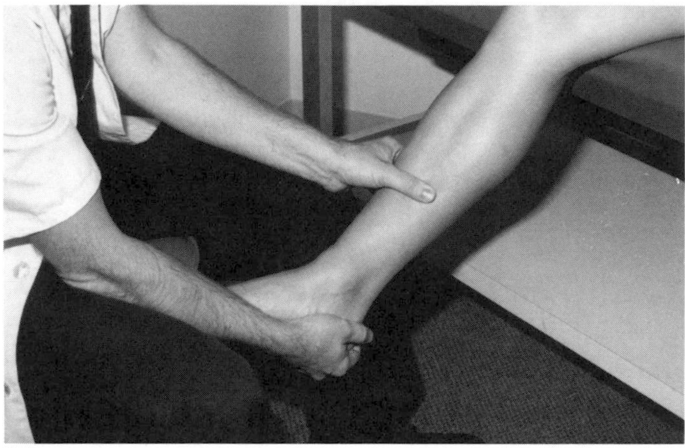

FIGURE 1. Anterior drawer test.

3. **Thompson squeeze test**
   a. Place the patient prone with the feet over the end of the table. Squeezing the calf should cause passive plantarflexion of the ankle (Fig. 3).
   b. Absence of plantarflexion (positive Thompson test) is due to a completely torn Achilles tendon.
4. **Syndesmosis squeeze test**
   a. Squeeze the distal fibular shaft toward the tibia.
   b. Localized pain usually indicates a fibular fracture or disruption of either the interosseus membrane or the distal tibia-fibula syndesmosis.
5. **External rotation stress test**
   a. Evaluate the patient seated with the knee flexed 90°. Stabilize the leg and externally rotate the foot and ankle.
   b. Pain over the distal tibia-fibula joint may indicate tear of its ligaments.
6. **Peroneal stress test**
   a. Evaluate the patient seated with leg over table, knee flexed 90°. Have the patient actively dorsiflex and evert the ankle against resistance.
   b. The peroneal tendons sublux or dislocate if unstable.

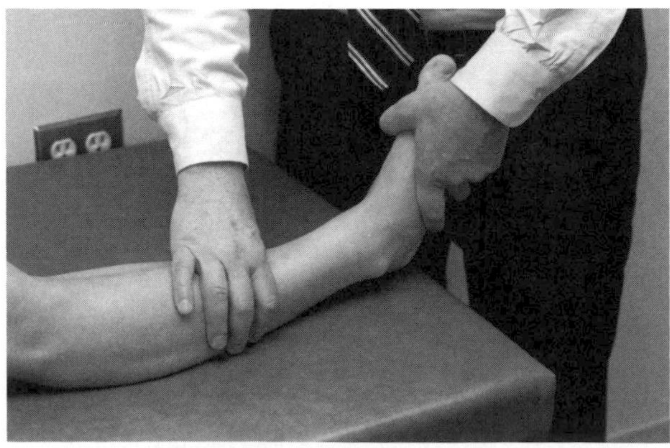

FIGURE 2. Talar tilt stress test.

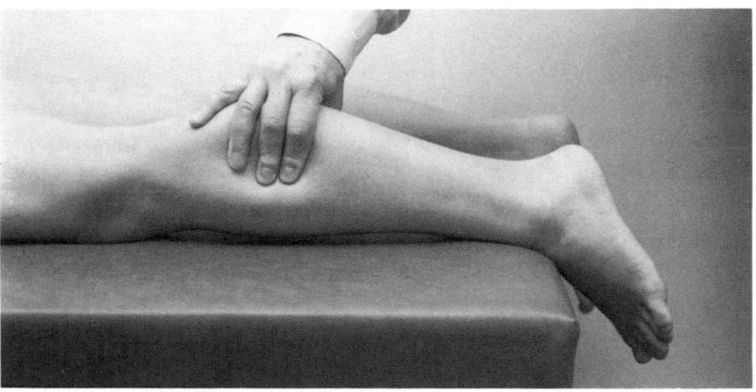

FIGURE 3. Normal Thompson test.

7. **Compartment pressure measurements**
   a. Intracompartmental pressures in all four leg compartments (anterior, lateral, superficial posterior, and deep posterior [Fig. 4]) are determined using either a slit-catheter or the solid-state intracompartment catheter (STIC).
   b. In an **acute** injury situation, the following values and recommendations are used:
      i. 0–10 mm Hg = normal
      ii. 10–30 mm Hg = elevated, but not dangerous
      iii. 30–40 mm Hg = watch closely, correlate with the clinical picture, and perform repeated pressure measurements until symptoms resolve
      iv. 40–60 mm Hg = usually dangerous, requiring compartment release
      v. > 60 mm Hg = consistently dangerous, requires urgent release
   c. In patients who are thought to have **chronic** compartment syndrome, measurements are first made at rest. The patient is then exercised until symptoms occur. Pressure measurements are made postexercise until they return to normal.
      i. In normal legs, resting pressures are below 12 mm Hg, rise quickly with exercise to levels as high as 80 mm Hg, and return to the resting level within 5 minutes.
      ii. Values greater than the above-listed are suspicious for a chronic compartment syndrome.
      iii. The most important finding is a failure to return to the resting pressure level within 5 minutes after cessation of exercise.

F. **Radiographic tests**
   1. **Plain x-rays**
      a. At least an anteroposterior and lateral view of the injured segment should be obtained.
      b. If the ankle is involved, a mortise view is also obtained.
      c. If clinically indicated by the exam, the joints above and below are visualized.
   2. **Stress x-rays** allow documentation of the degree of ankle instability.
      a. **Anterior drawer:** A lateral radiograph is made while the examiner manually performs the anterior drawer test. More than 8 mm of anterior displacement of the talus (compared to the unstressed lateral x-ray) indicates an incompetent anterior talofibular ligament (Fig. 5).
      b. **Talar tilt:** A mortise radiograph is made while the examiner performs the talar tilt test on both the injured and the normal ankles. The angle between the tibial plafond and the talar dome is measured. If the injured ankle has a tilt of 25° or is 10° greater than the normal side, the calcaneofibular ligament is incompetent (Fig. 6).

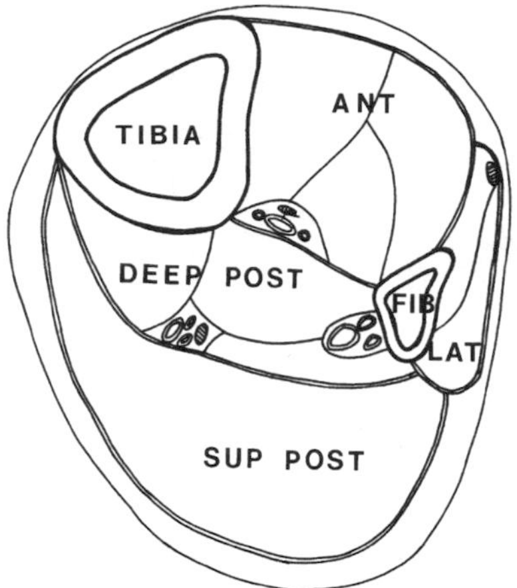

FIGURE 4. The four compartments of the leg.

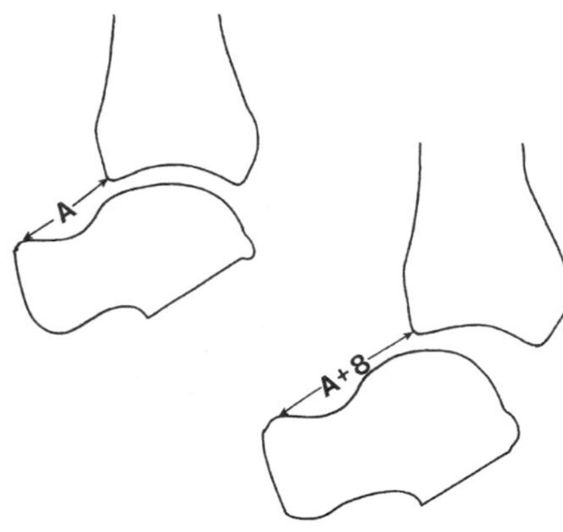

FIGURE 5. Anterior drawer sign is positive if there is > 8 mm displacement between the two fixed points.

   c. **External rotation stress test:** A mortise radiograph is performed when the examiner performs the external rotation stress test. Widening of the distal tibia-fibula clear space to 6 mm or greater indicates disruption of this joint.
3. **Technetium bone scan:** Detects stress fractures as early as 1–2 days after the onset of symptoms (plain x-rays commonly are negative for the first 2 weeks of symptoms). Because the scan is also more sensitive than plain x-rays, it can be used for earlier detection of infections or degenerative arthritis.
4. **Tomograms and computed tomography (CT):** Useful for evaluating the size and position of intra-articular fractures, such as talar dome osteochondral lesions
5. **Magnetic resonance imaging (MRI):** Sensitive in evaluating soft tissue pathology (partial tears of muscle and tendon, periosteal avulsion from the tibia, and soft tissue masses)

II. Specific Clinical Conditions

A. Acute lateral ankle sprains

1. **Description:** Complete or partial disruption of the talofibular, calcaneofibular, subtalar, or tibiofibular ligaments; may be associated tearing of the interosseous membrane
2. **Associated injuries**
   a. Fractures of the fibula, talus, calcaneus, or metatarsals
   b. Commonly peroneal tendon strains or subluxations and stretch neuropraxia of the sensory nerves of the foot
3. **History**
   a. Acute inversion of the ankle
   b. Amount of early swelling and presence of a "pop" at time of injury are good guides to severity of injury
   c. **Persistent pain after a sprain has been rehabilitated** requires a workup for:
      i. Chronic instability
      ii. Degenerative joint disease
      iii. Loose body
      iv. Occult fractures
      v. Intra-articular meniscoid lesions
      vi. Peroneal tendon injury

4. **Examination**
   a. Evaluate swelling, neurovascular status, and range of motion.
   b. Localize the tenderness to a specific anatomic structure.
   c. Perform the syndesmosis squeeze test and external rotation stress test.
   d. Determine the degree of ligament laxity with anterior drawer and talar tilt tests.
5. **X-rays**
   a. Should be obtained in any significant injury. Look for associated fractures.
   b. **Carefully assess the mortise view for widening**. Beware of the high fibular fracture or tibia-fibula diastasis.
   c. Consider stress x-rays.
6. **Grade the injury** (Table 1).
7. **Treatment of grades I–II**
   a. **Acute phase:**
      i. Ice for 20 minutes at least four times a day until all swelling is gone
      ii. Compression (horseshoe wraps, taping)
      iii. Elevation (48–72 hours)
      iv. Crutches if unable to bear weight without pain; advance weightbearing as tolerated by pain
   b. **Rehabilitation phase:**
      i. Support (tape, Aircast, canvas lacer)
      ii. Range of motion—plantarflexion and dorsiflexion
      iii. Strengthen evertors and dorsiflexors with resistive exercises
      iv. Proprioception training
      v. Agility drills
      vi. Endurance training
      vii. Return to sport
      viii. Support for 3–6 months

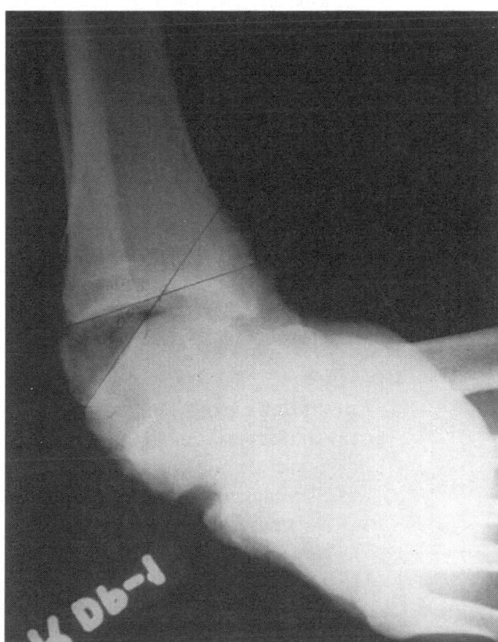

FIGURE 6. Positive talar tilt stress x-ray.

TABLE 1. Lateral Ankle Ligament Classification

Grade	Pathology	Examination
I	Partial tear	Minimal swelling No laxity
II	Partial tear ATFL or CFL	Mild-to-moderate swelling Mild-to-moderate laxity
IIIa	Complete tear ATFL	Substantial swelling Positive anterior drawer
IIIb	Complete tear ATFL and CFL	Substantial swelling Positive anterior drawer and talar tilt
IIIc	Complete tear ATFL and CFL Peroneal tendon tear or subluxation	Swelling Positive anterior drawer Positive talar tilt Tenderness or instability of peroneal tendons
IV	Complete tear ATFL and CFL Occult fracture	Swelling Positive anterior drawer Talar tilt, positive or negative Tender over involved bone

AFTL = Anterior talofibular ligament; CFL = Calcaneofibular ligament.

8. **Treatment of grade III and grade IV**
   a. Because of pain, swelling, and instability, this injury needs additional acute protection (short-leg cast, Aircast, or other rigid support) for 1–3 weeks.
   b. After completing acute phase immobilization, follow rehabilitation phase described previously.
   c. Some surgeons believe ligament repair is needed when there is gross instability in the high-performance athlete or in grade IIIc and grade IV injuries.
   d. Grade IIIc injuries usually need repair of the peroneal retinaculum.
   e. For grade IV injuries, see also the specific fracture section.
9. **Treatment of syndesmosis sprains:** In addition to the aforementioned methods, these patients need prolonged support (consider high Aircast). Patients often have pain for several months after injury.
10. **Treatment of tibia-fibula diastasis:** Open reduction and internal fixation with a syndesmosis screw

B. **Chronic lateral ankle ligament instability**
1. **History**
   a. Recurrent inversion injuries, often requiring several weeks to return to sport
   b. Athlete feels ankle is unstable on hills or uneven ground
   c. Pain and swelling with activity
2. **Examination:** Positive anterior drawer or talar tilt test
3. **X-rays**
   a. Repeat plain x-rays to evaluate for occult fracture.
   b. Perform stress x-rays.
4. **Classify**
   a. **Functional instability:**
      i. Ankle motion beyond voluntary control
      ii. Sense of instability
      iii. Normal range of motion
      iv. Normal or symmetric laxity exam
      v. Normal or equivocal stress x-rays
   b. **Mechanical instability:**
      i. Ankle motion beyond normal physiologic range
      ii. Abnormal laxity exam and stress x-rays

5. **Treatment**
   a. **Functional instability:**
      i. Eversion and dorsiflexion strengthening
      ii. Achilles stretching
      iii. Functional bracing and taping
   b. **Mechanical instability:**
      i. Rehabilitate as discussed previously for at least 3 months.
      ii. If rehabilitation is unsuccessful, perform repair (modified Brostrom) or reconstruction (Chrisman-Snook or similar).

C. **Traumatic fractures of the leg and ankle**
1. **Tibial shaft**
   a. **Description:** A fracture of the tibia below the tibial plateau and above the malleoli; does not involve the articular surfaces.
   b. **Mechanism of injury:**
      i. Results from direct impact or severe rotation on a fixed foot
      ii. Usually the result of high energy transmitted to the leg
      iii. Most common in skiers and soccer players
   c. **History:** The athlete recalls a sudden severe pain after the injury, is unable to bear weight, and often "heard the bone crack."
   d. **Examination:**
      i. **Determine if the fracture is open!** Even the smallest laceration or puncture site near the fracture should arouse concern for an open fracture.
      ii. Always note the distal neurovascular status before moving or manipulating the patient.
      iii. Deformity, gross bone motion at the suspected fracture site, crepitus, and extreme bone tenderness are usually present.
      iv. Examine the joints above and below the fracture site for additional injuries.
   e. **X-rays:** Anteroposterior, lateral, and oblique views of the whole tibia are necessary. If there is any concern for the nearby joints, obtain x-rays of those areas.
   f. **Treatment:**
      i. **Immediate** splinting using air, plaster, or preformed metal splints. Immobilize the joints above and below the site of injury.
      ii. **Open** fractures require irrigation, debridement, and antibiotic coverage.
      iii. **Stable** fractures with less than 5° of varus/valgus angulation may be treated in a long leg cast, with partial weight bearing for 2–4 weeks. This is followed by a fracture brace (which allows knee and ankle motion) until the fracture is completely healed.
      iv. If there is more than 5° malalignment, fracture reduction is indicated.
      v. Unstable comminuted or oblique fractures require longer periods of protection from weight bearing. As the fracture heals, it becomes more stable, allowing use of a fracture brace.
      vi. Fractures with an intact fibula tend to heal in varus and internal rotation. Therefore, the first cast should be applied with the fracture in mild valgus and external rotation.
      vii. Intramedullary nailing allows earlier weight bearing and rehabilitation of unstable fractures, but is more expensive and involves higher morbidity (infection, nonunion). Nevertheless, intramedullary nailing should be strongly considered for the unstable fracture. Early joint motion and weight bearing limit the amount and severity of a cast disease (joint stiffness and muscle weakness).
2. **Fibular shaft (intact tibia and ankle)**
   a. **Description:** An isolated fracture in midshaft, usually transverse
   b. **Mechanism of injury:** Direct blow to the side of the leg

c. **History:** The athlete can usually walk or even run but may note moderate pain over the fracture site.
d. **Examination:** Reveals tenderness and mild crepitus over the shaft of the fibula; ankle is normal
e. **Treatment:**
   i. **Protection** from activities that cause pain
   ii. May need crutches for several days to 2 weeks
   iii. Rarely requires a cast
   iv. Return to sports usually possible at 2–4 weeks

3. **Ankle fractures**
   a. **Description:** Fractures of one or both malleoli. Spiral fractures of the fibula regardless of position usually involve the ankle.
   b. **Mechanism of injury:** Usually is external rotation of the foot, combined with either pronation or supination.
   c. **History:** The athlete is unable to bear weight on the injured extremity, often heard a "crack," and is in considerable pain.
   d. **Examination:**
      i. Reveals tenderness and crepitus over the involved bone
      ii. May reveal gross instability or deformity of the ankle
      iii. **Check the distal neurovascular status**.
      iv. **Determine if fracture is open!**
   e. **X-rays:**
      i. Confirm the fracture location and displacement.
      ii. Carefully assess the mortise view. If the distance between the medial malleolus and the medial talus is greater than the distance between the superior talar dome and the tibial plafond, suspect a torn deltoid ligament. Although a widened mortise is most commonly seen with distal fibula fractures, widening may also occur without a fibula fracture or with high fibula fractures.
   f. **Treatment:**
      i. Splint immediately (see "Tibial Shaft," page 585).
      ii. Open fractures require urgent, thorough irrigation and debridement in the operating room, followed by antibiotic coverage.
      iii. **Nondisplaced fractures** with an intact mortise can be treated with cast immobilization for 4–6 weeks, followed by a functional brace until completely healed.
      iv. **Displaced fractures** are best treated with anatomic open reduction and internal fixation.

4. **Transchondral talar dome fractures**
   a. **Description:** A medial or lateral fracture of the superior dome of the talus
   b. **Mechanism of injury:** Inversion or eversion of the ankle
   c. **Predisposing factors:** Often seen with displaced ankle fractures or ankle ligament instability
   d. **History:** Usually noted acutely, but may present as chronic pain after an ankle "sprain"
   e. **Examination:**
      i. There is usually an ankle effusion and tenderness directly over the corner of the talus that is involved.
      ii. Mild crepitus may be present.
   f. **X-rays:**
      i. Anteroposterior, lateral, mortise, or plantarflexed mortise views may reveal the lesion (Fig. 7).
      ii. Tomograms or CT scans are frequently needed to confirm and better define the extent of the lesion.

g. **Treatment:**
   i. **Acute, nondisplaced**—immobilize for 6 weeks in cast or rigid brace. Once healed, rehabilitate as for ankle sprain.
   ii. **Acute or chronic, displaced**—perform surgical excision or replacement of the fragment and internal fixation, with curettage of the base of the lesion.
   iii. **Chronic, nondisplaced**—splint or cast for 4 weeks and reassess x-rays and clinical symptoms. Persistent symptoms require excision of the lesion.
   iv. In chronic cases, always assess for concomitant ligament instability. This may require reconstruction at the time of excision of the fragment.

5. **Posterior process fractures of talus, lateral process fractures of talus, and anterior process fractures of calcaneus**
   a. **Mechanism of injury:** Posterior process fractures (Fig. 8) occur with inversion and extreme plantarflexion, whereas the latter two occur with inversion alone.
   b. **Examination:** A careful exam is essential to make the diagnosis.
      i. Only the athlete with a lateral process fracture is tender over the lateral ligaments.
      ii. With a posterior process fracture, tenderness is localized to the posterior ankle just anterior to the Achilles.
      iii. The patient with an anterior process calcaneus fracture is tender 2–3 cm distal and anterior to the lateral malleolus.
   c. **X-rays:** Anteroposterior and lateral views of the ankle should reveal talus fractures, whereas the calcaneus fracture is best seen on an oblique foot view.
   d. **Treatment**
      i. **Posterior process of talus:**
         • Acute—short leg non–weight-bearing cast for 6 weeks
         • Chronic, symptomatic—excision
      ii. **Lateral process fracture of talus:**
         • Nondisplaced—short leg weight-bearing cast for 3–4 weeks
         • Displaced or neglected—open reduction, internal fixation or excision
      iii. **Anterior process calcaneus fracture:**
         • Acute—short leg non–weight-bearing cast for 6 weeks
         • Chronic—injection of corticosteroid using fluoroscopy; continued symptoms warrant excision

D. **Stress fractures of the tibia and fibula**
   1. **Description:** Tibial stress fractures occur most commonly at the junction of the mid and distal thirds of the tibia, the posterior medial tibial plateau, or just distal to the tubercle. Fibula stress fractures usually occur in the distal metadiaphyseal region.

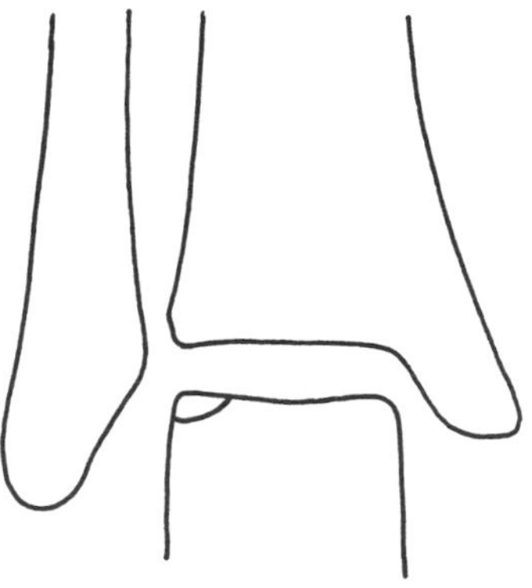

FIGURE 7. Transchondral lateral talar dome fracture.

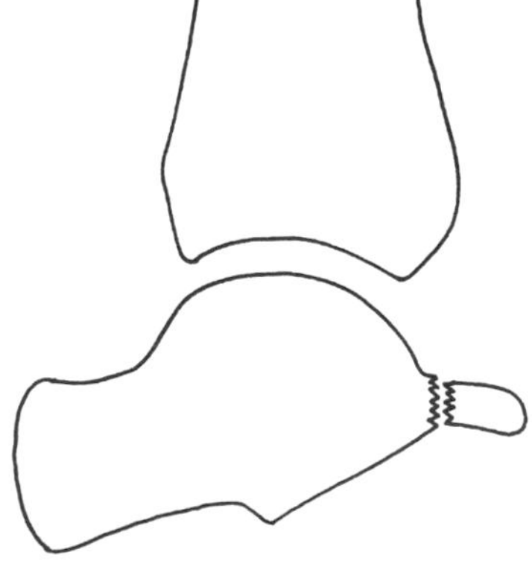

FIGURE 8. Posterior process talus fracture.

2. **Mechanism of injury:** Repetitive overload of the bone, usually caused by a change in training habits (increased intensity, duration or type of workout, a change in running surface or style of shoe), causes microfracture at area of excessive bone resorption.
3. **History:** Pain increases during the run and decreases or stops after completion. Often the athlete has a precipitous onset of pain.
4. **Examination:** There is localized bone tenderness. Ultrasound increases the pain when applied over the fracture site.
5. **X-rays**
   a. Rarely positive until 2 weeks after onset of symptoms
   b. Earliest finding is periosteal thickening or layering
6. **Special consideration**—beware of the **anterior tibial cortical stress fracture**. These frequently have delayed union, nonunion, and fracture completion.
7. **Treatment**
   a. Positive x-ray—use stress fracture protocol
   b. Negative x-ray but suspicious clinical picture—stress fracture protocol, repeat x-ray in 2–3 weeks. If you must know immediately or the athlete refuses to follow the protocol, obtain bone scan to confirm the diagnosis.
   c. **Stress fracture protocol:**
      i. Rest until all bone tenderness subsides.
      ii. Allow pain-free activities only. This may require crutches for a short time.
      iii. Start a flexibility and strength program.
      iv. Cross training—swim, bike, and "run" in pool with flotation vest; ice after workout.
      v. Begin the following running schedule when pain free (usually 4–8 weeks):
         (a) **Week 1**—run every other day, half the usual training distance, 1 minute per mile slower than usual training pace
         (b) **Week 2**—normal training frequency, ¾ usual training distance, same pace as week 1
         (c) **Week 3**—¾ usual training distance, 30 seconds per mile slower than usual training pace
         (d) **Week 4**—resume usual distance, 30 seconds per mile slower than usual training pace. After completing this week, if no pain, may resume full training schedule.
   d. Long-leg Aircast may allow earlier return to activity for competitive athletes. This device probably disperses forces over a greater area, resulting in decreased stress at the fracture site. Use must be pain free!

E. **Chronic exertional compartment syndrome**
   1. **Description:** Excessive pressure within an enclosed leg fascial compartment, causing reduction in blood flow to that compartment
   2. **History**
      a. These athletes typically have pain that begins at a consistent time into the exercise session. Symptoms then subside slowly after termination of the exercise.
      b. Pain is rarely present before exercise.
      c. There may be numbness on the dorsum of the foot with weakness of ankle dorsiflexion.
   3. **Examination**
      a. There may be firmness of the involved compartment while the athlete is symptomatic.
      b. The rest of the exam is usually normal.
      c. Compartment pressure measurements are the key in making the diagnosis. See "Compartment pressure measurements," page 581.
   4. **Treatment:** Surgical release of the offending compartment provides good results.

F. **Medial tibial stress syndrome**

1. **Description:** The periosteum is inflamed or avulsed from the posterior-medial distal tibia. If avulsed, fibrofatty tissue fills the defect.
2. **History**
   a. May be associated with the same training errors as stress fractures, but more likely to have an anatomic variation (heavy runner, cavus foot, overpronation) or poor running technique (increased leg rotation, leg cross-over).
   b. Most patients have had symptoms for a long time.
   c. Pain may eventually occur with minimal exertion or shortly after the onset of exercise.
3. **Examination**
   a. Pain and tenderness are localized to the area immediately posterior to the tibial ridge and extending for 6–10 cm.
   b. Obtain compartment pressure measurements because many of these patients have a concomitant deep posterior compartment syndrome.
4. **X-rays:** In chronic cases, there may be mild thickening or undulation of the posterior distal tibia. The bone scan is normal or shows a mild diffuse uptake along the painful area.
5. **Treatment**
   a. Rest—often for prolonged period
   b. Ice, stretch, and careful warm-up
   c. Correct anatomic variations with a semirigid foot orthosis
   d. A running shoe that provides both shock absorption and a firm heel counter
   e. Anti-inflammatory medication
   f. Resistant cases may require surgical cauterization of the tibial ridge with excision of the fibrofatty tissue.

G. **Overuse myositis (posterior tibialis, anterior tibialis, peroneals), alias "shin splints"**

1. **History:** Usually occurs early in season in inexperienced athletes; symptoms similar to periostitis but located over muscle-tendon units instead of along the tibial ridge
2. **Treatment:** Nonsurgical treatment is same as discussed previously, but condition resolves more quickly and consistently

H. **Acute compartment syndrome**

1. **Description:** Acute increase in tissue pressure within an enclosed anatomic space leads to increased local venous pressure, which causes decrease in arteriovenous gradient and decrease in blood flow
2. **History**
   a. Severe pain out of proportion to the clinical situation.
   b. Recent history of trauma, excess exercise, vascular injury, or prolonged, externally applied pressure.
3. **Examination**
   a. Weakness of muscles in the compartment
   b. Pain with passive stretch of these muscles
   c. Tenderness and tightness of compartment
   d. Hypesthesia of nerve traversing the compartment
   e. Compartment pressure measurements (at rest)
4. **Treatment**
   a. Remove circular dressings.
   b. Position leg at level of the heart.
   c. Decompress compartment if there is not **prompt** resolution of symptoms.
   d. Delay skin closure.

I. **Achilles tendon ruptures**
   1. **Description:** Complete disruption of the Achilles tendon, probably due to tendon degeneration and repeated microtrauma
   2. **History**
      a. Athlete feels "pop" and sensation of being kicked or cut in the heel
      b. Often occurs during the push-off phase of running
      c. Commonly seen in a 30–50-year-old athlete
   3. **Examination**
      a. Weak ankle plantarflexion and palpable defect in tendon
      b. Thompson test is positive (absent plantarflexion)
   4. **Treatment:** Casting for as little as 4 weeks causes permanent calf weakness. Options should be presented to the patient.
      a. Surgical repair is usually recommended in athletes because it offers lower risk of rerupture (< 2%) and better push-off strength:
         i. Repair technique—locking, nonabsorbable suture
         ii. Splint in equinus for 7–10 days
         iii. Cast boot in partial equinus 3–5 weeks, partial weight bearing, active and passive plantarflexion
         iv. Shoe with heel lift 4–6 weeks
      b. Nonoperative treatment requires cast immobilization for 8–12 weeks:
         i. Cast (some prefer long-leg) in full equinus for 4–6 weeks
         ii. Short-leg cast in partial equinus for 4–6 weeks
         iii. Follow with heel lift for 3 months
      c. Stretching and strengthening program

J. **Acute partial gastrocnemius tears**
   1. **Description:** Partial disruption in medial head of the gastrocnemius muscle at the musculotendinous junction
   2. **History:** Acute event while hill running, jumping, or other activity that requires forceful push-off
   3. **Examination:** No defect and negative Thompson test
   4. **Treatment**
      a. ½-inch heel lift, calf sleeve
      b. Avoid running, jumping, push-off
      c. Ice until pain and swelling subside
      d. Isometric calf contractions in plantarflexion followed by gentle stretching
      e. 3–6 weeks to full recovery

K. **Achilles tendinitis**
   1. **History:** Athletes with tight heel cords, overpronation, a recent change in shoes, or recent increase in training are most susceptible. Chronic cases are probably due to a partial tear of the tendon, tendon degeneration, or paratenon scarring.
   2. **Examination:** Tenderness, thickening, and fine crepitation are present either at insertion or 2–6 cm from insertion.
   3. **X-rays**
      a. Under penetrated lateral x-ray may show tendon thickening, insertion site calcification
      b. Magnetic resonance imaging or ultrasound demonstrates partial tear, degeneration, or fluid surrounding the tendon
   4. **Treatment**
      a. Correct anatomic variations (orthotics)
      b. Correct training errors
      c. Heel lift for several weeks
      d. Ice, anti-inflammatory medication, and phonophoresis to control inflammation

e. *Never* inject tendon with corticosteroid
f. Compulsive stretching program
g. Chronic symptoms may require surgical release of the peritenon with debridement of degenerative or partially torn tendon

L. **Retrocalcaneal bursitis**
1. **Description:** Inflammation and thickening of the retrocalcaneal bursa (immediately anterior to the insertion of the Achilles tendon)
2. **History**
a. Aching pain with exercise
b. Athlete's heel counter may be too constrictive, causing friction
c. Adolescent female skaters and runners most common
3. **Examination**
a. Tenderness and swelling localized anterior to the insertion of the Achilles tendon
b. Skin thickened, especially on lateral side
c. Hindfoot likely in varus
d. Examine athlete's shoes for excessive heel height, rigidity, or constrictive shape
4. **X-rays:** May demonstrate a prominent superior projection of the calcaneus or obliteration of the normal radiopaque space anterior to the tendon
5. **Treatment**
a. Nonsurgical treatment similar to that for Achilles tendinitis
b. For resistant symptoms, debridement of bursa and excision of superior projection of calcaneus

M. **Intra-articular meniscoid lesion**
1. **Description:** A localized fibrotic synovitis in the lateral ankle that may occur after inversion sprains
2. **History:** Persistent pain, swelling, catching in the anterolateral aspect of the ankle many months after a severe ankle injury
3. **Examination:** Mild swelling and tenderness localized to anterolateral ankle may be only abnormalities
4. **Treatment:** Arthroscopic debridement provides good relief.

N. **Posterior tibial tendinitis**
1. **History**
a. Diffuse pain and swelling posterior to medial malleolus or at its insertion into navicular
b. May be sequelae of an ankle sprain
c. Athletes at risk have planovalgus foot and play sports with sudden start-stop or push-off actions.
2. **Examination**
a. Tenderness localized to posterior tibialis tendon
b. Pain with passive pronation and active supination
c. Athlete may have pain and weakness when asked to stand on toes
3. **Treatment**
a. Rest, ice, anti-inflammatory medication
b. Acute—support strapping or cast if severe
c. Medial heel counter or medial posted orthosis to prevent pronation
d. Persistent—debride partial tears and proliferative synovium, decompress sheath, possibly add Kidner procedure
e. Complete rupture—reconstruct with contiguous long flexor tendons and/or subtalar fusion

O. **Flexor hallucis longus tendinitis**
1. **History**
a. Pain and swelling posterior to medial malleolus

b. Runners may have pain at sesamoids
c. Dancers and athletes involved in repetitive stop-start or push-off activities susceptible

2. **Examination:** Pain with hallux range of motion
3. **Treatment**
   a. Rest, ice, anti-inflammatory medication
   b. Rigid shoe, steel shank, heel lift
   c. Persistent—treat as for posterior tibialis

P. **Anterior tibialis tendinitis**

1. **History**
   a. Pain over dorsum of foot
   b. Runners doing hill work and skiers (owing to direct irritation from boots) most prone
2. **Examination:** Tenderness and swelling localized to the anterior tibialis tendon; pain increased by resisted ankle dorsiflexion
3. **X-rays:** Look for osteophytes on anterior distal tibia.
4. **Treatment**
   a. Rest, ice, anti-inflammatory medication, physical therapy modalities
   b. Persistent symptoms—excise osteophytes, debride peritenon

Q. **Peroneal tendon subluxation**

1. **Description:** The peroneal retinaculum is detached from its normal insertion on the posterior border of the fibula to the lateral surface of the fibula. This occurs during an acute dorsiflexion and inversion stress injury while the peroneal muscles are contracting forcefully. Peroneus brevis may tear longitudinally.
2. **History**
   a. Prior history of an ankle sprain
   b. Athlete may sense tendons subluxating with ankle range of motion
   c. Most common in skiers and basketball players
   d. If tendon tear present, pain behind lateral malleolus may be dominant symptom
3. **Examination**
   a. Subluxation of the peroneal tendons with active dorsiflexion and eversion against resistance
   b. If patient can relax, tendons may be subluxated manually by examiner
   c. May be mild, chronic swelling
4. **X-rays**
   a. May reveal a "rim" fracture of the lateral ridge of fibula
   b. In habitual dislocator, some authors recommend CT scan to evaluate depth of groove on posterior aspect of fibula
5. **Treatment**
   a. Acute
      i. Primary repair of retinaculum
      ii. Reconstruct retinaculum if inadequate
   b. Habitual—Reconstruct retinaculum with periosteal flap or autogenous tendon graft. Deepen groove if determined to be shallow. A sliding slot graft on the distal fibula is also effective.
   c. Short-leg cast for 3–6 weeks. A removable cast-boot may be used the final 3 weeks.

51

Stress Fractures

Keith L. Stanley, M.D.

Stress fractures are a common injury in athletics, recreation, and everyday life.

I. History

A. First recognized in military recruits
   1. Briethaupt in 1855 described a clinical syndrome of foot pain and swelling.
   2. Later recognized as a "march fracture," a stress fracture of the metatarsals. Also called "Deutschlander fracture." Noted to occur frequently in the first two weeks of training.
   3. The pattern of stress fractures in military recruits is changing.
      a. Likely due to changes in training and equipment
      b. Now more common in posterior tuberosity of the calcaneus, tibia, or femur

B. Stress fractures in athletes have become more of an issue in recent years.

II. Definition

Stress fractures are focal structural weaknesses that result from bone remodeling in response to repeated application of subthreshold stresses.

III. Epidemiology

A. Occurrences are usually **sports or activity specific**.
   1. **Running**
      a. Tibia
      b. Fibula
      c. Metatarsals
   2. **Football**
      a. Fifth metatarsal
      b. Tibia
      c. Pars interarticularis
   3. **Basketball**
      a. Tibia
      b. Fifth metatarsal
      c. Tarsal navicular
      d. Calcaneus
   4. **Gymnastics**
      a. Pars interarticularis
      b. Radius
   5. **Fast-pitch softball pitchers**—rib

B. Percentage of stress fractures pertaining to sports seen in the patient population[32]
   1. Running—69%
   2. Fitness class—8%
   3. Racket sports—5%

4. Basketball—4%
5. Other sports—14%

C. Male/female ratio about equal

D. Most common bones injured, reported as a percentage of all stress fractures:
1. Tibia—49.1%
2. Tarsals—25.3%
3. Metatarsals—8.8%
4. Femur—7.2%
5. Fibula—6.6%
6. Pelvis—1.6%
7. Sesamoids—0.9%
8. Spine—0.6%

E. Age relationship
1. **Femoral** and **tarsal** fractures more common in **older** patients
2. **Tibial** and **fibular** fractures more common in **younger patients**

IV. Bone Physiology

A. **Bone characteristics**
1. Bone is a viscoelastic, anisotropic tissue, i.e., a tissue whose properties depend on the direction and rate of loading.
2. Ninety percent of the organic tissue of bone is collagen.
3. Eight percent of the cortical weight of bone is made up of calcium hydroxyapatite crystals.
4. The **collagen phase** of bone resists **tensile stress** better than the mineral phase.
5. The **mineral phase** of bone resists **compression stress** better than the collagen phase.

B. **Mechanism of injury**
1. A compressive or tensile force when applied to bone generates stress $\left(\text{stress} = \frac{\text{force}}{\text{area}}\right)$.
2. The resulting deformation can be defined by the relative change in length $\left(\text{strain} = \frac{\text{length change}}{\text{length}}\right)$.
3. The relationship between stress and strain is linear until it goes beyond the yield strength.
4. At the breaking point, the **bone collapses in compression** or is **separated in tension**.
5. Bone is weaker in tension.
6. Muscle weakness may lessen the shock absorption capacity and cause redistribution of forces at focal points.
7. Concentrated concentric and eccentric muscle forces act on a specific bone and create injurious forces.
8. The **response to deforming strain** mechanically invokes **remodeling**.
9. **Bony adaptation** is a function of:
   a. Number of loading cycles
   b. Cycle frequency
   c. Duration of cycle
   d. Amount of strain
   e. Strain rate
   f. Strain duration per cycle
10. Osteoclastic activity results from the stress.
11. **If new bone formation falls behind the osteoclastic activity, microfractures develop**.
12. Each load cycle may propagate microfractures through the bone until a **symptomatic stress fracture arises**.

TABLE 1. Stress Fracture Etiologic Factors

Intrinsic Factors	Extrinsic Factors
Alignment abnormalities	Overt
Femoral neck anteversion	Continued self-abuse
Pronation/supination	Improper training
Tibial tension	Improper technique
Leg length discrepancy	Improper equipment
Muscle imbalance	Harsh environment
Muscle weakness	Covert
Flexibility	Joint instability
Genetic predisposition	Extrinsic pressure
Aging/hormonal	Biomechanical fault

C. **Other etiologic factors** (Table 1)
   1. Intrinsic factors
   2. Extrinsic factors
   3. Eating disorders

D. Summary of etiologic factors
   1. **Three basic factors in overuse injury**
      a. **Frequency**—how often
      b. **Duration**—how long
      c. **Intensity**—how hard
   2. Changing more than one of these factors at a time increases the risk of stress injury.

V. Diagnosis

Time to diagnose averages 5 to 16 weeks.

A. **History:** High index of suspicion when evaluating the facts (frequency, duration, intensity)
   1. Change in activity
   2. Change in equipment or playing surface
   3. Activities added to already demanding physical performance
   4. Training errors
   5. Onset of pain
   6. Pain localized
   7. Pain relief by rest and reduced activity
   8. Groin pain in femoral neck stress fractures

B. **Physical examination**
   1. Point tenderness, edema, warmth, and palpable callus in some cases
   2. Tenderness to percussion or to sound waves (tuning fork or ultrasound)
   3. Pain with trunk or hip extension in pars interarticularis stress fractures

C. **Radiologic studies**
   1. **Plain radiographs** usually negative early in course
      a. Two thirds of initial x-rays are negative, but half of these become positive.
      b. X-rays are specific but *not* sensitive.
   2. **Bone scan**
      a. Especially useful in tarsals, femur, pelvis, and tibial plateau
      b. Help to differentiate from periostitis (shin splints)
      c. Stress fractures are positive in all phases of triple-phase technetium bone scan. Periostitis is negative in the angiogram and blood pool phase and positive in the delayed image phase.

3. **Single-photon emission computed tomography (SPECT) imaging**
   a. More sensitive than planar bone scan
   b. Especially helpful in detecting stress fractures of the pars interarticularis, pelvis, and femoral neck
4. **Computed tomography (CT) scans**
   a. Useful in fractures of the tarsals
   b. Also helpful in spinal or linear stress fractures
5. **Tomography** may also be used, especially with tarsal fractures.
6. **Magnetic resonance imaging:** Newer high-resolution scanners detect many stress fractures extremely early. The radiologist must have the training and experience necessary to identify them.

VI. General Treatment

A. Usually takes 6–8 weeks but certain fractures take 3–4 months or longer
B. **Suggested phases of treatment**
   1. **Phase I: Pain control**, 10–14 days
      a. Nonsteroidal anti-inflammatory drugs
      b. Physiotherapy
      c. Flexibility and strengthening
      d. Rest
   2. **Phase II: Reintroduction of activity**. May last several weeks depending on the location and type of stress fracture. Initiation of phase II varies with size and type of stress fracture and level of symptomatic improvement.
      a. Continue phase I treatment.
      b. Begin training directed toward returning to sport (e.g., have a runner jog in a swimming pool).
      c. Modify playing surfaces or equipment if possible (e.g., begin jogging on grass rather than hard surface) later in phase II.
      d. Use alternating daily workouts.
   3. **Phase III: Preparation for return to competition**
      a. Increase sport-specific conditioning drills.
      b. Begin lower-level competitive challenges.

VII. Specific Stress Fractures

A. **Upper extremity**
   1. **Humerus**
      a. **Proximal** fractures and **medial epicondyle** fractures seen in younger throwing athletes and gymnasts. **Midshaft** fractures seen in adult throwing athletes and in workers doing heavy lifting.
      b. **History**—pain with throwing or lifting heavy weights; may involve entire upper arm
      c. **Examination**—may have pain on palpation or resisted motion
      d. Sometimes examination may appear normal.
      e. **Treatment:**
         i. Rest
         ii. May use immobilization such as a fracture brace
         iii. 6–8 weeks for healing
   2. **Ulna**
      a. Reported in softball pitchers, rodeo riders, and volleyball players
      b. **History**—pain with underhand maneuvers, especially after strenuous activity
      c. **Examination**—pain, edema, and local heat over involved areas. Pain with movement, especially resisted motion.

d. **Radiographic studies:**
   i. X-ray usually helpful
   ii. Bone scan to confirm, if x-ray is negative
e. **Treatment:**
   i. Rest
   ii. Modify biomechanics if an issue

3. **Olecranon**
   a. Occurs in throwing athletes; caused by intermittent extension overload
   b. **History**—pain as the arm extends in the throwing motion
   c. **Examination**—point tenderness to palpation and pain with triceps extension
   d. **Radiographic studies:**
      i. X-ray may be negative
      ii. If plain x-ray shows sclerosis around an area of lucence, be concerned about nonunion.
      iii. This is a *tension* lesion, so x-ray characteristics are unique to this type of stress fracture (transverse radiolucency extending from posterior nonarticular to articular surface).
   e. **Treatment:**
      i. Short-term immobilization to reduce the triceps pull may be necessary.
      ii. Surgery may be indicated if nonunion is evident.

4. **Radius**
   a. An uncommon location for stress fractures. Has been reported in military personnel as well as tennis, volleyball, and softball players and gymnasts and cheerleaders.
   b. **History**—pain in shaft of radius with exertional activity
   c. **Examination**—pain over the area involved
   d. **Radiographic studies:**
      i. X-rays may show contact thickening and even some bowing.
      ii. Bone scan confirmatory.
   e. **Treatment:**
      i. 6 weeks of rest
      ii. A longer period of rest may be needed in gymnasts and cheerleaders.

B. **Shoulder girdle and trunk**

1. **Coracoid process**
   a. Repeated impact in trapshooting
   b. **History**—aching in shoulder
   c. **Examination**—pain to palpation or resisted active adduction and forward flexion of the arm
   d. **Radiographic studies**—axillary view necessary for plain x-ray diagnosis
   e. **Treatment:**
      i. Rest
      ii. Avoid trapshooting 6–8 weeks

2. **First rib**
   a. Most commonly seen in baseball pitchers; also reported in basketball athletes
   b. **History**—may have insidious onset or a sudden event without preceding symptoms
   c. **Examination**—pain with arm motion over supraclavicular area
   d. **Radiographic studies**—x-ray usually positive over broad, flat, thick portion of first rib
   e. **Treatment:**
      i. Rest
      ii. Gradual return to activity

3. **Other ribs**
   a. Seen in softball pitchers, golfers, and rowers
   b. **History**—pain with rotation of trunk
   c. **Examination**—point pain over area involved
   d. **Radiographic studies:**
      i. X-rays many times negative
      ii. Bone scan helpful

C. **Spine**
1. **Spondylolysis:** Pars interarticularis stress fractures
   a. Most common in gymnasts, cheerleaders, and weight lifters. Has been seen in just about every type of athlete. L4 and L5 most common levels.
   b. **History:**
      i. Athlete usually involved in some repetitive **extension load** activity
      ii. Insidious onset of back pain
      iii. Ultimately complains of significant back spasms—many times misdiagnosed as a lumbar strain
      iv. Short periods of rest may temporarily relieve pain, but return to activity results in immediate exacerbation of symptoms.
   c. **Examination:**
      i. May have clinical hyperlordosis
      ii. Pain to palpation over transverse process areas
      iii. Exquisite pain and muscle guarding with the following maneuvers:
         (a) One-leg and two-leg standing **trunk extension test**
         (b) Trunk rotation and extension
         (c) Hip extension test (prone)
         (d) Trunk extension test (prone)
         (e) Combined hip and trunk extension test (prone)
      iv. Neurologic exam usually normal
      v. May occasionally have radiculopathy
   d. **Radiographic studies:**
      i. X-rays may be negative. If positive, the classic defect of a "collar" on the neck of the Scotty dog is seen on oblique views.
      ii. Bone scan is helpful but the SPECT scan is more sensitive.
   e. **Treatment:**
      i. Somewhat controversial
      ii. Some recommend just rest.
      iii. Some recommend rest with a corset brace.
      iv. Many believe a thoracolumbar sacral orthosis or a low profile antilordotic Boston brace is the best treatment.
      v. Healing usually takes 3–6 months.
      vi. Changes in biomechanics of the specific activity should be evaluated before return to activity (as a preventive measure).
      vii. Flexibility training is important as well as back stabilization rehabilitation.
2. **Spondylolisthesis**
   a. Bilateral pars defects allowing slippage of vertebral bodies (graded I–IV depending on amount of displacement):
      i. Grade I 0–25%
      ii. Grade II 25–50%
      iii. Grade III 50–75%
      iv. Grade IV > 75%
   b. **History**—similar to spondylolysis but may have radiculopathy
   c. **Examination**—similar to spondylolysis

d. **Radiographic studies:**
   i. X-rays show complete lysis of pars bilaterally. Lateral view shows defect as well as amount of slippage.
   ii. Adjunctive studies usually are not necessary.
e. **Treatment:**
   i. Intensive treatment similar to spondylolysis
   ii. If slippage progresses or if pain or radiculopathy persists, surgical stabilization should be considered.

D. **Pelvis**
1. Usually involves the **pubic ramus**. Not common and mostly found in long distance runners or joggers.
2. **History**—pain in the inguinal, perineal, or adduction region. Pain relieved by rest.
3. **Examination**
   a. Antalgic gait
   b. Full range of motion
   c. Pain over pubic ramus
   d. Positive "standing sign" (inability to stand unsupported on affected side)
4. **Radiographic studies**
   a. X-rays may take several weeks to be positive. Late in course, x-rays may show abundant callus.
   b. Many times a bone scan is needed for early diagnosis.
5. **Treatment**
   a. Rest
   b. Nearly 3–5 months to heal

E. **Femoral stress fractures**
1. **Femoral neck**
   a. Seen most frequently in runners and dancers. Complications can be severe (avascular neurosis, nonunion, varus deformity, displacement).
   b. **History:**
      i. Pain in groin, anterior thigh, or knee
      ii. Aching pain precipitated by weight-bearing activity
      iii. Usually a significant change in training
   c. **Examination:**
      i. Antalgic gait
      ii. Decreased hip motion, especially internal rotation
      iii. Axial compression on percussion over greater trochanter may elicit pain
   d. **Radiographic studies:**
      i. X-rays usually not positive early in course
      ii. Use bone scan or SPECT scan for early diagnosis
      iii. Plain x-rays and SPECT may help differentiate compression lesion (medial side) from tension lesion (lateral side)
   e. **Treatment:**
      i. Somewhat controversial
      ii. Most agree surgical treatment for tension (distraction) lesion
      iii. Blickenstaff criteria for compression lesion:
         (a) Type I, callus without a fracture line—treat conservatively
         (b) Type II, definite fracture line but no displacement—treat with immobilization or internal fixation
         (c) Type III, displaced—treat with internal fixation
      iv. Some authorities recommend surgery for all femoral neck stress fractures due to lack of patient compliance with bed rest and non–weight bearing.

2. **Femoral shaft stress fractures**
   a. Seen mostly in runners, especially female runners. Most common at the junction of the proximal and middle thirds of the femoral shaft.
   b. **History:**
      i. Sudden increases in frequency, intensity, or duration
      ii. Pain with running but progressing to pain with activities of daily living
   c. **Examination:**
      i. Physical findings may be few
      ii. Sometimes pain with palpation
      iii. Antalgic gait
   d. **Radiographic studies:**
      i. X-rays negative early, but in 2–6 weeks callus and lucent fracture line may be seen
      ii. Bone scans helpful for early diagnosis
   e. **Treatment:**
      i. Protected weight bearing with crutches for 1–4 weeks (length of time dependent on resolution of pain)
      ii. Resumption of athletic activity may take 8–16 weeks.

F. **Knee and lower leg stress fractures**

1. **Patella**
   a. Rare, but most commonly seen in basketball players. May be longitudinal or transverse.
   b. **History**—anterior knee pain
   c. **Examination:**
      i. Pain to palpation
      ii. Pain with resisted knee extension
   d. **Radiographic studies:**
      i. X-rays may show definite fracture lines.
      ii. Bone scans again helpful
   e. **Treatment:**
      i. Transverse fractures prone to displacement:
         (a) Nondisplaced fractures—immobilization
         (b) Displaced fractures—open reduction and internal fixation
      ii. Longitudinal fractures occur in lateral patellar facet; if displaced, excise lateral fragment.
2. **Tibial plateau fractures**
   a. Infrequent yet definitive site
   b. **History:**
      i. Pain in the anteromedial aspect of the proximal tibia
      ii. Weight bearing precipitates pain
   c. **Examination:**
      i. Localized tenderness
      ii. Localized edema
      iii. Need to differentiate from a pes anserinus tendinitis or bursitis
   d. **Radiographic studies**—x-rays usually positive 3–4 weeks after onset of symptoms
   e. **Treatment:**
      i. Conservative
      ii. Return to activity usually in 4 weeks
3. **Tibial shaft fractures**
   a. Need to differentiate between medial tibial stress syndrome, compression stress fracture, and tension stress fracture ("dreaded black line"):

i. **Compression stress fractures:**
   (a) Located in proximal or distal third or may develop as an extension of medial tibial stress syndrome
   (b) Located posteromedial
ii. **Tension stress fractures:**
   (a) Located in the central third of the tibia
   (b) Located in anterior or anterolateral cortex

b. **History:**
   i. Initially, pain occurs *after* activity.
   ii. Later, pain occurs *with* activity and activities of daily living.
c. **Examination:**
   i. Localized pain
   ii. May feel periosteal thickening
   iii. Positive "tuning fork test"
d. **Radiographic studies:**
   i. X-rays may be positive if symptoms have persisted 4–6 weeks.
   ii. Bone scans are helpful and show fusiform uptake, which differentiates from linear uptake of medial tibial stress syndrome.
e. **Treatment:**
   i. Local control of pain
   ii. Stop running; use crutches if necessary.
   iii. **Compression lesions** may take 6–12 weeks to heal.
   iv. **Tension lesions** best treated with intramedullary rod. If treated conservatively, may heal in 6 months, but there is a high rate of recurrence.

4. **Medial malleolar stress fractures**
   a. Extends in oblique fashion from plafond. Inherently unstable.
   b. **History**—pain with running
   c. **Examination:**
      i. Pain to palpation
      ii. Ankle effusion
   d. **Radiographic studies:**
      i. Some have positive x-rays
      ii. Many diagnosed by bone scan
   e. **Treatment:**
      i. If x-ray is positive, open reduction and internal fixation should be considered. Some respond well to a conservative approach.
      ii. If positive only on bone scan, immobilize 4–6 weeks.
5. **Fibular stress fractures**
   a. Most common in distal third just proximal to the distal tibiofibular syndesmosis
   b. **History:**
      i. Limp
      ii. Swelling
   c. **Examination:**
      i. Point tenderness
      ii. Localized edema
      iii. Hyperpronation common
   d. **Radiographic studies:**
      i. X-rays not positive for 3–4 weeks
      ii. Bone scan helpful
   e. **Treatment:**
      i. Conservative
      ii. For distal fractures, an ankle brace may be helpful.

G. **Stress fractures in the foot**

1. **Calcaneus**
   a. Seen in military personnel and runners
   b. **History**—presents with heel pain
   c. **Examination:**
      i. Positive "heel squeeze test"
      ii. Edema
   d. **Radiographic studies:**
      i. X-ray typically shows **endosteal callus** perpendicular to the long axis of the calcaneus.
      ii. Sometimes bone scans are needed.
   e. **Treatment:**
      i. Rapid healing with conservative treatment
      ii. Return to activity in 3–4 weeks
2. **Tarsal navicular stress fractures**
   a. Uncommon and challenging to diagnose. Many diagnosed late. An at-risk fracture for complications.
   b. **History:**
      i. Insidious onset of pain
      ii. Pain may be mild
      iii. Cramping sensation in midfoot
   c. **Examination:**
      i. Pain may be diffuse rather than localized.
      ii. Variable foot anatomy may contribute, but no one type is consistently prone to these fractures.
   d. **Radiographic studies:**
      i. X-rays usually not helpful
      ii. Bone scan can localize
      iii. CT scan helpful to determine state of healing
      iv. Tomograms an option
   e. **Treatment:**
      i. Difficult to treat conservatively
      ii. At least needs non–weight bearing casting 6–8 weeks
      iii. Internal fixation usually recommended
3. **Proximal diaphysis of the fifth metatarsal**
   a. Occur distal to the tuberosity and prone to nonunion
   b. **History:**
      i. Prodromal symptoms
      ii. Pain steadily worsens
   c. **Examination**—point tenderness distal to the tuberosity
   d. **Radiographic studies:**
      i. X-rays usually show sclerotic change around the fracture by the time patient presents.
      ii. Bone scans are only occasionally necessary.
   e. **Treatment:**
      i. Prolonged casting, although not considered optimal
      ii. Intramedullary screw is preferred treatment
4. **Other metatarsals**
   a. Second and third metatarsals most commonly fractured
   b. **History:**
      i. Localized pain
      ii. Edema

c. **Examination:**
   i. Point pain at the site
   ii. Edema
d. **Radiographic studies:**
   i. X-rays frequently positive
   ii. Bone scan if x-rays negative
e. **Treatment:**
   i. Rest
   ii. Uneventful healing usual

5. **Sesmoids**
   a. Difficult diagnosis. Differentiate from sesamoiditis and bipartite or tripartite sesmoids.
   b. **History:**
      i. Pain involving the first toe
      ii. Pain with "toe-off"
   c. **Examination:**
      i. Pain to palpation
      ii. Pain with resisted first toe plantar flexion
   d. **Radiographic studies:**
      i. X-ray may identify bipartite sesamoid but does not stand alone to diagnose stress fractures
      ii. Bone scan usually necessary
   e. **Treatment:**
      i. Initially conservative—restrict activity, cast, or use orthotics
      ii. Excision, but delayed or avoided if possible

VIII. Conclusions

A. **Always think stress fracture**!!!
B. Develop a systematic approach to the workup.
C. Treat aggressively.

Recommended Reading

1. Alfred RH, Belhobek G, Bergfield JA: Stress fractures of the tarsonavicular: A case report. Am J Sports Med 20:766–768, 1992.
2. Andrish J: The leg. In Delee J, Drez D (eds): Orthopedic Sports Medicine Principles and Practice. Philadelphia, W.B. Saunders, 1994, pp 1603–1631.
3. Barrick EF, Jackson CV: Prophylactic intramedullary fixation of the tibia for stress fractures in the professional athlete. J Orthop Trauma 6:241–244, 1992.
4. Baxter DE: The foot in running. Surg Foot Ankle 1225–1240.
5. Bingham JA: Stress fractures of the femoral neck. Lancet 2:13–15, 1945.
6. Blickenstaff MD, Morris JM: Fatigue fracture of the femoral neck. J Bone Joint Surg 45A:1031–1047, 1966.
7. Bollen SR, Robinson DG, Crichton KJ, et al: Stress fractures of the ulna in tennis players using a double handed back hand stroke. Am J Sports Med 21:751–752, 1993.
8. Boyer DW: Trapshooters shoulder: Stress fracture of the coracoid process. J Bone Joint Surg 57A:562, 1975.
9. Dahlstrom HA: Conservative management of distraction type stress fractures of the femoral neck. J Bone Joint Surg 68B:65–67, 1986.
10. Devas MB: Stress fractures of the femoral neck. J Bone Joint Surg 47B:728–738, 1985.
11. Eisomont FJ, Kitchel SH: Thoracic lumbar spine. In Delee J, Drez D (eds): Orthopedic Sports Medicine Principles and Practice. Philadelphia, W.B. Saunders, 1994, pp 1018–1062.
12. Engber WD: Stress fractures of the medial tibial plateau. J Bone Joint Surg 59A:767–769, 1967.
13. Farguharson-Roberts MA, Fulford PC: Stress fractures of the radius. J Bone Joint Surg 62B:194–195, 1980.
14. Fullerton LR: Femoral neck stress fractures. Sports Med 9:192–197, 1990.
15. Giladi M, Milgrom C, Simkin A, et al: Stress fractures. Am J Sports Med 6:647–652, 1991.
16. Glick JM, Sampson TG: Ankle and foot fractures in athletics. In Nicholas JA, Herschman EB (eds): Lower Extremity and Spine in Sports Medicine. St. Louis, C.V. Mosby, 1986.

17. Gross ML, Nasser S, Finerman GAM: Hip and pelvis. In Delee, Drez (eds): Orthopedic Sports Medicine Principles and Practice. Philadelphia, W.B. Saunders, 1994, pp 1063–1085.
18. Hamilton WG: Foot and ankle injuries in dancers. In Mann RA, Coughlin MJ (eds): Surgery of the Foot and Ankle, 6th ed. St. Louis, Mosby, 1993, pp 1241–1276.
19. Hershman EB, Lombardo J, Bergfeld JA: Femoral shaft stress fractures in athletes. Clin Sports Med 9:111–119, 1990.
20. Hershman EB, Mailly T: Stress fractures. Clin Sports Med 9:183–214, 1990.
21. Jackson D: Low back pain in young athletes. Am J Sports Med 7:364, 1979.
22. Jackson D, Wiltse L, Dingemen R, et al: Stress reactions involving the pars interarticularis in young athletes. Am J Sports Med 9:305, 1981.
23. Johansson C, Ekenman I, Tornkbiest H, et al: Stress fractures of the femoral neck in athletes: The consequence of a delay in diagnosis. Am J Sports Med 18:524–528, 1990.
24. Kadel NJ, Teitze CC, Kronman RA: Stress fractures on the tarsonavicular bone: CT findings in 55 cases. AJR 160:111–115, 1993.
25. Kahn KM, Fuller PJ, Brukner PD, et al: Outcome of conservative and surgical management of navicular stress fractures in athletes: 86 cases proved, computerized tomography. Am J Sports Med 20:657–666, 1992.
26. Kaine D, Roy S, Singer KM, et al: Stress changes of the distal radial growth plate: A radiographic survey of the literature. Am J Sports Med 20:290–298, 1992.
27. Kiss Z, Kahn KM, Fuller PJ: Stress fractures on the tarsonavicular bone: CT findings in 55 cases. AJR 160:111–115, 1993.
28. Kottmeier SA, Hanks GA, Kalenak A: Fibular stress fractures associated with distal tibial fibular synostosis in an athlete: A case report and literature review. Clin Orthop 281:195–198, 1992.
29. McBride AM: Stress fractures in runners. Clin Sports Med 4:737–752, 1985.
30. McBryde A: Stress fractures of the foot and ankle. In Delee, Drez (eds): Orthopedic Sports Medicine Principles and Practice. Philadelphia, W.B. Saunders, 1994, pp 1970–2021.
31. Mann RA, Coughlin MJ: Surgery of the Foot and Ankle, 6th ed. St. Louis, Mosby, 1993.
32. Matheson GO, Clement DB, McKinzie DC, et al: Stress fractures in athletes: A study of 320 cases. Am J Sports Med 15:46–58, 1987.
33. Meyer SA, Saltzman CL, Albright JP: Stress fractures in the foot and leg. Clin Sports Med 12:395–413, 1983.
34. Micheli L: Low back pain in the adolescent: Differential diagnosis. Am J Sports Med 7:363, 1979.
35. Mikawa Y, Kobori M: Stress fractures of the first rib in a weight lifter. Arch Orthop Trauma Surg 110:121–122, 1991.
36. Noakes TD, Smith JA, Lindberg G, et al: Pelvis stress fractures in long distance runners. Am J Sports Med 13:120–123, 1985.
37. Orava S, Kerpakka J, Julkko A, et al: Diagnosis and treatment of stress fractures located in the mid-tibial shaft in athletes. Int J Sports Med 12:419–432, 1991.
38. Pavlov H, Nelson TL, Warren F, et al: Stress fractures in pubic ramus. J Bone Joint Surg 64A:1020–1025, 1982.
39. Pavlov M, Tore JS, Freeberger RM: Tarsonavicular stress fractures: Radiographic evaluation. Radiology 48:641–645, 1983.
40. Pecina M, Bojanic I, Dubravcic S, et al: Stress fractures in figure skaters. Am J Sports Med 18:270–279, 1990.
41. Reddick AC, Shelbourne KD, McCarrol JR, et al: The natural history and treatment of delayed union stress fractures of the anterior cortex of the tibia. Am J Sports Med 16:250–255, 1988.
42. Schils JP, Andrish JT, Piraino DW, et al: Medial malleolar stress fractures in 7 patients: Review of the clinical and imaging features. Radiology 185:219–221, 1992.
43. Shelbourne KD, Fisher DA, Reddick AC, et al: Stress fractures of the medial malleolus. Am J Sports Med 16:60–63, 1988.
44. Teitze CC, Harrington RM: Patellar stress fracture. Am J Sports Med 20:761–765, 1992.
45. Vanhall ME, Keene JS, Lang TA, et al: Stress fractures of great toe sesmoids. Am J Sports Med 10:122–128, 1982.
46. Zogby RG, Baker BE: A review of non-operative treatment of Jone's fracture. Am J Sports Med 15:304–307, 1987.

52

Foot Problems

Stephen C. Hunter, M.D., Lawrence D. Powell, M.D., Craig K. Seto, M.D., and Paul D. Zawatsky, M.D.

I. Normal Anatomy (Figs. 1 and 2)

II. Anatomical Variants (Table 1 and Fig. 3)

III. Foot Problems

A. **Skin and nail problems** (Table 2)
B. **Tendinitis** (Table 3)
  1. **Etiology:** Stress causes macrotears (acute trauma) or microtears (chronic overuse) with resultant inflammation.
  2. **Common types:** posterior tibial, peroneal, Achilles
  3. **Radiographic assessment**
    a. Plain films usually not helpful—do not show tendon damage
    b. Occasionally see associated bony changes (e.g., avulsion of base of fifth metatarsal at peroneus brevis insertion, calcification, or erosion at Achilles tendon insertion)
    c. Computed tomography (CT), magnetic resonance imaging (MRI) may help detect complete tendon tear
C. **Plantar fasciitis** (Fig. 4A)
  1. **Etiology:** Excessive tightness of gastrocsoleus complex pulling into heelcord (Achilles) causes overload at plantar fascia origin on calcaneus during weight-bearing activities; microtears and inflammation ensue.
  2. **Symptoms/signs:** point tenderness/pain (particularly on first arising in morning)
    a. Specifically along medial tubercle of calcaneus
    b. Sometimes relieved with activity, returning at rest
  3. **Radiographic assessment:** Traction spurs off calcaneus may be seen (secondary findings and usually not a cause of pain).
  4. **Differential diagnosis**
    a. Entrapment of medial calcaneal branch of tibial nerve (calcaneal branch neurodynia—thought by some to be a component of plantar fasciitis syndrome)
    b. Plantar fascial tear—pain located directly under arch
    c. Tarsal tunnel syndrome (see page 614)
    d. Calcaneal stress fracture (see page 612)
    e. Central heel syndrome—heel pad deficiency
  5. **Treatment:** early intervention more efficacious than late intervention
    a. Heelcord stretching
    b. Nonsteroidal anti-inflammatory drugs (NSAIDs)
    c. Shock-absorbing heel pad and/or soft plantar arch orthotic (Fig. 4B)
    d. Decrease of weight-bearing activities initially with graduated return

Calcaneous
Talus
Navicular
Cuneiforms (2 visible)
Metatarsal
Cuboid
Phalanx
A
B

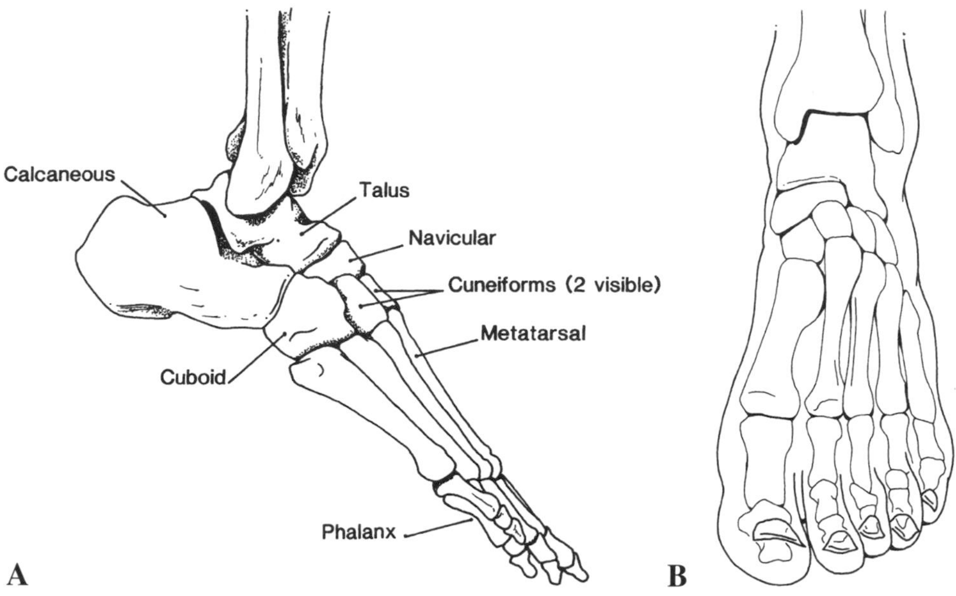

FIGURE 1. Normal bony anatomy of the foot. **A**, Lateral. **B**, dorsal.

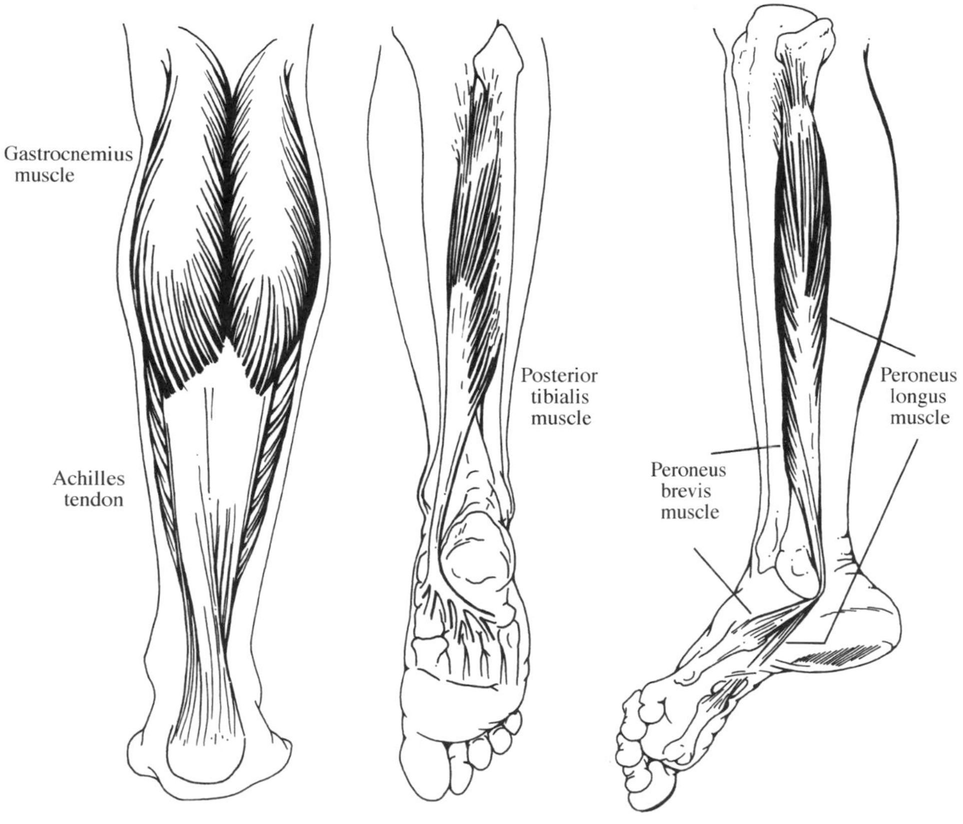

Gastrocnemius muscle
Achilles tendon
Posterior tibialis muscle
Peroneus longus muscle
Peroneus brevis muscle

FIGURE 2. Normal muscles and tendons of the lower leg and foot.

TABLE 1. Anatomic Variants of the Foot

Variants	Description	Etiology	Functional Consequence
Hyperpronation	A flat foot that is excessively dorsiflexed, abducted, and everted at subtalar joint	Structural abnormality. Compensation for tibia vara, Achilles tendon inflexibility, heel or forefoot varus	Excessive subtalar motion, stress overloading
Tarsal coalition	Bony or cartilaginous bar between bones of hindfoot and midfoot	Congenital	Limits eversion/inversion. Clinically may appear as rigid flat foot
Pes planus	Flat foot (see Fig. 3A)	Structural (e.g., tarsal coalition or neurologic disorder)	Abnormal stress loading (often associated with hyperpronation)
Pes cavus	High-arched foot, usually rigid (see Fig. 3B)	Structural or neurologic disorder	Less shock absorption; abnormal stress loading leads to overuse syndromes
Metatarsus primus adductus	Adduction of first ray	Structural abnormality	Difficulty fitting shoes; blister, callus, or bunion formation often complicated by claw or hammer toes
Morton's toe	Elongated second metatarsal compared with first	Congenital	Excessively mobile first metatarsal; abnormal stress loading from great toe to second toe; pain and callus formation; functional overuse syndromes

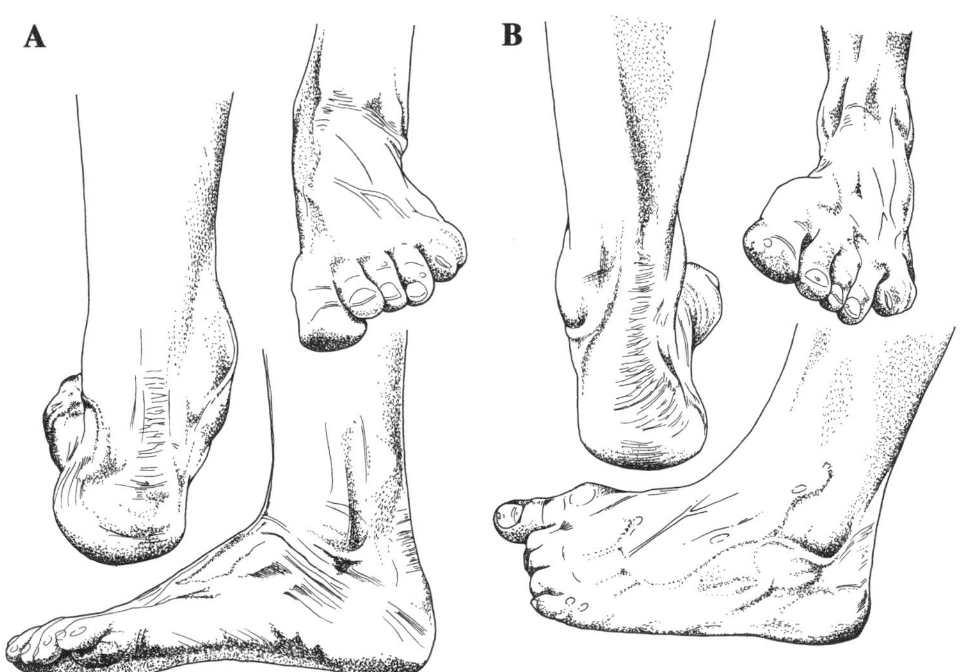

FIGURE 3. **A**, Pes planus (flat foot). **B**, Pes cavus (high-arched foot).

TABLE 2. Skin and Nail Problems

Type	Cause	Signs and Symptoms	Treatment
Calluses and corns (calluses of the toes)	Excessive localized friction or pressure from tight shoes or structural abnormalities of the feet, such as claw or hammer toes, dropped metatarsal head, loss of transverse arch	Pain; thickening and hardening of the skin (kept soft by moisture when between the toes)	Proper shoe fitting, padding (e.g., doughnut pad), debridement, bony resection, metatarsal pad, Boden splint
Blisters	Friction, pressure. Epidermal/dermal separation by serous fluid	Painful vesicles	Unruptured: sterile drainage (if painful), dressing. Ruptured: sterile cleansing, dressing (consider antibiotics for diabetic patient or for signs of secondary infection in any patient)
Warts	Virus (papilloma)	Pain at site; skin thickening with a central core; flat or raised	Trichloracetic acid or salicylic acid or other debridement, liquid nitrogen
Tinea pedis (athlete's foot)	Fungus	Dry or vesicular lesions; scaling, peeling, and cracking fissures in skin; deformed nails, hyphae and buds on KOH wet mount; iridescence by Wood's light	Dry: miconazole nitrate, clotrimazole, salicylic acid, tolnaftate, tar compounds. Vesicular: wet dressings with potassium permanganate or Burow's solution. Erythema or other signs of infection: consider antibiotics
Paronychia	Onychocryptosis with subsequent fungal/ bacterial infection	Inflamed nail margin with or without drainage	Antibiotics acutely (e.g., erythromycin); partial nail resection; proper nail cutting techniques
Subungual hematoma	Trauma	Dark blood under nail: pain/pressure at site	Drainage (insert no. 18 needle through nail or burn hole in nail with the tip of a heated paper clip) Note: ensure traumatic history to distinguish from subungual melanoma

e. Maintenance of aerobic, well-leg, and upper-body fitness
f. Tension night splints
g. Corticosteroid injection
h. Surgical release—only with failure of conservative measures

D. **Sever's disease** (calcaneal apophysitis)

1. **Etiology:** unilateral or bilateral heel pain in boys or girls at or just prior to growth spurt. Contributing factors include:
   a. Decreased heel cord and hamstring flexibility
   b. Microtrauma from running sports, especially soccer
   c. Biomechanical abnormality contributing to poor shock absorption, such as forefoot varus, hallux valgus, pes cavus, and pes planus
   d. Occasionally, acute trauma, such as a violent heel strike
2. **Symptoms/signs**
   a. Intermittent or continuous heel pain usually shortly after beginning of a new sport or season. Worse during and after activity. Improves with rest.

TABLE 3. Inflammatory Conditions

Type	Signs and Symptoms	Treatment
Posterior tibial tendinitis	Medial pain, swelling, pain with active inversion (hyperpronation could be a sign of complete posterior tibialis rupture)	Initial: rest, ice, NSAIDs, plantar arch orthotic. Rehabilitation:* plantar flexion and inversion strengthening exercises, heel cord flexibility
Peroneal tendinitis	Lateral pain, swelling, pain with active eversion; may complain of snapping sensation in cases of subluxation of tendon(s)	Initial: rest, ice, NSAIDs, orthotic to correct hyperpronation or heel pad to decrease tension on tendon. Rest: resistive eversion foot exercises. Surgery may be required for subluxation
Achilles tendinitis	Decreased gastrocsoleus flexibility. Pain, tenderness, swelling, and crepitus at site; pain with active plantar flexion	Initial: rest, ice, NSAIDs, orthotic to correct hyperpronation or heel pad to decrease tension on tendon. Rehabilitation: heel cord stretching and strengthening exercises. Possible surgical repair in chronic cases or with complete tendon rupture
Retrocalcaneal bursitis	Hindfoot pain in early phase of running. Tenderness and swelling anterior to Achilles tendon	Initial: rest, ice, NSAIDs. Rehabilitation: Heel cord stretching, modalities, heel lift, later add strengthening exercises
Calcaneal apophysitis (Sever's disease)	Similar to Achilles tendinitis, with tenderness, swelling, and crepitus at insertion in the skeletally immature athlete. Rule out posterior impingement of os trigonum with pain at site with extreme plantar flexion.	Initial: rest, ice, NSAIDs. Rehabilitation: Heel cord stretching, modalities, heel lift, later add strengthening exercises
Sesamoiditis	Local tenderness (tibial side most common). Pain worse with weight bearing. Rule out avascular necrosis, sesamoid fracture	Reduce weight-bearing stress at site: doughnut pad insert. Ice, NSAIDs, use of more rigid or fracture shoe. If conservative treatment fails: bone scan, computed tomography, or tomogram imaging to rule out stress fracture
Metatarsophalangeal joint synovitis	Pain at metatarsophalangeal joint (second most common), increased mobility (anterior-posterior translation), joint crepitus. Distinguish from interdigital neuroma	Metatarsal pad, figure-of-eight taping, Boden splint, NSAIDs, steroid injection (with caution), surgery

* Rehabilitation includes maintenance of aerobic, well-leg, and upper-body fitness. Physical therapy modalities, such as phonophoresis and iontophoresis, may also be useful.
NSAIDs = Nonsteroidal anti-inflammatory drugs.

b. Tender to palpation at or just anterior to Achilles insertion
c. Positive "squeeze" test—compression of medial and lateral aspects of calcaneal apophysis produces pain
d. Positive "Sever's test"—heel pain aggravated by standing on tip-toes

3. **Radiographic assessment:** Characterized by fragmentation, sclerosis and increased density of the apophysis. All of these are normal radiographic findings.
4. **Differential diagnosis**
   a. Achilles tendinitis/strain
   b. Heel pad pain
   c. Retrocalcaneal bursitis

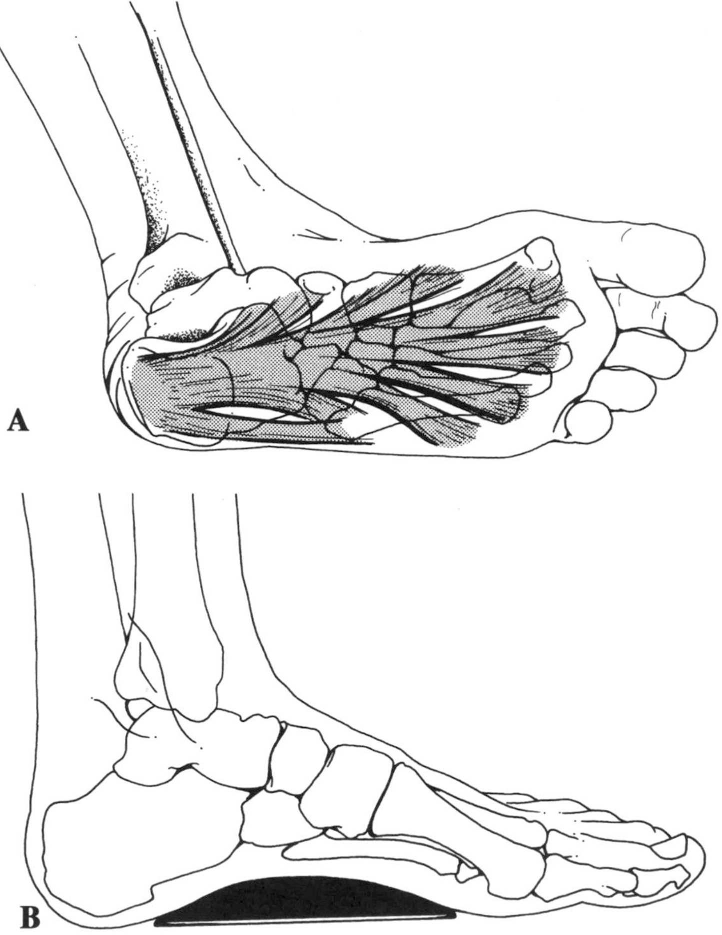

FIGURE 4. **A**, Plantar fascia. **B**, Orthosis for plantar fasciitis.

   d. Calcaneal stress fracture
   e. Plantar fasciitis
5. **Treatment**
   a. Initial treatment
      i. Rest (crutches in severe cases)
      ii. Ice
      iii. Heel lifts, cups, or pads
      iv. Stretching and strengthening
      v. NSAIDs
   b. Resistant cases
      i. Nighttime dorsiflexion splint
      ii. Rarely, short leg cast for 2 weeks
   c. Orthotics to correct significant biomechanical faults

E. **Turf toe**
1. **Etiology**
   a. Hyperextension of metatarsophalangeal (MTP) joint of great toe leads to ligament sprain, possible tearing of flexor tendon

   b. Often occurs in football linemen pushing off on artificial turf
2. **Symptoms/signs**
   a. Pain, tenderness, and swelling at great toe MTP joint
   b. Persistent symptoms with continued activity can lead to hallux rigidus.
   c. Pain with dorsiflexion
3. **Radiographic assessment**
   a. Usually normal, rule out bony avulsions
   b. May show degenerative changes of first MTP joint (chronic)
   c. May need additional imaging techniques to differentiate from sesamoid stress fracture. (*Note:* normally two sesamoid bones beneath MTP joint of great toe.)
4. **Differential diagnosis**
   a. Classic joint for presentation of gout
   b. Phalangeal or metatarsal fracture
   c. Osteoarthritis
5. **Treatment:** Rest and protection are key.
   a. Ice/NSAIDs acutely
   b. Taping to limit motion of MTP joint can assist in return to activity (Fig. 5)
   c. Metatarsal pad to unload first metatarsal may be helpful
   d. Rigid shoe or rigid metal or plastic forefoot plate provides forefoot support, limits MTP hyperextension

F. **Fractures**
1. **Talus** (Fig. 6A)
   a. **Etiology**
      i. Acute trauma
         (a) Rare in sports, usually surgical emergency
         (b) After radiographic confirmation, orthopedic referral mandatory
         (c) Talar neck fractures are associated with severe foot dislocation. *Note:* osteochondral fractures of the talar dome may occur with ankle sprains.
      ii. Stress fractures
         (a) Also rare
         (b) Symptoms—functional diffuse midfoot pain
         (c) Signs—anterior ankle tenderness on palpation, resistance to active and passive motion of subtalar joint. *Note:* subtalar joint allows eversion/inversion.

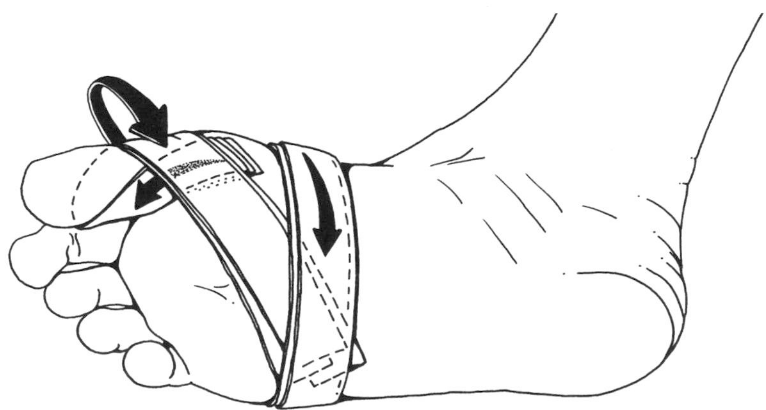

FIGURE 5. Taping to limit motion of metatarsophalangeal joint.

b. **Radiographic assessment—gives definitive diagnosis**
   i. Subtle or stress fractures usually require bone scan or CT.
   ii. Aseptic necrosis of talar head can occur after stress or traumatic fractures.

c. **Treatment of stress fractures of talus**
   i. Modified rest/cessation of weight-bearing activity; cast or support shoe, crutches. Healing process can take up to 6 months (repeat radiographs should document healing).
   ii. Progressive return to weight-bearing activity with confirmation of healing. Initial limitation of ankle and subtalar motion on return to activities (e.g., ankle brace).

2. **Calcaneus** (see Fig. 6)
   a. **Etiology**
      i. Traumatic—rare; orthopedic emergency
      ii. Stress—more common; usually related to endurance sports
   b. **Symptoms/signs**
      i. Localized pain in heel, accentuated by weight-bearing
      ii. Mild swelling
      iii. Pain with medial-lateral compression of calcaneus
   c. **Radiographic assessment, definitive**
      i. Plain film; Bohler's angle may be < 28° in traumatic fractures.
      ii. If negative, bone scan or CT
      iii. Assess for posterior process fractures of talus
   d. **Treatment** of stress fractures of calcaneus
      i. Modified rest and cessation of weight-bearing activities; cast or support shoe with crutches may be appropriate
      ii. Gradual return to activity when clinical symptoms abate and serial radiographic assessment documents healing. Full healing usually within 3 months. Ankle support to prevent subtalar motion and/or hindfoot shock-absorbing orthotic helpful on return to activity.

3. **Midfoot** (see Fig. 6)
   a. **Etiology**
      i. Major trauma—orthopedic emergency, Lisfranc fracture/dislocation (tarsometatarsal fracture/dislocation. If left untreated, permanent deformity/disability results.
      ii. Stress fractures—usually in tarsal navicular bone (common in jumpers, ballet dancers, equestrians)
   b. **Symptoms/signs of navicular stress fracture**
      i. Localized pain, swelling over navicular
      ii. Limited midfoot motion
   c. **Radiographic assessment**
      i. Plain films often negative
      ii. Bone scanning and/or CT are typically necessary with tarsal navicular fractures.
   d. **Treatment**
      i. Rest, cessation of weight-bearing activities, casting
      ii. Complications—high incidence of nonunion with tarsal navicular fractures; persistent symptoms and delayed union on x-ray studies beyond 3 months may indicate need for surgery.
      iii. Surgery—usually bone grafting with internal fixation; recovery can take up to 1 year.

4. **Metatarsal fractures** (see Fig. 6)
   a. **Etiology**
      i. Trauma—rare

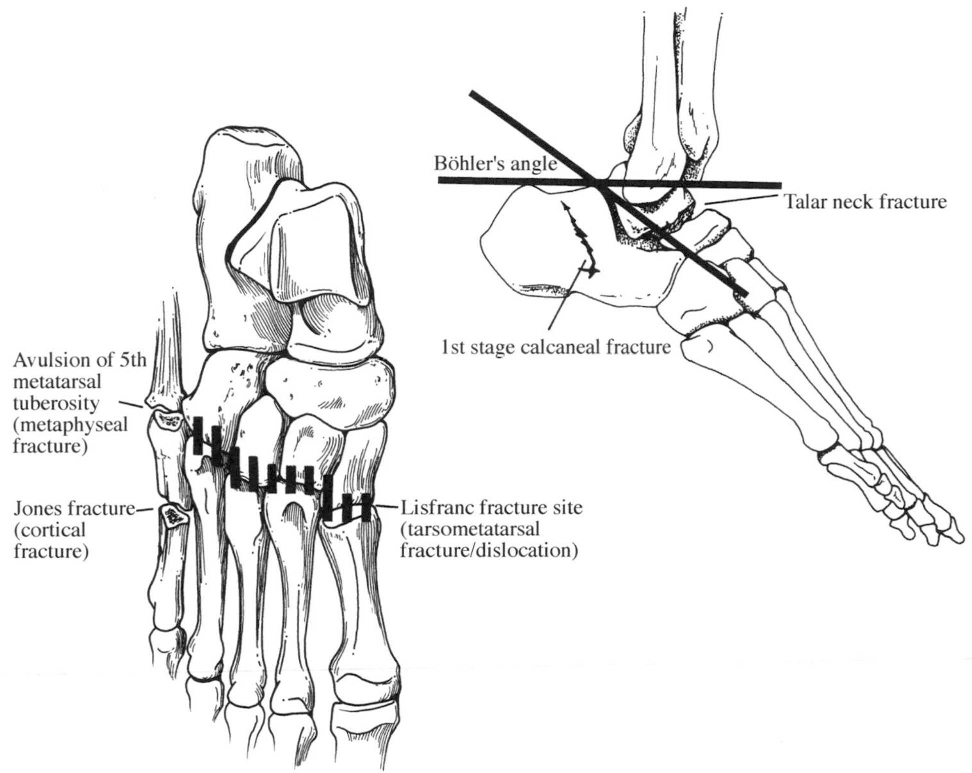

FIGURE 6. Fractures of the foot.

ii. Stress—common; seen in endurance running and jumping sports. *Note*: presence of stress fracture in adolescent female may alert you to look for other components of female triad.

b. **Symptoms/signs:** localized pain with weight-bearing, swelling, tenderness

c. **Radiographic assessment**
   i. Plain films are usually diagnostic.
   ii. Bone scan may be necessary to detect early lesions.

d. **Treatment**
   i. Second through fourth metatarsal stress fractures—nonoperative treatment (first metatarsal stress fracture rarely seen). Modified rest with cessation of weight-bearing activities (immobilization in cast or splint may be used, especially for pain control). Graduated return to activity when symptoms subside.
   ii. Avulsion of attachment of peroneus brevis tendon at the base of the fifth metatarsal (common with ankle sprains)—nonoperative treatment
   iii. Metaphyseal fracture—brief immobilization; reassess weekly
   iv. Jones fracture—stress fracture of proximal fifth metatarsal shaft (often seen in sprinters and jumpers):
      (a) Often have prolonged symptoms and delayed union or nonunion with nonoperative treatment
      (b) Treatment:
         • Cast until free of pain and swelling, then fracture shoe. May take 6–8 weeks.

- Initial surgical stabilization with intermedullary screw may allow earlier return to sports.

(c) Bone grafting and internal fixation indicated for athlete with delayed or nonunion

5. **Phalangeal fractures**
   a. **Etiology:** trauma such as crush injuries or jamming
   b. **Symptoms/signs:** pain, deformity, swelling, ecchymosis
   c. **Radiographic assessment:** plain films confirmatory
   d. **Treatment:** conservative unless open fracture
      i. Nondisplaced—buddy taping to adjacent toe and protection in stiff shoe; symptoms dictate activity restrictions
      ii. Displaced—reduced by manipulation; subsequent buddy-taping/splinting
      iii. Complications—intra-articular fractures can result in joint stiffness and arthritis; if resistant to closed manipulation, refer to orthopedist

G. **Dislocations**

1. **Subtalar/pantalar dislocations**
   a. Etiology: severe trauma, orthopedic emergency
   b. Immediate care indicated to avoid neurovascular damage
2. **Metatarsophalangeal/interphalangeal dislocations**
   a. **Etiology:** trauma, relatively common
   b. **Symptoms/signs:** pain, dysfunction, gross deformity of toes
   c. **Radiographic assessment:** done to rule out associated fracture
   d. **Treatment**
      i. Reduction with steady traction; if dislocation persists, orthopedic referral to rule out tendon entrapment, which can require surgical treatment
      ii. Splint/buddy-taping after reduction
      iii. Functional toe can usually be expected

H. **Neurologic injury**

1. **Tarsal tunnel syndrome** (Fig. 7): impingement of posterior tibial nerve beneath flexor retinaculum behind medial malleolus
   a. **Etiology:** hyperpronation that leads to stress/traction on nerve with impingement (a correctable cause)
   b. **Symptoms/signs**
      i. Aching pain at medial foot, aggravated by weight-bearing
      ii. Trigger point usually detectable by palpation at site of impingement (positive Tinel's sign: tapping over trigger point causes radiating pain along medial or lateral plantar nerve distribution)
   c. **Diagnostic measures**
      i. Radiographs not helpful
      ii. Electromyographic studies show fibrillation potentials in muscles in the foot innervated by the nerve (e.g., abductor hallucis, abductor digiti quinti).
      iii. Nerve conduction studies (chronic cases)
   d. **Differential diagnosis**
      i. Posterior tibial tendinitis
      ii. Calcaneal stress fracture
      iii. Gout
      iv. Plantar fasciitis
   e. **Treatment**
      i. Rest, NSAIDs, graduated return to activity
      ii. Orthotic with support, especially with hyperpronation or other contributory structural deformities
      iii. Surgical decompression for intractable cases

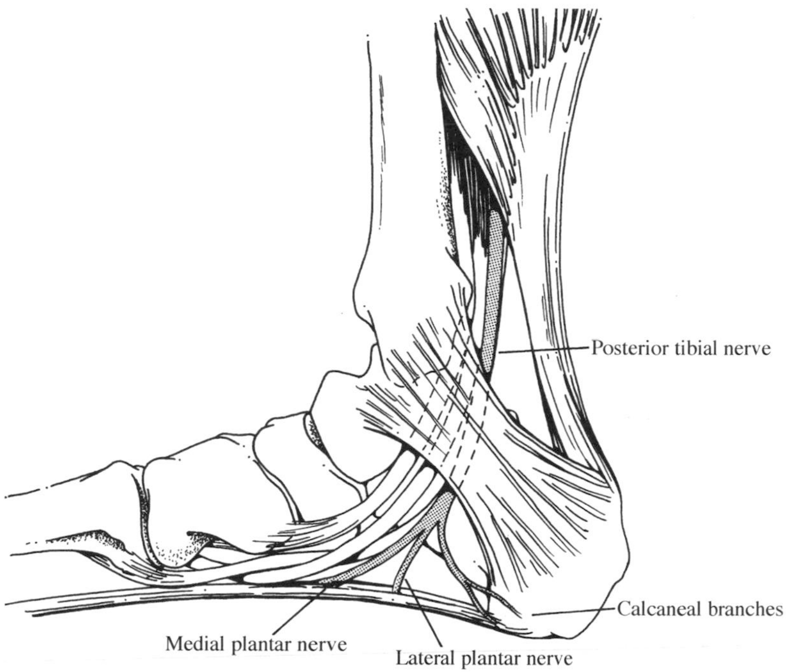

FIGURE 7. Tarsal tunnel syndrome.

2. **Morton's neuroma:** impingement of interdigital nerves as they bifurcate at metatarsal heads
   a. **Etiology**
      i. Trauma or repetitive stress leads to irritation of nerves as they cross under transverse metatarsal ligament to toes.
      ii. Swelling results, and a vicious cycle of swelling causing more pain and irritation causing more swelling occurs; "tumor" or inflammatory neuroma forms in chronic stages.
   b. **Symptoms/signs**
      i. Pain—typically burning neuralgia, worse with standing
      ii. Trigger point, tender to palpation between metatarsal heads; classically located between third and fourth metatarsals but can also occur between second and third (Fig. 8A)
      iii. Manual compression of metatarsals on either side of neuroma causes pain
   c. **Differential diagnosis**
      i. Metatarsalgia
      ii. Metatarsal stress fractures
   d. **Radiographic assessment:** not helpful
   e. **Treatment**
      i. Initial—NSAIDs, metatarsal pads to lift and spread metatarsal heads (Fig. 8B), sometimes corticosteroid injection
      ii. Chronic—surgical excision; patient left with permanent anesthesia between involved toes, but no functional deficits
      iii. Use of metatarsal pads on return to sports

I. **Reflex sympathetic dystrophy:** pain syndrome accompanied by evidence of autonomic dysfunction

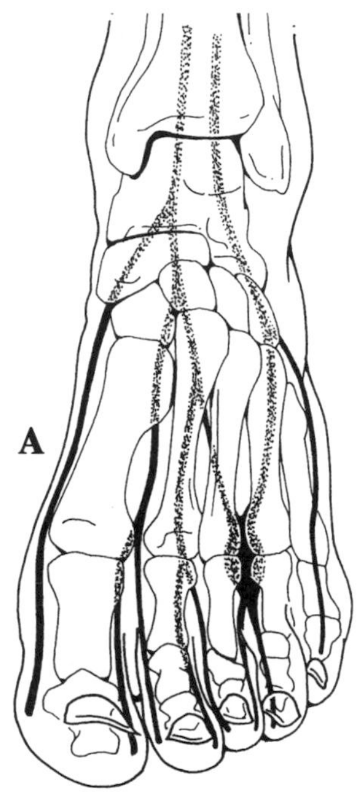

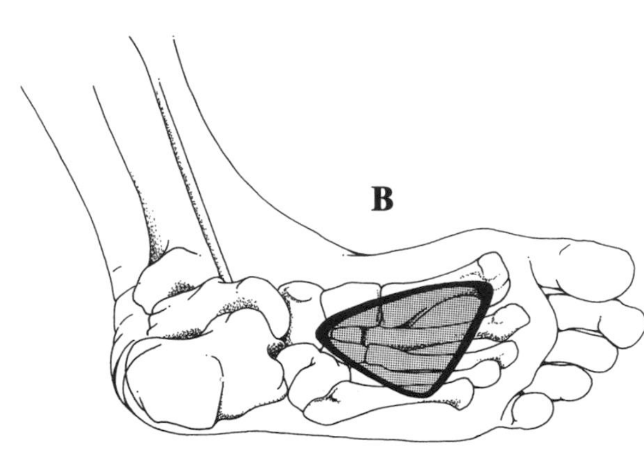

FIGURE 8. **A**, Morton's neuroma. **B**, Correct placement of metatarsal pad.

1. **Etiology**
   a. Can occur, regardless of patient's age, after an injury or trauma
   b. Cause currently unknown but believed to be dysfunction of the autonomic nervous system
2. **Symptoms/signs**
   a. Onset is heralded by severe, diffuse, unrelenting pain with exquisite tenderness to even light touch.
   b. Symptoms worsen with weight-bearing and improve by keeping the involved area motionless.
   c. Decreased range of motion and autonomic vasomotor signs, including warm or cool skin temperatures and decreased peripheral pulses. Skin may be moist to sweaty or dry to scaly with discoloration and swelling.
   d. Pain is usually out of proportion to the original injury.
3. **Radiographic assessment**
   a. May reveal diffuse osteoporosis of the involved part
   b. Bone scan may show delayed pattern of diffuse increased tracer throughout foot, with juxta-articular accentuation of tracer uptake
4. **Differential diagnosis:** peripheral nerve injuries, myofascial pain, polymyositis, systemic lupus erythematosis, Raynaud's disease, gout, thrombophlebitis
5. **Treatment**
   a. Prompt diagnosis and therapy improve the chance of permanent relief.
   b. Sympathetic blockade
   c. Physical therapy that includes vigorously active exercises, weight-bearing activities, and direct stimulation of the skin
   d. Adjuvant pharmacologic agents such as antidepressants, sedative-hypnotics, anxiolytics, anticonvulsants, narcotic analgesics, and corticosteroids
   e. Psychological evaluation is frequently required in more difficult cases.
   f. Occasionally, chemical or surgical sympathectomy is required.

53

Taping and Bracing

Denise Fandel, M.S., ATC, and Thomas Frette, M.A., ATC

I. Team Physician's Role in Taping and Bracing

A. **Determine appropriateness** of taping/bracing
B. **Facilitate selection process**
   1. **Identify** available options
   2. **Communicate** with treatment team
      a. Athletic trainer
      b. Coach
      c. Athlete
C. **Evaluate effectiveness** of selected support

II. Selection Considerations

A. **Diagnosis of injury**
   1. **Location**. Taping/bracing restricts undesired motion. It is contraindicated when restriction of motion may lead to decreased function or other problems.
   2. **Nature of injury**
      a. Taping/bracing provides support to acutely injured tissues.
      b. Taping/bracing decreases the effect of repetitive biomechanical forces resulting in chronic injuries.
   3. **Severity**. More severe injuries require more aggressive treatment.
B. **Goals of taping/bracing**
   1. **Prophylactic:** To reduce the incidence or severity of injury to uninjured normal anatomy or fully rehabilitated injuries
   2. **Rehabilitative:** To provide protection of healing injuries during their rehabilitation. **Taping/bracing does not substitute for or replace the need for complete rehabilitation**. It is only an adjunct to rehabilitation.
   3. **Functional:** To protect against reinjury following rehabilitation or surgical reconstruction
C. **Resources available**
   1. Taping
      a. Supplies are usually available.
      b. Requires application by athletic trainer or other skilled individual
      c. May become costly over repeated applications
   2. Braces
      a. Over-the-counter (OTC) braces instantly available
      b. Custom-made require time for fabrication
      c. Once instructed, athlete can self-apply
      d. Initially costly, but may be cost-effective over time; need to consult coaches and parents
   3. **If taping or bracing cannot provide any additional benefit, it is probably best to do without it**.

D. **Sport and position of athlete**
   1. **Physical requirements**. Taping is often tailored to allow the athlete to perform his or her skills.
   2. **Equipment**, including footwear, may need modification.
   3. **Environment** may affect choices.
      a. Temperature
      b. Humidity
      c. Aquatic
   4. **Rules**. Use materials that do not endanger other participants.

E. **Athlete's acceptance**
   1. Taping and bracing must not be uncomfortable or decrease performance.
   2. Involve the athlete in the decision-making process. Provide choices when possible.
   3. Realize the positive psychological effect of taping/bracing (assists the athlete's confidence on returning to competition).

F. **Research findings**
   1. Few studies are available.
   2. Many articles are supported only by clinical experience or tradition.
   3. New products should be viewed with an open but critical mind.

G. **Personal preferences**. Most physicians and athletic trainers develop a list of favorite techniques and devices, but each case should be viewed individually.

III. Implementation

A. **Communication.** Selection process, decision, and plan involves many individuals.
   1. Physician
   2. Athlete
   3. Coach
   4. Athletic trainer
   5. Sports physical therapist
   6. Orthotist
   7. Parent(s) or guardian(s)

B. **Education**
   1. **Taping**
      a. Teaching the trainer or coach the desired technique
      b. Prevention of skin problems (see at right)
   2. **Bracing**
      a. Instruction in the correct application of the brace
      b. Written directions on application and care
   3. **Promote concept of "earning the taping/bracing" by insisting on complete rehabilitation before resumption of sport**.

C. **Follow-up**
   1. Usually occurs at the conclusion of the athlete's season
      a. Reassess injured area; encourage "prehabilitation" of deficits before next season
      b. Reevaluate effectiveness of method of support
      c. May need to provide other alternatives for multisport athletes
   2. Provides opportunity to collect data for greatly needed research

IV. Principles of Taping

A. **Preparation**
   1. Decide on appropriate technique
   2. Gather needed tape supplies
   3. Position athlete's body part
      a. Position of function and/or protection
      b. Appropriate table height to optimize taper's body mechanics

B. **Tape selection**
   1. Qualities of a good athletic tape

a. Good adherence to athlete's skin
b. Adequate tensile strength to provide necessary support
c. Allows perspiration to escape
d. Easily unwinds and tears from roll
2. Size of body part determines appropriate width
3. Elasticity allows increased ease of application and desired movement, yet provides adequate injury protection.
a. More expensive
b. Many elastic tapes do not tear; require cutting with scissors

C. **Skin care**
1. **Preventive measures**
a. **Shave hair:**
i. Increases adhesion of tape
ii. Reduces irritation
iii. Reduces buildup of residue
b. **Apply a taping base** (e.g., tincture of benzoin):
i. Increases adhesion of tape
ii. Provides a protective layer between tape and skin
c. **Apply a tape underwrap** (e.g., thin polyester urethane foam):
i. Decreases skin problems
ii. Increases athlete's comfort
iii. May not be appropriate for all uses
d. **Apply a lubricant to possible areas of irritation** (e.g., lace and heel areas of the ankle).
2. **Proper tape removal**
a. Use scissors or cutters with blunt tip
b. Teach athlete proper removal technique
c. Cleanse skin to remove tape residue
d. Treat skin irritations and wounds promptly; these problems can prevent further taping.
3. **Allergic reactions to tape materials**
a. Recognize and treat problems.
b. Consider alternative tape supplies.
c. Investigate other forms of support and protection.

D. **Application**
1. **Requires a skilled individual—proficiency results from practice**
2. **Elements of proper taping technique**
a. Tearing tape is a basic skill; tape must be torn often.
b. Every piece of tape should have a distinct purpose.
c. Place anchor strips proximal and distal to the injured area directly on the skin.
d. Bridge across the injury, duplicating the anatomy needing support.
e. Weave the strips to add strength, overlapping by at least one half the width of the tape.
f. Adapt the two-dimensional tape to a three-dimensional body part.
g. Limit pressure around body prominences, especially when vascular and neural structures are superficial.
h. Use elastic materials over muscle bellies to allow normal muscle expansion.
i. Inspect for and tape over any gaps in the taping to prevent blisters and tape cuts.
3. **Avoid common problems that restrict circulation**.
a. Applying too much tape
b. Applying repeated circumferential strips without tearing between turns about the body part

c. Forcing the tape to go in a desired direction
d. Taping acute injuries (swelling causes tightness). *Do not tape acute injuries.*

V. Selected Taping Procedures

A. **Buddy taping** (Fig. 1A, B)
1. Common indications
a. Finger sprains
b. Minor fractures of proximal interphalangeal joint
2. Materials
a. ¼ inch tape
b. Felt or foam strip (optional)
3. Athlete position: felt or foam strip placed between injured and adjoining finger; avoid using index or little finger as a splint

B. **Thumb figure-of-eight** (Fig. 1C)
1. Common indications: hyperflexion injuries to the metacarpophalangeal (MCP) joint of the thumb
2. Materials
a. ¼ inch tape
b. Cloth or elastic
3. Athlete position: thumb abducted, wrist in slight extension
4. **Technique:** encircle wrist and thumb in a figure-of-eight pattern; repeat as necessary

C. **Thumb checkrein** (Fig. 1D)
1. Common indications: hyperextension or hyperabduction injuries to MCP joint of thumb; can result in injuries to MCP joint of index finger
2. Materials: ¼-inch and/or ½-inch tape
3. Athlete position: thumb slightly abducted
4. **Technique**
a. Encircle proximal phalanx of thumb and proximal phalanx of index finger
b. Press together adhesive surfaces between thumb and index finger
c. Anchor by taping around the checkrein

D. **Wrist taping** (Fig. 1E)
1. Common indications
a. Wrist sprains
b. Dorsal impingement
2. Materials
a. 1-inch or 1½-inch tape
b. Foam pad (for dorsal impingement)
3. Athlete position
a. Wrist slightly extended, pad on dorsum of wrist if needed to act as a "block" to extension range of motion
b. "Fan" of tape on volar or dorsal surface to prevent flexion or extension

E. **Elbow taping**
1. Common indications
a. Elbow hyperextension
b. Varus/valgus injuries
2. Materials: 1½-inch cloth tape or 2-inch elastic tape
3. Athlete position: slight flexion of elbow
4. **Technique for hyperextension injuries** (Fig. 2A)
a. Place anchor strips about the midupper arm and midforearm.
b. Criss-cross strips in an "X" pattern, creating a fan across the anterior aspect of the elbow.
c. Repeat anchors to close, taking care not to restrict circulation

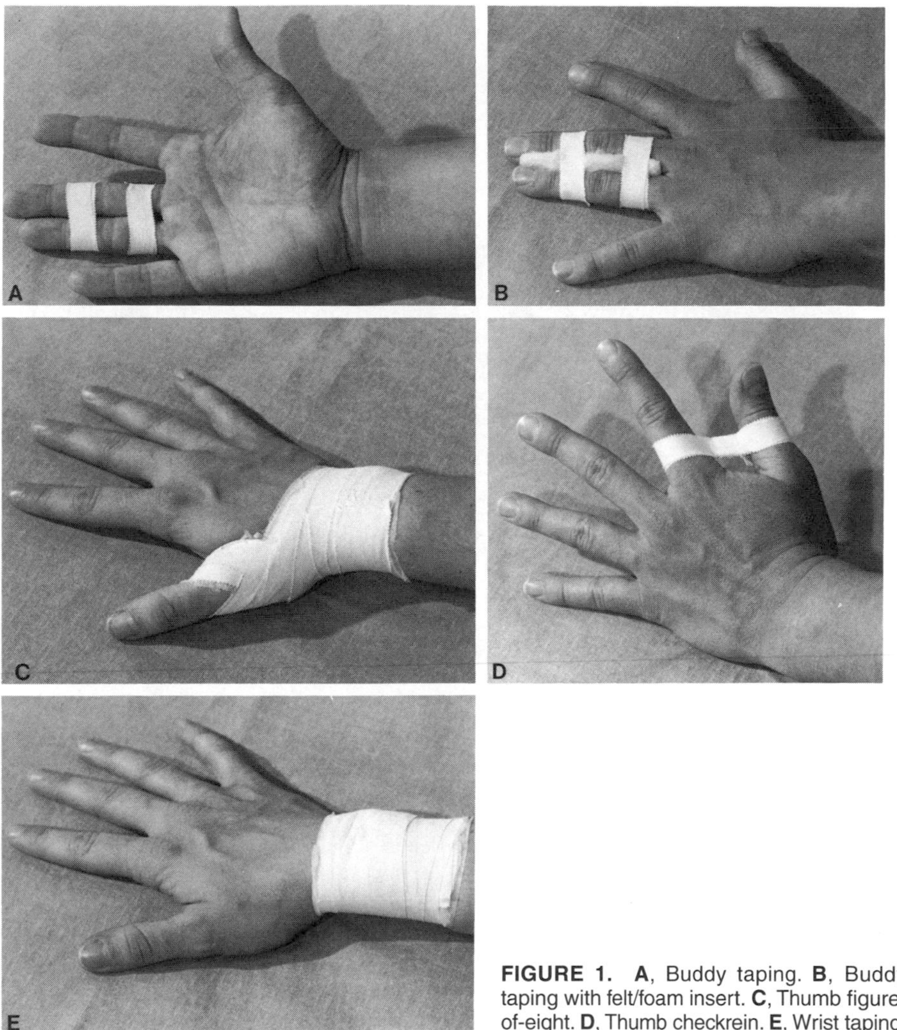

FIGURE 1. **A**, Buddy taping. **B**, Buddy taping with felt/foam insert. **C**, Thumb figure-of-eight. **D**, Thumb checkrein. **E**, Wrist taping.

5. **Technique for varus/valgus injuries:** modified to provide medial (Fig. 2B) lateral support

F. **Shoulder taping**
1. Restriction of motion required to provide adequate support decreases function
2. Suggest time and effort is probably better spent on rehabilitation

G. **Hip, hamstring, and groin taping**
1. Restriction of motion required to provide adequate support decreases function
2. Recommend use of elastic wraps in a figure-of-eight pattern about the waist and upper thigh, or neoprene thigh sleeves

H. **Anterior cruciate ligament taping**
1. Performance of custom-fitted and off-the-shelf braces far exceeds that of taping
2. Taping requires skilled practitioner

I. **Medial or lateral knee taping**

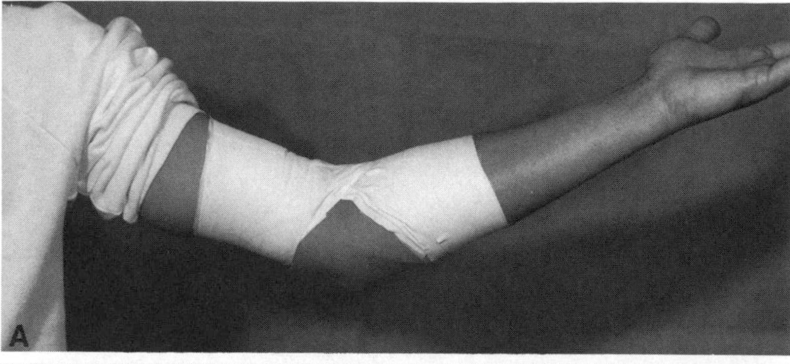

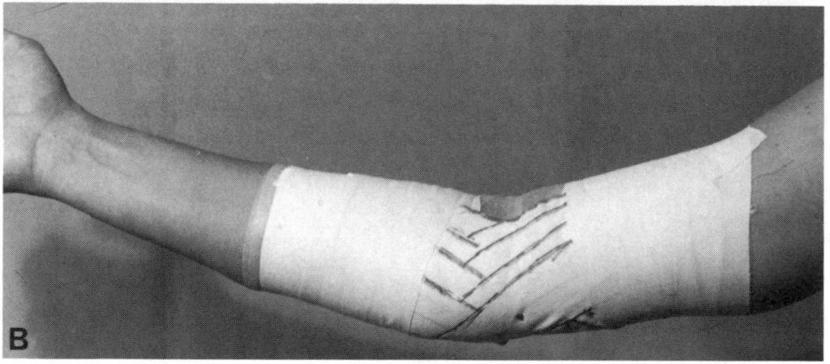

FIGURE 2. **A**, Elbow hyperextension taping. **B**, Medial elbow taping.

1. Common indication: collateral ligament sprain
2. Materials: 1½-inch or 2-inch cloth tape, or 3-inch elastic tape
3. Athlete position: standing with knee flexed about 15° by placing 1-inch to 1½-inch block under athlete's heel
4. **Technique for medial knee injuries** (Fig. 3)
   a. Place anchor strips about the midthigh and midcalf.
   b. Criss-cross strips in an "X" pattern, creating a fan across the medial aspect of the knee. Binding or crimping tape increases tensile strength.
   c. Repeat anchors to close, taking care not to restrict circulation.
   d. Cut the area posteriorly over the calf and close the gap.
5. **Technique for lateral knee injuries:** modified to provide lateral support

J. **Patellofemoral taping** (Fig. 4)
1. Common indications
   a. Patellofemoral pain syndromes
   b. Patellar tendinitis
2. Materials
   a. Hypafix*
   b. Sports Tape*
   c. Skin-prep wipes
3. Athlete position: knee slightly flexed; may vary depending on athlete symptoms
4. **Technique**
   a. Shave hair from anterior aspect of knee; clean with Skin-prep
   b. Apply three strips of Hypafix:

---

* Hypafix (2-inch roll, #4209) and Sports Tape (1½-inch roll, #1853A) available from Don Joy Co., 5966 LaPlace Court, Carlsbad, CA, 92008, 1-800-228-4421.

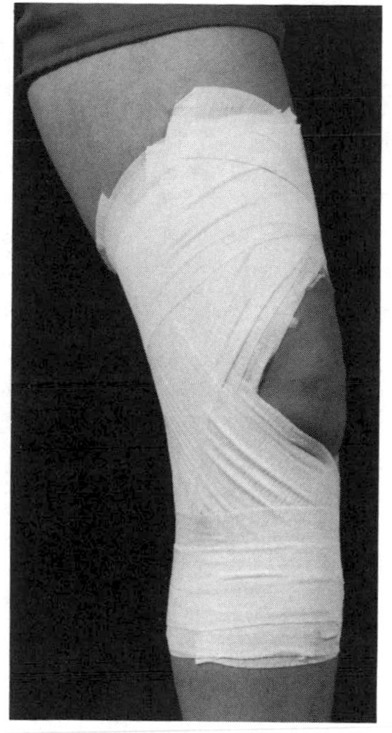

FIGURE 3. Medial knee taping.

   i. Starting laterally, place first strip over proximal half of patella, pushing knee cap distally, pulling medially, and puckering the skin (Fig. 4A).
   ii. Starting more laterally, place second strip over middle of patella, pulling patella medially and tilting medial edge downward, again puckering the skin (Fig. 4B).
   iii. Apply third strip over distal half of patella (Fig. 4C).
  c. Apply three strips of Sports Tape:
   i. Apply first and second strips in the same manner as Hypafix strips (Fig. 4D).
   ii. Starting laterally, place third strip over inferior pole of patella, rotating it medially and superiorly (Fig. 4E).
   iii. Apply optional anchor strip over all three previous strips, again pulling medially (Fig. 4F).

K. **Ankle taping** (Fig. 5)
 1. **Most researched taping procedure**
 2. Restricts extreme ranges of motion
  a. Does not increase the incidence of knee injuries or affect athletic performance
  b. Protective effect of taping due to increased proprioceptive input
  c. Prevents reinjury to ankles previously injured
  d. Some benefit provided by reusable cloth ankle wrapping or high-top shoes
 3. Common indications
  a. Prevention or treatment of ankle sprains
  b. Subluxing peroneal tendons and dorsal impingement by using appropriate padding
 4. Materials
  a. 1½-inch or 2-inch cloth tape
  b. Foam/felt as needed
 5. Athlete position: sitting on table, knee extended, ankle at a right angle of plantarflexion/dorsiflexion and neutral inversion/eversion

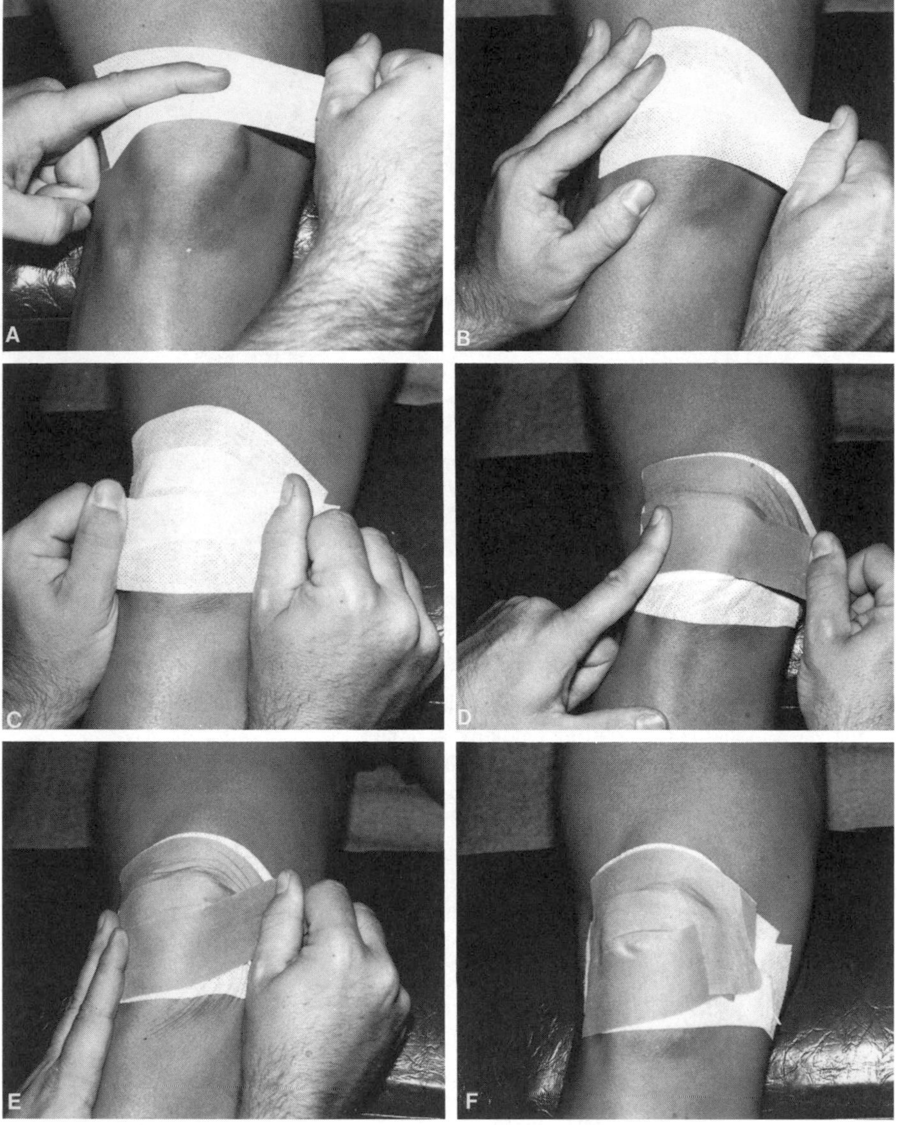

FIGURE 4. Patellofemoral taping.

6. **Technique:** specific application can be adapted by the experienced taper to achieve goal
   a. Shave skin and apply lubricated heel and lace pads (Fig. 5A)
   b. Place foam or felt padding for specific purposes:
      i. "J" pad posterior and distal to the lateral malleolus for subluxation of the peroneal tendons (Fig. 5B)
      ii. In cases of anterior ankle impingement, a square "dorsal block" pad on the lace area to restrict dorsiflexion (Fig. 5C)
      iii. "Horseshoe," "U," or "donut" pad about malleolus to place compression to the swelling of *subacute* injuries (Fig. 5D)

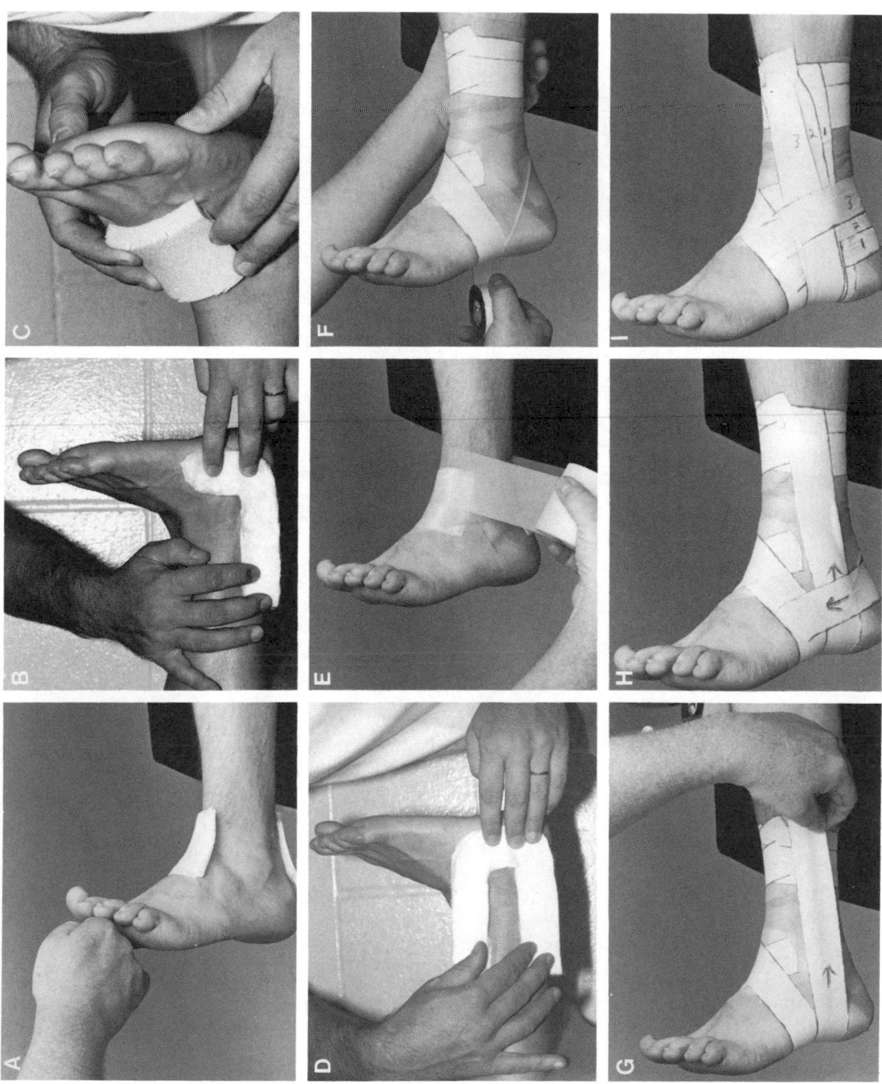

FIGURE 5. A–I, Ankle taping (*continued*).

c. Apply tape adherent and underwrap (Fig. 5E); underwrap may be omitted to provide additional support, especially to more acute injuries, but special care of the skin is required.
d. **Closed basketweave**, basic to most applications:
   i. Apply anchor strips around the calf at the level of the musculotendinous junction of the gastrocsoleus and around the arch proximal to the base of the fifth metatarsal (Fig. 5F).
   ii. Apply a "stirrup" strip, starting medially on the calf anchor medially, passing beneath the heel posterior to the malleoli, pulling laterally to the other side of the calf anchor (Fig. 5G); in eversion sprains, the stirrup is placed with equal tension medially and laterally.
   iii. Apply a "horseshoe" perpendicular to the stirrup, distal to the malleoli, starting and finishing on the arch anchor (Fig. 5H).
   iv. Repeat stirrups and horseshoes twice more, overlapping the previous strip by one half, completing the "basketweave" (Fig. 5I).
e. **Figure-of-eight** to restrict plantarflexion:
   i. Apply tape on the outside of the foot and angle under the foot (Fig. 5J).
   ii. Cross over the lace area and encircle the leg (Fig. 5K).
f. **"Heel locks"** to restrict inversion/eversion:
   i. Medial heel lock restricts inversion:
      (a) Apply tape on lace area (Fig. 5L).
      (b) Angle behind and across the medial aspect of the heel (Fig. 5M).
      (c) Continue under the heel and return to the lace area (Fig. 5N).
   ii. Lateral heel lock restricts eversion:
      (a) Apply in the opposite direction.
      (b) Angle across the lateral aspect of the heel (Fig. 5O).
   iii. Repeat heel locks to obtain desired support.
   iv. Place circular strips about the lower leg, overlapping distal to proximal, to cover remaining open spaces (Fig. 5P).
g. Repeat anchors to close (Fig. 5Q).
h. Remove taping by cutting along the medial aspect, posterior to the medial malleolus (Fig. 5R).

L. **Arch figure-of-eight** (Fig. 6)
1. Common indications
   a. Arch sprains
   b. Conditions resulting from excessive pronation
2. Materials: 1-inch or 1½-inch tape
3. Athlete position: same as ankle taping
4. **Technique**
   a. Eliminate underwrap to allow for foot perspiration.
   b. Apply anchor strip loosely around the metatarsal heads (Fig. 6A); allow for expansion of the foot on weight bearing.
   c. Apply a half figure-of-eight, starting at the base of the great toe, angling across the longitudinal arch, around the heel, and returning to the base of the great toe (Fig. 6B).
   d. Apply the other half figure-of-eight, starting at the base of the little toe, angling across the longitudinal arch, around the heel, and returning to the base of the little toe (Fig. 6C).
   e. Repeat steps "c" and "d" once or twice more (Fig. 6D).
   f. Apply horizontal strips, pulling medially, from the heel to the ball of the foot (Fig. 6E).
   g. Apply a "low dye" strip.

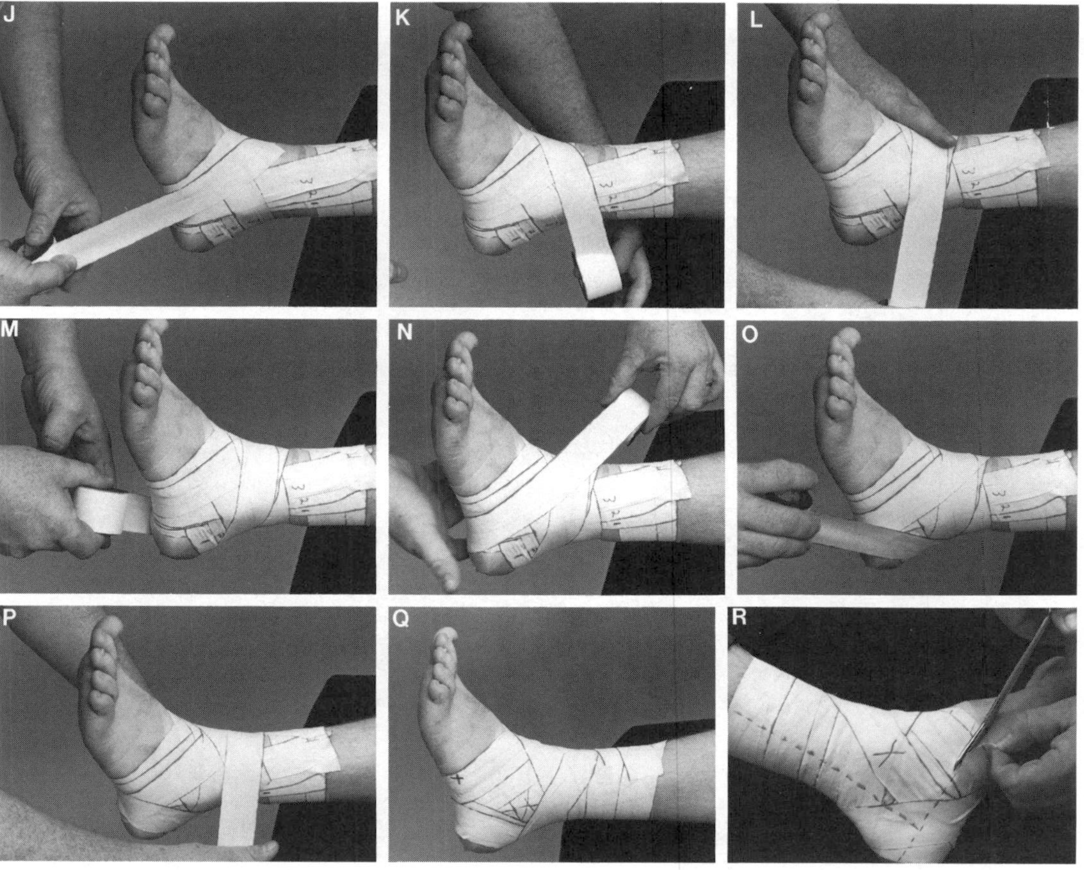

FIGURE 5. (*continuation*). **J–R**, Ankle taping.

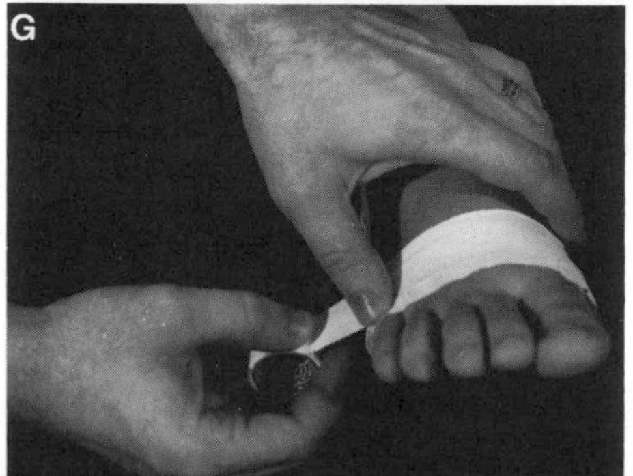

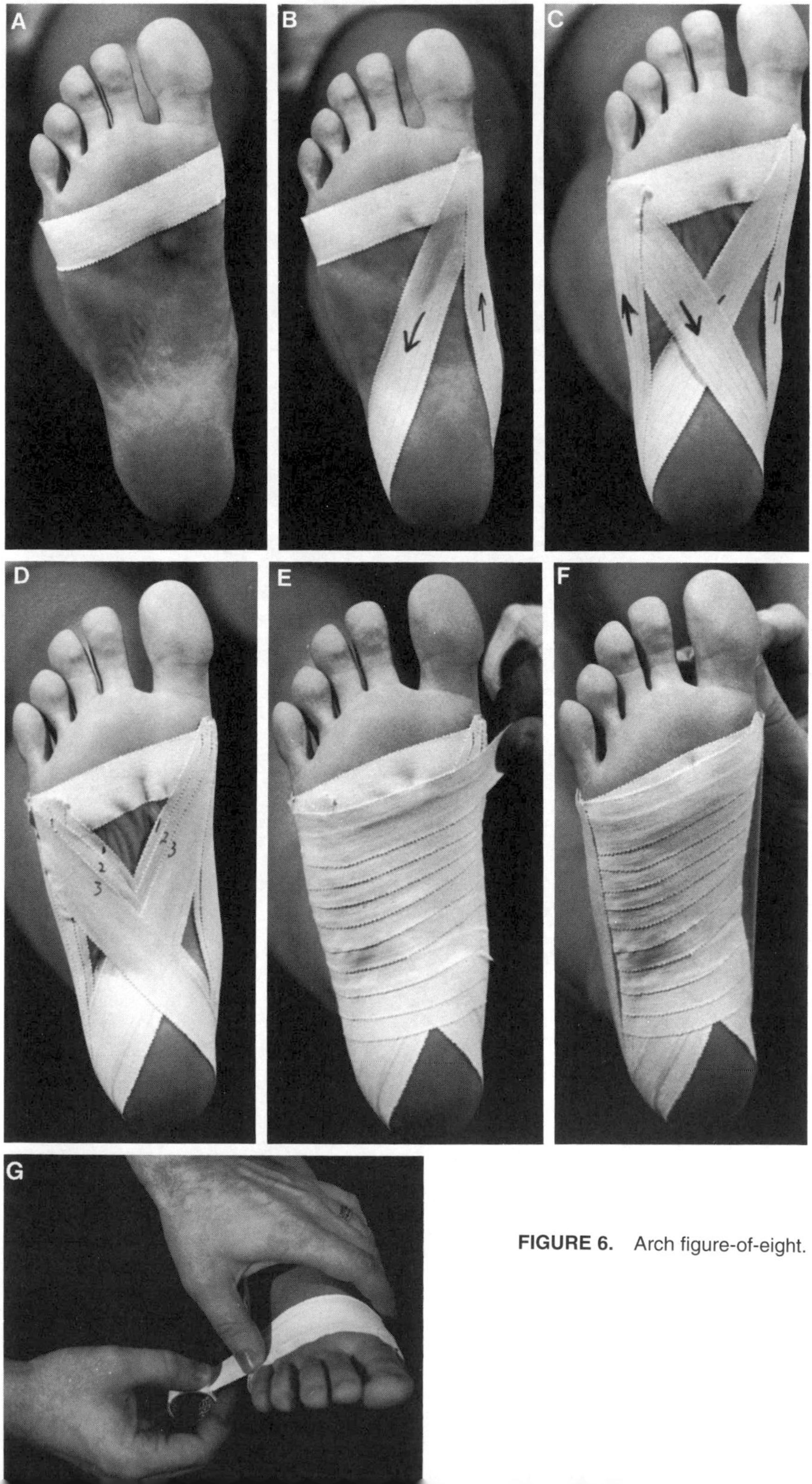

FIGURE 6. Arch figure-of-eight.

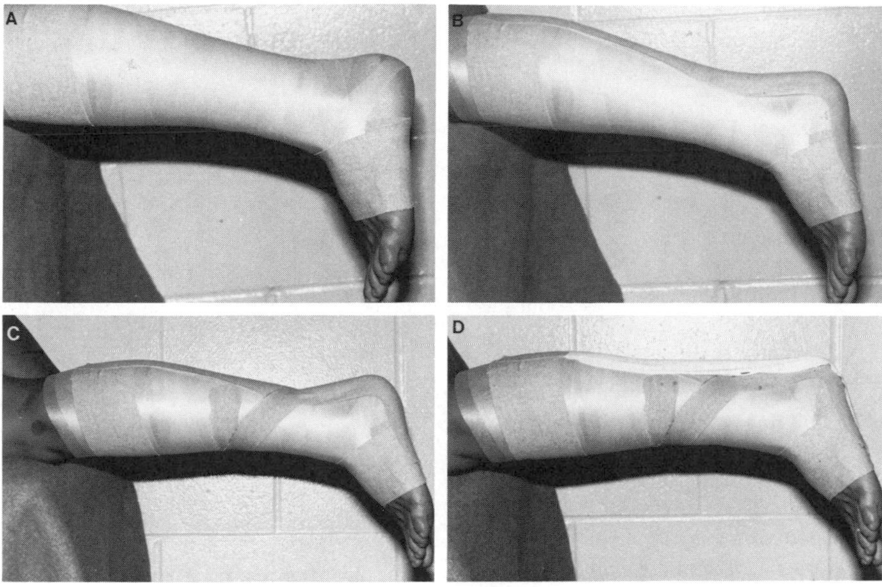

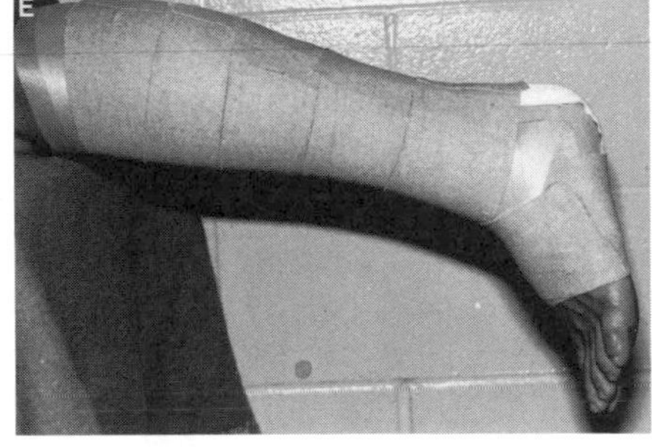

FIGURE 7. Achilles tendon taping.

   h. Close by applying a half anchor dorsum of the foot over the original anchor (Fig. 6G).

M. **Achilles tendon taping** (Fig. 7)
   1. Common indications
      a. Strain of the gastrocsoleus/Achilles tendon
      b. Achilles tendinitis
   2. Materials
      a. 3-inch elastic tape
      b. 1½-inch or 2-inch cloth tape (optional)
   3. Athlete position: prone with ankle plantarflexion
   4. **Technique**
      a. Apply anchors around the arch of the foot and the calf (Fig. 7A).
      b. Apply support strips, repeat as needed; may use any of the following alternatives:
         i. Start from the foot anchor, pull proximally to end at the calf anchor (Fig. 7B)
         ii. Start from the foot anchor, pull proximally, split tape in half to achieve better attachment to the anchors (Fig. 7C)
         iii. Using cloth tape, fan strips from calcaneus to achieve greater support (Fig. 7D)
      c. Close applying circular strips about the foot and calf (Fig. 7E).

N. **Turf-toe taping** (Fig. 8)
1. Common indications: sprains of the first metatarsophalangeal joint and sesamoiditis
2. Materials
   a. 1-inch tape
   b. Felt/foam (optional)
3. Athlete position: same as ankle taping, positioning great toe in direction opposite of injury.
4. **Technique**
   a. Place metatarsal pad with cut-out for base of first metatarsal for sesamoiditis (Fig. 8A).
   b. Apply anchor strips about the midarch of the foot and about the proximal phalanx of the great toe (Fig. 8B).
   c. Apply support strips from the distal anchor to the proximal; dorsal strips restrict flexion and ventral strips restrict extension (Fig. 8C).
   d. Repeat anchors to close (Fig. 8D).

VI. Bracing

A. **Comparisons of bracing to taping**
1. **Advantages of bracing**
   a. Do not require skilled application
   b. Sometimes more cost-effective
   c. Increased convenience
2. Disadvantages of bracing
   a. Migration of braces during active use:
      i. Failure to provide support
      ii. May lead to decreased performance
      iii. Migration may be reduced by use of tape adherent, or specially designed straps or undergarments.
   b. Athletes commonly complain about the weight of some braces, required to provide adequate protection.
   c. Brace parts wear out or may break, requiring untimely replacement.
   d. An athlete may be between sizes of OTC braces.
   e. Custom-made braces are more expensive and require time to be fabricated.

B. **Considerations of brace prescription**
1. **Brace market full of unsubstantiated claims and disclaimers of liability**
2. **Need to be knowledgeable about and critical of new devices**
3. **Often need to evaluate a currently used or "borrowed" device**
4. **Brace-related problems** (e.g., skin irritation, altered function) require attention.
5. **Discuss options with the treatment team**.

VII. Selected Braces

A. **Tennis elbow "counter-force" strap** (Fig. 9)
1. Common indications
   a. Lateral epicondylitis
   b. Medial epicondylitis (less often)
2. Description: OTC Velcro and elastic strap placed on proximal forearm, designed to reduce contractile force of wrist and finger extensors
3. Application and usage: worn during activities (sport or nonsport) that aggravate condition

B. **Silicone rubber wrist/hand cast** (Fig. 10)
1. Common indications: hand and wrist injuries requiring immobilization to participate in contact or collision sports, e.g., moderate sprains, healing nondisplaced or

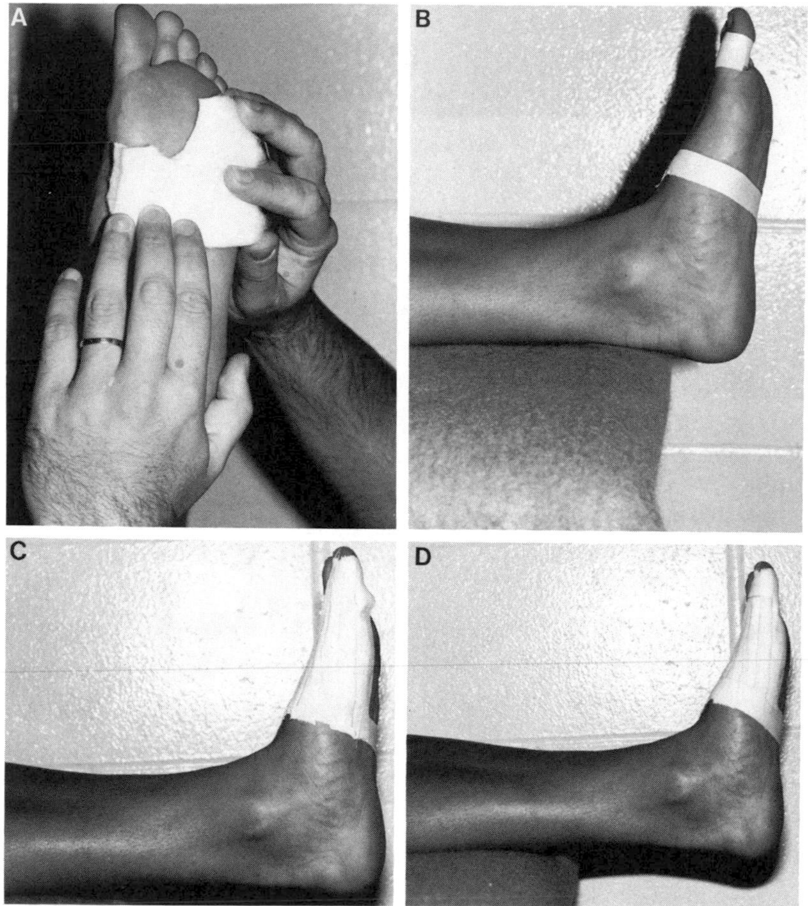

FIGURE 8. Turf-toe taping.

internally fixated fractures. Physician decides if injury can be adequately supported by silicone casting.

2. Description: custom-made (ScotchCast currently accepted by all high school and college/university athletic associations)
3. Application and usage: splint is univalved and secured by tape; bivalved cast maintains immobilization when not actively participating in sport

C. **Lateral prophylactic knee braces** (Fig. 11).
1. Common indications: decrease incidence and severity of valgus force injuries to the knee; most commonly used in football
2. Description: OTC hinged single lateral upright or hinged double upright device taped or otherwise strapped to the knee
3. Application and usage
   a. Brace migration prevention:
      i. Shave the skin, as for taping.
      ii. Use tape adherent.
   b. Maximal effectiveness requires team approach:
      i. Use of audiovisual aids (i.e., videotapes, posters) supplied by manufacturers to teach players proper application and daily reminders

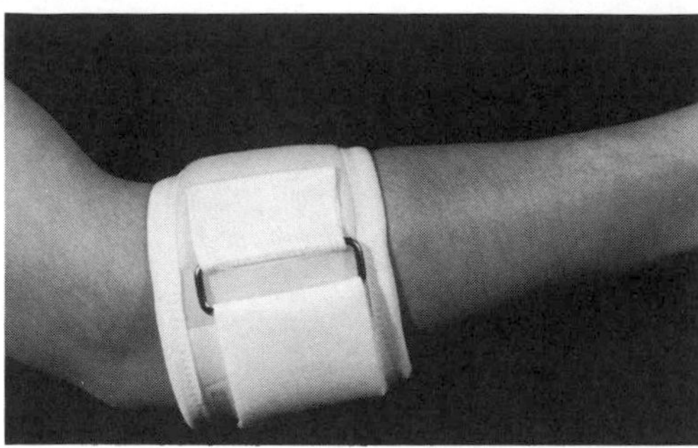

FIGURE 9. Tennis-elbow counter-force brace.

ii. Daily check of positioning by coaches and trainers
iii. Weekly check on upkeep by coaches, parents, equipment managers, trainers, and players

c. **Effectiveness debatable**

D. **Functional knee braces** (Fig. 12)
  1. Common indications
    a. Mild/moderate instability
    b. Postreconstructive surgery of moderate/severe instability
  2. Description: various designs using hinged double uprights with range-of-motion stops, straps, or fitted cuffs or shells; some OTCs, but most are custom-fitted; many use a neoprene sleeve undergarment
  3. Application and usage
    a. Migration and fit can be a problem (see "Lateral prophylactic knee braces").
    b. Exposed metal must be covered in contact-sport applications.
    c. Some studies have investigated the relative effectiveness of these braces.[1–3,5,7,12]

E. **Knee sleeves** (Fig. 13)
  1. Common indications
    a. Conservative management of many knee-pain complaints resulting from acute or chronic inflammation, including strains, cartilage tears, and patellofemoral problems
    b. May be used postoperatively for effusion control
  2. Description: OTC elastic or neoprene pull-over sleeve
  3. Application and usage
    a. Easily acquired and accepted
    b. Neoprene support increases sense of warmth, comfort

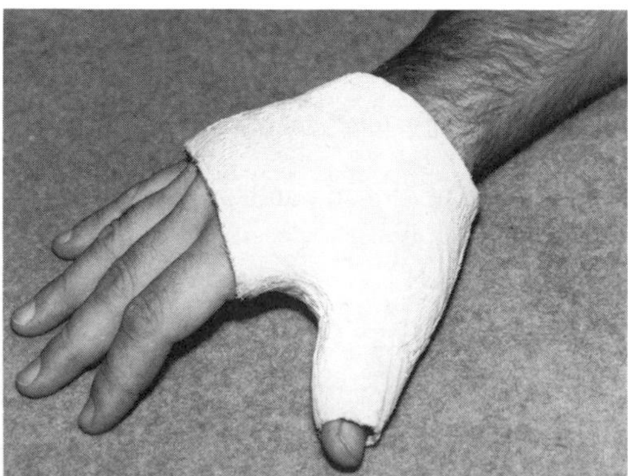

FIGURE 10. Silicone rubber wrist/hand cast.

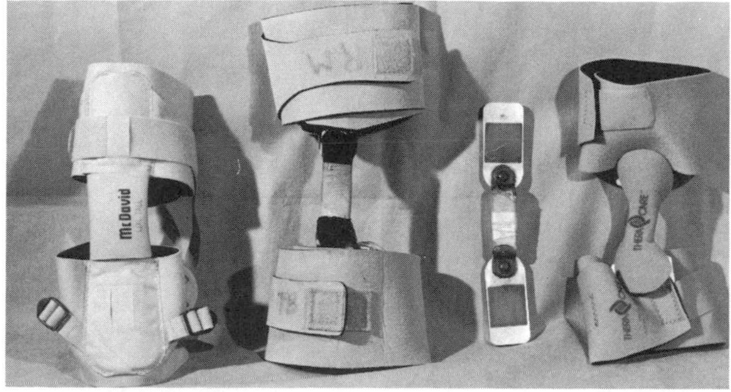

FIGURE 11. Examples of lateral prophylactic knee braces.

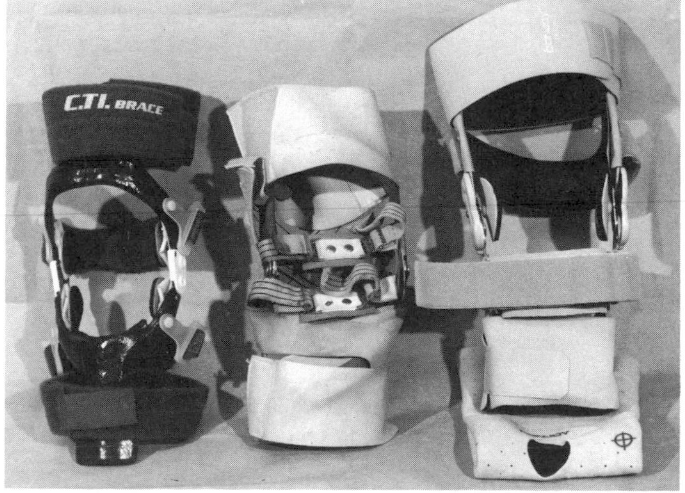

FIGURE 12. Examples of functional knee braces.

c. Patellofemoral problems usually require use of sleeve with patellar cut-out
d. Report of increased stability probably due to increased proprioceptive input
e. Similar braces with hinges rarely provide additional support.
f. **Similar devices available for other areas of the body—forearm, wrist, calf**

F. **Palumbo lateral patella stabilizing brace** (Fig. 14)
1. Common indications: conservative or postoperative management of patellofemoral joint problems
2. Description: OTC elastic or neoprene knee sleeve with patellar cut-out and a "Y"-shaped lateral buttress strap to dynamically decrease excessive lateral patellar tracking
3. Application and usage
   a. Usually place counterbalancing strap superiorly
   b. Cases of infrapatellar tendinitis may be aided by inferior placement of counterbalancing strap
   c. Cases of medial patellar subluxation (rare) may be aided by medial positioning of buttress strap

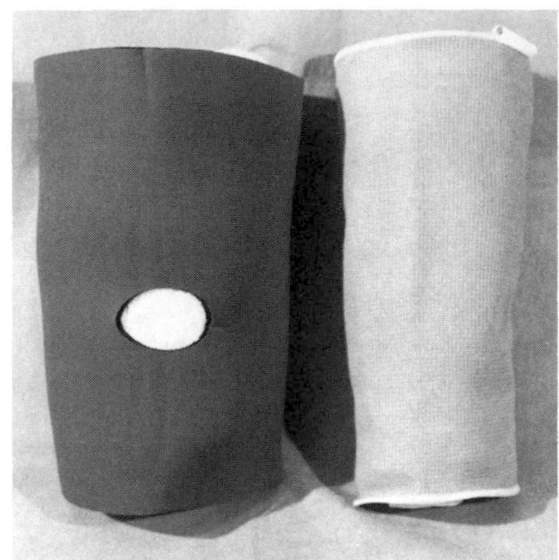

FIGURE 13. Knee sleeves, neoprene (*left*) and elastic (*right*).

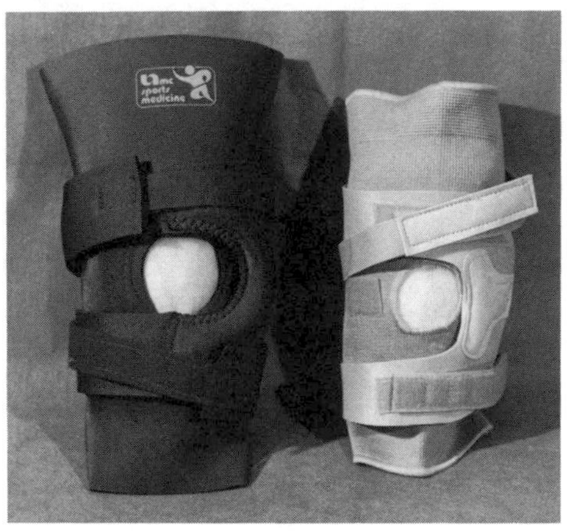

FIGURE 14. Palumbo braces, neoprene (*left*) and elastic (*right*).

G. **Ankle braces**
  1. Common indications
    a. Healed/healing ankle sprains or fractures
    b. Tendinitis about the ankle

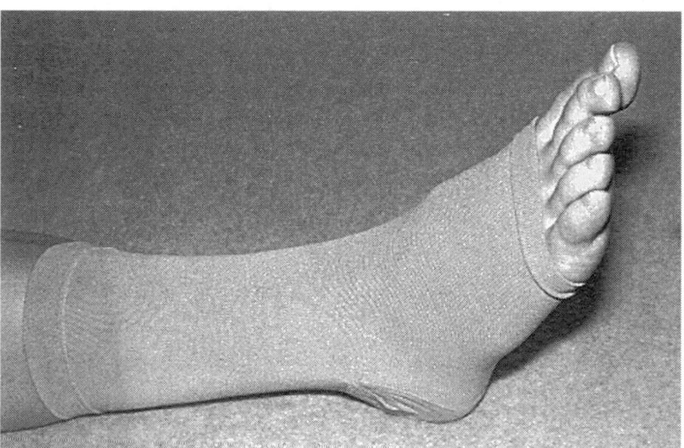

FIGURE 15. Slip-on elastic support.

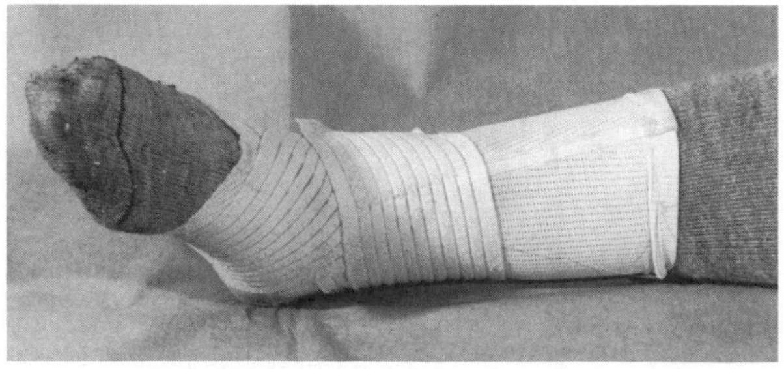

FIGURE 16. Slip-on Spandex sleeve with elastic and Velcro straps.

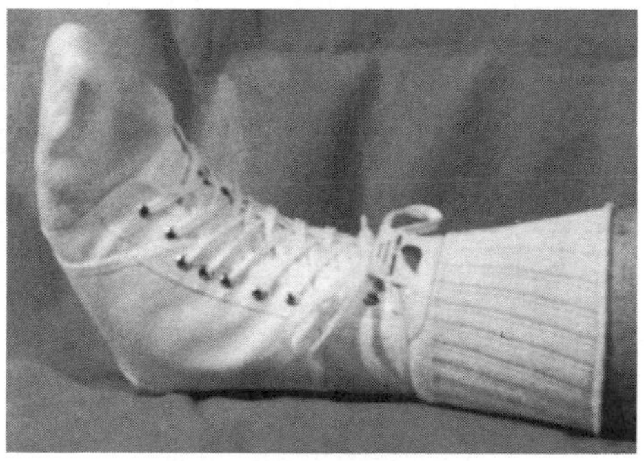

FIGURE 17. Lace-up ankle support.

2. Description, application, and usage
   a. **Slip-on elastic support** (Fig. 15) provides even compression to decrease edema; not a prophylactic support
   b. **Slip-on Spandex sleeve with elastic and Velcro straps** to restrict inversion/eversion (Fig. 16); good prophylactic support
   c. **Lace-up ankle support** (Fig. 17) uses medial and lateral stays to restrict inversion/eversion; best alternative to ankle taping; may be used as prophylactic or functional support
   d. **Stirrup splints**, based on semirigid orthosis, use Velcro straps to hold in place; designed for rehabilitative and functional uses:
      i. **Air Cast** (Fig. 18) uses adjustable air pressure linings to improve individual fit, decrease edema, and prevent excessive inversion/eversion.[29]
      ii. **Gel Cast** uses gel-filled linings to improve individual fit; can be placed in freezer to be used as one form of cryotherapy; holds in body heat for increased comfort and functional use.
      iii. Other devices use foam rubber linings or other materials; may be OTC or custom-made
      iv. **Hinged stirrup splint** has greater acceptance as a prophylactic brace.

H. **Orthotics—devices placed in athlete's shoe to balance the foot during activity**
   1. Common indications: lower extremity kinetic chain conditions resulting from excessive pronation, cavus foot, or other foot dysfunctions
   2. Description, application, and usage

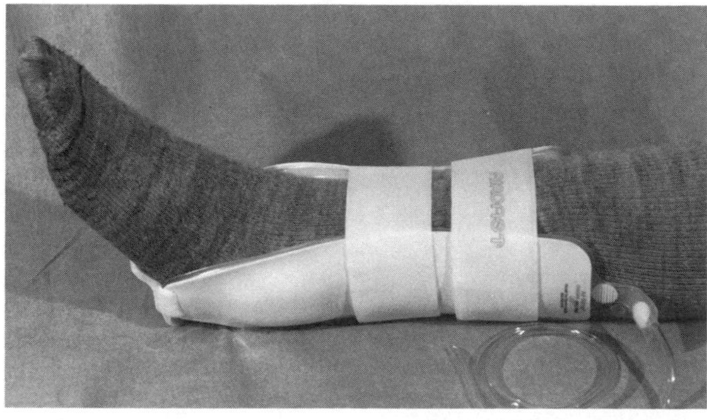

FIGURE 18. Air Cast with pressure adjustment tube attached. (Air Cast, Inc., Summit, NJ, 1-800-526-8785)

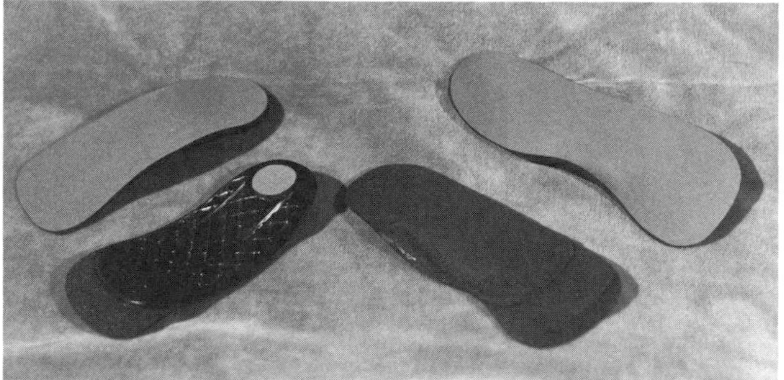

FIGURE 19. Spenco arch supports, rigid (*left*) and semirigid (*right*).

a. **Soft orthotics** provide OTC and cheaper solution; easy break-in
b. **Hard orthotics** provide customized solution for road runners not involved in agility activities
c. **Semirigid orthotics** (Fig. 19) provide support of hard orthotics for athletes involved in agility sports
d. **Sorbothane visoelastic insoles** (Fig. 20) reduce impact loading forces
e. **Steel shoe inserts** (Fig. 21) provide support to metatarsal fractures and "turf toe"
f. **Heel cups** (e.g., Tuli's, Fig. 22) decrease impact and improve shock absorption capabilities of calcaneal fat pad
g. **Longitudinal arch pads** (Fig. 23) provide symptomatic relief of painful foot conditions; may be held in place with tape or glue or may be self-adhesive to shoe
h. **Metatarsal arch pads** (Fig. 24) provide symptomatic relief of painful foot conditions; may be held in place with tape or glue or may be self-adhesive to shoe

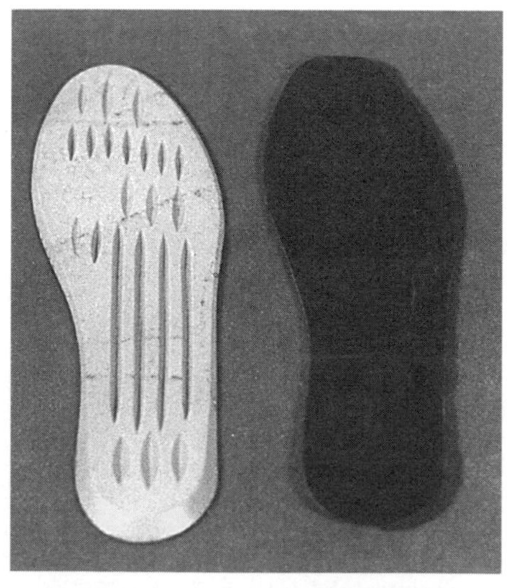

FIGURE 20. Sorbothane insoles.

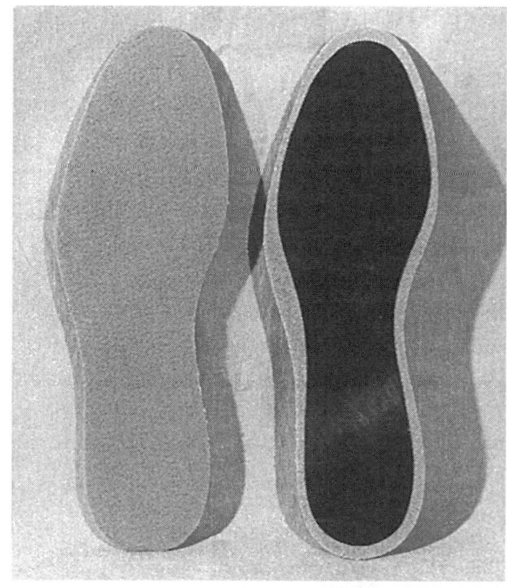

FIGURE 21. Steel shoe inserts.

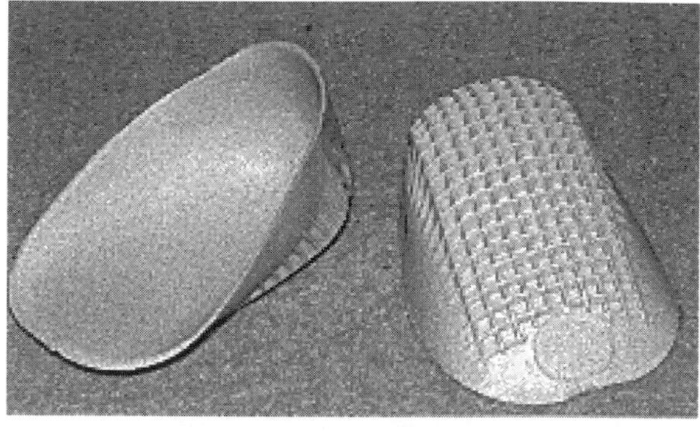

FIGURE 22. Tuli's heel cups.

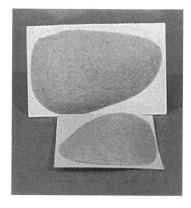

FIGURE 24. Metatarsal arch pads.

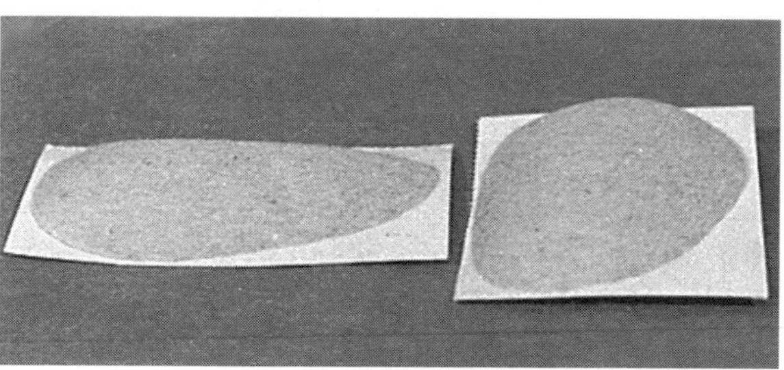

FIGURE 23. Longitudinal arch pads.

Recommended Reading

1. Albright JP, Powell JW, Smith W, et al: Medial collateral ligament sprains in college football: Brace wear preference and injury risk. Am J Sports Med 22(1):2, 1994.
2. Albright JP, Powell JW, Smith W, et al: Medial collateral ligament sprains in college football: Effectiveness of preventative braces. Am J Sports Med 22(1):12, 1994.
3. American Academy of Orthopaedic Surgeons Committee on the Knee: Prophylactic Knee Braces. Park Ridge, IL, American Academy of Orthopaedic Surgeons, 1987.
4. Bahr R, Karlsen R, Lian O, Ovrebo RV: Incidence and mechanisms of acute ankle inversion injuries in volleyball. Am J Sports Med 22(5):595, 1994.
5. Baker BE, VanHanswyk E, Bogosian S IV, et al: A biomechanical study of the static stabilizing effect of knee braces on medial stability. Am J Sports Med 15:556, 1987.
6. Bassett FH, Malone T, Gilcrist RA: A protective splint of rubber. Am J Sports Med 7:358, 1979.
7. Beck C, Drez D, Young J, et al: Instrumented testing of functional knee braces. Am J Sports Med 14:253, 1986.
8. Beriau MR, Cox WB, Manning J: Effects of ankle braces upon agility course performance in high school athletes. J Athletic Training 29(3):224–230, 1994.
9. Bradley JA: The modified rubber playing cast. Phys Sportsmed 10(11):168, 1982.
10. Bunch RP, Bednarski K, Holland D, Macinanti R: Ankle joint support: A comparison of reuseable lace-on braces with taping and bracing. Phys Sportsmed 13(5):59, 1985.
11. Cowell HR: College football: To brace or not to brace [editorial]. J Bone Joint Surg 69A:1, 1987.
12. Deppen RJ, Landfried M: Efficacy of prophylactic knee bracing in high school football players. J Sports Phys Ther 20(5):243, 1994.
13. Distefano V, Nixon JE: An improved method taping. J Sports Med 2:209, 1974.
14. Doughtie M: The use of RTV-11 silicone rubber for a carpal navicular fracture. Athletic Train 14:146, 1979.
15. France EP, Paulos LE, Jayaraman G, et al: The biomechanics of knee bracing: Part II. Impact response of the braced knee. Am J Sports Med 15:430, 1987.
16. Functional knee braces help stabilize medial collateral ligament. Orthop Today 6(8):1, 1986.
17. Garrick JG, Requa RK: Role of external support in the prevention of ankle sprains. Med Sci Sports 5:200, 1973.

18. Grace TG, Skipper BJ, Newberry JC, et al: Prophylactic knee braces and injury to the lower extremity. J Bone Joint Surg 70A:422, 1988.
19. Gross MT, Ballard CL, Mears HG, Watkins EJ: Comparison of DonJoy ankle ligament protector and Aircast Sport Stirrup orthoses in restricting foot and ankle motion before and after exercise. J Sports Phys Ther 16(2):60, 1992.
20. Gross MT, Batten AM, Lamm AL, et al: Comparison of DonJoy ankle ligament protector and subtalar sling ankle taping in restricting foot and ankle motion before and after exercise. J Sports Phys Ther 19(1):33, 1994.
21. Hewson GF, Mendini RA, Wang JB: Prophylactic knee bracing in college football. Am J Sports Med 14:262, 1986.
22. Knee braces to prevent injuries in football: A round table. Phys Sportsmed 14(4):108, 1986.
23. Laughman RK, Carr TA, Chao EY, et al: Three-dimensional kinematics of the taped ankle before and after exercise. Am J Sports Med 8:425, 1980.
24. Libera D: Ankle taping, wrapping, and injury prevention. Athletic Train 7:73, 1972.
25. Lysholm J, Mordin M, Ekstrand J, Guilquist J: The effects of a patella brace on performance in knee extension strength test in patients with patellar pain. Am J Sports Med 12:110, 1984.
26. McConnell JS: The management of chondromalacia patellae: A long-term solution. Aust J Physiother 32:215–223, 1986.
27. Metcalf GR, Denegar CR: A critical review of ankle taping. Athletic Train 18:121, 1983.
28. Nirschl RP: The etiology and treatment of tennis elbow. J Sports Med 12:110, 1984.
29. Palumbo PM: Dynamic patellar brace: A new orthosis in the management of patello-femoral disorders: A preliminary report. Am J Sports Med 9:45, 1981.
30. Paulos LE, France EP, Rosenbergy TD, et al: The biomechanics of knee bracing: Part I. Response of the valgus strains to loading. Am J Sports Med 15:419, 1987.
31. Peppard A: Thumb taping. Phys Sportsmed 10(4):139, 1982.
32. Prentice WE, Toriscelli T: The effects of lateral knee stabilizing braces on running speed and agility. Athletic Train 21:113, 1986.
33. Rovere GD, Haupt HA, Yates CS: Prophylactic knee bracing in college football. Am J Sports Med 15:111, 1987.
34. Stover C: A functional semirigid support system for ankle injuries. Phys Sportsmed 7(5):71, 1979.
35. Stover CN: Air stirrup management of ankle injuries in the athlete. Am J Sports Med 8:360, 1980.
36. Teitz CC, Hermanson BK, Kronmal RA, et al: Evaluation of the use of braces to prevent injury to the knee in collegiate football players. J Bone Joint Surg 69A:2, 1987.
37. Thorndike A: Athletic injuries: Prevention, Diagnosis and Treatment. Philadelphia, Lea & Febiger, 1948.
38. Whitesel J, Newell SG: Modified low-dyestrapping. Phys Sportsmed 8(9):129, 1980.

VIII
SPECIFIC SPORTS

54: Football

Margot Putukian, M.D., FACSM, Neal Stansbury, M.D., and Wayne Sebastianelli, M.D.

I. Overview

A. Approximately 1.5 million athletes participate in American football in the United States.
B. American football involves discontinuous sprint activity and requires strength.
C. Football is a contact sport with increased risk of injury. Physician coverage for games is optimal.
D. A variety of medical as well as musculoskeletal issues need to be considered in treating football players at all competitive levels.

II. Injury Statistics

A. Estimated 1.2 million football-related injuries sustained per year; risk of injury increased as teams get older and decreased with more experienced coaching staff
B. National Collegiate Athletic Association (NCAA) Injury Surveillance System injury rate was 3.7–4.4 per 1000 athlete exposures between 1986 and 1994.
   1. **Injury rate between 1985 and 1994 much higher in games versus practice** (36.3 per 1000 athlete exposures versus 4.1 per 1000 athlete exposures)
   2. **Spring football injury rate higher than regular season football rate**
   3. **Preseason injury rate higher than both regular season and postseason injury rate** (7.7 versus 6.1 versus 3.0) between 1988 and 1994, suggesting that preseason is critical time to stress proper stretching, warm-up, fluid and nutritional replacements, technique, and supervision
   4. Injury rates compared to other NCAA sports given in Table 1. In 1994–1995, the knee, ankle, and shoulder accounted for most of the injuries (19%, 14%, and 13%), with sprains, strains, and contusions accounting for the most common mechanisms (28%, 20%, and 14%). Cervical spine injuries can have catastrophic potential, but have fortunately declined since rule modifications were made about tackling and blocking techniques, improved fitness, coaching, and equipment.

III. Medical Problems

A. **Preparticipation physical examination:** probably the most important part of the initial evaluation of any athlete. Essential that evaluation is performed properly, thoroughly, and with sport-specific objectives.
   1. Three areas of importance in preparticipation physical examination: cardiac, musculoskeletal, neurologic. These areas are stressed not only in history, but also on physical examination.
      a. Family history of sudden cardiac death, myocardial infarction before age 50, Marfan's syndrome, hypertrophic cardiomyopathy

TABLE 1. Injury Rates (per 1000 athletic exposures)

Sport	Practice	Game	Combined
Spring football	9.2	23.2	9.6
Football	4.0	35.3	6.6
Wrestling	7.1	31.4	9.4
Women's gymnastics	7.8	22.1	8.6
Women's soccer	5.5	16.7	7.9
Men's soccer	4.8	20.3	7.9
Men's gymnastics	4.6	16.0	5.1
Ice hockey	2.3	16.5	5.6
Men's basketball	4.5	9.8	5.6
Women's volleyball	4.5	5.2	4.8
Men's lacrosse	4.0	15.9	6.1
Women's basketball	4.1	8.8	5.1
Field hockey	3.9	8.6	5.0
Women's lacrosse	3.5	7.2	4.3
Women's softball	3.2	5.1	3.9
Baseball	2.1	6.0	3.4

b. History of syncope, chest pain, dizziness
c. History of prior injury or incomplete rehabilitation important
d. History of previous head or neck injury, stingers or burners, as well as any workup in past important
e. Other areas of importance:
   i. Exercise-induced asthma
   ii. Single organs
   iii. Heat intolerance
   iv. Appliances (e.g., dental plates)
   v. Medications
   vi. Allergies
   vii. Medical conditions
   viii. Immunizations

2. Historical questions to assess risk for sudden cardiac death, preexisting musculoskeletal injuries, or anatomic conditions that put the athlete at risk for injury. **Thorough history is essential**.
3. **Physical examination**
   a. Emphasize cardiac, musculoskeletal, and neurologic systems
   b. Ensure adequate cervical spine protection, joint stability, absence of cardiac abnormalities, neurologic integrity
   c. Screen for inflexibility, muscle imbalances, improper rehabilitation
4. **Nutrition issues**. Needs for strength gaining often put athlete at risk for abuse of performance-enhancing drugs. Use of protein supplementation should be discussed. Athlete should understand basics regarding good nutritional balance and risks of excessive protein load as well as additional costs of protein supplements. Emphasis should be on healthy, natural, well-balanced diet.
5. **Fluids.** Study in high school football players in 50-play scrimmage simulation demonstrated no difference in anaerobic performance with 7% glucose polymer beverage containing electrolytes compared to water, but the beverage did have a positive effect on maintaining plasma volume during recovery from anaerobic exercise.

B. **Strength and conditioning** are important in young athlete.
  1. Stress maintenance of good flexibility program in conjunction with strengthening
  2. Sport specificity in training; endurance work as baseline
  3. Interval training and hill training for explosive speed
  4. Supervision and proper technique in strengthening program, especially if using free weights

C. **Infections:** General guideline is to avoid exercise during acute infection; no participation if fever > 100°F. Avoid common source water outbreaks. To avoid spread of infection, athletes should not share water bottles.
  1. **Myocarditis** reported as cause of sudden cardiac death in athletes
  2. **Skin infections** (herpes gladiatorum, ringworm) often spread from person-to-person contact. Antiviral, antifungal, impetigo, and antibacterial treatment necessary with protective covering to avoid transmission.
  3. **Infectious mononucleosis** is an additional consideration for splenic rupture. No activity for initial 2–4 weeks of symptoms, then dependent on athlete's clinical condition and presence or absence of splenomegaly. Abdominal ultrasound recommended for accurate assessment and follow up. Additional protective padding helpful in minimizing risk.
  4. **Human immunodeficiency virus (HIV)**
    a. No reason to disallow competition. Study in professional football players found 3.7 bleeding injuries per game for each team involving 3.5 players and found that 88% of the bleeding injuries were abrasions, with the remainder lacerations. Risk for transmission of HIV estimated to be less than 1 per 85 million game contacts.
    b. Universal precautions should be used for all body fluids. More important to consider activities **off** the field rather than on the field regarding risk factors.
    c. More substantial risk for **hepatitis**. Same precautions apply. Hepatitis vaccination series recommended.

IV. Head Injuries in the Athlete

A. **Statistics**
  1. Causes of minor head injury (according to National Head Injury Foundation)
    a. Motor vehicle accident 46%
    b. Falls 23%
    c. Sports 18%
    d. Assaults 10%
  2. Minor head injury is the most common head injury, estimated to occur at a rate of 250,000 per year in contact sports.
    a. Estimated that 20% of football players sustain cerebral concussions
    b. Soccer players also at risk; "footballer's migraine" describes the headaches that occasionally develop in these athletes
    c. Tysvaer and Storli estimate that a typical career soccer player participates in approximately 300 games, sustaining 2000 blows to head
    d. Head injuries common for almost all athletes

B. **NCAA data, head and neck injury** (Table 2)
  1. Ice hockey had highest percentage of head injuries of sports monitored, followed by football, field hockey, women's lacrosse, men's soccer
  2. Injury rates in sports with no head protection, such as men's soccer, women's soccer, and field hockey, comparable to helmeted sports of ice hockey, football, and men's lacrosse
  3. Player contact was primary injury mechanism for all but four sports mentioned; contact with stick for field hockey, contact with ball in women's lacrosse, softball, baseball

TABLE 2. NCAA Data, Head and Neck Injury, 1984–1991

	Head		Concussion‡		Neck	
	%*	IR†	%	IR	%	IR
Sports with No Head Protection						
Field hockey	4.5	0.23	3.8	0.20	1.0	0.05
Women's lacrosse	4.1	0.17	3.9	0.16	0.7	0.03
Men's soccer	4.0	0.31	3.2	0.25	0.4	0.03
Women's soccer	3.7	0.29	2.8	0.24	1.0	0.08
Women's basketball	3.1	0.16	3.0	0.15	0.9	0.05
Men's basketball	2.5	0.14	2.1	0.12	0.8	0.04
Wrestling	2.9	0.28	1.8	0.20	5.4	0.51
Sports with Head Protection						
Ice hockey	5.4	0.30	4.5	0.25	1.7	0.09
Football	4.5	0.29	4.1	0.27	4.2	0.28
Men's lacrosse	3.2	0.22	3.0	0.19	1.7	0.12
Women's softball	2.9	0.11	2.9	0.11	1.6	0.06
Baseball	2.8	0.09	2.1	0.07	0.3	0.01

* Percentage of all reported injuries
† Injuries per 1000 athlete exposures
‡ Concussion = subset of all head injuries

C. **Definitions**

1. **Focal lesions** often present with loss of consciousness, focal deficits
   a. **Subdural hematoma:** three times more common than epidural hematoma. Result of venous injury, lower pressure. Often unconscious; may or may not give history of deterioration, focal neurologic deficits.
      i. **Simple subdural**—collection of blood in subdural space not associated with underlying cerebral contusion or edema; mortality 20%
      ii. **Complex subdural**—collection of blood in subdural space associated with obvious contusion on the surface of the brain and hemispheric brain injury with swelling; mortality > 50%
   b. **Epidural hematoma:** middle meningeal or other meningeal arteries. Often disrupted in association with skull fracture. Bleeding is arterial; thus accumulation occurs under high pressure. Classically see loss of consciousness at time of injury followed by recovery of consciousness in variable period of time with athlete becoming lucid. Followed by severe headache, decreased level of consciousness, dilation of one pupil, and decerebrate posturing and weakness. Only one third of patients present with this classic history. Computed tomography (CT) scan establishes diagnosis.
   c. **Cerebral contusions**
   d. **Intracranial hemorrhage:**
      i. **Subarachnoid**—confined to surface of brain
      ii. **Intracerebral**—within the substance of brain itself. Intracerebral hemorrhage and contusion can occur with loss of consciousness or focal neurologic deficits. Persistent headache or periods of confusion after head injury with posttraumatic amnesia common.
2. **Diffuse brain injuries** are those injuries **not** associated with focal intracranial lesions. Represent a continuum of progressively more severe brain dysfunction caused by increasing amounts of acceleration damage to the brain. Diffuse brain injury can be classified according to whether structural or anatomic disruption occurs.

a. **Nonstructural diffuse brain lesions** are typically less severe because anatomic integrity is maintained. A **cerebral concussion** is a "clinical syndrome characterized by immediate and transient impairment of neurologic function secondary to mechanical forces." (Congress of Neurological Surgeons, 1966)
   i. **Mild concussion**—temporary disturbance of neurologic function without loss of consciousness; mildest form of injury in spectrum of diffuse brain injuries
   ii. **Classic cerebral concussion**—temporary, reversible neurologic deficiency that results in temporary loss of consciousness lasting < 6 hours
b. **Structural diffuse brain injury:**
   i. With axonal disruption, most severe
   ii. **Diffuse axonal injury**—prolonged traumatic brain coma with loss of consciousness lasting > 6 hours. Residual neurologic, psychological, or personality deficits often result because of structural disruption of numerous axons in white matter of cerebral hemispheres and brain stem.

3. **There is no such thing as minor head injury**.

D. **Mechanisms**
1. **Direct injuries**
   a. Moving object striking a quiescent head (boxing, baseball, field hockey, ice hockey)
   b. Moving head striking a fixed or slow-moving object (football, soccer, basketball)
2. **Indirect injuries (uncommon):** trauma impact on another body part transferred to the cranium (fall on coccyx)

E. **Biomechanics**
1. **Degree and location of injury dependent on**
   a. Magnitude, direction of impact
   b. Structural features of the skull
   c. Position of head at impact
   d. Response to force, as well as force itself
2. **Cumulative effect**
   a. Decreased processing of information leading to disability
   b. Increased disability with previous concussion
   c. Fatal head injuries; associated with prior concussion

F. **On-site management**
1. **Recognition** of injury
2. ABCs (airway, breathing, circulation)
3. Associated injuries—cervical spine, skull fractures (see below)
4. History and physical examination
   a. General assessment:
      i. Loss of consciousness; amnesia (posttraumatic or retrograde); ability to register information, recall information, and communicate
      ii. Ability to do calculations, maintain concentration and attention
      iii. Memory of event, score, quarter, color of opponents' jerseys, position, plays, events before game, day before
      iv. Consider additional neuropsychiatric testing
   b. Detailed neurologic examination
   c. Determination of necessity of additional diagnostic tests and treatment, especially emergent CT scanning and neurosurgical evaluation/treatment
   d. Resuscitation of the brain:
      i. Recognition of focal brain injury (large hematoma requires surgical removal)
      ii. Establish adequate airway—provide oxygen, hyperventilate
      iii. Supplemental oxygen

TABLE 3. Glasgow Coma Scale

Eye opening	1–4
Motor response	1–6
Best verbal response	1–5
Total:	> 13 good ≤ 13 fair < 7 poor

iv. Corticosteroids useful if comatose following trauma—100 mg dexamethasone or 1 g methylprednisolone sodium succinate to average adult
v. CT scan as soon as possible

e. Glasgow coma scale (GCS) known, established (Table 3). Good prognosticator:
   i. If GCS 3–4, 80% die or remain in vegetative state
   ii. If GCS > 11, only 6% die or remain in vegetative state
   iii. Prognosis improves as GCS improves

f. Follow-up evaluations and return-to-play considerations

G. **Classification systems. There are many; embrace your own, and ensure that trainers and other professionals you work with understand the grading system you are using**. Consistency is important. It is often easier to use descriptive terms, e.g., no loss of consciousness but posttraumatic amnesia present.

1. **Torg grades of cerebral concussion, 1982**
   a. I—short-term confusion, no loss of consciousness, no amnesia
   b. II—confusion and amnesia, no loss of consciousness; posttraumatic amnesia
   c. III—confusion and amnesia, no loss of consciousness; posttraumatic amnesia, retrograde amnesia
   d. IV—loss of consciousness (immediate transient), posttraumatic amnesia, retrograde amnesia
   e. V—loss of consciousness (paralytic coma), coma vigil, respiratory arrest
   f. VI—loss of consciousness (paralytic coma), death
2. **Nelson classification of concussion, 1984**
   a. 0—no complaints initially; subsequent complaints of headache, difficulty with sensorium
   b. I—stunned or dazed, no loss of consciousness, no amnesia, clears quickly (< 1 minute)
   c. II—headache, cloudy sensorium (> 1 minute), amnesia, no loss of consciousness
   d. III—loss of consciousness (< 1 minute), not comatose, grade II signs during recovery
   e. IV—loss of consciousness (> 1 minute), not comatose, grade II signs during recovery
3. **Cantu grading system for concussion, 1986**
   a. I—mild, no loss of consciousness, posttraumatic amnesia < 30 minutes
   b. II—moderate, loss of consciousness < 5 minutes, or posttraumatic amnesia > 30 minutes but < 24 hours
   c. III—severe, loss of consciousness > 5 minutes, or posttraumatic amnesia > 24 hours
4. **Colorado Medical Society, guidelines for the management of concussion in sports, 1991**
   a. **Grade I: confusion without amnesia, no loss of consciousness**
      i. Remove from contest
      ii. Examine immediately and every 5 minutes for development of amnesia or postconcussive signs at rest and with exertion
      iii. Permit return to contest if no amnesia and no signs appear for at least 20 minutes
   b. **Grade II: confusion with amnesia, no loss of consciousness**
      i. Remove from contest and disallow return

ii. Examine frequently for signs of evolving intracranial pathology
iii. Reexamine the next day
iv. Permit return to practice after 1 full week without signs

c. **Grade III: loss of consciousness**
i. Transport from field to nearest hospital by ambulance (with cervical spine immobilization if indicated)
ii. Perform thorough neurologic evaluation emergently
iii. Admit to hospital if signs of pathology detected
iv. If findings normal, instruct family for overnight observation
v. Permit return to practice only after 2 full weeks without signs

H. **Return-to-play decisions**

1. **Cantu guidelines, return to play after concussion**

a. **Grade I**
i. **First concussion:** May return to play if asymptomatic (no headache, dizziness, or impaired orientation, concentration, or memory during rest or exertion) for 1 week.
ii. **Second concussion:** Return to play if asymptomatic for 2 weeks
iii. **Third concussion:** Terminate season; may return to play next season if asymptomatic

b. **Grade II**
i. **First concussion:** May return to play after asymptomatic for 1 week
ii. **Second concussion:** Minimum of 1 month; may return to play then if asymptomatic for 1 week; consider terminating season
iii. **Third concussion:** Terminate season; may return to play next season if asymptomatic

c. **Grade III**
i. **First concussion:** Minimum of 1 month; may then return to play if asymptomatic for 1 week
ii. **Second concussion:** Terminate season; may return to play next season if asymptomatic

2. **Colorado Medical Society guidelines, return to play**

a. **Grade I**
i. **First concussion:** Remove from contest. Examine immediately and every 5 minutes for development of amnesia or postconcussive signs at rest and with exertion. May return to contest if no amnesia and no signs appear for at least 20 minutes.
ii. **Second concussion:** If in same contest, eliminate from competition that day. Otherwise treat as grade I.
iii. **Third concussion:** Terminate season. No contact sports for at least 3 months and then only if asymptomatic at rest and exertion.

b. **Grade II**
i. **First concussion:** Remove from contest and disallow return. Examine frequently for signs of evolving intracranial pathology. Reexamine the next day. May return to practice after 1 full week without signs.
ii. **Second concussion:** Defer return to play for 1 month. Consider termination of season.
iii. **Third concussion:** Termination of season mandated (also terminate season if any abnormality on CT or magnetic resonance imaging [MRI]).

c. **Grade III**
i. **First concussion:** Transport from field by ambulance (with cervical spine immobilization if indicated) to nearest hospital. Thorough neurologic evaluation emergently. Hospital confinement if signs of pathology are detected. If findings normal, instructions to family for overnight observation. May return to

no-contact practice only after 2 full weeks without signs. Return to full-contact activity at 1 month only if athlete has been asymptomatic at rest and exertion for at least 2 weeks.

ii. **Second concussion:** Terminate season (also terminate if any abnormality on CT or MRI). Return to contact sports should be seriously discouraged.

3. **Bottom line is close follow-up with individualization of management issues. Cookbook treatment not effective**.

I. **Differential diagnosis**
   1. Vasovagal syncope
   2. Migraine seizures
   3. Focal brain lesions (subdural hematoma, epidural hematoma, intracranial hemorrhage)
   4. Trauma-induced migraine ("footballer's migraine)
   5. Syncope secondary to other causes (cardiac, neurologic)
   6. Cerebrovascular accident

J. **Complications**
   1. **Postconcussive syndrome**
      a. Signs: persistent headache, inability to concentrate, irritability, fatigue
      b. Can last for several weeks to months postinjury
      c. Return to participation should not occur as long as signs present
      d. Treat symptomatically with frequent monitoring
   2. **Posttraumatic seizures** can be immediate or delayed
      a. Early seizures (within 1 week):
         i. Often associated with
            (a) Prolonged posttraumatic amnesia (> 24 hours)
            (b) Depressed skull fracture
            (c) Intracranial hematoma
         ii. Tend to be focal in onset
         iii. 50% of patients with early epilepsy have first seizure within first 24 hours; in 50% of these within first hour. Seizures associated with depressed skull fracture often occur within first hour and less often after 24 hours; tend to be single.
      b. Late seizures (after 1 week):
         i. Often associated with
            (a) Presence of acute hematoma
            (b) Depressed skull fracture
            (c) Development of early seizures
         ii. Most occur within 1 year
         iii. No consistent correlation between electroencephalogram abnormalities in first year after head injury and development of late epilepsy
         iv. If associated with intracranial hematoma, often occur after 24 hours; recurrent seizures common
         v. In absence of acute hematoma, depressed skull fracture, or history of early seizures, risk of late epilepsy roughly 1%
   3. **Long-term minor head disability**
      a. Neuropsychologic assessment raises question of chronic disability; 50% experience difficulties 3 months or more after injury
      b. Significant injury for the student athlete
      c. Important reason to have serial follow-up examinations
   4. **Skull fracture**—consider basilar skull fracture if see:
      a. Positive Battle's sign (postauricular hematoma)
      b. Otorrhea (cerebrospinal fluid leaking from the ear canal)
      c. Rhinorrhea (cerebrospinal fluid leaking from nose)

   d. Raccoon eyes (periorbital ecchymosis caused by leakage of blood from anterior fossa into periorbital tissues)
   e. Hemotympanum (blood behind eardrum)
   f. Cranial nerve injuries (especially facial)
   g. Palpable malalignment of calvarium
5. **Cervical spine injuries** are associated with fatal injuries.
6. **Recurrent head concussion:** After a player has suffered a first concussion, the chance of incurring a second concussion is more than four times greater than for the nonconcussed player.
7. **Second impact syndrome**—fatal brain swelling following minor head contact in players who still have symptoms from a prior concussion
8. **Dementia pugilistica**—chronic traumatic encephalopathy and premature loss of normal central nervous system function
   a. The cumulative effect of multiple blows to the head results in pathologic changes in brain substance even in boxers who experienced no knockouts.
   b. One cannot always predict the significance of head trauma or determine how many head impacts an athlete can safely sustain.

K. **Psychometric testing** of individuals who had suffered concussions yielded decline in performance compared to preinjury levels and sometimes remained depressed for 3 months or longer. Whether these results indicate long-term health risk to the injured person remains to be determined.

L. **Implications for the future:** May need to revise return-to-play guidelines if new data provide better insights into natural history of head injury, long-term sequelae, and risk of recurrent injury or complications with continued participation. Exciting research is ongoing in this area.

V. Cervical Injuries

Neck pain and radiating arm pain, paresthesias, weakness, or loss of cervical motion are criteria for removal from the game and further workup

A. **Myofascial sprains**
1. Muscular or ligamentous injury to the neck—most common form of neck injury
2. Presents with paravertebral spasm, decreased range of motion, usually without radicular or neurologic symptoms
3. X-rays to rule out fracture or ligamentous instability
4. Treatment includes nonsteroidal anti-inflammatory drugs (NSAIDs), rest, physical therapy
5. Return to play when full active range of motion with little or no pain, absence of neurologic findings, and negative work-up for more severe injury

B. **Brachial plexus injuries ("burner" or "stinger")**
1. Usually occur with blow to or distraction of the neck and shoulder, stretching the brachial plexus
2. Transient numbness or paralysis in the involved upper extremity; beware of bilateral symptoms, which may represent transient quadriparesis or spinal cord involvement
3. With first occurrence, consider cervical spine films to evaluate for congenital anomalies or spinal stenosis
4. Treatment includes NSAIDs, rest, and physical therapy
5. Return to play with full clinical strength and resolution of neurologic symptoms, especially in C5, C6 nerve distribution (not dependent on electromyographic findings); use protective equipment, including a neck roll

C. **Fractures and dislocations**
1. Less frequent after installation of rules banning "spearing" and use of the top of the helmet to strike another player

2. If neurologic injury present or fracture or dislocation suspected, spine must be immobilized until properly assessed, including x-rays
3. Do not remove helmet or shoulder pads until the spine is properly immobilized and protected; cut or remove face guard if airway management is necessary. If removal of shoulder pads and helmet is necessary, remove both at the same time to maintain a neutral alignment of the cervical vertebrae.
4. Be aware of emergency personnel guidelines that may advocate helmet removal—protect your players!

D. **Return-to-play criteria after cervical injury**
1. Absolute contraindications to return to collision sports
    a. **Congenital**
        i. Odontoid hypoplasia
        ii. Atlanto-occipital fusion
        iii. Klippel-Feil anomaly with occipital-cervical instability or mass fusion
    b. **Developmental**
        i. Spinal stenosis with episode of cervical cord neurapraxia and ligamentous instability or cord edema by MRI or more than one recurrence
        ii. "Spear tackler's spine" (stenosis with persistent straightening of cervical spine, often rigid in flexion and extension)
    c. **Traumatic conditions**
        i. Any C1–C2 injury with ligamentous laxity or C1–C2 fusion
        ii. Unstable ligamentous injuries of C2 to C7
        iii. Vertebral body fractures with sagittal component of displacement into the canal
        iv. Healed fractures with residual instability, neurologic finding, limitation of motion
        v. Disk herniation with neurologic findings or limited motion
        vi. Status postfusion of more than three levels
2. Relative contraindications
    a. **Developmental**—episode of central cord neurapraxia (with resolution) and vertebral body-to-canal ratio of ≤ 0.8
    b. **Traumatic**—full pain-free range of motion and neurologically intact with healed displaced body compression fracture or neural ring fracture; two- or three-level fusion
3. No contraindication
    a. **Congenital**—Klippel-Feil anomaly with stable one- to two-level fusion and full range of motion
    b. **Developmental**—stenosis ratio ≤ 0.8 in an otherwise asymptomatic patient
    c. **Traumatic**—full, pain-free range of motion and neurologically intact with healed stable compression fracture or healed spinous process fracture; solid one-level fusion after disk excision at C3 or below
    d. Study of collegiate football players found that players with Torg ratio < 0.8 had three times risk of incurring stingers

VI. Upper Extremity

A. **Shoulder girdle (clavicle fractures)**
1. Mechanism: direct blow (most common) or impact onto point of the shoulder
2. Conservative treatment usually successful with figure-of-eight strap or sling for 6–8 weeks; surgery if danger of skin necrosis or soft tissue interposition
3. Return to play with resumption of strength, healed fracture, and special shoulder pads for protection

B. **Acromioclavicular joint**
1. **Osteolysis of the clavicle**—usually secondary to repetitive or traumatic cause (weight lifting versus falling onto the point of the shoulder)

a. Attempt conservative therapy with rehabilitation, injections, acromioclavicular padding during play
b. Distal clavicle excision if continued pain, dysfunction

2. **Incomplete acromioclavicular separations** (coracoclavicular ligaments intact)
   a. Acromioclavicular injuries most commonly occur by a fall onto point of shoulder
   b. Diagnosed by tenderness directly over the acromioclavicular joint, pain with resisted adduction of the arm across the chest; x-rays with weights helpful in determining severity
   c. Conservative treatment with RICE (rest, ice, compression, elevation), physical therapy; return to play with acromioclavicular padding after restoration of strength
3. **Complete acromioclavicular separations**
   a. Diagnosed by palpable step-off between clavicle and acromion
   b. Treatment controversial; mostly conservative unless extensive muscle stripping or penetration of the distal clavicle through trapezius is present
   c. Strength and endurance comparable in operative versus nonoperative results for grade III injuries
   d. Return to play after restoration of strength, motion, and with acromioclavicular padding

C. **Glenohumeral instability**. A common football injury, often classified as **t**raumatic, **u**nidirectional, **B**ankart's lesion; **s**urgically amenable (TUBS). May also be **a**traumatic, **m**ultidirectional, **b**ilateral; **r**ehabilitation, **i**nferior capsular shift if surgery is necessary (AMBRI).

1. **Traumatic**—anterior most common secondary to abduction-external rotation force; often a result of improper tackling technique
   a. Acute injury should be treated with gentle reduction, which can be performed on the field by an experienced physician, and a 3–4 week period of immobilization, followed by rehabilitation and bracing to control abduction-external rotation moments. (Immobilization and rehabilitation, however, have not been shown to affect the high redislocation rate in young people.)
   b. X-rays including apical oblique to evaluate for reduction, Hill-Sachs, or bony Bankart lesion
   c. Role of arthroscopy or acute stabilization in young people controversial; decision making should be tailored to each case depending on risk factors, career goals, timing
   d. Surgical stabilization of choice at our institution is open Bankart repair with capsular shift if indicated
   e. Posterior dislocation less common; can occur by direct anterior impact of internally and adducted arm:
      i. Diagnosis: prominent coracoid, arm adducted and internally rotated with minimal external rotation, adequate x-rays crucial to avoid missing diagnosis
      ii. Acute treatment consists of reduction, immobilization, rehabilitation; recurrent instability is difficult problem secondary to high recurrence rate with current surgical techniques, although recent reports using capsular shift procedures appear promising
2. **Atraumatic**—less common in football; may occur in players with generalized ligamentous laxity, quarterbacks
   a. Prolonged trial of physical therapy, including rotator cuff program, stretching of posterior capsule if contracted, and scapular stabilization; return to play as symptoms tolerate
   b. Surgical treatment—capsular shift, but beware that surgery may not allow elite thrower to return to previous level of competition

D. **Rotator cuff/biceps**

1. Uncommon in younger population but may occur in quarterbacks; important to rule out subtle instability presenting as impingement syndrome

2. Evaluate for supraspinatus weakness by testing resisted abduction with arm in 30° of forward flexion from 90° straight abduction, with internal rotation; impingement test by forward flexing arm in internal rotation (Hawkins's sign)
3. Look for "popeye" arm, weakness in forward flexion and supination (Speed's test), if long head of biceps rupture suspected
4. X-rays of shoulder including anteroposterior, supraspinatus outlet view (lateral scapula with 10° caudal tilt) to evaluate acromial morphology (hooked versus straight); MRI or arthrogram if complete tear is suspected. MRI of suspected biceps rupture helpful to rule out large intra-articular tendon fragment.
5. Impingement syndrome with rotator cuff tendinopathy usually responsive to structured therapy program; surgical repair usually indicated if full-thickness tear in young population
6. Biceps tendon tendinitis, proximal rupture usually responsive to rest followed by rotator cuff program; surgical tenodesis for selected high demand positions, arthroscopic debridement of symptomatic intra-articular tendon fragment. Distal rupture most commonly treated by surgical reattachment.

E. **Contusions/exostosis**
1. Common, especially in linebackers; occurs from direct blow to the shoulder resulting in an injury similar to a hip pointer
2. Periosteal stripping in region of deltoid insertion may lead to "dotted veil" appearance on x-ray and eventual formation of mature exostosis
3. Initial treatment for contusions similar to treatment for quadriceps contusion—ice, rest, aspiration of hematoma if present, avoidance of heat and other modalities that may exacerbate bleeding and subsequent hematoma formation

VII. Elbow and Forearm

A. **Valgus injuries (overuse)**
1. Occurs occasionally in quarterbacks; diagnosed by pain and tenderness distal and posterior to medial femoral condyle with valgus stress and occasional ulnar nerve symptoms. MRI is becoming the study of choice to verify diagnosis.
2. Conservative treatment includes rehabilitation, protective function; may take 4–6 months to return to sport
3. Surgery if patient failed adequate rehabilitation and desires to continue as high demand thrower; arthroscopy to remove loose bodies and examine degree of medial laxity followed by ulnar collateral ligament if needed

B. **Hyperextension/dislocation injuries**
1. Occurs with fall onto outstretched hand, often with forced extension during tackling
2. Dislocations can be reduced with gentle traction with elbow in semiflexed position (for posterior dislocations—most common)
3. Both hyperextension and dislocation injuries require x-ray to rule out fracture and neurovascular assessment of hand and forearm
4. Treat both injuries with early protected range of motion; return to play with protected bracing after strength and motion restored (usually 3–6 weeks for dislocation, often sooner with hyperextension injury)

C. **Olecranon bursitis**
1. Traumatic bursitis common secondary to impact with tackling
2. Examination of the skin important to rule out open communication with bursa; x-ray to evaluate for bony spurs
3. Aspiration for persistent or large collection; consider sclerosing agent or excision with recurrence
4. Return to play with protective pad

VIII. Wrist and Hand

A. Wrist sprains and fractures

1. Injuries of the wrist must be evaluated carefully for location of tenderness and pain with movement; fractures and ligament injuries must be ruled out clinically and radiographically before diagnosis of wrist sprain.
2. Scaphoid fractures
   a. Acute nondisplaced fracture can be treated with long arm thumb spica cast for 4–6 weeks, followed by short arm thumb spica until healed. These fractures are occasionally treated with Herbert screw fixation in high demand athlete who cannot afford the prolonged healing period.
   b. Return to play dependent on position; for example, linemen can often return quickly with appropriate outer cast padding
   c. Displaced or symptomatic nonunion needs open fixation, often with bone grafting; return to play with protective splinting after adequate healing and strength restoration
3. Distal radius and ulna fractures
   a. Conservative versus operative treatment dependent on fracture pattern and stability
   b. Return to play dependent on fracture stability and player position; may take 2–3 months before sufficient healing and strength
4. Carpus fractures other than scaphoid
   a. Most common—avulsion fractures, which can often be treated with immobilization and early return to play if position allows
   b. Important to rule out carpal dislocations (e.g., lunate/perilunate) or ligamentous injuries (e.g., scapholunate) with appropriate stress x-rays; wrist arthrogram if plain films are inconclusive

B. Injuries to the thumb

1. Collateral ligament injuries
   a. Common injuries occur by adduction (radial) or abduction (ulnar ligament) forces applied to the metacarpophalangeal joint. Diagnosis by reproduction of pain with stress testing, tenderness to palpation over radial or ulnar aspect of metacarpophalangeal joint.
   b. Radial ligament injuries and incomplete ulnar ligament injuries can be treated with protective splinting, early return to play in most positions
   c. Complete tear of ulnar collateral ligament (as confirmed by stress radiography) most commonly treated by open ligament repair secondary to high prevalence of Stener lesions
2. Fractures and dislocations of the thumb
   a. Fractures and dislocations at the metacarpophalangeal joint are also common secondary to the precarious position of thumb.
   b. Metacarpophalangeal dislocations are most commonly volar; important to differentiate simple (reducible) from complex (irreducible, requiring open reduction secondary to interposition of the volar plate). Can return to play early with protective splint for 4–6 weeks.
   c. Intra-articular fractures (Bennett's) are usually unstable and require fixation. Phalanx fractures, if stable, can be treated with protective splinting and early return to play.

C. Hand fractures/dislocations excluding the thumb

1. Occur frequently from direct impact; diagnosis confirmed by x-ray
2. Fractures of the fourth and fifth metacarpals can usually be reduced to acceptable position and treated with protective splinting. Less tolerance for displacement with second and third metacarpals; require operative fixation more frequently.
3. Proximal phalanx fractures often require operative fixation to maintain length, proper rotation

4. Middle phalanx fractures more commonly amenable to closed reduction, buddy taping
5. Distal tuft fractures should be treated as soft tissue injuries; if suspected, examination of the nail bed and meticulous repair if damaged or removal from the fracture site if incarcerated. The time-honored hot paper-clip or electrocautery relieves painful subungual hematomas.
6. Most hand fractures, if stable, can be treated with protective splinting, early return to play
7. Dislocations are most commonly dorsal and can be treated by closed reduction, continuous buddy taping for 3–6 weeks, early return to play
   a. X-rays after the game important to rule out bony injury
   b. If dislocation of proximal interphalangeal joint is volar (rare), need to treat in same manner as rupture of the central slip of the extensor tendon

D. **Tendon/capsular injuries**

1. Flexor tendon injuries usually occur when attempting to grab another player's jersey, with resultant pain and inability to flex the distal interphalangeal joint of the involved finger.
   a. Important to determine level of retraction of the tendon; if retracts into the palm, blood supply is significantly compromised, and repair should be performed as soon as possible (within 7 days). Lower level retraction injuries can be repaired later (blood supply from vincula maintained, but best results with early diagnosis and repair).
   b. Always obtain x-ray because bony avulsion injuries, which usually limit the amount of retraction of the tendon, can occur. Early repair of bony injury also yields the best result.
2. Extensor tendon avulsions off the distal phalanx (mallet finger) usually occur by "jamming" the finger, causing forced flexion of the distal interphalangeal joint.
   a. Exam reveals inability to extend distal interphalangeal joint
   b. Always obtain x-ray to determine if bony avulsion has occurred; subluxation of distal interphalangeal joint (usually occurs with fragment involving more than ⅓ of the joint surface) requires more aggressive treatment
   c. Mallet fingers should be treated with continuous extension of distal interphalangeal joint with splint, free range of motion of proximal interphalangeal joint, early return to play
3. Extensor tendon avulsions of the central slip (insertion into the proximal aspect of the middle phalanx) also occur by "jamming" the finger and are often misdiagnosed as a capsular sprain.
   a. With other fingers held in extension and metacarpophalangeal joint flexed on involved finger, test for ability to extend proximal interphalangeal joint. If ability absent, suspect central slip rupture.
   b. X-rays important to rule out fracture
   c. Treat with proximal interphalangeal joint held in continuous extension for at least 6 weeks with distal interphalangeal joint free. Failure to recognize and treat these injuries results in a boutonniere deformity.
4. Capsular sprains and lateral collateral ligament injuries can be treated by continuous buddy taping for 6 weeks and return to play.

IX. Chest and Abdomen

A. **Rib fractures**

1. Occur by direct blow to the ribs with resultant pain, especially when breathing
2. X-rays important to rule out presence of pneumothorax (collapsed lung)
3. Return to play with protective "flak jacket" when symptoms are tolerable

B. **Sternoclavicular joint**
  1. Dislocations or injuries caused either indirectly by blow to shoulder or directly by injury to upper chest
  2. Diagnosed by pain and swelling at sternoclavicular region with exacerbation during arm range of motion
  3. X-rays important to rule out posterior dislocation, which often requires surgical reduction to avoid injury to major vessels
  4. Anterior dislocations most common and usually treated conservatively with return to play when strength and motion restored

C. **Pectoralis major ruptures**
  1. May occur with forceful extension/external rotation of the arm. Pain and ecchymosis most commonly along the anteromedial aspect of the arm (most ruptures occur near the insertion onto the humerus) and an inability to flex the pectoralis with adduction and internal rotation.
  2. Suspected incomplete injuries can be treated with rest and ice, with return to play upon restoration of motion and strength
  3. Complete ruptures are usually treated surgically secondary to significant loss of strength if treated conservatively.

D. **Rectus abdominis strain**
  1. Forceful resisted contraction of the abdominal musculature can lead to an intramuscular strain or avulsion from the iliac crest or pubis. Diagnosed by area of tenderness and pain with attempted flexion of the trunk.
  2. Treatment is usually conservative, with ice, stretching, and taping of the trunk to limit flexion and rotation on return to play.

X. Thoracolumbar Spine

A. **Thoracic or low back strain**
  1. Most common injury to spine in contact sports; muscle spasm or ligamentous strain usually occurs with bending or twisting during forceful activities
  2. Often secondary to fatigue or inadequate conditioning of the paraspinal muscles
  3. Most commonly occurs without radicular symptoms; suspect disk pathology if radiation of pain into lower extremities
  4. Plain anteroposterior, lateral, and oblique x-rays helpful to rule out any osseous injury or neural arch involvement
  5. Treatment consists of control of initial inflammatory phase with ice, rest; progression to back rehabilitation program when tolerated
     a. Most uncomplicated sprains respond in 7–10 days
     b. Flexibility and conditioning program during season and in off-season important to prevent recurrence

B. **Herniated nucleus pulposus**
  1. Injury pattern often similar to that of strain, but with radiculopathy into one or both lower extremities, weakness, with or without diminished reflex
     a. Straight leg raising often abnormal
     b. Often with complaints of paresthesias and pain in leg, which is more bothersome than back complaints
  2. Plain films of lumbar spine and MRI often helpful in documenting injury
  3. Initial treatment is same as for lumbar strain—consider epidural steroids or disk excision if no improvement with conservative care or if progressive neurologic insult

C. **Spondylolysis/spondylolisthesis**
  1. Common in linemen secondary to repetitive loading on posterior elements in an extended position

   a. Complaints similar to low back strain, but also commonly exhibit hamstring spasm and pain with resisted extension
   b. Previous history of spondylolisthesis or significant back pain important to determine chronicity
2. Anteroposterior, lateral, and oblique **x-rays** necessary to evaluate for "broken neck on Scotty dog" to confirm spondylolysis and to evaluate for presence of translation of vertebral body (spondylolisthesis). A bone scan is often helpful if x-rays are equivocal or to differentiate acute neural arch injury from low back strain with previously healed spondylolysis.
3. **Treatment** consists of restriction from play, abdominal and lumbar stretching, strengthening activities, and occasional use of lumbar orthosis.
   a. Resolution of hamstring spasm is often a reasonable gauge to begin functional progression in rehabilitation as tolerated
   b. Clinical progress more reliable indicator than x-rays, which often do not demonstrate bony healing even when patient becomes symptom free
   c. Known presence of spondylolysis or spondylolisthesis in an asymptomatic player is not a contraindication to play
   d. A symptomatic, skeletally immature individual with high-grade spondylolisthesis (slippage greater than half width of vertebral body) is a candidate for fusion.

D. **Thoracolumbar fractures**
1. Infrequent injuries that can occur with severe direct impact to the spine or violent muscle contractions
   a. If a fracture is suspected, important to maintain spine precautions before any movement of patient
   b. Neurologic assessment important in initial exam
   c. Generally complain of severe back pain, exacerbated with any attempted movement
2. **X-rays** of the spine, including anteroposterior, lateral, and oblique views to evaluate injury
   a. MRI if any neurologic injury is present with the fracture
   b. Consider CT scan or MRI of abdomen if suspect visceral injuries (rare)
3. **Treatment** dependent on fracture pattern and stability
   a. Isolated stable transverse process or spinous process fractures usually amenable to brief period of rest with return to play when symptoms tolerate (3–6 weeks)
   b. Fracture treatment should follow accepted guidelines for particular fracture pattern (for example, individuals requiring lumbar fusion should not be allowed to return to contact sports)

XI. Hip and Pelvis

A. **Soft tissue injuries**
1. **Hip pointers**
   a. "Hip pointer" is common term applied to injuries of iliac crest, including contusions from direct injury, muscle avulsions from violent contractions, and periostitis from repetitive abdominal muscular contractions or contusions
   b. Skeletally immature players should be evaluated radiographically to rule out displaced apophysis in avulsion-type injuries.
   c. **Treatment** consists of rest, ice, stretching, and NSAIDs:
      i. Most apophyseal injuries and muscle avulsions treated conservatively except for widely displaced apophyseal fractures and large muscle avulsions, which should be surgically repaired
      ii. Return to play when symptoms tolerate with padding, heat, and stretching before play and ice afterwards

d. Trochanteric bursitis from direct blow also a common injury in this region; treatment involves same protocol with judicious use of steroid injections if necessary

2. **Groin pull**
   a. Common term for injury to the iliopsoas or adductor group of the leg, usually caused by forced abduction, external rotation:
      i. Common in older and deconditioned athletes
      ii. Symptoms include pain with resisted adduction of leg or passive adduction, located along border of pubic ramus
   b. X-rays of the hip and pelvis to rule out avulsion fracture caused by the iliopsoas (lesser trochanter) or adductor group
   c. **Treatment** initially includes ice and rest, followed by stretching and strengthening when symptoms allow:
      i. Muscle spans two joints and is at increased risk for injury—best treatment is preventive by preseason strengthening program
      ii. Symptoms can be persistent depending on severity—adequate strength necessary before play to prevent exacerbations
      iii. Most avulsion injuries treated similarly, if not widely displaced
3. **Osteitis pubis**
   a. Common in football players, weight lifters. Exact etiology unknown, but thought to be secondary to overuse of adductors and gracilis with gradual resorption of bone at muscular attachment sites (medial aspect of pubic bones).
   b. Symptoms include gradual onset of groin pain exacerbated by resisted adduction and tenderness along inferior and medial borders of pubic bones
   c. X-rays may reveal resorption of bone at the pubic symphysis with resultant widening and sclerosis of the inferior pubic rami. Bone scans reveal diffuse uptake in the involved areas of the pubic rami.
   d. Relative rest and anti-inflammatories most successful for this overuse injury, which often takes 2–3 months to resolve

B. **Fractures/dislocations**

1. **Hip subluxation/dislocation**
   a. Unusual but potentially devastating injury secondary to possible osteonecrosis of the femoral head:
      i. Player experiences severe pain in hip with any attempted movement
      ii. Posterior dislocation most common; leg appears shortened, externally rotated
   b. X-rays before reduction necessary to rule out femoral neck fracture
   c. Gentle reduction should be performed urgently in controlled setting after neurovascular status and x-rays are assessed
2. **Lesser trochanter avulsion/other apophyseal avulsions**
   a. Most common under age of 20 and results from severe contraction of iliopsoas muscle (or other muscular attachment)
   b. Symptoms include immediate severe groin pain exacerbated by attempts to flex hip joint or pain and tenderness to palpation in suspected apophyseal location with exacerbation on resisted muscular contraction
   c. Treatment involves bed rest followed by gentle range of motion and partial weight bearing when tolerated when x-rays reveal nondisplaced or minimally displaced fractures. The role of open reduction for these injuries based on degree of displacement is controversial.

XII. Lower Extremity

A. **Thigh**

1. **Quadriceps contusions/exostosis**

a. Direct impact onto quadriceps muscle belly with resultant pain, decreased range of motion, and occasional palpable mass
b. Initial treatment of flexion, ice to minimize hematoma (not heat), followed by pain-free range of motion and functional rehabilitation (avoid heat, ultrasound, painful exercise)
c. Conservative treatment for myositis ossificans unless functional impairment
d. Return to play with extra thigh padding when full strength, function, and range of motion are achieved

2. **Hamstring injuries**
a. Sudden pain in posterior thigh with rapid hamstring contraction; associated with fatigue, poor conditioning, inadequate stretching. Short head of biceps is most common.
b. Prophylaxis with off-season conditioning, baseline hamstrings-to-quadriceps strength ratio of 0.6 or greater
c. Initial treatment of RICE, jogging, and pain-free functional rehabilitation when hamstrings 70% of baseline
d. Return to play when isokinetic strength ratio approximately 0.6

B. **Knee and leg**
1. **Ligament injuries**
a. **Medial collateral ligament:**
i. Most commonly caused by direct impact onto the lateral aspect of the knee with applied valgus stress
ii. Pain on the medial aspect of the knee with tenderness to palpation along the course of the medial collateral ligament: increased laxity to valgus stress at 30° of flexion. Increased laxity when knee at full extension indicates a more severe knee injury (often cruciate ligament disruption).
iii. Usually treated nonoperatively with protected weight bearing, inflammation control, range of motion at 30–60°, followed by progression to full range of motion, progressive resisted exercises, and return to play with functional knee brace when tolerated

b. **Anterior cruciate ligament:**
i. Most commonly occurs from noncontact twisting injury, but can occur from direct blow to the knee as well
ii. History of hearing or feeling a "pop" in the knee, rapid effusion (within a few hours) highly suggestive of an anterior cruciate ligament disruption; exam reveals positive Lachman's sign, pivot shift
iii. X-rays usually negative or may show a small bony avulsion
iv. Treatment for cruciate-dependent individuals or those who plan to continue to participate in high-risk sports is surgical in most instances; delaying surgery by at least 3 weeks is currently believed to reduce incidence of arthrofibrosis. Concomitant injuries most commonly treated by conservative medial collateral ligament management with delayed anterior cruciate ligament reconstruction.
v. Functional knee bracing on return to play remains a controversial topic.

c. **Posterior cruciate ligament:**
i. Mechanism of injury most commonly a hyperflexed knee or direct blow to the anterior tibia while foot is firmly planted
ii. Injury is often missed and a high index of suspicion is necessary. Exam reveals increased posterior tibial translation at 90° of flexion. Suspect more severe injury if posterior sag does not improve with internal rotation of the tibia.
iii. X-rays often negative or may reveal bony avulsion at tibial insertion

iv. Treatment for isolated posterior cruciate ligament is controversial; conservative approach most common with focus on functional restoration before play. Surgical proponents recommend reconstruction secondary to high incidence of patellofemoral and medial arthritis with this injury, although current studies fail to show improved outcome with operative intervention.

d. **Posterolateral instability:**

i. Isolated injury to this complex uncommon; usually accompanied by a cruciate ligament injury. Direct blow to the anteromedial tibia or severe twisting with the foot planted are the most common mechanisms.

ii. Exam shows increased laxity at 30° with varus stress, increased rotatory instability. Effusion often absent with combined cruciate and posterolateral injuries secondary to capsular tear. Important to assess peroneal nerve function at the time of injury.

iii. X-rays often negative but necessary to rule out avulsion fractures; MRI is helpful to delineate structures injured.

iv. Treatment involves direct surgical repair of posterolateral structures (or biceps tenodesis if tissues severely compromised) and reconstruction of cruciate injury when present.

2. **Meniscal injuries**

a. Common injuries that can occur by contact or noncontact mechanisms; often a twisting-type injury with joint line and/or posterior pain and complaints of locking, catching, or buckling. Unless the tear is peripheral, effusion is usually not noticed by the player until the evening or the next day.

b. Exam often reveals joint line tenderness, an effusion, pain with extremes of flexion, lack of full extension (or a "locked" knee) if a displaced bucket-handle is present. Nonspecific pain may be present with circumduction maneuvers.

c. X-rays are negative; MRI is the diagnostic test of choice when exam is equivocal.

d. Arthroscopy is indicated when symptoms do not respond to rest and control of inflammation; repair instead of excision of the meniscus should be attempted whenever feasible.

3. **Patellofemoral disorders**

a. **Patellar dislocation:**

i. Usually a noncontact, external rotation injury to the leg resulting in severe anterior knee pain with buckling or an inability to bear weight

ii. Knee diffusely swollen with significant tenderness along medial retinaculum, lateral trochlea, and patellar articular surfaces; apprehension with attempts at patellar translation (usually reduces spontaneously)

iii. X-rays, including merchant view, necessary to rule out patellar or trochlear ridge fracture or bone fragments in joint

iv. Treatment includes RICE, with progression to range of motion and quadriceps strengthening for initial injury; return to play usually requires 6–8 weeks. Repeat dislocators often require surgery to reconstruct medial structures and alter mechanical alignment.

b. **Patellar/quadriceps tendinitis** (jumper's knee):

i. Overuse injury common to football secondary to frequent stops and starts and eccentric loading of the extensor mechanism

ii. Most common areas of tendinitis are patellar tendon at inferior pole of patella and quadriceps tendon insertion into superior pole, but can occur anywhere along extensor mechanism

iii. Prevention is the optimal treatment, with conditioning including eccentric strength training and adequate stretching. Symptomatic players require relative rest (exercises that do not provoke symptoms) and anti-inflammatory modalities, with progression to concentric and isometric strength training, and finally eccentric training when asymptomatic during other therapy.

c. **Fat pad syndrome** (Hoffa's disease):
   i. Seen frequently secondary to contusions and resultant irritation to the anterior aspect of the knee
   ii. Tenderness to palpation usually present medial and lateral to patellar tendon and inferior patella—capsule in this region often feels "boggy"
   iii. Treatment involves relative rest, anti-inflammatory modalities, and stretching. Recalcitrant cases are uncommon, but usually respond to arthroscopic debridement.

4. **Medial tibial stress syndrome (shin splints)**
   a. Characterized by diffuse pain along the medial border of the tibia. Common in early season with increased training, exacerbated during exercise, and may persist for hours to days.
   b. Area of tenderness usually along the posteromedial border of the tibia—less well localized than a stress fracture. Should not be exacerbated with passive ankle or foot motion.
   c. X-rays are usually normal but may reveal mild cortical hypertrophy. Bone scan is helpful to distinguish from stress fracture and is negative or reveals diffuse linear uptake approximately one third the length of the tibia on posteromedial border.
   d. Rest is the most effective treatment; anti-inflammatory modalities and stretching by themselves do not resolve the condition. Gradual resumption of activities when pain free (usually 2–6 weeks). Orthotics may help prevent recurrence when significant pronation is present.

5. **Tibial stress fractures**
   a. Mechanism is most commonly a rapid increase in training, especially running activities.
   b. Point tenderness on the anteromedial aspect of the tibia is highly suggestive of the diagnosis.
   c. X-rays of a stress fracture are often negative or reveal only cortical thickening; if no fracture is seen on plain films, bone scan is the procedure of choice to make the definitive diagnosis.
   d. Treatment involves rest followed by gradual **pain-free** progression of activities; one study suggests that use of a pneumatic leg brace during rehabilitation protocol can shorten return-to-play time by several weeks.

C. **Ankle and foot**

1. **Ankle sprains**
   a. Most common ligamentous injury. Structures injured dependent on force and applied direction of injury; therefore, **history of injury important**.
      i. Plantarflexion and inversion stresses injure anterior talofibular ligament (ATFL), with progressive force injuring calcaneofibular, posterotalofibular, and tibiofibular ligaments in severe injuries
      ii. Inversion stress in neutral position injures calcaneofibular ligament
      iii. Dorsiflexion stresses tibiofibular ligaments
      iv. Eversion and external rotation injures deltoid ligament medially and tibiofibular ligament laterally, often accompanied by fibular fracture
   b. **Palpation and stress tests** are used to determine ligaments injured:
      i. Anterior drawer with 30° plantarflexion to assess ATFL; compare to contralateral side
      ii. Inversion test—grasp heel and apply inversion stress; ability to palpate talar head indicates complete tears of both ATFL and calcaneofibular ligament

   iii. Squeeze test—squeeze fibula and tibia together near ankle joint; pain indicates probable syndesmotic/tibiofibular ligament injuries
   iv. Evaluate for associated injuries, including peroneal tendon dislocation, fifth metatarsal fracture, posterior tibial tendon rupture, midfoot sprains
  c. **X-rays** are necessary to rule out fracture of medial malleolus, lateral malleolus, and talar dome:
   i. Stress x-rays helpful in chronic ankle instability to evaluate ligament integrity—anterior drawer assesses ATFL, talar tilt test (inversion stress) with > 5° asymmetry indicates instability, and loss of parallelism with Broden's view and inversion stress indicates subtalar instability. External rotation stress with mortise view to evaluate syndesmosis.
   ii. MRI useful to evaluate talar dome osteochondral injuries when suspected
  d. **Treatment** for acute injuries includes anti-inflammatory modalities, early restoration of range of motion, and functional management dependent on severity:
   i. Ankle braces to limit inversion/eversion stress used on grades II and III; cast immobilization rarely indicated in healthy athletes
   ii. Proprioceptive and peroneal strengthening immediately for grade I, immediate to 1 week for grade II, when tolerated in grade III (1 week to 1 month)
   iii. Return to play dependent on athlete's ability to demonstrate adequate performance in position-specific drills with little or no symptoms (usually < 1 week for grade I, 1–2 weeks for grade II, approximately 1 month for grade III)
   iv. Unstable fracture patterns, syndesmotic disruption require surgical stabilization
  e. **Functional instability:**
   i. Peroneal weakness, not ligamentous instability, responsible for approximately 50% of those with persistent functional instability
   ii. Brostrom lateral ligamentous repair currently most popular technique for ligamentous instability

2. **Midfoot sprains**
  a. Usually indirect injuries from forceful foot abduction when foot in fixed position or foot forced into severe plantarflexion
  b. Patient demonstrates pain or tenderness in midfoot region, unable to tiptoe, may have flattening of longitudinal arch
  c. Lateral and anteroposterior weight-bearing views—in normal anteroposterior view, medial border of second metatarsal base lines up with medial border of middle cuneiform; distance between second metatarsal base and lateral border of medial cuneiform should be symmetric on comparison views.
  d. **Treatment:**
   i. Conservative for normal x-rays. For severe medial sprain, use short leg non–weight-bearing cast 4–6 weeks followed by weight-bearing cast 2–3 weeks. Lateral midfoot sprains tend to resolve earlier.
   ii. For Lisfranc's dislocation, internal fixation to reduce second metatarsal base to medial cuneiform (weak link)
   iii. Return to sport with evidence of healing, such as ability to tiptoe, perform functional drills

3. **Fifth metatarsal base fractures**
  a. Three types:
   i. Tuberosity fractures from traction/avulsion-type injuries from the peroneus brevis or ligaments
   ii. Metaphyseal fractures by adduction and inversion forces

iii. Jones fracture (approximately 3 cm distal to tuberosity) by repetitive or single force by sharp turning

b. Tenderness to **palpation** over fifth metatarsal base and pain with eversion forces present with all fracture types

c. **X-rays** of foot determine fracture type; bone scans helpful to rule out Jones fracture when sclerosis, but no obvious fracture, present

d. Short leg cast or firm shoe with progression to weight bearing as tolerated for tuberosity and metaphyseal fractures. Treatment of Jones fracture controversial:

i. Conservative treatment—metatarsal support (cast, brace), weight-bearing versus non–weight-bearing debatable

ii. In high-demand professional athlete, percutaneous intramedullary compression screw hastens healing time. Screw fixation is also most common treatment when significant sclerosis present or delayed union with conservative treatment.

iii. Return to play with radiographic evidence of union and ability to perform functional tests

4. **Turf toe**

a. Hyperextension or, less commonly, hyperflexion injury to the first metatarsophalangeal joint, associated with flexible footwear and more common on artificial turf. Severity of injury can range from capsular or ligamentous strain, to axial compression with resultant chondral injury, or metatarsophalangeal dislocation.

b. Exam reveals tenderness about the metatarsophalangeal joint, pain with passive dorsiflexion and often with decreased range of motion, and difficulty with push-off.

c. **X-rays** to evaluate for bony injury to metatarsophalangeal joint. May see avulsions secondary to capsular injury; rarely, may have chondrolysis with repeated injuries. If plantar tenderness is present, obtain sesamoid views to rule out fractures in these structures.

d. **Treatment** dependent on severity of injury:

i. Capsular or ligamentous strains (characterized by localized tenderness) treated with ice, continuous play with taping to restrict

ii. Significant swelling, ecchymosis, and restricted range of motion indicate partial or complete capsular tear—treat with anti-inflammatory modalities, protective footwear, and restriction of play until clinical symptoms allow (usually 3–6 weeks)

iii. Chondral injuries or dislocation requires treatment similar to less injuries, as well as limited weight bearing and immobilization. Return to play dependent on clinical symptoms (often prolonged).

XIII. Protective Equipment

A. **Football helmet** must meet National Operating Committee on Standards for Athletic Equipment (NOCSAE) specifications

1. **Construction**

a. Outer shell is made of a polymer plastic (polycarbonate or acryl butadiene syrene) that is both lightweight and able to withstand high impacts.

b. Padding or suspension systems include pads, air and fluid-filled cells, a combination of cells and pads, and suspension:

i. Air cells can be inflated or deflated to provide better fit.

ii. Suspension types offer inferior protection and are being phased out.

iii. Important to check for cracks in the outer shell (especially at the locations of the face mask attachments), leaks, or other damage to the padding system to insure proper protection

iv. Helmet should have a NOCSAE label on outer shell warning of potential head or spine injury with improper helmet size

2. **Helmet fitting**
   a. Helmet should be donned by spreading the ear holes apart with the thumbs; helmet should turn minimally with attempts to rotate on head:
      i. No space between pads and face or back of head
      ii. One to two fingerbreadths above the eyebrows; helmet should not come over eyes even with firm pressure on top of the helmet
      iii. Base of skull should be covered, but helmet should not impinge on cervical spine with full extension
      iv. Jaw pads should provide snug fit and prevent lateral rocking
   b. Hair should be the same length at the time of fitting as it will be throughout the season. Long hair should be wet when fitting to simulate sweaty conditions.
   c. Chin strap (four-point more secure than two-point) helps to prevent forward and backward helmet motion; improper tension or strap failure can cause helmet to come off, or result in laceration to the bridge of the nose.
   d. Face masks used depend on position—ball carrying positions require a mask that protects yet allows for an unobstructed view, whereas linemen need additional protection to prevent eye and facial injuries.
   e. Plexiglas shields are also worn for those seeking additional eye protection.
   f. Mouth guards (required in college and high school) can be custom-made, mouth formed by heating, or obtained in standard sizes. They are helpful in dissipating blows to the chin, reducing intraoral and mandible injuries.

B. **Shoulder pads**
   1. Cantilever and flat are the two basic types:
      a. **Flat pads** are worn by those positions requiring greater glenohumeral motion.
      b. **Cantilever pads** (named for the bridge extending across the shoulder) are worn by players in constant contact and requiring additional protection.
      c. Modifications depend on position and preference; e.g., linebackers and other players hit in a standing position have pads that are larger anteriorly and slanted forward.
   2. **Shoulder pad fitting**
      a. Measure from acromioclavicular joint to acromioclavicular joint, and compare to manufacturer's chart to approximate fit
      b. Neck opening should be large enough to prevent neck impingement when lifting arm overhead but not large enough to allow excessive sliding about (1 to 2 fingerbreadths between neck and inside padding)
      c. Lateral aspect of pad should be just lateral to shoulder, with flaps or epaulets large enough to cover deltoid region
      d. Elastic axilla straps should be adjusted snugly but comfortably, to allow for blows to be distributed across pads
      e. Anterior pads should meet but not overlap when laced up
      f. Pads should extend below nipple line anteriorly and approximately 1 inch below the scapula posteriorly
      g. Important to inspect frequently for strap fraying or breakage, loose rivets, or cracks

C. **Other protective equipment**
   1. **Standard equipment**
      a. Hip pads are used to protect the iliac crest and tailbone from injury.
      b. Thigh pads and knee pads are inserted into the pants snugly and should not slip easily.
   2. **Special equipment**
      a. Neck rolls and collars are used frequently by those players who have previously experienced "burners and stingers" or on a prophylactic basis; efficacy of these devices in preventing further injury remains debatable.

b. Shoulder restraint devices are used to restrict abduction and external rotation in chronic shoulder dislocators, but these limitations may affect a player's capabilities in many positions.
c. Gloves and upper extremity pads are worn by linesmen and other players to prevent finger injuries, contusions, and myositis ossificans.
d. Rib pads or vests are commonly worn by quarterbacks to prevent injuries to the thorax.
e. The value of the prophylactic knee brace in preventing injury remains questionable; therefore, it is not a mandatory protection device.

Recommended Reading

1. Alves WM, Rimel RW, Nelson WE: University of Virginia prospective study of football-induced minor head injury: Status report. Clin Sports Med 6(1):211–218, 1987.
2. Borczuk P: Predictors of intracranial injury in patients with mild head injury. Ann Emerg Med 25:731–736, 1995.
3. Bradley JP: Management of lower extremity injuries in the NFL Foot/Heel/Toes, presented at American Orthopedic Society for Sports Medicine meeting, Palm Desert, CA, 1995.
4. Brown LS, Drotman DP, Chu A: Bleeding injuries in professional football: Estimating the risk for HIV transmission. Ann Intern Med 122(4):273–274, 1995.
5. Bruno LA, Gennarelli TA, Torg JS: Management guidelines for head injuries in athletics. Clin Sports Med 6(1):17–29, 1987.
6. Calabrese LH, LaPerriere A: Human immunodeficiency virus infection, exercise, and athletics. Sports Med 15:6, 1993.
7. Cantu RC, Micheli J (eds): American College of Sports Medicine's Guidelines for the Team Physician. Philadelphia, Lea & Febiger, 1991.
8. Chang CJ, Lombardo JA: Protective equipment: Football. In Mellion MB (ed): The Team Physician's Handbook. Philadelphia, Hanley & Belfus, 1990, pp 99–109.
9. Clare PE: Football. In Mellion MB (ed): The Team Physician's Handbook. Philadelphia, Hanley & Belfus, 1990, pp 489–505.
10. Colorado Medical Society: Guidelines for the Management of Concussion in Sports. Colorado Medical Society, Sports Medicine Committee, 1990 (rev 1991).
11. Criswell D, Powers S, Lawler J, et al: Influence of a carbohydrate-electrolyte beverage on performance and blood homeostasis during recovery from football. Int J Sport Nutr 1(2):178–191, 1991.
12. Epstein SE, Maron BJ: Sudden death and the competitive athlete: Perspectives in preparticipation screening studies. J Am Coll Cardiol 7:220, 1986.
13. Gerberich SG, Priest JD, Boen JR, et al: Concussion incidence and severity in secondary school varsity football players. Am J Public Health 73:1370–1375, 1983.
14. Griffin LY, et al: Orthop Knowl Update Sports Med. Chicago, American Academy of Orthopedic Surgeons, 1994.
15. Heidt RS: Ankle sprains in the NFL. Presented at American Orthopedic Society for Sports Medicine meeting, Palm Desert, CA, 1995.
16. Huston TP, Puffer JC, Rodney WM: The athletic heart syndrome. N Engl J Med 313:24, 1985.
17. Irrgang JJ, Miller MD, Johnson DL: Football. In Fu F (ed): Sports Injuries. Baltimore, Williams & Wilkins, 1994, pp 349–374.
18. Jordan BD, Zimmerman RD: Computed tomography and magnetic resonance imaging comparisons in boxers. JAMA 263:1670–1674, 1990.
19. Kelly JP, Nichols JS, Fillewy CM, et al: Concussion in sports: Guidelines for prevention of catastrophic outcome. JAMA 266:2867–2869, 1991.
20. Lawless D, Jackson CG, Greenleaf JE: Exercise and HIV-1 infection. Sports Med 19(4):235–239, 1995.
21. Levin HS, Amparo E, Eisenberg JM, et al: Magnetic resonance imaging and computerized tomography in relation to the neurobehavioral sequelae of mild and moderate head injuries. J Neurosurg 66:706–713, 1987.
22. Lillegard WA, Terrio JD: Appropriate strength training. Med Clin North Am 78(2):457–477, 1994.
23. Lombardo J, Nelson M, Smith D: Preparticipation Physical Evaluation. American Academy of Family Practice, American Academy of Pediatrics, American Medical Society for Sports Medicine, American Orthopaedic Society for Sports Medicine, American Osteopathic Academy of Sports Medicine, 1992.
24. McCaffrey FM, Braden DS, Strong WB: Sudden cardiac death in young athletes. Am J Dis Child 145:177, 1991.
25. McKeag DB, Kinderknecht J: A basketball player with infectious mononucleosis. In Smith NJ (ed): Common Problems in Pediatric Sports Medicine. Chicago, Year Book Medical Publishers, 1989.

26. Meyer SA, Schulte KR, Callaghan JJ: Cervical spinal stenosis and stingers in collegiate football players. Am J Sports Med 22(2):158–166, 1994.
27. Myers TJ, Yoganandan N, Sances A, et al: Energy absorption characteristics of football helmets under low and high rates of loading. Biomed Mater Engineer 3(1):15–24, 1993.
28. NCAA Injury Surveillance System (ISS) Head and neck injury data from 1984–1991. Overland Park, KS, National Collegiate Athletic Association.
29. Nelson WE, Jane JA, Gieck JH: Minor head injury in sports: A new classification and management. Phys Sports Med 12(3):103–107, 1984.
30. Rimel RW, Giordani B, Barth JT, et al: Moderate head injury: Completing the clinical spectrum of brain trauma. Neurosurgery 11(3):344–351, 1982.
31. Saal JA: Common American football injuries. Sports Med 12(2):132–147, 1991.
32. Saunders RL, Harbaugh RE: The second impact in catastrophic contact-sports head trauma. JAMA 252:538–539, 1984.
33. Speer KP, Bassett F: The prolonged burner syndrome. Am J Sports Med 18:591–594, 1990.
34. Torg JS: Return to play criteria following injury/surgery of the cervical spine. Presented at American Orthopedic Society for Sports Medicine meeting, Palm Desert, CA, 1995.
35. Wilberger JE: Minor head injuries in American football: Prevention of long term sequelae. Sports Med 15(5):338–343, 1993.
36. Yesalis CE, Bahrke MS: Anabolic-androgenic steroids: Current issues. Sports Med 19(5):326–340, 1995.
37. Zeppilli P: The athlete's heart: Differentiation of training effects from organic heart disease. Pract Cardiol 14:61, 1988.

55

Volleyball

Denise Fandel, M.S., ATC, and Morris B. Mellion, M.D.

I. General Concerns

Volleyball was invented in 1895 in Holyoke, Massachusetts, as a recreational sport of modest intensity.

A. **Power volleyball** is an increasingly popular competitive men's and women's sport that requires:
   1. Explosive movement
   2. Quickness and agility (frequent changes in direction and intensity)
   3. Rapid reaction time (ball may travel at 75 mph)
   4. Total body control
   5. Aerobic and anaerobic fitness
   6. Mental toughness

B. Volleyball is a contact sport in which the player may be injured due to contact with:
   1. The ball
   2. The floor
   3. Other players
   4. The nets and supporting apparatus

C. Certain aspects of volleyball **predispose the athlete to specific types of overuse injuries.**
   1. The **underhand passing position** of volleyball stresses the patellofemoral joint as well as the low back.
   2. Jumping and landing with **recurrent intense deceleration forces** further stress the patellofemoral joint as well as the patella tendon and its origin and insertion into the tibial tubercle.
   3. The **hitting motion of volleyball in serving and spiking (hitting)** subjects the shoulder to several overuse injuries.
   4. Repetitive, intense **hyperextension of the lumbosacral spine in hitting and blocking** subject the low back to injury.

D. Highly competitive volleyball players tend to be **lean and angular**. Height is a marked advantage for hitting and blocking on the front line (Fig. 1A). Agility and quickness are critical for defense.
   1. Similar characteristics as front court and back court basketball players
   2. Volleyball requires both **strength and endurance**.
   3. **Weight management** may be a problem for some athletes.

II. Volleyball Injuries

A. **General patterns**
   1. **Overuse injuries are more frequent than trauma.** Of traumatic injuries, highest number are due to contact with floor, especially sprains and strains occurring with body rotation over or around a planted foot.

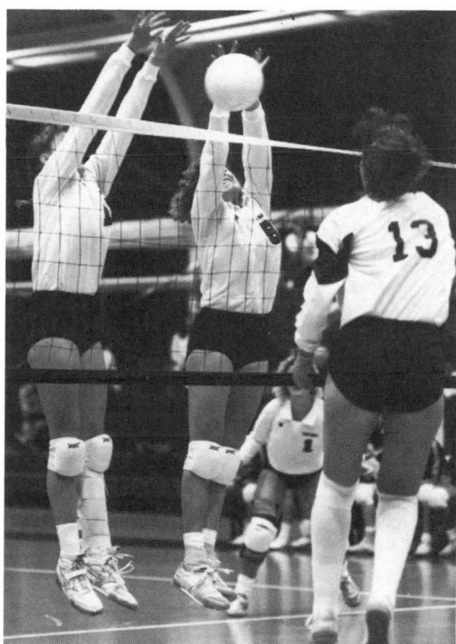

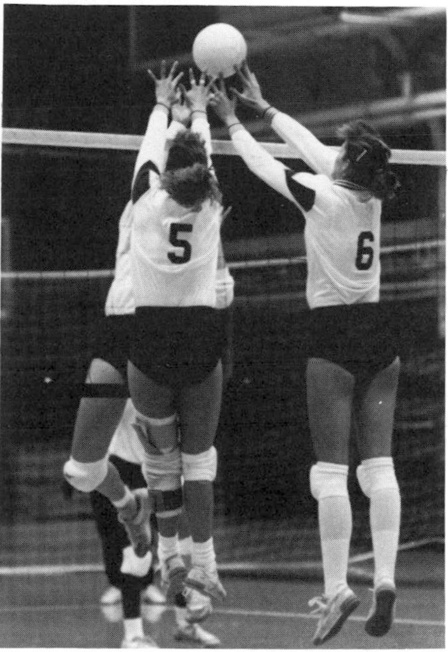

FIGURE 1. **A**, Height is a marked advantage for hitting and blocking on the front line. **B**, Finger injuries are common in volleyball from contact with the ball.

2. College freshmen and sophomores are injured more frequently than juniors and seniors. Higher conditioning and skill level appear to be protective.
3. Injuries in college volleyball generally result in players missing 1–6 days per injury.

B. **Traumatic injuries**
1. **Contact with the ball** (Fig. 1B)
   a. **Finger injuries**
      i. "Jammed fingers" (tenosynovitis)
      ii. Mallet finger and boutonniere deformity from poor blocking technique
      iii. Hyperextension injuries from poor setting technique (flexor tendon strain and volar plate injuries)
      iv. Fingertip contusions
   b. **Hands, wrists, and forearms**
      i. Contusions from recurrent ball trauma
         (a) Frequent in inexperienced players but occur at all levels
         (b) Occasionally severe
      ii. **Traumatic aneurysms** have been reported in small arteries of the hand.
   c. **Facial injuries:** The volleyball "six pack" can cause nasal fractures.
2. **Contact with the floor** produces a wide variety of trauma (Fig. 2), but certain injuries are relatively common.
   a. **Shoulder:** Acute rotator cuff strains (traumatic tendinitis) occur in digging and diving motions. There may be an underlying problem that is "asymptomatic" or "subclinical" before trauma in some cases:
      i. Contusions
      ii. Acromioclavicular separations
      iii. Glenohumeral dislocations
   b. **Knee**
      i. **Prepatellar bursitis** ("housemaid's knee")

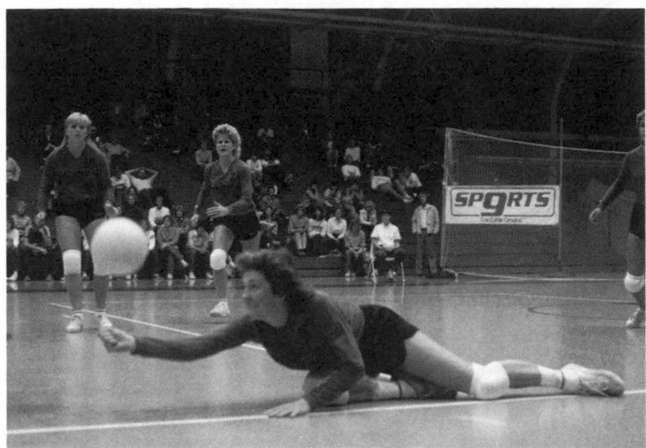

FIGURE 2. Contact with the floor produces a wide variety of traumatic injuries.

- ii. Ligament sprains
- iii. Meniscal tears

c. **Ankle—most often injured**
- i. **Sprains**
- ii. **Strains**

d. **Foot**—metatarsal arch
e. **Elbow**—olecranon bursitis
f. **Hand**—sprain of the thumb ulnar collateral ligament ("gamekeeper's thumb")
g. **Skin**—abrasions resulting from wet skin and the use of protective devices

3. **Contact with other players**
   a. Occurs when more than one player is digging or diving for the ball
   b. Jumping and landing on other player's foot during hitting and blocking
4. **Contact with the net and support apparatus**

C. **Overuse**

1. **Knee:** most common site for overuse injuries. Problems of the extensor mechanism due to jumping and landing.
   a. **Mechanism:** landing with quadriceps mechanism contracted and allowing it to absorb an intense load while the muscle is lengthened. Microtrauma results at the quadriceps tendon, the patellofemoral interface, the patellar origin of the patella tendon, and the insertion of the patella at the tibial tubercle.
   b. Predisposing factors
      i. Intrinsic (anatomic) factors
      ii. Extrinsic factors:
         (a) Incidence varies directly with number of practices and games per week (Table 1). Increase in volume and intensity of participation adds to the risk.
         (b) Hard playing surfaces raise incidence and shock-absorbing surfaces lower risk (Table 2).
   c. **Common syndromes**
      i. "Jumper's knee"—patellar tendinitis; term is also occasionally used to include all extensor mechanism problems in jumping sports:
         (a) Most common extensor mechanism problem in jumping sports
         (b) Somehow related to weakness of ankle dorsiflexor muscles, but mechanism is not clear
         (c) High incidence of patella alta

TABLE 1. Knee Extensor Mechanism Injuries: Relationship Between Incidence and Frequency of Practices/Games

Weekly Practices/Games	Volleyball Players Affected (%)
2	3.2
3	14.6
4	29.1
> 4	41.8

Adapted from Ferretti A, et al: Jumper's knee: An epidemiological study of volleyball players. Phys Sportsmed 12(10):97–106, 1984.

ii. Patellofemoral pain
iii. Quadriceps tendinitis
iv. Osgood-Schlatter disease—pubertal and peripubertal athletes

d. Other knee overuse—semimembranosis tendinitis

2. **Ankle/foot**
   a. Achilles tendinitis
   b. Plantar fasciitis
3. **Shoulder**
   a. **Etiology:** repetitive overhead hitting, blocking, serving, and setting (Fig. 3)
   b. **Rotator cuff tendinitis and impingement syndromes** include:
      i. Rotator cuff tears—acute and chronic
      ii. Supraspinatus tendinitis
      iii. Biceps tendinitis
      iv. Subdeltoid bursitis
      v. Glenoid labrum avulsion
      vi. Suprascapular nerve injuries
   c. **Predisposing factors**
      i. Poor technique
      ii. Lack of sport-specific conditioning:
         (a) Strength (Fig. 4), especially of the shoulder girdle muscles, which act as decelerators
         (b) Flexibility
         (c) Endurance:
            • Emphasis often on lifting heavy weights when endurance work necessary
            • No need to lift more than 8 pounds with rotator cuff muscles
      iii. Improper or inadequate warm-up
4. **Lumbosacral spine**
   a. **Etiological factors**
      i. Flexed hip posture of underhand passing position stresses lumbosacral spine (Fig. 5)

TABLE 2. Knee Extensor Mechanism Injuries: Relationship Between Incidence and Playing Surface

Playing Surface	Volleyball Players Affected
Cement	24/64 (37.5%)
Linoleum	55/237 (23.2%)
Wood parquet	3/64 (4.7%)
Other surfaces	11/42 (26.2%)

Adapted from Ferretti A, et al: Jumper's knee: An epidemiological study of volleyball players. Phys Sportsmed 12(10):97–106, 1984.

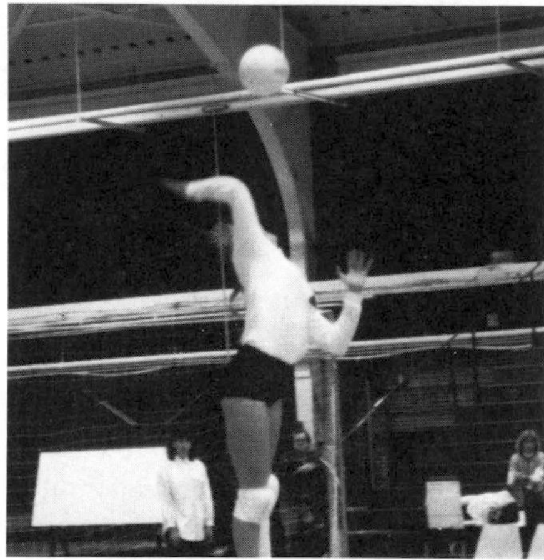

FIGURE 3. Repetitive overhead hitting, blocking, and serving can cause impingement and overuse syndromes.

ii. Forced hyperextension of low back in hitting, blocking, and setting stresses pars interarticularis of lower lumbar vertebrae

b. **Common syndromes**

i. Low back strain

ii. Intravertebral disk herniation

iii. Spondylolysis/spondylolisthesis

iv. Sacroiliac joint sprain/contracture

5. **Shin splints and stress fractures**

a. **Etiological factors**

i. Flexed hip posture of underhand passing position stresses lumbosacral spine

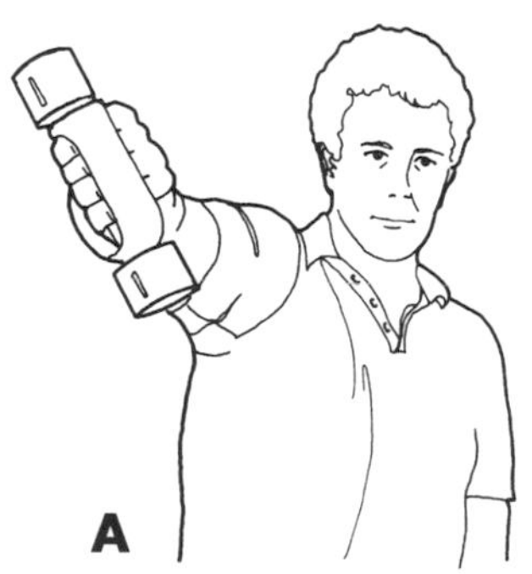

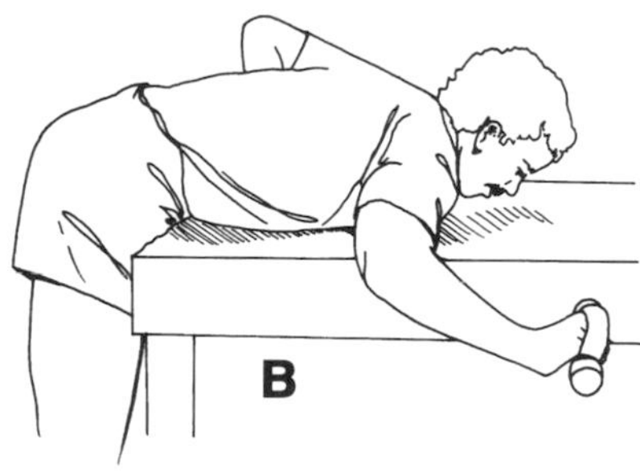

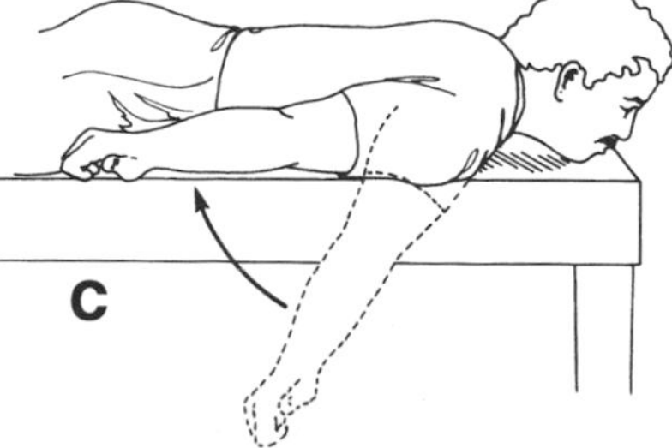

FIGURE 4. Shoulder strengthening exercises particularly useful in rehabilitating and preventing rotator-cuff injuries in volleyball players. **A**, Supraspinatus muscle is strengthened by internally rotating and abducting humerus. **B**, Strengthening exercise for posterior portion of deltoid muscle and rotator cuff. **C**, By elevating arm in an externally rotated position (with thumb pointed outward), the athlete exercises external rotators of shoulder and scapula stabilizers.

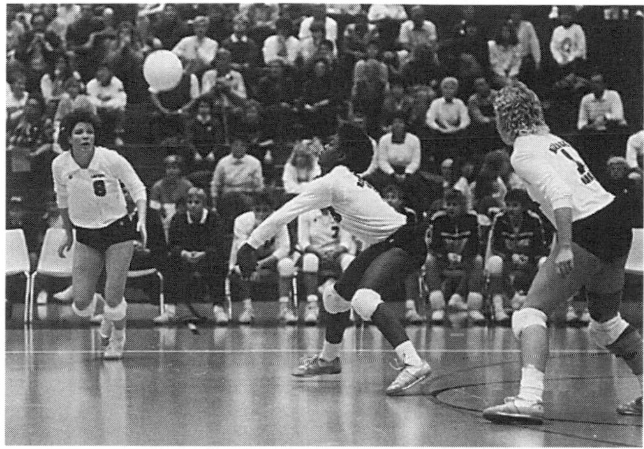

FIGURE 5. The flexed hip posture of the underhand passing position stresses the lumbosacral spine.

- ii. Common anatomic factors:
  - (a) Hyperpronating feet
  - (b) Genu varum (bowlegs)
- iii. Inadequate sport-specific conditioning:
  - (a) Inadequate flexibility
  - (b) Imbalance between anterior and posterior musculature
- iv. Increase in intensity or duration of participation

b. **Common stress fracture sites in volleyball**
- i. Metatarsals
- ii. Tibia
- iii. Fibula

c. **Bracing:** Some athletes may be able to participate with shin splints or mild stress fractures of the tibia or fibula after 10 or more days of rest by using an Air Cast leg brace including an anterior buttress.

d. **Preventive strategies—special prehabilitation and rehabilitation**
- i. **Year-round conditioning**
  - (a) Sport specific
  - (b) Strength, endurance, flexibility, agility, reaction time
  - (c) **Avoid plyometrics in athletes until a high level of strength, endurance, and flexibility have been attained.**
- ii. Employ a **gradual progression of skill** training
  - (a) Allow athlete time to build body awareness while learning new skill
  - (b) Chart number of foot contacts per training session to plan gradual increase in intensity
  - (c) **Do not allow plyometric training until athlete can lift a minimum of two times body weight in hip sled-squat**
- iii. **Diving and digging drills:** special tumbling drills to prepare player to dive and dig for the ball without injury
- iv. **Proprioception training**
  - (a) Body position awareness is vital to lower extremity landings and to the diving and digging movements in volleyball.
  - (b) **Proprioception drills can reduce injuries:**
    - • Lower extremity drills (see Box)
    - • Diving and digging drills have a proprioceptive component.

FOOTSPEED DRILLS

These drills are done 3 times a week. If done correctly and intensively, you will **help yourself and your team by:**

1. Increasing your footspeed
2. Increasing your quickness
3. Improving your coordination
4. Improving and increasing your lower leg strength

The entire drill takes only 12 minutes a day.

Materials

1. A piece of chalk or carpet
2. A flat, firm surface
3. A timing device

Choose an area where you can lay out a figure such as the one below:

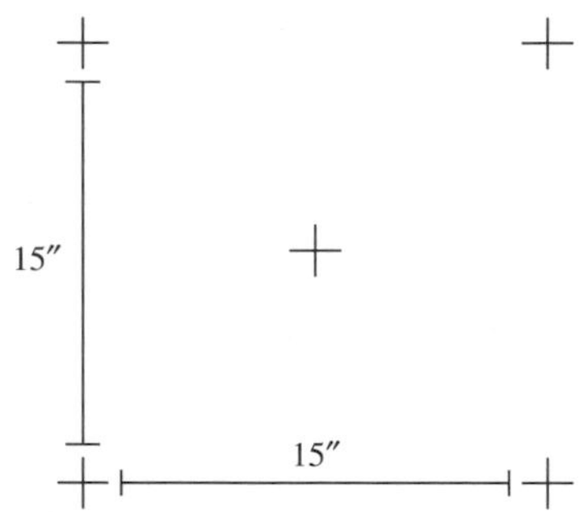

Set 1. Double Foot—Clockwise 4 corner
Set 2. Double Foot—Counterclockwise 4 corner
Set 3. Double Foot—Left clockwise triangle
Set 4. Double Foot—Counterclockwise left triangle
Set 5. Double Foot—Clockwise right triangle
Set 6. Double Foot—Forward triangle
Set 7. Double Foot—Backward triangle

The goal is to do one more repetition each time you do these drills. Each set lasts 30 seconds. Rest 45 seconds between sets. Record the number of attempts.

III. Sport-Specific Facilities and Protective Equipment

A. **Playing surface**
   1. Softer, more shock-absorbent surface reduces incidence of injuries (see Table 2). Suspended wooden (parquet) floor is currently best.
   2. Sweat on floor should be wiped up. At higher competition levels, rules are being tightened to prevent abuse of time-out to wipe the floor.

B. **Padded apparatus**
   1. Net supports and cables
   2. Officials' stand

C. **Uniforms**
   1. Padded hip briefs
   2. Knee pads

D. **Footwear**
   1. Court shoes required. Special volleyball shoes available.

2. High-tops may provide added ankle support if the lacing on the upper part of the shoe is tied separately from the lacing over the foot. This arrangement provides a looser tension over the foot and more support from higher tension over the ankle and lower leg.

IV. Taping and Bracing

A. General policy regarding taping and bracing

1. Ankles are a common site of injury in volleyball with a majority of injuries occurring at the net. Lace-up braces are preferred, even over adhesive taping. Some programs are experimenting with more rigid ankle braces.
2. Knees can require patellofemoral joint supports, e.g., Palumbo brace (neoprene style), but generally there is not a need for ligamentous braces.

B. Specific taping

1. **Fingers:** Use buddy tape for proximal interphalangeal and distal interphalangeal joint injuries, caused most commonly by blocking.
2. **Thumb:** For gamekeeper's thumb, use check-rein tape or modified figure-of-eight tape to prevent hyperextension. Injury occurs from contact with the floor and improper blocking with the thumbs facing forward toward the opponent.

V. Rules to Protect the Athlete

A. No hard materials on extremities—braces must have all hard-exposed surfaces padded and all metal covered.
B. No penetration completely over the centerline
C. Wiping the floor. At collegiate and interscholastic level of play, players are allowed to wipe the floor. At Olympic level, players must carry wiping cloth and cannot delay the game to wipe perspiration off the floor.

Recommended Reading

Bahr R, Karlsen R, Lian O, Ovrebo RV: Incidence and mechanisms of acute ankle inversion injuries in volleyball. Am J Sports Med 22(5):595–600, 1994.

Black JE, Alten SR: How I manage infrapatellar tendinitis. Phys Sportsmed 12(10):86–92, 1984.

Black KP, Lombardo JA: Suprascapular nerve injuries with isolated paralysis of the infraspinatus. Am J Sports Med 18(3):225–228, 1990.

Conlee RK, McGowan CM, Fisher AG, et al: Physiological effects of power volleyball. Phys Sportsmed 10(2):93–97, 1982.

Feretti A: Epidemiology of jumper's knee. Sports Med 3:289–295, 1986.

Feretti A, Guglielmo C, Ruso G: Suprascapular neuropathy in volleyball players. J Bone Joint Surg 69-A(2): 260–263, 1987.

Feretti A, Papandrea P, Conteduca F, Mariani PP: Knee ligament injuries in volleyball players. Am J Sports Med 20(2):203–207, 1992.

Feretti A, Puddu G, Mariani PP, Massimo N: Jumper's knee: An epidemiological study of volleyball players. Phys Sportsmed 12(10):97–103, 1984.

Goodwin-Gerberich S, Luhmann S, Finke C, et al: Analysis of severe injuries associated with volleyball activities. Phys Sportsmed 15(8):75–79, 1987.

Ho PK, Dellon AL, Wilgis EF: True aneurysms of the hand resulting from athletic injury. Am J Sports Med 13(2):136–138, 1985.

Lund PM: Marathon volleyball: Changes after 61 hours of play. Br J Sports Med 19(4):228–229, 1985.

Panariello RA: Arm deceleration training for the baseball pitcher. NSCA J 14(6):19–25, 1992.

Rosi G, Pichot O, Bosson LJ, et al: Echographic and Doppler screening of the forearm arteries in professional volleyball players. Am J Sports Med 20(5):604–606, 1992.

Schafle MD, Requa RK, Patton WL, Garrick JG: Injuries in the 1987 national amateur volleyball tournament. Am J Sports Med 18(6):624–631, 1990.

Toriola A, Adeniran SA, Ogunremi PT: Body composition and anthropometric characteristics of elite male basketball and volleyball players. J Sports Med 27(2):235–239, 1987.

Yi ZR, Lian HY, Peng WK, Nan Zy: A biomechanical study of suprascapular nerve injuries in volleyball. International Series on Biomechanics, vol 6B. Champaign, IL, Human Kinetics, 1987, pp 951–954.

56

Soccer

Karl Lee Barkley II, M.D.

Soccer is known to be the most popular sport in the world. It has been steadily increasing in popularity in the United States. The World Cup Championship, held in the United States in the summer of 1994, exposed even more Americans to the sport.

I. General Concerns

A. **Participation in the United States.** One out of every six Americans (42 million) is involved in soccer in some capacity. Participants include those in youth, recreational, high school, college, and professional leagues. Coaches, parents, referees, officials, and spectators contribute substantially to the number of people interested and involved in soccer in the United States. Participation increased by 11% in 1994.

B. **International participation.** Soccer is the world's most popular sport with an estimated 200 million or more participants according to the international governing body of soccer, the Fédération Internationale de Football Association (FIFA). The World Cup championship is the most viewed television sporting event on a global basis.

C. **The game of soccer**

1. Eleven players to a side (one goalkeeper)
2. Ball may be advanced by kicking or by heading
3. Goalkeeper may use his or her hands to control the ball in the designated penalty area. Use of the hands or arms is not allowed by the field players (an exception would be the "throw in," in which the player initiates play after the ball has gone over the sidelines). The player may "trap" or stop the ball with chest or thighs.
4. Two 45-minute periods are played with a 15-minute halftime in between. Youth soccer matches may vary in length depending on the age of the participants.
5. Soccer is a contact sport. The game is controlled by the referee and his or her interpretation of the rules.
6. Basic strategy in soccer has evolved from a position-specific approach to more of a total team approach, in which every player may be involved in offense and defense.

II. Soccer Equipment, Facilities, and Safety Issues

A. **Footwear**

1. **Three types of cleats**
   a. Metal studs—good for wet fields; have longer cleats than the molded plastic type
   b. Molded plastic—all purpose and most common, but not good on wet fields
   c. Turf cleats—designed for better traction on artificial turf or extremely hard or dry fields
2. **Importance of feel**
   a. Soccer shoes lack support found in some traditional athletic shoes because of the player's desire to have as much feel of the ball as possible. This may increase the risk of ankle injuries.

   b. Players sometimes take new shoes, wet them, and allow them to dry while on their feet to get as tight a fit and as much feel as possible. Some players wear soccer cleats a full size smaller than their sneaker size.

B. **Shinguards**
   1. Protective against injury
      a. Can prevent tibial fractures by dispersion of forces
      b. Soft tissue injuries lessened
      c. Ideal shinguard covers the length of the tibia and the malleoli as well
   2. Shinguards required by most leagues
      a. Requirement varies in youth and recreational leagues
      b. National Collegiate Athletic Association (NCAA) mandates this as the only required equipment for men's and women's soccer players. Many NCAA players often wear as small a shinguard as possible so as not to feel constrained. This obviously limits the protective value of the shinguard. Most players, if given the choice, would not wear shinguards at all.

C. **Field conditions**
   1. Normal dimensions include 110 m length and 75 m width. There is some variation.
   2. **Poor conditions correlated with or suspected of contributing to injuries**
      a. Holes and uneven ground predispose to ankle injury.
      b. Inadequate safety margins (fence or wall on the sidelines) can subject the player to collisions.
      c. Field size can affect collision potential (bigger bodies playing in a limited space brings greater chance of contact with other participants). This may be seen in high school setting where the soccer matches are played on the football field.
      d. Field hardness can be a factor in causing injuries (abrasions and contusions).
      e. Weather-related changes may play a factor (wet or muddy fields).
      f. Artificial surfaces may produce more injuries (as in football), but more research on this issue needs to be done for soccer.

D. **Soccer goal safety issues**
   1. During 1979–1993, 27 persons were injured or killed by falling soccer goals (18 of these incidents were fatalities).
   2. **Mechanism of death was blunt head trauma usually from the crossbar of the goal striking the victim.**
   3. The soccer goal typically was not properly anchored in these incidents, and the goalpost fell forward as a result of climbing on, swinging on, or doing chinups on crossbars. In one case, the wind blew the goalpost over.
   4. **Recommendations for prevention of injuries**
      a. Stake or counterweight goalpost properly when in use, including two stakes on rear and one on each side
      b. Store goalpost face down if not in use
      c. Goals not in use can be chained to a permanent structure such as a fence.
      d. Consider disassembly when not in use for long periods of time

E. **Soccer ball**
   1. Standard soccer ball is size 5; there are also sizes 3 and 4. The better soccer balls are hand-stitched leather.
   2. Weight: 400 to 450 g
   3. Plastic molded or coated to prevent water absorption
   4. Smaller sizes for youth soccer (under age 12 may use size 4)
   5. Inflation should be 8.5 to 15.6 psi

F. **Rules of soccer and safety**
   1. The referee has the responsibility for controlling foul play, which has been implicated as a risk factor for soccer injuries. Players are allowed shoulder-to-shoulder

contact and incidental contact. Deliberate holding, pushing, or tripping are not allowed, although these contacts do occur at higher levels of competition and are not always called or noticed by the referee. Contact obviously does occur in other ways (two players attempt to head the ball simultaneously) but it is up to the referee to decide what constitutes a foul versus a "play on" situation (contact deemed incidental or unintentional).

2. Several means of punishing excessive contact exist.
   a. A penalty kick from directly in front of the opponent's goal may be awarded to the team of the fouled player.
   b. A yellow card may be issued to a player as a warning for foul play. A second yellow card issued to the same player in the match results in expulsion of that player. The team of that player plays at a man disadvantage for the rest of the game.
   c. A red card may be issued for the first offense of foul play if the referee deems it serious enough. This carries with it immediate expulsion.

G. **Environmental concerns**

1. **Heat** has been a concern at some youth tournaments, including the 1988 USA Cup Youth Soccer Tournament in Blaine, Minnesota. The medical staff instituted some alterations in the rules in accordance with measured Wet Bulb Globe Temperatures. The following measures were used alone or in combination depending on the degree of temperature elevation.
   a. Establish alternate schedule for midday games to avoid maximum heat
   b. Allow unrestricted substitutions at all levels
   c. Shorten game times
   d. Add quarterly fluid breaks
   e. Allow fluid breaks during play or free access to fluids
2. Types of heat injuries and management (see Chapter 17, "Safe Exercise in the Heat and Heat Injuries")
   a. Injuries include:
      i. Heat cramps
      ii. Heat syncope
      iii. Heat exhaustion
   b. Recognition of high-risk conditions before beginning play or practice is essential.
3. **Lightning:** referee has the power to postpone or cancel the game if there is lightning sighted in the area.

III. Musculoskeletal Soccer Injuries

A. **Epidemiology.** Multiple studies and investigations try to establish the risk factors of soccer morbidity and injury. Most of these studies are retrospective and suffer from underreporting of injuries. Injury definitions vary from study to study, making some comparisons difficult (a common definition uses sporting time lost). Despite the limitations, these studies have produced some trends that are worth noting.

1. **Competition produces higher risk than practice.** There is generally more intensity and aggressiveness in competition.
2. Male senior soccer players (older than 19 years) have greater injury risk than youth. **A rise in injury rates is noted around age 14–16.**
3. **Girls are more than twice as likely to be injured as boys in the younger age groups.** This lacks satisfactory explanation and has not been shown in men's and women's groups.
4. Injuries involve the lower extremities 60–75% of the time. (There is variability here.) Ankle and knee injuries are most common.
5. **Injuries in players under 12 years of age are uncommon and usually do not involve much lost time.**

6. Soccer injuries for all groups increase with the intensity of play and the level of play or competition.
7. **Poor field conditions, faulty or absent equipment, and foul play have been correlated with higher injury rates.**

B. **Traumatic injuries, sprains, and strains**

1. **Contusions** are probably the most common injuries but generally do not result in lost time from practice or competition. Lower extremities are the most common site. Conservative management principles apply.
   a. **"Hip pointer"**—a hematoma at the iliac crest after a contusion
   b. **Myositis ossificans**—can be seen in the quadriceps after a contusion and hematoma formation. It involves calcification of the hematoma, which may limit leg range of motion later. Preventive treatment involves early application of the RICE principle (rest, ice, compression, and elevation), crutches, and bandaging the leg in a knee-flexed position. Early physical therapy and range-of-motion exercises help prevent limitation of motion later.
   c. **Acute compartment syndrome:**
      i. Seen in the lower leg following a contusion
      ii. Involves swelling and an increase in pressure in the enclosed fascial compartment(s) of the lower leg. Tissue hypoxia leads to progressing weakness and sensory changes, which vary according to which of the four compartments (anterior, lateral, posterior, and deep posterior) are involved.
      iii. Diagnosis involves suspicion and may need verification by measurement of intracompartmental pressure with a Wick catheter.
      iv. Treatment involves monitoring the player for development of numbness and paresthesias after a direct blow. If Wick catheter measurements indicate increased compartmental pressures, surgical release of the fascia is the definitive procedure. Ice is controversial because it may exacerbate the condition because of the potential for capillary constriction. Elevation is not advised because it is thought to decrease the local arteriovenous pressure gradient and aggravate the condition.
2. **Muscle strains** in thigh, adductor, and hamstrings are common. Strains may occur with or without avulsions.
   a. Sartorius from anterior-superior iliac spine
   b. Rectus femoris from anterior-inferior iliac spine
   c. Hamstring from ischial tuberosity
   d. Iliopsoas from lesser trochanter
   e. Piriformis from greater trochanter
   f. External oblique from the iliac crest
   g. Acute medial head of the gastrocnemius strain or tear:
      i. Occurs during sudden forceful push-off and is more common in older and middle-aged athletes
      ii. Physical exam
         (a) Pain on palpation at medial head of gastrocnemius, often quite exquisite and associated with some significant swelling
         (b) Thompson test negative (plantar flexion noted on squeezing the calf)
      iii. Treatment
         (a) Heel lift
         (b) Compression with calf sleeve
         (c) Ice
         (d) Avoidance of aggravating activities with gradual return to sport
         (e) Flexibility and stretching key in rehabilitation
         (f) Healing may be slow, sometimes 6–8 weeks

3. **Ankle sprains.** Usually the lateral ankle ligament complex is injured. This is the most common injury that results in lost time from practice and games (See Chapter 50, "Ankle and Leg Injuries").
4. **Tibia fractures.** The potential for direct kicks to the tibia is well known in soccer, and fractures are possible even with shin guards. These injuries warrant referral to an orthopedist.
5. **Knee injuries** (see Chapter 49, "Knee Injuries")
   a. **Anterior cruciate ligament (ACL)**—generally noncontact injuries in soccer from sudden deceleration or cutting
   b. **Medial collateral ligament (MCL)**—kicking motion using the inside of the foot can in a collision lead to excessive valgus forces on the knee, which can injure the medial capsular and ligamentous structures of the knee.
   c. **Posterior cruciate ligament (PCL)**—on an artificial turf field or a hard field, a player lands directly on the tibial tuberosity with the knee flexed at 90° causing rupture of the PCL.
   d. **Meniscal injuries**—seen alone or in combination with the aforementioned ligamentous disruptions
   e. **Osseous and osteochondral injuries**

C. **Overuse injuries**

1. **Achilles tendinitis**
   a. Overuse predisposes
   b. Tight heel cords, hyperpronators
   c. Physical exam—tenderness, possibly crepitance
   d. Treatment—RICE, correct anatomic faults, nonsteroidal anti-inflammatory drugs (NSAIDs), modified training, consider heel lift
2. **Achilles tendon rupture**
   a. Chronic tendinitis predisposes
   b. Middle-aged men most commonly injured, such as the older recreational league soccer player
   c. Steroid injection is risk factor
   d. Patient may report "pop" or feel as if he or she has been kicked or struck from behind in the Achilles tendon
   e. Physical exam—palpable defect, positive Thompson test, and inability to perform single toe raise due to lack of strength (some active plantar flexion may be preserved, however, because of contribution from posterior tibialis)
   f. Treatment—surgery usually, although casting can be tried
3. **Retrocalcaneal bursitis**
   a. A bursal inflammation anterior to Achilles tendon
   b. Athlete notes an aching pain with exercise
   c. Heel counter may be too tight in the soccer shoe
   d. Physical exam—local tenderness and swelling noted in the area anterior to the Achilles tendon. There may be a positive pinch test as opposed to tenderness at the Achilles insertion. It is, of course, possible to have both bursitis and tendinitis at the same time.
   e. Treatment:
      i. Usually involves similar treatment as for Achilles tendinitis
      ii. Corticosteroid injection can be considered for bursa but not for tendon
      iii. Surgical debridement an option for recalcitrant cases or when there is a significant superior projection of calcaneus noted on x-ray (Haglund's deformity)
4. **Peroneal tendinitis, subluxation, or dislocation**
   a. Mechanism usually involves dorsiflexion and inversion of the foot against an actively contracting peroneal group. The peroneal retinaculum can be torn allowing

the peroneal tendon to sublux or dislocate. The injury can often be a complication of recurrent ankle sprains. Athlete may report a bothersome, repetitive snapping and painful sensation over the lateral ankle with subsequent activity.

b. Pain is posterior to the lateral malleolus, and swelling and pain may extend along the course of the peroneal tendons.
c. Physical exam:
    i. Pain, swelling, and crepitance noted in the suggestive location
    ii. Pain with resisted dorsiflexion and eversion
    iii. Palpation for subluxation of peroneal tendons in an everted and dorsiflexed position should be attempted or athlete may be able to demonstrate subluxation to you if a chronic condition
d. Treatment:
    i. Acutely, the RICE principles of treatment should be followed.
    ii. A J-shaped pad may be applied in a compressive fashion with tape for tenosynovitis or subluxation/dislocation.
    iii. NSAIDs are useful.
    iv. In the acute stage, casting may be helpful for the injured retinaculum and the dislocated peroneal tendon.
    v. A lateral heel wedge insert may be helpful.
    vi. Surgery can be considered for chronic subluxation/dislocation not responsive to conservative measures.

5. **Posterior tibialis tendinitis**
    a. Forceful eversion, seen in the action of the kick when the foot is repeatedly forced into hyperpronation, can cause this tendon to be strained.
    b. Physical exam:
        i. Reveals pain beneath the medial malleolus, pain with resisted inversion, and sometimes difficulty standing on toes because of pain
        ii. Suspect rupture with inability to rise on toes (if Achilles tendon is intact)
        iii. Observe for the "too many toes sign." Examiner stands behind the patient and observes more toes visible on the injured side than the uninjured side. This is due to increased pronation in the patient with a ruptured posterior tibialis tendon.
    c. Treatment—Conservative measures including medial heel wedge apply unless rupture is suspected, in which case surgery may be considered in the active athlete.
6. **Plantar fasciitis.** Excessive traction at the insertion of the plantar fascia on the medial calcaneal tuberosity leads to inflammation and pain. Repetitive sprinting and the flexible sole of the toe box in the soccer shoe can exacerbate the problem. Historical features, physical exam, and treatment are covered in Chapter 52.
7. **Stress fractures**
    a. **Metatarsals** (second and third) are most common and easiest to diagnose. Calcaneus, navicular, talus, and malleoli can be involved.
    b. Repetitive activity during the heavy training schedule of the elite or professional can predispose to injury.
    c. Physical exam—localized tenderness is noted with palpation or weight bearing. Swelling may or may not be present.
    d. X-rays:
        i. Initially plain films may be negative, only to show callus formation later at 2–4 weeks.
        ii. Bone scan is the gold standard.
        iii. Computed tomography (CT) scan may be necessary in the workup of ankle pain of unclear origin.

e. **Treatment depends on site:**
   i. **Second through fourth metatarsal** can be treated with conservative measures, including restriction of activities and gradual return to practice. The athlete probably should be out 4–6 weeks. Immobilization can be considered if walking is painful.
   ii. **Fifth metatarsal proximally (Jones fracture):** Conservative measures often do not work as well, and many of these patients go to surgery because of the high rate of nonunion.
   iii. **Calcaneus:** Conservative measures can be employed.
   iv. **Navicular:** Nonunion is a problem, and open reduction, internal fixation (ORIF) with bone grafting may be necessary if conservative measures fail.
   v. **Avulsion at the base of the fifth metatarsal** may be seen in association with lateral ankle sprain and is not a stress fracture. Conservative measures can be employed.

8. **Turf toe**
   a. Hyperextension of first metatarsophalangeal joint with injury to the plantar capsule
   b. Associated with the advent of artificial turf and first noted in football linemen. The flexible soccer shoe and greater traction of artificial surfaces can contribute to this injury.
   c. Physical exam—pain on the flexor surface on palpation and with passive dorsiflexion of the first metatarsophalangeal joint
   d. Treatment—rigid shoe insert helpful along with taping; usual conservative principles apply (RICE)
9. **Reverse turf toe or "soccer toe"**
   a. **Acute and chronic damage of the dorsal capsular structures of the first metatarsophalangeal**
   b. **Repetitive forced hyperflexion of this joint involved in kicking with instep ball strike.** The supple soccer shoe is again a factor.
   c. Physical exam—pain is noted dorsally over this joint and with passive plantar flexion.
   d. Treatment—conservative measures apply, with taping to prevent plantar flexion. Usually responds better than turf toe.
10. **Footballer's ankle.** This is an impingement syndrome of the foot and ankle. Repeated kicking means repeated traction on the capsular ligaments where they attach to the talus and tibia. Anterior impingement is most common, but posterior impingement has been reported as well.
   a. Anterior tibiotalar osteophytes noted on radiograph
   b. Player may complain of diffuse anterior ankle pain and perhaps limited range of motion
   c. Treatment can include conservative rehabilitation, steroid injection locally, surgical debridement
11. **Flexor hallucis longus tendinitis** can occur from repetitive exaggerated plantar flexion of the foot during the kicking motion.
   a. Medial retromalleolar pain and swelling are noted.
   b. Physical exam—pain in the retromalleolar area with forced plantar flexion of the foot. Lidocaine 1% injection in this area may eliminate pain and prove diagnostic.
   c. Treatment
      i. Restrictive taping of the ankle and first metatarsophalangeal joint, NSAIDs, and the RICE principles
      ii. Recalcitrant cases may need immobilization and even debridement.

12. **Chronic compartment syndrome of the lower leg**
    a. Related to exertion
    b. Usually involves the anterior compartment and is more commonly bilateral
    c. Symptoms (numbness, pain, swelling) come with predictable amount of exertion and resolve within 1 hour after stopping exercise.
    d. Diagnosis can be confirmed with Wick catheter measurements. Consider stress fracture, periostitis, nerve compression, and venous thrombosis.
    e. Treatment (other than time off from sport) involves surgical release.
13. **Groin pain in the soccer player** can be caused by a variety of disorders. The term "athletic pubalgia" has been used to refer to the chronic causes of groin pain.
    a. **Groin strain:** Usually refers to strain of the adductors (longus, magnus, brevis) but has been used to describe injuries to the iliopsoas, rectus femoris, and sartorius. Management involves conservative principles.
    b. **Osteitis pubis:** Involves inflammation over the symphysis pubis. Management consists of rest and NSAIDs.
    c. **Inguinal hernias:** Can be overlooked as a cause of groin pain. Occult inguinal hernias can coexist with other causes of groin pain. Ultrasound or CT scan may be required to evaluate "groin strains" that do not heal.
    d. **Rectus abdominis strain/tendopathy:** Point tenderness at the insertion of the rectus on the pubis noted. Conservative measures emphasizing stretching along with NSAIDs are helpful. This can be more of a chronic and overuse problem rather than just an acute strain.
    e. **Adductor tendinitis:** Typically more insidious in onset, with pain in area of attachment of adductors associated with pain on resistance of adduction of thigh. Treatment is usually conservative.
14. **Overuse injuries about the knee.** Soccer players are susceptible to iliotibial band syndrome, patellar tendinitis, pes anserinus bursitis, plica syndrome, and popliteus tendinitis (see Chapter 49, "Knee Injuries").
15. **Sever's disease**—calcaneal apophysitis in the immature athlete and youth soccer player
16. **Metatarsalgia**—tenderness located over metatarsal heads from repetitive activity such as running
17. **Sesamoid problems**
    a. Inflammation or fracture may occur and is common in soccer players. It is difficult to distinguish between fracture and inflammation because of the common occurrence of the congenitally partite sesamoid. The incidence of partite sesamoids is higher in soccer players than the general population, possibly indicating an adaptive change to the repetitive stresses placed on the forefoot in soccer.
    b. The metal cleat or stud of the soccer shoe sits beneath this area, and the flexor hallucis brevis tendon (sesamoids contained within) is constantly loaded. This contributes to the sesamoids being injured or inflamed often.
    c. Conservative measures are usually sufficient. Surgery is rarely indicated. A custom-molded foot orthosis employing support proximal to the first metatarsal head can allow earlier return to activity. Casting and immobilization are sometimes required in sesamoiditis and stress fractures.
18. **Hallux rigidus.** Gradual onset of aching in the first metatarsophalangeal joint associated with limited movement of toe, stiffness, and enlargement at the metatarsophalangeal joint. Repetitive pushing off while cutting may predispose in the soccer player.

D. **Position-specific concerns**
1. **Goalkeeper injuries**
    a. **Collision injuries more common in goalkeeper**
    b. Head of goalkeeper can collide with goalpost, field, or another player

c. Being kicked by another player more common at goalkeeper position
d. Hand injuries are seen because goalkeepers use hands to block shots and because kicks intended for the ball often hit goalkeeper's hands. There have been case reports of finger avulsions from contact and entanglement with the net. None of these players were wearing gloves at the time.
e. Goalkeepers have more head, face, and upper extremity injuries than lower extremity injuries according to one study. They also seem to have a higher percentage of dislocations and fractures as compared to field players.
f. **Goalkeepers are allowed to wear padding of the knees, elbows, and flanks. Caps are permitted to shade from the sun. Mouthguards and athletic cups should be considered for the goalkeeper at higher levels of competition.**

2. Midfielders and center forwards have the highest injury rates according to some, but studies vary.

IV. Nonmusculoskeletal Injuries

A. Head injuries

1. **Mechanisms of head injury**
   a. **Heading the ball incorrectly** can lead to injury. A player who attempts to head the ball with the neck flexed or extended can experience more head motion, which some investigators believe can be a factor in causing concussions.
   b. **Being struck by a kicked ball at close range** where the ball often moves at high speeds can lead to head injury.
   c. **Head-to-head contact** is common in a play in which two players attempt to head the ball simultaneously. There is more risk for injury when one player is unaware of the other's approach.
2. **Types of head injuries** (see Chapter 39, "Head Injuries")
   a. **Concussions**
   b. **Skull fractures**
   c. **Epidural and subdural hematomas**
   d. **Nonspecific symptoms** have been reported after heading. **These symptoms may represent the sequelae of unrecognized Grade I–type concussions:**
      i. Headaches
      ii. Pain in the neck
      iii. Dizziness
      iv. Irritability
      v. Insomnia
      vi. Hearing disturbance
      vii. Memory disturbance
   e. **Chronic heading syndrome.** This concept is still the subject of some controversy. Studies have shown electroencephalographic changes, cerebral atrophy, deficits in psychological testing, and degenerative cervical spine changes in study groups of Norwegian soccer players versus controls. These changes have been attributed to the minor trauma involved in repetitive heading. A U.S. national team study revealed no chronic symptoms compared to age-matched elite track athletes. Further studies are needed.
3. **Prevention of head injuries**
   a. **Proper heading technique:**
      i. **Head with the eyes open.** Coaches at the youth level should teach this. This avoids having the ball strike the player in another part of the face or head besides the forehead. It also may lessen the potential for collisions with other players not seen if the player has his or her eyes closed.

ii. **Actively head the ball.** Attempt to contact the ball with the forehead in an active manner as opposed to accepting contact with the ball passively. This may decrease the number of concussions.

iii. **Good headers of the ball use the entire body and have strong neck muscles.** Using the entire body (especially the lower back and legs) dissipates the forces more effectively and decreases the risk of injury. The risk of injury is lowered by the good header when head-neck-torso rigidity is maximized at impact. This decreases the rotational acceleration of the head and limits injury.

b. **Soccer ball factors:**

i. **Proper ball size is important.** One source recommends no. 5 for adults, no. 4 for juniors, and no. 3 for smaller children. The smaller ball is lighter and thus less likely to cause head injury.

ii. **Plastic molded balls or urethane-coated, leather-stitched balls prevent the absorption of excessive water in wet conditions.** The noncoated leather ball can become up to 20% heavier due to water absorption. Fatalities have been reported with the use of a noncoated ball in wet conditions.

B. **Eye injuries**

1. Usually in adolescents and young boys
2. Most are ball induced but can involve contact with opponent's elbow, shoulder, foot, or head
3. **Younger athletes are at risk because of flat or less developed orbital rims, which give the eye more exposure to potential trauma.**
4. **Types of eye injuries** (see Chapter 41)
   a. Hyphema most common in two series
   b. Vitreous hemorrhage
   c. Corneal abrasion or laceration
   d. Angle recession
   e. Retinal tear
   f. Blowout fracture
   g. Secondary glaucoma
   h. Lid laceration
5. **Prevention**
   a. Ordinary lenses offer no protection and may increase risk of injury.
   b. Polycarbonate lenses offer the best protection and should be recommended and required (for players with refractive errors who do not wear contacts) according to some sources. Their acceptance for racquet sports has been slow, and it may be slower for soccer.

C. **Dental and maxillofacial injuries**

1. 6.4–20% of soccer injuries involve the teeth, alveolar process, or nasal bones according to two studies.
2. **Factors associated with injury**
   a. Most injured are over 20 years of age.
   b. Competition is a greater risk than practice.
   c. Goalkeepers are more susceptible to dental injuries.
   d. Lacerations, abrasions, and contusions can be associated with many of these injuries.
3. **Prevention**
   a. **Mouthguards** should be considered for the goalkeeper and for the player with orthodontic devices, caps, or other dental work that needs protection.
   b. Field players have less risk but still should be encouraged to use mouthguards.

D. **Genitourinary**. Trauma to this region is possible through contact with a kicked ball or a direct kick. These injuries, uncommon and mostly found in male athletes, theoretically could be prevented with the use of an athletic protective cup. Many athletes find these devices objectionable because they are uncomfortable. Goalkeepers may be at higher risk for these types of injuries, which can include scrotal hematoma and testicular rupture, and are the most likely players to wear this equipment.

E. **Nonmusculoskeletal problems of the foot**
   1. **Calluses and corns:** Build-up of hyperkeratotic material at pressure point or bony prominence. Proper shoes, padding, and filing or sanding down with an emery board after soaking can be helpful.
   2. **Ingrown toenail with infection:** Consider trial of antibiotics and soaking followed by partial resection of nail with digital block technique with or without nail matrix ablation.
   3. **Blisters:** Do not rupture; if ruptured, keep clean and observe for signs of infection.
   4. **Subungual hematoma** is common among soccer players and is usually from direct trauma. Over the course of a career, a player may lose a nail many times and develop a dysmorphic nail. Some players elect to have their nail matrix ablated to avoid this. Acutely, a hot paper clip or 18-gauge needle may be used in a drill-like fashion to relieve pressure (the needle affords more control). There are also commercial cautery units available that work well.

V. Soccer Training

A. **Weights**—Upper body strength becomes more important at higher levels because shoulder-to-shoulder contact is allowed.

B. **Aerobic conditioning**—Soccer players in an adult match typically cover about 10 km.

C. **Anaerobic conditioning**—Of the 10 km covered by a soccer player, 10–15% is sprinted, so anaerobic reserve is important.

D. **Plyometrics**—Soccer requires explosive movements in the kicks, cuts, jumps, and sprints used during an average game.

E. **Agility drills**—ball handling drills, etc.

F. **Stretching and adequate warm-up**—Essential to lessen the occurrence of injuries. Younger players are more flexible than their older counterparts and may not require as much stretching, with adequate warm-up being all that is needed.

G. **Tactical strategy practice**

H. "**Economic training**" is the catch phrase used to denote practice activities that combine several of the above-mentioned types of training in one activity (one-on-two drills or soccer specific exercises are examples).

VI. Women's Soccer

A. **Injuries.** Typically, women sustain the same types and numbers of injuries as men, but there do appear to be some differences.
   1. Girls less than 12 are more than twice as likely to be injured as their male counterparts. Reasons are not clear.
   2. **NCAA data suggest that women sustain injuries to the ACL more than twice as often as men.** This has previously been seen in women's basketball (another sport that requires cutting, stopping, and pivoting quickly). However, NCAA data imply that overall injury incidence is similar between the two groups.
   3. One source reports a higher incidence of injuries in women soccer players during the premenstrual and menstrual period.

B. **Female athlete triad**. Sports medicine physicians, practitioners, trainers, and coaches should be aware of this concept. They need to recognize female athletes with signs and symptoms of these three entities (see Chapter 11, "Women in Sports"). Female soccer players are probably not at risk as much as athletes in sports that emphasize or require certain body types (gymnastics, dance, running sports).

1. Eating disorders
2. Oligomenorrhea or amenorrhea
3. Osteoporosis

VII. Indoor Soccer

This variation on outdoor soccer is growing in popularity. Typically five players to a side compete in an ice hockey rink–sized field surrounded by wooden dasher boards and plexiglass tops that enclose the field. The field surface is artificial carpet usually laid on top of concrete. Studies have been inconclusive as to whether injuries are higher in indoor soccer or outdoor soccer. One study of youth soccer players showed increased incidence of injuries among the indoor participants, whereas another study showed no difference in adult participants. More work needs to be done.

VIII. Soccer Organizations and Leagues

A. Organizations
   1. International—Fédération Internationale de Football Association (FIFA)
   2. United States
      a. United States Soccer Federation (USSF)—the national governing body and the U.S. representative to FIFA
      b. National Soccer Coaches Association of American (NSCAA)—the largest soccer coaches organization in the world
      c. United States Youth Soccer Association (USYSA)—the largest youth soccer organization in the United States and the official youth extension of the USSF, providing soccer opportunities from recreational to competitive for youth.
      d. American Youth Soccer Organization (AYSO)—another large soccer organization for youth that maintains an affiliation with the USSF and has more of a recreational emphasis.
   3. State, county, and local—Various soccer organizations exist at this level. They administer league play, register players, collect waivers for play, and in some cases provide liability insurance. Some state organizations have begun to offer sports medicine instruction at coaches' conventions.

B. Leagues and levels of play
   1. Major League Soccer—Ten-team pro league completed successful first season in 1996.
   2. U.S. International Soccer League—a grass roots professional soccer league of 90 teams
   3. "A" league—Another pro league of six teams
   4. Indoor professional soccer leagues
   5. U.S. National Teams—between five and nine active national teams administered by the USSF, including men's and women's at different age levels
   6. Intercollegiate—NCAA, NAIA (National Association of Intercollegiate Athletics)
   7. High school
   8. Youth leagues

Recommended Reading

1. Arendt EA, Dick RW: Gender specific knee injury patterns in college basketball and soccer. Am J Sports Med 23(6):694–701, 1996.
2. Backous DD, et al: Soccer injuries and their relation to physical maturity. Am J Dis Child 142:839–842, 1988.
3. Benson MT (ed): 1994–95 NCAA Sports Medicine Handbook. Overland Park, KS, National Collegiate Athletic Association, 1994, p 56.
4. Burke MF: Soccerball-induced eye injuries. JAMA 249(19):2682–2685, 1983.
5. Curtin J, Kay NRM: Hand injuries due to soccer. Hand 8(1):93–95, 1976.
6. Elias SR, Roberts WO, Thorson DC: Team sports in hot weather: Guidelines for modifying youth soccer. Phys Sportsmed 19(5):67–78, 1991.

7. Fields KB: Head injuries in soccer. Phys Sportsmed 17(1):69–73, 1989.
8. Hoff GL, Martin TA: Outdoor and indoor soccer: Injuries among youth players. Am J Sports Med 14(3):231–233, 1986.
9. Injuries associated with soccer goalposts—United States, 1979–1993. JAMA 271:1233–1234, 1994.
10. Inklaar H: Soccer injuries: Incidence and severity. Sports Med 18(1):55–73, 1994.
11. Inklaar H: Soccer injuries: Aetiology and prevention. Sports Med 18(2):81–93, 1994.
11a. Jordan SE, et al: Acute and chronic brain injury in U.S. national team soccer players. Am J Sports Med 24(2):205–210, 1996.
12. Keller CS, Noyes FR, Buncher R: The medical aspects of soccer injury epidemiology. Am J Sports Med 15(3):s-105–112, 1987.
13. Kibler WB: Injuries in adolescent and preadolescent soccer players. Med Sci Sports Exerc 25:1330–1332, 1993.
14. Leach RE, Corbett M: Anterior tibial compartment syndrome in soccer players. Am J Sports Med 7:258–259, 1979.
15. Lohnes JH, Garrett WE, Monto RR: Soccer. In Fu FH, Stone DA (eds): Sports Injuries: Mechanisms, Prevention, Treatment. Baltimore, Williams & Wilkins, 1994, pp 603–624.
16. Martens MA, Hansen L, Mulier JC: Adductor tendinitis and musculus rectus abdominis tendopathy. Am J Sports Med 15:353–356, 1987.
17. McCarroll JR, Meaney C, Sieber JM: Profile of youth soccer injuries. Phys Sportsmed 12(2):113–117, 1984.
18. McMater WC, Walter M: Injuries in soccer. Am J Sports Med 6(6):354–356, 1978.
19. Moller-Nielsen J, Hammer M: Women's soccer injuries in relation to the menstrual cycle and oral contraceptive use. Med Sci Sports Exerc 21(2):126–129, 1989.
20. Nielsen AB, Yde J: Epidemiology and traumatology of injuries in soccer. Am J Sports Med 17:803–807, 1989.
21. Nysether S: Dental injuries among Norwegian soccer players. Commun Dent Oral Epidemiol 15:141–143, 1987.
22. Orlando RG: Soccer-related eye injuries in children and adolescents. Phys Sportsmed 16(11):103–106, 1988.
23. Sane J, Ylipaavaliniemi P: Maxillofacial and dental soccer injuries in Finland. Br J Oral Maxillofac Surg 25:383–390, 1987.
24. Scerri GV, Ratcliffe RJ: The goalkeeper's fear of the nets. J Hand Surg 19B(4):459–460, 1994.
25. Schmidt-Olsen S, et al: Injuries among young soccer players. Am J Sports Med 19:273–275, 1991.
26. Slagle C: Personal communication, 1995.
27. Smodlaka VN: Groin pain in soccer players. Phys Sportsmed 8(8):57–61, 1980.
28. Smodlaka VN: Medical aspects of heading the ball in soccer. Phys Sportsmed 12(2):127–131, 1984.
29. Soccer Industry Council of America: 1995 National soccer participation survey. West Palm Beach, FL, American Sports Data, 1995.
30. Sullivan JA, et al: Evaluation of injuries in youth soccer. Am J Sports Med 8(5):325–327, 1980.
31. Taylor DC, et al: Abdominal musculature abnormalities as a cause of groin pain in athletes: Inguinal hernias and pubalgia. Am J Sports Med 19:239–242, 1991.
32. Tysvaer AT, Lochen EA: Soccer injuries to the brain: A neurophysiologic study of former soccer players. Am J Sports Med 19:56–60, 1991.
33. Tysvaer AT, Storli O: Soccer injuries to the brain: A neurologic and electroencephalographic study of active football players. Am J Sports Med 17:573–578, 1989.

57

Basketball

Peter J. Bruno, M.D., FACSM, W. Norman Scott, M.D., and Gordon Huie, PA

In 1891, Dr. James Naismith, while working as an instructor in the Springfield, Massachusetts, YMCA, wanted an indoor activity for his pupils during the long New England winters. He set about nailing two peach baskets to the gymnasium balcony and hence, basketball was born (Fig. 1).

Basketball is probably the most popular sport in the United States. In an economical sense, it requires only one ball and the baskets are in abundance in every community. Its recent popularity in the Olympics as well as the emergence of superstars has gained basketball a strong following. Unfortunately, increasing injuries also accompany this competitive sport.

Historically, the game was intended to be a noncontact sport, but it has since evolved into a contact sport. As a contact sport, injuries may inadvertently be caused by collision with other players, or with the floor, rim or backboard, or the ball. Since 1891, professional as well as amateur basketball players have evolved into bigger, stronger, more agile, and faster athletes. The potential for injuries is now even greater.

I. Head and Facial Injuries

A. **Lacerations**
   1. Most frequent to head and facial area; common areas are eyebrows, lips, chin
   2. **Mechanism** of injury
      a. Collision with another player's bony prominences (elbows, knees, head, hand)
      b. Fall with a forward velocity against the floor
   3. **Treatment**—generally these measures are sufficient for return to play
      a. Focal pressure
      b. Sutures
      c. Adhesive dressing
      d. Further treatment rarely necessary
      e. May return to game

B. **Fractures**
   1. Rare
   2. **Nasal fractures** sometimes encountered
      a. Ascertain any airway obstructions
      b. Hard face masks may permit player to resume activity
      c. X-rays
      d. Closed reduction may be performed in a few days if:
         i. No bleeding
         ii. No nasal hematoma

C. **Concussions**
   1. More frequent than casually assumed but relatively rare
   2. Require more intensive medical treatment

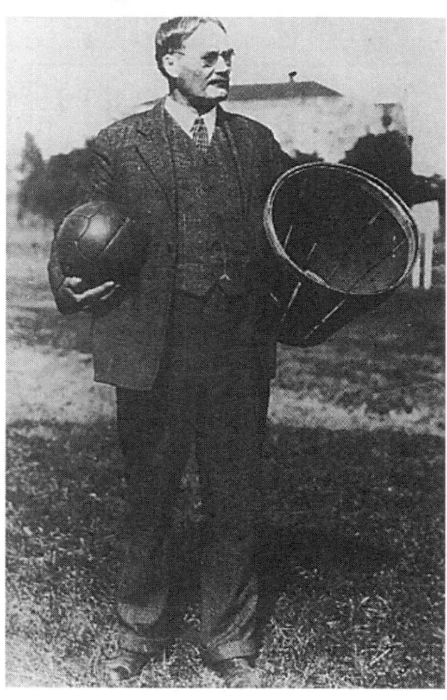

FIGURE 1. Dr. James Naismith, inventor of basketball. (From Sachare A: Laying the foundation. In Sachare A (ed): The Official NBA Basketball Encyclopedia, 2nd ed. New York, Villard Books [Div. of Random House, Inc.], 1994, with permission.)

3. Severe concussions
   a. Employ emergency resuscitative measures if necessary. Equipment should be readily available.
   b. Transport to designated medical facility
   c. Document neurologic deficits at all times. Observe for any neurologic deterioration, including changes in personality and cognitive thinking.
   d. Consult neurologist

D. **Eye injuries**
   1. Most common is corneal abrasion
   2. Trauma from fingers or fingernails
   3. Resolves spontaneously within 48–72 hours
   4. Full ophthalmologic exam warranted if severe pain present

II. Cervical Spine Injuries

A. Majority are **cervical strain**
   1. Nerve root stretching—player complains of "stingers" or "burners" extending along upper extremity
   2. **Mechanism** of injury
      a. Diving after a loose ball
      b. Blow to the head with a force greater than the cervical musculature can withstand, stretching the brachial plexus
   3. **Treatment**
      a. Rest
      b. Nonsteroidal anti-inflammatory drugs (NSAIDs)
      c. Muscle relaxants
      d. Immobilization
   4. **Radiographs** to rule out any fractures or dislocations

B. **Compression fractures and dislocations**
   1. Rare

2. Immobilize immediately
   a. The structure of the cervical spine serves as a protective conduit for the spinal cord and cervical nerve roots.
   b. Immobilization prevents further insult.
3. Observe for paresthesia and any neurologic deficits.

C. **Equipment must be readily available at courtside or in locker room**
1. Neck collars
2. Emergency resuscitative equipment
3. Spinal board

D. **Returning to activities**—condition specific
1. No contraindication
2. Relative contraindication
3. Absolute contraindication

III. Lumbar Spine Injuries

A. **Low back strain (musculature)**
1. Mechanism—jumping/impact activities combined with lateral rotation
2. **Examination**—palpation
   a. Point tenderness
   b. Muscle spasm
3. **Radiographs** to rule out spondylolysis, spondylolisthesis, fractures (Fig. 2A)
4. **Treatment**
   a. Rest
   b. NSAIDs
   c. Muscle relaxants
   d. Heat (cold for acute injuries)
   e. Physical therapy

B. **Degenerative disk disease and herniation**
1. Presentation
   a. Radiating pain to lower extremities
   b. Decrease range of motion
   c. Paresthesia
   d. Loss of bodily functions
2. **Examination**
   a. Neurologic changes
      i. Motor/sensory deficits
      ii. Absent or diminished reflexes of the lower extremities
   b. Often cannot straight-leg raise
3. **Radiographs**
   a. Routine x-rays may demonstrate disk space narrowing, vacuum phenomenon, or osteophytic spurring.
   b. Computed tomography (CT) or myelogram may demonstrate a bulge or herniation at the suspected level (Fig. 2B).
4. **Treatment**
   a. Heat/ice
   b. Rehabilitation
   c. Rest
   d. NSAIDs
   e. If symptoms are persistent, surgery may be indicated.

C. **Spondylolysis/spondylolisthesis**
1. **Spondylolysis**—a defect of the pars interarticularis due to repeated microtrauma, usually involving the posterior aspect of the spine

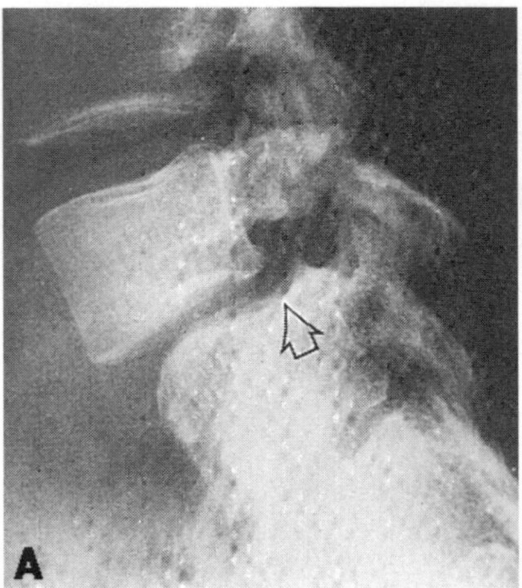

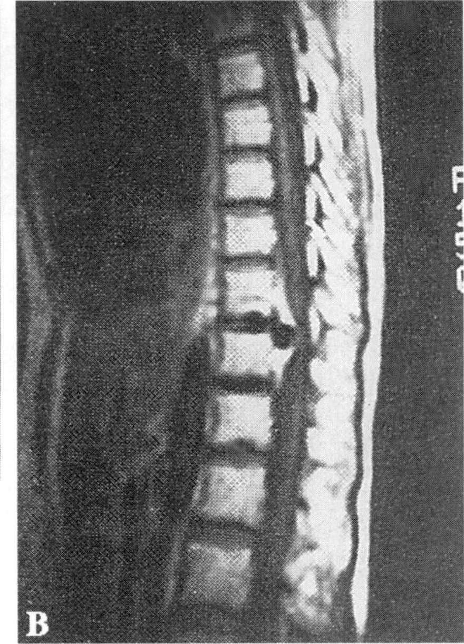

FIGURE 2. Radiographs for lumbar spine injuries. **A**, Spondylolisthesis from low back strain. **B**, Myelogram shows herniation.

2. **Spondylolisthesis**—anterior translation of one vertebral body on an adjacent vertebral body in the coronal plane
   a. Diagnosed most frequently in the evaluation of young people with back pain
   b. Mean age is between 15 and 16 years
   c. 85% of lesion occurs around L-5 vertebral level
   d. Onset of symptoms often coincides closely with the adolescent growth spurt. Adolescents and skeletally immature teens should be observed for any progression of slippage.
3. Repetitive sustained stresses can induce fatigue fractures in the lumbar spine.
4. Pain is localized and can radiate to the buttocks.
5. **Radiographs** can confirm the diagnosis on lateral view. Radiologic changes may not be apparent for weeks to months.
6. **Treatment** is somewhat controversial.
   a. Some advocate exercise and stretching.
   b. Some advocate bracing and rest:
      i. Immobilization for 23–24 hours a day for 6 weeks if diagnosis is made early
      ii. Immobilization for 6 months with well-established fractures
   c. In extreme circumstances, surgical intervention with internal fixation

IV. Shoulder Injuries

The shoulder joint has the greatest range of motion of all the joints in the human body. Bone restraints to motion are minimal; therefore, a greater amount of restraint is stressed on the capsule and rotator cuff. Most common injuries are shoulder subluxation/dislocation and tears of the rotator cuff.

A. **Dislocations**
   1. Require immediate attention; must be reduced. Pain and muscular spasm may interfere with reduction if treatment is delayed.
   2. Anterior instability accounts for 98% of all shoulder instabilities.
   3. **Mechanism** of injury is external rotation and forward elevation.

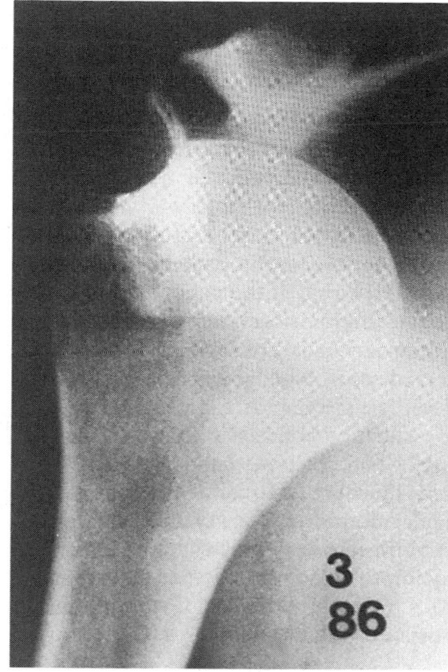

FIGURE 3. Dislocated shoulder. (From Pagnani MJ, Galinat BJ, Warren RF: Glenohumeral instability. In DeLee JC, Drez D (eds): Orthopedic Sports Medicine: Principles and Practice. Philadelphia, WB Saunders, 1994, with permission.)

   a. Occurs more in players taking defensive positions
   b. Rate of recurrence more common under the age of 20
4. Diagnosis apparent on physical examination (humeral head is palpable)
5. Decreased range of motion (full abduction and internal rotation not possible)
6. **Radiographs** (Fig. 3)
7. Reduction
   a. Slight abduction, forward flexion, and gentle internal rotation
   b. Intravenous sedation
   c. Stimson's maneuver[28]; if unsuccessful, try Kocher's maneuver[18]
   d. As a rule, reduction requires experience and should not be attempted by personnel unfamiliar with the above-mentioned techniques.
   e. A neurovascular exam should be done before and after reduction.
8. Postreduction immobilization is controversial.
   a. Some advocate 3 weeks.
   b. Some advocate 4–6 weeks.
9. Player may return to sports after progressive rehabilitation
10. Surgical procedure is indicated for recurrent dislocating player

B. **Rotator cuff injuries**—tears in the musculature of the shoulder
1. **Mechanism**
   a. Traumatic
   b. Repetitive minor trauma
2. Differential diagnosis—biceps tendinitis may develop with overhead activities.
3. Radiographs not of much benefit; magnetic resonance imaging (MRI) extremely helpful
4. **Treatment**
   a. NSAIDs
   b. Rest
   c. Aggressive rehabilitation after the shoulder quiets down

d. Gradual resumption of activities
e. Surgery if pain is persistent and with decreasing ability to elevate arm

V. Elbow Injuries

A. Elbow and forearm injuries are frequent, but rarely result in fractures and dislocations.
B. Common injuries
1. Abrasions
2. Lacerations
3. Olecranon bursitis
a. Due to chronic repetitive trauma
b. May result in neuropathies
C. Causes
1. Diving after a loose ball
2. Defending against a "posted up" opponent
3. "Pulling down" a rebound with elbows flailing

VI. Wrist Injuries

A. Common **mechanism**—falling on outstretched hand
1. Fractures of carpal bones
2. Fractures of ulna and radius bones
B. **Evaluation**—difficult for the primary care physician
1. Wrist **sprains and strains** result in microtears to supporting ligaments and tendons.
a. **Radiographs** indicated if:
i. Swelling
ii. Ecchymosis
iii. Extreme tenderness
b. **Treatment:**
i. Splinting
ii. Ice
iii. Elevation
iv. NSAIDs
c. Gradual return to activities in 3–4 weeks
2. **Fractures**
a. Distal ulna/radius fractures are not the most common, but the potential injury is great.
b. Colles fracture involves the distal metaphysis of the radius, which is dorsally displaced and angulated:
i. Requires immediate immobilization/reduction to preserve neurovascular structures
ii. Treatment (uncomplicated)—immobilization for 6–8 weeks with serial x-rays
iii. Treatment (complicated)—surgery if reduction not achieved in closed reduction attempt
c. Scaphoid bone is most commonly fractured:
i. Deep palpation of "snuff box" area results in extreme tenderness
ii. Radiographs
iii. Treatment:
(a) Surgery for displaced fractures
(b) Thumb spica cast (controversial)
C. Other commonly missed wrist injuries
1. Dislocation of lunate bone
2. Scapholunate dissociation
3. Both require surgical intervention

VII. Finger Injuries

A. Common in basketball players
B. Due to repetitive trauma
   1. Blocking shots
   2. Catching hard passes
C. **Boutonniere deformity**—hyperextension of the distal interphalangeal joint with flexion of the proximal interphalangeal joint (Fig. 4A) caused by the disruption of the extensor tendon insertion (central slip) into the base of the middle phalanx
D. **Swan neck deformity**—hyperextension of the proximal interphalangeal joint with flexion of the distal interphalangeal joint (Fig. 4B)
E. **Mallet finger**—flexion deformity of the distal interphalangeal joint (Fig. 4C) resulting from unrecognized or untreated volar plate injury of proximal interphalangeal joint. Trauma to tip of extended finger results in avulsion of the insertion of the extensor tendon dorsally of the distal phalanx.
F. Treatment
   1. Strict immobilization with a splint for 6 weeks. Compliance is poor.
   2. Surgical repair and/or reconstruction may be required.

VIII. Injuries of the Chest

A. Most common are contusions due to contact with bony prominences, such as the elbow
B. Rarely results in rib fractures
C. Treatment with NSAIDs

IX. Cardiac Considerations

A. **Athletic heart syndrome**
   1. Benign condition
   2. Biventricular hypertrophy
   3. Normal systolic and diastolic function

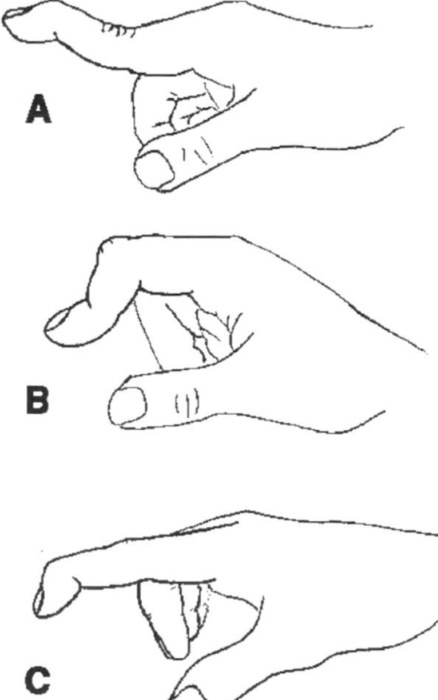

FIGURE 4. **A**, Boutonniere deformity. **B**, Swan neck deformity. **C**, Mallet finger.

4. **Cardiac hypertrophy and bradycardia as a consequence of normal physiologic adaptations to training**
    a. Predominantly endurance training—heart responds with increase in left ventricular chamber size, measured as left ventricular end-diastolic volume
    b. Isometric strength training—increase in left ventricular mass, primarily due to increased wall thickness
    c. Bradycardia frequently associated with irregularity of pulse owing to sinus arrhythmia
    d. Frequently S4 gallop, systolic ejection murmur (secondary to increase in stroke volume). The murmur should be distinguished from a pathologic murmur with maneuvers that increase left ventricular filling (e.g., Valsalva).
    e. Electrocardiogram:
        i. Increased P wave amplitude and notching
        ii. Left ventricular hypertrophy and right ventricular hypertrophy
        iii. Sinus bradycardia secondary to increased vagal tone after training
        iv. Wandering atrial pacemaker
        v. First-degree atrioventricular block
        vi. Mobitz type I second-degree block
        vii. Junctional bradycardia
        viii. All the above-listed changes are secondary to increase in vagal tone.
        ix. ST changes due to early repolarization ST elevation > 0.5 mm in two consecutive leads localized to the precordium, often with slurring of the R wave and giant T waves or T wave abnormalities
        x. Also may have J-point depression of biphasic T waves
    f. Echocardiogram—left ventricular wall thickness < 13 mm (no normal is > 16 mm)
    g. Chest x-ray:
        i. Cardiothoracic ratio frequency exceeds 0.5
        ii. Increased caliber and distribution of pulmonary vessels
5. **Preparticipation physical stress**
    a. Cardiac symptom review
    b. Family history—look for relative with familial hypertrophic cardiomyopathy, sudden death, syncope
    c. Past medical history—look for high blood pressure, valvular disease
    d. Physical examination—check wing span, pectus, arachnodactyly
    e. Molecular basis—blood testing for genetic screening of inherited diseases

B. **Sudden death**
1. Less than 30 years of age
    a. Familial hypertrophic cardiomyopathy is most common cardiovascular disorder.
    b. Coronary artery abnormalities
    c. Marfan's syndrome
2. Older athletes (over 30 years of age)—coronary artery disease
3. Refer to the Bethesda Conference 1994 recommendation.

X. Injuries of the Groin

A. Direct trauma
1. Testicular area
2. Adductor muscle group (adductor longus/magnus, "groin pull"—resumption of immediate activities not recommended

B. Treatment
1. Rest; may gradually resume activities
2. Ice (severe injuries)
3. Scrotal support (severe injuries)

XI. Injuries of the Quadriceps and Hamstring

A. Mechanism—excessive tension on contracted muscles
   1. Diminished range of motion
   2. Complains of point tenderness
B. Preventable
   1. Warm up muscles adequately.
   2. Stretch out muscles before competing.
C. Treatment
   1. Ice/heat
   2. Rest
   3. Gradual resumption of activities as symptoms lessen

XII. Knee Injuries

A. **Meniscal injuries**
   1. Function of medial and lateral menisci
      a. Act as shims that distribute torsional and compressive forces
      b. Act as shock absorbers
      c. Limit extremes of flexion and extension
      d. Facilitate complex movements
      e. Assist in controlling instability
   2. **Mechanism**
      a. Often occurs in flexion with an abnormal force applied
      b. Caused by a compressive trapping of the semilunar cartilage between the femur and tibia
      c. Once elasticity of cartilage is overcome, meniscus tears
   3. **Examination**
      a. Player hears a "pop"
      b. Swollen
      c. Joint line tenderness
      d. Possible positive pivot shift test
      e. Apley's grind test
      f. McMurray's test (medial meniscus)
   4. **Radiographs**
      a. Rule out fractures; do not demonstrate a tear
      b. MRIs extremely helpful
   5. **Treatment**
      a. Ice
      b. Non–weight bearing
      c. NSAIDs
      d. Arthroscopic surgery
         i. If torn meniscus is resected, player may return to activities in 72 hours.
         ii. If torn meniscus is repaired, player is non–weight bearing for 3 weeks.
B. **Ligament injuries**
   1. Function is to provide stability and constraints
      a. Anterior cruciate ligament
      b. Posterior cruciate ligament
      c. Lateral collateral ligament
      d. Medial collateral ligament
   2. **Mechanism of injury**
      a. Most common is a valgus force applied with external rotation resulting in anterior cruciate ligament tear

   b. Hyperextension injuries can lead to both anterior and posterior cruciate ligament tears.
   c. Common cause is player landing on foot of another player.
3. **Radiographs**
   a. Rule out fractures; do not demonstrate tear
   b. MRI helpful—be careful of overreading
4. **Specific exams**
   a. Anterior drawer test
   b. Posterior drawer test
   c. Pivot shift
   d. Reverse pivot shift
5. **Treatment**
   a. Partial tears:
      i. Physical therapy
      ii. Bracing
      iii. Strengthening
      iv. Gradual resumption of activities depending on stability of the knee
   b. Surgical reconstruction may be indicated if player wishes to continue competitive sports. Professional athlete will miss a season before returning to NBA standards.

C. **Patella subluxation**
1. More numerous than dislocations
2. Occurs with a combination of twisting the knee and strong contracture of the quadriceps muscle
   a. May or may not have a direct blow
   b. Usually a lateral force
   c. Knee in the flexed position
3. **Examination**
   a. Player complains of a "slipping" sensation
   b. Knee effusion
   c. Hypermobility of patella
   d. Positive "apprehension" sign
4. **Treatment**
   a. Bracing
   b. NSAIDs
   c. Patella taping for 6 weeks
5. Return to sports depends on evidence of adequate healing.
   a. Lack of effusion
   b. Absence of pain
   c. Return of symmetry of the performance of the lateral hypermobility test

D. **Patella dislocation**
1. Patella usually moves to the lateral aspect of the distal femur.
2. **Examination**
   a. Medial tenderness
   b. Knee held in flexion (Fig. 5)
   c. If player or coach inadvertently straightens leg, a loud "clunk" can be heard and felt
3. Radiographs demonstrate patella resting in lateral gutter
4. **Treatment**
   a. NSAIDs
   b. Immobilization in cylinder cast for 6 weeks
   c. Recurrent dislocators require surgery.
5. Criteria for return to sports similar to subluxating patella mentioned previously

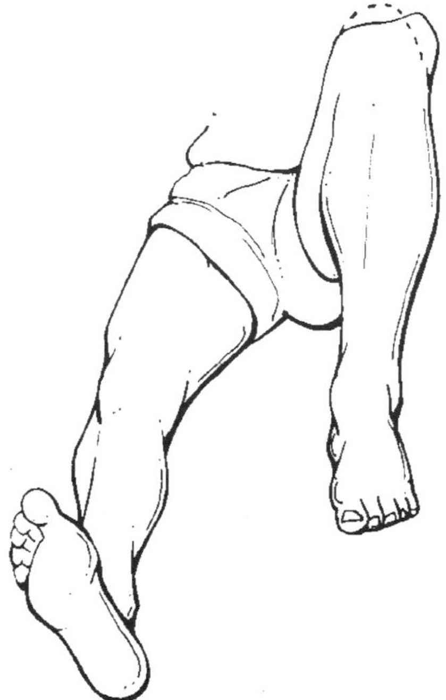

FIGURE 5. Dislocated left patella in flexion. (From Walsh MW: Patellofemoral joint. In DeLee JC, Drez D (eds): Orthopaedic Sports Medicine: Principles and Practice. Philadelphia, WB Saunders, 1994, pp 1163–1248, with permission.)

E. **Chondromalacia patella**
   1. Described as fibrillation, fissuring, or blistering of the articular surfaces
   2. Due to repetitive trauma or impaction activities, or direct blow to the patella. Most players have some form of this in their career.
   3. **Examination**—mild effusion that resolves spontaneously
   4. Treatment
      a. Ice
      b. NSAIDs
      c. Arthroscopic surgery in severe injuries:
         i. Removes the offending flap
         ii. Removes loose bodies about the knee joint

XIII. Leg Injury—Medial Tibial Stress Syndrome

A. Also referred to as shin splints
B. Due to overuse and found in the overconditioned athlete
   1. Athlete usually ignores early signs of pain in anteromedial aspect of tibia
   2. Jumping and running on hard surface
C. **Examination**
   1. Diffuse pain over the mid to distal third of tibia
   2. Differential diagnosis of stress fractures
D. **Treatment**
   1. NSAIDs for 7–10 days
   2. Rest
   3. Gradual return to activities

XIV. Ankle and Foot Injuries

A. **Ankle sprains**

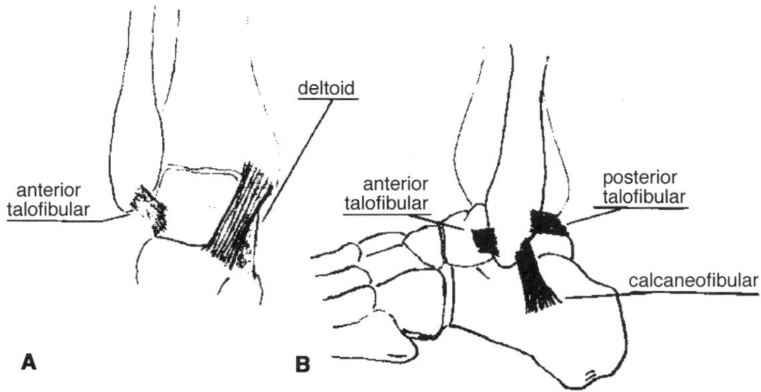

FIGURE 6. Ligaments most commonly injured in the ankle. **A**, Medial aspect and **B**, Lateral aspect.

1. **Most common injury**
   a. Reported in 45% of players
   b. Usually an inversion injury:
      i. Player landing on foot of another player
      ii. Sudden lateral movement
      iii. Player with a history of ankle sprains
2. Medial aspect—deltoid ligament (Fig. 6A)
3. Lateral aspect (Fig. 6B)
   a. Calcaneofibular ligament
   b. Anterior talofibular ligament
   c. Posterior talofibular ligament
4. **Classification**
   a. Grade I (mild)—stretching of ligament without any tears
      i. Little swelling or tenderness
      ii. Minimal or no function loss
   b. Grade II (moderate)—demonstrates a partial macroscopic tear
      i. Moderate pain, swelling, and tenderness
      ii. Some loss of motion and stability
   c. Grade III (severe)—complete ligament rupture
      i. Marked swelling and tenderness
      ii. Abnormal joint motion and instability
5. **Radiographs** to rule out any fractures
   a. Lateral malleolus, medial malleolus, posterior malleolus, and talus
   b. Entire lower leg (proximal fibula)—Maisonneuve's fracture (Fig. 7).
6. **Treatment**
   a. Grades I and II:
      i. Rest, ice, compression, elevation
      ii. Immobilization with elastic bandage
      iii. Early motion and weight bearing
   b. Grade III (controversial):
      i. Surgery—primary repair
      ii. Cast immobilization
   c. Prophylactic taping of ankle highly recommended
7. **Criteria for return to sports**
   a. Full range of motion
   b. Ambulation without a limp

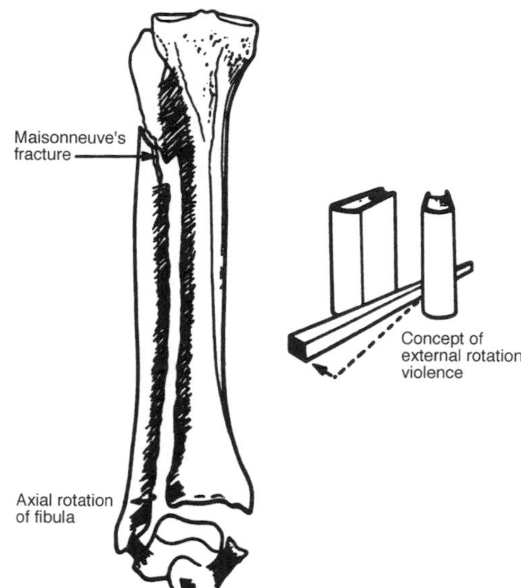

FIGURE 7. Maisonneuve's fracture. (From VanderGriend RA, Savoie FH, Hughes JL: Fractures of the ankle. In Rockwood CA, Green DP, Bucholz RW (eds): Rockwood and Green's Fractures in Adults, 3rd ed. Philadelphia, JB Lippincott, 1991, pp 1983–2039, with permission.)

c. 90% strength on Cybex testing
d. Must be able to reach maximum speed in running and cutting

B. **Fractures**
1. Malleoli are most common
a. Cause is similar to sprains but with a greater force
b. Variables:
i. Age
ii. Position/direction of foot
iii. Magnitude of deforming force
c. Lauge-Hansen classification—supination and external rotation injury most common, resulting in a fracture of the lateral malleolus as well as possible rupture of the anterior talofibular ligament
2. **Examination**
a. Player in excruciating pain
b. Sudden onset of swelling and tenderness
3. **Radiographs.** Mortise view demonstrates an unequal space between:
a. Talus and medial malleolus
b. Talus and lateral malleolus
c. Talus and distal tibia
4. **Treatment**
a. Acute phase
i. Immobilization with soft, bulky, Jones-type dressing supplemented with splints, which accommodates initial swelling for first 3–5 days
ii. Cold compresses
iii. Elevation
b. Stable or undisplaced fractures may be managed with closed reduction/casting:
i. Short leg cast for 4–6 weeks
ii. Long leg cast if there are rotational instabilities
c. Weight bearing permitted after initial symptoms subside
d. Surgery for:
i. Disruption of joint space
ii. Displaced fractures

C. **Ruptured Achilles tendon**
 1. Commonly occurs in third and fourth decades of life
 2. **Mechanism of injury**—hyperdorsiflexion of the foot with a contraction of the gastrocnemius muscles in the calf
 3. **Examination**
  a. Player complains of hearing and/or feeling a loud "pop" at the posterior ankle
  b. Excruciating pain
  c. Diminished plantar flexion of foot
 4. **Treatment** in initial phase
  a. Posterior splint for immobilization
  b. Ice
  c. NSAIDs
 5. Surgical repair
  a. Done within 1 week of injury to prevent shortening
  b. Cast in equinus—serial cast until ankle joint returns to 90°
  c. Rehabilitation
 6. May return to sports the following season

D. **Fractures and dislocations of the foot**
 1. Not common, but more common in basketball than any other sport. Usually involve base of fifth metatarsal.
 2. **Mechanism of injury**
  a. Direct trauma by another player landing on foot
  b. Repetitive stress of inversion and plantar flexion
 3. **Treatment**
  a. Immobilization for 6–8 weeks
  b. Non–weight bearing for 6 weeks
  c. If symptoms persist, surgery may be necessary.

E. **Soft tissue injuries**
 1. Common
 2. **Mechanism** for blistering of skin
  a. Sudden stops
  b. Twist
  c. Pivot
 3. **Prophylaxis**
  a. Moleskin to bony prominences
  b. Wear two pairs of socks

XV. Conclusion

Many basketball injuries can be prevented if the athlete permits adequate time for warming up and stretching prior to any competitive game. This allows the muscles to perform efficiently and, in some critical period, enables the player to move quickly out of harm's way. Prophylactic taping of the ankle and any other weakened joint is encouraged. Use of protective equipment such as high-top shoes, elbow pads, and knee pads also contributes to the player's safety.

Recommended Reading

1. American Society for Surgery of the Hand: Fractures and dislocation of the hand. In The Hand: Examination and Diagnosis, 2nd ed. New York, Churchill Livingstone, 1983, pp 53–63.
2. American Society for Surgery of the Hand: Acquired deformities. In The Hand: Examination and Diagnosis, 2nd ed. New York, Churchill Livingstone, pp 64–83.
3. American Society for Surgery of the Hand: Major injuries requiring early treatment. In The Hand: Primary Care of Common Problems. Aurora, Co, American Academy of Orthopaedic Surgeons, 1985, pp 62–105.
4. Balduini FC, Tetzlaff J: Historical perspectives on injuries of the ligaments of the ankle. Clin Sports Med 1:3–12, 1982.

5. Bradford DS: Spondylolysis and spondylolisthesis in children and adolescents: Current concepts and management. In Bradford DS, Hensinger RM (eds): The Pediatric Spine. New York, George Thieme, 1985, pp 403–423.
6. Clare P: Football. In Mellion MB, Walsh WM, Shelton GL (eds): The Team Physician's Handbook. Philadelphia, Hanley & Belfus, 1990, p 493.
7. Cooney WP, Linscheid RL, Dobyns JH: Fractures and dislocations of the wrist. In Rockwood CA, Green DP, Bucholz RW (eds): Fractures in Adults, 3rd ed. Philadelphia, JB. Lippincott, 1991, p 586.
8. Eismont FJ, Kitchel SH: Thoracolumbar spine. In DeLee JC, Drez D (eds): Orthopaedic Sports Medicine: Principles and Practice. Philadelphia, WB Saunders, 1994, p 1058.
9. Garrick JM: The frequency of injury, mechanism of injury, and epidemiology of ankle sprains. Am J Sports Med 5:241–242, 1977.
10. Hawkins RJ, Mohtadi N: Controversy in anterior shoulder instability. Clin Orthop 272:152–161, 1991.
11. Hawkins RJ, Mohtadi N: Rotator cuff problems in athletes. In DeLee JC, Drez D (eds): Orthopaedic Sports Medicine: Principles and Practice. Philadelphia, WB Saunders, 1994, pp 623–656.
12. Hensinger RN: Back pain in children. In Bradford DS, Hensinger RN (eds): The Pediatric Spine. New York, George Thieme, 1985, pp 41–60.
13. Hensinger RN, Lang JR, MacEwen GD: Surgical management of spondylolisthesis in children and adolescents. Spine 1:207–216, 1976.
14. Huie G, Scott WN: Initial assessment of knee injuries: Anterior cruciate ligament tears. Phys Assistant 18:57–62, 1994.
15. Huie G, Scott WN: Initial assessment of knee trauma: Meniscal injuries. Phys Assistant 19:43–56, 1995.
16. Ireland ML, Micheli LJ: Bilateral stress fracture in the lumbar pedicle in a ballet dancer. J Bone Joint Surg 69A:140–142, 1987.
17. Jackson D: Low back pain in young athletes. Am J Sports Med 7:364, 1979.
18. Kocher ET: Eine Neue Reductionmedthode Fur Schulterverrenkung. Berl Klin Wocheschr 7:101–105, 1870.
19. Lauge-Hanson N: Ligamentous ankle fractures: Diagnosis and treatment. Acta Chir Scand 97:544–550, 1949.
20. Meyer AW: Chronic functional lesions of the shoulder. Arch Surg 35:646–674, 1937.
21. Micheli LJ, Steiner EM: Treatment of symptomatic spondylolysis and spondylolisthesis with the modified Boston brace. Spine 10:937–943, 1985.
22. O'Neil DB, Micheli LJ: Post-operative radiographic evidence for fatigue fracture as the etiology of spondylolysis. Am J Sports Med 17:196, 1989.
23. Pagnani MJ, Galinat BJ, Warren RF: Glenohumeral instability. In DeLee JC, Drez D (eds): Orthopaedic Sports Medicine: Principles and Practice. Philadelphia, WB Saunders, 1994, pp 580–622.
24. Renstrom AFH, Kannus P: Injuries of the foot. In DeLee JC, Drez D (eds): Orthopaedic Sports Medicine: Principles and Practice. Philadelphia, WB Saunders, 1994, pp 1705–1767.
25. Rowe CR: Prognosis in dislocations of the shoulder. J Bone Joint Surg 38A:957–977, 1956.
26. Sachare A: The Official NBA Basketball Encyclopedia, 2nd ed. New York, Villard Books, 1994.
27. Sitorius MA, Kwikkel M: Basketball. In Mellion MB, Walsh WM, Shelton GL (eds): The Team Physician's Handbook. Philadelphia, Hanley & Belfus, 2990, pp 530–541.
28. Stimson LA: An easy method of reducing dislocation of the shoulder and the hip. NY Med Rec 57:356–357, 1900.
29. Torg JS, Gennarelli TA: Head and cervical spine injuries. In DeLee JC, Drez D (eds): Orthopaedic Sports Medicine: Principles and Practice. Philadelphia, WB Saunders, 1994, p 445.
30. VanderGriend RA, Savoie FH, Hughes JL: Fractures of the ankle. In Rockwood CA, Green DP, Bucholz RW (eds): Rockwood and Green's Fractures in Adults, 3rd ed. Philadelphia, JB Lippincott, 1991, pp 1983–2039.
31. Walsh MW: Patellofemoral joint. In DeLee JC, Drez D (eds): Orthopaedic Sports Medicine: Principles and Practice. Philadelphia, WB Saunders, 1994, pp 1163–1248.
32. Yancey RA, Micheli LJ: Thoracic spine injuries in pediatric sports. In Stanitski CL, DeLee JC, Drez D (eds): Pediatric and Adolescent Sports Medicine. Philadelphia, WB Saunders, 1994, pp 162–174.

58

Wrestling

Timothy F. Kelly, M.A., ATC

I. General Considerations

A. Wrestling styles

1. **Greco-Roman** wrestling was developed in the 19th century by the French and is typified by upper-body throws in which one wrestler takes the opponent to the mat. It is a more restrictive style of wrestling, because wrestlers are prohibited from actively using their legs or grabbing their opponent below the waist. Points are awarded for the degree of skill a wrestler displays in throwing the opponent to the mat in a manner by which both shoulders touch the mat spontaneously.
2. **International freestyle** wrestling is the most popular style in the world. Unlike Greco-Roman, the legs play an integral part in the execution of many maneuvers. Holds below the waist are permissible, as are trips and throws. Participants wrestle a single period for 5 minutes. Points are awarded for takedowns, reversals, and exposure of the opponent's back to the mat. Pins are awarded when a wrestler holds the opponent to the mat for a 1-second count.
3. **Intercollegiate freestyle** wrestling is almost exclusive to high school and collegiate programs in the United States. It varies only slightly from international freestyle. Wrestlers are awarded additional points for controlling or "riding" the opponent and for escaping the opponent's control. Table 1 lists the various weight classes and divisions.

B. **Mechanisms of injury** in wrestling have been classified into six categories. The first five were identified by Snook.

1. **Direct blows** may occur during takedowns, clashing of heads, or from an errant elbow and usually result in contusions or lacerations.
2. **Friction** occurs with constant contact with the mat and/or the opponent and may result in abrasions, skin infections, and bursitis.
3. **Falls** can occur during takedowns, trips, or throws and can be exacerbated by the weight of the opponent landing on the bottom wrestler. The potential exists for serious injury with any type of fall.
4. **Twisting and leverage** mechanisms are common with various holds and maneuvers in wrestling and may lead to strains and sprains.
5. **Self-induced injuries** are uncommon and are usually caused by the wrestler's own exertion, such as back strain when attempting to lift a resisting opponent.
6. **Insidious mechanisms** may be observed in wrestlers with significant injuries. Many wrestlers may be unable to remember the exact mechanism or the onset of their injuries. Some of these injuries are likely to be attributed to overuse.

II. Wrestling Injuries

A. **Patterns of injury**

1. Because of the combative nature of wrestling and the heavy body contact, the incidence of injury is relatively high and has been compared to that of football,

TABLE 1. Weight Classifications in Wrestling

Senior International Greco-Roman and freestyle wrestling (20 years or older)	
48 kg or 105.5 lbs	74 kg or 163.0 lbs
52 kg or 114.5 lbs	82 kg or 180.5 lbs
57 kg or 125.5 lbs	90 kg or 198.0 lbs
62 kg or 136.5 lbs	100 kg or 220.0 lbs
68 kg or 149.5 lbs	130 kg or 286.0 lbs
Intercollegiate freestyle	
118 lbs	158 lbs
126 lbs	167 lbs
134 lbs	177 lbs
142 lbs	190 lbs
150 lbs	Hwt (177–275 lbs)
Interscholastic freestyle	
103 lbs	140 lbs
112 lbs	145 lbs
119 lbs	152 lbs
125 lbs	160 lbs
130 lbs	171 lbs
135 lbs	189 lbs
	275 lbs (188–275 lbs)

USA Kids Division

9–10 Years Old		***11–12 Years Old***		***13–14 Years Old***	
50 lbs	85 lbs	60 lbs	105 lbs	70 lbs	115 lbs
55 lbs	90 lbs	65 lbs	110 lbs	75 lbs	120 lbs
60 lbs	95 lbs	70 lbs	115 lbs	80 lbs	125 lbs
65 lbs	100 lbs	75 lbs	120 lbs	85 lbs	130 lbs
70 lbs	110 lbs	80 lbs	130 lbs	90 lbs	135 lbs
75 lbs	120 lbs	85 lbs	140 lbs	95 lbs	145 lbs
80 lbs	130 lbs	90 lbs	150 lbs	100 lbs	155 lbs
	Hwt	95 lbs	165 lbs	105 lbs	165 lbs
		100 lbs	Hwt	110 lbs	175 lbs
					Hwt

USA Wrestling

Cadets (15–16 years old)		***Juniors (17–18 years old)***		***Espoirs (19–20 years old)***
83.5 lbs	132 lbs	98 lbs	154.0 lbs	(Same weight classes as senior international)
88.0 lbs	143 lbs	105.5 lbs	165.0 lbs	
94.5 lbs	154 lbs	114.5 lbs	178.0 lbs	
103.5 lbs	167 lbs	123.0 lbs	191.5 lbs	
112.0 lbs	182.5 lbs	132.0 lbs	220.0 lbs	
121.0 lbs	209.0 lbs	143.0 lbs	275.0 lbs	
	242.0 lbs			

soccer, lacrosse, and ice hockey. The occurrence of serious injuries, however, appears low.

2. More injuries occur during practice than during competition because of the far greater time spent practicing; however, matches carry a much higher risk of injury.
3. The **knee** is the most frequently injured anatomic site, although injuries are distributed over the entire body.
4. **Ligament sprains and musculotendinous strains** are the most common injuries in wrestlers.
5. Younger wrestlers are injured less seriously and less often than older, more competitive wrestlers. Wrestling appears to be a relatively safe sport for preadolescent boys.
6. The **takedown process**, in which one wrestler takes the opponent to the mat, places wrestlers at high risk for injury. During a takedown, one wrestler is usually

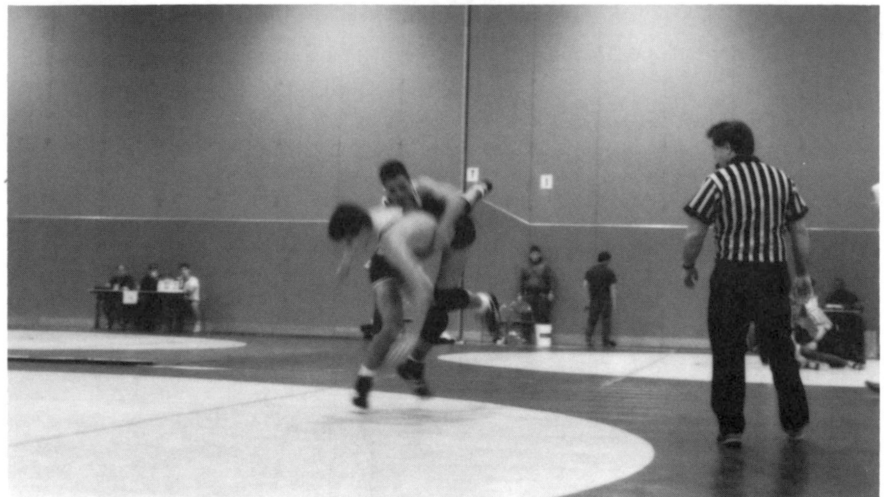

FIGURE 1. The takedown process places the wrestler at high risk for injury.

caught off guard and is taken to the mat in a manner over which he has little control (Fig. 1).

7. **Reinjuries** are often noted in wrestlers who attempt to return to activity before complete healing and rehabilitation has occurred.

B. **Specific injuries**

1. **Head and face injuries**

a. **Lacerations** occur frequently during wrestling and are usually the result of a direct blow, as in the clash of heads or an errant elbow. Lacerations are noted around the orbit, scalp, zygomatic arch, and lower mentum.

i. **Treatment**—application of Steri-Strips may provide a temporary closure of the wound and allow continued participation. Supportive dressings are usually warranted.

ii. **Precautions:**

(a) Lacerations should be cleaned, dressed, and monitored closely for signs of infection.

(b) Consideration should be given to the use of relatively heavy nylon (4–0 to 5–0) sutures, which may be deemed more appropriate when wrestlers continue to actively participate.

(c) Cosmetic suturing should be avoided. If needed, wrestlers may opt for cosmetic revision at the end of the wrestling season.

b. **Epistaxis** may occur with incidental contact to the nose. A direct blow or contact to the nose, as seen with a cross-face maneuver, can injure the highly vascular nasal septum. Epistaxis may present with mild to profuse bleeding from one or both nares.

i. **Treatment:**

(a) Mild epistaxis may resolve spontaneously with little intervention.

(b) Persistent cases of epistaxis should be treated with direct pressure over the affected nares while the head is tilted slightly forward, reducing the chance of blood traveling down the oropharynx. Ice application may prove beneficial.

(c) A **pledget or "nose plug"** treated with petroleum jelly may be inserted or gently screwed into the effected nostril. Pledgets soaked with vasoconstrictors, such as 1% phenylephrine or 4% cocaine, have been used for many years, but these substances are banned at many levels of competition.

ii. **Precautions:**
   (a) Allowing the end of the nose plug to slightly protrude from the naris facilitates easy removal on completion of activity.
   (b) Athletes should be instructed not to blow their noses following significant bouts of epistaxis.
   (c) If treatment fails to achieve hemostasis, proper referral to a medical facility for nasal packing may be indicated.
   (d) **Recurrent bouts** of epistaxis may be treated with nasal cauterization:
   - Chemically with silver nitrate sticks
   - Electrocautery under local anesthesia

c. **Nasal fractures** may occur following a blow to the nose. Wrestlers can often return to activity by wearing a protective face guard that adequately protects the nose.

d. **"Cauliflower ear"**

i. **Etiology:**
   (a) Continuous friction and/or direct trauma to the auricle producing bleeding into the soft tissue of the ear
   (b) Failure to wear protective headgear while wrestling

ii. **Diagnosis:**
   (a) Localized perichondral swelling with the disappearance of the normal convexities of the auricle, mild discomfort, and disfigurement
   (b) Differential diagnosis:
   - Cellulitis
   - Perichondritis

iii. **Treatment:**
   (a) Immediate aspiration with 25- to 27-gauge needle. Multiple aspiration sites may be necessary to drain the ear completely. Aseptic practices should be rigidly followed.
   (b) Compression dressing following aspiration to prevent reaccumulation of blood and serum
   (c) Methods of ear compression include:
   - Strips of gauze soaked in flexible collodion layered from the anterior to posterior aspect of the ear to form a small cast around the ear
   - Similarly, strips of plaster of Paris casting material to form a small cast around the ear
   - A commercial silicone that easily molds the contours of the ear
   - A fluffy, gauze mastoid dressing

iv. **Precautions:**
   (a) The ear canal should not be blocked or obstructed following application of the compressive dressing because it is imperative that the athlete be able to equalize ear pressure.
   (b) Monitor daily for signs of infection
   (c) Potentially disfiguring if left untreated

e. **Concussions** may occur with a hard fall or heavy contact to the head. Proper evaluation and treatment are essential.

2. **Neck injuries** occur infrequently due to enforcement of the rules prohibiting slams and certain types of throws and maneuvers. Common neck injuries observed in wrestlers include:
   a. Sprains/strains
   b. Degenerative disk changes
   c. Neurogenic pain syndromes

d. Cervical spondylosis
e. Facet syndrome
f. **Etiology**
   i. **"Bulling"** or spearing with the head held in slight hyperextension while attempting a takedown or blocking a takedown is common in wrestling. This technique is associated with the greatest number of neck injuries.
   ii. **Stretch and pinch** mechanisms are commonly noted during the takedown process, when the head and neck are forced laterally while the shoulder is depressed.
   iii. **Forced extension and axial compression** can be observed when one wrestler is taken directly to the mat in a manner by which the head is the first part of the wrestler to strike the mat.
   iv. **Combinations** of neck motion
g. **Prevention**
   i. Rule enforcement
   ii. Preseason x-ray examination of individuals with prior history of neck injury
   iii. Preseason neck strength conditioning program

3. **Chest and trunk injuries** common to wrestling
   a. **Rib and costochondral injuries**
      i. **Etiology:**
         (a) **Direct blows** can be observed when one wrestler lands with his arm or leg on the opponent's chest following the takedown maneuver.
         (b) **Forced compression** injuries may occur when one wrestler falls forcefully on top of his prone or supine opponent following a takedown.
         (c) **Torsional strain** is common to various wrestling maneuvers and can result in muscle strains and costochondral separations.
         (d) **Exertional injuries** can be noted when one wrestler expends enormous effort performing a maneuver against the resistance of the opponent.
      ii. **Diagnosis:**
         (a) Labored breathing, point tenderness, and mild to severe, debilitating pain mostly associated with trunk motion
         (b) X-ray examination
      iii. **Treatment:**
         (a) Any injury involving the ribs is usually quite painful and **self-regulating** to the participation of the wrestler.
         (b) **Rest and anti-inflammatory medication**
         (c) **Local corticosteroid injection** may be beneficial in highly competitive wrestlers.
         (d) **Padding and taping** for practice are advisable when symptoms have subsided. A commercial rib belt may offer additional support.
      iv. **Precautions:**
         (a) Careful evaluation of injury before moving the athlete with suspected rib injury
         (b) Pneumothorax, hemothorax
   b. **Muscle strains** may result from sudden torsional movements or rigorous exertion common to many wrestling maneuvers. The oblique and rectus abdominis muscles may become involved.
   c. **Contusions** are also common.
4. **Back injuries** occur infrequently in wrestling. Most injuries are observed during the takedown process.
   a. Back injuries include:
      i. Sprain
      ii. Strain

        iii. Spondylolysis/spondylolisthesis
        iv. Sciatica
        v. Sacroiliac sprain
    b. **Etiology**
        i. May occur when wrestlers "spar" for position, placing the back in **mild hyperextension**.
        ii. Torsional mechanisms
        iii. **Extension against resistance**, as when a wrestler attempts to lift an opponent
        iv. **Hyperflexion mechanisms** reported in various rolling maneuvers
    c. **Treatment** (general)
        i. Rest/modified activity
        ii. Reduction of pain and spasm
        iii. Patient education
        iv. Stretching and conditioning programs
        v. Strengthening exercises
5. **Shoulder injuries** occur frequently, usually when one wrestler is taken to the mat and lands forcibly on the tip of the shoulder. The mechanism usually results in a sprain of the acromioclavicular joint. Occasionally, a wrestler may subluxate or completely dislocate the shoulder. This is not surprising because the glenohumeral joint is subjected to considerable strain when used as a lever arm, and extreme ranges in motion are often applied during competitive wrestling. Common shoulder injuries include:
    a. Dislocation
    b. Subluxation
    c. Acromioclavicular sprain
    d. Sternoclavicular sprain
    e. Capsule strain
6. **Elbow injuries** may result when a wrestler "posts" or completely extends the elbow to break a fall when landing on the mat following a takedown. This maneuver may lead to hyperextension or a fracture-dislocation injury. Wrestlers should be instructed to flex the elbow slightly when it is to be used in this manner. Hyperextension taping is effective in preventing full extension of the elbow. Common elbow injuries include:
    a. Fracture
    b. Hyperextension
    c. Olecranon bursitis
    d. Epicondylitis
7. **Hand and wrist injuries** occur occasionally. Finger sprains can be buddy-taped to allow functional use during practice or competition. Finger dislocations can be properly splinted and padded to allow further competition. Frequent hand and finger injuries include:
    a. Sprain
    b. Dislocation
    c. Subluxation
8. **Thumb injuries** can be debilitating to the wrestler. Most involve the ulnar collateral ligament, which is injured when the thumb is forcefully abducted. This represents a serious injury if the wrestler lacks strong opposition of the thumb, which is needed to grasp and hold an opponent. Surgery and a thumb spica cast may be required.
9. **Knee injuries** account for a large portion of all injuries sustained in wrestling. Severe strain is often placed on the knee during certain maneuvers.
    a. Common knee injuries in wrestling include:
        i. Meniscal tears
        ii. Sprains
        iii. Strains

   iv. Subluxation/dislocation
   v. Bursitis

b. **Meniscal injuries** are common in wrestling. Wrestlers appear to injure the **lateral menisci** more frequently than do athletes in any other sport. The takedown is a highly vulnerable period for a meniscal injury. The lead leg, used during takedowns and defensive maneuvers, appears to be highly susceptible.
   i. **Etiology.** Although the exact pathomechanics of meniscal injuries are not always identified, Wroble and colleagues have cited the following mechanisms:
      (a) **Indirect forces**
      (b) **Torsion**
      (c) **Shearing/hyperextension**
      (d) **Insidious/overuse**
   ii. Diagnosis:
      (a) May present atypically in wrestlers
      (b) Lateral, rather than medial, meniscal injuries occur more frequently.
      (c) Minimal symptoms, other than complaint of "locking"
      (d) Many wrestlers may attempt to "wrestle through" meniscal injuries.

c. **Sprains and strains** are the most common knee injuries:
   i. Incidence of **anterior cruciate ligament** and other catastrophic injuries is low.
   ii. **Indirect force** accounts for most of these injuries.
   iii. The **takedown** is associated with most injuries.
   iv. **Leg wrestling** may carry a higher potential for medial collateral ligament and lateral collateral ligament injuries. Some wrestlers ride their opponents, almost exclusively using their legs for control (Fig. 2).

d. **Patellar subluxation/dislocation** injuries are sometimes observed in younger wrestlers, who may benefit from wearing a specialized neoprene sleeve designed to enclose and stabilize the patella or from McConnell patellar taping.

e. **Prepatellar bursitis** is a frequent knee problem in wrestlers. The lead leg used during takedowns is most often afflicted. Recurrences are not uncommon.

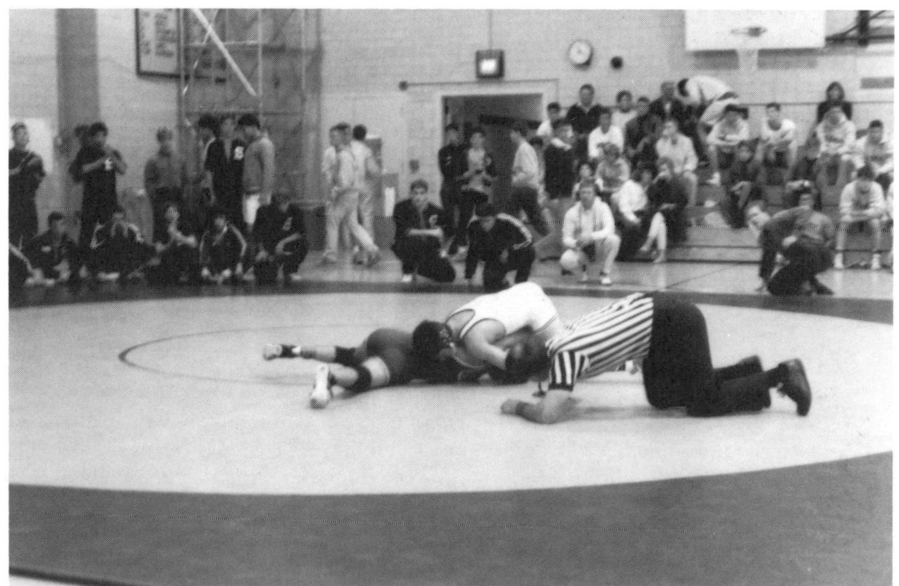

FIGURE 2. Extreme torsional forces on the back of the wrestler being pinned.

i. Etiology
   (a) Single traumatic event
   (b) Repeated bouts of irritation or trauma

ii. **Diagnosis:**
   (a) History of trauma or irritation
   (b) Superficial patellar swelling
   (c) May have normal range of motion, except with extreme flexion

iii. **Treatment:**
   (a) Immediate aspiration (culture and Gram stain) of all cases
   (b) Compressive wrap
   (c) Nonsteroidal anti-inflammatory agents
   (d) 1 week of immobilization in recurrent cases
   (e) Steroid injections produce variable results.
   (f) Repeated bouts of inflammation may necessitate a bursectomy.
   (g) Knee pads worn while wrestling

f. **Septic bursitis** may also afflict wrestlers.

i. Etiology—*Staphylococcus aureus* is usually the invading organism.

ii. **Diagnosis:**
   (a) Often **asymptomatic**
   (b) May show local signs of infection, including erythema, warmth, and fever
   (c) Culture and sensitivity of bursal aspirate
   (d) Laboratory tests (bursal glucose values, white blood cell count, Gram stain, and lactic acid tests) not always reliable in distinguishing traumatic from septic bursitis

iii. **Treatment:**
   (a) Same treatment as for prepatellar bursitis
   (b) Penicillinase-resistant penicillin is drug of choice until sensitivity tests are available

10. **Ankle injuries** occur infrequently in wrestlers. A sprain may occur when a wrestler's foot "sticks" in the mat while performing a maneuver. Sprains can be adequately taped for participation following a proper rehabilitation program. Ankle injuries include:
    a. Sprain
    b. Fracture
    c. Overuse injury

C. **Treatment on the mat**

1. **Time constraints**
   a. Injury time allotment is 1½ minutes for both high school and college wrestling.
   b. Physician/trainer must work quickly yet thoroughly in evaluating and treating the injured wrestler during the injury time-out.
2. **Epistaxis:** Treatment of epistaxis during a match does not count toward the allotted injury time.
3. **Rules regarding treatment**
   a. Taping is permissible during an injury time-out. Taping that substantially reduces the normal motion of a joint is prohibited.
   b. The use of braces or mechanical devices that do not permit normal range of motion of a joint or that prevent an opponent from applying a hold is prohibited.
   c. The use of medications during a match to relieve a preexisting condition such as asthma or diabetes is strictly prohibited.
4. **Return to wrestling**
   a. At the end of the allotted injury time, or any time prior, a decision about whether the athlete can continue participation must be rendered to the referee.

b. The referee has the authority to end the match when, in his or her opinion, a wrestler may be in danger of further injury.
c. Coaches, trainers, and parents cannot override the referee's decision.
d. The attending physician may prohibit an injured wrestler from returning to participation or, after careful examination, deem the wrestler fit to continue.
e. The referee may override a physician's opinion that an injured wrestler may continue participation.
f. The decision of the attending physician that a wrestler cannot continue participation may not be overruled by anyone, including the referee.

D. **Common skin conditions** (see Chapter 36)
  1. **Pyodermic infections**
    a. Staphylococcus
    b. Streptococcus
  2. **Viral infections**
    a. Herpes gladiatorum
    b. Herpes zoster
    c. Molluscum contagiosum
  3. **Fungal infections**
    a. Tinea pedis
    b. Tinea cruris
    c. Tinea corporis
  4. **Infestations**—scabies
  5. **General treatment strategies**
    a. **Proper hygiene**
      i. Frequent showering
      ii. Daily laundering of wrestling gear
      iii. Fingernails cut short and cleaned daily
    b. **Mat cleaning** done after every practice with an appropriate antiseptic solution
      i. Antibacterial
      ii. Antiviral
      iii. Antifungal
    c. **Medication** taken as directed
    d. **Isolation** of wrestler(s) with staphylococcal or streptococcal infections for 7–10 days
    e. **Proper wound care:** Mat burns and other open wounds should be meticulously cleaned and monitored daily for infection.
    f. **Visual inspection** of wrestlers at weigh-in for contagious skin conditions
      i. **Disqualification** if skin condition present
      ii. National Collegiate Athletic Association (NCAA) Guidelines permit participation with some solitary or localized lesions that can be securely and effectively covered (see Appendix A).

III. Prevention Strategies

A. **Medical supervision**
  1. **Physician** present at all meets and tournaments
  2. **Athletic trainer** or another qualified person at all practices and weigh-ins
  3. An **emergency plan**, including initial triage, first aid, communication, and transportation
  4. An accurate system of **record keeping** for thorough documentation of injuries

B. **Coaching.** Wrestlers should be aware of illegal holds and potentially dangerous maneuvers and learn proper defenses against them.

C. **Conditioning and strength programs**

APPENDIX A. NCAA Guideline 2B: Skin Infections in Wrestling (July 1981; Revised June 1994)

Data from the NCAA Injury Surveillance System (ISS) indicate that skin infections are associated with at least 10% of the time-loss injuries in wrestling. It is recommended that qualified personnel examine the skin over the entire body and the hair in the scalp and pubic areas of all wrestlers before any participation in the sport.

Open wounds and infectious skin conditions that cannot be adequately protected should be considered cause for medical disqualification from practice or competition. Categories of such skin conditions and examples include:

- I. Bacterial skin infections
  - A. Impetigo
  - B. Erysipelas
  - C. Carbuncle
  - D. Staphylococcal disease
  - E. Folliculitis (generalized)
  - F. Hidradenitis suppurativa
- II. Parasitic skin infections
  - A. Pediculosis
  - B. Scabies
- III. Viral Skin infections
  - A. Herpes simplex
  - B. Herpes zoster (chicken pox)
  - C. Molluscum contagiosum
- IV. Fungal skin infections—tinea corporis (ringworm)

Note: Current knowledge indicates that many fungal infections are easily transmitted by skin-to-skin contact. In most cases, these skin conditions can be covered with a securely attached bandage or non-permeable patch to allow participation.

Besides identification of infected individuals and their prompt treatment, prevention can be aided through proper routine cleaning of all equipment, including mats, and shared common areas, such as locker rooms.

Further recommendations developed by the NCAA Wrestling Committee regarding the disposition and treatment of skin conditions can be found in the NCAA Wrestling Championships Handbook.

References

1. Belongia EA, Goodman JL, Holland EJ, et al: An outbreak of herpes gladiatorum at a high-school wrestling camp. N Engl J Med 325(13):906–910, 1991.
2. Goodman RA, Thacker SB, Solomon SL, et al: Infectious disease in competitive sports. JAMA 271(11): 862–866, 1994.

From the National Collegiate Athletic Association: 1994–95 NCAA Sports Medicine Handbook. Overland Park, KS, National Collegiate Athletic Association, 1995, with permission.

1. Muscular endurance
2. Muscular strength
3. Aerobic fitness
4. Flexibility
5. Ideal wrestling weight

D. **Proper warm-up/cool-down**
   1. Jogging
   2. Stretching
   3. Rehearsal of wrestling skills

E. **Officiating.** It is vital that referees anticipate and position themselves to whistle or stop a potentially dangerous or illegal hold before an injury occurs (Figs. 3 and 4).

F. **Equipment**
   1. Properly fitted
   2. High quality
   3. Protective features

IV. Special Aspects of Prehabilitation and Rehabilitation

A. **Prehabilitation**
   1. **Strength assessment**
   2. **Cardiovascular assessment**

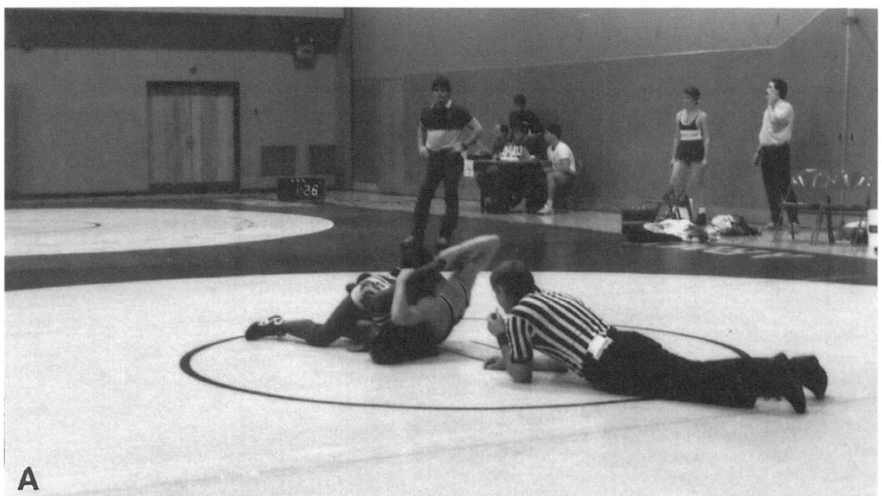

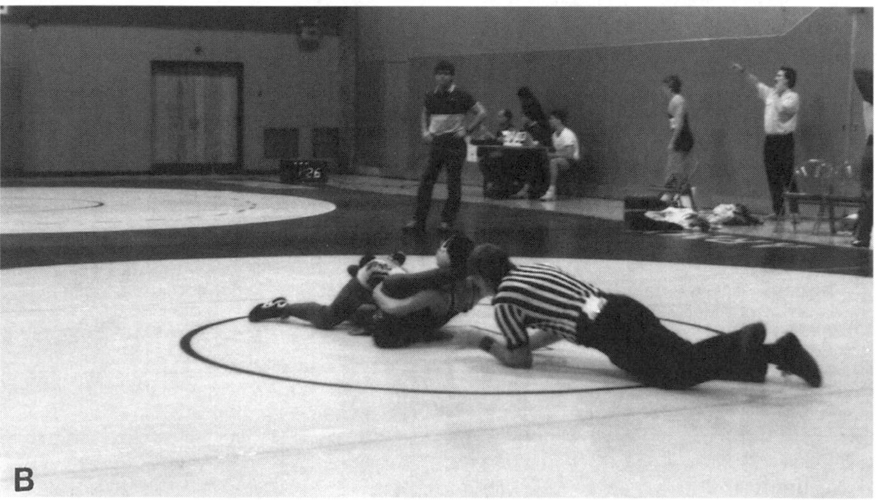

FIGURE 3. **A**, High torquing forces are applied to the shoulder of the wrestler on the left in what is known as the "guillotine maneuver." **B**, The official is in position to interrupt the match and bring the wrestlers back to the referee's position if the hold becomes potentially dangerous.

3. **Flexibility assessment.** Wrestling demands extensive joint mobility for optimal performance. Emphasis should be placed on the following areas:
    a. Heel cords
    b. Hamstrings
    c. Quadriceps
    d. Adductors
    e. Abductors
    f. Low back
    g. Shoulders
4. **Maturation assessment.** Evaluation of preadolescent wrestlers may be necessary for proper matching of younger competitors. Proper matching is important in reducing injuries as well as ensuring satisfaction in younger wrestlers.
5. **Previous injury assessment**—evaluation and rehabilitation of preexisting injuries

B. **Rehabilitation**

1. **Compliance:** Collegiate wrestlers are often noncompliant athletes who must be carefully monitored throughout the rehabilitation process.

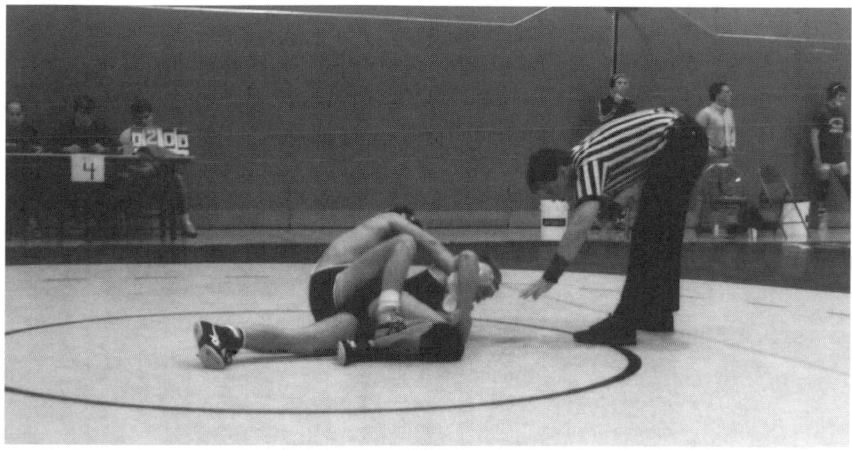

FIGURE 4. The left foot of the wrestler on top is trapped in a position that may lead to injury. The official is evaluating whether it is a potentially dangerous hold.

2. **Coach:** The coach can stimulate compliance by wrestlers by demanding adherence to the physician's or trainer's recommendations.
3. **Weight control:** Wrestlers must stay within a reasonable reach of their wrestling weight during the rehabilitation process.

V. Wrestling Facilities and Protective Equipment

A. **Facilities**

1. **Wrestling mats**—constructed from Ensolite foam with an outer vinyl coating that permits easy cleaning. The mat has properties of controlled compression and controlled recovery to provide shock absorption for the heavy impact that occurs in takedowns and throwing maneuvers.
2. **Wrestling room**—dimensions at least 50 square feet per wrestler to minimize the chance of injury from collisions with other wrestlers. Walls and pillars in the wrestling room should be padded at least 5 feet high.

B. **Equipment**

1. **Face guard:** Wrestlers with facial sutures or nasal fractures may benefit from wearing a protective face guard (Fig. 5A).
2. **Mouth guard:** All wrestlers, especially younger wrestlers with orthodontic braces, should wear mouthpieces.
3. **Knee and elbow pads** provide protection of previously injured areas. Pads of neoprene construction are currently popular.
4. **Footwear:** Soles are of a gum-rubber composition that allows ankle and foot mobility while maintaining adequate traction with the mat. **These shoes should never be used for running because they provide no shock-absorbing qualities.**
5. **Athletic supporters** provide protection of the testicles.
6. **Headgear:** The use of properly fitted headgear is essential for protection of the ears during wrestling (Fig. 5B).

VI. Rules to Protect Wrestlers

A. **Governing bodies**

1. Members of the NCAA Rules Committee and the National Federation of State High School Associations (NFSHSA) have established their own individual sets of wrestling rules.

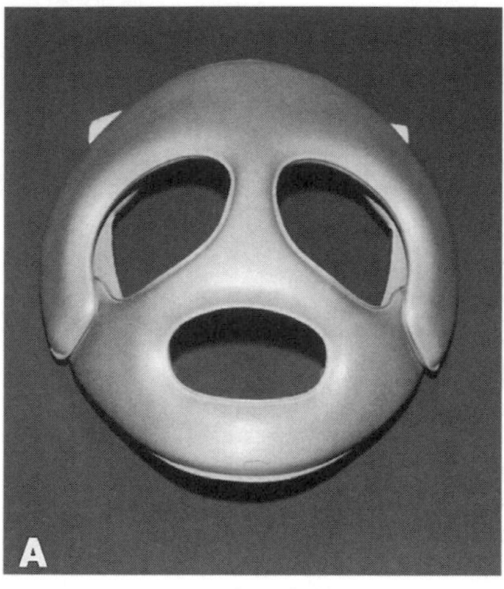
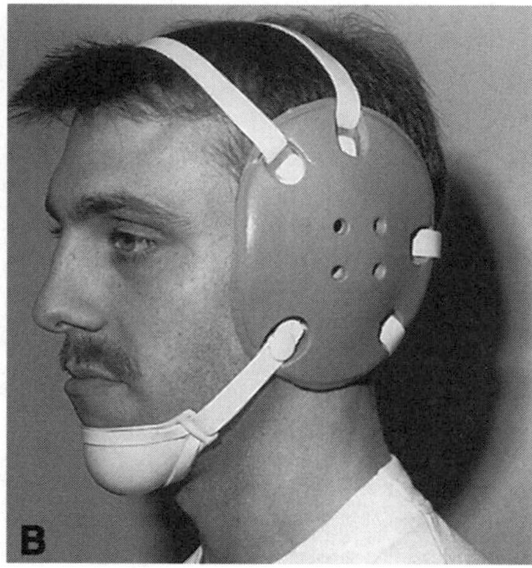

FIGURE 5. **A**, Face guard attached to the wrestler's headgear to protect from facial injuries. **B**, Protective headgear designed to prevent injuries.

2. International wrestling rules and regulations are set by the Federation Internationale des Luttes Amateurs (FILA). USA Wrestling is the national governing body for the sport of amateur wrestling in the United States. It oversees wrestlers seeking to qualify for national, international, and Olympic teams.

B. **Specific rules**

1. Most rules are the same or similar; however, subtle differences do exist between interscholastic and collegiate wrestling (see Table 2).
2. To ensure safety, the referee may temporarily halt a match for illegal holds, unnecessary roughness, or potentially dangerous situations.
   a. **Illegal holds** are maneuvers that inflict pain and are dangerous to the receiving wrestler, such as holds that cover the mouth, throat, and eyes. The offending wrestler is penalized.
   b. **Potentially dangerous** situations are those in which a hold or maneuver may place a wrestler in danger of injury. These moves usually force a joint beyond its normal mobility. The referee can break these holds before an injury is allowed to occur. No penalty is assessed because these are usually unintentional.

TABLE 2. Major Differences in Rules for Interscholastic and Intercollegiate Wrestling

Parameter	High School	Collegiate
Length of matches		
Period 1	2 min	3 min
Period 2	2 min	2 min
Period 3	2 min	2 min
Number of matches/day	5 full matches	No limit
Time between matches	45 minutes	1 hour recommended
Weigh-ins	1½ hours before meet	1½–5 hours before meet
Dehydrating equipment	Sauna, plastic suits, and other dehydrating devices strictly prohibited	No similar rule although highly discouraged
Certification	Wrestlers may be required to certify at the weight at which they intend to wrestle the majority of the season	Currently under review

c. **Unnecessary roughness** may be assessed when one wrestler uses more aggressiveness than is necessary, such as a forceful trip or an aggressive cross-face. A penalty is assessed.

VII. Special Concerns of the Team Physician

A. **"Making weight"** (see Appendix B)

1. **Certification of scholastic wrestlers**
   a. Each state is allowed to regulate the certification process by which wrestlers seek to qualify (make weight) for a given weight classification to compete in over the majority of the wrestling season.
   b. Predetermined dates are set by which the wrestler must make the requirements of the weight classification.
   c. A wrestler may not wrestle below certification weight, but may wrestle at a higher weight class.

APPENDIX B. NCAA Guideline 2D: Weight Loss–Hypohydration (July 1985; Revised June 1992)

There are two general types of weight loss common to student-athletes who participate in intercollegiate sports: loss of body water (at issue here) or loss of stored body lipid (fat) and body tissue. The loss of body water or the process of dehydration, which leads to a state of negative water balance (hypohydration), is brought about by withholding drinking fluids and carbohydrates; the promotion of extensive sweating; and the use of emetics, diuretics, or laxatives. The problem is most evident in those who must be certified to participate in a given weight class, but is also present in other athletic groups.

There are no valid reasons for subjecting the student-athlete's body to a hypohydrated state because of the variety of adverse physiologic effects and possible pathology that accompany hypohydration. These include reduced strength and local muscular endurance, smaller plasma and blood volume, modified cardiac functioning (including higher heart rate, smaller stroke volume, and less cardiac output), impaired thermoregulation, decreased kidney blood flow and filtration, reduced liver glycogen stores, and loss of electrolytes.

When hypohydration is extensive, attempts at rehydration usually are insufficient for body fluid and electrolyte homeostasis to be restored before competition. In wrestling, this is especially true between the official weigh-in and actual competition

The practice of fluid deprivation (dehydration) should be discouraged. To promote sound practices, student-athletes and coaches should be educated about the physiologic and pathologic consequences of hypohydration. The use of laxatives, emetics, and diuretics should be prohibited. Similarly, the use of excessive food and fluid restriction, self-induced vomiting, vapor-impermeable suits (e.g., rubber or rubberized nylon), hot rooms, hot boxes, and steam rooms should be prohibited.

Hypohydration constitutes an unnecessary potential health hazard that acts synergistically with poor nutrition and intense exercise to compromise health and athletics ability. The positive alternative is to minimize weight loss and maintain a desired weight over the course of the competitive season. To implement these policies, the use of standard measures of percent body fat and body weight is advisable to ascertain a reasonable weight status for the student-athlete. In wrestling, the official weigh-in should be scheduled an hour before match time.

References

1. American College of Sports Medicine, Position Stand: Weight Loss in Wrestlers. Indianapolis, American College of Sports Medicine, 1976.
2. Buskirk ER: Weight loss in wrestlers. Am J Dis Child 132(4):355–356, 1978.
3. Horwill CA: Does Rapid Weight Loss by Dehydration Adversely Affect High-Power Performance? Chicago, Gatorade Sports Science Institute, 3(30), 1991.
4. Swaka MN (chair): Symposium—Current concepts concerning thrist, dehydration, and fluid replacement. Med Sci Sport 24(6):643–687, 1992.

d. If a wrestler fails to make weight for a meet, he may become eligible to compete in the next higher weight classification.
e. Recertification at a lower weight classification should be strongly discouraged.
f. Physicians are urged to become actively involved in the certification process.
g. Certification weight should be based not only on visual assessment and current weight, but also on body composition assessment.

2. **Weight-cutting practices**
   a. Why wrestlers cut weight:
      i. Wrestlers seek to gain an advantage over their opponents by reducing body weight and body fat to a minimal level to compete in the lowest possible weight classification over a supposedly smaller and weaker opponent.
      ii. There may be two good wrestlers at one weight, which means one wrestler may not get the opportunity to compete unless he moves to another weight classification.
      iii. Most wrestlers believe they can make weight for a lower weight class with no loss in performance. This belief is often unsound.
   b. Methods of weight-cutting
      i. Thermal methods:
         (a) Plastic or rubber suits
         (b) Saunas or steam rooms
         (c) Excessive exercise
         (d) Combinations of the above methods
      ii. Nutritional methods:
         (a) Diet restriction
         (b) Fluid restriction
      iii. Other less common methods:
         (a) Excessive spitting
         (b) Self-induced vomiting
         (c) Diuretics
         (d) Laxatives
3. **The process of making weight**
   a. About 2 or 3 days before the official weigh-in, wrestlers begin to restrict their food and water intake while continuing to exercise and wrestle at vigorous levels.
   b. Several hours before the official weigh-in, wrestlers unable to meet the weight requirement may attempt acute dehydration to qualify.
   c. Wrestlers may lose up to 10% or more of their body weight following these methods.
   d. After the weigh-in, wrestlers frequently attempt to rehydrate themselves by consuming large quantities of fluid. Research has shown that a 5-hour rehydration period does not allow the body enough time to rehydrate and that most high school and college wrestlers are competing in a dehydrated state.
   e. This weight-cutting process is repeated many times throughout a wrestling season.
   f. Fellow wrestlers and coaches are most frequently consulted for information concerning making weight; physicians and parents are rarely consulted about these problems.
4. **Health consequences associated with making weight**
   a. **Thermal injuries:**
      i. Heat cramps
      ii. Heat exhaustion
      iii. Heat stroke
   b. **Renal and cardiac disturbances:**
      i. Lower plasma and blood volumes
      ii. Decreased cardiac output

iii. Decreased renal blood flow and urine output
iv. Electrolyte problems
v. Possible renal damage

c. **Other disturbances:**
   i. Learning ability is reduced.
   ii. Anxiety
   iii. Depression
   iv. Eating disorders:
      (a) Bulimia nervosa
      (b) Anorexia nervosa

d. **Decrements in physical performance:**
   i. 2% loss of body weight impairs thermoregulatory system
   ii. 3% loss reduces muscular endurance time
   iii. 4–6% loss reduces muscular strength and endurance time, and causes heat cramps.
   iv. > 6% loss can lead to heat cramps, exhaustion, stroke, coma, death

e. **Long-term studies** needed to examine dehydration in wrestlers:
   i. Delayed renal damage during the middle decades of the wrestler's life.
   ii. Possible stunting of growth and maturation in younger wrestlers

B. **Preventive strategies against weight reduction abuses**

1. **Education**
2. **Nutritional guidance**
3. **Preseason conditioning programs**
4. **Weight monitoring**—a daily record of each wrestler's weight before and after each practice
5. **Body composition assessment.** Following the preseason conditioning program, an assessment of body composition should be undertaken by qualified personnel.
   a. A 5% level of body fat should be considered the minimal percentage at which a wrestler can safely compete.
   b. Most wrestlers completing a 4–6 week preseason conditioning program are close to their actual wrestling weight.
   c. Any wrestler seeking to reduce weight further must get prior approval from the physician, so that an appropriate weight reduction plan can be set up.
   d. Caloric intake and expenditure should be monitored closely.
   e. Wrestlers should be discouraged from losing more than 2–3 pounds per week.
6. **Method of body composition**
   a. The Opplinger and Tipton regression equation is designed specifically for wrestlers (Table 3).

TABLE 3. Opplinger and Tipton Regression Equation for Prediction of a Minimal Wrestling Weight in Scholastic Wrestlers*

Opplinger and Tipton Model (r. 962)	
(0.49) × (current weight in lbs)	= ________
(1.65) × (height in inches)	= ________
(1.81) × (chest diameter)	= ________
(6.70) × (right wrist diameter)	= ________
(1.35) × (chest depth)	= ________
	Sum total – 156.56 = Minimal wrestling weight

* All measurements in centimeters unless otherwise noted.
From Opplinger RA, Tipton CM: Iowa wrestling study: Cross validation of the Tcheng-Tipton minimal weight prediction formulas for high school wrestlers. Med Sci Sports 20:310–316, 1988, with permission.

b. This equation uses various anthropometric measurements, obtained with an antropometer or similar body caliper device, to compute minimal wrestling weight.
c. Coaches, trainers, and physicians can easily use this equation for assessment of body composition.

C. **Blood-borne pathogens**
1. All medical personal working actively with wrestlers should have an institutional policy addressing hepatitis B virus and human immuodeficiency virus transmission for their own safety and that of the wrestlers. This is important because of the close body contact and the frequent episodes of bleeding often noted in competitive wrestling.
2. This policy should minimally include:
   a. Blood-borne pathogens exposure control plan
   b. Annual training and education
   c. Record keeping
   d. Personal protective equipment

Recommended Reading

1. American College of Sports Medicine: Position Stand on Weight Loss in Wrestlers. Madison, WI, American College of Sports Medicine, 1976.
2. Boring WJ: Science and Skills of Wrestling. St. Louis, CV Mosby, 1975.
3. Carson RF: Championship Wrestling. New York, AS Barnes & Co., 1974.
4. Estwanik JJ, Bergfield J, Canty T: Report of injuries sustained during the United States Olympic wrestling trials. Am J Sports Med 6:335–340, 1978.
5. Estwanik JJ, Bergfeld JA, Collins HR, Hall R: Injuries in interscholastic wrestling. Phys Sportsmed 8:111–121, 1980.
6. Gable D, Peterson JA: Conditioning for Wrestling: The Iowa Way. West Point, NY, Leisure Press, 1980.
7. Gibney R: Safety in Individual and Dual Sports. Sports Safety Monographs 4. Washington, D.C., American School and Community Safety Association, American Alliance for Health, Physical Education, and Recreation 12:43–46, 1977.
8. Gross CG: Treating "cauliflower ear" with a silicone mold. Am J Sports Med 6:4–5, 1978.
9. Hartmann PM: Injuries in preadolescent wrestlers. Phys Sportsmed 6:79–82, 1978.
10. Hecker AL, Wheeler KB: Impact of hydration and energy intake on performance. In Kaverman D (ed): Schering Symposium: Athletic Training Winter. 1984, pp 260–264.
11. Herbert WG, Ribisl PM: Effects of dehydration upon physical working capacity of wrestlers under competitive conditions. Res Q 43:416–422, 1972.
12. Hinkamp JF: High school athletic injuries. Ill Med J 148:127–129, 1975.
13. Hursh LM: Food and water restriction in the wrestler. JAMA 241:915–916, 1979.
14. Katch FL, McArdle WD: Nutrition, Weight Control and Exercise. Boston, Houghton-Mifflin, 1977.
15. Lok V, Yuceturk G: Injuries in wrestling. J Sports Med 2:324–328, 1974.
16. Morgan WP: Psychological effect of weight reduction in the college wrestler. Med Sci Sports 2:24–27, 1970.
17. Mysnyk MC, Wroble RR, Foster DT, Albright JP: Prepatellar bursitis in wrestlers. Am J Sports Med 14:46–54, 1986.
18. Opplinger RA, Tipton CM: Iowa wrestling study: Cross validation of the Tcheng-Tipton minimal weight prediction formulas for high school wrestlers. Med Sci Sports 20:310–316, 1988.
19. Porter PS, Baughman RD: Epidemiology of herpes simplex among wrestlers. JAMA 194:998–1000, 1965.
20. Rasch PG, Kroll W: What Research Tells the Coach About Wrestling. Washington, D.C., American Association of Health, Physical Education and Recreation, 1964.
21. Reek CC: A national study of incidence of accidents in high school wrestling. Res Q 10:72–73, 1939.
22. Requa R, Garrick JG: Injuries in intercollegiate wrestling. Phys Sportsmed 9:51, 1981.
23. Round Table: Weight reduction in wrestling. Phys Sportsmed 9:79–96, 1981.
24. Strauss RH, Lanese RR: Injuries among wrestlers in school and college tournaments. JAMA 248:2016–2019, 1982.
25. Snook GA: Injuries in intercollegiate wrestling. Am J Sports Med 10:142–144, 1982.
26. Snook GA: The injury problem in wrestling. Am J Sports Med 9:184–188, 1976.
27. Snook GA: Wrestling. In Schneider RC (ed): Sports Injuries: Mechanism, Prevention, and Treatment. Baltimore, Williams & Wilkins, 1985, pp 129–138.
28. Taylor HL, Herschel A, Mickelson O, et al: Some effects of acute starvation with hard work on body weight, body fluids, and metabolism. J Appl Physiol 6:613–623, 1954.

29. Tcheng TK, Tipton CML: Iowa wrestling study: Anthropometric measurements and prediction of a "minimal" body weight for high school wrestlers. Med Sci Sports 5:1–10, 1973.
30. Tipton CM: Physiological problems associated with the "making of weight." Am J Sports Med 8:449–450, 1980.
31. Tipton CM, Tcheng TK: Iowa wrestling study: Weight loss in high school students. JAMA 214:1269–1274, 1970.
32. Wheeler CE, Cabaniss WH: Epidemic cutaneous herpes simplex in wrestlers (herpes gladiatorum). JAMA 194:993–997, 1965.
33. Wroble RR, Albright JP: Neck injuries in wrestling. Clin Sports Med 2:295–324, 1986.
34. Wroble RR, Mysnyk MC, Foster DT, Albright JP: Patterns of knee injuries in wrestling: A six year study. Am J Sports Med 14:55–66, 1986.
35. Zambraski EJ, Tipton CM, Tcheng TK, et al: Iowa wrestling study: Changes in the urinary profiles of wrestlers prior to and after competition. Med Sci Sports 7:217–220, 1975.
36. Zambraski EJ, Foster DT, Gross PM, Tipton CM: Iowa wrestling study: Weight loss and urinary profiles of collegiate workers. Med Sci Sports 8:105–108, 1976.

59

Swimming and Diving

Richard W. Hammer, M.D.

I. General Considerations

A. **Perspective:** Both swimming and diving are popular recreational water activities as well as competitive sports.

B. **Scope:** All ages from infants to elderly persons swim. Divers are usually not as young or as old.

C. **Focus:** Competitive events begin in water sports around age 8 (sometimes earlier) and extend through college. Masters programs involve all ages beyond 25. This chapter does not discuss water polo or water skiing, although they share similar problems.

D. **Sports medicine concerns vary by age of swimmer or diver and specific activity involved.** Most concerns focus on practice and training; more time is spent in these situations. Safety programs should be introduced early to protect the athlete. Swimming is a sprint, middle distance, and endurance activity; diving is more a spatial orientation sport.

II. Traumatic and Overuse Injuries

A. **Shoulder**

1. **Injury generally develops during training. It can be related to overuse but sometimes develops during a change in stroke as a child matures, from changes in coaches, from adjustment of stroke to increase speed or power, or from using improper stroke technique.**
2. **Stroke changes as fatigue develops, and in the process pain develops and stroke efficiency decreases.**
3. **Anatomy.** Biceps tendon, rotator cuff, related muscles, and impingement of shoulder are often involved (Fig. 1).
4. **Muscles.** Detection of these small muscle injuries depends on attention to the location of each and knowledge of function.
    a. Subscapularis
    b. Upper trapezius
    c. Infraspinatus
    d. Rhomboids
    e. Deltoid—injury to a particular segment can be identified (usually middle and anterior). Differentiate from subacromial bursitis or rotator cuff injury.
    f. Serratus anterior
5. **Ligaments**
    a. Coracoacromial ligament
    b. Acromioclavicular ligament—more often injured during direct trauma applied to the shoulder.
    c. Coracoclavicular ligament—rarely involved in swimming

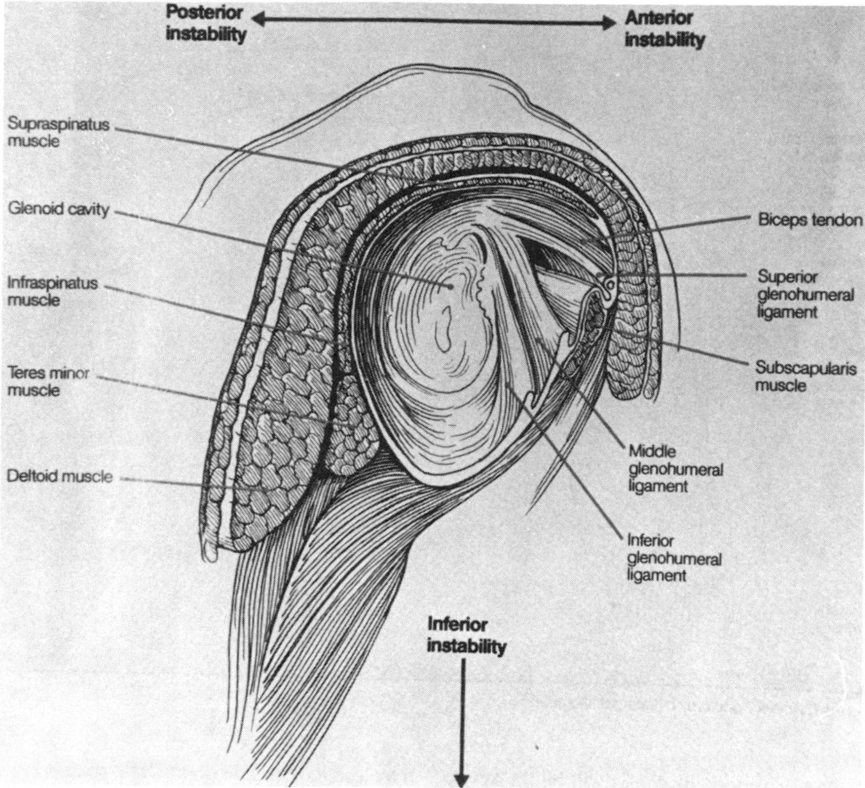

FIGURE 1. Anatomy of the shoulder showing parts that may be involved in overuse shoulder injuries. (From McMaster WC: Painful shoulder in swimmers: A diagnostic challenge. Phys Sportsmed 14(12):108–122, 1986, with permission.)

6. **Tendons**
   a. Biceps—most common tendon of shoulder to be involved in overuse injury
   b. Deltoid—need to differentiate from subdeltoid bursitis
7. **Bursae**
   a. Subacromial
   b. Subdeltoid—may become inflamed and swollen and limit motion through mechanical obstruction or pain
8. **Shoulder joint**
   a. Dislocation, subluxation
   b. Synovitis
   c. Capsulitis
9. **Other problems affecting the shoulder**
   a. **Neck:**
      i. Arthritis
      ii. Disk problems
      iii. Tumors, cord problems
   b. Miscellaneous
      i. Congenital problems
      ii. Thoracic outlet syndrome
      iii. Upper chest problems encroaching on shoulder or brachial plexus

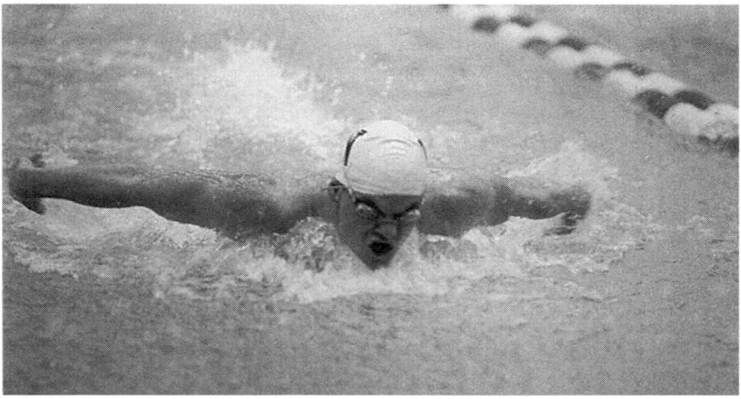

FIGURE 2. The butterfly stroke is one of the overuse mechanisms that may result in shoulder injuries. (Courtesy of Sports Information Office, University of Nebraska–Lincoln.)

10. **History and physical examination,** other evaluations
    a. Obtain **history** of:
        i. Mechanism of injury (Figs. 2 and 3)
        ii. Prior injuries
        iii. Current medications
    b. **Observe shoulder in relaxed position:**
        i. Notice depressions:
            (a) Torn ligaments
            (b) Acromioclavicular separations
        ii. Notice swellings:
            (a) Capsulitis
            (b) Bursitis

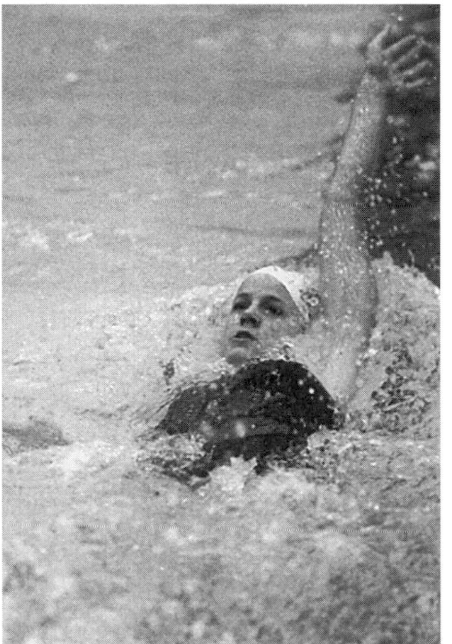

FIGURE 3. The backstroke may cause overuse injury to the shoulder as well as to the back. (Courtesy of Sports Information Office, University of Nebraska–Lincoln.)

c. **Observe abnormal movements:**
   i. Torn muscle
   ii. Contused muscles
   iii. Inability to raise shoulder laterally:
      (a) Injury to deltoid
      (b) Acromioclavicular separation
   iv. Painful flexion of elbow—biceps tendinitis
d. **Palpation** (point tenderness aids in localizing injury):
   i. Acromioclavicular joint
   ii. Joint capsule area
   iii. Biceps tendon
e. **Muscle loss of strength:**
   i. Estimate by appearance
   ii. Measure upper arm circumference
   iii. Specific strength measured by machines with digital readouts
f. **Neurologic evaluation:**
   i. Reflexes—biceps tendon
   ii. Sensory, pain perception—brachial plexus, local nerve
g. **Laboratory evaluations:**
   i. Uric acid—gout, pseudogout
   ii. Rheumatoid arthritis factor, antinuclear antibody, human leukocyte antigen—rheumatoid arthritis, other collagen vascular diseases
   iii. Serum iron—hemochromatosis
   iv. Serum copper—liver problems (Wilson's disease)
h. **Other confirming evaluations:**
   i. Electromyography—muscular damage or diseases or nerve damage
   ii. Arthrography—cuff deficits, damage to muscular capsular component of joint
   iii. Magnetic resonance imaging—may be done with or without enhancement, best for soft tissue visualization
   iv. Ultrasound—helps to see cuff structures
i. **Special treatments** (use principles outlined in Chapter 43, "Shoulder Injuries")
   i. Work with swimmer and coach to **adjust workout and/or stroke**
   ii. Give shoulder **adequate rest**; avoid continuing injury in other activities
   iii. Ensure adequate **warm-up; ice after workout**
   iv. **Complete rest of shoulder** if aforementioned does not help

B. **Back**

1. Most back problems for swimmers are in lower back and sacral areas. Approximately 15.8% of swimmers have some abnormalities in this area.
2. Back injuries occur from constant pounding, from turns at end of the pool, or from striking water at end of dive.
3. Severe injuries may result from improper technique, diving into shallow water, diving into another swimmer or diver, or falling on deck. Always enter unknown water feet first.
4. **Limitations of participation**
   a. **Defective atlanto-occipital structure:**
      i. Avoid diving.
      ii. Start races in the water.
      iii. Avoid water polo.
   b. **Arthritis, gout**—depends on stage, symptoms, and degree of control
   c. **Disk syndrome:**
      i. Avoid diving.

ii. Avoid flip turns and grab starts—lap swimming minus flip turns may be prescribed in some patients as therapy.

d. **Scoliosis:**
   i. Adaptation depends on degree of involvement
   ii. May lead to bracing, surgery
   iii. Some swimmers and divers remove braces during competition and do well.

C. **Head**
1. **Lacerations**
   a. Most common to divers in the water sports. Many will recall diver Greg Louganis' injury at the 1988 Olympics.
   b. Could also occur when head hits wall of the pool, most likely in backstroke.
2. **Contusions**
   a. From striking head against wall on turns, finishes
   b. On diving board
   c. Observe for further neurologic factors
   d. May have headache for several days
3. **Cervical spine injuries**
   a. May occur in diving—either in a specific dive or from chronic trauma to cervical spine
   b. May occur when diving into shallow water or onto another participant
   c. Swimmers less likely to have back or cervical spine problems than gymnasts

D. **Knee**
1. The knee may be injured as in other sports (see Chapter 49, "Knee Injuries").
2. **In swimmers, more likely to occur in breaststrokers**
   a. **An overuse/abuse problem (breaststroker's knee)**
   b. **One form occurs in medial aspect of knee:**
      i. Tibial collateral ligament
      ii. Medial retinaculum
      iii. Gracilis tendon
   c. **Extensor mechanism malalignment may be a form of breaststroker's knee.**
   d. Occurs when overtraining or adjusting stroke—a valgus stress with external rotation
   e. Treatment varies:
      i. Proper warm-ups, stretching
      ii. Ice after use
      iii. Aspirin or nonsteroidal anti-inflammatory drugs
      iv. Complete rest
      v. Physical therapy

E. **Groin injuries**
1. May be injured, as in other sports
2. **In swimmers, more likely to occur in breaststrokers**
   a. Can be an overuse problem or sudden stress on iliopsoas muscle
   b. Can occur when not properly warmed up
   c. Swimmer has trouble flexing hip; can palpate tenderness in groin area
   d. The iliopsoas is a muscle used in all strokes, so complete rest from swimming along with analgesics and physical therapy may be needed.
   e. Occasionally requires cortisone injection
   f. May ultimately require surgery

F. **Wrist injuries**
1. **Injuries to swimmers may occur on turns or finishes when striking the wall or getting hand or arm caught in gutter**
2. **Divers may injure wrist on entry into water**

a. More likely to occur if diver used overlapped hands with wrists extended and forearms pronated. Another technique is closed fists with one thumb grasped in other hand.
b. May result in radial styloid fracture, first metacarpal fracture, or wrist sprain
c. May be treated with strapping, stopping training, or surgery
d. **Wrist pain a frequent problem in divers** from repeated water entries or a bad entry. May use a restraining system for wrist when diving or make a splint.

G. **Miscellaneous injuries**

1. **Swimmer's ear**
   a. Swollen inflamed external ear canal (Fig. 4)
   b. Responds to combination antibiotic-corticosteroid drops or acetic acid with or without steroid drops
   c. May require oral antibiotics as well as local drops and/or analgesics
   d. May need long-term prophylaxis after each swim with 2% vinegar (acetic acid), 70% alcohol, 3% boric acid in isopropyl alcohol or aluminate sulfate–calcium acetate solution
   e. Ear plugs:
      i. Commercial ones not usually helpful
      ii. May require professionally produced plugs from an audiologist or otolaryngologist
   f. With adequate treatment and response, athlete may be able to participate in the water for short periods
2. **Other ear problems**
   a. **Barotrauma** may cause problems 3 feet or more below surface:
      i. Transudation of fluid into middle ear cleft
      ii. Perilymph fistula or rupture of round or oval windows
      iii. Otitis media

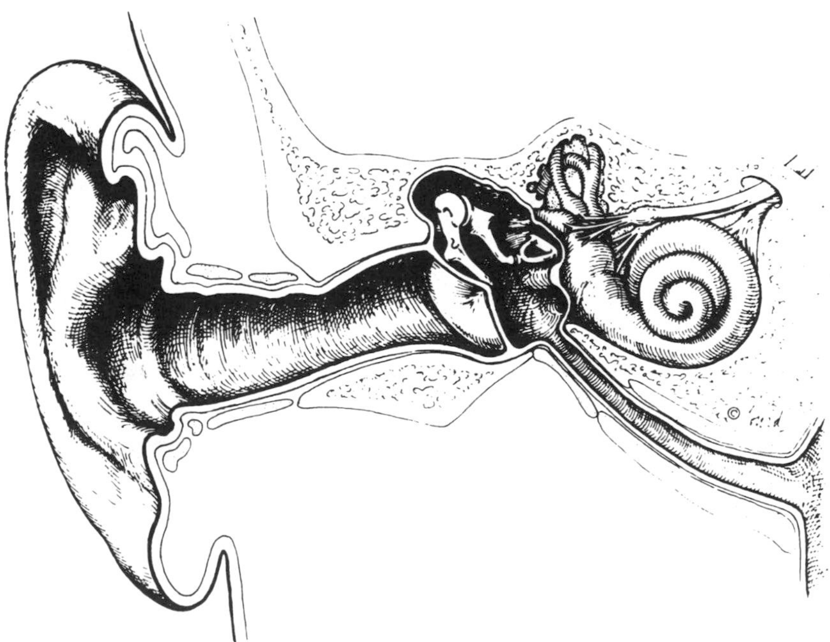

FIGURE 4. Anatomy of the ear. (With permission of the artist: © Jane Hurd, 1981.)

iv. Acute mastoiditis
v. High diving or deep underwater swimming not advised if athlete has secretory otitis media

b. **Participation with perforated drums:**
i. With tubes, use protective ear plugs or ear molds
ii. Bathing cap may help
iii. Avoid diving, deep underwater swimming, swimming in pond water
iv. Treat infection with combination ear drops
v. May occur with suppurative otitis media

3. **Conjunctivitis**
a. If infectious, treat appropriately
b. May be from **chlorine irritation:**
i. Use of goggles helpful
ii. Give trial of ophthalmic cromolyn sodium (also used in allergic conjunctivitis)
iii. May respond to over-the-counter eye drops or may require steroid ophthalmic preparations after viral infection ruled out

4. **Athlete's foot**
a. Restrict from pool or showers where patient may expose others
b. Treat with antifungal topically; if severe, may also need oral medication
c. Advise shower clogs for protection and prevention

5. **Warts**
a. Use quick method to get athlete back into action; liquid nitrogen or hyfrecation possibly.
b. Advise shower clogs for protection
c. If topical methods used, restrict from pool and shower areas until healed

6. **Lacerations**
a. May occur from sharp edges of starting blocks, from exposed bolts on deck or block, or from glass on pool decks
b. Repair appropriately using adherent strips or sutures.
c. Avoid water unless wound is properly protected (Greg Louganis completed another dive after repair and won again the next week).

7. **Ankle**
a. **Most likely overuse occurs from flutter kick and involves extensor retinaculum of the ankle**
b. Treat by adjusting stroke, stretching; use ice, anti-inflammatory medication
c. May require rest, physical therapy

III. Other Problems in Swimmers and Divers—unless otherwise noted, treat as in other sports

A. **Skin rashes**
1. Possibly caused by water, chemicals in the water, or rubdown materials
2. Visit with coach and respond according to findings; otherwise treat as other athletes

B. **Fractures** occur more often in divers.
1. Usually from striking diving platform while performing dive, particularly fingers, wrist, and nose
2. Sometimes may continue to participate if fiberglass cast is applied. More expensive but allows more normal lifestyle.
a. Undisplaced stable fractures
b. Severe sprains

C. **Pneumonia**—same as other athletes

D. **Asthma**
1. Water sports are less asthmagenic than cycling or running.

  a. Lower pollen count over water
  b. Higher hydrostatic pressure on chest
  c. Reduction of CO_2 from hyperventilation due to controlled breathing pattern; counteracts respiratory heat loss
2. Swimming makes asthma worse when parasympathetic drive is encouraged during immersion, or athlete is sensitive to chlorine
3. Athlete may need to take preexercise medication via inhaler to prevent exercise-induced asthma

E. **Gastroenteritis:** If epidemic among users of pool, ask pool manager to have pool tested (may be bacterial from *Shigella*, *Vibrio cholerae*, or others; viral from a rotavirus; or parasitic from *Giardia*, etc.)

F. **Sunburn, sunstroke, heat exhaustion**
1. Rare but can occur during long meets under just the right circumstances
2. Encourage adequate fluid intake as prevention
3. Encourage sunblock application. Water sports competitors get many hours of sun exposure, but rarely use sunblock protection except early in the season.

G. **Hypothermia**
1. More likely in long-distance swimmers but can also occur in early morning hours of meet or practice
2. Observe for alertness, coordination, skin color, shivering

H. **Nutrition**
1. Swimmers and divers tend to be low to medium body fat percentage.
2. **Otherwise, trained and fit long-distance swimmers may need extra body fat for buoyancy and insulation.**
3. "Pregame" meals are a problem for all or partial day meets. **Most important to stay hydrated; avoid "quick" energy sources such as sugars just before an event.**

I. **Menstruation**
1. Rarely causes absence from the pool
2. Early intense competition and practice may delay menarche.
3. If a problem involves menstruation, inquire about anorexia, thyroid, pregnancy, or personal difficulties as possible causes.

J. **Surfing injuries**
1. Also a popular water sport with some injuries peculiar to it
2. Lacerations—75% to lower extremity
3. Soft tissue injury
  a. Sprains, strains, dislocations
  b. Primarily to knee, lower back, shoulder, ankle, and neck, in descending order of frequency
4. Fractures are uncommon—primarily nose, feet, arms, ribs. Broken teeth also.
5. Cause—surfer's own board (80–90% fins, tails, or rails of board)

K. **Drowning**
1. Same problem as with other persons using water for sport, recreation, or commerce
2. May occur following inhalation of water and secondary laryngospasm
3. May result from "diving reflex" in swimmer, who hyperventilates, enters water, and while swimming stays at bottom of pool

IV. Warm-up, Cool-down, and Stretching

A. Controversial

B. Swimmers have traditionally **"stretched"** each other before competition, often with movements not used in swimming or diving.

C. Some authorities prefer more general warm-up activities.

1. Put joints through full range of swimming motion
2. Avoid harmful overstretching—may lead to some loss of strength

D. **Warm-up**
1. Length of time varies among swimmers
2. Start of warm-up is on deck to loosen muscle and increase heart activity
3. Move to water to get body ready for competition
4. Wear warm-up suit while waiting for event
5. In long meets, swimmer may need to repeat these phases to be ready

E. **Rubdowns**
1. Traditional for swimmer
2. Best in hands of practicing therapists
3. Avoid overrelaxing
4. Avoid abnormal absorption of chemicals from substances applied to skin

F. **"Swim down"**
1. Valuable for swimmer to cool down gradually after event
2. Usually done in adjoining pool to avoid tightening of muscles after event

G. **Taper**
1. Method to prepare body for competition
2. Usually once a season but may be useful for specific competition
3. Involves duration of taper, frequency of workouts, and exercise intensity.
   a. Training reduced in incremental and stepwise way
   b. Value is individual application
   c. 60–90% reduction in volume over 7–21 days (14 days seems best) and training frequency by less than 50% (20% is a conservative amount)
   d. Coaches and swimmers need to be aware of psychological and physical results of taper

V. Sport-specific Facilities and Protective Equipment

A. **Pool configuration**
1. Markings, blocks, and lane lines are specified by governing bodies.
2. Water temperature, acidity, and chlorine content should be monitored.
3. Diving boards and water depth are regulated for divers.
4. Pool depth regulated for safety, warm-up, and competition may be modified accordingly.

B. **Protective equipment**
1. Swimmers may use goggles to protect eyes from chlorine.
2. Rubdown oil is allowed unless judged excessive or not permitted by the pool operator.
3. Long-distance swimmers use lard or similar substance for insulation for some events.
4. Swimming caps may be used to reduce friction with water.
5. For additional speed, swimmers may "shave" body or head hair.

VI. Rules to Protect the Athletes

A. **Age group division, male and female**
1. Standards set for 8 years old as lowest age group
2. Age divisions rise by 2-year increments for equal competition
3. Competition further divided into male and female groups
4. Swimmers younger than 8 compete, but more for recreation and learning fundamentals.
5. Masters swimmers also divided by age groups and sex

B. **Coach certification**
1. Each governing body sets its own standards.
   a. Safety certified
   b. CPR certified
   c. May be required to be registered members

2. Levels of proficiency may be outlined.
3. Programs are established for the protection of athletes.

C. **Safety advisors**
1. Each club, pool, or swimming organization needs to set safety standards for use of pool and for competition.
2. United States Swimming has national chairperson and local sport committee safety chairperson and advises that a local swim/diving club use a safety person.

D. **Specified warm-ups**
1. Designated lanes for a club
2. Designated sprint lanes
3. Diving monitor to signal water clear
4. No diving by divers or swimmers unless supervised

E. **Water depth**
1. Swimmers start from blocks only in specified depth or deeper water
2. Divers require water of specified depth or deeper

F. **No jumping into pool** when race is in progress and, otherwise, only with referee's approval

G. **No interference** during diving or swimming competition

H. **Specifications** listed for starting block surfaces, composition, and structure of diving boards and towers; also for pool size, depth, wall surfaces, deck, lighting, and electrical cords or other apparatus on deck

I. Certified officials when possible

J. Clearing pool before each event starts

K. Giving each diver time between the announcement of a dive and its execution

L. Competition between those of similar abilities and time standards to separate abilities within an age group

M. In long-distance swimming, officials in boats following swimmers can order swimmer out of water if hypothermia is suspected.

N. Swimming officials should be alert to possibility of troubled swimmers with exercise-induced asthma, laryngospasm, or "diving reflex." Swimmers who do poorly may also have spontaneous pneumothorax or pneumonia.

O. Referees have authority to adjust, postpone, or cancel meets if conditions of the meet jeopardize the safety of the swimmers or divers.

P. Referees have authority to stop a meet when lightning or other severe weather threatens.

Q. **NOTE:** Complete rules may be obtained from the organization authorizing the competition. International competition is conducted under rules of Federation Internationale de Natation Amateur.

R. If a swimmer or diver is taking any prescribed or over-the-counter medication, make sure it is not a banned substance.

VII. Sport-specific Special Concerns of the Team Physician

A. Swimmer's shoulder
B. Swimmer's ear
C. Breaststroker's knee
D. Nutrition and hydration when dealing with long meets and multiple events per day
E. Water as the medium in which the sport takes place
F. Temperature problems ranging from hypothermia to heat stroke
G. Stretching activities specific to swimming or diving
H. Body type as predictor of success in female swimmers
I. Preparticipation physical exam—should be sport specific and include at least a 2-minute orthopedic exam

Recommended Reading

1. Ball RM: The sports participation evaluation. N J Med 88(9):629–633, 1991.
2. Bar-Or O, Inbar O: Swimming and asthma. Sports Med 14(6):397–405, 1992.
3. Burd B: Infant swimming classes: Immersed in controversy. Phys Sportsmed 14(3):238–244, 1986.
4. Davidson TM, Wolfe DP: Sunscreens, skin cancer, and your patient. Phys Sportsmed 14(8):65–79, 1986.
5. Dummer GM, Rosen LW, Heusner WW, et al: Pathogenic weight control behaviors in competitive swimmers. Phys Sportsmed 15(5):75–86, 1987.
6. Dyment PG: The orthopedic component of the preparticipation examination. Pediatr Ann 21(3):159–162, 1992.
7. Eichel BS: How I manage external otitis in competitive swimmers. Phys Sportsmed 14(8):108–116, 1986.
8. Goldstein JD, Berger PI, Windler GE, Jackson DW: Spinal injuries in gymnasts and swimmers. Am J Sports Med 19(5):463–468, 1991.
9. Higgins P, Simenski J, Pearson R: Near drowning—lap swimming [letter]. N Engl J Med 315:1551–1553, 1986.
10. Hoehelma RA: The preparticipation sports physical examination. Pediatr Ann 21(3):145–146, 1992.
11. Houmard JH, Johns RA: Effects of taper on swim performance. Sports Med 17(4):224–232, 1994.
12. le Viet DT, Lantieri LA, Loy SM: Wrist and hand injuries in platform diving. J Hand Surg 18A:876–880, 1993.
13. Levine M, Lombardo J, McNeeley J, Anderson T: An analysis of individual stretching programs of intercollegiate athletes. Phys Sportsmed 15(3):130–138, 1987.
14. Makintubee S, Millonee J, Istie G: Shigellosis outbreak associated with swimming. Am J Public Health 72:166–168, 1987.
15. McMaster WC: Painful shoulder in swimmers: A diagnostic challenge. Phys Sportsmed 14(2):108–122, 1986.
16. Peter G: Recommendations for swimming with ear infections and/or associated complications. Pediatr Infect Dis J 11(1):58–59, 1992.
17. Renneker M: Surfing: The sport and life style. Phys Sportsmed 15(10):156–162, 1987.
18. Rory S, Irvin R: Sports Medcine. Englewood Cliffs, NJ, Prentice Hall, 1983, pp 452–453.
19. Ross Laboratories: Nutrition and Hydration in Swimming: How They Can Affect Your Performance. Columbus, OH, Ross Laboratories, 1986.
20. Scvasso ML, Browne A, Pink M, et al: The painful shoulder during freestyle swimming. Am J Sports Med 19(6):577–582, 1991.
21. Selesnick H: A more comfortable cast. Phys Sportsmed 21(5):106–116, 1993.
22. Siders WA, Luhaski HC, Bolonchuk WW: Relationships among swimming performance, body composition and somatotype in competitive collegiate swimmers. J Sports Med Phys Fit 33:166–171, 1993.
23. Tonsoline PA: Chronic adductor tendinitis in a female swimmer. J Orthop Sports Phys Ther 18(5):629–633, 1993.
24. United States Swimming's Sports Medicine Informational Series: Diarrhea (#6). Colorado Springs, U.S. Swimming, 1987.
25. United States Swimming's Sports Medicine Informational Series: Eat to Compete (#2). Colorado Springs, U.S. Swimming, 1987.
26. United States Swimming's Sports Medicine Informational Series: Exercise Induced Asthma and the Competitive Swimmer (#3). Colorado Springs, U.S. Swimming, 1987.
27. United States Swimming's Sports Medicine Informational Series:Nutrition and Competition (#1). Colorado Springs, U.S. Swimming, 1985.
28. United States Swimming's Sports Medicine Informational Series: Strength Training for Age Group and Senior Swimmers. Colorado Springs, U.S. Swimming, 1985.
29. United States Swimming's Sports Medicine Informational Series: Swimmer's Ear (#8). Colorado Springs, U.S. Swimming, 1985.
30. United States Swimming's Sports Medicine Informational Series: Swimmer's Shoulder and Rehabilitation (#7). Colorado Springs, U.S. Swimming, 1985.
31. United States Swimming's Sports Medicine Informational Series: Training Considerations for the Female Athlete (#3). Colorado Springs, U.S. Swimming, 1985.
32. United States Swimming's Sports Medicine Informational Series: Training Concepts for the Age Group Swimmer (#4). Colorado Springs, U.S. Swimming, 1985.
33. United States Swimming's Sports Medicine Informational Series: Travel and Competition (#5). Colorado Springs, U.S. Swimming, 1985.

60

Baseball and Softball

Turner A. Blackburn, Jr., M.Ed., PT, ATC

I. Overview

A. Extremely popular sports—large number of participants at many levels
   1. Professional
   2. Amateur
   3. Recreational

B. Classified as "limited contact impact" sports

C. Common types of injuries
   1. High-speed collisions
      a. Between players
      b. With fences and other equipment
      c. Ball striking player
      d. Bat striking player
   2. Running injuries
   3. Throwing injuries

II. Biomechanical and Pathomechanical Considerations in Baseball and Softball

A. **Biomechanics of overhand throwing.** Efficient throwing depends on a coordinated **transfer of momentum** (momentum = mass × velocity) from larger, slower body segments to segments of smaller mass that can move faster, thus imparting a **high velocity** to the ball (in excess of 95 mph) at ball release.
   1. **Wind-up phase* establishes the rhythm**—variable among pitchers (Fig. 1A)
      a. Initiated by first movement of pitcher, usually with a downward swing of the arms, which are then raised overhead (**gathered position**)
      b. Weight shifts forward on the right foot and then back to the left foot during arm swing
      c. Shoulders and hips rotate as arms go overhead, body shifts from facing the batter to being perpendicular to the line of throw
      d. Right foot must move from its perpendicular position on top of the rubber to a position parallel to the rubber and just in front of it
      e. Pitcher must maintain balance on "stance leg" (right leg) as the "stride leg" (left leg) goes in the air, hip and knee flexed at approximately chest-high level
      f. Spine flexes with leftward rotation
      g. **Wind-up phase ends when the hands come apart from the gathered position**
      h. Wind-up lets pitcher hide the ball
      i. Lasts anywhere from 0.5 to 1.3 seconds
      j. Sequence is as follows: initiation, pivot foot, gather
      k. **Wind-up from the stretch**

* Description of phases assumes right-handed pitcher.

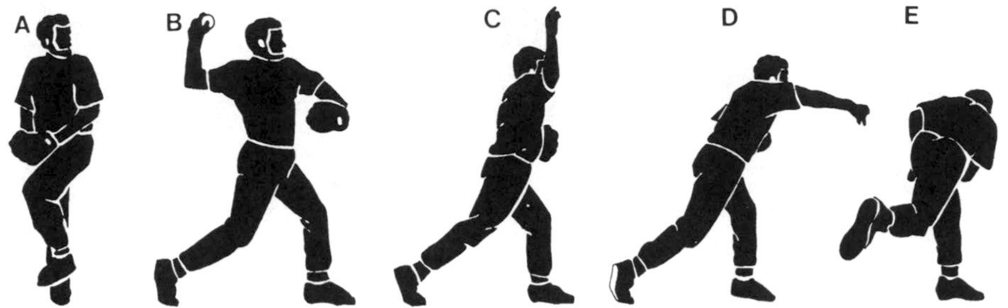

FIGURE 1. Phases of the overhand throw: **A**, Windup. **B**, Cocking, late phase before maximum external rotation. **C**, Late acceleration, near ball release. **D**, Deceleration. **E**, Follow-through.

   i. Used when runner is on base
   ii. Eliminates the first half of the wind-up
   iii. Pitcher may lose some rhythm

2. **Cocking phase** (Fig. 1B)
   a. Begins at hands apart
   b. Ends when the right arm is at its most extreme external rotation
   c. **Early cocking**
      i. Stride leg extends forward as the hips begin to derotate or "open up." Center of gravity is moved forward by the stance or "push" leg (takes approximately 0.5 second).
      ii. Right arm moves into external rotation and horizontal abduction:
         (a) Rotator cuff stabilizes humeral head and externally rotates humerus
         (b) Scapulothoracic muscles stabilize scapula
         (c) Posterior deltoid pulls humerus into horizontal abduction
      iii. Anterior chest muscles and humeral internal rotators are put on stretch:
         (a) Pectoralis major and minor
         (b) Latissimus dorsi
         (c) Subscapularis
         (d) Teres major
   d. **Late cocking**
      i. Stance leg pushes center of gravity forward
      ii. Stride leg plants with foot parallel to line to plate and just left of center. Quadriceps, hamstrings, and hip extensors decelerate the body from rotation and forward motion. **This allows the momentum transfer to begin its progression proximally through the trunk to the arm.**
      iii. Shoulder reaches maximum amount of external rotation/horizontal abduction, **"winding" the glenohumeral joint capsule like a spring** (Fig. 2A)
      iv. The glenohumeral joint is at approximately 90° abduction and 25–30° horizontal abduction. The wrist is supinated. The spine is hyperextended, and the elbow is flexed to approximately 90°.
3. **Acceleration phase** (Fig. 1C)
   a. Begins when the ball moves forward
   b. Ends when the ball is released
   c. **High constant forces** develop through momentum transfer from trunk to arm as glenohumeral capsule "unwinds"
   d. Occurs in approximately 0.1 second
   e. Burst of muscle action occurs:
      i. Latissimus

   ii. Pectoralis major and minor
   iii. Serratus anterior (to stabilize the scapula)
   iv. Triceps

f. Two distinct motions occur at the shoulder during the acceleration phase:
   i. Horizontal adduction (40 msec)
   ii. Internal rotation (40 msec); occurs at an angular velocity of approximately 6000° per second

g. The triceps extends the elbow from 90° to 25° at approximately 7000° per second. Valgus stress occurs across the elbow (Fig. 2B), stressing the anterior band of the ulnar collateral ligament and the origin of the flexor mass. The radiohumeral joint and olecranon fossa are compressed.

h. Pathomechanics during acceleration:
   i. **Midshaft spiral humeral fractures**—infrequent
   ii. **Muscle strains:** Muscles produce high forces, attempt to control high forces, protect the anterior capsule, and decelerate the arm.
      (a) Pectoralis major
      (b) Latissimus dorsi
      (c) Subscapularis
      (d) Biceps
      (e) Supraspinatus
      (f) Infraspinatus
   iii. **Glenohumeral joint laxity:**
      (a) **Extreme external rotation and horizontal abduction** of the glenohumeral joint stretches the anterior capsule and can cause anterior subluxation during the cocking phase.
      (b) **High force production by the accelerator muscles and the body's momentum** also stresses the anterior capsule during the acceleration phase. If there is joint laxity, the humeral head subluxes forward pulling the supraspinatus and infraspinatus tendons into the acromial arch and causing secondary impingement symptoms.

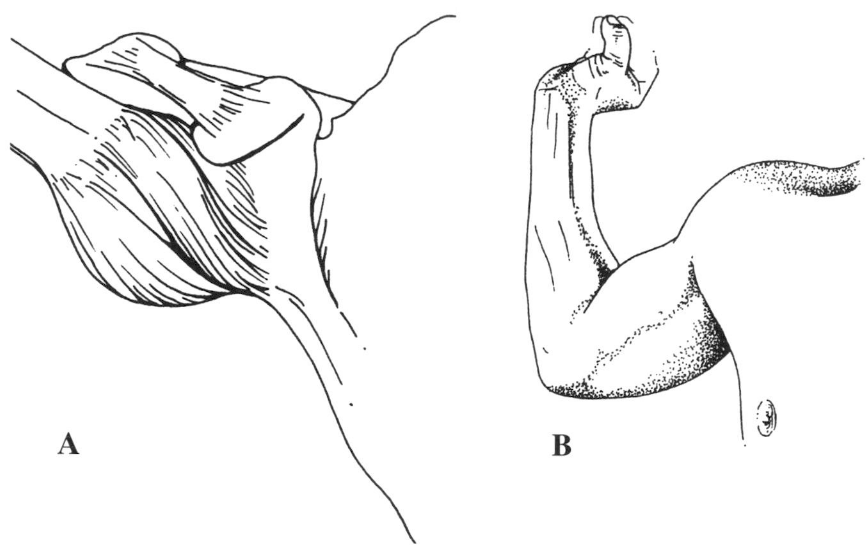

FIGURE 2. **A**, "Winding" of anterior capsule with external rotation and horizontal abduction during cocking phase. **B**, Valgus stress on the elbow during acceleration.

(c) **"Opening up too soon"** can aggravate this type of problem.
(d) **High, rapidly changing forces** during the deceleration phase stress the posterior capsule. The posterior rotator cuff is subject to high stress when stabilizing the humeral head, especially if there is posterior capsular laxity.

iv. **Superior glenoid labrum lesion:**
(a) **Laxity of the anterior capsule** allows the humeral head to sublux anteriorly and abrade the labrum, causing breakdown.
(b) **"Labrum grinding factor"** created by **internal rotation** and **horizontal abduction** of the humeral head may cause abrasion (grinding) of the labrum even in a stable shoulder.

4. **Release arc**
   a. Hand is moving at the speed of the pitch at release
   b. Ball must be released at a **critical point** to be effective
   c. Muscles about the shoulder are relatively quiet by electromyographic measurements at release
   d. Stride leg continues to decelerate trunk momentum
   e. **Variations in release:**

i. **"Bull whip" release**
(a) **Causes:**
- Pitcher locks stride leg in recurvatum rather than allowing it to flex
- This decelerates forward momentum to create trunk rotation and extra "whipping" motion through rest of body to the arm

(b) **Results of bull whip release:**
- Impact forces transmitted through lower extremity and pelvis
- Increased derotation forces at pelvis
- Increased stress on the shoulder during acceleration
- May lead to injury

ii. **Opening up too soon**
(a) **Causes:**
- Squaring shoulders to batter too soon before release
- Hips derotated too quickly
- Stride too short
- Stride leg too far left of midline
- Hip and knee of stride leg not flexed adequately during late cocking
- Rushing a pitch

(b) **Results of opening up too soon:**
- Arm lags behind body at release
- Increased stress on anterior shoulder and medial elbow during acceleration
- Elbow drops toward side while pitcher attempts to locate proper release point
- Increased injury potential

iii. **Opening up too late**
(a) **Causes:**
- Squaring shoulders to batter too late
- Stride leg too far right of midline
- Hips derotated too slowly

(b) **Results of opening up too late:**
- Arm ahead of body at release
- Body loses momentum
- Decreases effectiveness
- Relatively few injuries result

5. **Deceleration** (Fig. 1D)
   a. Begins at ball release
   b. Ends after strongest contraction phase of the rotator cuff muscles
   c. Strong but variable forces put on the posterior rotator cuff
   d. Posterior rotator cuff must slow the 6000–7000° per second internal rotation and horizontal adduction of humerus
   e. Stride leg aids in deceleration
   f. Biceps decelerates elbow extension and stabilizes anterior capsule
   g. **Scapulothoracic muscles are important during this phase for stabilizing the scapula, controlling scapula protraction, and providing a stable base** for the rotator cuff to decelerate the arm.
   h. **Pathomechanics during deceleration:**
      i. **Muscle strains**
         (a) **Posterior rotator cuff:**
            - High deceleration forces required of these small muscles cause breakdown in the tendons of the rotator cuff near their humeral attachment usually on the undersurface.
            - Pain causes the thrower to decrease speed because deceleration from higher speed cannot be tolerated.
         (b) **Biceps:**
            - Biceps **control deceleration of the elbow** via forces on its origin at the glenoid fossa and attachments to the glenoid labrum. The biceps tendon may also become inflamed.
            - **A weak rotator cuff** forces the biceps tendon to work harder during deceleration, causing more irritation to the biceps tendon and usually a rotator cuff problem as well.
      ii. **Glenoid labrum** may tear or degenerate because of deceleration forces and perhaps "shoulder grinding factor," especially if rotator cuff or biceps is weak or there is capsular instability
6. **Follow-through** (Fig. 1E)
   a. Begins following strongest contraction phase of the rotator cuff muscles
   b. Ends when stance or "push leg" or "trailing leg" contacts the ground
   c. Completes dissipation of the momentum of throwing motion
   d. Puts body in a position to field batted balls
7. **Types of deliveries.** All show glenohumeral joint to be at about 90° of abduction. The degree of **body lean** affects the way the delivery appears.
   a. **Overhead:**
      i. Similar to outfielder's throw
      ii. Better use of body
      iii. Mechanically allows for higher velocity with less prime mover activity and gives a much longer lever arm
      iv. Curve ball is much more deceptive because of angle of delivery
      v. More **control problems** with this type of pitch
   b. **Three-quarters:**
      i. Shorter lever arm—prime movers do more work
      ii. Flatter trajectory, so curve ball is not so deceptive
      iii. Pitcher usually has **better control**
   c. **Sidearm:**
      i. Increased elbow valgus stress and anterior shoulder stress
      ii. More "drag"—relies on whipping motion
      iii. Pitch is flat—easier to hit
      iv. Associated with more injuries

8. **Pathomechanics of overhand throwing**
   a. Most throwing injuries occur over a period of time and are termed **overuse injuries.**
   b. **Any factor** (sprained ankle, patellar tendinitis, low back dysfunction, shoulder pain, coaching, etc.) **that changes the form, rhythm, coordination, and timing of a pitcher can cause injury to the throwing arm.**

B. **Biomechanics of underhand pitching.** Little research has been done on the underhand fast pitch motion. **Few career-ending injuries** occur with this type of pitch, possibly explaining the lack of research. The **rotator cuff is not loaded** as it is in the overhand pitch, and **extreme external rotation is avoided.** The **anterior capsule** is not stressed as much as it is in the overhand pitch. **The medial elbow is stressed.**

1. **Wind-up and cocking:**
   a. Stride leg moves forward while stance leg pushes body forward
   b. Glenohumeral joint moves in arc of flexion, abduction, and then extension
   c. Radius and form of arc vary with pitcher's style
2. **Acceleration** begins with forward motion of the ball:
   a. Shoulder flexors, depressors, and horizontal adductors provide for speed of arm into the forward-flexed position. Muscles involved:
      i. Pectoralis major and minor
      ii. Subscapularis
      iii. Deltoid
   b. At the elbow and shoulder, the biceps contracts to propel the ball forward.
3. **Release** occurs in front of body
4. **Deceleration**—forces here are much **less stressful**, and the position of the arm allows **larger muscles** to absorb the shock:
   a. Triceps
   b. Latissimus dorsi
   c. Posterior rotator cuff
   d. Teres major
   e. Posterior deltoid
5. **Follow-through** puts body in position to field ball

C. **Biomechanics of sliding.** Sliding allows the base runner to reach a base (other than running from the batter's box to first base, usually!) at the fastest possible speed without going past the base and allows the runner to be as small a target as possible to prevent being tagged.

1. **Feet first:** runner slides in on either the right or left side, according to preference. The right-sided slide is described here. For left-sided slide, right and left designations are reversed.
   a. Right-sided slide has the runner flexing right knee as much as 90°
   b. Feet-first slide is timed to allow left foot to touch the base first. Sliding forces are usually absorbed over entire right thigh.
   c. Variations:
      i. **"Pop-up slide"**
         (a) Runner's weight never transfers entirely to thigh, but stays at leading edge of the **flexed shin and knee**
         (b) This allows runner to quickly assume a standing and running position
      ii. **Hook slide**
         (a) Runner attempts to slide away from area of base or plate where thrown ball may arrive, to avoid the tag
         (b) Runner is usually outside of direct path to base, but must still make contact with left foot during slide past base and deceleration

d. **Injuries**
   i. Abrasions
   ii. Cleat laceration to ankle and shin of opposing player as the player tries to make the tag
   iii. Fractures, dislocations, and sprains of runner's and possibly opposing player's foot or ankle
   iv. Ball striking player

2. **Head first**
   a. Many believe that this technique is a bit **faster** than the feet first slide.
   b. Landing occurs on the chest, with head up and arms outstretched.
   c. An even **smaller target** is available for the tag.
   d. **Injuries:**
      i. Abrasions
      ii. **Head and neck** much **more exposed** to injury from collision and from being hit by the ball
      iii. **Hands and fingers** at greater risk of injury by cleats and collisions

III. Common Injuries in Baseball and Softball

A. **Lacerations and abrasions**—etiology
   1. Sliding
   2. Spikes
   3. Field/stadium disrepair
   4. Collisions

B. **Ankle and foot injuries**
   1. **Types**
      a. Various fractures
      b. Medial and lateral sprains
      c. Contusions
      d. Great toe dysfunction in pitchers
   2. **Etiology**
      a. Sliding
      b. Running
      c. Ball impact
      d. Bases
      e. Pitching from mound

C. **Contusions/myositis ossificans**—etiology
   1. Collision between players
   2. Ball striking a player
   3. Collision with other objects

D. **Muscle strains**—etiology
   1. Inadequate conditioning
      a. Strength
      b. Flexibility
      c. Endurance
   2. Inadequate warm-up and maintenance of warm-up
   3. Overuse

E. **Knee injuries**—etiology
   1. Usual causes as in other running and contact sports
   2. Impact with baseball environment (bases, sprinklers, fences, grandstand, etc.)
   3. Cleats and spikes allow for more foot fixation, increased risk of knee injury

F. **Lumbosacral dysfunction**—etiology
   1. Injury rate not unusually high versus other sports

2. Pitching: sacroiliac joint and lumbar facets stressed
   a. Rotational components of the pitching act
   b. Height of pitching mound
   c. Landing forces on front leg

G. **Head and face injuries**—etiology
   1. Swinging bats
   2. Thrown and batted balls

IV. Management of Throwing Arm Injuries

A. **General considerations**
   1. Rather than simply treating the symptoms, a **careful clinical and biomechanical evaluation** of the athlete helps the examiner define the nature and cause of the injury. Basic treatment principles, modalities, rest, and rehabilitation are called for (see Chapter 38, "Comprehensive Rehabilitation of the Athlete"). Emphasis should be placed on the total athlete. Cardiovascular fitness, lower body strength and flexibility, and reconditioning of the throwing arm are essential to successful treatment and rehabilitation. The following sections focus on major injuries to the throwing arm that do not resolve with a few days of care.
   2. **An interval throwing program** provides a **gradual** increase in throwing intensity at a controlled pace based on symptoms (Table 1).

B. **Rotator cuff injuries** can vary from a mild case of tendinitis to partial- or full-thickness tears.
   1. **Etiology**
      a. Overuse
      b. Change in mechanics
      c. Weakness in rotator cuff
      d. Anterior capsular laxity

TABLE 1. Interval Throwing Program

Each phase consists of several throwing sessions. The athlete should work up to the parameters within each phase. Generally, the athlete throws daily. However, if soreness or stiffness develops after a throwing session and persists, then the next session should be reduced or skipped. Progression to the subsequent phase is based on achieving the phase goals without any symptoms.

Session sequence:

___ Warm-up (break sweat, stretch, "soft-toss" 10–15 feet until loose, work to long-toss distance)
___ Long-toss interval
___ Short-toss interval
___ Rest 10–30 minutes
___ Repeat warm-up
___ Long-toss interval
___ Short-toss interval
___ Cool-down (stretch, ice, monitor symptoms)

	Long-toss interval		Short-toss interval		
Phase	Distance (feet)	# throws*	Distance (feet)	# throws*	Speed/Pitch Type/Surface
1	90	25	30	50	½, straight, flat
2	120	25	60	50	½, straight, flat
3	150	25	60	50	¾, straight, flat
4	180	25	60	50	¾, straight, mound
4	210	25	60	50	½–¾, breaking, mound
6	240	25	60+	50	¾–full, all, mound
7	Work to game situations; number of pitches in game situation should be increased as able; monitor mechanics and accuracy (85% of pitches should be strikes)				

* In each phase, prescribed number of throws should be completed within a 5-minute time period.

2. **Symptoms**
   a. Pain when trying to pitch intensely, generally in the early phase of deceleration:
      i. May or may not have pain at rest or night
      ii. May have trouble even warming up when problem becomes severe
   b. Often the injury pattern falls into one of injury, rest, and return to full play, then reinjury, rest, return to full play, and so on. It may take the athlete 6–12 months before medical help is sought and a good diagnosis is made.
3. **Examination** (see Chapter 43, "Shoulder Injuries")
   a. **Weakness (and sometimes pain)** to manual muscle testing:
      i. Supraspinatus—"empty can" position
      ii. External rotation at 90° abduction
      iii. Abduction at 90°
      iv. External rotation at 0° abduction
   b. **Impingement tests:**
      i. Neer
      ii. Hawkins
   c. Pain on palpation of rotator cuff
   d. External rotation and abduction demonstrate increase in pain
   e. Biceps tendon and coracoid process tender to palpation
   f. Slow-motion analysis of throwing on video tape to identify **mechanical flaws**
   g. Relocation test
   h. Radiographic and other imaging techniques
4. **Differential diagnosis**
   a. Biceps tendinitis
   b. Glenoid labrum tear
   c. Subdeltoid bursitis
5. **Treatment**
   a. Rest: 1–6 weeks, depending on severity
   b. Modalities:
      i. Ice
      ii. Ultrasound
      iii. Electrical stimulation
      iv. Phonophoresis
      v. Iontophoresis
      vi. Anti-inflammatory medication
   c. Therapeutic exercise program based on physical exam
      i. Strength
      ii. Flexibility
   d. Surgery—**only after exhaustive conservative care:**
      i. Arthroscopic evaluation of the rotator cuff as well as the subdeltoid bursa. In partial tears, debridement of the lesion may be performed. If there are acromial abnormalities, acromioplasty may be performed.
      ii. **Difficult to return to competitive level after open surgery because of scarring**
   e. Return to throwing (see Table 1 and Chapter 38, "Comprehensive Rehabilitation of the Athlete")
6. **Prognosis**
   a. Tendinitis should clear with proper care.
   b. Partial and complete lesions of the rotator cuff may need surgical treatment and then a good rehabilitation and return to throwing program.
   c. May take a year, even with surgery, for complete return.

C. **Glenoid labrum injuries.** Injury to the anterior-superior glenoid labrum **does not result in glenohumeral instability**, as seen in anterior dislocations when the anterior-inferior glenoid labrum is torn. Occasionally, the posterior-superior labrum is damaged with overuse.

1. **Etiology**
   a. Falls on outstretched arm
   b. Anterior or posterior instabilities
   c. Rotator cuff weakness
   d. Heavy weight training
   e. Throwing technique changes
   f. Batting
   g. Shoulder grinding factor
2. **Symptoms**
   a. **Pain during acceleration phase** of throwing:
      i. Unable to move the arm briskly through full range of motion while throwing
      ii. Once through painful area (painful arc), it no longer hurts
   b. Usually no pain at rest and no night pain
   c. No swelling evident
   d. Biceps tendinitis possible
   e. History—either a one-pitch episode or a gradual buildup
3. **Examination**
   a. Pain with **overpressure in horizontal adduction** takes joint into extreme of motion, stressing joint capsule and creating joint compression, which may trap torn labrum and cause discomfort.
   b. **Labrum "clunk" test**—shoulder in external rotation and abduction, forcing an anterior and posterior motion of the humerus in an attempt to catch the torn labrum between the bony segments and create a "clunk." Athlete may have more pain with forced external rotation at 90° abduction than in a more abducted position.
   c. Palpation of biceps tendon
4. **Differential diagnosis**
   a. Rotator cuff tendinitis and tears (often seen in conjunction with one another)
   b. Biceps tendinitis
   c. Abnormal joint laxity
5. **Treatment**
   a. Rest for 7–10 days
   b. Therapeutic exercise program
   c. Review mechanics of throwing
   d. Modalities and medication not much help
   e. Return to throwing
   f. **Surgery after failure of exhaustive conservative care:**
      i. Arthroscopic debridement of superior labrum
      ii. Tendon of the long head of the biceps may be involved
6. **Prognosis**
   a. Conservative treatment may work in the majority of cases.
   b. Two to 6 weeks may be required of a rehabilitation program.
   c. If arthroscopic debridement is performed, throwing may start in 2–3 weeks, with full play by 12 weeks if all goes well.

D. **Anterior glenohumeral joint laxity**

1. **Etiology**
   a. Repetitive throwing
   b. Poor mechanics
   c. Trauma
   d. Congenital

2. **Symptoms**
   a. Pain during acceleration
   b. Impingement symptoms
   c. Inability to throw hard because of pain
3. **Examination**
   a. Relocation test
   b. Various laxity tests
   c. Overall body laxity tests
   d. May have labrum and rotator cuff pathology
4. **Differential diagnosis**
   a. Rotator cuff pathology
   b. Labrum tear
5. **Treatment**
   a. Rest
   b. Therapeutic exercise program with dynamic stability emphasis
   c. Review of mechanics
   d. Return to throwing
   e. Surgery:
      i. Arthroscopic debridement of rotator cuff and labrum
      ii. Open anterior capsule reefing and aggressive postoperative care, so athlete can regain full range of motion and return to throwing
6. **Prognosis:** more difficult to return from surgery to full potential

E. **Valgus extension overload of the elbow:** injuries to ulnar nerve, wrist flexor mass origin, medial elbow ligaments, radiocapitellar joint, and olecranon fossa.
1. **Causes**
   a. **Poor mechanics:**
      i. Opening up too soon
      ii. Bull whip release
   b. Overuse
   c. Occurs during **acceleration phase**
2. **Symptoms**
   a. Ulnar nerve:
      i. Transient radiating pain is present in early phase.
      ii. In chronic cases, pain is more constant.
   b. Wrist flexors—pain at medial epicondyle at rest and during performance, depending on severity
   c. Elbow medial compartment laxity—instability during the throwing act
   d. Osteochondritis dissecans may develop at radiocapitellar joint:
      i. Pain at joint on throwing
      ii. Locking and clicking
   e. Olecranon fossa degeneration:
      i. Pain on medial side of joint
      ii. Spur formation
      iii. Loss of extension in chronic cases
3. **Examination**
   a. Ulnar nerve:
      i. Positive Tinel's sign
      ii. Sensory changes to pinprick in hypothenar eminence
      iii. Tenderness over ulnar groove
      iv. Electromyography/nerve conduction velocity changes
   b. Wrist flexors:
      i. Weakness of grip

   ii. Pain or weakness on manual muscle testing of the wrist flexors
   iii. Pain to palpation of medial epicondyle area
  c. Medial compartment laxity:
   i. Opening on valgus stress test
   ii. Tenderness over medial collateral ligament
  d. Radiocapitellar joint:
   i. X-ray findings
   ii. Loss of extension

4. **Differential diagnosis.** Flexor mass pain and medial ligament pain are similar; care must be taken in palpation to discern between the two.
5. **Treatment**
  a. Acute:
   i. Relative rest
   ii. Modalities
   iii. Therapeutic exercise program
   iv. Return to throwing program
  b. Chronic:
   i. Arthroscopic surgery for loose body removal, radiocapitellar debridement, and posterior olecranon spur debridement:
    (a) Begin range-of-motion and strengthening program immediately.
    (b) Begin return to throwing program at 6 weeks. May take 6 months before full return.
   ii. Open surgery for medial ligament reconstruction and posterior olecranon spur excision:
    (a) 10 days immobilization
    (b) Cast brace at 30–90° until 6 weeks
    (c) At 6 weeks, aggressive range-of-motion and strengthening program
    (d) Return to throwing program
    (e) Full play at 6–12 months after surgery
6. **Prognosis**
  a. **If this problem is identified early, mechanical problems are corrected,** and the overuse situation is changed, it should clear easily.
  b. **When allowed to progress, it can become quite difficult to manage.** Surgical intervention may allow the athlete to return to play, but **advancement in the sport may not be possible.** That much stress may still cause problems at the elbow.

V. Prevention of Injuries

A. Proper conditioning

1. Off-season programs
  a. Aerobic foundation
  b. General strengthening
  c. Flexibility
  d. Isolated rotator cuff and scapular stabilizer exercises (Fig. 3)
  e. Throwing program
2. In-season program, maintenance program
  a. Running—anaerobic training
  b. Isolated rotator cuff and scapular stabilizer exercises
  c. Flexibility:
   i. Hamstrings
   ii. Gastrocnemius
   iii. Quadriceps

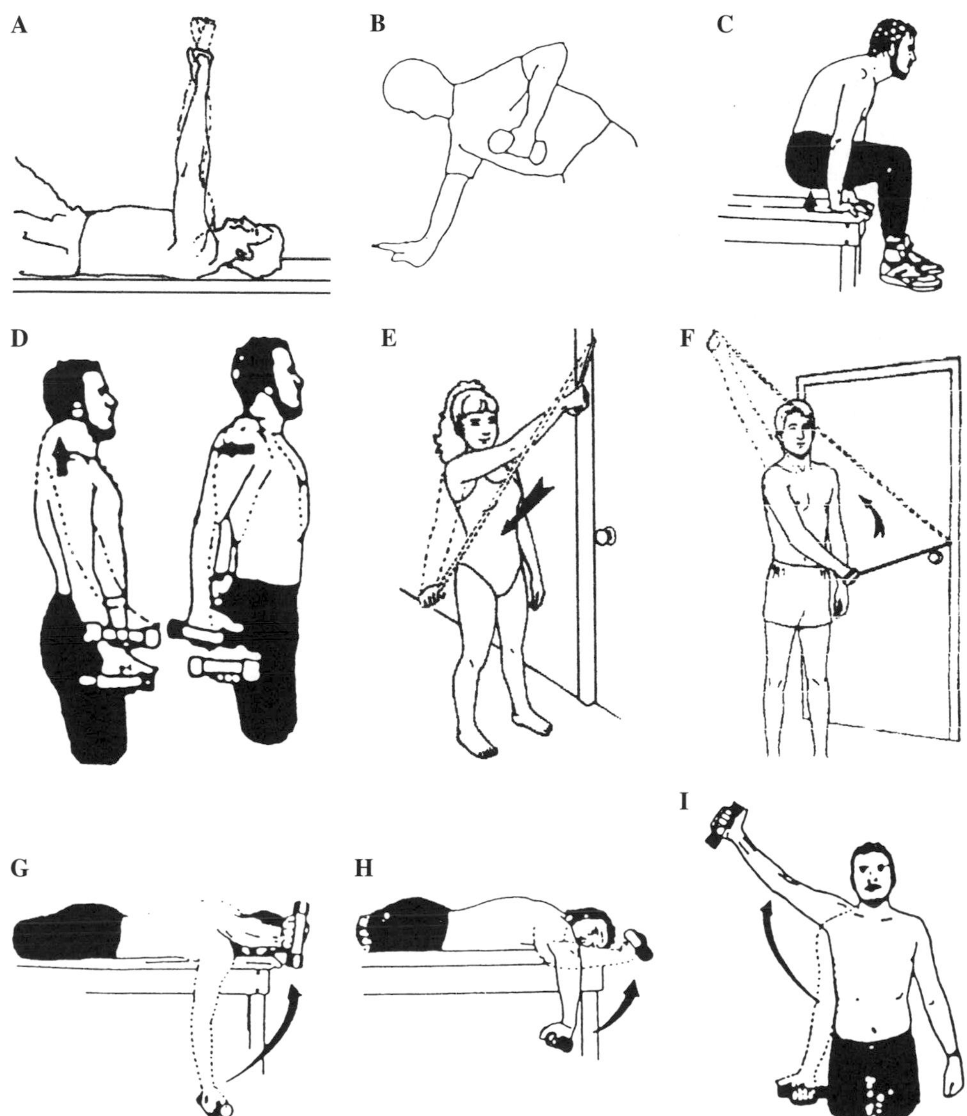

FIGURE 3. Core scapula and rotator cuff exercises—"Voight's Majik Three" (three positions, three exercises, three sets). **A**, Shoulder punches for serratus anterior. **B**, Bent row for posterior scapula stabilization. **C**, Sitting dip, also for scapula stabilization. **D**, Shoulder shrugs with scapular retraction for trapezius. **E**, D–1 PNF with rubber tubing for coordinated neuromuscular training to shoulder girdle. **F**, D–2 PNF. **G**, Prone horizontal abduction for supraspinatus. **H**, Prone external rotation for infraspinatus and teres minor. **I**, Arm elevation for scapula stabilization.

iv. Rectus femoris
v. Spine
vi. Elbow **"Super 7"** exercises
  (a) Wrist extension
  (b) Wrist flexion
  (c) Pronation/supination
  (d) Biceps curl

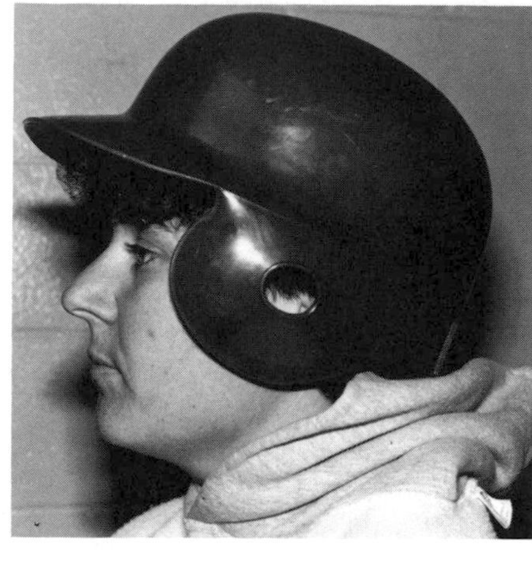

FIGURE 4. Batting helmet.

(e) Triceps curl
(f) Stretch extensors/flexors
(g) Grip

3. **Recreational** softball and baseball participants often have a **poor level of conditioning.**

B. **Technique training is important. Emphasis should be put on proper mechanics.**
   1. Pitching instruction
   2. Batting
   3. Sliding

C. **Overuse**
   1. Base young players' pitching limits on **pitches thrown** (games and practices), not on innings thrown.
   2. Coaches must pay particular attention to pitchers, no matter at what level.

D. **Umpires:** Conscientious and quality umpiring cuts down on injuries.

E. **Playing surfaces**
   1. Warning track located between field and fences

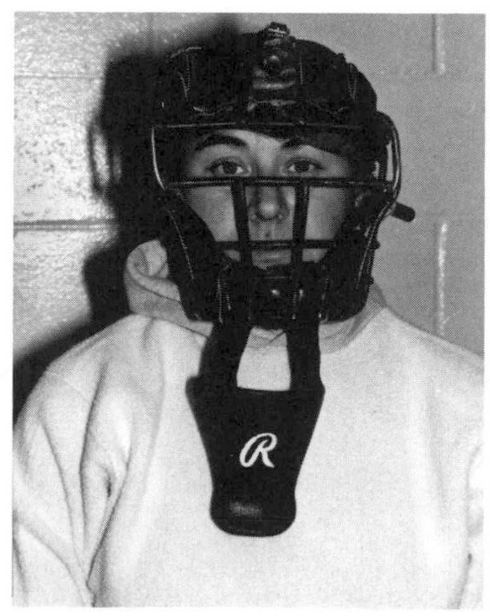

FIGURE 5. Face mask with throat protector.

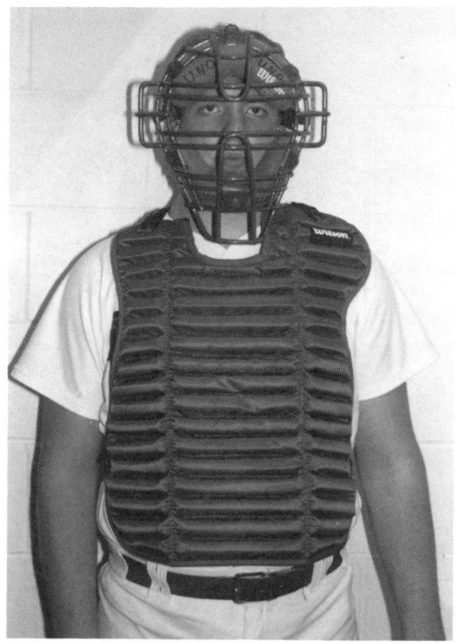

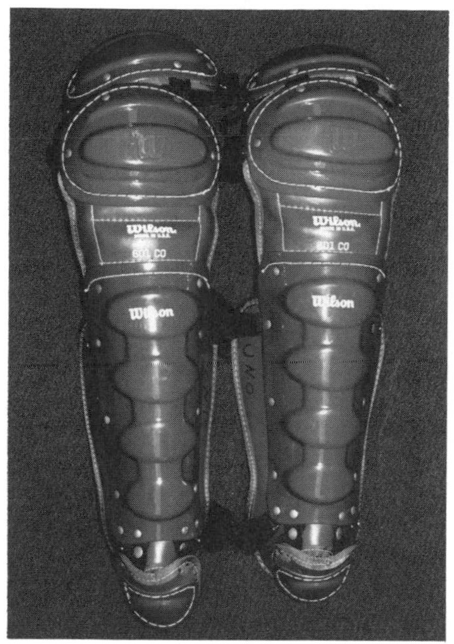

FIGURE 6 *(Left).* Face mask with metal extension throat protector and padded chest protector.
FIGURE 7 *(Right).* Rigid shin guards.

2. Fencing around entire field in good repair and **padded** where appropriate
3. Line markings not of lime (irritates eyes and skin)
4. Batter's box and pitcher's mound kept in good repair
5. Smooth infield
6. Breakaway bases to decrease sliding injuries
7. Appropriate screening to protect fans

F. **Equipment**

1. Batting helmets (Fig. 4)
   a. Jaw and ear protection
   b. Plastic eye guards
2. Metal or hard plastic cup inside athletic supporter
3. Nonmetal spikes/soccer-style shoes
4. Batting gloves
5. Sliding pads to prevent abrasions ("strawberries")
6. Ankle and shin protectors for catchers and those with injuries
7. Catcher's and umpire's protective equipment—face mask equipped with throat protector (Fig. 5), chest protector (Fig. 6), and shin guards (Fig. 7)
8. Trunk protectors for batters in youth leagues
9. Sunglasses
10. Sunscreen
11. Unbreakable aluminum bats to reduce injury potential
12. Toe guard to prevent pitchers from damaging shoes and possibly their toes

G. **Other problems in baseball and softball**

1. Oral cancer from chewing tobacco
2. Blisters on fingertips of pitchers

61

Track and Field

Margot Putukian, M.D., FACSM

I. Overview

A. History of track and field dates back to ancient times.
   1. Ancient Greeks believed in a "whole man" concept—development of the body as well as the mind and soul.
   2. Involvement in running, jumping, and throwing sports trained individuals for combat. Track and field events such as javelin, discus, and running parallel war activities and emphasize both strength and accuracy.

B. Track and field often attracts multisport athletes.

C. Year-round competition and training

D. Events
   1. Different demands depending on nature of event in which athlete participates. Changes the types of training as well as types of injuries commonly seen.
   2. Explosive events, power events, and endurance events
      a. Sprints (100 m, 200 m, 400 m)
      b. Middle distance (800 m, 1500 m)
      c. Distance (3000 m; 5000 m; 10,000 m; marathon)
      d. 100 hurdles, 400 hurdles
      e. Relays (4 × 100 m, 800 m, 4 × 400 m, 4 × 800 m, 4 × 1500 m, distance medley, sprint medley)
      f. Long jumps
      g. High jump
      h. Triple jump
      i. Shot put
      j. Javelin
      k. Discus
      l. Hammer
      m. Heptathlon
      n. Decathlon
      o. Pole vault
      p. Steeplechase

II. Statistics

A. Difficult to look at injury statistics given lack of denominator (player hours or athlete exposures) as well as variability in methodology of studies

B. No National Collegiate Athletic Association (NCAA) data collected for track and field

C. 35% of participants in the 1985 Junior Track Olympics reported need for performance-related medical treatment.

D. In general, **most injuries are overuse injuries that occur during training.**

1. Acute injuries often muscle strains or avulsions, or completion of stress fractures; other acute injuries uncommon
2. Majority of injuries involve lower extremities
3. Some risk for head or neck injury during high jump; risk of blunt trauma with javelin, hammer, discus
4. Of particular concern are acute medical problems such as cardiovascular collapse secondary to underlying cardiac problem, dehydration, or other abnormalities related to environmental conditions. Medical concerns otherwise primarily related to chronic training.

E. **Site of injury**
1. **Knee most common site of injury in runners,** constituting 48% of all injuries
2. Lower leg 20%
3. Foot 17%
4. Hip 6%
5. Upper leg and thigh 4%
6. Lower back 4%

F. **Specific diagnoses**
1. Anterior knee pain accounts for 24% of running injuries in men and 30% of running injuries in women
2. Medial tibial stress syndrome 7.2% of injuries in men and 11.4% in women
3. Iliotibial band syndrome 7.2% of injuries in men and 7.9% in women
4. Patellar tendinitis 5.1% of injuries in men and 3.1% in women
5. Metatarsal stress syndrome 3.1% of injuries in men and 3.8% in women
6. Achilles tendinitis 4.7% of injuries in men and 27% in women

III. Medical Problems

A. **Preparticipation physical examination**
1. Stress importance of cardiac, musculoskeletal, and neurologic systems.
2. History of sudden cardiac death, Marfan's syndrome, hypertrophic cardiomyopathy, or premature atherosclerotic disease
3. Screen for possible anatomic abnormalities that may predispose to injury; consider orthotics and flexibility/strengthening program.
4. Assess for nutritional or training errors.
5. Rule out significant medical or orthopedic problem that would preclude activity or require restrictions.
6. In female athletes, special attention to menstrual dysfunction, potential for eating disorders, stress fractures (see Female athlete triad, page 747).

B. **Nutrition issues.** Sports nutrition is an area of increased interest. Important to consider nutrition when an athlete presents with symptoms of fatigue, burnout, or recurrent minor injuries.
1. Ideal nutritional intake:
   a. 6–10 g carbohydrate/kg body weight
   b. 0.8–1.5 g protein/kg body weight
   c. Remainder of calories from fat
2. This translates into a diet of 60–70% carbohydrate, 10–15% protein, and 25–30% fat. More recently, protein component increased to 20–25%, and fat decreased to 10–15%.
3. If an athlete eats adequate caloric intake from a variety of wholesome foods, nutritional needs are met. Proper food selection, not supplementation, is the ideal form of nutrition.
4. **Iron deficiency** is common in young athletes. Iron loss can be due to hemolysis with hemoglobinuria, gastrointestinal losses, and loss of iron through excessive sweating. Female athletes at increased risk because of additional loss that occurs

with menses. Athletes not immune from other medical problems; thus complete workup of iron-deficient athlete important.

a. Iron deficiency or decreased iron stores can occur without anemia in as many as 9.5–57% of athletes, depending on study.
b. Girls, more than boys, take in less than the recommended dietary allowance (RDA) of 18 mg/day of iron.
c. Pseudoanemia: increase in plasma volume of 6–25% with training results in hemoglobin and hematocrit appearing falsely low
d. Screening hemoglobin with follow-up ferritin reasonable for assessing iron deficiency. Ferritin is storage form of iron, but can be falsely elevated in acute inflammation (is an acute phase reactant) and can be decreased with high-intensity training. Iron and total iron binding capacity can also be helpful in differentiating pseudoanemia from true anemia.
e. Supplementation of 324 mg ferrous gluconate two to three times daily if truly iron deficient. Intake of iron-rich foods important as well as adequate vitamin C intake. Daily multivitamin with iron otherwise reasonable supplement.

5. **Calories:** adequate total caloric intake obviously essential, yet often neglected
   a. In attempt to eat "healthy," many athletes restrict fat intake, such that fat-soluble vitamins also at risk for being deficient
   b. Some athletes experiment with caloric restriction as a means of affecting body weight. Unfortunately, if associated with a distorted body image, risk for eating disorder along with its concomitant medical problems increases.
   c. Risks of eating diet containing < 10% fat include low energy intake and low levels of vitamins A, D, E, and K.
   d. Additional deficiencies noted in athletes include zinc, magnesium, folate, and vitamins B_6, C, and B_{12}.
6. **Protein intake:** often an issue in vegetarian athletes and those that restrict food intake
   a. Nutritionist helpful to ensure adequate intake
   b. If vegetarian, protein complementarity (legumes and grains) can ensure adequate protein intake, but still important to assess iron intake
   c. Protein intake of 1.0–1.5 g protein/kg body weight/day adequate for both strength and endurance athletes
   d. Protein intake, along with fat and total energy intake, has been shown to be lower in amenorrheic athletes than in normally menstruating athletes.
7. **Calcium:** intake often far less than the RDA
   a. In one study, 51% of cross country runners consumed less than two thirds the RDA for calcium.
   b. Calcium, along with estrogen, necessary in women for normal bone deposition and, if depleted, can lead to a lower bone density. Peak bone density reached in women in their early 20s to 30s; thus, adequate intake in childhood and adolescence of increased importance.
8. **Nutritional supplements and ergogenic aids**
   a. Because athletes do whatever it takes to gain a competitive advantage, they are at risk for use and abuse of supplements as well as ergogenic aids. Some of these are restricted under U.S. Olympic Committee and NCAA drug testing. Examples of nutritional ergogenic aids include amino acids, medium-chain fatty acids, vitamins, minerals, herb extracts, special proteins, and enzyme complexes. Often marketed to target individual sports.
   b. **Supplements:** Positive effects unproven in controlled studies if individual not deficient. Amino acid supplementation may be detrimental if kidney function is marginal, especially in setting of dehydration. Protein and vitamin supplementation in great excess can be dangerous. Excesses of most vitamins are eliminated from the

body. Fat-soluble vitamins (A, D, E, and K) are stored within the body, and thus toxicity is possible. Most methods of supplementation are expensive.

c. **Ergogenic aids** include erythropoietin, human growth hormone, and anabolic steroids
   i. Difficult to detect erythropoietin and human growth hormone with current drug testing regimens
   ii. Anabolic steroids detectable with urine drug testing
   iii. All associated with significant side effects. Erythropoietin associated with hyperviscosity syndrome, even death. Hyperviscosity syndrome made worse with dehydration that can occur with prolonged exercise. Human growth hormone also associated with side effects, including acromegaly-like features. Anabolic steroid side effects well-known.
   iv. For up-to-date information, contact U.S. Olympic Committee drug information hotline (800-233-0393).

9. **Fluid considerations**
   a. During prolonged exercise, 2–4 lb body weight loss/hour, equivalent to 1–2 L/hour
   b. Rate of dehydration can be estimated by changes in nude body weight; each pound weight loss = 450 mL of dehydration
   c. Dehydration can incur physiologic changes; increase in core body temperature of 0.3°C, increase in heart rate of 8 beats/minute, and decrease in cardiac output of 1 L/minute, for every liter of water (2.2 lb) lost while exercising in the heat
   d. Proper rehydration essential during, after, and in between events
   e. Thirst not good indicator of fluid status
   f. For athlete with weight of 68 kg (150 lb), carbohydrate requirement is 30–60 g/hour. This requirement as well as fluid needs can be met by drinking 625–1250 mL/hour of beverages with 4–8% carbohydrate.
   g. Some studies relate decrease in gastric emptying once glucose concentration > 6%. Water still excellent source for short distance events.
   h. For on-site evaluation and management of syncope or presyncope, measurement of orthostatics most reliable
   i. Cannot assume every runner is dehydrated without proper assessment. Differential diagnoses include significant cardiac problems as well neurologic, metabolic, and electrolyte disturbances (see Syncope, page 749)

10. **Nutritional needs are different for the female athlete.**
   a. Societal influences have made constant dieting acceptable for girls and women, and athletes are even more likely to attempt to change their body appearance if they think it will improve performance.
   b. This puts them at increased risk to suffer from nutritional deficiency as well as eating disorders.

C. **Female athlete triad.** Disordered eating, menstrual dysfunction, and osteoporosis have become known as "the female athlete triad." Most commonly seen in sports that select for lean body weight (swimming, cross country skiing, cross country running) or in sports scored subjectively (gymnasts, figure skaters, divers), but **present in every sport**.

1. **Eating disorders**
   a. Origins multifactorial:
      i. Identity
      ii. Self-esteem
      iii. Family dynamics
      iv. Coping skills
      v. Control issues
      vi. Alterations of body image

vii. Often history of sexual or physical abuse
viii. Societal pressures increase risk

b. Women account for 90% of eating disorders.
c. Increased incidence in athletes compared to the general population. Characteristics associated with some of our best athletes that put them at additional risk for developing eating disorders:
   i. Perfectionism
   ii. Goal setting
   iii. Overachieving
d. Subtle messages by coach, parents, or teammates, which are often unintentional, can add to pressures that lead an athlete to experiment with pathogenic weight control behaviors:
   i. Misconception that lower body weight improves performance
   ii. Messages such as "your times have gotten slower—have you gained weight?" or "you had a great race, have you lost weight?"
   iii. Education of coaches essential in recognition and prevention of eating disorders
e. Difficult to identify; team approach often necessary for proper treatment
f. Treatment team usually includes physician, psychiatrist, and ultimately nutritionist. Additional support system can include coach, sport psychologist, athletic trainer, and family. Psychological counseling is cornerstone.
g. Treatment not very successful, emphasizing need for prevention through education and early identification
h. Screen for concomitant depression. Preliminary studies suggest favorable response to antidepressants such as fluoxetine.

2. **Menstrual dysfunction**
   a. Common in female athletes, especially endurance athletes
   b. Etiologies multifactorial—menstrual dysfunction, shortened luteal phase, anovulation, oligomenorrhea, and amenorrhea all can occur in response to chronic exercise and in association with decreased bone mineral density (BMD).
   c. Exercise-associated menstrual dysfunction remains diagnosis of exclusion
   d. Must rule out other conditions:
      i. Pregnancy
      ii. Thyroid disorders
      iii. Adrenal disorders
      iv. Prolactin-secreting tumors
      v. Ovarian disorders
   e. Important to initiate workup and treatment because of long-range consequences of menstrual dysfunction. Treatment must be individualized.
   f. "Progesterone challenge" helpful in functionally differentiating estrogen-deficient state from estrogen- and progesterone-deficient state:
      i. Positive challenge—if progesterone is given to individual with amenorrhea and this produces bleeding, then estrogen is present and only progesterone is lacking.
      ii. Negative challenge—if no bleeding is produced, then body lacks both estrogen and progesterone.
   g. If exercise-associated amenorrhea is diagnosed and no contraindication exists, estrogen and progesterone supplementation should be considered. Many use age 16 as younger cutoff for initiating treatment.
   h. Oral contraceptive pill has good side effect profile, is well tolerated, and has convenient packaging. If positive progesterone challenge, can use monthly progesterone alone.
   i. Other considerations:
      i. Decrease training intensity
      ii. Increase body weight if underweight

iii. Assess nutritional intake
iv. Maintain high index of suspicion for eating disorders

3. **Osteoporosis and stress fractures**
   a. Amenorrheic runners have lower estrogen levels and lower BMD than runners with normal menstrual cycles.
   b. History of menstrual dysfunction correlated with BMD in runners; those with always normal cycles had highest BMD, and those with history of amenorrhea and current amenorrhea had the lowest BMD.
   c. Low BMD risk factor for early osteoporosis and stress fractures. Increased incidence of stress fractures seen in runners with amenorrhea.
4. **Recognition and treatment—detection and education critical**
   a. The preparticipation physical examination offers a good opportunity to address these issues with female athletes.
   b. It provides an opportunity to educate young athletes about the importance of maintaining normal menstrual function, the risks of eating disorders, and the relation of both of these to the incidence of stress fractures and early osteoporosis.
   c. Ask athletes who present with stress fractures about their current and past menstrual history.
   d. A supplemental history for the female athlete is a helpful screening tool during the preparticipation physical exam (Fig. 1).

D. **Overtraining**
1. Often difficult to recognize and treat effectively
2. Symptoms nonspecific
   a. Fatigue
   b. Irritability
   c. Sleep difficulty
3. Common in endurance athletes with increase in training volume or intensity
4. Often see depression, anger, and fatigue as well as decrease in performance (i.e., "staleness")
5. Laboratory testing normal. Important to assess for:
   a. Anemia
   b. Hypothyroidism
   c. Infection
   d. Collagen vascular disease
   e. Glucose abnormalities
6. Assess for depression
7. Treatment
   a. Decrease in training
   b. Increase in carbohydrate intake
   c. Gradual return to activity
8. Use of sports psychologist can be helpful
9. Overtraining contributes to:
   a. Burnout
   b. Overuse injuries
   c. Stress fractures
   d. Menstrual dysfunction
   e. Iron deficiency

E. **Syncope—common medical problem with multiple etiologies**
1. Need to be rigorous in excluding serious medical problem, especially if syncope occurs in the midst of full exertion.
2. Ask about history of associated chest pain, palpitation, shortness of breath, dizziness.
3. Differential diagnosis includes:

Supplemental History for the Female Athlete

1. At what age did you have your first menstrual cycle? ________
2. How many days does your cycle last? ________ How many days between cycles? ________
3. How many periods have you had in the past 12 months? ________
4. What is the date of your last menstrual cycle? ________
5. Do you ever have cramping with your period? ________
6. If so, what do you do to lessen your symptoms? ________
7. Have you ever had "irregular" cycles (shorter than 21 days, or with more than 35 days between cycles)? ________
8. Have you ever had heavy bleeding? ________
9. Have you ever stopped having a period? ________
   If so, when and for how long? (Give *details*)
10. Have you ever had a stress fracture? If so, please list sites, dates, method of diagnosis (X-ray, bone scan). ________
11. Is there any family history of osteoporosis (thinning of the bones)? ________
12. When was you last pelvic exam? ________ Last breast exam? ________
13. Have you ever had an abnormal pelvic exam or PAP smear? ________
14. Do you/have you ever taken birth control pills or hormones? ________
    If yes, why were they prescribed? (circle) birth control / irreg. menses / no menses / painful menses
15. Has a physician ever told you that you had anemia (low hematocrit or iron)? ________
16. What is your present weight? ________ Present height?________
17. Are you happy with your present weight? ________ If not, what is your desired weight? ________
18. Does your weight fluctuate? ________ Highest weight ________ Lowest weight ________
19. Do you have trouble maintaining your optimal weight? ________
20. Do you diet regularly? ________
21. Do you ever feel out of control of your eating patterns? ________
22. Have you ever tried to control your weight by Dieting/fasting? ________ Diet pills? ________
    Diuretics? ________ Laxatives? ________ Vomiting? ________ Excessive exercise? ________
23. Have you ever had an eating disorder? ________
24. Do you take vitamins or supplements? ________
25. In an average 2 days, how many servings of each do you eat? (please circle)

Grains (cereal, bread, rice, pasta)	0 1 2 3 4 >4	Fruits	0 1 2 3 4 >4
Dairy products (milk, yogurt, cheese)	0 1 2 3 4 >4	Red meat	0 1 2 3 4 >4
Beans, nuts, tofu	0 1 2 3 4 >4	Vegetables	0 1 2 3 4 >4
Chicken, fish	0 1 2 3 4 >4	Eggs	0 1 2 3 4 >4

26. How many meals do you eat each day? ________
27. How much alcohol do you drink at one time? (avg.) ________ Per week (avg.)? ________
28. Do you smoke cigarettes? ________ Would you like to see the sports nutritionist? ________

FIGURE 1. A supplemental history assists in early detection of eating disorders, menstrual dysfunction, and osteoporosis in female athletes.

a. Dehydration
b. Cardiac sources:
   i. Long Q-T interval
   ii. Arrhythmias
   iii. Hypertrophic cardiomyopathy
   iv. Anomalous coronary arteries

v. Aortic stenosis or other valvular abnormalities
vi. Neurocardiogenic syncope

c. Neurologic sources:
i. Seizures
ii. Arteriovenous malformations
iii. Aneurysms

d. Hematologic (anemia) or electrolyte abnormalities (red flag for eating disordered individuals)

4. History essential—if occurs during exertion, much more concerning than if occurs after full exertion and standing still (common in neurocardiogenic syncope)
5. Further workup and testing as indicated by history, family history, and physical examination
6. Often difficult to differentiate pathologic cardiac condition from "athlete's heart"
   a. Athlete's heart represents physiologic changes that occur in response to training.
      i. Hypertrophy
      ii. Prolonged electrocardiographic intervals
      iii. Functional heart murmurs that are not pathologic
   b. Echocardiography, maximal exercise testing, and tilt-table testing are often useful adjuncts to history and physical examination in differentiating normal athlete from an athlete with a pathologic condition.

F. **Gastrointestinal problems**

1. **Alterations in gastrointestinal function**—25% of runners experience abdominal cramps, diarrhea, nausea, and abdominal pain.
2. **Gastrointestinal bleeding**
   a. Severe gastrointestinal bleeding after endurance running reported, with rare occurrences of death secondary to acute hemorrhage
   b. Milder forms of gastrointestinal bleeding common
      i. Studies have reported anywhere from 8–22% clinically detectable bleeding in marathoners after a race.
      ii. If more sensitive assays are used, an increase in fecal heme concentrations is seen in 83% of marathoners.
      iii. Thus, runners have an increase in stool heme after a race, and in approximately 20% this is detectable clinically.
   c. Bleeding self-limited and resolves in roughly 72 hours
   d. Bleeding can be associated with excessive iron loss and resultant iron deficiency. Must differentiate from runner's anemia.
   e. Pathophysiology unclear, but must consider NSAID use, bowel ischemia, traumatic shearing effect from running, underlying gastrointestinal abnormalities
   f. After gastrointestinal pathology ruled out, treatment issues surround presence/absence of iron deficiency and consideration of antimotility agents for diarrhea
3. **Reflux/delayed gastric emptying**—common complaint in endurance athletes
   a. May result in nausea or vomiting
   b. Exercise increases acid secretion and in some athletes may lead to heartburn-type symptoms.
   c. Symptoms exacerbated by precompetition nervousness
   d. Thorough workup indicated to rule out gastrointestinal pathology
   e. Treatment centers on alteration in eating patterns, trials with magnesium or aluminum hydroxide and simethicone (Maalox), or H_2 blocker trial (used 1 hour before events).

G. **Exercise-induced asthma**—common in athletes, especially when exercising in the cold

1. Symptoms variable, occurring with exercise

  a. Wheezing
  b. Tightness
  c. Chest pain
  d. Shortness of breath
2. Symptoms sometimes vague—poor exercise tolerance or cough or tightness after exercise
3. Symptoms aggravated by:
  a. Allergens
  b. Upper respiratory infections
  c. Environmental conditions (humidity, cold air)
4. Provocative testing helpful in making diagnosis and assessing response to bronchodilators.
  a. Spirometry before exercise challenge
  b. Adequate exercise challenge (can use whatever athlete describes as a "typical" precipitant)
  c. Postexercise spirometry. Look for decrease in forced expiratory volume in the first second (FEV_1) and decrease in FEV_1 as a fraction of total forced vital capacity.
5. Treatment
  a. Beta-agonist, such as albuterol, often helpful as preexercise medication to prevent exercise-induced asthma
  b. Other medications include sodium cromolyn (Intal) or nedocromil sodium (Tilade) as premedication
  c. Inhaled corticosteroids or 3–4 times daily use of medications helpful if acute flare of symptoms, baseline asthma (not only exercise-induced asthma), or allergen-induced asthma
6. Avoid known precipitants.
7. Proper cardiovascular warm-up can lessen symptoms and allow athlete to "run through" asthma
  a. 15–20 minutes at approximately 70% $\dot{V}O_2max$
  b. Series of 40–50-yard sprints
8. Minimize symptoms
  a. Use scarf or other methods to warm inspired air
  b. Breathe through nose
9. Drug testing concerns—drugs allowed change frequently. All medication questions should be addressed to the U.S. Olympic Commission Drug Information Hotline (800-233-0393).

H. **Renal issues**
1. **Pseudonephritis—proteinuria, hematuria, and cellular elements in urine after exercise**
  a. Exercise associated with decreased renal blood flow
  b. Decreased glomerular filtration rate results, with dehydration, as exercise continues playing role as well
  c. Proteinuria, hematuria, and pyuria, as well as cellular elements seen after intense exercise, are transient and resolve after rest.
  d. Workup indicated if abnormalities persist after discontinuing exercise, or if other symptoms or risk factors exist
2. **Gross hematuria**—reported in runners
  a. Often occurs without warning and without symptoms, as painless clots of blood or grossly bloody urine
  b. Possibly due to traction effect on bladder with bleeding
  c. Cystoscopy can sometimes detect bleeding source, but often negative

d. Further workup indicated if abnormalities persist despite stopping exercise or if other symptoms or risk factors are present

IV. Musculoskeletal Issues

A. Basic running mechanics

1. Important to understand normal biomechanics of running to understand abnormal biomechanics and how they can affect incidence of injury
2. **Foot strike**—at lower speeds occurs with heel, but at higher speeds occurs with forefoot
3. Ground strike occurs 800 to 2000 times/mile for average runner, or 5000 foot strikes per hour of running
4. **Reaction forces at foot strike are usually 1.5 to 5 times body weight.** Joint shear forces during running increase to almost 50 times that of walking, underscoring importance of proper biomechanics of running in preventing overuse injuries.
5. At initial rearfoot contact, foot in supination. This is associated with "closed-pack," rigid position of the tarsal bones, increasing stability.
6. Foot then pronates with tarsal joints assuming "open-packed" position, which is more accommodating and less rigid, allowing for partial absorption of reaction forces. Internal rotation of tibia on talus.
7. As progress to pushoff, subtalar joint supinates with external rotation of tibia. Foot remains in supination during airborne phase and forward swing of leg.
8. Major muscle groups all show increased electromyographic activity during running, and all lower extremity joints show increased motion during running.
9. In stance phase of running, ankle generates 60% of the power generation, whereas the knee and hip generate 40% and 20%, respectively.
10. **The knee is the principal shock absorber during running, absorbing twice as much energy as the ankle and hip.**
11. **Abnormal biomechanics can lead to overload of other structures.** For example, abnormal amount of rearfoot varus or pronation can abnormally load structures higher in the biomechanical chain, leading to increased valgus stress at the knee. This is an important etiologic factor in patellofemoral dysfunction (see page 756)
12. **Orthotics** or shoe inserts may help in preventing injury if significant rearfoot, forefoot, or biomechanical abnormalities present. Should be screened for in the preparticipation physical examination.

B. Physiologic issues—demands depend on type of activity

1. **Sprinters:** energy requirements provided primarily by anaerobic energy pathways. Glucose major fuel source.
2. **Long distance events:** energy requirements provided primarily by aerobic energy pathways, with fat and glucose derived from glycogen stores
3. **Middle distance and combination events:** combination of both aerobic and anaerobic pathways
4. Specificity of training to demands based on types of energy pathways used

C. Strengthening and conditioning—key in track and field is sport specificity in training. This differs for each event.

Much of training continues year round. Need to emphasize variability in training and avoid overtraining.

1. **Endurance and sprint athletes:** Strengthening of muscle fiber types (fast twitch versus slow twitch) demonstrates specificity, i.e., endurance-type training leads to changes in slow-twitch fiber morphology as well as enzyme metabolism specific for endurance-type activities. Similarly, explosive all-out–type strengthening programs specifically train fast-twitch muscle fibers and the metabolic functions used to sustain these activities. It is more beneficial to train with sport specificity in mind with strengthening and conditioning program.

2. **Use of entire range of motion for strengthening important.** Strength gains seen are specific to the range and speed at which strengthening exercises are performed.
3. **Field events:** Maintain quadriceps-hamstring balance. Again, sport specificity helpful. Shoulder scapular stabilization and rotator cuff strengthening program helpful for shot-put, javelin, hammer, and discus. Reproduction of shoulder movement with manual resistance. Proprioceptive work helpful in hurdles, discus, javelin, and triple and long jump.
4. **Develop smaller supporting muscles.** Strengthening prevents development of shin splints, plantar fasciitis, patellofemoral dysfunction, and other overuse injuries.

D. **Flexibility:** Despite lack of reliable data on effects of increased flexibility in preventing injury, most agree that a flexibility program helps avoid acute muscle strains. If muscle length at which maximal stretch felt is greater, it takes a larger acute overload to "stretch" the muscle past this length leading to injury. Flexibility remains essential tool in treatment of muscle strains and joint protection.
1. Flexibility program should be worked into strengthening program such that strength is improved throughout range of motion without loss of motion.
2. Ballistic stretching should be avoided.
3. Flexibility exercises are best performed after muscles warmed up as well as at end of practice or competition.
4. Stretch larger muscle groups first, followed by smaller groups.
5. Hamstring flexibility important in mechanical low back injuries. If hamstring flexibility is limited, trunk flexion is limited, and increases in stress are seen in low back.

V. Common Mechanisms of Injury

A. **Precipitating factors**
1. **Training errors account for majority of injuries (approximately 80%)**
   a. Changing to harder running surface
   b. Abrupt increase in training mileage (> 10%)
   c. Abrupt increase in training intensity
   d. Hill running
   e. Running on crowned roads
   f. Previous injury
   g. Inadequate rest/nutrition
2. **Anatomic problems**
   a. Hip
   b. Pelvis
   c. Back
   d. Knee
   e. Foot and ankle

B. **Overuse injuries** are most common mechanism in track and field injuries. Classified according to the timing of pain in relation to the onset of activity.
Type 1—pain after activity
Type 2—pain during activity, not restricting activity
Type 3—pain during activity, restricting activity, which restricts performance
Type 4—chronic, unremitting pain

VI. Specific Musculoskeletal Injuries

A. **Upper extremity**
1. **Shoulder impingement**
   a. Common in field events:
      i. Javelin

   ii. Discus
   iii. Shot-put
  b. Etiologies:
   i. Rotator cuff pathology
   ii. Labral tear
   iii. Biceps tendinitis
   iv. Multidirectional instability with muscular compensation or overuse
  c. After assessment and exclusion of problems requiring surgical intervention, initial treatment usually similar:
   i. NSAIDs
   ii. Ice
   iii. Decrease in training
   iv. Flexibility
   v. Evaluation of biomechanics
  d. If no response, assess need for further diagnostic studies, specialist evaluation
 2. **Acromioclavicular injuries**
  a. Most commonly occur after fall on shoulder with arm by side
  b. Pain and swelling directly over joint
  c. Pain with adduction (crossover test)
  d. Treatment:
   i. Ice
   ii. NSAIDs
   iii. Relative rest
 3. **Fractures**
  a. Usually occur from direct fall
  b. Treatment varies depending on fracture site and type.
 4. **Medial epicondylitis**
  a. Seen in throwers
  b. Evaluation and treatment no different than in other sports:
   i. Need to exclude fracture, valgus instability, and neurologic involvement
   ii. Treatment:
    (a) Biomechanical evaluation
    (b) Ice
    (c) NSAIDs
    (d) Physical therapy modalities
    (e) Relative rest
   iii. Consider arm brace (reversal of lateral epicondylitis strap)

B. **Lower extremity—knee accounts for 30–50% of all injuries**
 1. **Iliotibial band friction syndrome**
  a. Common in runners. Iliotibial band inserts into Gerdy's tubercle along the lateral tibia. Often seen in conjunction with greater trochanteric bursitis.
  b. Athlete presents with lateral knee pain, often in midrange of knee flexion, from 20–70°, when iliotibial band rubs across lateral femoral condyle.
  c. Contributing anatomic factors (should be corrected if possible):
   i. Leg length discrepancy
   ii. Abnormal foot biomechanics (especially hyperpronation)
   iii. Tibia vara
   iv. Scoliosis
  d. Tightness of musculature or muscle imbalances often seen—important in treatment
  e. Can reproduce on examination by resisting knee extension and looking for painful arc. This is sometimes difficult to differentiate from trochlear articular surface or osteochondral defect.

f. Treatment:
    i. Stretching
    ii. Ice
    iii. Oral NSAIDs
    iv. Phonophoresis
    v. Iontophoresis
    vi. Avoid running on beveled surfaces.
    vii. Consider corticosteroid and anesthetic agent at region of femoral condyle if other measures fail.

2. **Greater trochanteric bursitis**
    a. Tight lateral structures often compress the bursa and cause an irritative force to occur with repetitive sliding of the iliotibial band over the greater trochanter.
    b. Athlete often presents with:
        i. Lateral hip pain
        ii. No pain with passive hip rotation
        iii. Pain with active abduction, passive adduction
    c. Need to assess:
        i. Biomechanics of hip, knee, and foot and ankle
        ii. Leg length discrepancies
        iii. Training errors
    d. Treatment:
        i. NSAIDs
        ii. Ice massage
        iii. Iliotibial band stretching
        iv. Phonophoresis
        v. Iontophoresis
        vi. Corticosteroid injection if not responsive
3. **Patellofemoral dysfunction**
    a. Abnormal tracking of the patella with resultant patellofemoral irritation and pain
    b. **Contributing factors:**
        i. Increased Q angle
        ii. Deficient vastus medialis obliquus (VMO) or tight vastus lateralis musculature
        iii. Patella alta
        iv. Pronation—increases functional Q angle
        v. Genu valgum and recurvatum
    c. Characterized by anterior knee pain, often made worse by climbing or usually descending stairs or prolonged sitting ("theater sign")
    d. Understanding static and dynamic orientation of the patella important in understanding the nature of tracking dysfunction as well as in guiding rehabilitative tools
    e. **Treatment:**
        i. Mainstay remains strengthening of the VMO along with improved flexibility of lateral structures
        ii. Various patellar taping methods to allow the patella to track more normally and facilitate pain-free strengthening of the VMO
        iii. Correction of leg length discrepancy or excessive pronation or other abnormal foot biomechanics if present
        iv. Closed chain kinetic exercises, such as partial squats, one-legged squats, or step-downs, are excellent rehabilitative exercises. Used in combination with physical therapy modalities to decrease inflammation. Biofeedback as part of rehabilitative exercises often helpful.

4. **Leg-length discrepancy**
   a. Up to 5 mm normal. Can contribute to iliotibial band friction syndrome, greater trochanteric bursitis, patellofemoral dysfunction, or muscular imbalances.
   b. **Physical examination:** measurement from anterior-superior iliac spine to medial malleolus bilaterally. Pelvic obliquity, reproducibility of measurement can make this method imprecise.
   c. **Radiographic measurements:** standing postural studies; standing anteroposterior view of the pelvis to include the femoral heads and iliac crests. Then measure from bottom of film to measure discrepancy (more accurate). Does not discern exact location of discrepancy (tibia versus femur), but this is usually of little consequence in management.
   d. Once discrepancy defined, **heel lift** incorporated into shoe to correct. **Usually correct for approximately 60–75%.** If leg length much greater than 1.5 cm, need to modify shoe externally.
5. **Patellar tendinitis**
   a. **Common, especially in activities requiring jumping**
   b. Pain along infrapatellar tendon, inferior pole of patella, or insertion of infrapatellar tendon into tibial tubercle
   c. Pain during knee extension, especially terminal extension
   d. Treatment:
      i. Ice
      ii. Stretching
      iii. NSAIDs
      iv. Modalities (phonophoresis, iontophoresis)
      v. Decreased activity
   e. Can use alternate cardiovascular equipment (bicycle, aqua arc, swimming) to maintain fitness while allowing for relative rest. Zuni unloader (Soma Systems, Inc., Austin, Texas) extremely useful—harness system that "unloads" and allows athlete to run with lower body weight and thus minimize forces yet maintain normal running biomechanics.
   f. Avoid activities that aggravate pain, such as jumping and plyometrics.
6. **Meniscal lesions**
   a. Most common mechanism is twisting injury in association with jumping
   b. Athlete presents with:
      i. Joint line pain
      ii. Lack of full extension
      iii. Joint effusion that occurs slowly (versus immediate effusion seen in cruciate ligament tears)
      iv. Inability to go down into a squat or duck walk
   c. On examination:
      i. Positive joint line pain
      ii. "Bounce home" test
      iii. Hyperflexion
      iv. Circumduction maneuvers (figure-of-eight movement of foot with knee in hyperflexion)
      v. McMurray's maneuver
      vi. Apley's maneuver
   d. Magnetic resonance imaging sometimes helpful in determining extent of tear, associated injuries, likelihood of repair versus meniscectomy
   e. **Treatment** (if not causing mechanical obstruction):
      i. Non–weight bearing (weight bearing if pain free)
      ii. Decrease in activity

iii. NSAIDs
iv. Ice
v. Maintenance of quadriceps and hamstring strength

f. Gradual reintroduction of activity with pain and swelling as well as mechanical symptoms (clicking, catching, locking) as guide regarding further conservative versus surgical management. Sport specificity and individualization necessary for proper management.

7. **Hamstring, adductor, quadriceps strains**
   a. Common, especially in sprinters
   b. Sudden pain in belly of affected muscle
      i. Often describe "pulling" or "tearing" sensation
      ii. Athletes often run through this initial discomfort only to experience increasing pain and disability later.
   c. Variable amounts of swelling and ecchymoses depending on extent of muscle damage as well as exact location of injury
   d. Short head of biceps most common hamstring injury:
      i. Most often occurs at proximal musculotendinous junction.
      ii. Injuries more likely to occur at higher speeds because less time spent in support phase and thus greater velocities and forces at heel strike on hamstring.
      iii. Although data speculative, appear to see increased incidence of hamstring strains with:
         (a) Inadequate flexibility
         (b) Quadriceps-hamstring muscle imbalances
         (c) Inadequate warm-up
         (d) Prior injury
         (e) Poor proprioception
   e. **All of these extremely difficult to treat**
      i. Initial management:
         (a) Compressive wrap
         (b) Ice
         (c) Stretching
      ii. Subsequent management:
         (a) NSAIDs
         (b) Possibly ultrasound if scarring occurs
      iii. Rehabilitation should emphasize:
         (a) Eccentric activity
         (b) Reproduction of sport-specific demands
         (c) Maintenance of adequate range of motion
   f. Return to activity gradually as long as have full motion, full strength, and normal functional testing
   g. Recurrence common and often frustrating for athlete. Progression back to full activity therefore must be slow. Use of sport-specific progression helpful (i.e., if athlete is sprinter, must slowly incorporate high-speed activities into rehabilitation program).

C. **Lower extremity—lower leg, foot, ankle**

1. **Medial tibial stress syndrome**
   a. Pain over the medial third of the posteromedial tibia
   b. Association with excessive pronation
   c. **Area of tenderness often located in soleus muscle, which is involved in inversion of the subtalar joint and plantar flexion of the ankle joint.**
   d. Thickening of the medial tibial cortex common on plain radiographs; myositis and tendinitis evident on scintigraphy (differentiated by an increased blood pool phase).

e. **Scintigraphy can help differentiate from stress fracture. Plain radiographs may show evidence of stress fracture after 14 days.**
f. Progression from medial tibial stress syndrome to stress fracture is a concern; treatment is aimed at preventing this.
g. **Treatment:**
  i. Ice
  ii. Assess biomechanical abnormalities, specifically need for orthotics
  iii. Eccentric strengthening of antagonistic muscle groups and flexibility exercises
  iv. Avoid NSAIDs.
  v. Relative rest with alternative methods of training useful (cycle, swim, running in the pool, Zuni unloader)
  vi. Pain useful guide in management. Day-to-day, week-to-week adjustments in training regimen often necessary.

2. **Fractures and stress fractures**
  a. Treatment varies depending on site, extent, and circumstances.
  b. Proximal fifth metatarsal fractures are common.
  c. **Tuberosity avulsion fractures** (Table 1):
    i. **Most common fracture of the proximal fifth metatarsal**
    ii. Often occurs where plantar aponeurosis or peroneus brevis attaches
    iii. Fracture displacement rare
    iv. **Look for associated lateral malleolus fracture.**
    v. **Differentiate from unfused tuberosity apophysis by smoothness and orientation of fracture line (fracture often perpendicular to shaft of bone).**
    vi. **Differentiate from os peroneum by smoothness of edges and often bilaterality.**
    vii. **Treatment:**
      (a) **Symptomatic**
      (b) Can immobilize with cast or molded hard-soled shoe for 1–2 weeks, followed by protected weight bearing to tolerance and close follow-up.
  d. **Jones fracture:**
    i. **Acute forefoot injury without prodrome**
    ii. Occurs at junction of metaphysis and diaphysis, without intermetatarsal extension.
    iii. Treatment varies:
      (a) Conservative management with casting for 6–8 weeks
      (b) Medullary cannulated screw fixation

TABLE 1. Foot Fractures

Fracture Types	Mechanism	Location	Chronicity	Prognosis
Avulsion	Hindfoot inversion	Tuberosity	Acute	Excellent
True Jones	Forefoot adduction	Metaphyseal-diaphyseal junction	Acute	Good
Diaphyseal stress	Cyclical loading	Proximal diaphyses		
Torg type I		Narrow fracture line, no medial sclerosis	Acute or chronic	Fair–good
Torg type II		Wide fracture line, some medial sclerosis	Delayed union	Variable
Torg type III		Complete medullary sclerosis	Nonunion	Variable

Adapted from Quill GE: Fractures of the proximal fifth metatarsal. Orthop Clin North Am 26:353–361, 1995.

(c) Many favor medullary cannulated screw fixation in athletes because of earlier return to competitive athletics as well as more favorable fixation with increased healing rate.
(d) Individualization necessary in management

e. **Proximal fifth metatarsal diaphyseal stress fractures:**
   i. Fracture resulting from repetitive cyclic forces applied to the foot
   ii. Can have prodromal symptoms or acute or chronic presentation. Torg has established a classification that helps differentiate stress fractures by their potential to heal (see Table 1):
      (a) Acute, early diaphyseal stress fracture (periosteal reaction)
      (b) Delayed union (lucent fracture line and medullary sclerosis)
      (c) Nonunion
   iii. Treatment depends on patient's needs and expectations:
      (a) Type I—Treat as acute nondisplaced Jones fracture.
      (b) Type II—Treat operatively with bone graft or medullary screw fixation.
      (c) Type III—Treat operatively; some prefer closed cannulated medullary screw fixation, others open methods.

f. **Other stress fractures:**
   i. Runners account for 69% of all stress fractures.
   ii. Increased stresses on normal bone
   iii. Normal to increased stresses on weakened bone
   iv. Occur throughout the lower extremity:
      (a) Tibia (34%)
      (b) Fibula (24%)
      (c) Metatarsals (18%)
      (d) Femur (14%)
      (e) Pelvis (6%)
   v. If occur where vascular supply poor or on the tension side of the bone, prognosis poor:
      (a) Anterior tibia
      (b) Femoral neck
      (c) Proximal fifth metatarsal
      (d) Tarsal navicular
   vi. Associated with:
      (a) Gait abnormalities
      (b) Leg length discrepancy
      (c) Poor surface
      (d) Incompletely rehabilitated prior injuries
      (e) Reduced bone mineral density
      (f) Training errors

3. **Peroneal, anterior tibialis, and posterior tibialis strains**
   a. Common overuse injuries as well as acute overload injuries and strains
   b. **Usually caused by:**
      i. **Training errors**
      ii. Increase in training
      iii. Change in shoes
      iv. Poor flexibility
   c. Treatment
      i. Ice
      ii. Stretching
      iii. Addressing training errors or foot and ankle biomechanics
   d. Can see avulsions or partial tears, especially of peroneal tendons

e. Peroneal tendons run in common tendon sheath, just posterior to the lateral malleolus. They then bifurcate and run in own tendon sheaths, with peroneus brevis attaching to base of fifth metatarsal and peroneus longus extending below arch and attaching to first metatarsal and medial cuneiform.
f. Magnetic resonance imaging (MRI) helpful in evaluation of significant tendon injuries. Tendinitis rarely detected by MRI.

4. **Plantar fasciitis**
   a. Microtears caused by traction of plantar fascia and associated structures at calcaneal insertion
   b. Present with heel or arch pain, often worst with first steps after getting out of bed
   c. Seen in both pes planus and pes cavus, although latter more common
   d. Tight plantar flexors and gastrocsoleus complex as well as excessive pronation increase risk of developing plantar fasciitis
   e. Pain to palpation along plantar fascia, often at insertion into calcaneus. Pain with resisted toe flexion and passive toe extension.
   f. Radiographs may demonstrate heel spur, but this often presents bilaterally despite unilateral symptoms (i.e., radiographs do not always correlate with symptoms).
   g. **Treatment:**
      i. NSAIDs
      ii. Ice massage
      iii. Arch stretches
      iv. Heel cushioning (Visco heels, Baverfeind, Germany)
      v. Counterforce taping can help.
      vi. Phonophoresis or iontophoresis
      vii. Corticosteroid injection useful if other modalities not helpful
   f. **Night splints** useful to keep plantar fascia at length. Stretching of gastrocsoleus complex and hamstrings also important as well as intrinsic strengthening of the foot musculature.
   g. **Arch supports or orthotics if other rearfoot abnormalities present**
5. **Heel pain—fat pad contusion, heel spurs**
   a. Common in hurdlers, jumpers, and endurance runners
   b. Pain along fat pad or at insertion of plantar fascia into calcaneus. Often have history of increased training or increased wear of shoes without replacement.
   c. Exaggerated heel strike in gait common
   d. **Treatment:**
      i. Ice massage
      ii. NSAIDs
      iii. Shoe modification including soft cushioning:
         (a) Visco heels useful
         (b) Cushioning incorporated into orthotics if other foot abnormalities present
         (c) Replacement of shoes if worn
6. **Achilles tendinitis and tendinosis**
   a. Common in events involving jumping or landing as well as sprinting. Tendinitis represents an inflammatory process, whereas tendinosis refers to chronic intratendinous degenerative changes that occur without acute inflammation.
   b. Pain often approximately 2 cm proximal to insertion of Achilles tendon into calcaneus or distal tendon
   c. Palpation of nodularity may signify mucinous degeneration of tendon and partial tear.
   d. Can palpate crepitus along tendon sheath with passive or active motion—"squeaking tendon"
   e. Pain along tendon, with resisted plantar flexion and with passive dorsiflexion

f. Positive **Thompson test** signifies complete tear. Should test with knee in full extension as well as 90° of flexion.
g. **Treatment:**
    i. Ice
    ii. Relative rest
    iii. NSAIDs
    iv. Bilateral heel lifts to put tendon at rest
    v. Modify activities to pain tolerance
    vi. Eccentric rehabilitation program that emphasizes stretching, return to functional activities, slow progression
    vii. Assess for training errors or anatomic precipitants.
h. Treatment of Achilles rupture should be individualized:
    i. For competitive athlete, surgical treatment may be better option for earlier functional recovery
    ii. Surgical debridement sometimes considered for recalcitrant tendinitis or tendinosis

7. **Ankle sprains:**
    a. Common in cross country runners
    b. Evaluation and treatment no different than any other sport
    c. Inversion mechanism most common with involvement of anterior talofibular ligament, calcaneofibular ligament, and posterior talofibular ligament, progressively
    d. Watch for associated foot or metatarsal injury.
    e. Deltoid ligament less commonly involved. Distal anterior tibiofibular ligament involvement (syndesmotic sprain) portends more extensive injury with longer recovery time.
    f. **Acute treatment:**
        i. Ice
        ii. Elevation
        iii. Compression wrap
        iv. Immobilization if severe
        v. NSAIDs
        vi. Weight bearing as tolerated by pain as long as normal gait biomechanics maintained.
        vii. X-rays to assess for fracture
        viii. Consider repeat films 7–10 days later if initial films negative and symptoms persist or worsen to avoid missing occult fracture.
    g. **Chronic treatment:**
        i. Rehabilitation important for early return of motion and strength as well as proprioception and functional activity.
        ii. Bracing or taping often allows return to sport early on.

8. **Ankle injuries—chondral and osteochondral lesions**
    a. Occur in conjunction with ankle sprains
    b. Ankle most stable in dorsiflexed position. At risk for injury when in plantar flexion.
    c. Chondral or osteochondral injuries can occur, most commonly at the talar dome, less commonly the tibial plafond. Can also develop loose bodies.
    d. Athletes present with:
        i. Pain
        ii. Swelling
        iii. Locking with activity
    e. Often discovered when presumed ligamentous injury fails to respond to appropriate treatment

f. Plain radiographs often negative initially. Lesions better seen on computed tomography or magnetic resonance imaging.
g. Treatment depends on location and size of lesion or fragments and amount of pain and disability.
h. Arthroscopic debridement, drilling, or removal of loose bodies sometimes necessary

D. **Hip and spine account for close to 20% of all injuries.**
1. **Spondylolysis and spondylolisthesis:**
a. Defect in pars interarticularis
b. Athlete presents with:
i. Acute-onset back pain, usually worse with activity and specifically extension
ii. Pain to palpation along spine or often paraspinally
iii. Pain with extension, aggravated by one-legged extension
c. Initial films may be negative. Flexion and extension views to assess for presence and severity of spondylolisthesis.
d. Bone scan with single-photon emission computed tomography imaging helpful if initial films negative and clinical picture consistent
e. Treatment:
i. Bracing if caught before x-ray evidence present
ii. Limitation of activity
iii. Ice
iv. Neutral spine stabilization strengthening
f. Gradual increase in sport-specific activity as tolerated with pain as guide. Follow-up bone scans not helpful because scans remain positive for several months.

2. **Muscular imbalance**
a. **Common cause of muscular strains and overuse injuries**
b. Unclear etiology but can see in association with:
i. Old injury
ii. Response to overload
iii. Response to muscular weakness
iv. Response to leg length discrepancy or other asymmetric anatomic abnormalities
c. Treatment:
i. Most difficult aspect of treatment is recognition of muscular imbalances.
ii. Treatment rests on flexibility of tight structures in addition to strengthening of weak structures.
iii. Correction of anatomic abnormalities or gait abnormalities is essential.

3. **Herniated nucleus pulposus**
a. Less common injury in runners, more common in track athletes
b. Often present with central back pain, worse with flexion
c. Pain over disk space, positive straight leg raise
d. Careful neurologic exam to exclude neurologic compromise
e. Plain radiographs may show degenerative changes and disk space narrowing. Flexion and extension views to assess for presence or absence of spondylolysis or spondylolisthesis.
f. MRI helpful in assessing soft tissue and disk itself. Can demonstrate compromise of cord or nerve roots and assess for spinal stenosis.
g. MRI also helpful in ruling out spinal cord tumor, multiple sclerosis, or other space-occupying lesion
h. Diskogram or myelogram may be helpful if surgery under consideration
i. Treatment:
i. Relative rest
ii. NSAIDs

iii. Ice
iv. Physical therapy modalities
v. Consider epidural steroid injections or oral steroids, depending on individual situation.

j. Activity may be allowed if no neurologic compromise, full strength and motion, and pain controlled. Every situation must be individualized, taking into account extent of injury and the athlete's level of compromise and pain.

4. **Paraspinal muscular strains**
   a. Common, especially in hurdlers. Often secondary to acute overuse or injuries related to strengthening program.
   b. Athlete presents with paraspinal pain, often with limitation of motion
   c. Pain with activity, minimal pain if lie still. Pain with active and resisted motion.
   d. Assess for presence of disk, spondylolysis or spondylolisthesis by history as well as exam.
   e. Additional diagnostic studies indicated if no response to initial treatment or guided by history or physical examination.
   f. Treatment:
      i. Initial treatment:
         (a) Ice
         (b) NSAIDs
         (c) Stretching
      ii. Heat after 48 hours before activity, followed by ice and physical therapy modalities after activity
      iii. Abdominal as well as neutral spine strengthening program once acute pain subsides
      iv. Flexibility program

VII. Environmental Issues

A. **Heat injuries**
   1. Common issues in outdoor competition during summer months
      a. **Heatstroke:**
         i. Temperature > 104°F
         ii. Altered mental status
         iii. Sweating absent
         iv. Seizures and coma
         v. Can be fatal, accounting for hundreds of deaths in the United States annually
         vi. Treat as medical emergency
         vii. Assess renal, neurologic, hepatic systems, and hospitalize
      b. **Heat exhaustion:**
         i. Temperature does not exceed 104°F.
         ii. Mental status changes absent
         iii. Symptoms:
            (a) Profound weakness
            (b) Dizziness
            (c) Syncope
            (d) Muscle cramps
            (e) Nausea
         iv. Risks similar to heatstroke if unrecognized
         v. Treatment often similar—assessment by physician, rest in cool environment out of the sun, oral fluids
         vi. Activity should be restricted for the remainder of the day, and the athlete should be reevaluated the following day.

c. **Heat cramps:**
   i. Cramps often in abdomen and lower extremities
   ii. Often related to fluid or electrolyte deficiency
   iii. Treat with fluid and electrolyte replacement
d. **Heat syncope:**
   i. Decrease in vasomotor tone and venous pooling (especially immediately after stopping exercise), which leads to syncope
   ii. Dehydration and increased temperature contribute
e. **Heat tetany:** spasm, often in the wrist, seen with heat and exacerbated by hyperventilation
f. **Heat edema:**
   i. Swelling of the hands and feet in response to heat
   ii. Often worst in initial phases of accommodation to new environment
   iii. Self-limited
   iv. Often resolves with cold compresses and elevation
   v. Diuretics not indicated and may exacerbate dehydration

2. **Risk factors for heat injury**
   a. Very young or very old age
   b. Preexisting dehydration
   c. Obesity
   d. Previous history of heat-related illness
   e. Heart disease
   f. Alcohol use
   g. Drugs (tricyclic antidepressants, amphetamines, LSD, PCP, cocaine, anticholinergics, antihistamines, diuretics, beta-blockers)
   h. Increased humidity, temperature, no clouds, no wind
   i. Poor physical conditioning
   j. Presence of acute febrile illness
3. **Treatment** focuses on rapid cooling and transport to medical facility.
   a. If rectal temp > 104°F, cooling should occur immediately, with ideal to reach temperature of 102°F within 30–60 minutes.
   b. Electrolyte abnormalities common

B. **Cold weather injuries**
   1. Common in winter months, or if windy or wet conditions
   2. Heat production in the body maintained by:
      a. Basal heat production:
         i. Produced by metabolic processes
         ii. Ineffective in maintaining body temperature when exposure to cold environment occurs
      b. Muscular thermoregulatory heat:
         i. Produced by shivering
         ii. Blood flow preferentially shunted to vital organs
         iii. Can increase heat production threefold to fivefold, but requires energy
         iv. Also increases cooling of distal extremities and skin
      c. Mild-to-moderate exercise-induced heat:
         i. Produced by low-intensity exercise
         ii. Can increase heat production fivefold
         iii. Uses low-energy requirements and can thus be sustained for long period of time
      d. High-intensity exercise-induced heat:
         i. Produced by body during high-intensity exercise
         ii. Can increase heat production 10-fold, but because of higher energy requirements cannot be maintained long

3. **Specific cold weather injuries**
   a. **Frostnip:**
      i. Reversible without permanent tissue damage
      ii. Blanching of skin; slow, painless crystal formation on ears, face, toes, and fingertips
      iii. Commonly seen in windy conditions
   b. **Chilblains:**
      i. Repeated exposure to cold water or wet cooling
      ii. Red, hot, tender swollen extremity with numbness or tingling
      iii. Irreversible damage can occur to capillaries, muscles, nerves serving extremity
      iv. Can progress to gangrene
   c. **Frostbite:**
      i. Freezing of soft tissue
      ii. Commonly involves nose, fingertips, ears, and toes
      iii. Symptoms:
         (a) Local pain
         (b) Numbness
         (c) Redness
         (d) Superficial blistering
         (e) With increased severity of exposure, deeper blistering and involvement of deep soft tissue and bone
4. **Hypothermia**
   a. Occurs when core temperature < 95°F
   b. Significant cause of mortality
5. **Treatment of cold injuries**
   a. **Best treatment is prevention**
   b. Rewarming slowly, after warm environment secured
   c. Removal of all wet clothing, proper measurement of core body temperature
   d. Use of warm whirlpool, analgesics, skin protection
   e. Other preventive measures:
      i. Layered clothing
      ii. Covering the head
      iii. Protecting hands (mittens better than gloves) and toes
      iv. Avoid wetness
      v. Proper nutrition and hydration
      vi. Adequate warm-up before activity
      vii. Breathe through nose to warm inspired air
      viii. Avoid alcohol, nicotine, and other drugs
      ix. Never train alone

C. **Guidelines about environmental issues—American College of Sports Medicine Guidelines remain standard.**
   1. Use of wet bulb globe temperature (WBGT) ideal
   2. WBGT = (0.7 Twb) + (0.2 Tg) + (0.1 Tdb)
      where Twb = wet bulb thermometer temperature
      Tg = black globe thermometer temperature
      Tdb = dry bulb thermometer temperature
   3. Color-coded flag system (Table 2)

VIII. Safety and Equipment Issues

For all events, need to maintain proper supervision of surface and runways. When multiple events are going on at one time, safety issues are paramount. This is especially true for javelin, hammer, discus, and shot put, in which injury to spectators (impalement) is significant.

TABLE 2. Color-Coded Flag System

Color	Risk	Comments	Restrictions
Black	Extreme risk	WBGT > 82°F	Cancel race
Red	High risk	WBGT 73–82°F	Be aware, high-risk athletes should not run
Yellow	Moderate	WBGT 65–73°F	Heat-sensitive athletes should slow pace
Green	Low risk	WBGT 50–65°F	No restrictions
White	Risk for hypothermia	WBGT < 50°F	Hypothermia possible, especially if wet or windy

A. **Track surface**
 1. **Equipment issues**
  a. Tracks generally oval with inner length equal to ¼ mile, 440 yards, or 400 m
  b. Cinder, clay, or all-weather synthetic track often used for track surface itself
  c. Proper maintenance of surface as well as adequate drainage
 2. **Safety issues**
  a. Depending on surface used, varying amounts of shock absorption and damping characteristics
  b. These factors may play a role in injury.
  c. Banking of track may alter biomechanics of both inside and outside leg. Banking is increased in smaller tracks.

B. **Jumping events**
 1. **Equipment issues**
  a. Ramps for long jump, triple jump, pole vault, and javelin often use rubberized synthetic surfaces.
  b. Maintenance issues same as for track surface
  c. Takeoff boards need to be replaced frequently
  d. Landing pits usually contain slightly moist sand, which needs to be turned and maintained at a minimum of 12–18 inches deep.
  e. Pits extend from 10 feet in front of and at least 20 feet beyond the takeoff board.
 2. **Safety issues**
  a. If ramps not wide enough, can cause injury, especially inversion ankle sprains.
  b. Runways must be kept clear of foreign objects, spectators, and other obstacles.

C. **Pole vault**—sprinter with a pole
 1. **Equipment issues**
  a. Foam rubber padding around planting box as well as underneath bar
  b. Planting box with sawdust or sand inside
  c. Crossbar usually fiberglass
  d. Poles usually fiberglass (lighter, more expensive) or metal, up to 18 feet long
 2. **Safety issues**
  a. Poles can break during takeoff or from contact with vaulting box.
  b. Landing mats should cover vaulting box on all sides.
  c. Thickness of mat should range from 28–36 inches.
  d. Risk of injury to cervical spine or head and risk of fracture can occur secondary to incorrect fall mechanism.
  e. Missing pole plant into vaulting box can lead to shoulder subluxation, dislocation, and acromioclavicular joint injuries.
  f. Proper technique and supervision are important.

D. **Hurdles**—consider as sprint event with obstacles
 1. **Equipment issues**
  a. Hurdle designed to tip over forward

   b. Soft top hurdles minimize contact injuries with hurdle during practice.
   c. Protection of ankle, heel, and knee with padding minimizes injuries in practice.
2. **Safety issues**
   a. Lanes clear of foreign objects, obstacles, spectators
   b. Injuries can occur secondary to direct contact with hurdles on inside of trailing leg.

E. **Throwing events**
1. Raise biggest concern regarding injuries to both athletes and spectators
2. Examples:
   a. Shot put
   b. Discus
   c. Hammer
   d. Javelin
3. Proper technique and supervision
4. Proper warm-up helpful in preventing overuse injuries
5. Concern for spectators being struck by discus, javelin, hammer, or shot put

Recommended Reading

1. Clark N : Nutritional problems and training intensity, activity level, and athletic performance. In Pearl AJ (ed): The Athletic Female. 1993, pp 165–168.
2. Costill D: Carbohydrates for exercise: Dietary demands for optimal performance. Int J Sports Med 9:1–18, 1988.
3. Coyle EF: Fluid and carbohydrate replacement during exercise: How much and why? Sports Science Exchange 7(3), 1994.
4. Drinkwater BL, Bruemmer B, Chestnut CH III: Menstrual history as as determinant of current bone density in young athletes. JAMA 263:545, 1990.
5. Drinkwater BL, Nilson K, Chestnut CH III, et al: Bone mineral content of amenorrheic and eumenorrheic athletes. N Engl J Med 311:277, 1984.
6. Drinkwater BL, Nilson K, Ott S, et al: Bone mineral density after resumption of menses in amenorrheic athletes. JAMA 256:380, 1986.
7. Eichner ER: Infection, immunity, and exercise. Phys Sportsmed 21:125, 1993.
8. Herzog DB, Copeland PM: Eating disorders. N Engl J Med 313:295–303, 1985.
9. Kaiserauer S, Snyder AC, Sleeper M, et al: Nutritional, physiological, and menstrual status of distance runners. Med Sci Sports Exerc 21:120–125, 1989.
10. Knapik JJ, Bauman CL, Jones BH, et al: Preseason strength and flexibility imbalances associated with athletic injuries in female collegiate athletes. Am J Sports Med 19:76–81, 1991.
11. Lillegard WA, Terrio JD: Appropriate strength training. Med Clin North Am 78:457–477, 1994.
12. Lombardo J, Nelson M, Smith D: Preparticipation Physical Evaluation. Kansas City, MO, American Academy of Family Practice, American Academy of Pediatrics, American Medical Society for Sports Medicine, American Orthopaedic Society for Sports Medicine, American Osteopathic Academy of Sports Medicine, 1992.
13. Macintyre JG, Taunnton JE, Clement DB, et al: Running injuries: A clinical study of 4,173 cases. Clin J Sports Med 1:81–87, 1991.
14. Martin RK, Yesalis CE, Foster D: Sports injuries at the 1985 Junior Olympics, and epidemiological analysis. Am J Sports Med 15:603–608, 1987.
15. Nickerson HJ, Holubets MC, Weiler BR, et al: Causes of iron deficiency in adolescent athletes. J Pediatr 114:657–663, 1989.
16. Nickerson JH, Holubets M, Tripp AD, et al: Decreased iron stores in high school female runners. Am J Dis Child 139:1115, 1985.
17. Nickerson HJ, Tripp AD: Iron deficiency in adolescent cross-country runners. Phys Sportsmed 11:60–66, 1983.
18. Poortmans JR: Exercise and renal function. Sports Med 1:125–153, 1984.
19. Puffer JC, Zachazewski MS: Management of overuse injuries. Am Fam Phys 38:225–232, 1988.
20. Putukian M: The female triad: Eating disorders, amenorrhea, and osteoporosis. Med Clin North Am 78:345–356, 1994.
21. Quill GE: Fractures of the proximal fifth metatarsal. Orthop Clin North Am 26:353–361, 1995.
22. Rowland TW, Deisroth MA, Green GM, et al: The effect of iron therapy on the exercise capacity of nonanemic iron deficient adolescent runners. Am J Dis Child 142:165, 1988.
23. Sevier T: Infectious diseases in athletes. Med Clin North Am 78:389–412, 1994.

24. Stewart JC, Ahlquist DA, McGill DB, et al: Gastrointestinal blood loss and anemia in runners. Ann Intern Med 100:843–845, 1984.
25. Torg JS: Fractures of the base of the fifth metatarsal distal to the tuberosity: A review. Contemp Orthop 19:497–505, 1989.
26. Wadler GI: Drug use update. Med Clin North Am 78:439–455, 1994.
27. Waller BF, Harvey WP (eds): Cardiovascular Evaluation of Athletes: Toward Recognizing Young Athletes at Risk of Sudden Death. Newton, MA, Laennec Publishing, 1993.
28. Yesalis CE, Bahrke MS: Anabolic-androgenic steroids: Current issues. Sports Med 19:326–340, 1995.
29. Zeppili P: The athlete's heart: Differentiation of training effects from organic heart disease. Pract Cardiol 14:61, 1988.

62

Gymnastics

Jerry Weber, M.S., PT, ATC

I. General Discussion

A. **Participation.** The wide popularity of gymnastics as a sport has greatly increased the participation by members of both sexes over the past decade. The benefits of gymnastic training for a prospective athlete in the formative years are evidenced by the large number of children's gymnastics clubs and instructional programs. The strenuous requirements of this sport in strength, flexibility, agility, and physical size tend to eliminate most early participants from becoming truly competitive at the high school and most certainly at the college level. A physician working with competitive-level gymnasts must be familiar with the basic requirements of the sport and the different individual events in male and female programs (Table 1).

B. **Forces involved**
   1. Gymnastics events exert tremendous forces on the bodies of the participants.
   2. Dismounts may entail great rotational or twisting forces from great heights, causing severe injury to the lower body, or, if improperly performed, a fall on the side, back, head, or neck.
   3. Forces involved in the swinging apparatus (horizontal bar, rings, uneven bars) exert many times the weight of the body on the shoulders, elbows, and wrists, with the potential for distraction and stress injuries.

C. **Medical concerns.** The physician working with gymnasts must be knowledgeable about potential acute injuries as well as chronic overuse problems.

II. Overview of Injury Patterns—Body Survey

A. **Head and neck injuries**
   1. **Concussion**
      a. **Mechanism:** Striking head on mat or apparatus in a fall or dismount.
      b. **Evaluation:** General neurologic screen; medical observation is recommended for unconsciousness.
      c. **Treatment:** Physician should follow standard head injury guidelines for severity and follow-up.
   2. **Cervical subluxation/dislocation/fracture**
      a. **Mechanism**
         i. Fall from apparatus
         ii. Overrotation or underrotation on a dismount from apparatus or in a floor tumbling pass
         iii. Failure to clear the vaulting horse
         iv. Striking head on end of horse
         v. Being driven into landing mat
      b. **Evaluation and treatment:** Emergency evaluation of airway, breathing, and circulation and life-saving measures instituted

TABLE 1. Gymnastic Events for Men and Women

Men's Events	Women's Events
Floor exercise	Vault
Pommel horse	Uneven bars
Still rings	Balance beam
Vault	Floor exercise
Parallel bars	
Horizontal bar	

Note: The trampoline is no longer a competitive event at high school, collegiate, or international levels.

3. **Neck strain or sprain**—extensor or flexor muscle mass injuries, whiplash, ligamentous injuries
   a. **Mechanism:** Fall on head or neck with neck flexed or extended. Injuries to these muscles can occur without contact by use of the head and neck to provide lead momentum in a specific maneuver.
   b. **Evaluation**
      i. Neurologic status
      ii. Active and passive ranges of motion
      iii. Strength levels
      iv. Pain levels
   c. **Treatment**
      i. Ice in acute stage
      ii. Soft neck collar to provide support if indicated
      iii. Encourage early active motion and isometric strengthening
      iv. Physical therapy as indicated
4. **Lacerations** to scalp, forehead, orbit, or chin
   a. **Mechanism:** Lacerations may occur any time the head strikes the hard surface of a mat or strikes any part of the apparatus.
   b. **Evaluation and treatment:** physician's discretion
5. **Nerve root irritation**
   a. **Mechanism:** Acute episode of neck strain or sprain of insidious onset with pain or numbness in a specific neurologic pattern
   b. **Evaluation**
      i. History of injury in the neck area
      ii. Neurologic examination of involved area
   c. **Treatment**
      i. Avoidance of irritating activities
      ii. Physical therapy includes cervical traction once bony injury eliminated
      iii. Appropriate strength maintenance exercises

B. **Shoulder injuries**
1. **Glenohumeral dislocation**—acute episode
   a. **Mechanism:** Forced external rotation of the abducted shoulder causing anterior dislocation (most common)—usually from a fall or failure to maintain proper swing on rings or high bar with torsion to arm that maintains grip
   b. **Evaluation**
      i. History
      ii. Physical examination of shoulder to evaluate loss of deltoid "roundness"
      iii. On involved side, palpation of head of humerus in anterior-lateral chest wall
      iv. Neurovascular status of distal extremity

c. **Treatment**
   i. Reduction of joint if no fracture is suspected
   ii. Immobilization with arm at side and hand across abdomen
   iii. Ice or medication for pain
   iv. X-ray

2. **Glenohumeral subluxation**
   a. **Mechanism:** Same as dislocation.
   b. **Evaluation**
      i. History—athlete may describe shoulder slipping out of joint and back in place.
      ii. Physical examination to determine joint stability
      iii. Apprehension test
   c. **Treatment:** Immobilization until discomfort is gone then early motion and strengthening, especially of rotator cuff musculature. Repeated episodes of shoulder instability, whether dislocations or subluxations, may effectively eliminate any gymnast from competing in the swing events, either due to pain and failure of the shoulder, or with repair, because of the inherent loss of external rotation.

3. **Acromioclavicular sprain/separation**
   a. **Mechanism:** Fall on the shoulder to mat or apparatus
   b. **Evaluation**
      i. History and comparative clinical exam to determine appearance, clavicular mobility at the acromioclavicular joint, and pain
      ii. Comparative x-rays with and without distracting weights for degree of separation
   c. **Treatment** depends on degree of injury:
      i. **First degree**
         (a) Ice
         (b) Return to activity as tolerated by pain and motion
      ii. **Second degree**
         (a) Ice and physical therapy
         (b) Immobilization (sling) only if dictated by pain. Motion as tolerated.
         (c) May be able to return to certain events earlier than others
         (d) Short course of anti-inflammatory medication at discretion of physician
      iii. **Third degree**
         (a) Ice and immobilization.
         (b) Moist heat therapy at 72 hours.
         (c) Sling for comfort and stabilization for 10–14 days.
         (d) NSAIDs
         (e) Begin range of motion (ROM) exercises at 2 weeks, followed by resistive motion exercises as tolerated.

4. **Chronic acromioclavicular inflammation**
   a. **Mechanism:** Irritation of acromioclavicular joint from constant stress from swing maneuvers and handstand activities. Acromioclavicular joint can become tender to palpation and painful with full active ROM activities.
   b. **Treatment**
      i. Inflammations usually respond well to local physical therapy, rest, avoidance of irritating activities, and anti-inflammatory medications.
      ii. Resistant or acutely tender inflammations may respond well to local corticosteroid injection.

5. **Internal derangement**
   a. **Mechanism:** Labrum tears and rotator cuff impingement syndromes are common in gymnasts from stress on the shoulder girdle. Internal derangements may be associated with some degree of glenohumeral instability.

b. **Evaluation:** Proper evaluation and diagnosis are important to management.
c. **Treatment**
   i. The majority of these problems respond well to conservative measures:
      (a) Physical therapy
      (b) Medication or injection therapy
      (c) Appropriate strengthening activities (rotator cuff)
      (d) Rest and avoidance of sport-related and weight training–related activities (e.g., overhead lifts or tricks that compromise stability)
   ii. The athlete who does not respond to conservative measures may require arthroscopic intervention.

6. **Thoracic outlet syndrome**
   a. **Mechanism:** Thoracic outlet syndromes may occur in athletes as a result of repeated overhead rotatory stress.
   b. **Evaluation:** Pain in shoulder and arm with numbness and tingling of hand and swelling or cyanosis of upper extremity with overhead activities suggest thoracic outlet syndrome.
   c. **Treatment:** See Chapter 43, "Shoulder Injuries"

C. **Elbow injuries**
1. **Dislocation**
   a. **Mechanism:** Fall on outstretched hand with semiflexed elbow
   b. **Evaluation**
      i. History
      ii. Physical examination of bony landmarks
      iii. Check neurovascular status distal to injury.
      iv. Reduction followed by x-ray examination. Obtain x-rays before reduction if fracture is suspected.
   c. **Treatment**
      i. Ice and pressure wrap from hand to midbiceps
      ii. Immobilization in posterior 90° elbow splint for 10 days to 3 weeks
      iii. **Active** motion in flexion and extension important
      iv. Passive mobilization to be avoided
      v. Early strengthening of elbow extensors encouraged
2. **Epicondylitis—medial or lateral**
   a. **Mechanism:** Strain of forearm flexor or extensor muscles from varus or valgus stress on the elbow or torsion stress of elbow from specific pivotlike maneuvers in handstand positions
   b. **Evaluation**
      i. History
      ii. Active and passive ROM
      iii. Palpation to determine areas of point tenderness
      iv. X-ray to determine possibility of avulsion fractures or hypertrophic bony changes at the epicondyle
   c. **Treatment**
      i. Physical therapy and strengthening exercises to emphasize resisted supination and pronation
      ii. Neoprene elbow sleeve for compression, support, and warmth may be of some benefit to the athlete.
      iii. Anti-inflammatory medications or corticosteroid injection may be indicated.
3. **Valgus or varus sprains**
   a. **Mechanism:** Falls from or on the apparatus may result in stress to the collateral ligaments, most commonly the medial collateral ligament. This ligament may also be stressed by certain moves on any of the specific events.

b. **Evaluation**
   i. History
   ii. Palpation to determine point tenderness
   iii. Comparative valgus stress test to determine ligament stability
c. **Treatment**
   i. Ice
   ii. Compression
   iii. Early tolerated motion to maintain full flexion
   iv. Physical therapy and appropriate strengthening with eccentrics (to include the flexor and pronator group) to ensure full return to activity

4. **Ulnar neuritis**
   a. **Mechanism:** Insidious overuse problem in which ulnar nerve becomes stretched, contused, or otherwise irritated at the ulnar groove
   b. **Evaluation:** History—complaints of pain, tingling, and numbness down medial forearm to include outside of the hand and fifth finger
   c. **Treatment**
      i. Avoidance of irritating positions or repetitious elbow movements
      ii. Protection from further insult
      iii. Physical therapy to relieve swelling
      iv. May require surgical intervention in extreme cases

D. **Forearm injuries**
   1. **Fracture**
      a. **Mechanism:** An injury specific to gymnasts in which the leather grip that the athlete is wearing for the horizontal bar "catches" or grabs onto the bar and, instead of allowing the athlete to complete the "giant swing," holds the hand in position on the bar as the body continues around the circle, causing the forearm to "wrap around" and sustain multiple fractures. This serious injury requires the coach or whoever is present to get the athlete off the apparatus without inflicting further damage to the arm.
      b. **Evaluation and treatment** as appropriate for the fracture(s)
   2. **Forearm splints:** The athlete reports pain and aching in one or both forearms during and after workout. It is caused by interosseous inflammation, usually of the wrist extensors.
      a. **Mechanism:** Stress to the interosseous region of the forearm from the athlete being in a weight-bearing position on the hands much of the time during floor exercise, vault, and especially the pommel horse and parallel bars
      b. **Evaluation**
         i. History—usually atraumatic pain with and without palpation and resisted gripping
         ii. X-ray to rule out stress fracture to the ulna or radius
         iii. If unresolved pain persists, a bone scan may be indicated.
      c. **Treatment**
         i. Ice massage to the area during and after workouts
         ii. Anti-inflammatory medication as indicated by level of disability
         iii. Pressure wrap or taping of the area for added support

E. **Wrist.** The wrist is an area of special concern in gymnastics because of the tremendous stress placed on this joint in all events.
   1. **Navicular fracture—acute or stress-induced**
      a. **Mechanism:** Fall on the extended wrist or maneuver in which the weight of the body comes down sharply on one or both wrists. Stress fractures of this bone occur from constant pounding that the wrist undergoes in this sport.
      b. **Evaluation**
         i. Classic signs of navicular fracture

ii. Point tenderness over the anatomic snuff box
iii. Painful and limited wrist extension
iv. History may or may not be specific.
v. X-ray in acute episode may not be positive.
vi. If symptoms persist, x-rays must be repeated after 10–14 days, or bone scan may be indicated.

c. **Treatment:** Positive navicular signs even in the absence of radiographic evidence should be treated with immobilization until it is proved that there is no fracture present.

2. **Dorsal wrist and hand pain**
   a. **Mechanism:** The insertion of the extensor carpi radialis brevis tendon into the base of the second metacarpal can become raised and point tender (carpal boss) because of the resisted wrist extension required in body support in many gymnastic events.
   b. **Evaluation:** Lateral x-ray view of the wrist may reveal an actual avulsion or lifting of the bony surface in extreme cases. The athlete experiences pain in this area while working out as well as after practice.
   c. **Treatment**
      i. Limitation of wrist extension
      ii. Ice
      iii. Physical therapy modalities to lessen inflammation
      iv. Tape for support
      v. Extreme cases of actual avulsion may require immobilization for a limited amount of time.

F. **Hand, fingers, and thumb injuries**
   1. **Dislocations:** The most common hand injuries in gymnastics are dislocations of the interphalangeal joints of the fingers. Metacarpophalangeal joint dislocations may also occur. Most competitive gymnasts do not tolerate even a 10-day period of immobilization or splinting except for a fracture, but the finger should be splinted in slight flexion during their time out of the gym, with "buddy taping" of the finger for protection during workouts.
   2. **Soft tissue injuries, blisters, and "rips"**
      a. **Mechanism:** A gymnast's hands are subjected to severe abuse in the sport. Even with the use of leather grips and chalk, the friction between skin and apparatus at times causes even callused skin to tear away in patches or "rips."
      b. **Treatment:** Soft tissue wounds should be treated to avoid infection. Appropriate protective padding and wrapping should be applied to prevent irritation until the athlete can tolerate friction in the area. Typical blister treatment such as moleskin or second skin to protect the wound site usually does not work on gymnasts' hands and still allow them to practice.

G. **Chest injuries**
   1. **Rib injuries**
      a. **Mechanism:** Falls on or from the apparatus can cause rib contusions or costochondral sprain or separation injuries. Rib fractures are rare but, if warranted, x-rays should be performed to rule out this possibility.
      b. **Evaluation:** History, palpation, lateral and anteroposterior compression tests to localize injury site and help determine if x-rays are needed
      c. **Treatment:** Rib binder, medication, activity as tolerated, and appropriate cold or moist heat therapy
   2. **Sternoclavicular sprain**
      a. **Mechanism:** Acute fall or blow to the sternoclavicular area or overuse injury with insidious onset from "swing" stress or strength moves on rings

b. **Evaluation**
   i. History (acute or chronic), palpation, and inspection to determine degree of separation if any
   ii. X-ray if indicated
c. **Treatment**
   i. Local cold or hot applications for swelling and discomfort
   ii. Medication as indicated
   iii. Rest and progressive return to activities as tolerated

3. **Sternocostal sprain or separation**
   a. **Mechanism:** Fall through the parallel bars that allows the body to drop below shoulder level while the hands are still holding onto the bars puts distractive force on the pectoral muscles and the ribs at the sternum. This extensive chest injury may incapacitate the athlete for up to 4 weeks.
   b. **Evaluation:** The athlete presents with a specific history of the aforementioned mechanism and extensive chest and possibly shoulder pain and tenderness with associated limitation of ROM.
   c. **Treatment**
      i. Rest
      ii. Compression binder
      iii. Medication for discomfort
      iv. Early return of motions as tolerated
      v. Physical therapy and strengthening as indicated

H. **Lower abdomen, hip, and pelvic injuries**
   1. **Muscle strain**
      a. **Mechanism:** The lower abdominal and hip flexor musculature in both male and female gymnasts is typically strong from training efforts that require these muscle groups to be strenuously worked at all times. Injuries to this region are not common in the competitive gymnast. Younger gymnasts may strain these muscle groups in training to achieve higher strength levels.
      b. **Treatment:** Relative rest and therapeutic exercise
   2. **Contusion to the anterior pelvis**
      a. **Mechanism:** Female gymnasts may incur severe bruises to the anterior superior iliac spine region on uneven bars when swinging down from the high bar to the low bar by slamming the anterior pelvic region into the lower bar. Repeated trauma to this poorly padded area can cause extreme tenderness and bruising.
      b. **Treatment**
         i. Avoidance of the maneuver or padding of anterior bony area
         ii. Ice to reduce swelling and decrease tenderness

I. **Lumbar spine.** Low back pain is a common complaint in both male and female gymnasts. Many gymnasts, especially females, have a pronounced lordotic curve. This abnormal curvature can be attributed to years of back flexion and extension flexibility exercises, "extension walkovers," and abnormal strengthening of the iliopsoas muscles. A gymnast who presents with low back symptoms needs to be examined thoroughly to identify the cause of pain.
   1. **Acute low back pain**
      a. **Mechanism**
         i. Sudden explosive overrotation
         ii. Hard landings on the feet with the knees locked, causing the back to be jammed
         iii. Falls to the mats, floor, or apparatus
         iv. Pain associated with spasm of the extensor muscles on one or both sides of the spine, swelling, and loss of normal motion

b. **Treatment**
   i. Ice
   ii. Pain and anti-inflammatory medication
   iii. Sacral belt for support
   iv. Physical therapy to include lumbar traction and flexibility and strengthening exercises
   v. If problem resolves in a few days, gymnast may return to limited activities
   vi. Gymnasts should be cautioned against stressing their backs too soon, and should be observed to be sure that further symptoms do not occur that may warrant other measures.

2. **Chronic low back pain.** Many gymnasts have a certain level of chronic back pain because of the nature of their sport. This chronic soreness and pain usually responds to appropriate stretching and physical therapy. When these measures do not control the pain or other symptoms arise, measures need to be taken to evaluate for more serious conditions.
3. **Radiculopathy**
   a. **Evaluation:** Unilateral pain down into the buttock and hamstring with associated tingling may be caused by nerve root irritation or sciatic nerve irritation. Pain, tingling, and numbness further down the leg into the foot may represent specific nerve root irritation or a possible disk lesion. Depending on the severity of symptoms, diagnostic measures should include:
      i. Complete clinical examination
      ii. X-ray
      iii. Computed tomography scan or magnetic resonance imaging, if indicated
   b. **Treatment:** See Chapter 48, "Pelvis, Hip, and Thigh Injuries."
4. **Spondylolysis and spondylolisthesis**
   a. **Evaluation:** X-rays should always be obtained in an athlete with persistent low back pain. Many gymnasts have positive radiographic evidence of posterior lamina defects or spondylolisthesis. These may be unilateral or bilateral and typically represent an old injury, especially in a gymnast who has been in the sport since childhood.
   b. **Treatment:** This condition is considered fairly benign and may or may not cause symptoms. When spondylolisthesis is present, or anterior slippage of the superior vertebral body occurs, the athlete may have more pronounced symptoms. Depending on the degree of slippage and physical symptoms, the gymnast will have to be advised as to activity level or counseled to quit the sport altogether. The muscle strain and associated muscle spasm often respond favorably to physical therapy.

J. **Knee injuries**
1. **Mechanism:** Gymnasts are vulnerable to all the various knee injuries common to athletes in all sports that involve running and jumping but with the added stress, rotation, and twist associated with landing from heights. The majority of knee injuries in gymnasts occur on dismounts or during floor exercise passes that involve tumbling passes. The team physician who is working with gymnasts can expect to see the full complement of knee injuries from infrapatellar tendinitis to anterior cruciate ligament tears.
2. *Note:* Gymnasts who have suffered a torn anterior cruciate ligament should have full reconstruction of this ligament to prevent further knee deterioration and to allow for eventual return to the sport.

K. **Leg injuries**
1. **Shin splints**
   a. **Mechanism:** Repeated stress to the lower leg from running, jumping, and dismounts. May be intensified in female gymnasts from beam workouts. Often associated with stress to the medial longitudinal arch, which causes strain on the tibialis posterior muscles.

b. **Evaluation:** Typical history of shin splint complaints. Pain in anterior shin along interosseous region of tibia and fibula during activities, and deep aching afterward and without activity.
c. **Treatment**
   i. Ice before, during, and after workouts
   ii. Aspirin therapy or other anti-inflammatory medications
   iii. Physical therapy in extreme cases to include electrical stimulation, heat, and ultrasound
   iv. Anterior shin stretching exercises, lower leg strengthening exercises, and arch supports indicated in all cases
   v. Typical orthotic-type arch supports do not work during workouts because shoes are not worn; however, they may be of benefit when worn while out of the gym. Proper supportive arch taping should be used during time in gym.

2. **Calf strains**
   a. **Mechanism:** Injuries to the triceps surae muscle group do occur in gymnastics during the floor exercise events. The forcible, explosive plantar flexion or "punch" required by the gymnast to be "launched" on tumbling passes or dismounts is stressful and may cause damage, especially to the gastrocnemius group.
   b. **Evaluation**
      i. History
      ii. Clinical evaluation to determine comparative muscle shape and palpable defects or masses
      iii. Strength tests to determine whether the gastrocnemius or soleus muscles are involved
   c. **Treatment**
      i. Ice with pressure wrap to control effusion
      ii. Crutches may be necessary until acute tenderness has subsided.
      iii. Heel lift may be used if weight bearing or partial weight bearing
      iv. Gentle early stretching and strengthening exercises depending on severity of the injury
3. **Strain or rupture of Achilles tendon**
   a. **Mechanism:** The same mechanism that causes calf muscle strains is responsible for injuries to the Achilles tendon. Actual ruptures or partial tears of the Achilles tendon usually occur in older athletes but may occur in high school and college age competitors.
   b. **Evaluation**
      i. History—tenderness is more distal in the calf to the musculotendinous junction or in the tendon itself.
      ii. A palpable, visible defect may be present and the ability to actively plantar flex the ankle is absent or diminished.
      iii. A common test (Thompson's test) for complete rupture is to squeeze the muscle mass proximal to the injury. In a compete tear, the foot does not plantar flex with this passive movement, thus indicating rupture of the Achilles tendon.
   c. **Treatment**
      i. Ice and compression are the immediate concern.
      ii. Non–weight-bearing crutch walking is required.
      iii. The decision as to surgical versus nonsurgical treatment is up to the experience of the physician.
4. **Fibular stress fracture**
   a. **Mechanism:** Fibular stress fractures in gymnasts are not uncommon owing to the frequency of activity that stresses the lower leg. The possibility of a stress fracture should not be overlooked when treating the athlete for chronic shin splints.

   b. **Evaluation:** Ongoing symptoms that include painful walking outside the gym, extreme isolated point tenderness, or pain with interosseous compression should prompt the physician to order x-ray studies and possibly a bone scan to rule out this possibility.
   c. **Treatment:** Most gymnasts are able to continue modified workouts with a fibular stress fracture because they can work the upper body on the various apparatus and avoid the dismounts, running, and landings necessary in floor and vault. Once healing has begun, the gymnast can slowly return to full activity with support as dictated by tolerance and the physician's discretion.

L. **Ankle injuries**
1. **Mechanism**
   a. In their competitive careers, most gymnasts experience some type of ankle injury. The ankles absorb a tremendous amount of force when the gymnast lands perfectly, and with a rotational or twisting component involved in many dismounts, the ankle is placed in even more jeopardy. Lateral ankle injuries (inversion–plantar flexion) occur quite often not only from improper landings, but also from the foot hitting a seam between mats.
   b. Acute anterior impingement of the tibia against the talus is a special problem in gymnasts caused by landing "short," in which the athlete underrotates a somersault and lands in a deep squatted position, jamming the anterior ankle. Over a course of time, this situation can lead to a chronic inflammatory condition with exostosis of the anterior talar lip. Because of these problems, it is not unusual for many competitive college gymnasts to exhibit early arthritic changes in the ankle that lead to arthroscopic or surgical intervention.
2. **Evaluation**
   a. History (acute or chronic)
   b. Check for:
      i. Effusion
      ii. Tenderness
      iii. Joint laxity
   c. X-rays when indicated to determine extent of bony changes.
3. **Treatment**
   a. Acute severe sprains:
      i. Pressure and ice
      ii. The ankle should be wrapped from the toes to above the ankle to avoid pitting edema of the foot.
      iii. Extreme injuries may require a bulky dressing or even a cast for proper healing and weight bearing.
      iv. In most cases, early motion and strengthening are important to ensure proper return to activity.
   b. Less severe sprains:
      i. Physical therapy
      ii. Strengthening
      iii. Support
      iv. Anti-inflammatory medications
      v. A fracture boot is commonly used in early stages of management in conjunction with crutches or alone to protect the joint.
      vi. It is highly recommended that competitive gymnasts protect their ankles with athletic tape or lace-up braces that allow full function while protecting against abnormal ROM.

M. **Foot injuries:** The same forces that are exerted on the ankle affect the foot structures as well.

1. **Medial longitudinal arch sprain**
   a. **Mechanism:** Pain in the medial aspect of the foot and along the course of the posterior tibialis tendon may or may not be associated with shin splints. Arch pain may be acute or result from chronic overuse syndrome.
   b. **Treatment**
      i. Proper management includes supporting the medial arch with tape and padding. Modification of footwear does not work because no rigid foot support is worn in gymnastics.
      ii. Appropriate physical therapy to control pain and swelling along with rest or modification of activity
2. **Heel bruising**
   a. **Mechanism:** In working dismounts from a somersault, athletes may overrotate the maneuver, which causes them to land with full weight on their heels. This can cause significant injury to the heel pad of one or both feet.
   b. **Evaluation**
      i. History
      ii. Physical exam reveals diffuse or specific point tenderness, localized heel pad swelling, and perhaps ecchymosis
   c. **Treatment**
      i. Ice massage
      ii. Padding for comfort
      iii. Solid plastic heel cup
      iv. Avoidance of reinjury is important to avoid chronic problems
      v. Physical therapy after 3–4 days to include moist heat, ultrasound, and electrical stimulation
      vi. Heel taping or heel cup draws natural padding of heel fat pad together.

III. Traumatic and Overuse Injury

A. Traumatic injuries in gymnastics, although many times quite serious, may be easier to deal with for everybody concerned than chronic overuse conditions. Typically the acute injury has a specific onset with predictable diagnosis and prognosis. Ground rules can be laid out in a specific manner.

B. Overuse syndromes can be hard to document, with symptoms coming and going until the athlete finally mentions them and usually wants something done immediately. Many gymnasts attempt to work through most injury situations and often are successful, so that by the time the resistant injury is reported, it will have become a full-blown chronic problem with a frustrating, lengthy return to activity. It is important that the team physician allow the athlete to remain as active as possible without compromising treatment of the injury in question.

IV. Injury Prevention

A. **Prevention of gymnastics injuries is directly related to organization and supervision in the gym itself.**

B. **Proper coaching and spotting techniques** are vital in preventing many serious injuries.

C. **Recognition of the gymnast's abilities** by the coach is important to make sure that the athlete is not attempting maneuvers before going through the proper learning sequence.

D. **Strengthening and flexibility training** along with proper warm-up are also essential in assuring lower incidence of injury.

V. Special Aspects of Prehabilitation and Rehabilitation

A. At the competitive level, it is important that the athlete be allowed to continue working on flexibility, strength, and cardiovascular conditioning as permitted.

B. Skill training can also continue within limits with lower extremity injuries, such as allowing modified swinging skills on apparatus, even though wearing a brace or even a short leg cast.
C. Other activities that may be permitted include swimming and cycling.

VI. Sport-Specific Facilities and Protective Equipment

A. Properly maintained and safe gymnastics apparatus are important in preventing injuries.
B. The use of tumbling pits and spotting belts where possible can decrease the incidence of injuries while the athlete is learning tumbling sequences, dismounts, and vaults.
C. Properly fitted, well-maintained hand grips are necessary in preventing injury.
D. It is up to the gymnast and coach to recognize and correct any possible problems before they occur.

VII. Sport-Specific Taping and Bracing

A. It is highly recommended that ankle taping or bracing be routine for competitive gymnasts.
B. Support at the wrist with various wraps, straps, compression sleeves, and athletic tapes is the norm for gymnasts. Every gymnast develops his or her own method of wrist support that may be different for each event or hand grip combination.
C. Taping the ankle to prevent extremes of dorsiflexion may help to prevent problems in landing short and anterior ankle impingement.

VIII. Special Concerns of the Gymnastic Team Physician

A. **Compliance**
   1. Compliance with physician's requests and orders may be a problem with some athletes, and gymnasts are no different. Coaches, parents, teammates, and the athletes themselves at times may resist orders for rest or modification of activities to allow an injury to heal.
   2. It is important that the physician discuss specific problems directly with not only the athlete but also the parents and coach to ensure that the entire story gets back to them to avoid this problem.

B. **Burnout**
   1. Gymnasts may begin their sport career as early as 4 or 5 years of age and continue past college, working out 5 to 6 days a week every week of the year. Even a highly successful young gymnast can develop signs of burnout and may continue in the sport only to please the coach or parents.
   2. **Injury and illness can be a way for the athlete to find a way out of the dilemma.** When this problem is suspected, it may be up to the physician to approach this problem and bring it out in the open for discussion by all concerned.

C. **Eating disorders**
   1. For gymnasts at any level to be successful, many have to control their body weight. If gymnasts are overweight, their sport can be much more difficult for them and may even lead to stress injuries.
   2. In an effort to control weight, both male and female gymnasts, but especially females, may develop eating disorders such as anorexia nervosa and bulimia, which can lead to serious physical and mental health problems and, if identified, should be dealt with by the physician for proper referral.

Recommended Reading

1. American Physical Therapy Association: Latest Techniques in Anterior Cruciate Ligament Surgery and Rehabilitation. JOSPT 15:256–322, 1992.
2. Andrews M, Noyes FR, Barber-Westin SD: Anterior cruciate ligament allograft reconstruction in the skeletally immature athlete. Am J Sports Med 22:48–54, 1994.

3. Arnheim DD, Prentice WE: Principles of Athletic Training (8th ed). St. Louis, Mosby Year Book, 1993.
4. Bale P, Goodway J: Performance variables associated with the competitive gymnast. Sports Med 10:139–145, 1990.
5. Barron JL, Yocum LA: Unrecognized Achilles tendon rupture associated with ipsilateral medial malleolar fracture. Am J Sports Med 21:629–631, 1993.
6. Biedert R: Dislocation of the tibialis posterior tendon. Am J Sports Med 20:775–776, 1992.
7. Dalldorf PG, Bryan WJ: Displaced Salter-Harris type I injury in a gymnast: A slipped capital humeral epiphysis? Orthop Rev 23:538–541, 1994.
8. DeSmet L, Claessens A, Fabry G: Gymnast wrist. Acta Orthop Belg 59:377–380, 1993.
9. Dixon M, Fricker P: Injuries to elite gymnasts over 10 years. Med Sci Sports Exerc 25:1322–1329, 1993.
10. Dobyns JH, Gabel GT: Gymnast's wrist. Hand Clin 6:493–505, 1990.
11. Goldstein JD, Berger PE, Windler GE, Jackson DW: Spine injuries in gymnasts and swimmers: An epidemiologic investigation. Am J Sports Med 19:463–468, 1991.
12. Hoppenfeld S: Physical Examination of the Spine and Extremities. Norwalk, CT, Appleton and Lange, 1976.
13. Howse C: Wrist injuries in sport. Sports Med 17:163–175, 1994.
14. Kerr G: Preventing gymnastic injuries. Can J Sport Sci 15:227, 1990.
15. Lane V: Gymnastics. Practitioner 234:752–755, 1990.
16. Ledbetter WB, Buckwalter JA, Gordon SL (eds): Sports-Induced Inflammation. Park Ridge, IL, American Academy of Orthopaedic Surgeons, 1991.
17. Lindner KJ, Caine DJ: Injury patterns of female competitive club gymnasts. Can J Sports Sci 15:254–261, 1990.
18. Maffulli N, Chan D, Aldridge MJ: Overuse injuries of the olecranon in young gymnasts. J Bone Joint Surg Br 74:305–308, 1992.
19. Markoff KL, Shapiro MS, Mandelbaum BR, Teurlings L: Wrist loading patterns during pommel horse exercises. J Biomech 23:1001–1011, 1990.
20. Meeusen R, Borms J: Gymnastic injuries. Sports Med 13:337–356, 1992.
21. Proffer DS, Patton JJ, Jackson DW: Nonunion of a first rib fracture in a gymnast. Am J Sports Med 19:198–201, 1991.
22. Ruggles DL, Peterson HA, Scott SG: Radial growth plate injury in a female gymnast. Med Sci Sports Exerc 23:393–396, 1991.
23. Sands WA, Shultz BB, Newman AP: Women's gymnastic injuries: A 5-year study. Am J Sports Med 21:271–276, 1993.
24. Stinson JT, Wiesel SW (eds): Spine Problems in the Athlete. Clin Sports Med 12(3):entire issue, 1993.
25. Stuart PR, Briggs PJ: Closed extensor tendon rupture and distal radial fracture with use of a gymnast's wrist support. Br J Sports Med 27:92–93, 1993.
26. Sward L, Hellstrom M, Jacobsson B, Karlsson L: Vertebral ring apophysis injury in athletes: Is the etiology different in the thoracic and lumbar spine? Am J Sports Med 21:841–845, 1993.
27. Tolat AR, Sanderson PL, DeSmet L, Stanley JK: The gymnast's wrist: Acquired positive ulnar variance following chronic epiphyseal injury. J Hand Surg Br 17:678–681, 1992.
28. Victor J, Mulier T, Fabry G: Refracture of radius and ulna in a female gymnast: A case report. Am J Sports Med 21:753–754, 1993.
29. Wadley GH, Albright JP: Women's intercollegiate gymnastics: Injury patterns and "permanent" medical disability. Am J Sports Med 21:314–320, 1993.
30. Watson JT, Bergfeld JA (eds): Fractures. Clin Sports Med 9(1):entire issue, 1990.
31. Weiker GG: Hand and wrist problems in the gymnast. Clin Sports Med 11:189–202, 1992.
32. Woo SL-Y, Buckwalter JA (eds): Injury and Repair of the Musculoskeletal Soft Tissues. Park Ridge, IL, American Academy of Orthopaedic Surgeons, 1991.

63

Bicycling

Morris B. Mellion, M.D.

I. Bicycling and Bicycle Racing

A. **General concerns.** Stimulated by four American bicycle racing gold medals in the 1984 Olympics and Greg Le Mond's victory in the 1986 and 1989 Tour de France, bicycling has experienced an explosive increase in popularity in the United States. The total number of U.S. bicyclists has risen from 72 million in 1983 to 99 million in 1992, and racing, touring, and off-road riding are among the fastest-growing sports. The number of mountain bike riders alone increased from 200,000 in 1983 to 25 million in 1992. Consequently, physicians should understand how to prevent, evaluate, and manage the wide variety of traumatic and overuse injuries commonly experienced by the cyclist. **To treat bicyclists effectively, physicians must know the basic design and function of the bicycle, the relationship of proper and improper bicycle "fit" to injuries, and the potential of the various forms of serious riding and racing for injury**.

1. **Road racing** is a term used to describe all forms of bicycle racing on the open road as well as a specific event.
   a. The **time trial** is a race against the clock in which riders start at intervals of generally 1 minute.
      i. A short race, generally 9–50 miles (15–80 km)
      ii. Intense test of physical and mental strength
      iii. **Relatively trauma-free** because of distance between riders
      iv. **Variation: team time trial**—four cyclists per team riding in a pace line
   b. The **criterium** is a fast race of many laps around a short course beginning with a mass start.
      i. Distance usually 15–65 miles (24–104 km)
      ii. **Many fast racers in a pack** making tight turns at close range
         (a) **Many spills** occur.
         (b) **Skill and experience are paramount.**
   c. The **road race event** is a 1-day race over a long stretch of open road beginning with a mass start.
      i. Distance generally > 40 miles (64 km); > 100 miles (160 km) typical for high-level riders
      ii. **Grueling endurance event. Medical concerns include:**
         (a) **Trauma**
         (b) **Overuse**
         (c) **Dehydration and heat illness**
         (d) **Nutritional problems**
         (e) **Hypothermia in cooler weather**
   d. A **stage race** is a set of various road race events on consecutive days.
      i. Generally scored both as individual stages and as a collective single race
      ii. Two short stages may be held on single day.

e. **"Ultra races"** are multiday distance races that generally continue through the night.
   i. Examples: Race Across America (RAAM) and Paris-Brest Paris Race
   ii. **Medical concerns:**
      (a) **Extreme fatigue and sleep deprivation**
      (b) **Fluids and nutrition**
      (c) **Hyperthermia and hypothermia**
      (d) **Overuse and trauma**

2. **Track racing** includes a variety of individual and team events in which **specialized bicycles, generally without brakes,** are ridden on steeply banked indoor and outdoor tracks.
   a. **Medical concerns: trauma** related to riding at close quarters through tight turns on a narrow track
   b. There are few velodromes in the United States, and most have rough, poor-quality surfaces.
3. **Triathlon** is an endurance competition consisting of swimming, bicycling, and running portions in immediate succession.
   Medical concerns:
   a. **Hyperthermia and hypothermia**
   b. **Dehydration and nutrition**
   c. **Overuse and trauma**
4. **All-terrain bicycle racing** involves heavier, lower-geared bicycles with wide balloon tires and upright handlebars in competition in rough or hilly terrain. These bicycles are also popular for recreational riding in similar terrain as well as on the open road and in urban areas. They are usually ridden without toe clips.
   Medical concerns:
   a. **Overuse on flat or uphill terrain**
   b. **Trauma on the downhills**
5. **Cyclo-cross** is an off-road race in which the competitor who covers the greatest distance in laps around a 1–2 mile course of rough terrain in a set amount of time wins. The type of bicycle used varies with the course. The racer may have to carry the bicycle around or over obstacles.
   Medical concerns:
   a. **Trauma**
   b. **Overuse**

B. **Bicycle touring** is open-road riding for recreation.
   1. **Light touring:** Riding with only a handlebar bag or seat bag; may be supported by vehicles (often called **"sag wagons"**), especially for multiday trips
   2. **Loaded touring:** Carrying large amounts of luggage in panniers (saddle bags) attached to racks mounted adjacent to the front and rear tires
   3. **Medical concerns**
      a. **Overuse**
      b. **Trauma**
      c. **Thermoregulation**
      d. **Dehydration**
      e. **Sun exposure**

C. **Rules to protect the cyclist**
   1. Helmet requirements
   2. Gearing limitations by age of racer (U.S. Cycling Federation, e.g., young racers may not have extremely high gears on their bicycles)
   3. Prerace equipment checks by officials
   4. Requirement for water and aid stations at races
   5. Riding conduct rules

II. The Bicycle

A. Anatomy and terminology of the modern bicycle

1. A bicycle consists of a **frame** ("frameset") with various **components**, such as handlebars, brakes, and wheels, attached (Fig. 1).
2. The frame is shaped like a diamond lying on its side (Fig. 2)
   a. Racing bicycles have more upright geometry with steeper angles to the diamond making a stiffer frame that is more responsive in the turns.
   b. Touring bicycles have somewhat flatter geometry, producing more shock absorption with some sacrifice in cornering.
   c. All-terrain bicycles have somewhat flatter geometry that absorbs shock on rough surfaces with greater sacrifice in cornering.

B. **Proper fit of the bicycle to the rider** is critical for prevention and treatment of overuse injuries in cyclists.

1. The most efficient, accurate method to fit a bicycle for a racer or serious rider is with a **commercial system such as a Fit Kit or ProBike Fit.** This service is generally provided for a fee by bicycle mechanics at shops that cater to racers and other serious riders. Riders using cleated shoes or step-in pedals may have their cleat adjustment checked and set using the **rotational adjustment device** associated with the Fit Kit.
2. Frame size selection and the basic fit adjustments may be made by estimates using these guidelines:
   a. **Frame size.** To determine the proper frame size of a bicycle, the rider should straddle the top of the bicycle with both feet, in riding shoes, flat on the ground (Fig. 3):
      i. For racing, triathlon, criterium, and touring bicycles, there should be a 1–2 inch space between the crotch and the top tube.
      ii. For mountain bikes and hybrids, the clearance should be 3–6 inches, with the higher end of the scale being safer for extremely rough terrain.

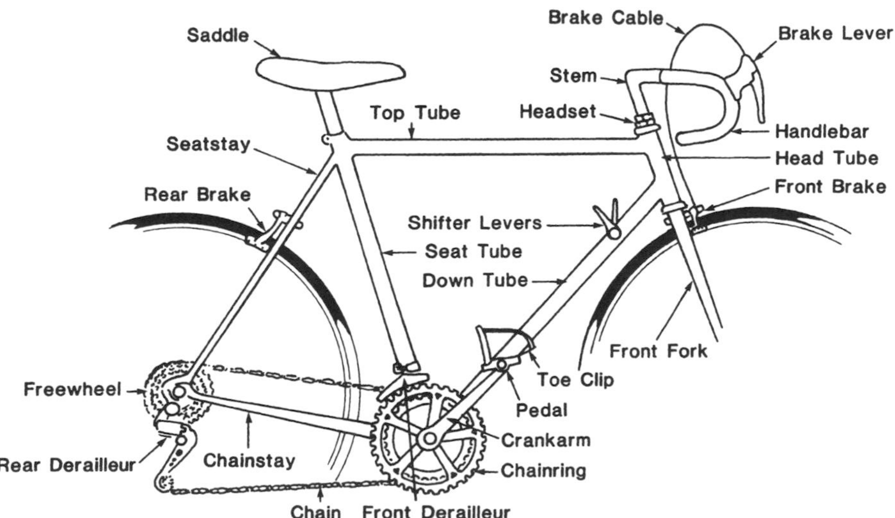

FIGURE 1. Anatomy and terminology of a modern bicycle. (From Mellion MB: Bicycle injuries: Prevention, diagnosis, and treatment. In Mellion MB (ed): Office Sports Medicine, 2nd ed. Philadelphia, Hanley & Belfus, 1996, pp 355–374.)

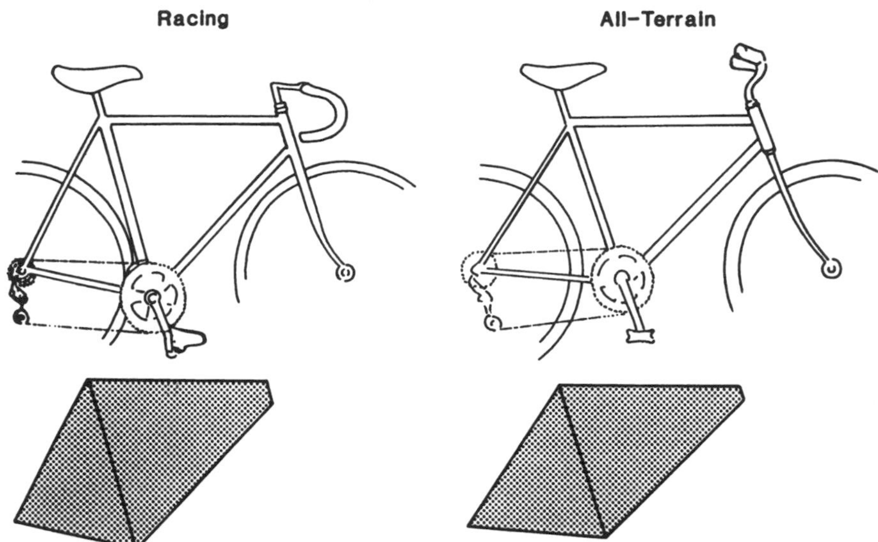

FIGURE 2. The bicycle frame is shaped like a diamond lying on its side. Racing bicycles have more upright geometry with steeper angles to the diamond. All-terrain bicycles have somewhat flatter geometry with more shallow angles. Touring bicycles are generally in between.

iii. Another technique for determining frame size is to measure inseam height (Fig. 4) and multiply by 0.65 for road bikes and 0.52 for mountain bikes.

b. **Seat height.** Several scientific and quasiscientific methods exist:

i. **Inseam method.** With rider wearing cycling shoes, measure inseam (floor to crotch) (Fig. 4) and multiply by 1.06–1.09 to obtain seat height measured from the top of the saddle to the top of the pedal when the crank arm is at 6 o'clock ("dead-bottom center").

ii. **Knee flexion measurement method.** With the bicycle on a wind trainer or positioned next to a wall or a vehicle for support, saddle height is set so that there is 25–30° of knee flexion when the saddle is in a neutral fore-aft position and the pedal is at dead-bottom center (Fig. 5).

iii. **Bone length method.** With the rider standing upright, back flat against a wall, and legs spread 6 inches, measure upper leg length from greater

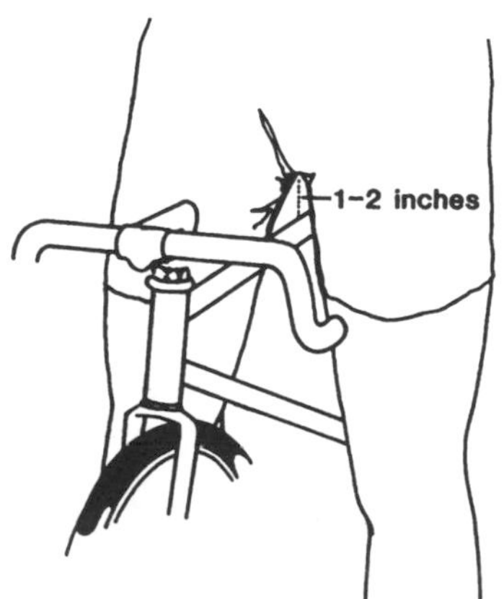

FIGURE 3. Proper frame size. Allow 1–2 inches between the crotch and the top frame tube. For mountain bikes and hybrids, the clearance should be 3–6 inches with the higher end of the scale safer for extremely rough terrain. (From Mellion MB: Bicycling injuries: Prevention, diagnosis and treatment. In Mellion MB (ed): Office Sports Medicine, 2nd ed. Philadelphia, Hanley & Belfus, 1996, pp 355–374.)

trochanter to lateral femoral condyle and lower leg length from lateral femoral condyle to tip of lateral malleolus. Seat height equals the sum of upper and lower leg length multiplied by 0.96 (Fig. 6).

iv. **Estimation from leg length.** With the bicycle on a wind trainer or positioned next to a wall or vehicle for support, the rider sits with the pedals in the 6 and 12 o'clock positions with the heels on the pedals. The seat should be raised or lowered until the leg on the 6 o'clock pedal is barely straight (Fig. 7).

v. **"Rocking in the saddle" method.** Raise the seat to the point at which the rider must rock from side to side to pedal; then lower it until the rocking disappears.
   (a) Roughest estimate, although many coaches swear by it
   (b) Not as reliable in less experienced cyclists who may pedal in toe-down position
   (c) Excellent method for setting exercycle height in a gym or athletic club

vi. **All seat height formulas are estimates.**
   (a) Adjustments of ¼ inch at a time, usually upward, may be made after a trial of several rides.
   (b) More experienced riders may make adjustments as small as ⅛ inch.

vii. **Pitfalls of seat height formulas**
   (a) They do not account for foot length or riding style. An individual with a foot disproportionately large for leg length who rides with a predominantly toe-down style might require a larger frame.

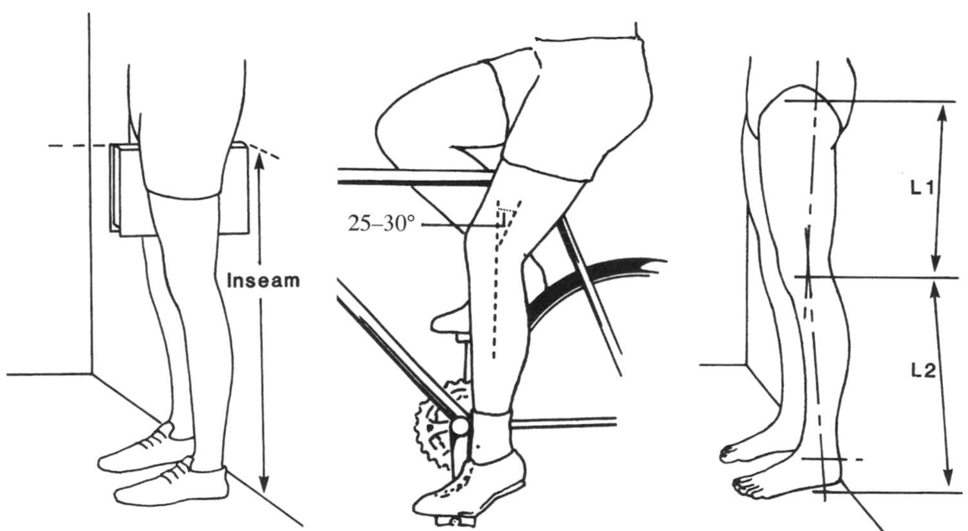

FIGURE 4 *(Left).* Seat height by inseam method. With rider wearing cycling shoes, measure inseam (floor to crotch) and multiply by 1.06 inches to obtain seat height.

FIGURE 5 *(Middle).* Seat height by knee flexion method. Measure the amount of knee flexion with the foot at dead-bottom center of the pedaling stroke (6 o'clock). There should be 25–30° flexion of the extended leg. The rider's ankle should be at the same angle that it usually is at dead-bottom center in the cyclist's normal riding position. (From Mellion MB: Bicycle injuries: Prevention, diagnosis, and treatment. In Mellion MB (ed): Office Sports Medicine, 2nd ed. Philadelphia, Hanley & Belfus, 1996, pp 355–374.)

FIGURE 6 *(Right).* Seat height by bone length method. With the rider standing upright, back flat against a wall, and legs spread 6 inches, measure upper leg length from greater trochanter to lateral femoral condyle and lower leg length from lateral femoral condyle to tip of lateral malleolus. Seat height equals the sum of upper and lower leg length multiplied by 0.96.

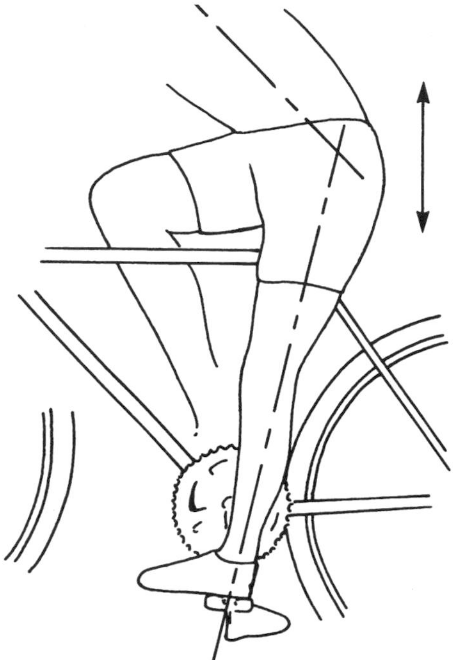

FIGURE 7. Seat height estimation from leg length. With the bicycle positioned next to a wall or vehicle for support, the rider sits with the pedals in the 6 and 12 o'clock positions with the heels on the pedals. The seat should be raised or lowered until the leg on the 6 o'clock pedal is barely straight.

(b) Saddle compressibility and rider weight vary so that a heavier rider on a more compressible saddle might have an effectively lower seat height than that obtained by measurement.

(c) The distance between the sole of the riding shoe and the pedal spindle differs significantly among the wide variety of available clipless pedals.

c. **Fore and aft saddle position.** The bicycle saddle is built on a pair of rails that are connected to the seat post and allow approximately 1.5 inches of adjustment range. With the rider in the saddle and the pedals at the 3 and 9 o'clock positions, the seat should be adjusted so that a plumb line dropped from the front edge of the patella should fall to the end of the crank arm (Fig. 8). This is virtually the same position as previous recommendations that a plumb line dropped from the tibial tubercle intersect the axle of the pedal.

d. **Saddle angle**

i. Saddle angle should be set using a carpenter's level placed along the longitudinal axis of the saddle.

ii. **One anatomic difference between male and female riders is the angle of the pubic arch in relation to the saddle angle.**

(a) In the **male**, the arch of the pubic symphysis is higher and allows enough clearance above the nose of the saddle that the rider can tolerate a saddle that is level or angled slightly upward in front.

(b) The shallower **female** pubic arch may cause the soft tissue of the perineum to press against the nose of the saddle. Consequently, most women may prefer to have the saddle level or tilted slightly downward. Others attempt to compensate by riding with a more upright posture to take the weight off the anterior perineum.

e. **Reach.** Handlebar reach is the distance from the saddle to the transverse part of the handlebars. A rough estimate of proper reach may be obtained by placing the elbow at the front of the seat with the fingers fully extended (Fig. 9).

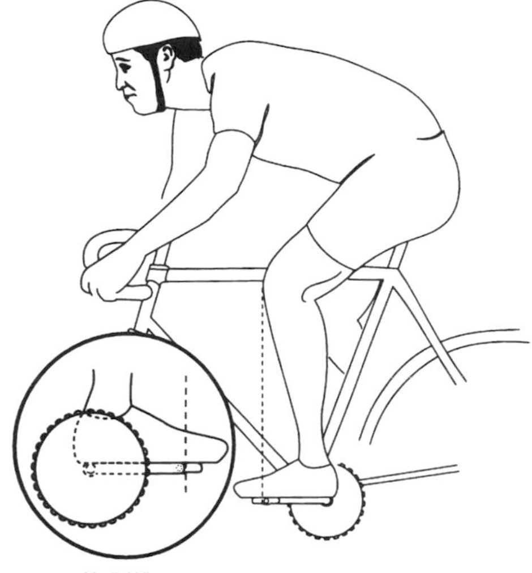

FIGURE 8. Seat position relative to the pedals is determined by putting the pedals at the 3 o'clock and 9 o'clock positions, with the ball of the foot firmly on the pedal. A plumb line dropped from the middle of the anterior surface of the patella should fall at the front edge of the crank arm. (From Mellion MB: Bicycle injuries: Prevention, diagnosis, and treatment. In Mellion MB (ed): Office Sports Medicine, 2nd ed. Philadelphia, Hanley & Belfus, 1996, pp 355–374.)

i. More accurate determinations of reach may be made using trunk measurements with the Fit Kit or according to formulas in the bicycle literature.

ii. The reach is adjusted by replacing the stem with one having more or less extension (Fig. 10).

f. **Handlebar height.** The handlebar height should always be at or lower than seat height.

i. For racing, it should always be lower than seat height. How low depends on individual characteristics of the rider and specific type of race.

(a) More experienced riders may want a lower position to improve aerodynamics.

(b) Time trialists and other short distance racers may place the stem 3–4 inches or more below the saddle height.

ii. Taller riders may want the difference between saddle height and the top of the handlebars to be greater to accommodate longer arms.

iii. Handlebars on mountain bikes should be 1–2 inches below the top of the saddle to help put weight on the front wheel.

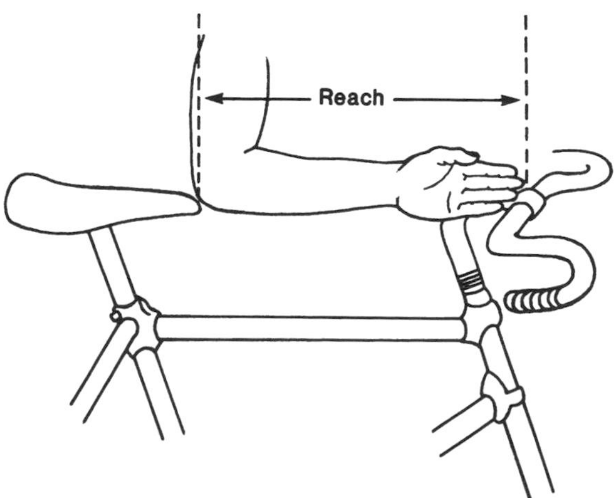

FIGURE 9. Handlebar reach is the distance from the saddle to the transverse part of the handlebars. A rough estimate of proper reach may be obtained by placing the elbow at the front of the seat with the fingers fully extended. (From Mellion MB: Bicycle injuries: Prevention, diagnosis, and treatment. In Mellion MB (ed): Office Sports Medicine, 2nd ed. Philadelphia, Hanley & Belfus, 1996, pp 355–374.)

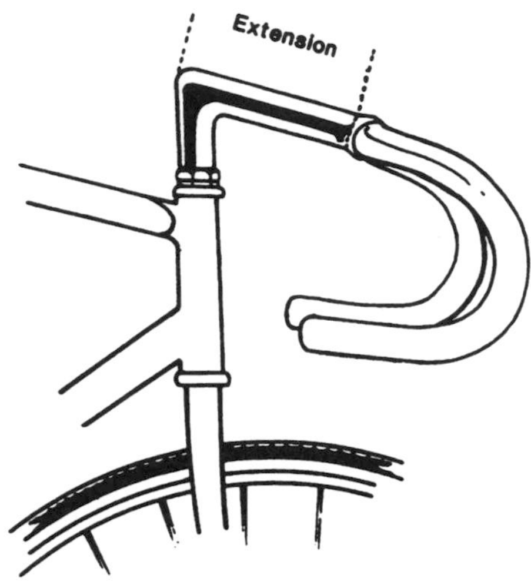

FIGURE 10. Extension is the horizontal length of the handlebar stem. The reach is adjusted by replacing the stem with one having more or less extension. (From Mellion MB: Bicycling injuries: Prevention, diagnosis, and treatment. In Mellion MB (ed): Office Sports Medicine, 2nd ed. Philadelphia, Hanley & Belfus, 1996, pp 355–374.)

g. **Handlebar width**
   i. Handlebar width on the **road bike** should equal shoulder width measured between the lateral borders of the acromions.
   ii. **Mountain bike** handlebar width should be determined empirically by comfort of the rider.
   iii. Narrower handlebars provide quicker steering, and wider bars give more control at slower speeds.

h. **Aero bar**
   i. Aerodynamic body position, much like a downhill ski racing tuck, for long periods of time (Fig. 11)
   ii. Takes rider's weight off hands, thus protecting against nerve root entrapment in wrists
   iii. Extensive use in :
      (a) Triathlon
      (b) Time trials
      (c) Touring
      (d) Ultramarathon

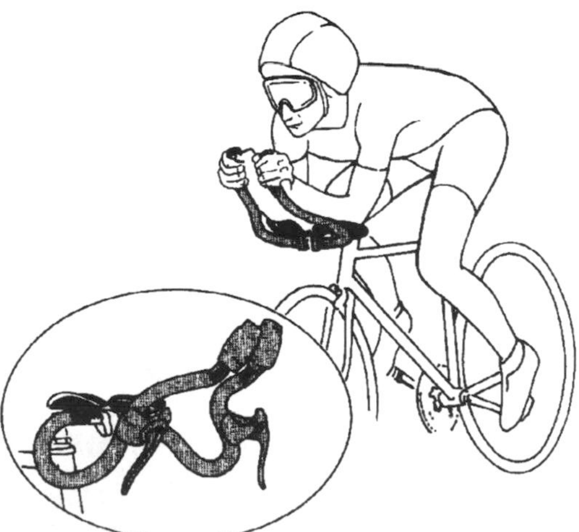

FIGURE 11. The aero bar is designed to permit the rider to maintain a highly aerodynamic position for a prolonged time. (From Mellion MB: Common cycling injuries: Management and prevention. Sports Med 11:52–70, 1991, with permission.)

TABLE 1. Treatment of Leg Length Discrepancies with Bicycle Fit Adjustments

Rule 1: Always adjust the bicycle first to the long leg
Rule 2: Corrections for length should always slightly undercompensate the total difference because many cyclists adapt by increased "ankling" (dorsiflexion or plantar flexion) while pedaling.

Example A: Tibial Length Discrepancy of 6 mm
Adjust saddle height to allow 25–30° of knee flexion at dead-bottom center of the pedaling stroke on the long leg
Correct for the length difference on the short leg using approximately 4 mm of a lift or leather shim that is placed between the shoe and the cleat
Use cycling orthotics to correct for active pronation

Example B: Femoral Length Discrepancy of 6 mm
Adjust saddle height to allow 25–30° of knee flexion at dead-bottom center of the pedaling stroke on the long leg
Place a 2- or 3-mm lift or shim between the shoe and the cleat on the short leg
Move the foot of the short leg back 2 mm on the pedal
Move the foot of the long leg forward 2 mm on the pedal

From Holmes JC, Pruitt AL, Whalen NJ: Lower extremity overuse in bicycling. Clin Sports Med 13:187–203, 1994, with permission.

iv. Aero bar height set lower than seat height in attempt to flatten rider's back to a position parallel to the ground

i. **Leg length discrepancy.** Riders with leg length discrepancies have special fit needs (Table 1).
   i. In general, the bicycle should be fit to the long leg with special corrections for the short leg.
   ii. **Tibial leg length discrepancies** can be corrected with lifts or shims installed between the pedal and the shoe and/or with cyclist orthotics.
   iii. **Femoral leg length discrepancies** require a combination of lifts, shims, and orthotics with a modification of the foot position on the pedal. The long leg should be moved a few millimeters forward and the short leg a few millimeters back.

C. **Pedaling and gearing.** Riding with too much pedal resistance at too low a cadence (pedal revolutions per minute) is second only to improper bicycle fit as a cause of overuse problems in cyclists.
   1. **General principles.** The human body functions most effectively and safely in a narrow range of pedal resistance to effort.
      a. **Sources of resistance to bicycle movement:**
         i. **Inertia of bicycle and rider**
         ii. **Uphill grade** (gravity)
         iii. **Wind**
         iv. **Friction of air.** Approximately 90% of the energy expended riding 20 mph on a calm day is used to overcome the friction of the bicycle and the rider against the still air.
         v. **Rolling resistance** of tires on road surface
         vi. **Fatigue.** Strength, force, and efficiency are all reduced in fatigued muscles.
      b. **Gearing.** A method of overcoming resistance that allows the cyclist to pedal comfortably with a relatively constant pedal resistance at a generally uniform cadence by shifting through a range of 10–24 "speeds" or gears (Fig. 12):
         i. **Chainwheels** are the relatively large front gears attached to the "crank," or axle, around which the rider pedals.
            (a) **Large chainwheel** and **small chainwheel** used on virtually all road bicycles and all-terrain bicycles
            (b) **"Granny":** a small chainwheel used for hill climbing on touring bicycles and all-terrain bicycles

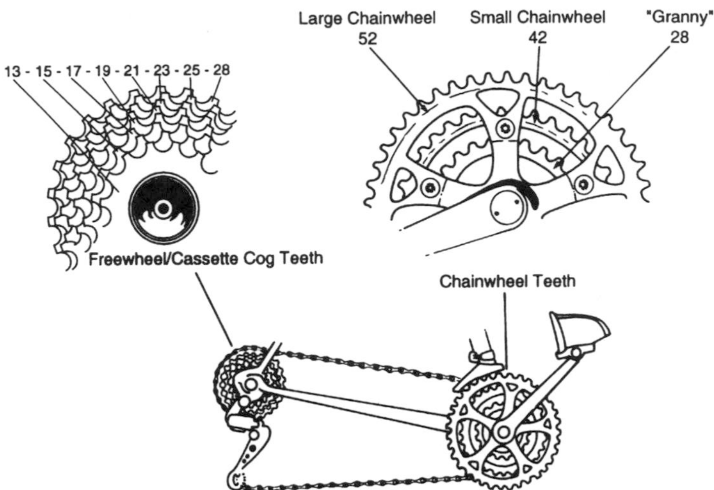

FIGURE 12. Modern bicycle gearing. This example is from a touring bicycle with three chainwheels on the crank and eight cogs on the cassette/freewheel. (From Mellion MB: Bicycling injuries: Prevention, diagnosis, and treatment. In Mellion MB (ed): Office Sports Medicine, 2nd ed. Philadelphia, Hanley & Belfus, 1996, pp 355–374.)

ii. The **cassette** or **freewheel** is a cluster of 5–9 gears ("cogs") mounted to the right of the rear wheel on the same axle.

iii. A **chain** composed of evenly spaced links connects one of the chainwheels to one of the cassette or freewheel cogs to drive the rear wheel of the bicycle. Because the gear teeth must be evenly spaced and of uniform size to mesh with the links of the chain, the size of the gears may be expressed by the number of teeth they have.

(a) The front derailleur shifts the chain from one chainwheel to another.

(b) The rear derailleur shifts the chain from one cog of the cassette or freewheel to another.

iv. **Gear ratio** is the ratio of the size of the chainwheel in use to that of the freewheel cog in use:

$$\text{Gear ratio} = \frac{\text{\# of teeth on chainwheel}}{\text{\# of teeth on freewheel cog}}$$

(a) Higher gear ratios result in higher pedal resistance in given riding conditions. Riding safely with higher gear ratios requires strength, endurance, and better technique.

(b) Lower gear ratios may result in lower pedal resistance and may permit pedaling, or "spinning," at a higher cadence.

v. Generally, racers and other serious bicyclists in the United States multiply the gear ratio by the diameter of the rear wheel to obtain a ratio known as **gear number** or **gear inches:**

(a) **Gear number** (gear inches) = Gear ratio × rear wheel diameter, expressed in inches

(b) Table 2 indicates the ranges of gear ratios generally available on road and all-terrain bicycles and describes the uses of these gear ratios.

2. **Optimal cadence** (pedal revolutions per minute) varies with the type of riding and the skill, strength, and endurance of the athlete.

a. **May be expressed in terms of several variables:**

TABLE 2. Ranges and Uses of Gear Ratios

Examples	Gear Ratio = # of teeth on chainwheel / # of teeth on freewheel cog	Gear Inches = gear ratio × wheel diameter
Very high gear	$\frac{52}{13} = 4$	4 × 27 = 108
Lower gear	$\frac{52}{26} = 2$	2 × 27 = 54
Very low gear	$\frac{28}{28} = 1$	1 × 27 = 27

Gear Inches	Uses
27–35 (or lower)	Very low gears. Used for climbing steep hills. Also used for touring hilly terrain with a heavily loaded bicycle
36–44	Low gears. Used for climbing hills or riding into a severe headwind
45–60	Slightly low gears. Used for gentle hills or mild headwind
61–85	Standard gears. Used for riding on level ground. Effort may be maintained for a long time
86–108	High gears. Used for high-speed riding. Used when riding downhill or riding with a tailwind
> 108	Special gearing, not available on most bicycles. Used by competitive racers

i. **Gross efficiency** (work performed/energy cost)
   (a) 60–80 rpm optimal for moderate-to-high workloads
   (b) Up to 100 rpm for exceptionally high workloads
   (c) Falls off sharply > 100 rpm

ii. **Heart rate**
   (a) 80 rpm optimal peak
   (b) 60–100 rpm optimal range

iii. **Perceived exertion**
   (a) 80 rpm optimal peak
   (b) 60–100 rpm optimal range

iv. **Lactate concentration**
   (a) 80 rpm optimal peak
   (b) 60–100+ rpm optimal range
   (c) At 110–120 rpm, lactate rises steeply

v. **Generation of power for effective racing**
   (a) 90–110 rpm optimal range (may be mechanically more efficient)
   (b) Short bursts at higher rpm

b. **Racers must often sacrifice efficiency for speed.**

c. **An individual rider's percent of fast-twitch and slow-twitch muscle fibers may influence optimal cadence.**

d. **Relatively high cadence/low resistance pedaling reduces the incidence of overuse injuries. Racers and serious cyclists should begin their seasons with 500–1000 miles of this kind of riding.**

III. Bicycle Injuries

A. General injury data

1. More than 600,000 bicycle injury visits per year to U.S. emergency rooms

2. **Approximately half of hospital admissions from cycling accidents involved motor vehicles. Most often, the vehicle driver fails to see the bicyclist,** especially in low-light dawn and dusk hours and at night.
3. **Road surface damage and obstacles often involved:**
   a. Road cracks and potholes
   b. Damaged shoulders
   c. Trash on road
   d. Gravel on surface (often left from previous winter's snow control)
   e. Railroad crossings
   f. Sewer openings and rain drainage gates
   g. Cattle guards
   h. Curbs

B. **Traumatic injuries**
1. **Head injuries**
   a. Account for most of bicycle-related deaths
   b. Generally preventable
   c. Victims rarely wearing helmets
2. **Face injuries**
   a. Most often abrasions and contusions
   b. **Good helmet offers substantial protection**
3. **Musculoskeletal injuries**
   a. Contusions, sprains, and fractures
   b. Common sites
      i. Hand
      ii. Wrist and lower arm
      iii. Shoulder
      iv. Ankle and lower leg
4. **Abdominal and genital injuries**—from handlebar trauma when stopping short
5. **Skin injuries**
   a. Lacerations
   b. Abrasions: **"road rash"**
      i. Grading system similar to burns:
         (a) First degree: superficial
         (b) Second degree: partial thickness
         (c) Third degree: full thickness
      ii. Treatment
         (a) First degree, second degree, and small third degree:
            • Hydroactive dressings (DuoDerm, Tegasorb)
            • Silvadene cream, three times per day
         (b) Larger third degree
            • Silvadene cream, three times per day
            • Wet-to-dry soaks
         (c) Tetanus prophylaxis
6. **Spoke injuries**
   a. Loose spikes must be tightened or removed.
   b. If a spoke must be removed, loosen the two adjacent spokes. Ride slowly home or to assistance until the wheel is either replaced or fixed.
   c. Spoke injuries are often caused by getting a finger, foot, or piece of clothing caught in the wheel while riding. These injuries are almost always avoidable.
7. **Bicycle-mounted child seat injury**
   a. Riding in a bicycle-mounted child seat exposes the child to adult-level forces.
   b. Most injuries involve head and face; therefore, **helmet use is critical.**

C. **Strategies to prevent trauma**
   1. **Use proper protective clothing and safety equipment** (see page 802).
   2. **Maintain bicycle in top mechanical condition**
      a. **Check brakes frequently.** Ensure that there is no lubricant on the brake pad surface or on the adjacent braking surface of the wheel. Clean wheel braking surface with acetone if necessary.
      b. **Check tires and tubes frequently;** repair or replace if even slightly damaged.
      c. **Perform a preride check routinely.** Check quick-release levers on wheels whenever getting on bicycle.
   3. **Anticipate the errors of others.**
      a. Assume that the other riders or vehicle drivers do not see you.
      b. Watch the eyes of motor vehicle drivers.
   4. **Riding strategies**
      a. Control speed. Reduce speed when brakes are wet.
      b. Anticipate obstacles and road damage.
      c. Practice with extra clothing in a protected area:
         i. Diverting around obstacles
         ii. Jumping over obstacles
         iii. Braking technique
         iv. Forced turns and tight downhill turns

D. **Overuse injuries**
   1. **Neckache and backache**
      a. Common problem; up to 60% of riders
      b. **Upper left trapezius and levator scapula** muscles also common sites.
         i. Caused by muscle tension from watching for overtaking traffic, either by turning head or by looking through helmet mirror.
         ii. Trigger point spasms may develop.
      c. **Mechanism of injury**
         i. Increased load on arms and shoulders to support rider
         ii. Increased handlebar "reach" causing hyperextension of neck and exaggerated flexion of low back—accentuated by dropped handlebars
         iii. Road shock transmitted through handlebars, arms, and shoulder girdle to neck. Cumulative effect in long rides, especially in ultramarathon.
      d. **Management**
         i. **Mechanical:**
            (a) Raise handlebars
            (b) Use stem with shorter extension
            (c) Move seat forward
            (d) Use handlebars with less drop
            (e) Ride with "unlocked" elbows
            (f) Change hand position frequently
            (g) Change mirror placement
            (h) Switch to upright handlebar
         ii. **Medical:**
            (a) Strength and flexibility exercises: dynamic cervicothoracic and lumbar muscular stabilization
            (b) Ice massage
            (c) Nonsteroidal anti-inflammatory drugs (NSAIDs)
            (d) Skeletal muscle relaxants (not benzodiazepines)
      e. Evaluate **treatment failures** for:
         i. Degenerative disk disease—radiculopathy
         ii. Degenerative arthritis

f. **Scheuermann's disease**
   i. Increased incidence reported in adolescent bicycle racers
   ii. Attributed to anterior end plate damage from pulling hard on handlebars while pedaling too large a gear

2. **Handlebar problems**
   a. **Ulnar neuropathy** ("cyclist's palsy" or "handlebar palsy")
      i. Gradual onset of numbness, tingling, and/or weakness in the ring and little fingers. Generally occurs after several days of long or intensive rides.
      ii. Duration: several days to months
      iii. Etiology:
         (a) Ulnar nerve compression at the wrist in or near Guyon's canal
         (b) Nerve traction due to hyperextension of wrists while riding
      iv. **Management**
         (a) **Mechanical:**
            - Check bicycle fit. Improper fit may increase the forces at the wrists.
            - Decrease the length or intensity of rides.
            - Wear padded gloves.
            - Add handlebar padding.
            - Change hand position frequently
            - Avoid hand positions with marked wrist hyperextension.
         (b) **Medical:**
            - Generally resolves spontaneously
            - Rarely, surgical decompression
   b. **Carpal tunnel syndrome**
      i. Rarely result of handlebar trauma alone
      ii. Management similar to ulnar neuropathy
   c. **de Quervain's syndrome**
      i. Anecdotal reports related to shifting in intense mountain bike riding
      ii. Technical advances in shifters should prevent

3. **Saddle problems**
   a. **Ischial tuberosity soreness**
      i. Tenderness associated with infrequent riding occurs at beginning of riding session
      ii. Generally self-limited
   b. **Skin problems**
      i. **Chafing**
         (a) **Mechanical management:**
            - Padded riding shorts
            - Seat position and height adjustment
            - Saddle pad
            - Saddle change to different shape or padded saddle
         (b) **Medical management:**
            - Change out of sweat-soaked shorts and shower immediately after riding
            - Talcum powder; effective only for short rides
            - Lubricating ointments, e.g., Cramer's Skin Lube or Mueller's lubricant
            - Anusol or Anusol HC creams
            - Nonfluorinated corticosteroid creams
            - Shave perineum prophylactically to prevent irritation caused by traction on hairs
      ii. **"Saddle sores" management** (folliculitis, furuncles, carbuncles)
         (a) Warm soaks
         (b) Incision and drainage
         (c) Antibiotics—may involve coliforms in this area

iii. **Callus formation** over ischial tuberosities
(a) Adaptive response to friction and pressure
(b) Management—trim back with pumice stone if thick enough to be a problem
iv. **Subcutaneous perineal nodules**
(a) Necrotic fascial "pseudocyst"
(b) Racers and serious riders
(c) May appear as "accessory testicles"
c. **Pudendal neuropathy**
i. Numbness and tingling in scrotum and penile shaft
ii. Etiology—compression of dorsal branch of pudendal nerve between bike seat and pubic symphysis
iii. **Mechanical management:**
(a) Adjust saddle angle to horizontal or only slightly upward in the front.
(b) Use wider saddle.
(c) Wear padded cycling shorts.
(d) Add saddle padding.
d. **Traumatic urethritis**
i. Varies from silent hematuria to marked dysuria with hematuria and pyuria; predisposes outflow tract to obstruction and infection.
ii. Easily mistaken for benign prostatic hypertrophy
iii. Management—similar to pudendal neuropathy
e. **Vulva trauma**
i. Superficial abrasions
ii. Lacerations
iii. Contusions
iv. Hematomas
v. Management:
(a) Similar to pudendal neuropathy
(b) Lower front end of saddle slightly
f. **Torsion of testes**
i. Described in association with bicycling
ii. No definite cause-and-effect relationship
g. **Male impotence**
i. Inability to attain an erection documented in cyclists after repeated or multi-day rides
ii. Incidence low
iii. Management
(a) Stop riding until symptoms resolve.
(b) Bicycle adjustments:
• Fit Kit recommended
• Padded shorts and seat

4. **Hip problems**
a. **Trochanteric bursitis**
i. **Mechanism:**
(a) Repetitive sliding of fascia lata over greater trochanter
(b) Generally occurs when rocking from side to side while pedaling because seat is too high
ii. **Management**
(a) **Mechanical:**
• Lower seat height
• Change frame size if too large to adjust

(b) **Medical:**
- Iliotibial band stretching
- Ice massage
- NSAIDs
- Occasional local steroid injection into bursa

b. **Iliopsoas tendinitis**

i. Pain in medial, proximal aspect of thigh

ii. **Management**

(a) **Mechanical**—same as trochanteric bursitis

(b) **Medical:**
- Stretching
- Ice massage
- Rest
- NSAIDs

5. **Knee problems**

a. **Anterior knee pain ("biker's knee" or "cyclist's knee" = extensor mechanism malalignment)**

i. Includes:

(a) Patellofemoral pain syndrome

(b) Quadriceps tendinitis

(c) Chondromalacia patella

(d) Patella tendinitis

(e) Osgood-Schlatter disease

(f) Single entity or in combination

ii. Etiology

(a) **Training errors:**
- Inadequate training base for workload
- Overly aggressive hill climbing
- Pedaling big gears
- Inadequate rest
- Deep squats and heavy knee extensions in weight room

(b) **Bicycle fit problems:**
- Seat too low
- Seat too far forward
- Improper cleat position
- Lack of "float" in cleats
- Crank too long

(c) **Anatomic variants:**
- Severe foot hyperpronation and hindfoot valgus
- Genu varum
- Genu valgus
- Internally or externally rotated feet

iii. **Treatment**

(a) **Correct training errors**

(b) **Correct bicycle fit problems**

(c) **Compensate for anatomic variants:**
- Hyperpronating feet, hindfoot valgus—external medial wedge or medial shim and/or cyclist's orthotic
- Genu varum—spacers between pedal and crank arm
- Genu valgum—medial wedges or cants
- Internally or externally rotated feet—floating cleats

(d) **Aggressive rehabilitation program:**

- Vastus medialis obliquus strengthening
- Hamstring, quadriceps, and heel cord stretching
- McConnell taping
- Phonophoresis or iontophoresis
- Ice, NSAIDs

(e) **Occasionally, surgery required**

b. **Medial knee pain**
   i. Occurs only among high-level competitors
   ii. Irritation and fibrosis of **plica** or **medial patellofemoral ligament**
   iii. **Treatment:**
      (a) Rehabilitation as for anterior knee pain
      (b) Corticosteroid injection
      (c) Plica excision or medial patellofemoral ligament release

c. **Lateral knee pain: iliotibial band friction syndrome**
   i. Represents 24% of knee pain problems in cyclists. More prevalent since introduction of fixed step-in cleat in 1985.
   ii. Etiology
      (a) **Bicycle fit problems:**
         - Improper cleat adjustment
         - Saddle too high
         - Saddle too far aft
      (b) **Anatomic factors:**
         - Hyperpronating foot
         - Prominent lateral femoral condyle
         - Leg length discrepancy
         - Genu varum
         - Tight iliotibial band
   iii. **Treatment:**
      (a) **Correct fit:**
         - Use floating pedals with a fixed end point that matches cyclist's anatomic alignment while preventing excessive internal rotation.
         - Set saddle height so rider's knee has 30–35° flexion at dead-bottom center (lower than standard seat height in Fig. 5).
      (b) **Compensate for anatomic factors:**
         - Hyperpronating foot—cycling orthotics
         - Genu varum—spacers between pedal and crank arm
         - Leg length discrepancy ¼ inch or greater (see Table 1)—shims, orthotics, foot positioning
      (c) **Medical treatment:**
         - Rest, occasionally prolonged
         - Iliotibial band stretching
         - Ice, NSAIDs, and phonophoresis or iontophoresis
         - Corticosteroid injections
         - Partial excision of overlying iliotibial band

d. **Posterior knee pain**
   i. Includes:
      (a) Biceps femoris tendinitis
      (b) Semimembranosis tendinitis
      (c) Posterior capsule strain
   ii. Etiology
      (a) Competitive cyclists training too aggressively or off bike
      (b) **Training errors:**
         - Too much aggressive riding out of saddle
         - Overinvolvement of hamstrings in upstroke

- Excessive hamstring curls in weight room
- Too much running or rollerblading as cross training

(c) **Bicycle fit problems:**
- Saddle too high and/or too far aft
- Cleats set with excessive toe-in
- Leg length discrepancy with bicycle set for long leg with inadequate correction for short leg

iii. **Treatment**
(a) Relative or complete rest
(b) Refit bicycle as appropriate
(c) Correct for leg length discrepancy
(d) Medical treatment:
- Hamstring, quadriceps, and heel cord stretching
- Ice, NSAIDs, and phonophoresis or iontophoresis
- Tenolysis and debridement

6. **Foot and ankle problems**

a. **Paresthesias**
i. Common when riding long distance; self-limited
ii. Etiology:
(a) Tight shoe straps and clips
(b) Increased pedal pressure
iii. **Mechanical management:**
(a) Loosen toe straps and clips
(b) Ride at higher cadence with lower pedal resistance
(c) Switch to newer "step-in" shoe-pedal combination

b. **Metatarsalgia**
i. Etiology:
(a) Poor foot position
(b) Improperly placed shoe cleats
(c) Increased pedal pressure from riding high gears at low cadence
ii. **Treatment:**
(a) **Mechanical:**
- Proper size toe clips
- Proper cleat adjustment
- Metatarsal pad
- Ride at higher cadence with lower pedal resistance

(b) **Medical**—if marked pes planus or hyperpronation, consider cycling orthotics

c. **Achilles tendinitis**
i. Etiology:
(a) Low saddle height causing pronounced ankle dorsiflexion during pedal rotation
(b) Toe clip too short or cleat positioned so that foot is too far behind pedal spindle, causing excessive "ankling" (dorsiflexion/plantar flexion) with increased stress to Achilles tendon
(c) Cleats set with excessive toe-in increasing torquing stress on Achilles tendon
ii. **Management**
(a) **Mechanical**—correct fit problems:
- Raise seat higher
- Proper toe clip size or cleat position
- May move foot position 1–3 mm forward of neutral to overcompensate for Achilles tendinitis while healing
- Accommodate bike fit to leg length discrepancy (see Table 1)

(b) **Technique**—reduce out of saddle riding, especially on mountain bike
(c) **Medical:**
- Heel cord stretching
- Ice massage
- NSAID therapy
- **Avoid local corticosteroid injections.**

d. **Plantar fasciitis**
i. Pain in sole at origin of plantar fascia on anterior calcaneus
ii. **Management**
(a) **Mechanical**—same as Achilles tendinitis
(b) **Medical:**
- Heel cord stretching
- Ice massage
- NSAID therapy
- Iontophoresis
- Corticosteroid injection

7. **Other common problems**
a. **Dehydration**
i. Rapid sweat evaporation causes the rider to underestimate fluid needs.
ii. Thirst is an inadequate guide.
iii. **Prevention and management:**
(a) Undertake conscious hydration several days before event.
(b) Keep two bottles of fluid on bicycle. *Note:* **Standard bicycle water bottles hold only 20 oz, and large bicycle bottles hold 27–28 oz.**
(c) Adequate hydration if passing clear urine every 1–2 hours

b. **Sunburn**
i. Common problem relating to exposure time
ii. Common areas:
(a) Arms
(b) Thighs
(c) Lips
iii. Prudent use of sunscreen advised

E. **Mountain bike injuries**
1. Increased incidence of trauma. Few studies are available, but two reports provide reliable data.
2. Chow and colleagues surveyed 459 members of two Southern California off-road bicycle clubs, and 268 (58.4%) responded.
a. **255 (84%) injured during previous year:**
i. Most injuries minor
ii. 26% required professional care
iii. 4% hospitalized
iv. 201 (90%) had soft tissue injuries (abrasions, lacerations, contusions)
v. 27 (12%) sustained fracture or dislocation
vi. 12% had head and/or neck injuries—low incidence attributed to the fact that 88% used helmets

b. 87.6% of injuries occurred **off of paved roads**
c. 74.2% of injuries occurred **while descending a grade**
d. 36% thought **excessive speed** contributed to injury
e. 34.7% attribute injury to riding **unfamiliar terrain**
f. 22% admitted **inattentiveness** as a factor
g. 19.6% admitted **riding beyond their ability**
h. Most injuries occurred in falls without preceding collision

TABLE 3. Mountain Bike Injuries by Type

	Male: 47 Riders, 208 Injuries (%)	Female: 14 Riders, 91 Injuries (%)
Wound (laceration, abrasion, puncture)	36.5	35.2
Bruise	21.6	33.0
Strain	16.3	15.4
Tendinitis	10.1	5.5
Sprain	8.2	6.6
Fracture	4.3	4.4
Dislocation	2.9	0.0

Adapted from Pfeiffer RP: Off-road bicycle racing injuries—the NORBA Pro/Elite category: Care and prevention. Clin Sports Med 13:207–218, 1994.

3. Pfeiffer surveyed 47 male and 14 female National Off-Road Bicycle Association **Pro/Elite riders** retrospectively for **injuries sustained in the 1992 competitive season.**
   a. **47 men, 208 injuries = 4.43 per rider/year**
   b. **14 women, 91 injuries = 6.5 per rider/year**
   c. Tables 3 and 4 list the injuries by type and body part.
   d. No significant head injuries but a few minor concussions with significant helmet damage

IV. Safety Equipment and Protective Clothing

A. **The bicycle helmet is generally very effective in preventing serious head injuries because of the relatively low speed at impact in bicycle injuries compared with motorcycle injuries.**
   1. **Required**
      a. All U.S. Cycling Federation–sanctioned events
      b. All Triathlon Federation USA competitions
      c. All National Off-Road Bicycle Association competitions
      d. Most local club and charity races and rides
   2. **Mechanism of action**
      a. **High-density, expanded polystyrene (EPS) or polyurethane foam crushes to absorb the shock of a severe impact.**
      b. **More resilient materials may produce a recoil that may add to the trauma.**

TABLE 4. Mountain Bike Injuries by Body Region, 1992 Survey

Body Region	Men (%)	Women (%)	Body Region	Men (%)	Women (%)
Ankle/foot	4.3	6.6	Shoulder	7.2	8.8
Lower leg	12.3	9.9	Collarbone	1.9	0.0
Knee	22.6	13.2	Upper arm	0.0	5.5
Thigh	8.2	6.6	Elbow	8.2	12.1
Hamstring	1.9	3.3	Forearm	4.8	4.4
Groin	0.96	0.0	Wrist	5.8	3.3
Pelvis	2.9	0.0	Hand/fingers	5.3	5.5
Abdomen	0.0	0.0	Neck	1.9	0.0
Low back	3.8	16.5	Face dental	0.96	3.3
Chest	3.4	0.0	Head	0.96	1.1
Upper back	2.4	0.0	Eye	0.0	0.0

From Pfeiffer RP: Off-road bicycle racing injuries—the NORBA Pro/Elite category. Clin Sports Med 13:207–218, 1994, with permission.

3. **Three types**
   a. **"Hard shell" helmet** consists of a hard shell that spreads the shock over a wider area and a crushable foam liner to absorb the shock.
      i. Advantage: proven safety record in actual use
      ii. Disadvantage: bulkier and heavier
      iii. No longer mass produced
   b. **"No shell" helmet** generally consists only of a single, molded, EPS layer with a Lycra cover.
      i. Advantages: light and attractive
      ii. Disadvantages: greater sliding friction against pavement in a crash might predispose to neck injury.
   c. **"Mini-shell" helmet** is similar to "no-shell" helmet, but it has a thin, smooth, hard outer shell layer.
      i. Advantages: light and attractive
      ii. Smooth, hard surface glides on pavement causing a more glancing impact and, consequently, less head and neck trauma.
4. **Standards**
   a. **American National Standards Institute Z90.4 standard** is minimum required for racing.
   b. **Snell Memorial Foundation B95 standard** is more stringent:
      i. Higher test impact
      ii. Likely to become even more stringent in the near future
   c. **American Society for Testing and Materials standard** may become industry favorite because is likely to cost manufacturers less for certification than Snell.
5. Other important features
   a. **Good retention system (straps and buckle)**
   b. Aerodynamically designed to reduce drag
   c. Air flow entrained to avoid thermal stress

B. **Mirrors** allow cyclist to observe overtaking vehicles without turning head. Various models mount on:
   1. Helmet
   2. Eyeglasses (sunglasses)—best option
   3. Handlebars

C. **Protective eyewear**
   1. Protects rider from:
      a. Radiation of sun
      b. Flying objects such as bugs, dust, and stones
      c. Irritants such as wind, rain, cold air, and allergens
   2. Wraparound or semiwraparound preferred—goggles for extreme conditions
   3. Polycarbonate or other unbreakable material

D. **Cycling gloves**
   1. Functions
      a. Cushion hands from road shock
      b. Provide good handlebar grip
      c. Prevent blisters
      d. Protect hands in a fall
      e. Some have terry backing to wipe sweat from face
      f. Protect from cold injury (winter gloves)
   2. Palms padded with shock-absorbent elastopolymer or neoprene
   3. Summer gloves—fingerless, leather palms, mesh or lightweight fabric backing
   4. Winter gloves—full fingers and insulation

E. **Handlebar tape and padding**
   1. Most racers use colorful, lightweight tape to enhance handlebar grip.
   2. Padded handlebar tape and slip-on foam rubber pads may be used for greater shock absorption.

F. **Saddle pads and padded saddles may provide extra shock absorption.**
   1. Saddle pads
      a. Elastopolymer in closed-cell neoprene cover
      b. Air bladder construction
      c. Fleece
      d. May reduce pedaling power slightly
   2. Padded saddles—elastopolymer or other high-tech material incorporated into the saddle itself

G. **Reflectors**
   1. **Bicycle reflectors**
      a. Generally removed by racers to reduce drag
      b. Wheel-mounted reflectors should be removed for high speeds or windy conditions because they may cause the bicycle to vibrate and become unsteady.
      c. Important for night and urban riding
   2. **Reflective tape**
      a. Most important on back of shoes
      b. On helmet
      c. On wheels
   3. **Reflective clothing**

H. **Lights**
   1. Halogen headlights
   2. Flashing light or strobe behind rider

I. **Protective clothing**
   1. **Bright tight cycling clothing**
      a. **"Advertises" presence of cyclist to other riders and motor vehicle drivers**
      b. Special materials keep cyclists cool in hot weather and warm in cold windy weather.
      c. Reduces drag
   2. **Reflective tape** may be added for riding at dawn, dusk, or night.
   3. **Cycling shorts** protect inner thighs, groin, and buttocks from chafing and pressure trauma.
      a. Seamless crotch pad traditionally natural chamois that requires lubricating with lanolin
      b. New synthetic padding only needs washing

J. **Bicycle shoes**
   1. **Stiff midsole distributes pedaling forces over entire foot and helps prevent foot and ankle overuse syndromes.**
   2. **Racing shoes connect to pedals with slotted cleats and toe clips or with step-in cleats.**
      a. Designed to transmit force to the pedal throughout the full revolution
      b. Roomy toe box necessary to prevent toe trauma
      c. Tight lacing or firm Velcro fastener high up on arch to anchor foot in proper position and prevent toe trauma
      d. **Cleat adjustment critical for smooth pedaling and overuse prevention. Rotational adjustment device is most accurate adjustment system** (see page 785).
      e. Racers with biomechanical foot problems may require:
         i. **Orthotics in shoes. Cycling orthotics are different from running orthotics**—rigid orthotic extends under metatarsal heads to control foot position over the pedal spindle.

ii. Canted shims between shoe and cleat
iii. Adjustable pedals (Biopedal)

f. **Rotational freedom** with step-in cleats:
i. Initially, step-in cleats provided a tight union without rotation freedom (laxity). Many knee and leg overuse problems resulted, especially if the cleat angle was improperly set.
ii. Newer "floating" cleats allow 5–10° of rotational freedom.
iii. **Replacement cleats** are available for many of the earlier fixed, step-in bindings to provide "float."

3. **Touring shoes** resemble court shoes with roomy toe box still small enough to fit in toe clips.
   a. More freedom of movement than racing shoes
   b. Fewer overuse problems
   c. Less force transmitted to pedals
4. **Mountain bike shoes** are heavier-duty touring shoes. Step-in bindings may be attached or inset into shoes.

Recommended Reading

1. Brownlie LW, Gartshore I, Chapman A, Banister EW: The aerodynamics of cycling apparel. Cycling Sci 3(3&4):44–50, 1991.
2. Burke ER: Proper fit of the bicycle. Clin Sports Med 13:1–14, 1994.
3. Chow TK, Bracker MD, Patrick K: Acute injuries from mountain biking. West J Med 159:145–148, 1993.
4. Cohen GC: Cycling injuries. Can Fam Phys 39:628–632, 1993.
5. Easterbrook M, Knuttgen HD, Pashby TJ, et al: Eye injuries and eye protection in sports: Position statement for the International Federation of Sports Medicine. Phys Sportsmed 16(11):49, 1988.
6. Ellis TH, Streight D, Mellion MB: Bicycle safety equipment. Clin Sports Med 13:75–98, 1994.
7. Gisolfi CV, Rohlf DP, Navarude SN, et al: Effects of wearing a helmet on thermal balance while cycling in the heat. Phys Sportsmed 16(1):139–146, 1988.
8. Grandjean AC, Ruud JS: Nutrition for cyclists. Clin Sports Med 13:235–247, 1994.
9. Helzer-Julin M: Sun, heat and cold injuries in cyclists. Clin Sports Med 13:219–234, 1994.
10. Holland SP: Medical care delivery on a 150-mile bicycle tour. Clin J Sports Med 3:242–250, 1993.
11. Holmes JC, Pruitt AL, Whalen NJ: Cycling knee injuries: Common mistakes that cause injuries and how to avoid them. Cycling Sci 3(2):11–14, 1991.
12. Holmes JC, Pruitt AL, Whalen NJ: Iliotibial band syndrome in cyclists. Am J Sports Med 21:419–424, 1993.
13. Holmes JC, Pruitt AL, Whalen NJ: Lower extremity overuse in bicycling. Clin Sports Med 13:187–205, 1994.
14. Kyle CR: Energy and aerodynamics in bicycling. Clin Sports Med 13:39–73, 1994.
15. Lofthouse GA: Traumatic injuries to the extremities and thorax. Clin Sports Med 13:113–135, 1994.
16. Mellion MB: Bicycling injuries: Prevention, diagnosis and treatment. In Mellion MB (ed): Office Sports Medicine, 2nd ed. Philadelphia, Hanley & Belfus, 1996, pp 355–375.
17. Mellion MB: Common cycling injuries: Management and prevention. Sports Med 11:52–70, 1991.
18. Mellion MB: Neck and back pain in bicycling. Clin Sports Med 13:137–164, 1994.
19. Montalto NJ, Janas TB: Medical coverage of recreational cycling events. Clin Sports Med 13:249–258, 1994.
20. Pfeiffer RP: Off-road bicycle racing injuries—the NORBA pro/elite category. Clin Sports Med 13:207–218, 1994.
21. Richmond DR: Handlebar problems in bicycling. Clin Sports Med 13:165–173, 1994.
22. Ryschon TW: Physiologic aspects of bicycling. Clin Sports Med 13:15–38, 1994.
23. Weiss BD: Bicycle-related head injuries. Clin Sports Med 13:99–112, 1994.
24. Weiss BD: Clinical syndromes associated with bicycle seats. Clin Sports Med 13:175–186, 1994.
25. Weiss BD: Nontraumatic injuries in amateur long distance bicyclists. Am J Sports Med 13:187–192, 1985.

64

Golf

Mark Amundson, M.S., PT, ATC

I. Golf and Special Sports Medicine Concerns

A. The invention of golf is hard to pinpoint. A variety of stick and ball games were played in Northern Europe as early as the twelfth century.

B. Golf, as we know it, made rapid developments in Scotland during the nineteenth century, and championship golf was inaugurated in 1860.

C. The National Sporting Goods Association estimates that 18–20 million Americans golf at least twice each year.

D. Because of the vast number of golfers in the United States and other countries, injuries are inevitable, and the primary care physician needs skills in the care of these injuries.

II. Overuse and Traumatic Injuries Related to the Golf Swing

A. **Lumbar strain and sprain**

1. **Definition:** an injury, either acute or chronic, involving the muscles or ligaments (or both) of the low back region
2. **Evaluation**
   a. History of violent muscular contraction against resistance
   b. History of overstretching
   c. History of overuse or repeated positioning
   d. Pain on palpation of the lumbar musculature
   e. Pain with movement of the lumbar spine
   f. Pain with resistance to movement of the lumbar spine
   g. Pain with prolonged sitting or standing
   h. Pain in the buttocks and hip region
   i. Lack of neurologic signs or symptoms
   j. History of stress and tension
3. **Mechanisms**
   a. Low back strain/sprain during the take-away phase of the swing results from the rotation of the lumbar spine on a relatively fixed lower body.
   b. Low back strain/sprain during the impact phase of the swing results from the uncoiling of the lumbar region and from the jarring force of contact with the ground.
   c. Low back strain/sprain during the follow-through phase of the swing results from the hyperextension and rotation of the lumbar spine (reverse "C").
4. **Frequency:** In a 5-year analysis of injuries to professional golfers, 26% of the injuries were to the lumbar spine.
5. **Treatment**
   a. Rest in the acute stage
   b. Physical therapy procedures (see page 812)

c. Flexibility exercises for the low back, hips, and hamstring muscles
d. Strengthening exercises for the low back, abdominal, and hip muscles
e. Proper posture and lifting techniques

6. **Prevention**
a. Proper swing mechanics
b. Proper conditioning (see page 813)
c. Education in proper body mechanics
d. Lumbar support during activity

B. **Lumbar disk injury**

1. **Definition:** an injury, either acute or chronic, involving one or more intervertebral disks in the lumbar spine. The injury can be to the annulus portion of the disk or a herniation or bulging of the nucleus pulposus.
2. **Evaluation**
a. History of twisting or overlifting
b. History of repeated poor body mechanics
c. Sharp pain in the center of the back
d. Pain with forward bending
e. Pain with hyperextension of spine
f. Positive straight leg raise test
g. Pain radiating into one or both legs
h. Lateral shift of pelvis when standing
i. Positive neurologic tests
3. **Mechanisms**
a. During the take-away phase of the swing, the disk can be injured due to the rotation and forward bent posture of the spine.
b. During the impact and follow-through phases of the swing, the disk can be injured because of the hyperextension and rotation of the spine.
c. Disk injuries can result from forward bending improperly when picking up the golf bag or retrieving the ball from the hole.
4. **Frequency:** Disk injuries are included in all lumbar spine injuries, which make up 26% of the total injuries.
5. **Treatment**
a. Rest in the acute phase
b. Physical therapy procedures (see page 812)
c. Flexibility exercises for the low back, hips, and legs
d. Pelvic stabilization exercises for strengthening the hip, abdominal, and low back muscles
e. Proper body mechanics
f. Consultation with appropriate physician for further tests and/or surgical intervention
6. **Prevention**
a. Proper body mechanics
b. Proper conditioning (see page 813)
c. Proper swing mechanics
d. Lumbar support during activity
e. Opposite-handed swinging to reverse the mechanics of the spine

C. **Thoracic strain/sprain**

1. **Definition:** an injury, either acute or chronic, involving the muscles or ligaments (or both) of the thoracic region
2. **Evaluation**
a. History of muscular contraction against resistance
b. History of repeated poor posture
c. Pain on palpation of muscles

   d. Pain with deep breathing, coughing, or sneezing
   e. Pain with resistance to trunk rotation
3. **Mechanisms**
   a. Thoracic strain/sprains during the take-away phase of the swing result from rotation of the thoracic spine while the hips remain relatively stationary.
   b. Thoracic strain/sprains during the impact phase of the swing result from the contraction of the muscle to unwind the spine and from the force created by impacting the ground.
   c. Repeated performance of the golf swing results in hypertrophy and limited flexibility of the right-sided back muscles (right-handed golfer), which may result in injury.
4. **Frequency:** A 5-year analysis of injuries to professional golfers showed that thoracic strain or sprains make up 21% of the total number of injuries.
5. **Treatment**
   a. Rest in the acute phase
   b. Physical therapy procedures
   c. Flexibility exercises for the midback and shoulder girdle muscles
   d. Strengthening exercises for midback and shoulder girdle muscles
   e. Mobilization of the thoracic spine to minimize the common hyperkyphotic curve of the golfer
6. **Prevention**
   a. Proper body mechanics
   b. Proper conditioning
   c. Proper swing mechanics
   d. Rib belt during activity
   e. Opposite-handed swinging to reverse the mechanics of the spine and minimize one-sided hyperdevelopment

D. **Cervical strain/sprain**
1. **Definition:** an injury, either acute or chronic, involving the muscles or ligaments (or both) of the neck region
2. **Evaluation**
   a. History of muscle contraction against resistance
   b. History of movement beyond the normal range
   c. History of chronic positioning or repeated movement patterns
   d. Palpation of spasms in the neck muscles
   e. Pain with movement of the neck and head
   f. Pain into the shoulder or arm
3. **Mechanisms**
   a. Left-sided cervical strain or sprains during the take-away phase of the swing result from the head remaining fixed while the upper back turns to the right (right-handed golfer).
   b. Right-sided cervical strain or sprains during the impact phase of the swing result from the contraction of the right cervical and thoracic muscles while the head remains steady.
   c. Repeated swinging results in chronic irritation of the left cervical paraspinals, levator scapulae, and left trapezius muscle as well as irritation of the ligaments and joint capsules of the cervical spine.
4. **Frequency:** A 5-year analysis of injuries to professional golfers shows that cervical strain or sprains account for 5% of the total injuries.
5. **Treatment**
   a. Rest in the acute phase
   b. Physical therapy procedures

   c. Flexibility exercises for the muscles of the neck, upper back, and shoulder girdle
   d. Strengthening exercises for the above-mentioned muscles
   e. Range-of-motion exercises for the cervical spine
   f. Proper body mechanics
6. **Prevention**
   a. Proper body and spine mechanics
   b. Proper conditioning
   c. Proper swing mechanics
   d. Opposite-handed swinging to reverse the mechanics of the spine

E. **Impingement syndrome of shoulder**
1. **Definition:** an overuse injury resulting in the impingement (squeezing) of the soft tissue structures of the shoulder between the coracoacromial arch and the greater tuberosity of the humerus
2. **Evaluation**
   a. History of repeated use of the arm for internal and external rotation activities
   b. History of repeated use of the arm for overhead activities
   c. Pain with abduction of arm, especially from 80–130° of motion (**painful arc syndrome**)
   d. Pain with resisted movement of internal or external rotation
   e. Pain when lying on involved arm
   f. Pain when sleeping and difficult to get into comfortable position
   g. Tenderness over anterior-lateral aspect of the shoulder, just distal to the tip of the acromion
3. **Mechanisms**
   a. **Right shoulder impingement** results from abduction of the shoulder during the take-away phase of the swing.
   b. **Left shoulder impingement** results from hyperabduction of the shoulder during the follow-through phase of the swing.
4. **Frequency:** A 5-year analysis of professional golfers indicates that 8% of the total injuries occur to the shoulder.
5. **Treatment**
   a. Flexibility exercises for the rotator cuff, latissimus dorsi, and pectoral muscles
   b. Strengthening exercises for the rotator cuff, latissimus dorsi, and pectoral muscles
   c. Physical therapy procedures
   d. Decompression surgery
6. **Prevention**
   a. Proper swing mechanics
   b. Proper conditioning

F. **Medial epicondylitis (golfer's elbow)**
1. **Definition:** an overuse injury of the medial aspect of the elbow involving the epicondyle of the humerus, the wrist and finger flexor muscles, and the pronator muscles
2. **Evaluation**
   a. History of sudden overload to contractile units of the medial elbow
   b. Tenderness over medial epicondyle of humerus
   c. Pain with flexion of wrist or fingers
   d. Pain with resistance to flexion of wrist or fingers
   e. Loss of function or palpable gap in muscle
   f. History of chronic use of wrist flexors or pronators
3. **Mechanisms**
   a. Right medial epicondylitis in the right-handed golfer due to extension of the right elbow during the impact phase of the swing while the right wrist remains dorsiflexed

b. Left medial epicondylitis in right-handed golfer because of supination of the left forearm during the follow-through phase of the swing

4. **Frequency:** A 5-year analysis of professional golfers indicates that 6% of all injuries occur to the elbow.
5. **Treatment**
   a. Flexibility exercises for wrist and finger flexor muscles and pronator muscles
   b. Strengthening exercises for wrist and finger flexor muscles and pronator muscles
   c. Physical therapy procedures
6. **Prevention**
   a. Proper swing mechanics
   b. Proper conditioning
   c. A "tennis elbow" band around proximal forearm

G. **Lateral epicondylitis**

1. **Definition:** an overuse injury involving the lateral epicondyle of the humerus, the wrist and finger extensor muscles, and the supinator muscles
2. **Evaluation**
   a. History of sudden overload to the wrist or finger extensors or the supinators
   b. Tenderness over the lateral epicondyle of the humerus
   c. Pain with use of the wrist or finger extensors or supinators
   d. Pain with resistance to the finger or wrist extensors or the supinator muscles
   e. Loss of function of wrist or finger extension or palpable gap in the muscle
   f. History of chronic overuse of the wrist or finger extensors or supinators
3. **Mechanisms**
   a. **Left lateral epicondylitis** in right-handed golfer due to forceful contraction of the left elbow extensors during the impact phase of the swing
   b. **Right lateral epicondylitis** in right-handed golfer due to pronation of forearm during the follow-through of the swing
4. **Frequency:** A 5-year analysis of professional golfers indicates that 6% of all injuries occur to the elbow.
5. **Treatment**
   a. Flexibility exercises for the wrist and finger extensors and supinator muscles
   b. Strengthening exercises for the wrist and finger extensors and supinator muscles
   c. Physical therapy procedures
6. **Prevention**
   a. Proper swing mechanics
   b. Proper conditioning
   c. Wear a "tennis elbow" band around the proximal forearm

H. **Wrist tendinitis**

1. **Definition:** an overuse injury resulting in inflammation and irritation of the tendons of the wrist flexors and extensors and the tendons of the finger flexors and extensors
2. **Evaluation**
   a. History of violent contraction against resistance
   b. History of overstretching or chronic overuse
   c. Pain with wrist motion
   d. Pain with movement against resistance
   e. Palpable or audible click in the wrist
   f. Tenderness in the wrist
   g. Loss of function
3. **Mechanisms**
   a. **Left wrist tendinitis** in right-handed golfer due to repeated radial deviation of the wrist during take-away phase of the swing

   b. **Right wrist tendinitis** in right-handed golfer due to repeated dorsiflexion of the wrist during the take-way phase of the swing
   c. **Left wrist tendinitis** in the right-handed golfer due to forceful contact with the ball and ground during the impact phase of the swing
4. **Frequency:** A 5-year analysis of professional golfers shows wrist injuries accounting for 6% of the total number of injuries.
5. **Treatment:** physical therapy procedures
6. **Prevention**
   a. Proper swing mechanics
   b. Tape or wrap wrist or wear wrist brace

I. **Carpal fractures**
1. **Definition:** any fracture of one or more carpal bones caused by the golf swing
2. **Evaluation**
   a. History of direct blow or fall on wrist or hand
   b. History of forceful hyperextension of wrist
   c. Acute pain in the wrist
   d. Pain with palpation of involved area
   e. Pain with movement of wrist
   f. Swelling in the wrist area
   g. Positive roentgenogram
3. **Mechanisms**
   a. **Hamate fracture** of the left wrist in a right-handed golfer due to the force of the wrist and hand being thrust into the ball during the impact phase of the swing
   b. **Scaphoid (navicular) fracture** of the right wrist in a right-handed golfer due to the compressive force of hitting the ground during the impact phase of the swing
4. **Frequency:** No specific frequency was noted for carpal fractures.
5. **Treatment**
   a. Cast for 4–6 weeks; if a navicular fracture, casting may be necessary for up to 6 months. May also require surgical intervention.
   b. Postcast
      i. Restoration of normal range of motion
      ii. Strengthening exercises for all muscles of the forearm
      iii. Physical therapy procedures
6. **Prevention:** proper swing mechanics

J. **Degenerative arthritis of the metacarpophalangeal (MCP) joint of the thumb**
1. **Definition:** a degenerative process occurring at the MCP joint of the thumb due to repetitive stress from the golf swing
2. **Evaluation**
   a. History of jamming injury to thumb
   b. History of repeated stress to MCP joint
   c. Pain with use of thumb
   d. Pain with pressure of MCP joint
   e. Swelling of MCP joint
   f. Loss of function and stiffness of MCP joint
   g. Crepitation with passive motion
3. **Mechanism: left MCP degenerative arthritis** in right-handed golfer due to repeated hyperabduction of the thumb during the take-away phase of the swing
4. **Frequency:** A 5-year analysis of professional golfers shows that 7% of all injuries are to the hand or fingers.
5. **Treatment**
   a. Physical therapy procedures
   b. Arthroscopic debridement of joint

6. **Prevention**
   a. Proper swing mechanics
   b. Proper-sized grips
   c. Range-of-motion exercises for joint
   d. Splint or taping for support

III. Treatment of Overuse Injuries (Physical Therapy Procedures)

A. Complete rest of the injured area for a period of 3–10 days. This may require the involved joints to be restricted in a sling or splint.
B. Ice packs or ice massage for 20–30 minutes, three to four times per day for the first 3–5 days
C. Heat packs or warm whirlpool for 15–20 minutes one to two times per day after the initial 3–5 days of cold therapy
D. Anti-inflammatory medication for 7–14 days
E. Ultrasound with the use of 10% hydrocortisone cream as the medium (phonophoresis) for 8–10 minutes, one to two times per day for 8–10 days
F. Iontophoresis—transportation of dexamethasone sodium phosphate (4%, 1 mL) and lidocaine (4%, 2 mL) ions through the skin with the use of electrical stimulation (4 mA). Treatment is for 20 minutes on an every-other-day basis for a total of three to five treatments.
G. Cortisone injection
H. Appropriate supportive device (such as lumbosacral corset or neoprene elbow sleeve)

IV. Other Golf-Related Problems

A. **Ocular trauma** in golf is rare.
   1. It has been reported that chemical injuries to the eye have taken place when persons have cut into a liquid-center golf ball and been squirted in the eye with the chemical.
   2. A player may be struck in the eye with a golf ball in flight or by a club while someone is swinging it.

B. **Head injuries** have been reported in golf when a person is struck in the head with a golf ball or club. A study done in England showed that of 52 head injuries that occurred in sport and were serious enough to be reported to a regional neurologic center, 14 (27%) were golf related.

C. **Skin cancer** has been reported to be more prevalent among golfers than nongolfers and has been reported to occur at a younger age in golfers than nongolfers. In a study of women professional and amateur golfers, the professionals received five times as much sun as the amateurs, and five professional players had developed basal cell carcinomas at an average age of 25.5 years.

D. **Psychomotor difficulties**, known as the "yipps," have been reported by great players such as Ben Hogan, Bobby Jones, and Sam Snead. The "yipps" attack golfers on short putts and totally disable the player from hitting the putt properly. Most often the player either strikes the ball with a sudden forceful jerk or stubs the putter on the ground before ever hitting the ball. No successful treatment has ever been found for the "yipps," and this disability has been the undoing of many great golfers.

E. **Oculophysical disability** occurs when a golfer who suffers from refractive errors such as astigmatism or muscle imbalance has difficulty with the short game in golf. The long game appears to rely heavily on physical action rather than oculophysical coordination, whereas the short game relies heavily on oculophysical coordination. Thus, some persons have problems with chipping and putting owing to eye dysfunction.

F. **Sudden death** does occur in golf. It is rare, but some of the causes that have been reported include cardiac events, lightning, and heatstroke. Accidents such as a shaft of the club being broken around a tree and plunging into the body have also been reported.

V. Conditioning Program for Golf

A. **Flexibility exercises.** All flexibility exercises should be repeated 5–10 times on each side of the body, and each repetition should be held for 10–20 seconds. Each stretch should be gradual in nature with no bouncing.

1. **Neck:** turn head to look over each shoulder, bend chin to chest and look to ceiling, tilt ear toward shoulder without elevating the shoulder
2. **Shoulder**
    a. Lie on back with arm out to side at 90° and elbow bent to 90°; let arm rotate backward.
    b. Pull arm across chest and under chin without rotating torso.
    c. Reach arm overhead with elbow bent completely; place behind head and pull with other hand.
3. **Forearm**
    a. Extend elbow completely while flexing wrist and fingers as far as possible.
    b. Extend elbow completely while extending wrist and fingers as far as possible.
4. **Chest**
    a. Stand in a corner; place forearm of each arm on wall and lean into corner.
    b. Grasp hands behind back and pull arms up backward.
5. **Trunk**
    a. Clasp hands above head and lean body sideways.
    b. Lie on back with arms at shoulder level and flat on ground, roll onto one hip while keeping back flat, and pull the top leg toward chest while keeping bottom leg straight.
6. **Low back and hip**
    a. Lie on back, and pull one knee to chest.
    b. Lie on back, and pull both knees toward chest.
    c. Lie on back, and keep one leg straight while pulling other leg to waist and then across chest.
7. **Hamstring**
    a. Sit with both legs out straight, knees flat on floor, and toes pointed toward ceiling. Bend forward at hips, keeping the back straight.
    b. Stand with knees bent and touch toes, and keep touching toes while straightening knees.
8. **Calf**
    a. Stand facing wall; keep knees straight, heels flat, and toes straight ahead; and lean into wall by bending arms.
    b. Stand facing wall, bend knees, keep heels flat and toes straight ahead, and lean into wall.

B. **Muscle-strengthening exercises.** Strengthening exercises should be done with light weights to increase strength gradually. The exercises should be done with both sides of the body, and the weights should be gradually increased over a period of time. Initially a person should do 1–2 sets of 10 repetitions and increase to 2–3 sets of 10 repetitions.

1. **Neck:** Start with head in neutral position, place hand against forehead, and try to bend head down. Resist with hand so no movement takes place. Hold contraction for 3–5 seconds. Repeat for extension, lateral side bending, and rotation each direction.
2. **Rotator cuff**
    a. Hang arm by side with elbow straight, turn hand inward as far as possible, then raise arm up at 45°. Rotate arm so the hand is pointing toward the ceiling.
    b. Lie on side, rest top arm on body, and bend elbow to 90°, and rest hand on floor. Rotate arms so hand turns up toward ceiling.
    c. Lie on side, place bottom arm under the body, bend elbow to 90°, and rest hand on floor. Rotate arm so hand turns up toward stomach.

3. **Latissimus dorsi**
   a. Lie on stomach with arm by side, and lift arm up backward as far as possible.
   b. Sit in chair with arm rests, place hands on arm rests, and push down so the body is lifted off the chair.
   c. Stand with arms above head, grasp pulleys or rubber tubing, and pull down and back as far as possible.
4. **Forearm**
   a. Sit with forearm resting on table and wrist hanging over edge with palm up; bend wrist up as far as possible.
   b. Sit with forearm resting on table and wrist hanging over edge with palm down; bend wrist up as far as possible.
   c. Sit with forearm resting on table and wrist hanging over edge with palm up; rotate forearm so palm faces down.
   d. Sit with forearm resting on table and wrist hanging over edge with palm down; rotate forearm so palm faces up.
   e. Stand with arm hanging by side, and bend wrist laterally toward thumb side.
   f. Stand with arm by side, and bend wrist laterally toward little finger.
5. **Chest:** Lie on back with arms out to side at 90° at shoulder; raise arms toward the midline until hands touch.
6. **Abdominal muscles:** Lie on back on floor, knees bent and feet flat on floor, place arms by side or across chest, and raise torso off floor until shoulder blades come off floor.
7. **Back**
   a. Lie on stomach with arms by side, and raise one leg up backward, keeping knee straight.
   b. Get on hands and knees, and raise one arm and opposite leg up backward to level of body.
8. **Hip**
   a. Lie on side with top leg straight and bottom knee bent for stability; raise top leg up sideways as far as possible.
   b. Lie on stomach with one leg hanging over edge of table; lift the leg up backward as far as possible keeping the knee straight.

C. **Cardiovascular exercises**
1. Cardiovascular fitness is an integral component of a person's overall fitness. Golfers need cardiovascular fitness to walk 18 holes or more and not become fatigued.
2. There are many different modes for developing cardiovascular endurance. Biking, swimming, walking, and jogging are a few of the more common. Initially a person should exercise for 10–15 minutes three times per week and then gradually build up to 20–30 minutes three times per week of aerobic exercise at an intensity level of 70–80% of their target heart rate.

VI. Equipment and Technique

A. Equipment

1. Length of club—determined by the length of the golfer's arm and the distance of the finger tips from the ground
2. Grip size—an individual preference. A standard size is when the fingertip of the long finger of the left hand just touches the palm of the left hand when the club is gripped properly.
3. Shaft flexibility—differs for each individual. Usually the shaft flexibility is determined by the direction that the golfer consistently hits the ball.
4. Swing weight of club—also individual for each golfer. The size of the individual as well as the direction of the normal shot help determine the proper swing weight.

B. **Technique**—a complex issue that goes beyond the scope of this chapter. Proper technique is one way of preventing the many overuse injuries that have been described. The best advice for developing proper technique is to take lessons from a PGA Golf Professional.

VII. Special Rules for Protection

Rule 6-8a of the U.S. Golf Association Rules of Golf states that when a golfer believes that he or she is in danger from lightning, the golfer may make the decision to discontinue play.

Recommended Reading

1. Duda M: Golf injuries: They really do happen. Phys Sportsmed 15(7):191–196, 1987.
2. Farley KG: Ocular trauma resulting from the explosive rupture of a liquid center golf ball. J Am Optom Assoc 56:310–314, 1985.
3. Hanke WC, Zollinger TW, O'Brian JJ, Bianco L: Skin cancer in professional and amateur female golfers. Phys Sportsmed 13(8):51–52, 61–63, 66–68, 1985.
4. Jobe FW, Yocum LA, Mottram RE, Pink MM: Exercises for Better Golf. Inglewood, CA, Human Kinetics, 1994.
5. Lindsay KW, McLatchie G, Jennett B: Serious head injury in sport. BMJ 281:789–791, 1980.
6. McCarroll JR: Golf. In Schneider RC, et al (eds): Sports Injuries: Mechanism, Prevention, and Treatment. Baltimore, Williams & Wilkins, 1985, pp 290–294.
7. PGA and Senior PGA Tour: A 5 year injury analysis. Inglewood, CA, Centinela Hospital, 1990–1994.
8. Roberts J: Injuries, handicaps, mashies, and cleeks. Phys Sportsmed 6:121–123, 1978.
9. Stover CN, Wiren G, Topaz SR: The modern golf swing and stress syndromes. Phys Sportsmed 4:42–47, 1976.
10. Vaupel GL, Andrews JR: Diagnostic and operative arthroscopy of the thumb metacarpophalangeal joint. Am J Sports Med 13:139–141, 1985.

65

Tennis

Terry L. Nicola, M.D.

I. Tennis-Specific Conditioning and Body Mechanics

A. **Combined endurance and strength sport**

1. A typical match requires 300 to 400 bursts of effort, necessitating strength and efficiency of form for each burst, without fatiguing during the final games and points.
2. **Aerobic performance level** averages 60–70% of the predicted maximum heart rate during a singles match and 40% for a doubles match.
3. Given the high demands of lower extremity endurance for repeated bursts of running, a focus on lower extremity conditioning is recommended:
   a. Stationary bicycling at 90 rpm with 1-minute high-intensity bursts alternated with 4-minute light pedaling may simulate the intensity of tennis play.
   b. 30-minute sessions, three times per week, are a necessary minimum for a conditioning effect.
   c. The desired result is a consistent level of performance for an entire match.
4. Specificity of strength and coordination training necessitates that athletes play tennis to be good at tennis. A progressive resistance strengthening program to key muscle groups (e.g., the rotator cuff) serves to increase the body's tolerance for the progressive tennis drills and match play.
   a. Prepare needed muscles for each tennis stroke.
   b. Balance conditioning of agonist and antagonist muscles for skeletal joint stability.

B. **Tennis form—evaluation of specific components for injury prevention**

1. **General concepts**
   a. **Service stroke phases**
      i. **Wind-up phase:** lower extremity preparation with hips, knees, and ankles flexed for recoil; abdominal muscles set
      ii. **Cocking phase:** ball toss and recoil of service arm, shoulder muscles on maximum stretch
      iii. **Acceleration phase:** energy release from lower extremity drive, abdominal flexion, and finally upper extremity swing and ball contact
      iv. **Deceleration phase of the service arm:** primarily from the shoulder and upper trunk
   b. **Backhand and forehand stroke phases**
      i. **Preparation phase:** trunk rotation, running or jumping to planned set-point with "stop" foot planted, racquet drawn back
      ii. **Acceleration phase:** lower extremity and trunk lean into the stroke, motion of arm-racquet lever primarily from shoulder, finally racquet contact with the ball
      iii. **Deceleration phase:** lower extremity and trunk rotation toward the net
   c. **Return strokes at the net**—quick lower extremity and trunk movements similar to those described for backhand and forehand stroke phases, abbreviated by short punch strokes.

2. **Back and trunk motion**
   a. **Primary concern is lower back (lumbar spine) hyperextension during service and overhead strokes.** This stress can be minimized by tossing the ball slightly ahead of the service line and launching into the service driving from the lower extremities, with less back and neck hyperextension.
   b. Thoracic spine flexibility for rotation is necessary for the ground strokes.
   c. There may be excessive back motion in an attempt to compensate for shoulder and lower extremity inflexibility.
3. **Shoulder motion**
   a. **Primary concern is loading of the shoulder structures during service and overhead strokes**
   b. From wind-up to cocking phases, the combined glenohumeral and scapular motion is responsible for 90° abduction and another 30° by thoracic lateral tilt (Fig. 1).
   c. The abducted glenohumeral joint also externally rotates up to 120°, which may overstretch the anterior joint capsule.
4. **Elbow and wrist motion**
   a. These joints are a relatively fixed part of the arm-racquet lever, responsible for reach and conduction of energy generated by motion of the lower extremities, trunk, and shoulder.
   b. **Error in form is generally due to unwanted wrist-snapping motion during the backhand stroke.** Wrist motion should not occur except in the service stroke during acceleration phase of wrist flexion.
   c. **Grip mechanism** involves the wrist extension muscles as stabilizers for the wrist and finger flexor tendons as they cross the wrist:
      i. The grip should be as relaxed as possible to minimize stress on the above wrist muscles and their origin at the elbow epicondyles (see "Traumatic and Overuse Injuries," next page).
      ii. The racquet handle should have a "sticky" grip.
      iii. **Correct handle circumference** is equal to the distance from the tip of the ring finger to the proximal palmar crease, measured along the radial border of the ring finger.
5. **Hip, knee, and ankle motion**
   a. The lower extremity stresses seen in sprinting events are present in pursuits that are part of a tennis volley. Stresses on quadriceps, hamstrings, patella, and calf muscles are **similar to the stresses of sprinting.**

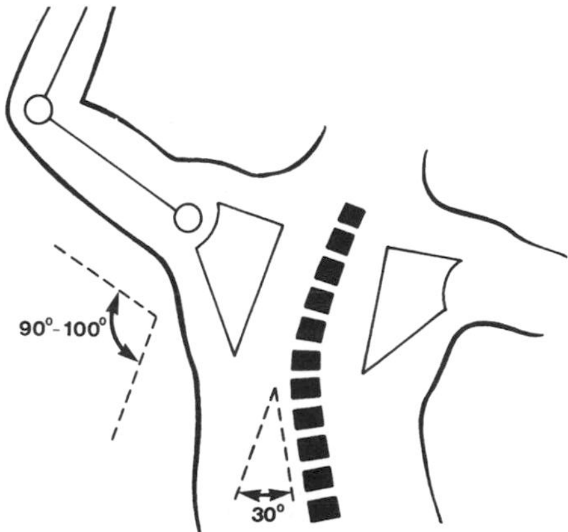

FIGURE 1. This view of the service wind-up illustrates the addition of 30° lateral thoracic tilt to the 90°–100° of scapulohumeral abduction.

b. **Lower extremity set and preparation** for each stroke involves predominantly a partial squat (hip flexion, knee flexion, and ankle dorsiflexion) to drive into the stroke with spring from the legs rather than compensatory back and arm motion.
c. The triceps surae muscles (posterior calf) are stressed during ankle and foot push-off in service strokes and jumps when hip and knee are fully extended.

C. **Equipment and force transmission**
1. **Upper extremity injuries are closely associated with the forces transmitted from the racquet to the upper extremity and trunk.** The ball may reach speeds of more than 100 mph. In cases of poor control or recent upper-body injuries:
a. Reduce string tension by 3–5 lb from that recommended by the manufacturer.
b. Use natural gut strings.
c. The weight of the racquet is a factor, especially the racquet head, situated at the distal end of the lever formed by arm and racquet. Consider large ceramic composite racquets, which are lighter and dissipate energy well.
d. Technique and incorrect off-center ball impact with the racquet head increases vibration intensity to the wrist threefold.
e. Check for fitted grip.
f. Use only new tennis balls.
2. **Footwear**
a. Important for shock absorption and dissipation of ground reaction forces
b. A stable shoe must have a **good heel counter** and **snug fit** with a flexible forefoot to allow a base of support for rapid directional changes on the court. **Such side-side stability may not be seen in other sport shoes such as running shoes.**
c. A lighter tennis shoe may be used for clay courts.
d. Shoes and orthotic devices should be considered in someone who has already corrected for errors in tennis form or conditioning.
3. **Court surfaces may be clay, composition, hard court, grass, or carpet.**
a. In rehabilitation of tennis injuries, carpet, composition, and clay are more forgiving to the lower extremities.
b. Slower ball velocity on clay courts is more forgiving to the upper extremities.

II. Traumatic and Overuse Injuries

A. Severe disruptive injuries, such as tendon ruptures, completed stress fractures, and adolescent physeal plate injuries, present as sudden loss of motion and strength, with pain increasing in severity on repeated attempts to keep playing.

B. The predominant mode of tennis injury is overuse stress to bone, ligament, muscle, tendon, and nerve.
1. **Lateral tennis elbow**
a. Pain at the lateral elbow—an estimated 50% of all tennis players suffer injury to the extensor carpi radialis brevis at the common wrist extensor tendon origin at the lateral epicondyle.
b. Risk factors:
i. Player age > 30 years
ii. Improper grip size
iii. Use of a metal racquet
iv. Duration of average practice > 2 hours per day
v. Tight strings
vi. Incorrect wrist-flexed backhand or tight grip:
(a) Both technique errors cause contraction and pull of the extensor carpi radialis brevis on the lateral epicondyle.

(b) Symptoms can be elicited by resisted wrist extension or tight grip.
(c) Passive wrist flexion range, with elbow extended and forearm pronated, may be restricted.

2. **Medial tennis elbow**
   a. Pain at the medial elbow is generally attributed to strain at the common flexor tendon origin at the medial epicondyle.
   b. This injury, common to elite or highly ranked recreational players, is due to repeated wrist flexion overload during the service or to a powerful forehand top spin (pronation stress).
   c. Diagnosis—local tenderness is present over the medial epicondyle, with pain on active wrist flexion and passive, supinated, elbow-extended wrist extension.
3. **Other concomitant elbow injuries**
   a. Other rare disorders found with classic elbow injuries include **triceps tendinitis** (posterior tennis elbow), **medial collateral ligament injury** elicited by valgus stress to the elbow, and **osteochondral articular loose bodies**.
   b. **Concomitant neurologic injury** may include ulnar nerve (cubital tunnel), median nerve (pronator teres syndrome, carpal tunnel syndrome), or radial nerve entrapment (radial tunnel syndrome).
   c. Occasional anterior elbow compartment pain with flexion contracture can represent **elbow synovitis** from service overuse (biceps in acceleration phase) and is responsive to rest and flexibility exercises.
   d. Medial and lateral **elbow tendinosis** are conditions of experienced tennis players with degenerative changes at the epicondyle rather than inflammatory changes. These conditions respond more to physical rehabilitation than to injections:
      i. Suspect these conditions in refractory tennis elbow
      ii. Magnetic resonance imaging may be helpful in differential diagnosis
4. **Shoulder injuries (tennis shoulder)**
   a. **Adaptive changes to the dominant shoulder (King Kong arm)** include a drooped and hypertrophied shoulder girdle with chronic overstretch to the trapezius, levator scapulae, and rhomboid muscles. There may also be a reversible upper thoracic scoliosis.
   b. **Lateral scapular glide test** of Kibler detects loss of normal scapular glide (scapular droop) with abduction of the proximal arm (Fig. 2). Without lateral scapular glide, impingement of the rotator cuff may occur with overhead arm movements.
   c. **Overuse of the rotator cuff muscles** (supraspinatus, infraspinatus, teres minor, subscapularis) leads to glenohumeral joint instability. Combined with scapular

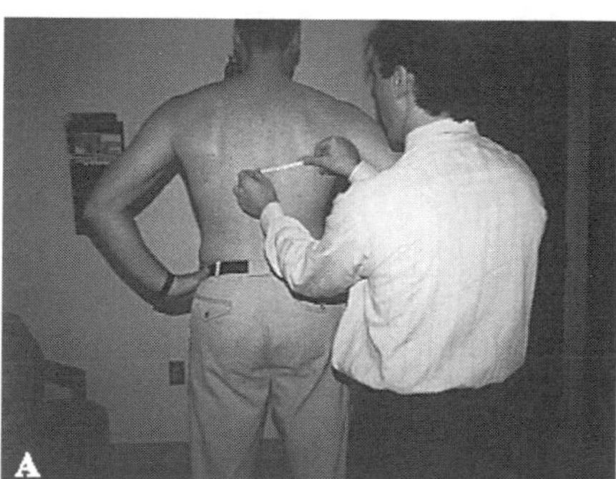

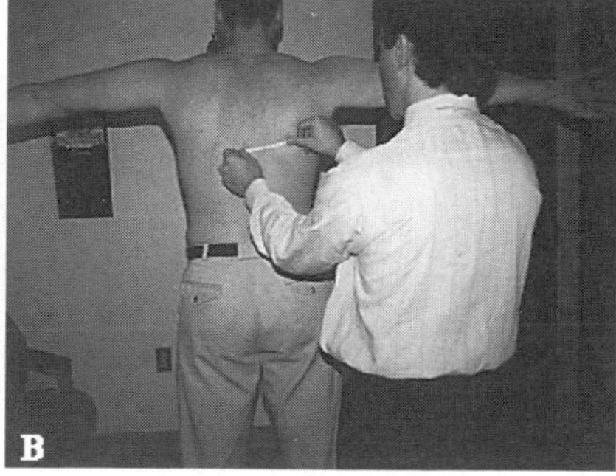

FIGURE 2. Lateral scapular glide test. Three postures used to compare symmetry of scapular glide, as measured from a reference point on the thoracic spine to the inferior angle of each scapula: arms at side (not shown); **A**, hands on hips; **B**, shoulders abducted 90° with arms internally rotated.

droop, joint instability may subject the cuff muscles to impingement under the coracoacromial arch during service and overhead strokes.

   i. Injury may also occur to other subacromial structures such as the subacromial bursa and biceps long-head tendon.
   ii. In younger athletes, overuse to these muscles is possible without actual impingement.

d. The athlete typically presents with subacromial pain and pain referred to the lateral arm.
e. The athlete reports the **involved arm "feels dead" during tennis play**.
f. Passive shoulder abduction–internal rotation by the examiner or simulation of service motion reproduces symptoms.
g. Tenderness in the bicipital groove may be present.
h. Rotator cuff muscles may not be weak on exam in early injury.
i. **Neurologic exam** should look for ancillary nerve traction injury with deltoid muscle weakness and lateral shoulder hypesthesia. Winged scapula from weakness of the serratus anterior caused by traction injury to the long thoracic nerve may be missed. This nerve, as it arises from the C5, C6, C7 nerve roots, is susceptible to traction from shoulder depression during the service stroke or chronic tennis shoulder droop.

5. **Wrist and hand injuries—relatively uncommon in tennis.** Relate to **repetitive direct trauma from the racquet handle**.
   a. Examples include fracture to the hook of the hamate or injury to the digital nerve from pressure over the metacarpophalangeal heads.
   b. Focal tenderness, numbness, and dysesthesias in wrist or hand should raise suspicion of local trauma.
   c. Racquet grip should be evaluated and adjusted for fit and padding after the injury has resolved.
6. **Lower extremity injuries**
   a. **Rupture of the medial head of the gastrocnemius muscle (tennis leg)** may occur because of repetitive push-off from service and jumping overload to a knee-extended, ankle–plantar flexed leg (see Chapter 48, "Pelvis, Hip, and Thigh Injuries").
   b. **Achilles tendinitis** and rupture may follow a similar mechanism of injury, with strain or rupture at the tendon component of the triceps surae mechanism (see Chapter 50, "Ankle and Leg Injuries").
   c. **Patella and quadriceps tendinitis:**
      i. May be associated with aggressive side-to-side and vertical jumps
      ii. Patellofemoral loads are also high during deep knee bends in preparation for ground-stroke returns (see Chapter 49, "Knee Injuries").
   d. **Plantar fasciitis:**
      i. Believed to be due to repetitive forefoot push-off during volleys. As the long arch of the foot depresses, traction occurs to the fascia at its origin on the medial tubercle of the os calcis, with heal pain and tenderness over the area.
      ii. The majority of injuries are shoe related with poor heel fit (necessitating addition of a heel cup) or inadequate arch to support a cavus foot.
      iii. A hyperflexible (pronating) foot should be evaluated for heel fit and a medial heel counter addition to the midsole.
   e. **Lateral ankle sprains:**
      i. See Chapter 50, "Ankle and Leg Injuries."
      ii. Inadequate heel counter and worn outsole should be suspected causes.
      iii. This injury is more likely to occur on hard rather than clay court. The clay court allows foot slippage; fixed foot inversion stress is possible on hard courts.

7. **Back injuries**
   a. Tennis players may develop painful spine vertebral body wedge deformity or Schmorl's nodes from overdevelopment of dominant side paraspinal muscles.
   b. **Cervical and interscapular pain:**
      i. In association with drooped or protracted shoulder posture, there may be compensatory cervical hyperextension. Findings may include:
         (a) Cervical paraspinal tenderness
         (b) Decreased cervical motion
         (c) Tender and fatigued scapular support muscles (levator scapulae, trapezius, and rhomboid)
         (d) Constricted flexibility of pectoralis minor muscles (with protracted shoulder posture)
      ii. There may be an upper thoracic scoliosis and King Kong arm.
      iii. The overuse pattern is associated with the downward motion (acceleration and deceleration phases) of the service and overhead strokes.
      iv. Cervical symptoms may be aggravated by a service ball toss too far behind the baseline, causing excessive cervical hyperextension (Fig. 3).
      v. Sequelae secondary to cervical hyperextension include:
         (a) Facet joint injury
         (b) Brachial plexus traction injuries
         (c) Thoracic outlet syndrome (ulnar nerve)
   c. **Injuries to the lumbosacral spine:**
      i. Such injuries may be due to **service-related back hyperextension mechanism**, as discussed for cervical spine
      ii. Majority of injuries are referable to the facet joints of the lower lumbar segments, less commonly the disks
      iii. Low back may be stressed from compensatory rotation when thoracic spine rotation is constricted by poor flexibility
      iv. Combined lumbar lateral rotation/extension on examination may worsen facet joint symptoms

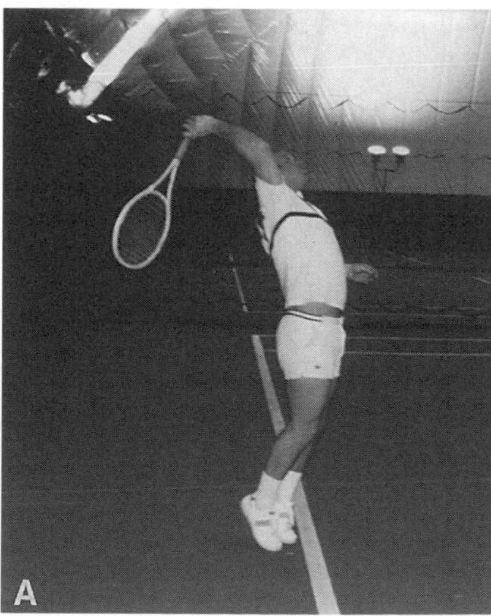

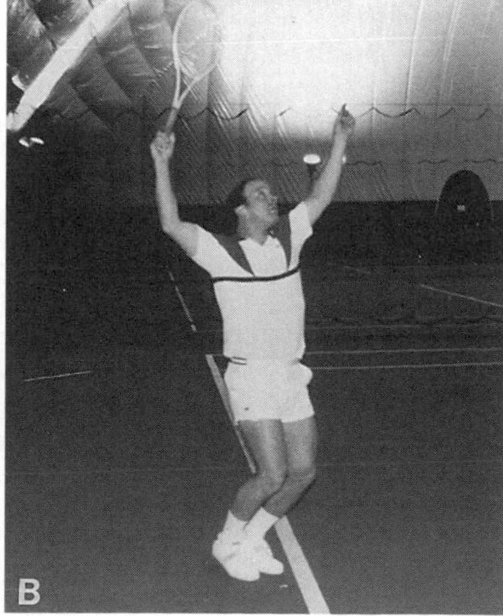

FIGURE 3. **A**, Back and neck hyperextension should be avoided during the service motion. **B**, Service ball toss in front of the service line ensures hyperextension is avoided.

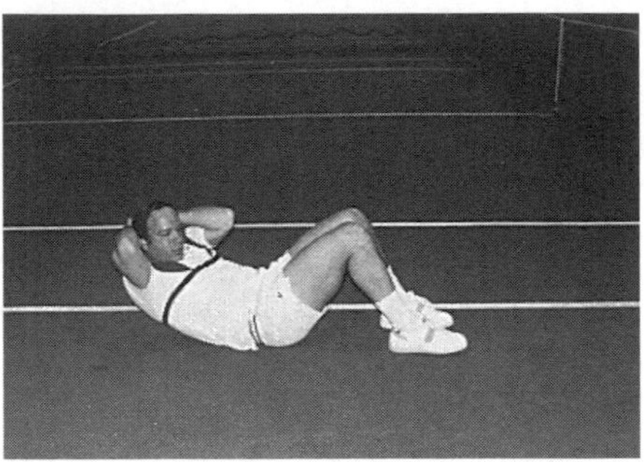

FIGURE 4. Sit-ups with hips and knees flexed in a "hook-lying" position avoids unwanted use of hip flexors and emphasizes abdominal muscle groups, preferably opposite elbow to opposite knee to focus on abdominal oblique muscles.

v. Loss of hip flexor (iliopsoas) flexibility increases load to spine
vi. If sitting worse than standing, suspect disk injury
vii. Secondary L-5 or S-1 root impingement possible
viii. Examine for lower extremity signs of neuropathy

d. **Abdominal wall strain:**
i. Muscles involved include rectus abdominis and internal and external oblique muscles. If symptoms are more toward the groin, consider iliopsoas strain.
ii. Diagnosis can be **confirmed by hook-lying sit-ups.** Cross elbow to opposite knee sit-up is specific for oblique muscle injury (Fig. 4).
iii. Other differential diagnoses for abdominal symptoms are listed in Table 1.

8. **Eye injuries**
a. Given tennis ball velocities greater than 100 mph, sport goggles are recommended.
b. For tennis, the safety of open versus closed goggles needs further research (see Chapter 41, "Eye Injuries in Sports: Evaluation, Management, and Prevention").

9. **Tennis and the adolescent athlete**
a. The U.S. Tennis Association guidelines from Key Biscayne, Florida, provide normative data for flexibility, strength, agility, and endurance to match young athletes fairly who may differ in physical maturity levels.
b. **Poor flexibility is a concern.** The bones may grow faster than the muscles and tendons. Aggressive flexibility program for tight muscles in the back and extremities is essential.
c. **Growth plate (physis) injuries** may include:
i. Slipped capital femoral epiphysis
ii. Supraspinatus traction to the apophysis at the humerus lesser tuberosity
iii. Osgood-Schlatter disease
iv. Sever's disease
v. Humeral medial epicondyle apophysitis (adolescent medial tennis elbow)

III. Rehabilitation

A. Acute injuries

1. See general guidelines in Chapter 38, "Comprehensive Rehabilitation of the Athlete."
2. No return to formal tennis training and competition should be allowed until strengthening, flexibility, and equipment modification have arrested symptoms.

TABLE 1. Differential Diagnosis for Nonmuscular Abdominal Pain

Acute abdominal process	Inguinal hernia
Epididymitis	Testicular torsion
Herniated disk	Osteitis pubis
Stress fracture	Entrapped intercostal nerve

3. Initiate tennis-specific drills to the recovering body part before formal participation in training and competition.
4. Aerobic fitness through cross training should be maintained, with protection of the injured body part.

B. **Protection, strength, and flexibility**
   1. **Shoulder**
      a. **Protect the injury** by avoidance of daily overhead motions and activities such as pitching, volleyball, and crawl or butterfly swimming. Refractory symptoms may require a part-time sling.
      b. **Active range-of-motion program** of glenohumeral joint:
         i. Internal and external rotation with the shoulder positions at 0° abduction
         ii. Progress gradually to 90° shoulder-abducted position for these exercises
      c. **Muscles of particular concern:**
         i. Rotator cuff and serratus anterior muscles for all strokes
         ii. Latissimus dorsi and deltoid muscles for overhead and backhand strokes
         iii. Rhomboid muscles to counter effects of shoulder droop
      d. Shoulder rehabilitation, especially in younger athletes, should correct for rotator cuff weakness of the external rotators relative to the stronger internal rotators—a so-called muscle strength imbalance of less than 2:3 ratio.
         i. Loss of glenohumeral internal rotation flexibility should also be corrected.
         ii. Rotator cuff strengthening is associated with increased ball service velocity.
      e. In general, **full scapulohumeral rhythm** must be returned before return to formal training and competition.
   2. **Elbow**
      a. **Protect the injury** by avoiding use of manual tools that require a firm grasp (hammer, screwdriver) or heavy household utensils.
         i. A cock-up wrist splint protects daily overuse of wrist flexors and extensors during early healing period (Fig. 5A).
         ii. A forearm counterforce bank ("tennis elbow splint") may be used when the athlete resumes tennis-related drills and practice or for mild (inconsistent symptoms) tennis elbow (Fig. 5B).
         iii. If injury is complicated by elbow swelling, medial-lateral instability, or articular lesion, an elbow flexion splint may be necessary.
      b. **Progressive resistance program** should include ordered sequence of isometric to isotonic strengthening of grip and wrist flexion and extension. Pronation-supination and flexion-extension of elbow may be added as symptoms allow.

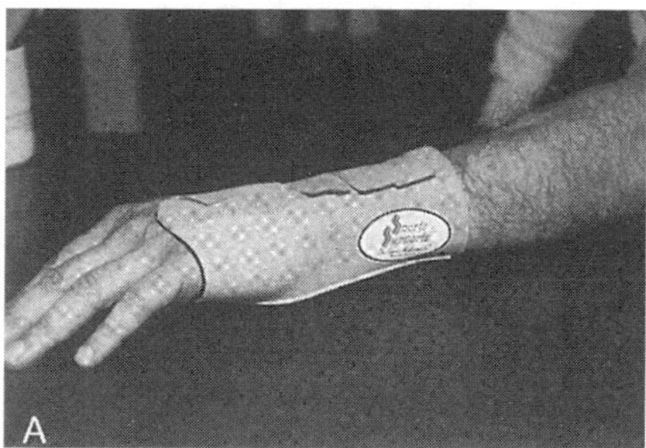

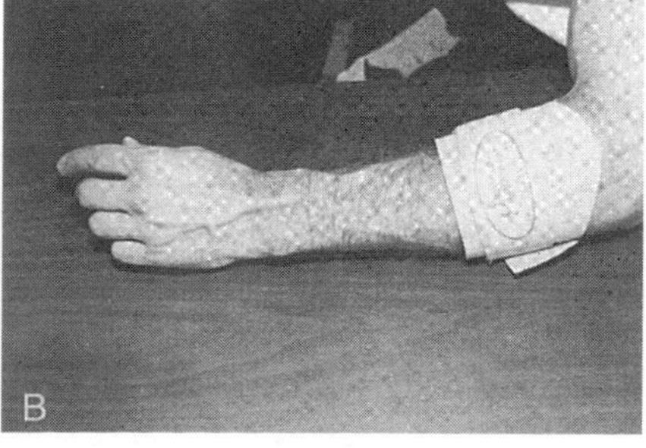

FIGURE 5. **A**, The neutral position wrist splint and **B**, the forearm counterforce brace reduce the load to an injured wrist extensor.

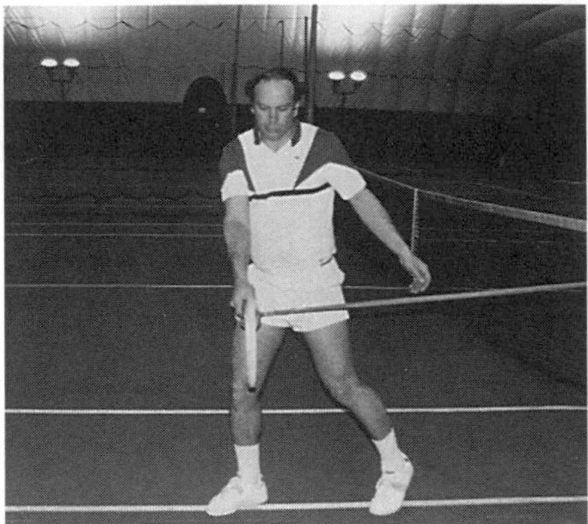

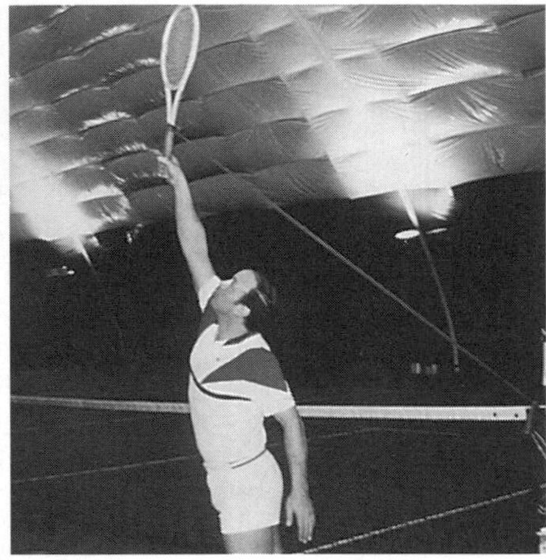

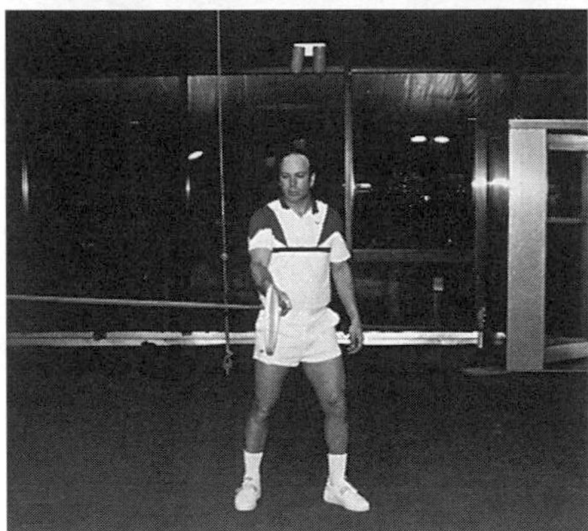

FIGURE 6. Tennis strokes such as the backhand may be practiced during later phases of injury rehabilitation by "anchoring" of the racquet with elastic tubing to any fixed handle, knob, or pole.

c. **Stretching:**
   i. Wrist flexor tendon injury (medial tennis elbow)—wrist extension stretch with forearm supinated, elbow extended
   ii. Wrist extensor tendon injury (lateral tennis elbow)—wrist flexion stretch with forearm pronated, elbow extended

3. **Functional skills rehabilitation for the upper extremity**
   a. Start with **"anchored racquet" exercises,** with racquet secured by rubberized tubing to a wall post or door. The athlete should simulate backhand, forehand, and overhead strokes against this elastic resistance (Fig. 6).
      i. Any postinjury incoordination patterns can be corrected at this time.
      ii. Backhand simulation is most important for lateral tennis elbow.
      iii. Overhead stroke simulation is most important for shoulder injuries and medial tennis elbow.
   b. Overhead stroke–related injuries can progress from anchored racquet exercises as tolerated to **"windmill" simulation of service** without racquet, then with racquet. There is no contact made with a tennis ball during these full-service simulations—hence, the term "windmill."
   c. The asymptomatic athlete then can begin ball contact service, starting with high-arc service lobs from behind baseline, progressing to full-speed service.
   d. **Lateral tennis elbow** should follow a similar pattern of easy, high-arc backhand strokes, progressing to full-speed, short-arc strokes.
      i. Backboard volleying drills may provide high-level endurance and also test the stroke.

    ii. The wrist should be neutral or slightly extended, **not flexed,** at time of backhanded ball strike.
  e. **Refractory lateral tennis elbow may require learning a two-handed backhand technique.**
4. **Back**
  a. Rehabilitation by a medical team skilled in back disorders is essential, given that the spine is multiarthrodial, has multiple motor functions and flexibility patterns, and protects the spinal cord.
  b. See Chapters 40 and 47 for protection of the acutely injured spine, basic rehabilitation program, and avoidance of aggravating daily activities and sports.
  c. Functional drills outlined in this chapter for the upper and lower extremities should be tolerated without back symptoms before formal training and competition.
  d. **Back hyperextension should be avoided** during the service stroke.
5. **Lower extremity**
  a. Refer to Chapter 52, "Foot Problems" and Chapter 61, "Track and Field" for fundamental rehabilitation of sprinters' injuries.
  b. **Patellar taping** to redirect patellar tracking (McConnell taping) may inhibit pain from injury to patellofemoral glide mechanism.
  c. When full strengthening and flexibility are attained and endurance is intact for a 3-mile jog, the rehabilitation program may progress to a **plyometric and sprint agility program** before sports participation.
    i. An average 2-hour match includes approximately 30 minutes of actual play, each point 10 seconds in duration, with more than 20 seconds of rest.
    ii. Sprinting and side-to-side jumping plyometric drills should gradually approach these parameters.
  d. **The athlete should display full range of motion at the hip, knee, and ankle during jumps, service, and low ground strokes.**
  e. Initial entry into tennis volleying:
    i. For ankle injury—should include ankle taping, air splint, or similar mediolateral stabilizer for ankle injury
    ii. For knee injury—rarely requires bracing other than simple neoprene patellar knee sleeve

C. **Proprioceptive neuromuscular facilitation**—methods proposed to enhance flexibility and motor coordination via sensorimotor pathways
1. **Contract-relax stretching** is a form of proprioceptive neuromuscular function in which contraction of a given muscle group allows for greater postcontraction passive stretch.
2. Proprioceptive neuromuscular facilitation may describe the hands-on technique by which trained therapists place inhibitory and facilitatory resistance to key muscle groups and limbs to alter incorrect movement patterns learned during the postinjury period.
  a. In tennis, this technique may consist of slowly simulated strokes, with a therapist manually controlling a given body part, such as the shoulder or back.
  b. One example would be a therapist facilitating better abduction and elevation of the scapula during a service stroke.
3. **Other forms of motor awareness enhancement**
  a. Use of **plyometric techniques** in which lower extremity muscles are put through a horizontal or vertical jump drill to augment responsive power output and decrease reaction time
  b. For upper extremity, lightly weight tennis racquet with a 1-lb racquet necklace during simulated volleying drills

c. **Injury prevention and effects on performance by these techniques are uncertain.** If done incorrectly, they may increase the risk of overload injury.

IV. Facilities

A. See page 818 and Chapter 19, "Sports Surfaces" for information on tennis court surfaces.

B. **Year-round facilities** allow for continued endurance base to be maintained during the off-season by indoor tennis and tennis drills, bicycling for lower extremity conditioning, swimming for upper extremity conditioning, and rowing for back conditioning.

C. **Tennis camps:** For those athletes seeking off-season coaching or who do not have access to a coach, there are many quality tennis camps available and publicized in the major tennis magazines.

V. Team Safety and Sportsmanship

A. **Practice session injuries: Racquet and ball missile injuries can be avoided** by clearly defined rules about boundaries on tennis courts where players are warming up or volleying in close parallel files. In doubles matches, team partners should have a clear strategy or strict playing zone agreement.

B. **Unsportsmanlike aggression**

1. A direct tennis ball return to the face of an opponent should be considered unsportsmanlike aggression until decided otherwise.
2. Overhead return should have a planned trajectory, specifically *away* from an opponent's face.
3. No player should return a volley at an opponent's feet unless control is adequate to miss other parts of an opponent's body. The player should also be held accountable for the safety of the opponent in such risky shots.
4. Any throwing of a racquet during a match should be considered unsafe and prohibited, preferably with a penalty rule included. Of course, throwing the racquet *vertically* in the air *after* victory is just plain fun!

Recommended Reading

1. Atwater AE: Biomechanics of overarm throwing movements and throwing injuries. Exerc Sport Sci Rev 7:43–85, 1979.
2. Blackwell JR, Cole KJ: Wrist kinematics differ in expert and novice tennis players performing the backhand stroke: Implications for tennis elbow. J Biomech 27(5):509–516, 1994.
3. Chandler TJ, Kibler WB, Stracener EC, et al: Shoulder strength, power, and endurance in college tennis players. Am J Sports Med 29(4):455–458, 1992.
4. Elliott BC: Tennis: The influence of grip tightness or reaction impulse and rebound velocity. Med Sci Sports Exerc 14:348, 1982.
5. Giangarra CE, Conroy B, Jobe FW, et al: Electromyographic and cinematographic analysis of elbow function in tennis players using single and double-handed backhand strokes. Am J Sports Med 21(3):394–399, 1993.
6. Grabiner MD, Groppel JL, Campbell KR: Resultant tennis ball velocity as a function of off-center impact and grip firmness. Med Sci Sports Exerc 15:541, 1983.
7. Hatze H: The effectiveness of grip bands in reducing racquet vibration transfer and slipping. Med Sci Sports Exerc 24(2):226–230, 1992.
8. Ilfeld FW: Can stroke modification relieve tennis elbow. Clin Orthop Rel Res 276:182–186, 1992.
9. Kelley JD, Lombardo SJ, Pink M, et al: Electromyographic and cinematographic analysis of elbow function in tennis players with lateral epicondylitis. Am J Sports Med 22(3):359–363, 1994.
10. Kibler WB: The role of the scapula in the overhead throwing motion. Contemp Orthop 22:525, 1991.
12. Lehman RC (ed): Racquet sports [entire issue]. Olin Sports Med 14(1), 1995.
13. Mont MA, Cohen DB, Campbell KR, et al: Isokinetic concentric vs. eccentric training of shoulder rotators with functional evaluation of performance enhancement in elite tennis players. Am J Sports Med 22(4):513–517, 1994.
14. Murakami Y: Stress fracture of the metacarpal in an adolescent tennis player. Am J Sports Med 16:419, 1988.

15. Regan W, Wold LE, Conrad R, Morrey BF: Microscopic histopathology of chronic refractory later epicondylitis. Am J Sports Med 20(6): 746–749, 1992.
16. Rettig AC, Beltz HF: Stress fracture in the humerus in an adolescent tennis tournament player. Am J Sports Med 13:55, 1985.
17. Ryu RKN, McCormick J, Jobe FW, et al: An electromyographic analysis of shoulder function in tennis players. Am J Sports Med 16:481, 1988.
18. Saal JA (ed): Rehabilitation of sports injuries. Phys Med Rehabil State Art Rev 1(4):597–638, 1987.
19. Sward L, Hellstrom M, Jacobsson B, Peterson L: Back pain and radiologic changes in the thoracolumbar spine of athletes. Spine 15(2):124–129, 1990.
20. Sward L, Svensson M, Zetterberg C: Isometric muscle strength and quantitative electromyography of back muscles in wrestlers and tennis players. Am J Sports Med 18(4):382–386, 1990.
21. Snijders CJ, Volkers ACW, Mechelse K, et al: Provocation of epicondylalgia lateralis (tennis elbow) by power grip or pinching. Med Sci Sports 19:518, 1987.
22. Wadsworth TG: Tennis elbow: Conservative, surgical, and manipulative treatment. BMJ 294:621, 1987.

66

Alpine Skiing

William I. Sterett, M.D., and J. Richard Steadman, M.D.

I. Overview

A. **Injury rate**
   1. Two to three per 1000 skier days, lower than competitive football or basketball
   2. Higher percentage of ski injuries require surgical intervention

B. **Level of competition**
   1. Secondary school
   2. Regional team
   3. National team
   4. Olympic/World Cup (physician required to be present on hill during competition)
   5. Disabled ski team

II. Preparation of Athlete

A. **Clothing and equipment**
   1. Layered clothing for warm-up and warm-down
   2. Reliable bindings, with multimode adjustable toe and heel releases
   3. Quality skis do not delaminate under the stress of binding loads
   4. Well ventilated goggles to protect the eyes from ultraviolet radiation as well as injury
   5. Pads, to protect the slalom skier against injury from slalom poles
      a. Padded gloves and uniforms
      b. Additional arm pads
   6. Helmets, required for downhill
   7. Breakaway poles for slalom and giant slalom—must have optimum strength and flexibility

B. **Cardiovascular**
   1. The competitive Alpine skier is characterized by a significantly increased $\dot{V}O_2max$, an increased stroke volume, and an increased blood volume.
   2. The lactic acid threshold is increased with training.
   3. Fluid loss occurs rapidly at high altitude and low humidity and if not replaced promptly results in decreased performance. Water or hypotonic sugar or salt solutions are preferable.

C. **Musculoskeletal strength, endurance, and agility**
   1. Must be gained preseason and maintained in season. "Peaking" is important and sometimes must be obtained two to three times per season.
   2. Overtraining is difficult to evaluate and recognize. An increasing pulse rate is sometimes helpful in diagnosis. Overtraining seems to occur more often in women athletes.
   3. Agility can be taught.
      a. Simple drills are available in the coaching manuals, and in addition to these, soccer, water-skiing, and mountain biking may be components of an agility program.

b. The "SAID" principle (*s*pecific *a*daptation to *i*ndividual *d*emands) must be recognized so that some of the conditioning, both aerobic and anaerobic, is attained "on slope."

4. Rule of 3's
   a. Quit before 3 o'clock.
   b. Decrease intensity every third day.
   c. Increased incidence of problems at 3000 m and above

III. Competition Responsibilities

A. **Precompetition responsibilities**

1. **Dry land endurance**
   a. Basic principles:
      i. Low intensity, low pulse
      ii. Long duration
      iii. Short, complete breaks
   b. Typically overuse injuries:
      i. Muscle strain
      ii. Patellofemoral pain
2. **Quickness**
   a. Basic principles:
      i. High intensity, short duration
      ii. Incomplete breaks (pulse greater than 120 beats/minute)
   b. Ruptures and strains common
   c. Check for cardiac disease preconditioning.
3. **Flexibility**
   a. Prestretched muscle:
      i. Greater strength
      ii. Greater power
      iii. Injury protection
   b. Most injuries occur from **lack** of flexibility
4. **Strength and power**
   a. Overload
   b. Isotonic
   c. Isometric, e.g., a downhill tuck
   d. Isokinetic:
      i. Best for strengthening
      ii. May induce injuries
   e. Principles:
      i. High intensity, short duration
      ii. Incomplete breaks
      iii. With weights

B. **"On the mountain" responsibilities**

1. **Skiing ability.** The ski team physician should ski well enough to attend practices and competition on the ski mountain itself.
   a. **On the mountain experience is necessary to:**
      i. Supervise preparations for event coverage.
      ii. Develop preventive strategies.
      iii. Ensure proper first aid and evacuation procedures.
      iv. Develop rapport with athletes and coaches.
   b. **Ski patrol training helpful:**
      i. Physician as trainee
      ii. Physician as trainer

2. **Radio communication**
   a. Mandatory for event coverage:
      i. With coach and team
      ii. With ski patrol and mountain manager
   b. Is highly recommended both at home and away
3. **Event coverage at home**
   a. **Coordination** with:
      i. Mountain manager or ski area manager:
         (a) General planning and logistics
         (b) Grooming and condition of course
      ii. Ski patrol leader:
         (a) Personnel, supplies, and equipment on hill
         (b) Ski traffic patterns and crowd control
         (c) Evacuation plan
         (d) Physician availability on hill and at base
         (e) Spectator medical support
      iii. Support medical personnel:
         (a) Assign duties to assisting physicians, trainers, and medical support personnel.
         (b) Coordinate availability of medical facility at mountain or local hospital.
         (c) Coordinate ambulance availability if appropriate.
      iv. Medical support personnel or coaches from attending teams
      v. Personal equipment:
         (a) Ski equipment well maintained
         (b) Warm clothing for "standing and waiting" by race course
         (c) "Fanny pack" or backpack with emergency supplies
   b. **United States Skiing medical kit (to be carried by trainer)**
      i. Equipment:
         (a) Cryotherapy
         (b) Elastic tubing
         (c) Blood pressure cuff and stethoscope
         (d) Ultrasound
      ii. Bandaging:
         (a) Peroxide and povidone-iodine (Betadine)
         (b) Wound closure kit
         (c) Gauze pads
         (d) Ace wrap
      iii. Taping
      iv. Bracing and splinting
      v. Casting
      vi. Padding
      vii. Injection or aspiration
      viii. Miscellaneous
      ix. Drug inventory
         (a) Nonsteroidal anti-inflammatory drugs
         (b) Antibiotics
         (c) Antihistamine
         (d) Other

C. **Postcompetition responsibilities**
1. **Emergent problems**
   a. Closed head injury
   b. Open fractures and dislocations:

   i. Coordinate local care
   ii. Transport to hospital immediately
2. **Nonemergent problems**
   a. Minor fractures
   b. Ligament injuries
   c. Coordinate care and follow-up with physician in athlete's home town
   d. Communicate with treating physician

IV. Specific Injuries

A. **Closed head injuries**
1. Common
   a. Aerialists
   b. Mogul skiers
   c. Ballet skiers
2. Recognition
   a. On-hill testing:
      i. Orientation
      ii. Follow three-part commands
      iii. Amnesia
   b. Mild:
      i. Minimal or no loss of consciousness
      ii. Posttraumatic amnesia lasting < 15 minutes
   c. Moderate:
      i. Loss of consciousness < 5 minutes
      ii. Posttraumatic amnesia > 20 minutes
   d. Severe:
      i. Loss of consciousness > 5 minutes
      ii. Posttraumatic amnesia > 12 hours
3. **Return to competition (first head injury)**
   a. Mild—1 week *after* completely asymptomatic
   b. Moderate—2 weeks *after* completely asymptomatic
   c. Severe—1 month *after* completely asymptomatic with normal head computed tomography scan

B. **Spine trauma**
1. Particularly cervical spine and thoracolumbar junction
2. "Downed" skier should not be moved until spine palpated and neurologic function checked

C. **Knee ligaments**
1. **Medial collateral ligament (MCL) tear**
   a. Catching inside edge of ski leads to forceful external rotation/valgus load
   b. Level of injury:

Grade I	2–5 mm opening
Grade II	5–10 mm opening
Grade III	> 10 mm opening relative to other side

   c. Treat nonoperatively in hinged orthosis for Grade II to Grade III tears
   d. Return to competition when skier has full pain-free range of motion and normal laxity profile
2. **Anterior cruciate ligament (ACL)**
   a. **Mechanism:**
      i. Hyperextension leads to isolated injury.
      ii. Valgus/external rotation leads to combined injury.
      iii. Hyperextension is common in ski racers.

b. **Presentation:**
   i. Skier hears a "pop" or tear
   ii. Sense of "giving way" or instability while standing
   iii. Effusion within 24 hours

3. **Treatment**
   a. Ice, compression, elevation, early range of motion
   b. Orthopedic consultation
   c. Nonoperative treatment roughly doubles the number of future knee injuries

D. **Lower extremity fractures**
   1. **Femur**
      a. Direct impact, high-energy injury
      b. Advanced skiers at greater risk
      c. Immediate traction to avoid significant blood loss within the thigh
   2. **Tibial shaft:** mid/distal one-third junction most common
   3. **Tibial plateau:** high association with ligament and meniscal pathology
   4. **Ankle:** twisting injury may occur despite tightened ski boot.

E. **Upper extremity injuries**
   1. **Thumb**
      a. Acute tear of ulnar collateral ligament most common
      b. Caused by catching thumb on ski pole or hard-packed snow
      c. Cast for Grade I to II (< 35° opening or < 15° greater than other thumb)
      d. Open repair for Grade III
   2. **Shoulder**
      a. Dislocation:
         i. Anterior—high recurrence rate in skiers younger than 25
         ii. Posterior—uncommon
      b. Fracture:
         i. Proximal humerus—common, requires orthopedic consultation
         ii. Clavicle—usually nonoperative, treated in a sling or figure-of-eight bandage
      c. Acromioclavicular separation
   3. **Elbow**
      a. Dislocation:
         i. Usually posterior
         ii. Low risk of recurrence, high risk of stiffness
      b. Fracture:
         i. Olecranon
         ii. Radial head

F. **Environment—weather-related injuries**
   1. **Cold**
      a. Frostbite of the nose, ears, and cheeks is common.
         i. If caught early, in frostnip stage, massage usually restores circulation and reverses damage.
         ii. Rapid rewarming (40–44°C) key to treatment of extremity frostbite.
      b. Skiers should check each other for frostbite, and the physician should be alerted to the risk.
      c. The wind-chill factor should be known to the physician, who should add this to the skier's speed.
      d. Hypothermia may be a problem if frostbite injury is severe and evacuation delayed.
   2. **Sun**
      a. **Ultraviolet rays** can be intense with altitude and reflected light. The eyes need protection, and ordinary glasses may not be enough because 10% of ultraviolet light may enter from the top and sides.

b. Maximum protection sunscreen should be liberally used on exposed parts:
   i. **Formerly frostbitten areas are particularly vulnerable to ultraviolet damage.**
   ii. Carelessness in protecting the skin leads to an increased incidence of basal cell carcinoma in later life.
c. **Herpes labialis** is common and should be treated preventively with protective screens.
d. Visibility is critical to racers. Snow, fogging, flat light, and glare all impair performance and jeopardize safety.

V. Diagnosis and Treatment

A. On the hill

1. The history surrounding the fall usually reveals the injury.
   a. Knee—heard a "pop" in hyperflexion injury, suspect ACL tear
   b. Hand—fell on abducted thumb, think ulnar collateral ligament injury
2. "Common injuries occur commonly"
   a. ACL tear
   b. Fractured tibia or ankle
   c. Dislocated shoulder
   d. Ulnar collateral ligament tears
   e. Occasionally concussion
3. Inspect obvious deformities and painful areas.
4. **Palpation is the essence of on-the-slope diagnosis.** Palpate the entire spine first, then the pelvis and hip joints, then long bones for tenderness and deformity.
5. Splint all fractures and joint injuries on site. When in doubt, use a backboard/cervical collar.
6. Coordinate evacuation to a definitive treatment center appropriate to the injury. Whenever possible, stay with the patient until definitive care is arranged.
7. **Do not allow evacuation until preliminary diagnosis by history and manual examination is accomplished, and all long bone fractures are splinted. Protect against hypothermia.**

B. Off the hill

1. Palpate spine, pelvis, and all extremities
   a. Neurologic evaluation of sensation and strength in C5–T1 and L2–S1 motor groups
   b. Evaluate for rib fracture and pneumothoraces.
   c. Dislocation and vascular compromise occur and need to be recognized and treated immediately.
2. Extremities with crepitation pain or tenderness need to be excluded for fracture.
   a. X-ray in two planes required
   b. Splint until definitive care available

Recommended Reading

1. Feagin JA, Lambert KL, et al: Consideration of the anterior cruciate ligament injury in skiing. Clin Orthop 13–17, 1987.
2. Sterett WI, Krissoff WB: Femur fractures in alpine skiing: Classification and mechanisms of injury in 85 cases. J Orthop Trauma 8:310–314, 1994.
3. Sterett WI, Steadman JR: The surgical treatment of knee injuries in skiers. Med Sci Sports Exerc 27:328–333, 1994.
4. Sterett WI, Steadman JR, Roalstad M: The management of head injuries in alpine skiing. U.S. Skiing Association Training Manual. Park City, Utah, USSA, 1994.

67

Cross Country Skiing

David C. Thorson, M.D.

Cross country skiing was "invented" 4000 to 5000 years ago in the Scandinavian countries. The earliest skis were transportation aids made of large animal bones attached to the feet with leather straps. Skis were used in warfare during the battle of Oslo in 1200 A.D. Modern sports skiing began in the mid–nineteenth century in Norway and quickly spread throughout Scandinavia. It was introduced into the United States by Norwegian immigrants who lived in Minnesota in the mid–nineteenth century. The Féderation International de Ski (FIS), the governing body of Nordic (cross country, jumping, biathlon, and Nordic combined), Alpine (slalom, giant slalom, super G, downhill) and freestyle (moguls, ballet, and aerials) skiing, was formed in 1924. Cross country skiing became an Olympic sport that year.

Cross country ski racing, sanctioned by the FIS, covers distances from 5 km to 50 km. Even longer distances are raced in numerous citizen races held throughout the world. Advances in technique and technology have decreased race times. Racers routinely hit speeds of 30–40 mph on the downhill portions of the course. The newer skating techniques have allowed racers to attain higher speeds along the flats and uphill sections. The newer waxes and composite skis with faster bases and better weight distribution have increased glide by reducing friction. Boots and bindings now couple the ski to the boot more effectively and allow the skier to transfer energy to the snow more efficiently. Sports nutrition has allowed athletes to maintain glycogen stores better, and athletes routinely take fluids and other nourishment during the longer races. Races are either **classic (diagonal stride, skating minimized) or freestyle (skating)**. Racers are started sequentially in most events; however, in the longer "marathon" events, pack starts are routine.

Injuries can be related to one or a combination of mechanisms, including environment, overuse, and overstress (includes trauma). Good injury data are hard to find because most injuries are not severe enough to demand immediate attention, which makes tracking and identification difficult. Medical personnel taking care of these athletes have noted some injury pattern changes associated with changes in technique and technology (e.g., hip adductor muscle strain and anterior tibialis overuse associated with skating techniques).

I. Equipment

A. **Diagonal stride equipment**
   1. **Skis**
      a. Longer than skating skis
      b. More curved tip
      c. More camber
      d. Synthetic bases designed for temperature ranges and to hold kicker wax
   2. **Boots**
      a. Usually cut below the ankle with "inner sock" snow cuff extending above
      b. Less rigid midsole with softer heel counters
   3. **Bindings**

   a. Flex determined by binding and is adjustable with flex plates
   b. Toe attachment with less solid heel fixation when heel is resting on ski
4. **Poles**
   a. Usually shorter than skating poles
   b. Carbon fiber and composite technology with aerodynamic shafts
   c. Traditional grip and retention strap

B. **Skate ski equipment**
1. **Skis**
   a. Usually shorter
   b. Less rounded tip
   c. Less camber
   d. Bases designed for glide and higher speeds, not to hold kicker wax
2. **Poles**
   a. Usually longer and stiffer
   b. Construction similar to diagonal stride poles
   c. Ongoing research regarding pole grip design to improve performance (i.e., T handles)
3. **Boots**
   a. Higher, cut above the ankle
   b. More rigid midsole and heel counter
   c. Increased lateral stiffness
   d. Upper and lower cuff with an ankle hinging system
4. **Bindings**
   a. Less flex, designed to keep the foot and ski in close contact
   b. Rigidity to linkage between boot and ski that allows for edging and steering of ski

II. Environmental Factors

A. **Temperature (20% of injuries are related to the cold)**
1. FIS minimum is –4°C on any part of the course
   a. FIS-sanctioned races cannot be started if the temperature is below –4°C on any part of the course.
   b. Combination of temperature and speed produce wind-chill (see Table 1).
   c. Athletes wearing metal jewelry increase risk of frostbite to contact area
   d. Eye protection needed for corneal frostbite, ultraviolet exposure, and snow particles
2. Increased risk due to hypothermia or hyperthermia
3. Increased risk due to dehydration or hypovolemia—high-intensity exercise in low humidity
4. **Frostbite and frostnip**
   a. Exposed skin
   b. Thin clothing
   c. Low body fat
   d. Wind-chill (with no wind, the wind-chill at –4°C on downhill sections easily reaches –35 to –40°C)
   e. Humidity
5. **Exercise-induced bronchospasm**
   a. Cold dry air
   b. Elevation of heart rate 8–12 minutes

B. **Altitude**
1. Altitude sickness, associated with prolonged stays at > 6000 feet
   a. Acute mountain sickness
   b. High-altitude pulmonary edema
   c. High-altitude cerebral edema

TABLE 1. Determination of Wind Chill

Actual thermometer reading	Estimated wind speed in mph (and kph)									
	calm	5 (8)	10 (16)	15 (24)	20 (32)	25 (40)	30 (48)	35 (56)	40 (64)	(Wind speeds greater than 40 mph have little additional effect.)
	EQUIVALENT TEMPERATURE IN °F (AND °C)									
50°F (10°C)	50 (10)	48 (8.9)	40 (4.4)	36 (2.2)	32 (0)	30 (-1.1)	28 (-2.2)	27 (-2.8)	26 (-3.3)	LITTLE DANGER for properly clothed person. Maximum danger from false sense of security
40°F (4.4°C)	40 (4.4)	37 (2.8)	28 (-2.2)	22 (-5.6)	18 (-7.8)	16 (-8.9)	13 (-10.6)	11 (-11.7)	10 (-12.2)	
30°F (-1.1°C)	30 (-1.1)	27 (-2.8)	16 (-8.9)	9 (-12.8)	4 (-15.6)	0 (-17.8)	-2 (-18.9)	-4 (-20)	-6 (-21.1)	
20°F (-6.7°C)	20 (-6.7)	16 (-8.9)	4 (-15.6)	-5 (-20.6)	-10 (-23.3)	-15 (-26.1)	-18 (-27.8)	-20 (-28.9)	-21 (-29.4)	
10°F (-12.2°C)	10 (-12.2)	6 (-14.4)	-9 (-22.8)	-18 (-27.8)	-25 (-31.7)	-29 (-33.9)	-33 (-36.1)	-35 (-37.2)	-37 (-38.3)	INCREASING DANGER from freezing of exposed flesh
0°F (-17.8°C)	0 (-17.8)	-5 (-20.6)	-24 (-31.1)	-32 (-35.6)	-39 (-39.4)	-44 (-42.2)	-48 (-44.4)	-51 (-46.1)	-53 (-47.2)	
-10°F (-23.3°C)	-10 (-23.3)	-15 (-26.1)	-33 (-36.1)	-45 (-42.8)	-53 (-47.2)	-59 (-50.6)	-63 (-52.8)	-67 (-55)	-69 (-56.1)	
-20°F (-28.9°C)	-20 (-28.9)	-26 (-32.2)	-46 (-43.3)	-58 (-50)	-67 (-55)	-74 (-58.9)	-79 (-61.7)	-82 (-63.3)	-85 (-65)	GREAT DANGER
-30°F (-34.4°C)	-30 (-34.4)	-36 (-37.8)	-58 (-50)	-72 (-57.8)	-82 (-63.3)	-88 (-66.7)	-94 (-70)	-98 (-72.2)	-100 (-73.3)	
-40°F (-40°C)	-40 (-40)	-47 (-43.9)	-70 (-56.7)	-85 (-65)	-96 (-71.1)	-104 (-75.6)	-109 (-78.3)	-113 (-80.6)	-116 (-82.2)	
-50°F (-45.6°C)	-50 (-45.6)	-57 (-49.4)	-83 (-63.9)	-99 (-72.8)	-110 (-78.9)	-118 (-83.3)	-125 (-87.2)	-129 (-89.4)	-132 (-91.1)	
-60°F (-51.1°C)	-60 (-51.1)	-68 (-55.6)	-95 (-70.6)	-112 (-80)	-124 (-86.7)	-133 (-91.7)	-140 (-95.6)	-145 (-98.3)	-148 (-100)	

2. Tendency is recurring; affects up to 25% of people
3. Treatment
    a. Gradual increase in elevation, spend first night at < 7000 feet (**"Climb high, sleep low"**)
    b. Identify at-risk populations
    c. Acetazolamide (Diamox) for at-risk patients
    d. Evacuate to lower altitude patients who are worsening

C. **Wax room**
1. New fluorocarbon waxes vaporize during ironing and can cause lung damage if used in poor ventilation.
2. Allergic reactions to waxes and wax removers

III. Overuse Injuries

A. **Diagonal stride**
1. Biceps/triceps tendinitis associated with double poling
2. Low back pain
3. Iliotibial band syndrome
4. Hamstring strain
5. Posterior tibial/peroneal tendinitis
6. Achilles tendinitis
7. Skier's toe—first metatarsophalangeal joint overuse

8. Sacroiliac joint dysfunction
9. Plantar fasciitis
10. Patellofemoral pain syndrome

B. **Skating technique**
1. Biceps/triceps tendinitis
2. Low back pain
3. Hip abductor and adductor overuse
4. Wrist overuse
5. Achilles tendinitis
6. Posterior tibial/peroneal tendinitis
7. Skier's toe—first metatarsophalangeal joint overuse
8. Low back pain or sacroiliac joint dysfunction
9. Plantar fasciitis
10. Morton's neuroma
11. Calcaneal bursitis
12. Sever's disease in adolescents
13. Patellar tendinitis
14. Patellofemoral pain syndrome
15. Anterior tibialis overuse
16. Puncture wounds from ski pole tips of other skiers (most common during pack starts, but may happen in passing situations along the course)

IV. Overstress (Traumatic) Injuries

A. **Hand injuries**
1. **Skier's thumb**
   a. Be aware of Stener's lesion, which may need surgical repair.
   b. Know how to make hand-based thumb spica cast (fit to ski pole).
2. Navicular fracture may require a cast
3. Metacarpal fractures
4. Phalangeal fractures
5. de Quervain's tenosynovitis
6. Colles' fracture

B. **Concussion**—contact with ground or other objects around the course (see Chapter 39, "Head Injuries" for classification of concussion)

C. **Abrasions and contusions** secondary to falls and collisions

D. **Fractures of extremities**

E. **Knee injuries**
1. Anterior cruciate injury
2. Medial collateral injury
3. Lateral collateral injury
4. Meniscal injuries
5. More common with skating technique because of more rigid fixation of boot and binding

F. **Ankle injuries**
1. Medial and lateral sprains
2. Disruption of tibiofibular interosseous membrane (high sprain)
3. Avulsion fracture distal fibula
4. Other ankle fractures (often associated with widened mortice)
5. Dislocation of peroneal tendon from behind lateral malleolus

G. **Metatarsal fractures**
1. Jones fracture of proximal fifth metatarsal
2. Avulsion fracture of proximal fifth metatarsal
3. Stable second, third, and fourth midshaft fractures

H. **Elbow injuries**
   1. Fractures related to falls
   2. Ulnar and radial collateral ligaments strain or tear

I. **Shoulder injuries**
   1. Acromiclavicular separations
   2. Dislocations
   3. Subluxations
   4. Clavicular fractures

V. Fitness Demands

A. Aerobic fitness often exceeds that of distance runners or cyclists
B. Need power and upper extremity fitness of swimmers
C. Elite athletes often have $\dot{V}O_2max > 80$ mL O_2/kg/min.
D. Diagonal stride requires higher oxygen demands and offers less speed (19% higher O_2 consumption, 5% higher heart rates, and 36% higher ventilation rates) than skating technique
E. Double pole technique with skating V1 or V2 techniques most efficient
F. Cardiovascular changes are similar to other endurance athletes with changes seen with the "athletic heart." There is increased left ventricular wall thickness associated with increased pressure load from upper extremity work.
G. High caloric needs of endurance athlete and cold stress environment
H. Susceptible to overtraining or staleness as are other endurance athletes
I. Women at risk for amenorrhea, associated stress fractures, and disordered eating

VI. Injury Data

A. Numbers are likely biased due to underreporting
B. Cross country 0.72 injuries/1000 skier days versus Alpine 3.4–7.4 injuries/1000 skier days
C. The downhill sections of a trail are most risky, accounting for 88% of injuries
D. Upper and lower extremity injury rates almost even (41% upper extremity versus 49% lower extremity)
E. As cross country skiers become more experienced, the likelihood of injury decreases, and the injury is more likely to be an overuse injury.
F. Severe, season-ending or career-ending injuries are rare in experienced or elite-level cross country skiers.

Recommended Reading

1. Boyle JJ, Johnson RJ, Pope MH: Cross-country injuries: A prospective study. Iowa Orthop J 1:41, 1981.
2. Grover RF, Tucker CE, McGroarty SR, et al: The coronary stress of skiing at altitude. Arch Intern Med 150:1205, 1990.
3. Hoffman MD: Physiological comparisons of cross-country skiing techniques. Med Sci Sports Exerc 24:1023, 1992.
4. Hoffman MD, Clifford PS: Physiological responses to different cross country skiing techniques on level terrain. Med Sci Sports Exerc 22:841, 1990.
5. Hoffman MD, Clifford PS, Foley PJ, Brice AG: Physiological responses to different roller skiing techniques. Med Sci Sports Exerc 22:391, 1990.
6. Houston CS: Trekking at high altitudes: How safe is it for your patients? Postgrad Med 88:56, 1990.
7. Johnson RJ: Skiing and snowboarding injuries: When schussing is a pain. Postgrad Med 88:36, 1990.
8. Renstrom P, Johnson RJ: Cross-country skiing injuries and biomechanics. Phys Sportsmed 8(6):346, 1989.
9. Stray-Gunderson J, Denke MA, Grundy SM: Influence of lifetime cross-country skiing on plasma lipids and lipoproteins. Med Sci Sports Exerc 23:695, 1991.
10. Street GM: Technological advances in cross-country ski equipment. Med Sci Sports Exerc 24:1048, 1992.
11. Suominen H, Rahkila P: Bone mineral density of the calcaneus in 70–81-yr-old male athletes and a population sample. Med Sci Sports Exerc 23:1227, 1991.

68

Ice Hockey

Robert Johnson, M.D.

I. History of Hockey

A. **Shinty ("shinny")**—historically, a game resembling field hockey played by British soldiers. A similar game played on ice with pucks was introduced in 1860.

B. **First hockey game played in Montreal in 1879 by McGill University Hockey Club** with 30 players on a side.

1. Rules of the game first established in 1881, permitting nine players per side
2. Hockey sticks and skates specifically made for hockey in early 1880s
3. One-foot boards around perimeter of ice surface first used in 1880

C. **In 1892, Lord Stanley donated a cup to serve as the trophy for the best amateur team in Canada.**

D. **Professional hockey was first established in the United States in 1917.**

II. Hockey Organization and Participation

A. **USA Hockey**, located in Colorado Springs, Colorado, is the national governing body for ice hockey in the United States. USA Hockey is the official representative of the U.S. Olympic Committee and the International Ice Hockey Federation and works with the National Hockey League (NHL) and the National Collegiate Athletic Association (NCAA).

B. In 1968–1969, 3800 teams were registered with USA Hockey. In 1993–1994, 21,150 teams were registered with approximately 340,000 players.

C. Women's hockey is rapidly growing. Of the 21,150 teams registered by USA Hockey, 352 represent about 6000 girls and women. In 1995–1996, 38 women's teams competed in interscholastic competition in Minnesota; 58 teams are expected to compete 1996–1997. The first state high school tournament for girls was held in Minnesota in 1995. In many states, girls are still competing on boy's youth hockey teams.

D. **Age range of organized competition—5 to over 50**

E. **Age group divisions** (Table 1) are determined by birth date as of August 31 of each year.

F. More than 500,000 men and boys participate in Canada.

III. The Game of Ice Hockey

A. **Regarded by most to be the fastest competitive team sport**

B. **Structure**

1. **Professional, college, adult**—three 20-minute periods
2. **High school**—three 15-minute periods
3. **Youth**—three 12–15-minute periods

C. **The team**

1. **Composition**
    a. Eighteen players and two goalkeepers (usual position distribution)
    b. Six players compete at one time

TABLE 1. Age Group Divisions Determined by USA Hockey

Level	Boys	Girls
Mites	≤ 8	
Squirts	≤ 10	6–12
PeeWees	≤ 12	13–15
Bantams	≤ 14	
Junior Midgets	≤ 19	16–19
Junior	≤ 19	
Senior	> 19	> 19

i. Three forwards
ii. Two defensemen
iii. One goalie

2. **Goalkeeper (goalie)**—player who tends the goal to catch or deflect the puck and prevent the opponent from scoring
3. **Forwards (left wing, center, right wing)**—offensive-minded players who attack the opponent with the intent to score a goal. These position players also assist the defensemen in protecting their goal.
4. **Defensemen (left and right)**—primary responsibility is to protect their goal and goalie to prevent opponent from advancing to net to score
5. **Substitution** may occur during play ("on the fly") or during time stoppages for violations, goals, or penalties.

D. **The rink**
1. A rink should be 200 feet × 100 feet. The smallest recommended dimensions are 185 feet × 85 feet.
2. The rink should be surrounded by wooden or fiberglass boards 40–48 inches high with a yellow or light-colored kickplate at the bottom. It is recommended that safety glass or other protective screen encircle the rink.
3. The goal should have dimensions 4 feet high × 6 feet wide with metal goalposts and crossbar and a net surrounding the metal framework.

E. **Special equipment of the game**
1. **Puck** is Vulcanized rubber 1 inch thick and 3 inches in diameter, weighing 5.5–6 oz.
2. **Hockey stick**
   a. Forwards and defensemen—usually made of wood (the shaft may be made of other materials) with a shaft < 60 inches, a blade < 12.5 inches long × 3 inches wide, and a curve not to exceed 0.5 inch
   b. Goalie—wood shaft < 60 inches with a blade < 15.5 inches long × 3.5 inches wide, and a curve not to exceed 0.5 inches

F. **Skills of the game**
1. **Skating**—three factors in skill
   a. Angle of propulsion (angle formed by the skate blade in the direction of skate)
   b. Angle of forward inclination (body lean)
   c. Length of stride
2. **Shooting**
   a. Types of shots:
      i. Standing wrist shot (sweeping action with the stick terminating in a wrist snap and follow-through)
      ii. Skating wrist shot (similar to the standing wrist shot except the player has forward momentum while skating; most accurate)

iii. Standing slap shot (stick and blade are brought back a variable distance followed by a vigorous forward motion, "slapping" at puck much like a golf swing; least accurate)
iv. Skating slap shot (greatest velocity)

b. Maximal velocity is a result of strength of arm and shoulder muscles and full trunk rotation.

3. **Passing**
4. **Stick handling:** the ability to advance the puck while maneuvering on the ice
5. **Checking:** intentional contact with an opponent who is in possession of the puck, using the hip or shoulder. A player may check from the side, diagonally or frontally, approaching with no more than two skating strides.
6. **Goal tending:** the goalkeeper (goalie) tends the goal. The goalie is protected by special equipment and pads to catch or deflect pucks from the goal.

G. **Safety and protection within the game of hockey**

1. **Protective equipment**

a. Goalie:
i. Helmet
ii. Mask
iii. Throat protector
iv. Chest protector
v. Cup
vi. Thick padded shin guards
vii. Blocker (worn on one hand)
viii. Trapper (device to catch the puck worn on the opposite hand)
ix. Skates that are unique to protect the goal and goalie

b. Forward and defense:
i. Helmet
ii. Shoulder pads
iii. Elbow pads
iv. Padded gloves
v. Cup
vi. Breezers (padded hockey pants to protect the sacrum, coccyx, and pelvis)
vii. Shin guards
viii. Skates

c. **Face masks**
i. Full face masks required at youth and high school levels in 1975
ii. Eastern Collegiate Athletic Conference mandated use in 1977
iii. National Collegiate Athletic Association required use in 1980
iv. Helmets required in NHL but face masks remain optional. This level of play accounts for most of serious eye injuries.

2. **Rules to protect the players**

a. Penalties:
i. 2-minute (minor), 5-minute (major), 10-minute (major), or a combination of these
ii. Offending player must sit in a designated penalty box and his or her team must play with one less player on the ice ("shorthanded"). If two penalties are assessed against a team, the team must play two players short. A team never has to play more than two players short.
iii. For 10-minute penalties, the offending team does not have to play shorthanded. They lose the services of that player for that time interval.
iv. Single or multiple game disqualifications may be assessed depending on the severity of the infraction.

b. Goaltender protection:
   i. No unnecessary body contact with the goalie
   ii. "Crease"—a goalie-protected area in front of the goal where opposing players cannot enter without puck
c. Common penalties enforced for protection of players:
   i. **Cross-checking**—using the shaft of the stick with both hands to check an opponent
   ii. **Hooking**—using the blade of the stick on the opponent's body to block or impede the progress of the opponent
   iii. **Slashing**—striking or attempting to strike an opponent by swinging the stick
   iv. **Spearing**—poking or attempting to poke an opponent with the blade of the stick
   v. **Interference**—impeding the progress of an opponent not in control of the puck
   vi. **Charging**—using more than two skating strides to check an opponent
   vii. **Checking from behind**
d. Officiating: Two or three officials enforce rules, assess penalties, award goals

IV. Physiology of Ice Hockey

A. **Skating stride**
   1. **Three phases**
      a. Glide during single support
      b. Propulsion during single support
      c. Propulsion during double support
   2. **Propulsion**
      a. When extending knee joint in skating thrust, quadriceps develop largest contractile force
      b. Hamstrings and gastrocnemius stabilize knee during weight shift and push-off
   3. **Stride rate is related to skating velocity.** Stride length is unrelated except in young hockey players.
   4. Faster skaters show better timing in push-off mechanics with resultant push-off in direction perpendicular to skating direction. Elite skaters sustain gliding phase longer.
   5. In players ages 8–15, increases in velocity are accompanied by increases in stride length and no significant change in stride rate.
   6. To accelerate quickly, players should attempt full extension of hip, knee, and ankle.
   7. With fatigue, decrease in skating velocity is caused by decreased stride rate (slower leg extension and longer glide phase) and excessive forward lean.
   8. Typical game skating behavior is a complex activity involving repeated accelerations, decelerations, turning, and stopping. Complicating the skating behavior are the upper body activities of stick handling, shooting, passing, and checking.

B. **Physical characteristics of hockey players**
   1. **Professional players** are taller and heavier on average than college and junior players.
   2. **Defensemen** are taller and heavier than forwards.
   3. **Body composition (% fat)**
      a. Junior—8.6% to 13.6%
      b. College—8.6% to 10.7%
      c. Professional—9.7% to 14.2%
      d. Forwards and defensemen have equal body composition
      e. Goalies, on average, have higher body composition than forwards and defensemen

C. **Energy expenditure.** Most study of physiology has been performed on adult, elite hockey players, which underscores the uncertainty of applying this science to youth hockey.

1. **Game**
   a. Shifts:
      i. One shift averages 45–90 seconds with an average of two to three play stoppages per shift lasting an average of 27 seconds.
      ii. Average playing time per shift is 40 seconds with a recovery of 225 seconds between shifts.
      iii. One shift plus recovery averages work capacity of 32 mL/kg/min (66% of $\dot{V}O_2max$).
      iv. The average player plays 14 to 21 shifts each game with average playing time of 21–28 minutes per game (based on usual practice of alternating three "lines").
   b. Energy requirement estimated two thirds anaerobic metabolism and one third aerobic metabolism
   c. On-ice heart rate averages 152 beats/min
   d. On-ice energy requirements of college players estimated at 70–80% $\dot{V}O_2max$ and youth hockey players estimated in excess of 80% $\dot{V}O_2max$.
2. **Time-motion analysis**
   a. Adult players at the elite level average 6400–7200 m per game (3.9–4.4 miles per game).
   b. Forwards demonstrate more anaerobic activity than other positions. Aerobic system used primarily for recovery.
   c. Defensemen have longer playing time (+33%), more shifts (+17%), and longer playing time per shift (+21%)— but less recovery time between shifts (–35%). Defensemen average about 62% of skating velocity of forwards.
   d. Goalie's quick, explosive movements of short duration with rest periods of submaximal activity use primarily ATP-PC energy system.
   e. Although few, physiologic studies of youth hockey (older age groups) had similar findings.
   f. Adult recreational hockey players tend to stay on ice much longer per shift.
   g. Time-motion analyses are based on the use of alternating three lines:
      i. In adult recreational leagues, only two lines may be used.
      ii. At the collegiate and professional levels, four lines may be used.
   h. Heart rate telemetry estimates on-ice intensity averaging 70–80% $\dot{V}O_2max$ during a 60-minute stop-time game:
      i. For 30 minutes of each game, players' $\dot{V}O_2max$ exceeds 90%.
      ii. Adult recreational players average heart rate intensity in excess of 70%.
3. **Muscle glycogen stores (energy source)**
   a. Glycogen stores decline an average of 60% for forwards and defensemen after one game.
   b. All muscle fibers (types I, IIa, and IIb) contribute glycogen; type I depletes (contributes) most
   c. Two-fold increase in plasma free fatty acids suggests a small glycogen-sparing effect in muscle
   d. Consecutive-day games usually do not allow complete repletion of glycogen stores (based on diet as desired).
4. **Lactate accumulation**
   a. Because anaerobic glycolysis is the major energy contributor, lactate accumulates over the course of a game:
      i. 8- to10-fold increase in lactate during games
      ii. Because about 10 minutes are required to remove lactate from the exercising muscle, there is inadequate time between shifts for full recovery. Result is mild metabolic acidosis.

   b. Lactate values usually higher in first and second periods. Forwards and defensemen have similar levels.
   c. Levels actually lower than predicted because each shift is interrupted by an average of two to three play stoppages, averaging 27 seconds. This usually allows about 60–65% of phosphocreatine to be resynthesized before the next shift.
5. **Muscle fiber type**
   a. Wide range of fiber composition
   b. No difference from general population
   c. No position-to-position variation
6. **Anaerobic power and endurance**
   a. When tested, forwards, defensemen, and goalies have similar results in peak power and endurance.
   b. Similar results occurred when younger, less experienced players were tested.
7. **Aerobic endurance**
   a. Although hockey is largely anaerobic, improving aerobic capacity reduces fatigue and may enhance performance. Involvement of the anaerobic system may depend on the efficiency of the aerobic system.
   b. $\dot{V}O_2max$ ranges from 52–62 mL/kg/min. When youth hockey players are tested, their maximum aerobic capacities are similar to those of adult players when adjusted for size and weight.
   c. NHL players have shown consistent increase in aerobic capacities over the past 15 years presumably because of more effective off-season and in-season conditioning strategies.
8. **Muscle strength and endurance**
   a. Professional players were stronger than amateurs on each of six tests used for comparison.
   b. Comparing defensemen and forwards at similar levels, data relative to body weight showed them to be equal.
   c. In comparison to other sports, hockey players obtained high levels for total and relative leg force. Only elite canoeists and athletes from power events scored higher (Finnish study).
9. **Flexibility**
   a. Forwards and defensemen have similar flexibility.
   b. Goalies have significantly better flexibility, a key element for that position.
   c. Generally, the flexibility of hockey players exceeds that of other elite athletes in wrist, hip, knee, and ankle flexibility.
   d. Other elite athletes exceed hockey players in flexibility on neck rotation, all shoulder and elbow actions, trunk extension-flexion, and lateral flexion.
10. **Fatigue**
   a. A sport at risk for fatigue:
      i. Activities of ice skating require use of all major muscle groups.
      ii. Hockey has heavy metabolic demands for energy *and* removal of waste products of that energy metabolism.
   b. Studies of fatigue in hockey show a failure of return of maximal muscle contractions to preexercise levels at 24 hours. Loss of ability to generate maximal force affects the athlete's ability to perform peak-force activities to accelerate, stop, and turn.
11. **Detraining:** On-ice practice and game play may not provide sufficient stimulus to maintain or improve fitness among hockey players. Studies suggest additional aerobic activities may be necessary during the competitive season.
12. **Practical application of training studies**
   a. Programs that have **failed** to improve skating speed:

i. Leg squats using weights
ii. Pushing a partner as a technique of resistance skating
iii. Speed skating with instruction
iv. Skating with ankle weights

b. 6-week preseason training program consisting of continuous running, stair running, flexibility, and strength training resulted in 11% increases in $\dot{V}O_2max$. During the subsequent season, the gains in oxygen consumption were lost in the absence of any specific in-season aerobic training program.

c. Hockey training stimulates cardiovascular conditioning improvement similar to that of continuous training programs in untrained players. In fit, elite players, there were no improvements in cardiovascular fitness over the course of the season.

d. Hockey practice observations show 20 minutes of actual skating during a 60-minute practice. Heart rate monitoring did, however, provide sufficient stimulus to provide aerobic training effects.

e. Anaerobic endurance did improve over the course of a season by about 16%, but not associated with increases in glycolytic enzymes

f. Muscular fatigue over a 6-day routine of practices and games showed decrements in maximal voluntary muscle contractions implying fatigue. Levels decreased through the first 3 days, then reached a plateau at a level lower than baseline. Following a hockey practice, muscle output remains diminished over a practice-game cycle.

13. **Nutrition of hockey players**
    a. Dietary composition:
        i. Protein 14–20.5%
        ii. Carbohydrate 38–44%
        iii. Fat 34–43%
    b. Average daily intake is 2800–4900 calories/day.

14. **Environmental factors**
    a. Ice arenas usually have lower ambient temperatures than other athletic settings, which minimizes risk of heat-related injury.
    b. Hockey protective equipment reduces ability to dissipate heat.
    c. Despite hydration between periods and shifts, hockey players lose 2–3 kg body weight through sweat each game.

15. **Physiologic studies and their implications for shift length**
    a. Shorter shifts result in higher contribution of phosphocreatine and oxidative phosphorylation to ATP (energy source) turnover reducing the contribution of anaerobic glycolysis, which reduces the consumption of muscle glycogen.
    b. Shorter shifts result in less lactate accumulation in exercising muscles. Lactate accumulation causes muscles to be inefficient and fatigue more readily. If lactate levels are lower, lactate clears more quickly, and muscles recover more quickly.

V. Injuries in Ice Hockey (little data on girls' and women's injuries)

A. Epidemiology

1. **Incidence and rate**
    a. NHL—800 injuries per 1000 league games
    b. Injuries caused NHL players to miss 11% of all games.
    c. One injury every 7 hours of play for elite hockey players
    d. **Age group differences:**
        i. Age 11 to 14—1 injury/100 hours playing time
        ii. Age 15 to 18—1 injury/16 hours playing time
        iii. Age 19 to 21—1 injury/11 hours playing time
        iv. Professional—1 injury/7 hours playing time

TABLE 2. Practice Versus Game (Injuries/1000 Players): College Injury Comparison

Sport	Practice	Game	Total
Men's basketball	5.1	9.5	6.0
Men's gymnastics	4.7	14.8	8.9
Wrestling	6.8	28.1	8.9
Hockey	2.1	15.1	5.0

e. Average injury risk of *all* sports is 1.37%. Hockey has an average incidence of 2.71% compared to an average risk of 3.95% in soccer.
f. One study at the elite level showed 5% of all injuries were related to fighting.
g. **Catastrophic injury rate:**
   i. 2.55/100,000 compared to football rate of 0.68/100,000
   ii. Rules infractions related to 17% of all catastrophic injuries
h. **Injuries per player per year:**
   i. Youth hockey—0.02
   ii. Professional—3.0

2. **Descriptive injury data**
   a. 24–45% of all injuries occur during practice (Table 2)
   b. **55–76% of all injuries occur during games:**
      i. First period 27–31%
      ii. Second period 30–38%
      iii. Third period 28–36%
   c. **Acute versus overuse:**
      i. Acute, traumatic—80%
      ii. Overuse—20%
   d. **Location on the ice:**
      i. 40% in defensive zone
      ii. 35% in offensive zone
      iii. 25% in neutral zone
   e. **Injury by position:**
      i. Defensemen—107.8/1000 game hours:
         (a) 55% minor
         (b) 30% moderate
         (c) 15% severe
      ii. Forwards—71.8/1000 game hours:
         (a) 73% minor
         (b) 21% moderate
         (c) 6% severe
      iii. Goalies—39.2/1000 game hours:
         (a) 83% minor
         (b) 17% moderate
         (c) 0% severe
3. **Injury potential**
   a. **Collisions** with players, boards, goalposts
   b. **Skating velocity** (examples):
      i. Senior amateur players—30 mph (48 km/hour)
      ii. Peewee (ages 12 to 13)—20 mph (32 km/hour)
   c. **Sliding velocity** (after a fall) 15 mph (24 km/hour)
   d. **Hockey puck** (6 oz [170 g] hard rubber) shooting velocity:

TABLE 3. Mechanism of Injury

Mechanism	Biener et al. 1973 (%)	Lorentzon 1988 (%)
Stick	25	11.8
Puck	17	14.5
Collision*	17	57.9
Skate	5	2.6
Miscellaneous	36	13.2

* 33% injuries in adult hockey with 14% of collisions unintentional.
Note: Both studies examined elite level athletes.

i. Professional—120 mph (192 km/hour)
ii. Senior recreational—90 mph (144 km/hour)
iii. Peewee (ages 12 to 13)—50 mph (80 km/hour)
iv. Maximal impact force of puck at its terminal velocity—1250 lb (567.5 kg)
v. Hockey masks deform at puck speeds of 50 mph (80 km/hour).

e. **Hockey stick** velocity is measured at 100–200 km/hour during shooting.
f. **Hockey skates** often cause lacerations from sharp, steel blades
g. Nonimpact forces:
   i. Vertical reaction force during skating stride 1.5 to 2.5 times body weight compared with 3 to 4 times body weight in runners
   ii. Posterior push force during skating measured at 150 lb

4. **Mechanism of injury** (Tables 3 through 5)
5. **Anatomic sites** (Table 6)
   a. In Finland, youth hockey injuries occurred with incidence similar to youth soccer and alpine skiing.
   b. Under age 12, injury was infrequent. Beyond age 12, injuries increased evenly over the older age groups.
6. **Type** (Table 7)

TABLE 4. Mechanism of Injury (College)

Mechanism	%
Legal check	44.6
Accidental collision	28.8
Illegal stick check	12.2
Fighting	6.5
Illegal check	5.8
Noncontact	2.2

TABLE 5. Mechanism of Injury (Youth, Small Studies)

Mechanism	%
Collision*	50–86
Puck	14.3
Overuse	14.3
Stick	7.0
Skate	7.0

* 10% unintentional collisions. In one study, illegal checks and violations caused 66% of the injuries, but penalties were assessed only 14% of the time.

TABLE 6. Anatomic Sites

Site	%
Professional*	
Head, scalp, face	28.1–52.9
Eye	2.6
Shoulder	5.6–21.9
Hand	2.1–10.5
Thigh (groin)	15.3–35.7
Knee	11.6–17.0
Miscellaneous (back, foot/ankle, ribs)	3.8–23.3
College	
Knee	18.6
Face, eye, mouth, teeth	17.6
Shoulder, clavicle	14.9
Head, neck	10.6
Thigh, hamstring	9.0
Forearm, wrist, hand	6.9
Hip, groin, abdomen	6.4
Chest, back	4.8
Arm, elbow	3.7
Ankle	3.2
Youth†‡	
Head and neck	10–23
Upper body	23
Shoulder/arm	19–55
Trunk	13–17
Leg	17–19

* Range, four studies.
† Range, two studies
‡ At the Bantam level (ages 13 to 14), weight differences of 53 kg and height differences of 55 cm have been reported. Smaller players are more likely to be injured.

7. **Severity**
   a. **Minor (< 7 days' absence):** 61–73% (46% of all minor injuries caused by body checks)
   b. **Moderate (8–30 days' absence):** 19–22%
   c. **Severe (> 30 days' absence):** 8% (75% of all severe injuries caused by body checks)
8. Incidence and severity of injuries is increasing. Possible explanations:
   a. Increased participation
   b. Increase in speed of game and size of players playing it
   c. Longer seasons and more out-of-season participation at all levels
   d. Lack of proper training
   e. Inconsistency in rule enforcement

B. **Acute, traumatic injuries (80% of all injuries)**
   1. **Head**
      a. Full spectrum of injury due to closed head trauma including death
      b. **Concussions account for 8–14% of all hockey injuries.**
      c. Frequency of closed head trauma has decreased because of mandatory use of helmets.

TABLE 7. Types of Injury

Type	%
Adult (Elite)*	
Contusion	25–47
Laceration	28–50
Fracture†	4–15
Dislocation	1–8
Muscle, ligament	3–12
Other	3–5
College	
Sprains, dislocations	22
Contusions	20
Lacerations	13
Strains	11
Fractures	10
Concussions	8
General Trauma	6

* Range of three studies.
† Fractures are 12 times more common in leagues with checking.

d. Increased angular velocity of head and neck with helmet and face mask does not appear to increase head or neck injury risk.
e. See Chapter 39, "Head Injuries" for information on diagnosis and treatment.

2. **Neck (0.4–9.2% of all hockey injuries)**
   a. If player has loss of consciousness, assume cervical spine injury.
   b. **Since hockey helmets have been widely used, incidence of cervical spine trauma has increased. Attributed to more aggressive play associated with better and more complete protective gear.**
   c. **Increased incidence of severe cervical spine injury since early 1980s.**
      i. Before 1973, no spinal cord injuries caused by hockey were reported.
      ii. First published report in Canadian literature occurred in 1984.
      iii. **1981–1985, 15 major cervical spine injuries reported each year attributable to hockey. This annual frequency continues to the present day.**
   d. **Mechanism of serious injury:**
      i. **Axial load of cervical spine with head in neutral alignment**
      ii. **In most situations, player is pushed or checked from behind and slides head first into boards**
   e. **Cervical spine injury data**
      i. 96% men, 4% women
      ii. Of 117 cases, 5 died:
         (a) 48% had injuries to C4-5, C5, C5-6 with the spinal cord affected slightly over half the time.
         (b) 29 of 117 are permanently quadriplegic.
      iii. Causes:
         (a) Impact with boards—65.0%
         (b) Impact with player—10.3%
         (c) Impact with ice—7.6%
         (d) Impact with goalpost—0.9%
   f. Factors affecting high incidence of spinal cord injuries:
      i. Player taller and heavier, skating faster

ii. Increased aggressive behavior at all levels (imitating style of professionals)
iii. Rules not enforced consistently
iv. Insufficient emphasis on conditioning
v. Equipment problems (lack of shock absorption boards)

g. See Chapter 40, "Neck Injuries" for information on diagnosis and treatment.

3. **Eye and face**
   a. Significant injury reduction since mandatory face mask rule:
      i. Unilateral injuries reduced from 478 to 42 in one season; blindness reduced from 37 to 12 in one season.
      ii. Hockey still accounts for 37% of eye injuries and 56% of blindness in sports.
      iii. **Face masks have been estimated to save in excess of $10 million per year in injury costs.**
   b. Injury types (before face mask rule):
      i. Periorbital soft tissue trauma—43%
      ii. Hyphema—19%
      iii. Iris damage—13%
   c. Stick responsible for more eye injuries than puck
4. **Throat**
   a. Goalies particularly at risk for throat injuries (blunt trauma to larynx) from high-speed pucks
   b. Padded collars and other deflectors worn by both skaters and goalies to reduce injury risk
5. **Shoulder**
   a. **Acromioclavicular injuries:**
      i. Mechanism—direct blows to shoulder and falls on outstretched hand
      ii. Acromioclavicular separation common
      iii. In Norfray (1977, N = 77 hockey players) 45% had asymptomatic x-ray abnormalities, including osteolysis of acromioclavicular joint and callus from united and nonunited distal clavicle fractures.
      iv. In Lorentzon and colleagues, only one of four with acromioclavicular separations missed more than 1 week of practice or games.
   b. **Glenohumeral dislocation:**
      i. 8% incidence
      ii. Greater morbidity than acromioclavicular separations
      iii. High rate of recurrence
6. **Elbow, wrist, and hand**
   a. 20% of moderate-to-severe injuries due to wrist and hand problems
   b. **"Skier's thumb," "gamekeeper's thumb":**
      i. Associated with fall on outstretched hand while hockey stick is still in possession
      ii. Treatment same as that outlined for other sports
      iii. It is possible to fashion a splint of thermoplastic, plaster, or fiberglass to fit in the hockey glove. This may be prohibited by the rules or by the game officials.
      iv. Conservative versus surgical therapy recommendations are changing for early versus late repair of a grade III ulnar collateral ligament sprain. Check with your consultant.
   c. Scaphoid fractures—uncommon
   d. **Metacarpal fractures**—usually related to stick trauma ("slashing")
   e. **Lacerations** of forearm, wrist, and hand may occur after a fall if another player skates over the fallen athlete. Skate blades can cut through the thinner leather over the palm of the gloved hand. Frequently, wear and tear of the leather of the palm renders this paper-thin and affords little protection.

f. During fights and melees, the gloves are often dropped allowing other traumatic hand injuries plus the risk of human bites. Usual human bite precautions are necessary.

7. **Back (4.3–7.0%)**
   a. Infrequent site of injury
   b. Spondylolysis can occur acutely.
   c. Most back pain is probably of muscular origin and may be treated conservatively.
   d. Severe spinal injuries:
      i. T_{1-11} 9.2%
      ii. T_{11-12}/L_{1-2} 6.0%
      iii. L_2–S_5 5.1%
8. **Abdomen or groin**
   a. Common site of lower extremity injury because of forceful hip adductor contraction during the skating stride
   b. 10% of injuries in some studies
   c. Inguinal hernias, osteitis pubis, and pelvic or hip stress fractures have all been reported in hockey players.
   d. Rectus abdominis muscle injuries can also be debilitating and chronic in hockey players. When conservative treatment fails, surgical reinforcement has been necessary to permit the athletes to return to skating.
9. **Thigh contusions**
   a. Hockey players are at high risk because of the high incidence of collisions with players, goals, and boards.
   b. Generally the players are protected, but the protective padding may slide to one side.
   c. Treatment of quadriceps contusions is no different than for other collision sports.
10. **Knee (most common lower extremity injury)**
    a. **Medial collateral ligament sprain:**
       i. Most common serious knee injury in most series
       ii. Usually the result of varus or valgus and rotational stresses
    b. Anterior cruciate ligament sprains, less frequent than medial collateral ligament sprains
    c. Meniscal injuries usually occur in combination with ligamentous injuries.
    d. Hockey poses less injury risk to knee than soccer
11. **Ankle**
    a. Sprains are less common than in other sports because of the protection offered by the skate boot.
    b. Lacerations just above the boot do occur in hockey and often involve tendons. Insure that players tuck the tongue of the skate boot under the shin guards to minimize exposure of the anterior ankle to laceration.
12. **Foot**
    a. Fractures of bones in the foot occur as a result of a direct blow, usually from the puck.
    b. Other foot injuries are uncommon.

C. **Overuse injuries**
   1. Little data, other than incidence, about types of overuse injuries
   2. **Adductor tendinitis and patellar tendinitis are the most common overuse injuries, specifically related to the skating stride.**

D. **Special medical situations**
   1. **Commotio cordis**
      a. Manifestation of concussive injury to the heart resulting in ventricular dysrhythmia and cardiac asystole

   b. Despite protective equipment, rare case reports highlight the slight risk of such cardiac injury in hockey.
   c. Epidemiologic studies of this injury suggest pediatric and adolescent age groups may be predisposed.

2. **Indoor air quality problems ("ice-hockey lung")**
   a. Propane- or gasoline-propelled ice resurfacing machines (known as "Zamboni's") have been implicated in causing illness when their engines malfunction or ventilation within the arena is inadequate.
   b. Players are at increased risk to minimal exposures compared to spectators:
      i. Nitrogen dioxide gas is heavier than air and is found at higher concentrations at ice surface.
      ii. Thermic inversion occurs because of ice temperature.
      iii. Plexiglass shields along boards alter air circulation at playing level.
      iv. During games and practice, players have minute ventilation up to 30 times higher than at rest.
   c. **Nitrogen dioxide-induced respiratory illness:**
      i. Nitrogen dioxide is by-product of combustion
      ii. Recommended limits < 0.5 ppm (parts per million)
      iii. Common symptoms (acute onset following unknown indoor exposure after hockey practice or game):
         (a) Cough
         (b) Hemoptysis
         (c) Dyspnea
         (d) Chest pain
         (e) Headache
         (f) Weakness
         (g) Rarely, pulmonary edema
      iv. Treatment:
         (a) Withdrawal from toxic environment
         (b) Bronchodilators
         (c) Corticosteroids
         (d) Untreated, most symptoms resolve within 2 weeks
      v. Late complications of bronchiolitis obliterans may develop 2–6 weeks after initial symptoms.
   d. **Carbon monoxide poisoning:**
      i. Source—improper combustion of fuel of Zamboni; inadequate ventilation system for arena
      ii. Recommended limit— < 30 ppm (< 25 ppm in Canada; some researchers have suggested < 20 ppm)
      iii. Symptoms
         (a) Acute respiratory:
            • Hemoptysis
            • Dyspnea
            • Chest pain
            • Coughing spells
         (b) Central nervous system:
            • Headache
            • Dizziness
            • Sleepiness
            • Nausea and vomiting
      iv. Treatment—withdrawal from source of toxin; rarely requires emergency treatment

e. Safeguards:
   i. Thirteen states have tested indoor air quality of ice arenas.
   ii. Only three states have mandatory air quality testing in ice arenas.
   iii. Adequate ventilation of indoor arenas should be ensured.
   iv. Regular inspection and maintenance of ice resurfacing machines should be implemented.
   v. Regular monitoring of indoor air quality should occur.

E. **Injury prevention**
1. **Continue to update protective equipment.**
2. **Ensure use of mouth guards.**
3. **Fabric designs with a high coefficient of friction are being evaluated to reduce sliding speeds of fallen players.**
4. **Enforce the rules. One study suggested that 39% of all injuries were attributed to foul play.**
5. **Effective training and conditioning may minimize injury risk. Adequate nutrition, training, and hydration may reduce third-period fatigue and reduce fatigue in situations when several games are played on consecutive days as in tournaments.**

Recommended Reading

1. Agre JC, Casal DC, Leon AS, et al: Professional ice hockey players: Physiologic, anthropometric, and musculoskeletal characteristics. Arch Phys Med Rehab 69:188–192, 1988.
1a. Biener K, Muller P: Les accidents du hockey sur glace. Can Med 14(11):959–962, 1973.
2. Bjorkenheim JM, Syvahuoko I, Rosenberg PH: Injuries in competitive junior ice-hockey. Acta Orthop Scand 64(4):459–461, 1993.
3. Brust JD, Leonard BJ, Pheley A, Roberts WO: Children's ice hockey injuries. Am J Dis Child 146:741–747, 1992.
3a. Center for Disease Control: Nitrogen dioxide and carbon monoxide intoxication in an indoor ice arena—Wisconsin, 1992. MMWR 41 (21):383–385, 1992.
4. Cox MH, Miles DS, Verde TJ, Rhodes EC: Applied physiology of ice hockey. Sports Med 19(3):184–201, 1995.
5. Daly PJ, Sim FH, Simonet WT: Ice hockey injuries: A review. Sports Med 10(3):122–131, 1990.
6. Daub WB, Green HJ, Houston ME, et al: Specificity of physiologic adaptations resulting from ice-hockey training. Med Sci Sports Exerc 15(4):290–294, 1983.
7. Gerberich SG, Burns SR: Neurologic injuries in ice hockey. In Jordan BD, Tsairis P, Warren RF (eds): Sports Neurology. Rockville, MD, Aspen Publishers, 1989, pp 245–255.
8. Green HJ: Bioenergetics of ice hockey: Considerations for fatigue. J Sports Sci 5:305–317, 1987.
9. Greer N, Serfass RC, Picconatto W: The effects of a hockey-specific training program on performance of bantam players. Can J Sport Sci 17(1):65–69, 1992.
10. Hedberg K, et al: An outbreak of nitrogen dioxide-induced respiratory illness among ice hockey players. JAMA 262(21):3014–3017, 1989.
11. Kaplan JA, Karofsky PS, Volturo GA: Comotio cordis in two amateur ice hockey players despite the use of commercial chest protectors: Case reports. J Trauma 34(1):151–153, 1993.
12. Levesque B, Dewailly E, Lavoie R, et al: Carbon monoxide in indoor ice skating rinks: Evaluation of absorption by adult hockey players. Am J Public Health 80(5):594–598, 1990.
13. Lorentzon R, Wedren H, Pietila T: Incidence, nature, and causes of ice hockey injuries: A three-year prospective study of a Swedish elite ice hockey team. Am J Sports Med 16(4):392–396, 1988.
14. Lorentzon R, Wedren H, Pietila T, Gustavsson B: Injuries in international ice hockey: A prospective, comparative study of injury incidence and injury types in international and Swedish elite ice hockey. Am J Sports Med 16(4):389–390, 1988.
15. Montgomery DL: Physiology of ice hockey. Sports Med 5: 99–126, 1988.
16. Norfray JF, Tremaine MJ, Groves HC, et al: The clavicle in hockey. Am J Sports Med 5:275–289, 1977.
17. Pelletier RL, Montelpare WJ, Stark RM: Intercollegiate ice hockey injuries: A case for uniform definitions and reports. Am J Sports Med 21(1):78–81, 1993.
18. Pettersson M, Lorentzon R: Ice hockey injuries: A 4-year prospective study of a Swedish elite ice hockey team. Br J Sports Med 27(4):251–254, 1993.
19. Pforringer W, Smasal V: Aspects of traumatology in ice hockey. J Sports Sci 5:327–336, 1987.

20. Reid DC, Saboe L: Spine fractures in winter sports. Sports Med 7:393–399, 1989.
21. Reynen PD, Clancy WG: Cervical spine injury, hockey helmets, and face masks. Am J Sports Med 22(2): 167–170, 1994.
22. Sim FH, Simonet WT, Melton LJ, Lehn TA: Ice hockey injuries. Am J Sports Med 15(1):30–40, 1987.
23. Smith MD: Violence and injuries in ice hockey. Clin J Sports Med 1:104–109, 1991.
24. Stuart MJ, Smith AM, Nieva JJ, Rock MG: Injuries in youth ice hockey: A pilot surveillance strategy. Mayo Clin Proc 70:350–356, 1995.
25. Tator CH: Neck injuries in ice hockey: A recent unsolved problem with many contributing factors. Clin Sports Med 6(1):101–114, 1987.
26. Tator CH, Edmonds VE, Lapczak L, Tator IB: Spinal injuries in ice hockey players, 1966–1987. Can J Sports 34(1):63–69, 1991.
27. Twist P, Rhodes T: A physiological analysis of ice hockey positions. Natl Strength Conditioning Assoc J 15(6):44–46, 1993.

69

Martial Art Injuries

Leonard A. Wilkerson, D.O., FAAFP

I. Martial Arts

A. The term "martial arts" means those arts concerned with the waging of war, but in the 20th century they no longer have a military role. It is said that the study of the martial arts develops character or higher moral standards. As a result of this change, the term came to mean "the way."

B. An estimated 1.5–2 million Americans participate in the martial arts.
   1. Estimated ratio 5:1 male to female
   2. 20% are children

C. A wide cross-section of Americans participate in this activity, but little is known of the physical forces involved and little thought is given to potential morbidity and mortality.
   1. Information generated from a nationwide computer surveillance of emergency departments and from surveys mailed to martial arts instructors showed that no deaths and no serious weapon injuries were reported.
   2. From this information, the assertion is made that all forms of the martial arts are safe.
   3. Based on a review of some martial arts injuries, this assertion may not necessarily be true.

II. Common Martial Arts Practiced in the United States

A. **Karate:** means "the way of the empty hand."

B. **Tae kwon do:** means "foot, hand, way"
   1. An exhibition sport in the Olympics since 1988
   2. Scheduled to become an official sport in the year 2000

C. **Other martial arts**
   1. **Aikido:** means "the way of harmony"
   2. **Jujitsu:** means "compliance techniques"
   3. **Judo:** means "compliant way"
   4. **Kung fu:** These are nonsense words. Kung fu is a form of Chinese boxing.
   5. **Hapkido:** Korean martial art similar to aikido (Japanese) that includes kicks and hand strikes.

III. Popularity of the Martial Arts

A. Increased desire to know self-defense

B. Improved cardiovascular fitness and flexibility

C. Improved self-esteem and self-confidence

D. Need of a structured exercise program; also offers artistic expression

E. Need to compete. In older athletes beyond high school and college years, competitive spirit is still present.

IV. Understanding Injury Trends

A. **Tae kwon do tournament format**
   1. 2-minute rounds—fighter may fight new opponent in a single or double elimination
   2. 3-minute rounds in a single elimination

B. **Karate tournament format**
   1. Either single or double elimination
   2. Can be three 3-minute rounds

C. **Tournament rules**
   1. In both tae kwon do and karate:
      a. Kicks to head allowed
      b. Kicks to trunk allowed but not to back
   2. Punches to head prohibited in tae kwon do. In some karate tournaments, controlled contact to head with hands is allowed.
   3. In karate tournaments, leg sweeps allowed. No kicking below waist allowed in tae kwon do.

D. **Protective equipment**
   1. In tae kwon do
      a. Chest protectors
      b. Foot pads
      c. Shin and forearm pads
      d. Groin guard
      e. Head protector
   2. Optional in tae kwon do
      a. Mouth guard—physicians should push for this to be mandatory
      b. Hand covers
   3. In karate
      a. Shin and forearm pads
      b. No chest protector
      c. Hand covers optional; in some tournaments prohibited
   4. Protective gear decreases morbidity.
      a. Protective gear is available for:
         i. Forearms
         ii. Hands
         iii. Chest
         iv. Shin
         v. Feet
         vi. Mouth
         vii. Groin
         viii. Head
      b. Injury rate per 100,000 participants in various sports noted in Table 1

E. **Injury incidence—higher in tournament situation**
   1. McLatchie reported that some form of injury occurs every four contests.
   2. Incapacitating injury severe enough to cause withdrawal from competition occurs every 10 contests.
   3. Birrer and Birrer surveyed 6341 athletes.
      a. 50% of injuries sustained in tournaments
      b. 41% in nontournament settings

TABLE 1. Injury Rate per 100,000 Participants of Various Sports

Basketball	188.0	Wrestling	26.0
Football	167.0	Sledding	24.6
Aquatic activities	46.0	Dancing	18.8
Lacrosse	39.5	Martial arts	16.9

From Birrer RB, Halbrook SP: Martial arts injuries. Am J Sports Med 16:408–410, 1988, with permission.

4. Inverse relationship of injury rate and experience confirmed by Stricevic and associates
5. Stricevic reported:
   a. Punches have a higher injury ratio than kicks in karate tournaments.
   b. Protective gear for hands, head, chest, and limbs decreases morbidity.

V. Classification of Injuries

A. **Three groups**
   1. Injuries to the head and face
   2. Injuries to the trunk
   3. Injuries to the limbs

B. In all studies, the **most common injuries** were:
   1. Contusions
   2. Bruises
   3. Sprains
   4. Strains

C. **Orthopedic injuries**
   1. Result from direct impact
   2. Result from repetitive action—ballistic and torsional maneuvers

D. **Serious injuries**
   1. Concussions
   2. Paralysis
   3. Visceral rupture

E. Table 2 lists injuries at two national tae kwon do tournaments broken down by site of injury.

F. Table 3 is a summary of the injuries by anatomic site reported as percentages.

VI. Common Injuries to Head and Neck

A. **Lacerations**

B. **Epistaxis from a nose blow**

C. **Periorbital hematoma**
   1. From accidental strike in the face usually with a fist
   2. From a high kick

D. **Corneal abrasion—**scratch from a toenail or brushing by the eye with the toes

E. **Concussion**
   1. Commonly from a high kick or a spinning kick
   2. If the athlete is "knocked out":
      a. **Important to consider a possible cervical spine injury**
      b. Cervical spine injuries commonly are overlooked because associated head injuries and loss of consciousness seem to absorb all the attention.

F. **Fatality from a spinning hook kick**
   1. Oler and colleagues reported a fatality from a spinning hook kick to the face.
      a. Victim was immediately incapacitated, fell backward onto a hardwood floor, and died within 24 hours at a local hospital.
      b. Postmortem examination revealed an occipital skull fracture, bilateral acute subdural hemorrhage, contusions of frontal and temporal lobes, and hemorrhage and herniation of the brain stem.
   2. A back-spinning kick or back-hook kick cannot necessarily be thrown with control.
      a. If thrown too slowly, opponent may be able to deliver kick to back
      b. If thrown with proper speed, no control over impact
   3. Back-hook kick is a "kill" kick
      a. The back hook was designed to knock the enemy off his horse in ancient times.

TABLE 2. Injuries at Two National Tae Kwon Do Tournaments

Site of Injury	Adult	Junior
Head and neck		
Hematoma, contusion	9	17
Laceration	6	7
Mandible, temporomandibular joint strain, R/O fracture	3	10
Epistaxis, R/O fracture	4	6
Concussion without loss of consciousness	0	8
Neck strain, R/O fracture	1	6
Nasal fracture-dislocation	3	1
Loss of consciousness	3	1
Teeth avulsion	0	2
Corneal abrasion	0	1
Diplopia, R/O orbital fracture	0	1
Totals	29	60
Upper extremity		
Digit, hand strain, R/O fracture	5	8
Metacarpal fracture	2	3
Digit fracture-dislocation	2	0
Nail avulsion	0	2
Forearm contusion	0	1
Totals	9	14
Lower extremity		
Foot contusion	1	2
Digit sprain, R/O fracture	1	2
Contusion, hematoma	6	2
Knee contusion/synovitis	0	2
Knee strain	1	0
Shin hematoma	0	1
Ankle strain	1	0
Foreign body	1	0
Digit fracture	0	1
Laceration	0	1
Totals	11	11
Groin		
Contusion	2	5
Adductor strain	0	2
Totals	2	7
Torso		
Abdominal contusion	0	1
Solar plexus concussion	0	2
Costochondral separation	1	0
Low back spasm	0	1
Lumbosacral contusion, R/O fracture	0	1
Spinal cord contusion, R/O fracture	0	1
Totals	1	6
Other		
Panic reaction	0	3
Insulin reaction	0	1
Totals	0	4
Totals, all injuries	52	102
Grand total	154	

R/O = Rule out.
From Oler M, Tomson W, Pepe H, et al: Morbidity and mortality in the martial arts: A warning. J Trauma 31(2):251–253, 1991, with permission.

TABLE 3. Summary of Injuries by Anatomic Site (Reported as Percentages)

	Percentage of Adult Presentations (n = 47)	Percentage of Junior Presentations (n = 91)	Combined Presentations (n = 138)
Head and neck	49	54	52
Upper extremity	21	14	17
Lower extremity	23	13	17
Groin	4	8	6
Torso	2	7	5
Other (systemic)		4	3
Totals (rounding error)	99	100	100

From Oler M, Tomson W, Pepe H, et al: Morbidity and mortality in the martial arts: A warning. J Trauma 31(2):251–253, 1991, with permission.

On the ground, designed to inflict serious trauma to the head.

b. As a physician for many karate and tae kwon do tournaments, I have convinced some masters in some tournaments to remove this kick to the head because of potential injury.
   i. Front leg kicks to the head, such as round kicks, can be used in controlled fashion.
   ii. This markedly decreases the chance of serious injury.

G. **Head gear**

1. **Head gear prevents most soft tissue injuries to the face.**
   a. Lacerations
   b. Abrasions
   c. Injury to ear or scalp
2. **Unfortunately, head gear is not as protective to the brain as many in the martial arts believe.**
   a. Movement in the United States toward mandatory head gear
   b. Rhulen Insurance Company of New York, one of the largest insurers of the martial arts in the United States, has informed its policyholders that head gear is now required if insurance is to be in force during free-sparring.
   c. Because of this, mandatory head gear has now reached tournament circles and many schools and associations. From this movement, instructor and students are led to believe that they are "protected," and serious head injuries are prevented, but this is not the case.
3. Studies in the neurosurgical literature have compared peak acceleration of blows to the head, with and without head gear, using punches both to the front and to the side of the head.
   a. Punches were with:
      i. Bare hand
      ii. "Safety-chuck hand protectors"
      iii. 10-oz boxing gloves
   b. Kicks were delivered to the head, with and without head gear, using bare feet and "safety-kick" padding.
   c. Studies showed that **punches to the side of the head produced greater peak accelerations than kicks to the side**.
   d. **Kicks produced greater acceleration than did punches to the front of the head.**
   e. **Safety equipment failed to soften or lessen peak acceleration with or without**

head gear. Study subjects believed that safety equipment for hands or feet was protection for the wearer, rather than for the opponent.

4. Unequivocal evidence exists that **repeated brain injury of concussive or even subconcussive force results in characteristic patterns of brain damage and a steady decline in the ability to process information efficiently.**
   a. The effects of repeated blows to the head, punch or kick, are cumulative. Although some blows may be more severe than others, none are trivial, and each has the potential to be lethal.
   b. Blunt head blows cause shearing injury to nerve fibers and neurons in proportion to the degree the head is accelerated. These acceleration forces have an impact on the brain.
   c. Blows to the side of the head tend to produce greater acceleration forces than those to the face, whereas those to the chin, which acts as a lever of the head, produce maximal forces.
   d. Shearing of blood vessels may lead to bleeding within the brain and skull:
      i. Subdural hematoma
      ii. Bleeding within the brain, producing intracerebral hematoma with rapid death
   e. Head gear and protective padding to the hands and feet may lessen the force of brain acceleration, which seems to decrease the chance of a fatal bleed but increase nerve fiber shearing. Extra padding may reduce the chances of death, but it does not prevent brain damage due to tearing of brain substance.
5. **Demential pugilistica or punch-drunk syndrome is the medical term for traumatic encephalopathy.**
   a. Fight fans recognize the syndrome as:
      i. "Cuckoo"
      ii. "Goofy"
      iii. "Slug-nutty"
      iv. "Cutting paper dolls"
   b. **Traumatic encephalopathy may occur in anyone subjected to repeated blows to the head from any cause:**
      i. Football players
      ii. Rugby players
      iii. Soccer players
      iv. Wrestlers
   c. **Characteristic symptoms and signs:**
      i. Slow onset of an increasingly euphoric personality
      ii. Emotional lability
      iii. Little insight into his or her deterioration
      iv. Speech and thought becomes progressively slower
      v. Memory deterioration
      vi. Mood swings
      vii. Intense irritability and sometimes truculence leading to violent behavior (cheerfulness, however, is prevailing mood, with bouts of depression)
      viii. Tremor
      ix. Commonly, difficulty in speaking

VII. Injury to Extremities

A. Strains, sprains, fractures, dislocations, and tendon avulsions

1. Common sites:
   a. Forearm
   b. Thigh

c. Shin
d. Calf
e. Dorsum of the feet
2. In tournament situations where kicking is below the belt, **hematoma to the quadriceps** many times causes the competitor to retire from competition.

B. **Dislocation of the proximal interphalangeal joints** occurs when punches are poorly executed. Laceration of the fingers may occur from scratches if gloves are not worn.

C. Incidence of osteoarthritis in karate and tae kwon do experts
1. Studied in Britain, where karate is an established sport
2. The hands and wrists of 22 karate instructors who had practiced the sport for a minimum of 5 years were examined and x-rays obtained.
   a. There was no evidence that practice of the sport predisposed to the early onset of chronic tenosynovitis or osteoarthritis.
   b. Four activities seemed to have the greatest potential for damage:
      ii. Doing push-ups on the knuckles
      ii. Repeated punching of a firm target
      iii. Sparring
      iv. Breaking of objects
   c. Chronic synovitis of the metacarpal phalangeal joint from wood-breaking
   d. Avulsion of the extensor tendons of the distal fingers or dislocation of the proximal interphalangeal joints from hitting hard objects using "spear finger" technique

D. **Injuries about the elbow**
1. **Elbow dislocations**—mostly posterior
2. **Supracondylar and intracondylar fractures rare**
3. **Tendinitis**—medial and lateral epicondyles common

E. **Injuries about the shoulder**
1. **Dislocations** of shoulder
   a. 95% anterior
   b. 5% posterior
2. **Acromioclavicular sprain** seen if fall or roll is poorly executed

F. **Knee injuries**
1. Vulnerable in most sports
2. In martial arts, especially karate and tae kwon do, where ballistic and twisting moves are the rule, injury is usually from:
   a. Hyperextension
   b. Rotation
   c. Flexion
   d. Valgus or varus clipping
3. Other knee injuries that can occur:
   a. Meniscus tears
   b. Ligament sprains
   c. Patella tendinitis
   d. Patella subluxation or dislocation
   e. Epiphyseal fracture
   f. Osgood-Schlatter disease
4. Knee dislocation rare—true emergency
5. Hematoma can occur in any of the extremities and is the most common injury, with the quadriceps the most common site.
   a. In all studies, contestants had to stop fighting secondary to the pain.
   b. A late complication is myositis ossificans.

G. **Ankle sprains and fractures** are seen just as in any contact or collision sport.
H. **Injuries to the great toe, second toe, and fifth toe** are common. May develop osteoarthritis in later years.

VIII. Injuries of the Trunk

A. **Common** in the martial arts. Many martial artists aim at the region of the solar plexus surrounding the coeliac ganglion.
   1. This blow causes classic winding of the opponent and vulnerability to further attack.
   2. A blow to the solar plexus produces transient inspiratory difficulty with spontaneous recovery in 20–40 seconds.
B. **In tae kwon do, chest protectors are worn to disperse the penetration of the blow.**
   1. Tae kwon do practitioners kick 80% of the time, as opposed to punching.
   2. **In karate, however, chest protectors are not worn.** Karate instructors believe it decreases the student's ability to control the blow and thus decreases the discipline.
   3. Damage to the chest is usually by direct kick or punches.
      a. Costochondritis common
      b. Rib fractures common
      c. Pneumothorax seen
C. There have been **three reported cases of death from anterior chest trauma** from these types of blows.
   1. **The roundhouse kick**, also called "round kick," to the trunk usually damages the vulnerable organs.
      a. Liver
      b. Spleen
      c. Kidney
      d. Pancreas
   2. **Testicular injury** usually occurs from an uncontrolled kick.
      a. Many times causes forced retirement of the competitor
      b. Groin guards markedly decrease risk. Although there can be some pain, usually the competitor can continue to fight after a time-out.
   3. The most common trunk injuries, therefore, are to the **ribs** mainly from punches and to the **solar plexus** from kicks and punches (potential to cause pancreatitis).
   4. **Deaths from the martial arts**
      a. One from a spinning kick hitting the opponent in the face, knocking him out; upon hitting the floor, he expired.
      b. Three case studies of deaths from anterior chest trauma (see Figures 1–3 for examples of martial arts techniques involved):
      c. All three of the fatally injured had been training for a period of less than 1 year.
      d. Free-sparring training is recommended only for students who have undergone a period of adequate physical conditioning and have demonstrated competence in the basic free-sparring techniques.

Case study no. 1

A 26-year-old Caucasian male (Korean tae kwon do stylist) was practicing kumite (free-sparring) with his instructor when he received a kick to the left lower lateral aspect of the anterior chest. The patient was seen in the emergency room with fixed dilated pupils and had an isoelectric electrocardiogram, apnea, and cyanosis with bruise marks on the left anterior chest. External cardiac compression and endotracheal manual ventilation were performed. Administration of intracardiac adrenaline resulted in ventricular fibrillation, which subsequently converted to a ventricular tachycardia. In view of the prolonged dilated pupils, rescue efforts were stopped, and the patient was pronounced dead. Gross anatomic diagnosis revealed pulmonary

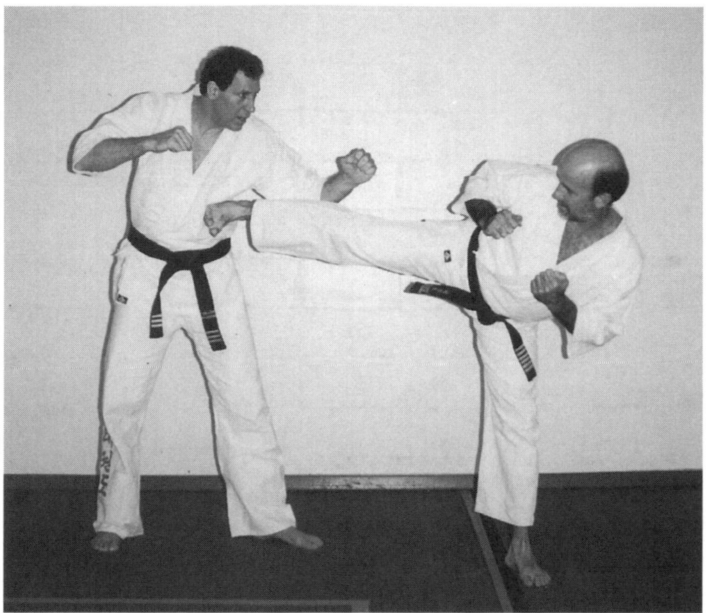

FIGURE 1. A kick to the left lower lateral aspect of the anterior chest (see case study no. 1).

edema and congestion, liver ecchymosis, rib fracture (fifth left), and aspirated food within the trachea, hypopharynx, and lungs. At autopsy, the suggested cause of death was aspiration and asphyxia secondary to the blow to the chest.

Case study no. 2

An 18-year-old Caucasian male (kempo stylist) was participating in his fifth bout of a competitive free-sparring tournament when he received a blow or multiple blows to the midsection that apparently ruptured his spleen. Later that evening the patient began to vomit and was in severe pain. He was transported to a hospital, where he was admitted with an admission diagnosis of a ruptured spleen. An exploratory laparotomy and splenectomy were subsequently performed. The patient, however, expired within 1 hour postsurgery. Gross and microscopic examination of the heart, liver, and spleen showed that the epicardium was normal, and the coronary vessels showed no lesions. Moderate numbers of myelocytes, occasional collections of lymphocytes, and a few polymorphonuclear cells were present in the interstitial tissue. Considerable numbers of atypical lymphocytes with moderately large nuclei and varying amounts of cytoplasm were found in the sinusoids and portal areas. A microscopic diagnosis of infectious mononucleosis involving the heart, liver, and spleen was determined from the examination.

Case study no. 3

An 18-year-old African-American male (Korean tae kwon do stylist) was practicing kumite with an advanced student when he received light contact from a roundhouse kick to the solar plexus. External cardiac compression and mouth-to-mouth resuscitation were administered by the instructor and another student. Although ambulance attendants continued resuscitative efforts, the patient was pronounced dead on arrival at a local hospital. Autopsy examination revealed the following gross anatomic diagnoses: hemorrhage into the soft tissue around the carotid sinus and vagus nerve at the level of the bifurcation of the innominate artery, multiple areas of ecchymosis in the liver, multiple petechial hemorrhages of all lobes of the lungs, hyperinflation of both lungs, and aspiration bronchitis.

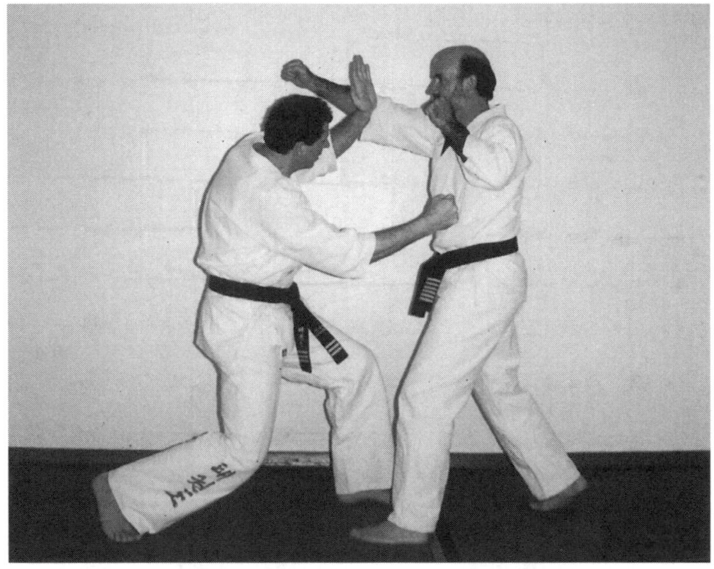

FIGURE 2. Multiple blows to the midsection (see case study no. 2).

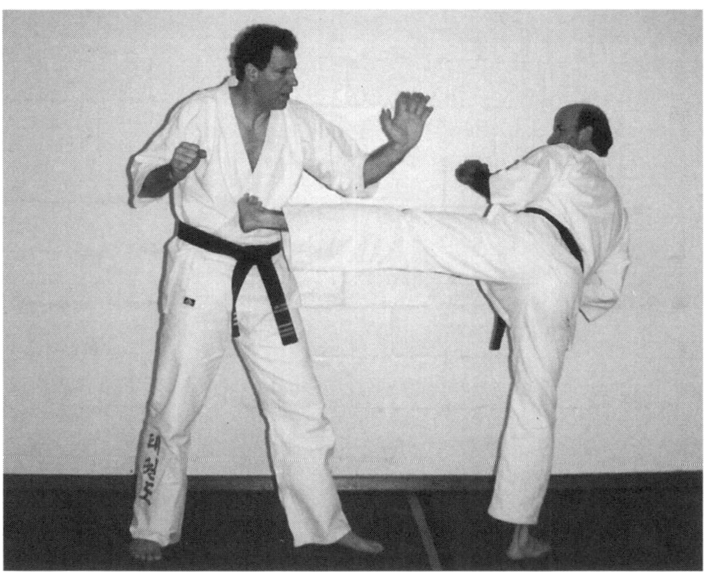

FIGURE 3. A roundhouse kick to the solar plexus (see case study no. 3).

IX. Common Medical Disorders Seen in Participants of Martial Arts

A. **Athletes with seizure disorders**

1. Studies have shown that a regular exercise program may have a beneficial effect on seizure control.
2. There are no reports of status epilepticus triggered by exercise.
3. It is a difficult decision for physicians, parents, and the martial arts instructor to give permission to the participant.

4. Reservations are based on the following concerns:
   a. Would a seizure during practice or tournament predispose the athlete to serious injury, particularly to the brain or spinal cord? Most data do not support this.
   b. Would single or cumulative head blows adversely affect seizure control or cause an immediate or early posttraumatic seizure? To date, reports suggest that this should not be a concern. However, because of inherent dangers, kicking or punching to the head should be excluded.
5. The Committee on Children with Handicaps and Sports Medicine of the American Medical Association recommends that children be allowed to participate in physical education and interscholastic activities, including contact and collision sports, provided there is:
   a. Proper medical management
   b. Good seizure control and proper supervision
   c. Avoidance of situations in which a dangerous fall could occur

B. **Asthma**
1. Asthma and exercise-induced asthma can usually be controlled with beta-agonists or cromolyn sodium (Intal) nedocromil (Tilade), or a combination of both.
2. If continued breakthrough occurs, reevaluate.
   a. Sometimes ipratropium bromide (Atrovent) helps prevent breakthrough.
   b. A sustained-release theophylline can be added.
3. A good warm-up before activity induces bronchodilation and resistance to exercise-induced asthma. This is helpful but should be in addition to beta-agonists.

X. Disorders Disqualifying an Athlete from Martial Arts

A. **Carditis**

B. **Severe uncontrolled hypertension**
1. Athletes with mild hypertension can be allowed a full range of physical activities.
2. Moderate-to-severe hypertension should be evaluated and treated accordingly by a physician.

C. **Severe congenital heart disease.** Physician assessment needed.

D. **Absence or loss of function in one eye.**
1. If the participant wants to do martial arts for self-defense, fitness, or flexibility, but not to participate in sparring with head contact, participation may be allowed.
2. Availability of eye guards approved by the American Society for Testing Materials may allow the competitor to participate.

E. **Absence of one kidney**

F. **Hepatomegaly**

G. **Splenomegaly**

H. **Poorly controlled seizure disorder**

I. **Pulmonary insufficiency.** The athlete may be allowed to compete if oxygenation remains satisfactory during a graded stress test.

J. **Atlantoaxial instability**

K. **Skin disorders**
1. Boils
2. Herpes simplex
3. Impetigo
4. Scabies
5. No contact until no longer contagious

L. **Absent or undescended testicle.** Groin guard required.

M. **Acute illness**
1. Needs individual evaluation so as not to worsen the illness
2. Careful not to put others at risk of being in contact with a contagious individual

XI. Physician's Responsibility at a Martial Arts Competition

A. **Examine the competitors before the competition if requested by officials.**
   1. Many times they will not ask you to do this.
   2. Your duty, as the physician, is to administer first aid while circulating on the floor during sparring matches. There could be a number of rings active at the same time.

B. **Inspect the fighting area to ascertain whether adequate flooring is used.**

C. **Treat minor injuries**, such as lacerations, strains, and sprains.
   1. In serious injuries, it is best to refer to a hospital emergency room.
   2. When requested, the physician advises the referees as to the fitness of a competitor to continue in a competition.

D. **Some injuries that exclude further participation are:**
   1. Fractures
   2. Concussion that results in disorientation or amnesia; any loss of consciousness
   3. Ocular injuries when sight is impaired, including periorbital injuries
      a. Hematoma
      b. Lacerations
   4. Testicular injury when recovery is not rapid; if scrotal hematoma present

Recommended Reading

1. Adams WM, Bruton CJ: The cerebral vasculature in dementia puglistica. J Neurol Neurosurg Psychiatry 52:600–604, 1989.

1a. American Academy of Family Physicians, American Academy of Pediatrics, American Medical Society of Sports Medicine, American Osteopathic Academy of Sports Medicine, American Orthopaedic Society for Sports Medicine: Preparticipation Physical Evaluation, 2nd ed. New York, McGraw-Hill, 1992.

2. Birrer RB, Birrer CD: Martial arts injuries. Phys Sportsmed 10(6):103–108, 1982.
3. Birrer RB, Birrer CD, Son DS, et al: Injuries in Tae Kwon Do. Phys Sportsmed 9(2):97–103, 1981.
4. Birrer RB, Halbrook SP: Martial arts injuries: The results of a five-year national survey. Am J Sports Med 16:408–410, 1988.
5. Crosby AC: The hands of karate experts: Clinical and radiological findings. Br J Sports Med 19:41–42, 1985.
6. Jaffe L, Minkoff J: Martial arts: A perspective on their evolution, injuries, and training formats. Orthop Rev 17:208–221, 1988.
7. Kurland HL: Injuries in karate. Phys Sportsmed 8(10):80–85, 1980.
8. Liebert PL, Buckley T: Providing medical coverage at karate tournaments. J Musculoskel Med Dec:23–28, 1992.
9. McLatchie GR: Analysis of karate injuries sustained in 295 contests. Injury 8:132–134, 1976.
10. McLatchie GR: Prevention of karate injuries—a progress report. Br J Sports Med 11: 78–82, 1977.
11. McLatchie GR: Recommendations for medical officers attending karate competitions. Br J Sports Med 13:36–37, 1979.
12. McLatchie GR: Karate and karate injuries. Br J Sports Med 15:84–86, 1981.
13. McLatchie GR, Davies JE, Caulley JH: Injuries in karate—a case for medical control. J Trauma 20(11): 956–958, 1980.
14. Mellion MD, Walsh WM, Shelton GL (eds): The Team Physician's Handbook. Philadelphia, Hanley & Belfus, 1990.
15. Oler M, Tomson W, Pepe H, et al: Morbidity and mortality in the martial arts: A warning. J Trauma 31:251–253, 1991.
16. Schmidt RJ: Fatal anterior chest trauma in karate trainers. Med Sci Sports 7:59–61, 1975.
17. Schwartz ML, Hudson AR, Fernie GR, et al: Biomechanical study of full-contact karate contrasted with boxing. J Neurosurg 64:248–252, 1986.
18. Stricevic MV, Patel MR, Okazaki T, et al: Karate: Historical perspective and injuries sustained in national and international tournament competitions. Am J Sports Med 11:320–324, 1983.

70

Dance Injuries

James G. Garrick, M.D.

I. General Considerations

A. **Ballet**

1. **Training**

   a. **The successful begin young.**

      i. **Novices in late teens prone to more problems.** Unique problems among college dance students.

      ii. Training may begin as early as age 5 (weekly).

      iii. Serious training (daily) begins early teens

      iv. Generally, professional status must be attained by late teens.

      v. Professionals may dance into their 40s and 50s. Ballet activities often continue into adulthood for the "recreational" dancer.

   b. **Training highly structured**

      i. **Practitioner MUST know what goes on in classes.**

      ii. Classes are precisely structured around a gradual warm-up (at the barre) with increasing speed and range of motion, concluding with actual "steps" and jumps carried out around and across the classroom.

      iii. Classes are taken daily, even during the performing season. Performance season days include classes, rehearsals, and performances.

   c. Year-round

      i. May perform only a few months

      ii. Classes continue virtually every day, throughout the entire year.

2. **Sex differences**

   a. The majority of dancers are female. Nevertheless, professional companies have nearly equal numbers of males and females.

   b. **Male dancers often begin later, in their teens.** Many have previous athletic experience (and injuries).

   c. Male/female differences:

      i. Female dancers dance en pointe (on their toes).

         (a) Usually begin pointe work at age 12

         (b) Going en pointe depends on training and strength, not musculoskeletal maturity.

      ii. Males dance on metatarsal heads, with metatarsophalangeal (MTP) joint dorsiflexion 90°.

      iii. Males responsible for lifting (partnering)

         (a) Lifting begins mid to late teens.

         (b) Boys frequently ill-prepared with respect to upper body strength.

3. **Psychology**

   a. **Pyramid system**

      i. Hundreds of thousands of little girls take ballet lessons.

ii. Only hundreds achieve professional status.
iii. Competition continues within professional companies.
(a) Corps de ballet
(b) Soloist
(c) Principal dancer

b. **Advancement based on subjective judgments**
i. Students must audition (compete) for entry into professional schools.
ii. Body type (dancer unable to alter)
iii. Weight
(a) Among the most weight-conscious of all athletes
(b) Anorexia nervosa and bulimia nervosa perhaps more common than in any other activity.

c. **Teenage dancers often separated from parents**
i. Live where training is appropriate
ii. Only adult input/supervision may come from teachers

d. Education usually ceases with high school; some do not complete high school.

e. Experience with medical care often bad:
i. Practitioners do not understand demands of continuous training.
ii. Treatment of injuries often superficial and expedient. Most injuries are of overuse variety, and cause must be found to prevent recurrence.

B. **Modern—from the artistic standpoint modern dance differs appreciably from ballet. From a medical standpoint the differences seem largely related to a few specific factors:**

1. Generally, modern dance is:
   a. Performed barefoot
   b. Does not emphasize external rotation of the hips
   c. Involves more movements requiring hyperextension of the knees
   d. Involves more abrupt movements
2. There are greater differences among the characteristics and demands of the various forms of modern dance than in ballet.
3. Most modern dancers (like all dancers) have some background in ballet.
4. Modern dance training usually begins later than ballet, often in late teens and 20s.
5. Modern dance companies are usually smaller than ballet companies and thus are less likely to have structured medical care systems.

C. **Jazz**

1. Among teenagers, jazz may be the most popular dance form.
2. Weight restrictions are not as demanding as in ballet.
3. Choreography does not demand external rotation of the hips as in ballet but generally requires better than average hip motion (splits and high kicks).

II. Medical Problems

A. **Menstrual abnormalities**

1. Both primary and secondary amenorrhea are common.
2. Delayed onset of menses is the rule rather than the exception in serious dance students.

B. Contagious diseases spread rapidly within a dance company or school because of daily, close contact of participants.

C. Smoking appears to be more common in the dance (ballet) community than in the general population.

D. **Nutritional disorders are common in the dance community.**

1. Bulimia and anorexia nervosa occur more frequently in the dance community than in the general population.
2. Found mainly in teenagers but can occur at any age

3. May enhance the problems associated with injuries (demineralization, slowed healing, worsened side effects with medications)

III. Injuries

While virtually any acute or overuse injury can be seen among dancers, **some injuries are so closely related to the specific demands of dance** (ballet in most instances) that their diagnosis and treatment merit special consideration.

A. **Types**
  1. **Acute**
    a. **Few are unique to ballet.**
    b. Generally same as seen with any running/jumping sport
    c. Occasionally, "environmental" injuries are seen:
      i. Falls from sets
      ii. Objects falling on dancers
  2. **Overuse**
    a. Vast majority of injuries are from overuse.
    b. **Frequently related to turn-out (external rotation of hips) or lack thereof**
    c. Related to activity variances:
      i. Following layoffs
      ii. New demands from new choreography
      iii. Increased activity during performance season
    d. Most difficult to treat
      i. Not totally disabling
      ii. Gradual onset and thus presented for treatment late in course

B. **Diagnosis**
  1. **Must be precise**
    a. Often related to the very specific demands of dance technique. Knowing the demands makes treatment easier.
    b. If vague, cause will not be found and reinjury will occur.
  2. **Must be immediate.** Little time available for reflection; dancer is de-training while waiting.
  3. Must be explained to dancer and often teacher or artistic director

C. **Treatment**
  1. Maintenance of conditioning (strength, flexibility, and endurance) is of paramount importance.
  2. Programs must allow continuation of as much training as possible. Must understand classwork and training in order to manipulate activities during treatment.
  3. Dancer must understand goals and rationale of treatment.
    a. Must actively participate in program
    b. Muscular rehabilitation (strength, endurance, and flexibility) is involved in the management of *every* injury.
  4. Program must be taught so dancer can carry it out away from medical facility.
  5. Frequent demands for expedient treatment (i.e., corticosteroid injection) must be tempered with long-term goals.
  6. Side effects of medications must be considered.
    a. Muscle relaxants—loss of timing and coordination
    b. Nonsteroidal anti-inflammatory drugs (NSAIDs)—food intake irregular

D. **Trunk and thoracic spine**
  1. **Parathoracic strains often actually involve the scapular stabilizing muscles** (rhomboids, trapezius, and levator).
    a. Cause is often related to lifting partner. Not uncommon to see males lacking in upper body strength.

b. Treatment is symptomatic and should include an upper body conditioning program.

2. **Scoliosis** has been reported to be more common in female ballet dancers than in the general population. May be related to a combination of delayed onset of menses and dietary anomalies.

E. **Lumbar spine—spondylolysis**

1. **Cause**
   a. May be prompted by lordosis secondary to inadequate external rotation of hips
      i. External rotation of the hips is increased by slight hip flexion.
      ii. In order to maintain an upright posture, increased lordosis is used to compensate for hip flexion.
   b. Condition may be more common in dancers than in general population.
2. **Diagnosis**
   a. Midline pain with hyperextension—arabesque position in ballet.
   b. Oblique x-rays to reveal defect
   c. Bone scan to reveal maturity of lesion
3. **Treatment**
   a. Pain-free activity is the keystone for management.
   b. Brace may be necessary for pain-free activities of daily living.
   c. Abdominal strengthening exercises are helpful.
   d. Gradual resumption of dance activities, with jumping and partnering resumed last.

F. **Hips—overuse**

1. **Piriformis syndrome**
   a. Cause is inadequate external rotation of hips or weak external rotators.
   b. Diagnosis
      i. Deep posterior hip (gluteal) pain
      ii. Pain when arising from a low chair or car seat
      iii. May be sciatic radiation
      iv. Pain on exam with increased internal rotation or external rotation against resistance
   c. Treatment—stretching and strengthening of external rotators of hip
2. **Degenerative joint disease**
   a. Cause is possibly long-term dance activities with repetitive microtrauma.
   b. Diagnosis
      i. May be seen in younger age groups than usually expected
      ii. Anterior hip pain, activity-related
      iii. Limitation of motion in rotation, pure flexion, and abduction
      iv. Weakness of musculature
   c. Treatment
      i. Strengthen hip musculature
      ii. Surgical treatment usually means an end to dancing.

G. **Thighs—sartorius tendinitis**

1. Cause is overuse as an external rotator of hip (weight-bearing or non–weight-bearing leg).
2. Diagnosis
   a. Tenderness at origin
   b. Pain with resisted hip flexion, external rotation, and abduction
3. Treatment
   a. NSAIDs
   b. Physical therapy local modalities for symptoms
   c. Stretching and strengthening exercises

H. **Knee**
1. **Acute**
a. **Sprains**
i. **Anterior cruciate ligament (ACL) injuries** do occur in ballet.
ii. Treatment—not necessarily surgical management, as a substantial number of dancers are known to be performing with an absent ACL, and no appreciable disability. Any surgical complication, even in small limitation of knee extension, is career-ending for a ballet dancer.
b. **Meniscal injuries**
i. Definitive diagnosis should be established early, as prolonged observation results in deterioration of conditioning. Early use of MRI or arthroscopy is often indicated.
ii. Treatment—meniscus repairs should not be mindlessly performed, because the period of immobilization may in itself be career-threatening.
2. **Overuse**
a. **Patellofemoral dysfunction is very common.**
i. Cause
(a) Inadequate quadriceps (vastus medialis) strength for demands of dancing
(b) External rotation of leg to compensate for inadequate hip external rotation (increase of quadriceps angle)
(c) Inadequate rehabilitation of prior knee injury
ii. Diagnosis
(a) Activity-related retropatellar or peripatellar pain, most often in region of medial retinaculum
(b) Occasional effusion if seen late in course
(c) Decreased tone or bulk of vastus medialis
(d) X-ray changes and crepitations are usually of confirmatory value only.
iii. Treatment
(a) Relative rest
(b) Avoidance of deep squats (grand plié)
(c) Physical therapy modalities if effusion present
(d) NSAIDs
(e) Quadriceps isometrics (full extension)
(f) Electrical muscular stimulation for vastus medialis if exercises are painful or ineffective
(g) Neoprene sleeve with lateral pad
(h) Surgical intervention should be considered only as a last resort and then only if the alternative is to stop dancing.
b. **Patellar tendinitis**
i. Cause may be repetitive jumping; relative quadriceps inflexibility (tight quadriceps not uncommon in ballet dancers).
ii. Diagnosis
(a) Activity-related infrapatellar pain
(b) Focal tenderness at origin of tendon fibers at inferior pole of patella
(c) Rarely swelling or x-ray changes
iii. Treatment
(a) Relative rest (no jumping)
(b) NSAIDs
(c) Ice
(d) Quadriceps stretching and strengthening
(e) Neoprene sleeve with lateral pad
(f) Steroid injections not indicated

I. **Leg**
  1. **Acute—Achilles tendon rupture**
    a. Cause often previous episode(s) of Achilles tendinitis
    b. Predominately in males
    c. Diagnosis
      i. Sudden, often loud, snap in distal calf
      ii. Dancer describes being struck in calf
      iii. Defect in tendon
      iv. Positive Thompson test
    d. Treatment—surgical treatment favored by most, but closed management has been effective in dancers.
  2. **Overuse**
    a. **Achilles tendinitis**
      i. Cause:
        (a) Usually overuse but may be minor sprain
        (b) May be mechanical from pressure
          • Ribbons on toe shoes tied too tightly
          • Footware used with character roles (e.g., cowboy boots)
      ii. Diagnosis
        (a) Achilles tendon pain with activities
        (b) Pain with passive dorsiflexion
        (c) Pain with (or inability to) arise on toes (relevé)
        (d) Swelling
        (e) Crepitation (uncommon)
      iii. Treatment
        (a) Physical therapy modalities
        (b) Relative rest. May have to avoid all dancing temporarily and use heel lift in shoes for daily activities.
        (c) Stretching and strengthening
        (d) Gradual return to dancing with avoidance of all pain
        (e) Steroid injections not appropriate
      iv. **Cautions**
        (a) Posterior ankle impingement often misdiagnosed as Achilles tendinitis
        (b) May enhance likelihood of rupture of Achilles tendon
    b. **Stress fractures** may involve distal tibia or fibula or (more uncommon) anterior border of mid-shaft of tibia with transverse fracture line through anterior cortex on x-ray (the "dreaded black line" of Hamilton).
      i. Cause is usually change in activity.
      ii. Diagnosis
        (a) Activity-related, localized pain at site of fracture
        (b) Focal tenderness
        (c) X-rays may not reveal if seen early in course
        (d) Bone scan
      iii. Treatment
        (a) Rest until **activities of daily living are pain-free** for 7–10 consecutive days
        (b) Gradual resumption of dancing activities—must remain pain-free
        (c) Stress fracture of anterior border of mid-tibia must be treated with extreme caution, as this lesion has a propensity to go on to overt fracture. Surgical drilling of the fracture site hastens safe return to dancing activities.

J. **Ankle—acute**
  1. **Sprains—usually lateral (inversion)**

a. Treatment
   i. With grade III sprains, some advocate surgical repair because instability in plantarflexed position (de riguer in ballet) is so disabling
   ii. Active, aggressive rehabilitation
   iii. Cast immobilization results in needless time loss.
b. **Cautions**
   i. **Peroneal tendon dislocations are often mistaken for lateral ankle sprains.**
      (a) Tenderness localized to posterior distal fibula
      (b) Ecchymosis may be extensive along course of peroneal tendons.
      (c) Flake of bone off lateral malleolus (x-ray)
      (d) Should be managed surgically when acute
   ii. **Avulsion fracture of base of the fifth metatarsal styloid**
      (a) Similar mechanism of injury
      (b) Pain and tenderness at base of fifth metatarsal
      (c) Usually may be treated as ankle sprain

2. **Ankle impingement**
   a. **Posterior**
      i. Cause: impingement of posterior process of talus or os trigonum.
      ii. Diagnosis
         (a) Posterior ankle pain with plantar flexion
         (b) Pain reproduced with active or passive plantar flexion
         (c) Presence of large posterior process of talus or os trigonum on x-ray
      iii. Treatment
         (a) First (few) episodes
            - NSAIDs
            - Physical therapy modalities for swelling
            - Contrast baths
            - Ankle strengthening (invertors and evertors)
         (b) Recurrent episodes
            - Surgical removal of posterior process of talus or os trigonum
   b. **Anterior**
      i. Cause: usually osteophytes of anterior tibia and/or anterior articular margin of dome of talus.
      ii. Diagnosis
         (a) Anterior ankle pain with extreme of dorsiflexion
         (b) X-rays reveal impingement of osteophytes
      iii. Treatment
         (a) First episodes—as for posterior ankle
         (b) Recurrent episodes—surgical excision of osteophytes

K. **Foot**
1. **Acute—spiral fracture of shaft of fifth metatarsal (dancer's fracture)**
   a. Cause is inversion injury while on toes.
   b. Diagnosis by x-ray
   c. Treatment—short period of immobilization followed by protection with taping and attenuated dance activities
2. **Overuse**
   a. **Stress fractures**
      i. Cause is usually activity change.
         (a) May involve **metatarsal shaft** (metatarsals 2–4)
         (b) May involve base of second metatarsal
            - A "ballet-specific" injury often resulting in long-term disability

- Usually requires bone scan for diagnosis
- Uncommon

(c) **Sesamoids**—utilize bone scan to assist in differentiating from bipartite sesamoid or sesamoiditis

ii. Diagnosis
(a) Activity-related pain, often well-localized
(b) Tenderness (focal) at fracture site
(c) X-rays (may not reveal if patient is seen early)
(d) Bone scan

iii. Treatment
(a) Activity attenuation until activities of daily living are pain-free for at least 7 consecutive days (longer for base of second metatarsal)
(b) Gradual resumption of dance activities—must remain pain-free

b. **Degenerative joint disease of first MTP joint**

i. Cause is frequent dorsiflexion of this joint, especially required in male dancer positions. Most often seen in male dancers.

ii. Diagnosis
(a) Pain at dorsum of MTP joint with hyperdorsiflexion, worsened with weight-bearing in this position
(b) Loss of dorsiflexion at MTP joint
(c) Tenderness at dorsum of joint
(d) X-rays reveal osteophyte at articular margin of dorsum of metatarsal head.

iii. Treatment
(a) Early—NSAIDs, contrast baths, taping to restrict motion of toe (which also compromises dancing)
(b) Late—surgical excision of osteophytes

c. **Morton's neuroma**

i. Cause
(a) May be related to constrictive footwear
(b) Usually at 3–4 interspace
(c) Can be seen with barefoot dancing (rare)

ii. Diagnosis
(a) Weight-bearing, activity-related pain
(b) Often "shock-like" sensation in involved toes
(c) Usually relief with removal of footwear

iii. Treatment
(a) Metatarsal pad placed just proximal to metatarsal heads
(b) Local injections of corticosteroid, three or fewer
(c) Surgical excision, probably successful in no more than 80% of cases

71

Administration and Medical Management of Mass Participation Endurance Events

William O. Roberts, M.D., FACSM

I. General Considerations

This chapter develops an algorithm for the management of mass participation endurance events. The medical director of an event is the safety and health advocate for the athletes who participate in the race. The safety of the athletes is the primary purpose of the race medical operation.

A. **Events**
   1. Road running
   2. Cycling
   3. Cross country skiing
   4. Triathlon
   5. Wheelchair
   6. Swimming

B. **Planned disaster**
   1. Mass gatherings always have the potential for medical illness or injury.
   2. Potential casualties occur in two groups of people
      a. Participants:
         i. Literature review allows estimate of injury type and incidence
         ii. Individual race experience allows more accurate estimate
      b. Spectators
   3. Event risks are unique and shared.
   4. Safety
      a. Primary goal of race committee
      b. Medical operation equals watchdog

C. **Incidence and risk**
   1. Estimating casualties
      a. Anticipated starters × casualty incidence
      b. Project needs: staff, supplies, equipment
      2. Risk ranges
      a. Running (41 km)—1% to 20%:
         i. Twin Cities Marathon (Minnesota)—0.5% to 2% (1.89% of entrants for 1983–1994)
         ii. Boston Marathon—5% to 12%
      b. Running (< 21 km)—1% to 5%: Falmouth Road Race (Massachusetts)— < 1% but severe casualties
      c. Triathlon (225 km)—15% to 30%
      d. Cross county skiing (55 km)—5%
      e. Triathlon (51 km)—2% to 5%
      f. Cycling (variable)—5%
   3. Variables and unknowns
      a. Weather
      b. Event distance
      c. Event type
      d. Condition of participants

D. **Anticipating casualty types**
- 1. Exercise-associated collapse (EAC)
    - a. Hyperthermic
    - b. Normothermic
    - c. Hypothermic
- 2. Trauma
    - a. Macrotrauma
        - i. Musculoskeletal:
            - (a) Fracture
            - (b) Dislocation
            - (c) Sprains and strains
            - (d) Contusions
        - ii. Vascular:
            - (a) Closed
            - (b) Open
        - iii. Head and neck:
            - (a) Concussion
            - (b) Intracerebral bleed
            - (c) Fracture-dislocation
        - iv. Visceral organs:
            - (a) Contusions
            - (b) Laceration
            - (c) Rupture
    - b. Microtrauma:
        - i. Tendinitis
        - ii. Stress fracture
        - iii. Fasciitis
    - c. Dermatologic:
        - i. Blisters
        - ii. Abrasions
        - iii. Lacerations
- 3. Random medical emergencies:
    - a. Cardiac arrest
    - b. Insulin shock
    - c. Asthma
    - d. Anaphylaxis
- 4. Drowning and near drowning

E. **Race medical operations purpose**
- 1. Prerace
    - a. Improve competitor safety
    - b. Injury prevention
- 2. Race day
    - a. Primary
        - i. Stop progression of injury or illness
        - ii. Evaluation of casualties:
            - (a) Triage
            - (b) Treatment
            - (c) Transfer
    - b. Secondary—prevent emergency room overload

F. **Role in race operations**
- 1. Event safety
- 2. Medical decisions
- 3. Medical spokesperson
- 4. Executive committee

II. Prevention Strategies

A. **Primary**
- 1. Definition
    - a. Prevent occurrence of casualties
    - b. Reduce severity of casualties
- 2. Types
    - a. Passive
        - i. Do not require cooperation of participants
        - ii. Examples:

            (a) Start times
            (b) Course modifications
            (c) Traffic control
      b. Active
         i. Require cooperation or behavior change
         ii. Examples:
            (a) Education
            (b) Safety advisories
         iii. Enforced active: helmets, wetsuits

B. **Secondary**
   1. Definition
      a. Early detection of injury or illness
      b. Intervention protocols to stop progression
   2. Examples
      a. Impaired runner policy
      b. Advanced Cardiac Life Support (ACLS), Advanced Trauma Life Support (ATLS), or EAC protocol
      c. On-course ambulance
      d. Finish line triage

C. **Tertiary**
   1. Definition
      a. Treatment of illness or injury
      b. Rehabilitation of illness or injury
   2. Examples
      a. Emergency room transfer
      b. Hospital admission
      c. Rehabilitation center

III. Preparation

A. **Race scheduling**
   1. Location
   2. Season
   3. Start time
   4. Finish time

B. **Competitor safety**
   1. Athletes' safety first
   2. Safest start and finish times
      a. For the elite competitor
      b. For the regular citizen
   3. Hazardous conditions
      a. Define:
         i. Heat
         ii. Cold
         iii. Traction
         iv. Wind
         v. Wind-chill
         vi. Lightning
      b. Alternatives:
         i. Alter
         ii. Postpone
         iii. Cancel
      c. Publish protocol in advance
      d. Announce risks at start
      e. Volunteer safety
   4. **Impaired competitor policy**
      a. Approach to athlete who appears ill or injured during competition, especially with regard to heat or cold stress
      b. No disqualification for medical evaluation—old rules about medical evaluation during competition resulting in automatic disqualification from event have been changed to allow assessment of athletes who appear ill before they are allowed to continue. This is especially important for citizen-class runners.
      c. Criteria to proceed (continue event)

i. Oriented to person, place, and time
ii. Straight line progress toward finish
iii. Good competitive posture
iv. Clinically fit appearance
d. Publish policy in advance
5. Emergency Room (ER) notification
a. Notify local emergency rooms of possibility of casualties from the race
b. Give date, time, and duration of event
c. Estimate casualty numbers and types
6. Preparticipation screening
a. Decide if the event should require pre-event medical screening:
i. Will it be cost-effective?
ii. Will it protect the event and its volunteer staff from liability?
b. Generally not recommended
7. Competitor education
a. Safety measures
b. Risks
c. Fitness
d. Hydration
e. Volunteer identification: standard colors, visibility

C. **Course**
1. Course survey
a. Hills, turns, immovable objects
b. Traffic control
c. Altitude changes
d. Open water
2. Start
a. Downhill
b. Variations: wave, split
3. Aid stations
a. Major:
i. Full medical care
ii. Equipped and staffed for most of the anticipated problems
b. Minor:
i. Comfort care
ii. Fluids
iii. First aid
iv. Shelter
c. Location
i. Every 15 to 20 minutes
ii. Increase number for large fields
iii. Finish line
d. Rolling aid:
i. Vehicle equipped to deliver medical care along the course
ii. Requires an open lane on the course for the vehicle(s)
iii. Bus or van
iv. Medical equipment and staff to deliver care for expected injuries
e. First-response teams
i. Motorcycles or bikes
ii. Automatic defibrillator
4. Finish area
a. Triage:
i. Chute triage
ii. Postchute triage
iii. Area triage (sweep teams)
b. Field hospital

        i. Major aid station
        ii. Subdivisions:
            (a) Triage
            (b) Intensive medical
            (c) Intensive trauma
            (d) Minor medical
            (e) Minor trauma
            (f) Skin
            (g) Medical records
    c. Ambulance support for ER transfer
    d. Shelter for well finishers
    e. Dry clothes shuttle or clothes dryer for wet or cold conditions
5. Ideal course
    a. Asymmetric hourglass
    b. Start, high-risk mark, and finish in the same area

D. **Transportation**
1. Well dropout competitors
    a. Prevent new or increased previous injury:
        i. Hypothermia
        ii. Stress fracture
        iii. Strain
    b. Examples:
        i. Vans
        ii. Buses
        iii. Snowmobiles
        iv. Snowcats
        v. Public transportation
        vi. Sled
        vii. Toboggan
        viii. Boat
2. Ill or injured competitors
    a. Prevent progression of illness or injury—overuse and acute injury or illness that precludes completion of the event without increasing morbidity or mortality
    b. Access care for illness or injury:
        i. Minor injury can use the well dropout transportation
        ii. Casualties requiring medical care need transport by ambulance to the nearest ER or event medical station
    c. Examples
        i. Ambulance:
            (a) Advanced Life Support (ALS)
            (b) Basic Life Support (BLS)
        ii. Helicopter
        iii. Vehicles listed above for well dropout competitors; medically equipped
3. Finish area
    a. Access care in finish area
    b. Examples:
        i. Wheelchair
        ii. Litter
        iii. Stretcher
        iv. Manned carries
    c. Access tertiary care by ambulance:
        i. ALS
        ii. BLS

E. **Communications**
1. Type
    a. Phone: portable, hard wire
    b. Ham radio systems
2. Location
    a. Start
    b. Course:
        i. Aid stations
        ii. Pick-up vans
        iii. Course spotters
        iv. Ambulance

    c. Finish area
        i. Field hospital: central dispatch for course
        ii. Triage teams
  3. 911
    a. Any volunteer
    b. Summon ambulance

F. **Fluids and fuel**
  1. Type
    a. Water
    b. Carbohydrate-electrolyte solutions
    c. High-carbohydrate foods and fruits
  2. Location
    a. Start
    b. Aid stations
    c. Finish area:
        i. Postchute area
        ii. Medical area
  3. Amount
    a. 6–12 oz each competitor every 20 minutes; every 10 minutes for large fields
    b. Double for start, finish, and transition areas
    c. Can be estimated from similar events or past race needs
  4. Publish in advance
    a. Fluid types
    b. Food types
    c. Locations

G. **Equipment**
  1. Shelter
    a. Tents
    b. Vehicles
    c. Buildings
  2. Security fencing
  3. Cots, chairs, tables
  4. Heating and cooling equipment
  5. Generator
  6. Defibrillator
  7. Back boards
  8. Lights
  9. Portable sink
  10. Toilet

H. **Supplies**
  1. Medical
  2. Trauma
  3. Intravenous fluids
    a. <4 hours 5% dextrose in half NS
    b. >4 hours 5% dextrose in NS
  4. Medications
    a. Albuterol
    b. Epinephrine
    c. Diazepam (Valium)
    d. Other
  5. Dextrose 50% in water
  6. Oxygen

I. **Staffing**—personnel located at start, over course, at finish
  1. Physicians
  2. Acute care nurses:
    a. Intensive care unit
    b. Coronary care unit
    c. ER
  3. Paramedics
  4. Emergency medical technicians
  5. Trainers
  6. First-aid personnel
  7. Nonmedical assistants
  8. Sources for volunteers: hospitals, clinics, American Red Cross, National Ski Patrol, National Guard, Armed Forces Reserves

J. **Medical and race records**
   1. Document care
   2. Calculate incidence of casualties
   3. Project future needs
   4. Research
   5. Document environmental conditions

IV. Medical Protocols

A. **First aid**
   1. Do no harm
   2. Stay within training level

B. **Basic problems**
   1. Exercise associated collapse
   2. Random medical emergencies
   3. Trauma

C. **Initial assessment (ABCDE)**
   1. *A*irway (cervical spine control)
   2. *B*reathing
   3. *C*irculation (hemorrhage control)
   4. *D*isability—neurologic status
   5. *E*xposure and exam

D. **Initial disposition**
   1. Race medical facility
   2. Transport to emergency facility

E. **Treatment and transfer protocols**
   1. Determine in advance
      a. Automatic transfers:
         i. Cardiac arrest
         ii. Respiratory arrest
         iii. Shock
      b. Delayed transfers
   2. Keep protocols simple.
   3. Integrate into Emergency Medical Services
   4. First aid versus treatment

F. **Medical precautions**
   1. Exposure to body fluids (blood, stool; *not* sweat) can transmit disease.
   2. Modified universal precautions are most frequently used.
      a. Hand washing
      b. Gloves
      c. Masks, gowns, goggles?
   3. Risks
      a. Hepatitis B
      b. Acquired immunodeficiency syndrome (AIDS)
   4. Disposal of contaminated waste
      a. Red Bag
      b. Sharps containers

G. **Adverse event protocol**
   1. If there is a medical event with an adverse outcome resulting in death or catastrophic injury, a predetermined protocol should be in place to communicate with the public and the press.
      a. Event is reported to the medical director and the head of the event administration
      b. Event should not be discussed outside of the immediate need for medical care
      c. Medical director or designated alternate should present incident to press
   2. Detailed records should be kept by the event administration and the medical director.

V. Exercise Associated Collapse (EAC)

A. **Classification and treatment system**
   1. Based on Twin Cities Marathon casualties
      a. Symptoms and signs of collapsed finishers

    b. Treatment protocols
    c. Weather
  2. Clinical classification system
    a. Varied presentation within each temperature class
    b. Symptoms did not reflect body temperature
    c. Similar treatment for all classes
    d. Rapid recovery for most casualties

B. **Definition of EAC**
  1. Requiring assistance during or after endurance activity
  2. Not orthopedic or dermatologic

C. **Etiology**
  1. Undetermined
  2. Hypotheses
    a. Dehydration
    b. Depletion of energy store
    c. Vasovagal response
    d. Internal fluid shifts
    e. Temporary malfunction of temperature regulation
    f. Central nervous system failure

D. **Diagnosis**
  1. Presence of signs or symptoms
  2. Major criteria
    a. Body temperature
    b. Mental status
    c. Ambulation status

E. **Clinical picture**
  1. Derived from clinical presentations of Twin Cities Marathon casualties
  2. Symptoms
    a. Exhaustion
    b. Fatigue
    c. Hot
    d. Cold
    e. Nausea
    f. Stomach cramps
    g. Lightheaded
    h. Headache
    i. Leg cramps
    j. Palpitations
  3. Signs
    a. Abnormal body temperature
    b. Unconscious
    c. Altered mental status
    d. Central nervous system changes
    e. Unable to walk unassisted
    f. Leg muscle spasms
    g. Tachycardia
    h. Vomiting
    i. Diarrhea
  4. EAC *includes*
    a. Heatstroke:
      i. Exertional
      ii. Possibly classic
    b. Heat exhaustion
    c. Heat cramps
    d. Heat syncope
    e. Exhaustion
    f. Exertion leg cramps
    g. Hypothermia
  5. EAC *excludes*
    a. Cardiac arrest
    b. Insulin shock
    c. Chest pain
    d. Asthma
    e. Anaphylaxis
    f. Seizure disorder
    g. Trauma

F. **Classification scheme**
  1. Classes

a. Hyperthermic—body temperature ≥ 103°F (39.5°C)
b. Normothermic—temperature between 97°F (36°C) and 103°F (39.5°C)
c. Hypothermic—body temperature ≤ 97°F (36°C)

2. Severity rating
   a. Mild
      i. Any symptom or sign
      ii. Walk with or without assistance
   b. Moderate:
      i. No oral intake
      ii. Extra fluid loss
      iii. Unable to walk
      iv. Severe muscle spasm
      v. Temperature ≥ 105°F (40.5°C) or ≤ 95°F (36°C)
   c. Severe:
      i. Central nervous system changes
      ii. Temperature ≥ 106°F (41°C) or ≤ 90°F (32°C)

G. **Management protocol**

1. Diagnosis and documentation
   a. Initiate medical record
   b. Record presenting symptoms and medical history
   c. Record vital signs
      i. Temperature
         (a) Rectal recommended
         (b) Tympanic membrane:
            - Shell temperature
            - Not accurate for core in athletes
            - Not recommended
      ii. Blood pressure
      iii. Pulse
      iv. Respirations
   d. Record mental status and orientation
   e. Record walking status
   f. Record other physical exam findings
   g. Record treatment and log times
2. Fluid replacement and redistribution
   a. Supine position (nonambulatory):
      i. Elevate legs and buttocks
      ii. Restore pooled blood to circulation
      iii. If ambulatory, assisted walking
   b. Oral fluids (preferred method of hydration):
      i. All mild cases
      ii. All moderate cases, if tolerated
   c. Intravenous fluids
      i. All severe cases
      ii. Moderate cases:
         (a) No response to oral fluids
         (b) Unable to tolerate oral fluids
   d. Recommended fluids
      i. Oral:
         (a) Simple glucose-electrolyte drinks
         (b) Fruit juices
         (c) Water

- ii. Intravenous:
  - (a) 5% dextrose in half NS when event duration less than 4 hours
  - (b) 5% dextrose in NS when event duration greater than 4 hours
  - (c) Lactated Ringer's:
    - Contains K+
    - Avoid until K+ known
    - Do not use in hypothermic individual—cold liver does not metabolize lactate

- e. Intravenous fluid debate
  - i. "Yes" camp:
    - (a) Finishers are dehydrated
    - (b) Improve rapidly with intravenous fluids
    - (c) Small amounts do not cause harm
  - ii. "No" camp:
    - (a) Invasive
    - (b) Electrolyte imbalance: hyponatremia risk, water intoxication
    - (c) Vasovagal etiology—leg-raising therapy
    - (d) Overhydrated
  - iii. "Compromise" camp:
    - (a) Continuum
    - (b) Clinical guess
    - (c) Needs clinical study
    - (d) Difficult to do
- f. Hyponatremia
  - i. Etiology:
    - (a) Water excess and dilution
    - (b) Sodium loss
    - (c) Redistribution
  - ii. Incidence:
    - (a) Low frequency
    - (b) Ultramarathon distances
    - (c) Marathon—few reports
  - iii. Significance:
    - (a) Reason for poor response to treatment
    - (b) Reason to transfer

3. Temperature correction
   - a. Hyperthermic EAC
     - i. Move to cool or shaded area
     - ii. Face cooling or fanning
     - iii. Remove excess clothing
     - iv. Active cooling (temperature > 105°F):
       - (a) Ice packs in neck, axilla, and groin
       - (b) Ice water tub immersion
       - (c) Fan sprayed, atomized mist
     - v. Control continued muscle contractions:
       - (a) Shivering
       - (b) Muscle cramping
       - (c) Medications:
         - Diazepam—1–5 mg slow intravenous push, repeat as needed
         - Thorazine—no longer recommended, inhibits sweating, hypotension
         - Dantrolene—may increase cooling rate, not generally recommended
     - vi. Monitor temperature every 5–10 minutes:

(a) Prevent missing delayed temperature rise
(b) Assess efficacy of treatment
(c) End active cooling at 102°F
(d) Monitor for rebound or overcooling
vii. Precool intravenous fluids
viii. Consider intravenous dextrose 50% in water
ix. Leg cramps:
(a) Fluid and fuel replacement
(b) Assisted walking
(c) Avoid massage until well hydrated
(d) Consider diazepam—1–5 mg intravenous push
(e) Consider magnesium sulfate—5 g intravenous loading dose
b. Hypothermic EAC
i. Handle gently
ii. Move to warm area
iii. Remove wet clothing (clothes dryer)
iv. Dry skin
v. Insulate with prewarmed blankets (clothes dryer)
vi. Breathe warmed, humidified air:
(a) Bennett respirator
(b) Bird respirator
vii. Warm packs in neck, axilla, and groin:
(a) Hot water bottles
(b) Warmed intravenous bags
viii. Prewarm intravenous fluids
ix. Monitor temperature at regular intervals
x. Walk to generate intrinsic heat—temperature > 95°F
xi. Consider intravenous dextrose 50% in water
c. Normothermic EAC
i. Maintain temperature
ii. Monitor temperature if not improving:
(a) Delayed hyperthermia
(b) Postrace hypothermia
4. Fuel supply
a. Oral glucose solutions
b. Intravenous glucose solutions—dextrose 5%; stock intravenous solutions
c. Dextrose 50%, indications
i. Low blood glucose: measure (home glucose meter) at toe, ear lobe
ii. Slow response to intravenous hydration
iii. Slow response to temperature correction
iv. Severe EAC
v. Cardiac arrest
5. Transfer or discharge
a. Transfer to emergency facility:
i. Not responding to usual treatment
ii. Severe casualties not responding rapidly
iii. Automatic transfers
b. Discharge from race medical facility:
i. Clinically stable and normothermic
ii. Instruct in fluid and energy replacement
iii. Reevaluate if change in status
iv. Recommend follow-up exam for severe casualties

VI. Random Medical Emergencies

A. **Cardiac arrest**
   1. Equipment and supplies
      a. Defibrillator
      b. Intubation equipment
      c. ACLS drug kits:
         i. Oxygen
         ii. Epinephrine
         iii. Atropine
         iv. Lidocaine
         v. Procainamide
         vi. Bretylium
         vii. Verapamil
         viii. Sodium bicarbonate
         ix. Morphine
         x. Dextrose 50% in water
      d. Oxygen delivery system
      e. Intravenous kits
   2. ACLS protocol
      a. Standard protocol:
         i. ABCs (airway; breathing; circulation)
         ii. Cardiopulmonary resuscitation
         iii. Cardiac monitor
         iv. Defibrillate if indicated
         v. Intravenous access
         vi. Intubate
         vii. Medications
      b. Twin Cities Marathon modifications
         i. Sustrate replacement:
            (a) Glucose has been depleted by the physical activity and should be replaced for the heart to respond to treatment.
            (b) Dextrose 50% in water intravenous push
         ii. High-dose epinephrine:
            (a) High-dose epinephrine seems a reasonable alternative to the low-dose regimen in the face of arrest after activity that depletes catecholamine.
            (b) 5–10 mg intravenous push
         iii. Acidosis:
            (a) Metabolic acidosis of activity must be reversed.
            (b) Sodium bicarbonate
   3. Death in road racing
      a. Estimate 1/50,000 to 1/100,000 entrants:
         i. Twin Cities Marathon and Boston Marathon—1 death/200,000 to 400,000 hours of participation
         ii. Sedentary men—1 death/100,000 hours
         iii. Active men, resting—1 death/200,000 hours
         iv. Active men, exercising—1 death/50,000 hours
      b. Road racing by trained individuals is safer than a sedentary lifestyle.
      c. Preventable
         i. With prescreening? Cost is a problem.
         ii. Close attention to symptoms
      d. Resuscitation successful:
         i. Twin Cities Marathon and others—no
         ii. London Marathon—yes for 3 of 4
         iii. New York Marathon—yes for 1 of 4

B. **Anaphylaxis**
   1. Types: atopic, exercise induced
   2. Treatment: epinephrine, antihistamine

C. **Asthma**
   1. Inhalers—albuterol metered-dose inhaler with extender
   2. Oxygen high flow

3. Nebulizer—albuterol
4. Subcutaneous terbutaline or epinephrine

D. Insulin shock
1. Dextrose 50% in water
2. Glucagon

VII. Trauma

A. **High-velocity activity collisions and falls**
1. Biking
2. Skiing
3. Wheelchair racing

B. Vehicle on course (collision)

C. **ATLS protocol**
1. Equipment
a. Back boards
b. Neck collars (semirigid)
c. Splints
d. Cricothyroidotomy kit
e. Oxygen
f. Intravenous fluids
2. Transportation
a. Type:
i. ALS
ii. BLS
b. Access:
i. Ambulance
ii. Helicopter
iii. Snowmobile and toboggan
3. Protocol
a. Primary survey
i. Airway and cervical spine control:
(a) Helmet on if airway okay
(b) Helmet off if unable to establish airway and breathing
ii. Breathing and ventilation
iii. Circulation and bleeding control
iv. Disability or neurologic status
v. Expose and examine
b. Initial resuscitation
i. High-flow oxygen
ii. Shock management:
(a) Fluid therapy
(b) Position
iii. Cardiac monitor
c. Secondary survey—look for other problems
d. Definitive field care:
i. Temperature maintenance
ii. Pain control
iii. Splint
iv. Other
e. Triage:
i. Race medical facility
ii. Emergency medical facility

VIII. Postrace Review

A. **What went right**
B. **What went wrong**
C. **Proposed changes**

IX. Costs

A. **Donations**
1. Volunteer time
2. Supplies

B. **Borrow**
1. Defibrillators
2. Glucose monitor

C. **Rent**
1. Tent
2. Heater

D. **Purchase**
1. Ambulance time
2. Special equipment

Index

Entries in **boldface type** indicate complete chapters.